Melvin A. Shiffman, Sid J. Mirrafati, Samuel M. Lam (Editors)
Chelso G. Cueteaux (Associate Editor)

Simplified Facial Rejuvenation

Melvin A. Shiffman · Sid J. Mirrafati
Samuel M. Lam (Editors)
Chelso G. Cueteaux (Associate Editor)

Simplified Facial Rejuvenation

With 884 Figures and 40 Tables

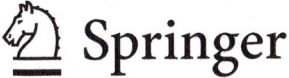

Melvin A. Shiffman, M.D., J.D.
Chairman, Surgery Section, Tustin Hospital and Medical Center, Tustin, California
Private Practice: 17501 Chatham Drive
Tustin, CA 92780-2302
USA

Sid J. Mirrafati, M.D.
Private Practice: President, Mira Aesthetics: 1101 Bryan Avenue, Suite G
Tustin, CA 92780
USA

Samuel M. Lam, M.D., F.A.C.S.
Private Practice: Director, Willow Bend Wellness Center
Lam Facial Plastic Surgery Center & Hair Restoration Institute
6101 Chapel Hill Boulevard, Suite 101
Plano, Texas 75093
USA

Chelso G. Cueteaux, M.D.
Presidente: Asociación Nacional de Medicina Estética
Federación Iberoamericana Cirugía Cosmética
and Federación Iberoamericana Medicina Estética y Cosmética
Private Practice: 412 Santa Ana
Rancho Viejo, Texas 78575
USA

Library of Congress Control Number: 2007923875

ISBN   978-3-540-71096-7   Springer Berlin Heidelberg New York

Springer is a part of Springer Science+Business Media
springer.com

Editor: Gabriele Schröder, Heidelberg, Germany
Desk Editor: Ellen Blasig, Heidelberg, Germany
Reproduction, typesetting and production: LE-TeX Jelonek, Schmidt & Vöckler GbR, Leipzig, Germany
Cover design: Frido Steinen-Broo, EStudio, Calamar, Spain

Printed on acid-free paper 24/3180/YL 5 4 3 2 1 0

Dedication

This book is dedicated to a family that has put up with my years of practicing medicine 7 days a week, 18 h per day, as well as taking on almost everything that has been asked of me by individuals and societies. As Editor of three different cosmetic surgery journals over 10 years, Chief of Surgery at one hospital, and now Chairman of the Surgical Section of another hospital, teaching internationally for the past 20 years, completely writing and formatting the International Board of Surgery examination and running these examinations over the past 3 years, writing over 350 papers, and authoring or editing over six books, including this seventh book, I have rarely been at home or "too busy when I am home." I am now on the Board of Governors of the American College of Legal Medicine as Treasurer and destined to be President in 2 years. My wife, Pearl, has taken all of this without complaint and my children, Scott, Karen, and Denise, have missed my presence to support their activities. Now three grandchildren, Ben, Greg, and Evan, have to put up with my infrequent presence at a variety of their events (sports, etc). At my age it is hard to change, I enjoy what I do and I only hope that all of them will continue to understand.

Melvin A. Shiffman

Foreword

It is a great pleasure for me to provide a foreword for this new book *Simplified Facial Rejuvenation*. I congratulate the editors, who selected a great number of aesthetic surgeons, working in different parts of the world, all of them with great experience in the art and science of aesthetic surgery. Such a book is needed at the present time.

Aesthetic surgery and especially facial aesthetic surgery is requested today by many. We already have plenty of books about aesthetic surgery. Most of them are excellent, but not all of them describe simple procedures for embellishment or rejuvenation. Major procedures are developed in detail but are not for all the patients of the present time.

Today, many patients who want to improve their facial appearance are young or mature. They want to stay young and are asking us to correct the first "weak point" of facial ageing, to treat a minor defect, or to enhance the beauty of a normal feature. Also, we have many senior citizens who do not want to have a major operation and who wish only for a mild improvement of their face. Many senior citizens do not want to change; they want to stay as they are and such simple procedures may be very helpful for them. Older patients very often want to have several simple procedures together instead of a major one. The satisfaction of the patient may be the same as that which he or she should have with a major procedure. Simple techniques alone or associated with other techniques give a natural look and not a postsurgical look, which is sometimes the result of a major procedure. *Beauty has no age.*

It is the aim of this book to inform aesthetic surgeons about conventional, new, or improved techniques, all of them reliable and simple and recommended by the authors. This group of aesthetic surgeons have great experience of such techniques and also of their indications. Prevention is better than cure and mini invasive techniques are frequently indicated.

In aesthetic surgery as in other surgical specialities, it is necessary to know *how* and also *why* a procedure has to be selected. All the problems of patient selection are discussed as well as minor surgical details about all the procedures used on the face, neck, and scalp (threads, section of muscles, superficial peelings, artificial fillers as well as biological fillers, suture lift, short access facial elevation, mesotherapy technique, partial removal of the buccal fat, etc.). A patient said once: "Why go under the knife when you can go through the needle?"

All of the procedures are reliable but should be done only by experienced aesthetic surgeons. A simple procedure does not mean an easy procedure and complications may happen in inexperienced hands. Simple does not mean minimal results. The results are often as good as those for a major procedure. We should not forget that the face is the public relations organ by excellence, the clock of age, the barometer of feelings. The face, in surface area, is very small compared with the body. A defect on the body can be easily concealed. On the face, it is not possible. This remark underlines how important is the work of the aesthetic surgeon on the face.

Everybody at any age would like to have a pleasant face or at least a normal one, without any blemish due to nature, to an accident, to a disease, or to ageing. It is well known that minor imperfections of the skin or aesthetic anomalies can cause much distress.

As Mario Gonzales Ulloa, the famous Mexican plastic surgeon, used to say: "A defect of 1 mm on the face is 1 km in the heart and in the mind." Since the beginning of humanity, man has tried to improve his condition and his appearance. Today, human culture is at its highest level in all fields, and aesthetic medicine and aesthetic surgery have made tremendous advances technically as well as in reliability. All over the world men and women are aware of such advances thanks to the media and the desire to improve one's appearance is strong. If health is the first thing that is indispensable in life, the second one is a pleasant appearance. Having a good look is not being vain, it is a culture and it is even a need in many professions.

Aesthetic surgery today is not only rejuvenation but it is also embellishment and maintenance of youth—face maintenance rather than radical surgery is the way to beat facial ageing. Simple procedures are very often enough. Aesthetic surgery as it has been said can put back what Father Time took away or what Mother Nature forgot.

Aesthetic surgery today is more accessible to many. A lot of very valuable improvements of the face can be achieved by simple techniques and they are described in detail in this book.

It is well known that a simple procedure on one element of the face can embellish or rejuvenate a whole face and *it will also improve the mind.*

All the simple techniques described in this book will allow the aesthetic surgeon to democratize even more beauty, which is as necessary as health. We live in a world which is refined in all fields. Being clean is not enough; today having a good look is a duty towards oneself as well as for the other individuals sharing our environment. It is a culture.

A good book is the best university and I congratulate the authors for their excellent contributions. Mel Shiffman, the main editor, deserves special gratitude. He decided to produce this book and tackled the hard work indispensable for this unusual and very useful tool to be published (he is also the father of several other books on aesthetic surgery) and he spent many hours at his computer when at home but also when travelling to teach, to attend meetings, and to discuss with his co-authors all over the world like an evangelist to spread generously his wide knowledge and collect the most recent and reliable techniques or ideas making possible the publication of this very useful book. He knows that the transmission of knowledge is a duty of the present towards the future.

He is a fountain of knowledge and a not cistern and is the living proof of a sentence used by Mario Gonzales Ulloa in his book *Man*:

The essential lies:
not in having but in giving,
not in knowing but in teaching,
not in being able but in accomplishing.

Thank you again, Mel.
Pierre F. Fournier

Preface

Facial rejuvenation is the art and science of improving the aesthetics of the face, scalp, and neck areas to give a more youthful appearance. For many years the standard has been a full facelift with various methods of superficial musculoaponeurotic system tightening as well as chemical peels or laser. More recently deep-plane facelift has been utilized to improve the results. However, some of these procedures have been associated with some significant risks and complications as well as prolonged recovery time.

There is a growing tendency for physicians to use less invasive procedures that reduce the risks and complications. Patients are more likely to select a less aggressive procedure not only for the reduced risks of injury but also because of reduced time of disability with early return to work and social activities. Patients wish to look younger but also want fewer scars and a less painful recovery. Newer less aggressive procedures, such as suture facelifts, are being developed to decrease complications and recovery time.

This book is an attempt to bring together some of the simpler procedures in facial, scalp, and neck rejuvenation. Some of these procedures are reinventions of older procedures with some variations and some are newer procedures.

The contributors to this book are international experts with extensive experience in facial cosmetic surgery and bring to the reader a variety of advances. Students as well as experienced surgeons can benefit from the information imparted for possible use in their own practices.

Melvin A. Shiffman

Contents

List of Contributors

Manoj T. Abraham, M.D.
Department of Otolaryngology—Head & Neck Surgery, New York Medical College
Valhalla, NY 10595, USA, and Facial Plastic, Reconstructive & Laser Surgery PLLC
P.O. Box 2179, Poughkeepsie, NY 12601
USA
E-mail: info@nyfacemd.com

Natale Fereira Gontijo de Amorim, M.D.
Pontifical Catholic University of Rio de Janeiro and the Carlos Chagas Institute
of Post-Graduate Medical Studies, Rio de Janeiro, Brazil, and Rua Dona Mariana 65
Rio de Janeiro 22280-020
Brazil
E-mail: ceip@visualnet.com.br

Patricio Andrades, M.D.
University of Alabama, Birmingham,
510 20th Street South, FOT 1102, Birmingham, AL 35294
USA

David Armstrong, M.D.
University of Tennessee Health Science Center, Memphis, TN 38163
USA

Pier Antonio Bacci, M.D.
Surgery School of the University of Siena, Siena, Italy, and Via Monte Falco 31, 52100
Arezzo
Italy
E-mail: baccipa@ntc.it

Benjamin A. Bassichis, M.D.
Department of Otolaryngology—Head and Neck Surgery, University of Texas
Southwestern Medical Center, Dallas, TX 75390, USA, and Advanced Facial Plastic
Surgery Center, Suite 110, 14755 Preston Road, Dallas, TX 75254
USA
E-mail: drbassichis@advancedfacialplastic.com

Kenneth Beer, M.D.
The Palm Beach Esthetic Center
Suite 303, 1500 North Dixie Highway, West Palm Beach, FL 33401
USA
E-mail: kenbeer@aol.com

Gary Dean Bennett, M.D.
7 Pelican Hill Circle, Newport Coast, CA 92657
USA
E-mail: dasseen@cox.net

George Bitar, M.D.
Suite 500, 8501 Arlington Blvd., VA 22031
USA
E-mail: gbitar007@aol.com

Dominic A. Brandy, M.D.
The Skin Center, Suite 2400, 2275 Swallow Hill Road, Pittsburgh, PA 15220
USA
E-mail: kym412@aol.com

David S. Chrzanowski, M.D.
Suite 201, 55 Highland Avenue, Salem, MA 01970
USA
E-mail: davidchrzanowski@yahoo.com

Ross A. Clevens, M.D.
Center for Facial Cosmetic Surgery
1344 South Apollo Blvd., Melbourne, FL 32901
USA
E-mail: info@drclevens.com

George Commons, M.D
Suite C, 1515 El Camino Real, Palo Alto, CA 94306
USA
E-mail: georgecmd@aol.com

Chelso G. Cueteaux, M.D.
412 Santa Ana, Rancho Viejo, TX 78575
USA
E-mail: chelso@anme.com.mx

Jorge de la Torre, M.D.
University of Alabama, Birmingham
510 20th Street South, FOT 1102, Birmingham, AL 35294
USA

Alberto Di Giuseppe, M.D.
Institute of Plastic and Reconstructive Surgery, School of Medicine
University of Ancona, Italy, and Via Simeoni 6, 60122 Ancona
Italy
E-mail: adgplasticsurg@atlavia.it

Zoe Diana Draelos, M.D.
Department of Dermatology, Wake Forest University School of Medicine
Winston-Salem, NC 27157, USA, and 2444 North Main Street, High Point, NC 27262
USA
E-mail: zdraelos@northstate.net

Giorgio Fischer, M.D.
Via della Camiluccia 643, 00135 Rome
Italy
E-mail: giorgiofischer@flashnet.it

Pierre F. Fournier, M.D.
55 Boulevard de Strasbourg, 75010 Paris
France
E-mail: pierre.fournier27@wanadoo.fr

James E. Fulton Jr., M.D., Ph.D.
Vivant Skin Care, Suite 300, 1801 Coral Way, Miami, FL 33145
USA
E-mail: dr.fulton@vivantskincare.com

Vincent Giampapa, M.D., F.A.C.S.
Department of Surgery, University of Medicine and Dentistry of New Jersey
Newark NJ 07103-2714, USA, and Plastic Surgery Center Internationale
89 Valley Rd., Montclair, NJ 07042
USA
E-mail: giampapamd@aol.com

Alvin I. Glasgold, M.D.
Robert Wood Johnson Medical School, University of Medicine & Dentistry of New
Jersey, Piscataway, NJ 08854-5635, USA, and 31 River Road, Highland, Park, NJ 08904
USA
E-mail: dralvin@glasgoldgroup.com

Mark J. Glasgold, M.D.
Robert Wood Johnson Medical School, University of Medicine & Dentistry of New
Jersey, Piscataway, NJ 08854-5635, USA, and 31 River Road, Highland, Park, NJ 08904
USA
E-mail: drmark@glasgoldgroup.com

Robert A. Glasgold, M.D.
Robert Wood Johnson Medical School, University of Medicine & Dentistry of New
Jersey, Piscataway, NJ 08854-5635, USA, and 31 River Road, Highland, Park, NJ 08904
USA
E-mail: rglasgold@hotmail.com

Mitchell P. Goldman, M.D.
Volunteer Professor of Dermatology/Medicine, University of California, San Diego
Medical Director, La Jolla Spa MD
7630 Fay Avenue, La Jolla, California 92037
USA
E-Mail: mgoldman@Spa-MD.com

Jorge Orlando Guerrissi, M.D.
Service of Plastic Surgery, Argerich Hospital, Buenos Aires, Argentina, and Medicine
Faculty and Plastic Surgery Unit, Buenos Aires University, Buenos Aires
Argentina
E-mail: guerrisi@speedy.com.ar

Charles D. Hasse, M.D., D.D.S.
Center for Oral Facial Reconstruction
Suite 711, 16300 Sand Canyon Avenue, Irvine, CA 92618
USA
E-mail: osurgn@cox.net

Enrique Hernández-Pérez, M.D.
Club VIP No. 369, 7801 NW 37th Street, Miami, FL 33166-6559
USA
E-mail: enrimar@vip.telesal.net

Mitchell V. Kaminsky, M.D.
369 Northwest Highway, Palatine, IL 60016
USA

Emina Karamanovski, M.D.
Lam Institute for Hair Restoration
6101 Chapel Hill Boulevard, Suite 101, Plano, TX 75093
USA
E-mail: emina@hairtx.com

Hassan Abbas Khawaja, M.D.
Cosmetic Surgery and Skin Center, 53 B II, Gulberg III, Lahore
Pakistan
E-mail: drhassan@nexlinx.net.pk

Yang-Che Kim, M.D.
192-3 Puchun2-dong Busanjin-gu, Busan 614-845
South Korea
E-mail: kimlaser@yahoo.co.kr

Young-Kyoon Kim, M.D.
5050 Clinic, 306 Megaplus, 541-1 Sangdong, Wonmigu, Bucheon 420-030
South Korea
E-mail: clinic5050@hotmail.com

Donald W. Kress, M.D.
1560 Opposumtown Pike, Frederick, MD 21702
USA
E-mail: info@plasticsurgeryone.com

Oh Sook Kwon, M.D.
2nd Floor, DongGung Town Building, ChungDam-dong, KangNam-gu, Seoul
Korea
E-mail: drnature5@hanmail.net

Samuel M. Lam, M.D., F.A.C.S.
Lam Facial Plastic Surgery Center & Hair Restoration Institute, Willow Bend Wellness
Center, 6101 Chapel Hill Boulevard, Suite 101, Plano, TX 75093
USA
E-mail: drlam@lamfacialplastics.com

Phillip R. Langsdon, M.D., F.A.C.S.
Chief, Division of Facial Plastic Surgery, University of Tennessee Health Science Center
Memphis, TN 38163, USA, and The Langsdon Clinic
7499 Poplar Pike, Germantown, TN 38138
USA
E-mail: langsdon@bellsouth.net

Héctor Leal Silva, M.D.
Centro de Dermatología y Cirugía Cosmetica, Belisario Dominguez 2309, Obispado
Monterrey, Nuevo Leon, 64060 Mexico
E-mail: hleal@ultralaser.com.mx

Jean-Paul Lintilhac, M.D.
10450 Wilshire Blvd., Los Angeles, CA 90024
USA
E-mail: simonelintilhac@adelfia.net

Mary P. Lupo, M.D.
Lupo Center for Aesthetic and General Dermatology
Suite 302, New Orleans, LA 70124
USA
E-mail: drlupo@drmarylupo.com

Pier Francesco Mancini, M.D.
Aesthetic Plastic Surgery, Clinica Mancini, C/ Padilla 40, 28006 Madrid
Spain
E-mail: fmancini@terra.es

Sergio Mancini, M.D.
Surgical Department and Surgery School of Siena University, Siena
Italy

Guy G. Massry, M.D.
Ophthalmic Plastic and Reconstructive Surgery, Spalding Dr. Cosmetic Surgery
and Dermatology, Suite 315, 120 South Spalding Dr., Beverly Hills, CA 90212
USA
E-mail: massrymd@aol.com

Sid J. Mirrafati, M.D.
Mira Aesthetics, Suite G, 1101 Bryan Avenue, Tustin, CA 92780
USA
E-mail: drmirrafati@youngerlook.com

Harry Mittelman, M.D.
Stanford University Medical Center, 795 Altos Oaks Drive, Los Altos, CA 94024
USA
E-mail: hmittelman@yahoo.com

David J. Narins, M.D.
222 Westchester Avenue, White Plains, NY 10604
USA
E-mail: dnarins@mac.com

Rhoda S. Narins, M.D.
School of Medicine, New York University, , New York, NY 10016, USA, and 222
Westchester Avenue, White Plains, NY 10604
USA
E-mail: rsnmd@worldnet.att.net

Joseph Niamtu III, M.D.
Cosmetic Facial Surgery, 10230 Cherokee Rd., Richmond, VA 23235
USA
E-mail: niamtu@niamtu.com

Susanna Nikitina, M.D.
15-1-108 Sikeirosa, 194000 St. Petersburg
Russian Federation
E-mail: nikiya@mail.wplus.net

Omer Refik Ozerdem, M.D.
Baskent University, Ankara
Turkey
E-mail: omerozerdem@yahoo.com

Eugenio Pacelli Chapa, M.D.
Plastika Surgery Center
Belisario Dominguez No. 2485 Pte., Col. Obispado, Monterrey, Nuevo Leon
Mexico
E-mail: epacelli.plastika@gmail.com

Djenane Pamplona, Ph.D.
Pontifical Catholic University of Rio de Janeiro, Rio de Janeiro
Brazil
E-mail: djenane@civ.puc-rio.br

Dae-Hwan Park, M.D.
Plastic and Reconstructive Surgery, Catholic University of Daegu, Daegu Catholic
Medical Center, 3056-6 Daemyung 4-dong, Namgu, Daegu, 705-034
Korea
E-mail: dhpark@cu.ac.kr

Bhupendra C.K. Patel, M.D.
Division of Facial Plastic Reconstructive and Cosmetic Surgery, University of Utah
Salt Lake City, UT 84132, USA, and 50 North Medical Drive; Salt Lake City, UT 84103
USA
E-mail: bhupendra.patel@hsc.utah.edu

Curtis Perry, M.D.
Tufts University School of Medicine, Boston , MA 02111, USA, and Artist Surgical
Center, 1567 South County Trail, East Greenwich, RI 02818
USA
E-mail: curtisperrymd@cox.net

Ivo Pitanguy, M.D.
Plastic Surgery Departments, Pontifical Catholic University of Rio de Janeiro and the
Carlos Chagas Institute of Post-Graduate Medical Studies, Rio de Janeiro, Brazil, and
Rua Dona Mariana 65, Rio de Janeiro
Brazil
E-mail: pitanguy@visualnet.com.br

Henrique N. Radwanski, M.D.
Plastic Surgery Departments, Pontifical Catholic University of Rio de Janeiro and the
Carlos Chagas Institute of Post-Graduate Medical Studies, Rio de Janeiro, Brazil, and
Pilos Botafogo Medical Center, Rua Dona Mariana 143 s. F22, Rio de Janeiro 22280-020
Brazil

Oscar M. Ramírez, M.D.
Johns Hopkins University School of Medicine, Baltimore, MA 21205-2196, USA, and
Esthétique Internationale, Suite 100, 2219 York Road,Timonium, MA 21093
USA
E-mail: drramirez@ramirezmd.com

Adam D. Schaffner, M.D.
Suite 311, 25 LeRoy Place, New Rochelle, NY 10805-2863
USA
E-mail: adamdavidschaffner@yahoo.com

Melvin A. Shiffman, M.D.
Surgery Section, Tustin Hospital and Medical Center, Tustin, CA, USA, and 17501
Chatham Drive, Tustin, CA 92780-2302
USA
E-mail: shiffmanmdjd@yahoo.com

Michel Siegel, M.D.
Facial Center for Plastic Surgery, Suite 420, 7700 San Felipe,, Houston, TX 77063
USA
E-mail: drsiegel@houstonfaces.com

Jared Spencer, M.D.
Stanford University Medical Center, 795 Altos Oaks Drive, Los Altos, CA 94024
USA
E-mail: jared.spencer@yahoo.com

Matthew R. Stumpe, M.D.
University of Tennessee Health Science Center, Memphis, TN 38163, USA, and 956
Court Avenue, B 226, Memphis, TN 38163
USA

Edward O. Terino, M.D.
Plastic Surgery Institute of Southern California
327 S Moorpark Rd, Thousand Oaks, CA 91361
USA
E-mail: terino@pixelgate.net

Thomas L. Tzikas, M.D.
Suite 160, 190 Congress Park Drive, Delray Beach, FL 33445
USA
E-mail: tzikasfps@aol.com

Luis Vasconez, M.D.
University of Alabama, Birmingham
510 20th Street South, FOT 1102, Birmingham, AL 35294
USA
E-mail: luis.vasconez@ccc.uab.edu

Longin Zurek, M.D.
St. George Private Hospital, 1, South Street, Kogareh, Sydney, NSW 2217
Australia
E-mail: zurek@ozemail.com.au

Part I
Anatomy and Anesthesia

CHAPTER 1

Anesthesia for Minimally Invasive Cosmetic Surgery of the Head and Neck

Gary Dean Bennett

1.1
Introduction

With progressive refinement of cosmetic and reconstructive surgical techniques, the development of less invasive surgical procedures, and the gradual demographic shift of the world's population toward older age, the popularity of cosmetic and restorative treatments continues to increase. While more than 50% of all aesthetic surgeries are performed in the office [1], the majority of the newer non-invasive and minimally invasive cosmetic and restorative procedures are performed in the office setting. As a consequence of this shift toward less invasive procedures and greater office-based surgery, the surgeon has assumed a greater role in the selection and management of the anesthesia administered during the procedure.

Decisions relating to the preoperative evaluation, the selection of the anesthesia to be administered, the intraoperative monitoring, the postoperative pain management, and the discharge criteria, which were previously performed by the anesthesiologist or the certified registered nurse anesthetist (CRNA), frequently become the responsibility of the surgeon. Evidence suggests that anesthesia-related deaths are significantly higher when the surgeon also administers the anesthesia [2]. Therefore, if the surgeon accepts the responsibility of the management of anesthesia, then it is incumbent on the surgeon to achieve an in-depth understanding of the concepts of anesthesia and to adhere to the same standards of care that are applied to the anesthesiologist or the CRNA [3]. This chapter should serve as an introduction to understanding the standards of care relating to anesthesia for the cosmetic surgeon.

1.2
Surgical Facility

When deciding where to perform surgical procedures requiring anesthesia, the surgeon should be aware that studies demonstrate a threefold mortality in surgeries performed in the office-based setting compared with similar surgeries performed at other facilities, such as free-standing surgical centers or hospitals [4]. Most states in the USA require that the surgical facility be accredited by one of the regulating agencies if general anesthesia or enough sedative medication is used which could potentially result in the loss of life-preserving protective reflexes (LPPRs) [5, 6]. All operating rooms where anesthesia is administered must be equipped with the type of monitors required to fulfill monitoring standards established by the American Society of Anesthesiologists (ASA) [7], and with resuscitative equipment and resuscitative medications [8, 9]. A transfer agreement should be established with a nearby hospital in the event that an unplanned admission is required. Preferably, the surgical facility should have convenient access to a laboratory in the event a stat laboratory analysis is required. Essentially, office-based surgical facilities should comply with the same standard of care as accredited outpatient surgical centers and hospital-based outpatient surgery departments.

1.3
Ancillary Personnel

The facility or office must be staffed by individuals with the training and experience required to assist in the care of the patient [9, 10]. Use of qualified and experienced operating room personnel has been shown to improve operating room efficiency and reduce surgical morbidity [11, 12]. All personnel assisting in the operating room and recovery area should maintain basic life support certification [13]. At least one health care provider in the facility must be certified to deliver advanced cardiac life support (ACLS) when anesthesia is administered [14]. The surgeon may prefer to enlist the assistance of an anesthesiologist or CRNA to provide intraoperative anesthesia and monitoring. If the surgeon elects to administer parenteral sedative or analgesic medication without the assistance of an anesthesiologist or a CNRA, then a second, licensed health care provider should be available to deliver the medications to the patient and monitor the patient throughout the perioperative period [15]. The use of untrained, unlicensed personnel to administer medication to the patient and to monitor the patient is associated with an increased risk of anesthesia-related complications to the patient. The nurse who has been assigned to monitor the patient during the administration of sedative and analgesic medication should not be required to double as a circulating or scrub nurse [16]. Preferably, the surgeon who chooses to administer anesthesia should also be ACLS-certified.

1.4
Preoperative Evaluation

Despite the development of minimally invasive non-surgical and surgical procedures, the importance of the preoperative anesthesia evaluation should not be minimized. An old adage within many anesthesia training programs is that while there may be minor surgical procedures, there is no such thing as a minor anesthetic. If the surgeon chooses to administer the anesthesia then he/she assumes the full responsibility for the preoperative assessment. Even if an anesthesiologist or a CRNA is to be involved on the day of surgery, a carefully performed preoperative evaluation by the surgeon is instrumental in reducing potential delays or cancellations of surgery and lowering the overall perioperative risk to the patient [17].

A comprehensive preoperative patient questionnaire is an invaluable tool to begin the initial assessment. Information contained in the history may determine the diagnosis of the medical condition in nearly 90% of patients [18]. Information requested by the questionnaire should include all current and prior medical conditions, prior surgeries and types of anesthesia received, adverse outcomes to previous anesthetics or other medications, eating disorders, prior or current use of antiobesity medications, current use of homeopathic or herbal supplements, and prior family history of severe reactions to anesthetics such as malignant hyperthermia. A complete review of systems, including questions about the presence of chest pain, shortness of breath, loss of consciousness, spontaneous bleeding or bruising, spontaneous weight loss, fever, or fatigue is crucial in identifying previously undiagnosed, untreated medical conditions, which could impact the outcome of anesthesia and sur-

Table 1.1 Guidelines for preoperative testing in healthy patients (ASA I–II)

Age	Test
12–40[a]	CBC
40–60	CBC, ECG
>60	CBC, BUN, glucose, ECG, CXR

Adapted from Roizen et al. [270]

CBC complete blood count, ECG electrocardiogram, BUN blood urea nitrogen, CXR chest X-ray

[a]Pregnancy test for potentially childbearing women suggested

gery. Obtaining a family history of sudden, unsuspected illness or death is also important in identifying patients with potentially undiagnosed medical conditions.

A routine physical examination may alert the surgeon to certain medical conditions such as undiagnosed or inadequately treated hypertension, cardiac arrhythmias, cardiac failure, or bronchial asthma, which could result in increased risk to the patient during the perioperative period. Preliminary assessment of the head and neck anatomy may be useful to predict possible challenges in the event endotracheal intubation is required even if general anesthesia is not planned. Obtaining preoperative history and physical examination has been shown to be superior to laboratory analysis in determining the clinical course of anesthesia and surgery [19–23].

For patients with complicated, unstable or previously unrecognized medical conditions, a consultation by the appropriate medical specialist is indicated to determine if the patient's medical conditional is optimally managed, if the medical condition may cause a significant increased in the perioperative risk to the patient, and to assist with the perioperative medical management of the patient if required. Additional preoperative testing may be considered medically necessary by the consultant.

Guidelines for the judicious use of preoperative laboratory screening tests for healthy patients not taking medications are presented in Table 1.1. Additional preoperative tests, noted in Table 1.2, may be indicated for patients with prior medical conditions or risk factors for anesthesia and surgery. Excessive or indiscriminately ordered preoperative laboratory testing for healthy patients not taking medications has limited value in predicting surgical or anesthesia-related morbidity and mortality [24–28].

One critical goal of the preoperative evaluation is the determination of a patient's overall level of risk related to the administration of anesthesia. By first establishing a patient's level of risk, strategies to reduce the patient's exposure may be considered. Compelling evidence suggests that certain coexisting medical conditions significantly increase the risk for perioperative morbidity and mortality [15, 29]. The risk classification system developed by the ASA in 1984 (Table 1.3) [30] has become the most widely accepted method of preoperative risk assessment. The value of the ASA system in predicting which patients are at higher risk for morbidity [31] and mortality [32–34] has been confirmed by numerous studies. Goldman et al. [35] established a risk assessment index based on cardiac disease, which has also been demonstrated to be effective in predicting perioperative mortality [36, 37]. Physicians should incorporate one of the acceptable risk classification systems as an integral part of the preoperative evaluation.

The type of surgery plays a key role in the overall risk of morbidity and mortality to the patient. The consensus of multiple studies confirms that more invasive

Table 1.2 Common indications for additional risk-specific testing

	Electrocardiogram	Chest X-ray	Electrolytes, glucose, liver function tests, blood urea nitrogen, creatinine	Urinalysis
History	Coronary artery disease, congestive heart failure, prior myocardial infarction, hypertension, hyperthyroidism, hypothyroidism, obesity, compulsive eating disorders, deep venous thrombosis, pulmonary embolism, smoking, chemotherapeutic agents chemical dependency, chronic liver disease	Bronchial asthma, congestive heart failure, chronic obstructive pulmonary disease, and pulmonary embolism	Diabetes mellitus, chronic renal failure, chronic liver disease, adrenal insufficiency, hypothyroidism, hyperthyroidism, diuretic use, compulsive-eating disorders, diarrhea	Diabetes mellitus, chronic renal disease, and recent urinary tract infection
Symptoms	Chest pain, shortness of breath, dizziness	Chest pain, shortness of breath, wheezing, unexplained weight loss, and hemoptysis	Dizziness, generalized fatigue or weakness	Dysuria, urgency, frequency, and bloody urine
Signs	Abnormal heart rate or rhythm, hypertension, cyanosis, peripheral edema, wheezing, rales, rhonchi	Cyanosis, wheezes, rales, rhonchi, decreased breath sounds, peripheral edema, abnormal heart rate or rhythm	Abnormal heart rate or rhythm, peripheral edema, jaundice	

Adapted from Roizen and Fischer [271]

surgeries, surgeries with multiple combined procedures, surgeries of prolonged duration, and surgeries with significant blood loss increase the risk of perioperative complications [38–42]. However, even with more minor procedures involving sedation or anesthesia, the physician should not neglect the preoperative evaluation and risk assessment.

1.5
Anesthesia and Patients with Preexisting Disease

Surgeons who perform outpatient surgery, especially office-based surgery, and particularly those surgeons who choose to administer sedative or analgesic medication, must appreciate how preexisting medical conditions may increase the risk of anesthesia in the surgical patient. Furthermore, the surgeon should maintain a reasonable understanding of the basic evaluation and

treatment of these medical conditions. The following sections contain an introduction to considerations of medical conditions which may have a significant impact on a patient during the course of anesthesia and surgery.

1.5.1
Cardiac Disease

The leading cause of perioperative anesthetic and surgical mortality is complications related to cardiac disease, including myocardial infarction and congestive heart failure [43, 44]. Fortunately, careful taking of preoperative history and physical examination can identify most patients with preoperative heart disease [45]. When assessing patients who are apparently asymptomatic for heart disease, but have risk factors for heart disease such as smoking, hypertension, diabetes mellitus, obe-

Table 1.3 The American Society of Anesthesiologists' physical status classification

ASA class I	A healthy patient without systemic medical or psychiatric illness
ASA class II	A patient with mild, treated, and stable systemic medical or psychiatric illness
ASA class III	A patient with severe systemic disease that is not considered incapacitating
ASA class IV	A patient with severe systemic, incapacitating, and life-threatening disease not necessarily correctable by medication or surgery
ASA class V	A patient considered moribund and not expected to live more than 24 h

sity, hyperlipidemia, or a family history of severe heart disease, the prudent physician should be aware that 80% of all episodes of myocardial ischemia are silent [46, 47]. Patients with known cardiac disease must be evaluated by the internist or the cardiologist to ensure the medical condition is optimally managed. Anesthesia and all except the most minor surgical procedures on patients with significant heart disease should preferentially be performed in a hospital setting.

Most studies have demonstrated a dramatically greater risk of reinfarction and death in patients undergoing surgery within 6 months after sustaining a myocardial infarction [48–50]. More recent studies suggest that if patients are monitored postoperatively in the hospital cardiac care unit with invasive hemodynamic monitoring, the rate of perioperative reinfarction and death is reduced [51, 52]. At this time, postponing all but the most minor elective cosmetic surgeries for at least 6 months after a myocardial infarction remains the most prudent decision.

The cardiac risk index established by Goldman et. al. [35] has proven extremely helpful in identifying patients with intermediate risk for perioperative cardiac complication [36]. Patients should be referred to a cardiologist for preoperative evaluation if the risk index score is greater than 13.

Dipyrdamole thallium scanning and dobutamine or adenosine stress echocardiography can predict potential perioperative cardiac complication [53]. A simple but reliable screening tool to evaluate the patient's cardiac status is the patient's exercise tolerance. The patient's ability to increase the heart rate to 85% of the age-adjusted maximal rate reliably predicts perioperative cardiac morbidity [54].

No one anesthetic technique or medication has ever emerged as the preferential method to reduce the incidence of perioperative complication in patients with cardiac disease [55, 56]. Most anesthesiologists agree that perioperative cardiac complications can be reduced through scrupulous patient monitoring and avoiding respiratory and hemodynamic fluctuations.

1.5.2
Obesity

With over 55% of the population of the USA afflicted, obesity has attained epidemic proportions [57]. In fact, obesity has emerged as one of the developing world's most prevalent health concerns. Assuredly, physicians who work with patients undergoing cosmetic surgery will routinely encounter patients with this preexisting medical condition. These physicians must be aware that obesity is associated with other risk factors, such as diabetes mellitus, heart disease, hypertension, sleep apnea, and occult liver disease [58]. A thorough preoperative evaluation must rule out these added risk factors prior to elective cosmetic surgery.

The body mass index (BMI), which is determined by weight (in kilograms) divided by height (in meters) squared, has become the standard method of quantifying the level of obesity. Patients with a BMI over 30 are considered obese, while a BMI over 35 indicates morbid obesity [59]. Morbidly obese patients (BMI greater than 35) undergoing major surgery or any surgery where a general anesthetic is planned should preferentially be referred to a hospital with health care providers experienced with the management of this high-risk group.

Airway control in morbidly obese patients may be particularly challenging owing to anatomical abnormalities of the airway [60]. The combination of higher gastric volume, lower gastric pH, and increased frequency of esophageal reflux elevates the risk of dreaded pulmonary aspiration [61]. The morbidly obese patient may have severe restriction in pulmonary function [62], which is further compromised in the supine position [63]. Pulmonary function may dangerously deteriorate when heavy sedation or general anesthesia is administered to the morbidly obese patient [64]. Hypoxemia may develop precipitously in this patient population while receiving heavy sedation or general anesthesia anytime in the perioperative period. Respiratory impairment may persist for up to 4 days after surgery or anesthesia [65].

Premedication with metaclopromide, or other dopamine-receptor antagonist, and ranitidine, or similar histamine type-2 (H2) receptor antagonist, should be administered the evening prior to and on the morning of surgery to reduce the risk of pulmonary aspiration pneumonitis [66]. Because of the increased risk of deep venous thrombosis (DVT) [67] and pulmonary embolism [68], prophylactic measures such as lower-extremity pneumatic compression devices and early ambulation should be used.

Fatal cardiac arrhythmias, sudden congestive heart failure, and intractable hypotension have developed in patients receiving anesthesia who have previously taken appetite-suppressant medications such as aminorex fumarate, dexfenfluramine (Redux), fenfluramine (pondamin) and phentermine (Ionam, Adipex-P, Fastin, Oby-Cap, Obenix, Oby-trim, or Zantryl). Some authors advocate a cardiac evaluation with an echocardiogram to rule out valvular disease associated with these medications, and continuous-wave Doppler imaging with color-flow examination for any patient who has previously taken any antiobesity medications. Sustained hypotension may not respond to ephedrine, a popular vasopressor. Phenylephrine is the treatment of choice for hypotension in this patient population [69].

anesthesia, or poor pain control, these cases of hypertension are usually accompanied by other signs, such as verbal complaints of pain during local anesthesia, patient movement during general anesthesia, tachycardia, or tachypnea. If the pain treatment, anxiolytics, and depth of anesthesia has been deemed appropriate, then initiating treatment of the blood pressure is indicated.

Beta-adrenergic receptor blocking agents, such as propranolol, judiciously administered intravenously in doses of 0.5 mg at 10-min intervals, are especially effective in treating perioperative hypertension, which is accompanied by tachycardia. Even small doses of beta-adrenergic blocking agents can reduce the incidence of cardiac ischemia [77]. Labetolol, an antihypertensive medication with combined alpha-adrenergic and beta-adrenergic receptor blocking properties, administered in 10-mg doses every 10 min, is also a safe and effective alternative for treating both hypertension and tachycardia [80].

For severe hypertension, hydralazine, a potent vasodilator may be useful in 2.5–5-mg doses intravenously at 15-min intervals. The effects of hydralazine may be delayed up to 20 min and sustained for hours. Hydralazine may cause tachycardia or hypotension, especially if the patient is hypovolemic [81].

1.5.3
Hypertension

Perioperative mortality is significantly increased in patients with untreated or poorly controlled hypertension [70, 71]. Satisfactory control of hypertension reduces the risk of mortality due to complications related to cardiovascular and cerebral vascular disease [72–74]. Most authors concur that preoperative stabilization of hypertension reduces perioperative cardiovascular complications such as ischemia [75–77]. Patients with undiagnosed or poorly controlled hypertension can easily be identified in the preoperative examination and referred to the family physician or internist for evaluation and treatment. Attributing severe hypertension to the patient's preoperative level of anxiety can be a deadly assumption. Considering that many effective medications are available for the treatment of hypertension, there is little defense for the physician who proceeds with surgery in a patient with uncontrolled hypertension.

Previously prescribed antihypertensive medications should be continued up to and including the morning of surgery. Abrupt withdrawal of these medications may result in dangerous rebound hypertension [78]. The only exception is the class of medications known as inhibitors of angiotensin-converting enzyme (ACE), which have been associated with hypotension during the induction of general anesthesia [79].

While mild to moderate perioperative hypertension may be a response to anxiety, an inadequate level of

1.5.4
Diabetes Mellitus

Patients with diabetes mellitus have a significantly increased rate of surgical morbidity and mortality compared with non-diabetic patients [82]. These complications are primarily related to the consequences of the end-organ disease such as cardiovascular disease, renal disease, and altered wound healing which is associated with diabetes mellitus [83–85]. The preoperative evaluation should identify diabetic patients with poor control as well as medical conditions associated with diabetes such as cardiovascular disease and renal insufficiency. The physician should keep in mind that diabetic patients have a greater incidence of silent myocardial ischemia [86].

The minimum preoperative analysis for the diabetic patient should include fasting blood sugar, glycosylated hemoglobin, electrolytes, blood urea nitrogen, creatinine, and electrocardiogram (ECG). If there are any concerns regarding the patient's medical stability, the patients should be referred to a diabetologist, cardiologist, nephrologists, or other indicated specialist. Patients with brittle diabetes or other severe medical conditions should preferentially undergo surgery in a hospital-based surgical unit.

The primary objective of the perioperative management of the stable diabetic patient is to avoid hypoglycemia. Although patients usually receive nothing by mouth after midnight prior to surgery, a glass of clear

Table 1.4 Grade of dyspnea while walking

Level	Clinical Response
0	No dyspnea
1	Dyspnea with fast walking only
2	Dyspnea with 1 or 2 blocks walking
3	Dyspnea with mild exertion (walking around the house)
4	Dyspnea at rest

Adapted from Boushy et al. [92]

juice may be taken up to 2 h prior to surgery to avoid hypoglycemia. To minimize the risk of perioperative hypoglycemia, patients should not take their usual dose of insulin or oral agents on the morning of surgery. Surgery of the diabetic patient should be scheduled as early as possible in the morning to further reduce the risk of perioperative hypoglycemia. After the patient arrives, a preoperative fasting glucose should be determined. An intravenous infusion of fluid containing 5% dextrose should be initiated and continued at 1–2 ml/kg/h until oral fluids are tolerated in the recovery room. Usually, half of the patient's scheduled dose of insulin is administered after the intravenous dextrose fluid infusion has begun [87].

At least one intraoperative glucose level should be measured for surgeries greater than 2 h, especially if general anesthesia is used. A final glucose level should be checked just prior to discharge. Glucose levels above 200 may be effectively managed with a sliding scale of insulin [88]. Treatment regimens directed toward tighter control of the blood glucose, such as insulin infusions, do not necessarily improve perioperative outcome, and recent data indicate that the risk of hypoglycemia may be greater with these regimens [89, 90]. It is imperative that diabetic patients tolerate oral fluids without nausea or vomiting prior to discharge.

1.5.5
Pulmonary Disease

An estimated 4.5% of the population may suffer some form of reactive airway disease which may influence perioperative pulmonary function [91]. These medical conditions include a recent upper-airway infection, bronchial asthma, chronic bronchitis, chronic obstructive airway disease, and a history of smoking. A thorough evaluation of the patient's pulmonary function is indicated if any of these medical conditions are identified in the preoperative history. Careful taking of history should help to separate these patients into low-risk and high-risk groups.

The degree of preoperative respiratory dyspnea correlates closely with postoperative mortality [92]. Using a simple grading scale, one can estimate the patient's preoperative pulmonary function (Table 1.4). Patients with level 2 dyspnea or greater should be referred to a pulmonologist for more complete evaluation and possibly further medical stabilization. Patients with level 3 and level 4 dyspnea are not suitable patients for outpatient surgery. The benefits of elective surgery in these patients should be carefully weighed against the increased risk.

Since upper-airway infection may affect pulmonary function for up to 5 weeks [93], major surgery requiring general endotracheal anesthesia should be postponed, especially if the patient suffers residual symptoms such as fevers, chills, coughing, and sputum production, until the patient is completely asymptomatic.

Multiple studies have confirmed that patients who smoke more than one pack of cigarettes daily have a higher risk of perioperative respiratory complications compared with non-smokers. However, cessation of smoking immediately prior to surgery may not improve the patient's outcome. In fact, the risk of perioperative complications may actually increase if smoking is abruptly discontinued immediately prior to surgery. Cessation of smoking for a full 8 weeks may be required to successfully reduce the risk of perioperative pulmonary complications [94].

If the preoperative physical examination reveals respiratory wheezing, reversible bronchospasm should be optimally treated prior to surgery, even if this treatment requires that the surgery be delayed. Therapeutic agents include inhaled or systemic selective beta-adrenergic receptor type-2 agonist (albuterol) as the sole agent or in combination with anticholinergic (ipratropium) and locally active corticosteroid (beclomethasone diproponate) medications [95]. Continuing the patient's usual asthmatic medications up to the time of surgery [96] combined with postoperative use of incentive spirometry [97] effectively reduces postoperative pulmonary complications.

With regard to medically stabilized pulmonary disease, there are no conclusive, prospective, randomized studies to indicate which anesthesia technique or medication results in improved patient outcome.

1.5.6
Obstructive Sleep Apnea

The National Commission on Sleep Disorders Research estimates that 18 million Americans suffer with obstructive sleep apnea (OSA). Unfortunately, the majority of patients with sleep apnea remain undiagnosed [98]. The incidence of OSA increases among obese patients [99]. Since the target population for many cosmetic surgery procedures includes patients with morbid obesity, concern about the diagnosis and safe treatment of patients with OSA becomes even more relevant.

OSA is a result of a combination of excessive pharyngeal adipose tissue and inadequate pharyngeal soft-tissue support [100]. During episodes of sleep apnea, patients may suffer significant and sustained hypoxemia. As a result of the pathophysiology of OSA, patients develop left and right ventricular hypertrophy [101]. Consequently, patients have a higher risk of ventricular dysarrythmias and myocardial infarction [102].

Most medications used during anesthesia, including sedatives such as diazepam and midazolam, hypnotics such as propofol, and analgesics such as fentanyl, meperidine, and morphine, increase the risk for airway obstruction and respiratory depression in patients with OSA [103]. Death may occur suddenly and silently in patients with inadequate monitoring [104]. A combination of anatomical abnormalities make airway management, including mask ventilation and endotracheal intubation, especially challenging in obese patients with OSA [105]. Perioperative monitoring, including visual observation, must be especially vigilant to avoid perioperative respiratory arrest in patients with OSA.

For patients with severe OSA, particularly those with additional coexisting medical conditions such as cardiac or pulmonary disease, surgery requiring sedation, analgesic, or general anesthesia performed on an outpatient basis is not appropriate. For these high-risk patients, monitoring should continue in the intensive care unit until the patient no longer requires parenteral analgesics. If technically feasible, local or regional anesthesia may be preferable in patients with severe OSA. Postoperatively, patients with any history of OSA should not be discharged if they appear lethargic or somulent, or if there is evidence of even mild hypoxemia [106].

During the preoperative evaluation of the obese patient, a presumptive diagnosis of OSA may be made if the patient has a history of loud snoring, long pauses of breathing during sleep, as reported by the spouse, or daytime somnolence [107]. If OSA is suspected, patients should be referred for a sleep study to evaluate the severity of the condition.

1.5.7
Malignant Hyperthermia Susceptibility

Patients with susceptibility to malignant hyperthermia can be successfully managed on an outpatient basis if they are closely monitored postoperatively for at least 4 h [108]. Triggering agents include volatile inhalation agents such as halothane, enflurane, desflurane, isoflurane, and sevoflurane. Even trace amounts of these agents lingering in an anesthesia machine or breathing circuit may precipitate a malignant hyperthermia crisis. Succinylcholine and chloropromazine are other commonly used medications which are known triggers of malignant hyperthermia. However, many non-triggering medications may be safely used for local anesthesia, sedation-analgesia, postoperative pain control, and

even general anesthesia [109]. Nevertheless, anesthesia for patients suspected to have malignant hyperthermia susceptibility should not be performed in an office-based setting. A standardized protocol to manage malignant hyperthermia (available from the Malignant Hyperthermia Association of the United States, MHAUS) and supplies of Dantrolene and cold intravenous fluids should be available for all patients.

Preferably, patients with malignant hyperthermia susceptibility should be referred to an anesthesiologist for prior consultation. Intravenously administered Dantrolene [110] and iced intravenous fluids are still the preferred treatment. MHAUS may be contacted at 800-98-MHAUS and the MH hotline is 800-MH-HYPER.

1.6
Selections and Delivery of Anesthesia

Anesthesia may be divided into four broad categories, local anesthesia, local anesthesia combined with sedation, regional anesthesia, and general anesthesia. The ultimate decision to select the type of anesthesia depends on the type and extent of the surgery planned, the patient's underlying health condition and the psychological disposition of the patient. For example, a limited procedure in a calm, healthy patient could certainly be performed using strictly local anesthesia without sedation. As the scope of the surgery broadens, or the patient's anxiety level increases, the local anesthesia may be supplemented with oral or parenteral analgesic or anxiolytic medication. As the complexity of the surgery increases, general anesthesia may the most appropriate choice.

1.6.1
Local Anesthesia

A variety of local anesthetics are available for infiltrative anesthesia. The selection of the local anesthetic depends on the duration of anesthesia required and the volume of anesthetic needed. The traditionally accepted, pharmacological profiles of common anesthetics used for infiltrative anesthesia for adults are summarized in Table 1.5 [111].

The maximum doses may vary widely depending on the type of tissue injected [112], the rate of administration [113], the age, underlying health, and body habitus of the patient [114], the degree of competitive protein binding [115], and possible cytochrome inhibition of concomitantly administered medications [116]. The maximum tolerable limits of local anesthetics have been redefined with the development of the tumescent anesthetic technique [117]. Lidocaine doses up to 35 mg/kg were found to be safe, if administered in conjunction with dilute epinephrine during liposuction [118]. With the tumescent technique, peak plasma levels occur 6–24 h after administration [118, 119]. More recently, doses up to 55 mg/kg have been found to be within the therapeutic safety margin [120]. However, recent guidelines by the American Academy of Cosmetic Surgery recommend a maximum dose of 45–50 mg/kg [14].

Certainly, significant toxicity has been associated with high doses of lidocaine as a result of tumescent anesthesia during liposuction [121]. The systemic toxicity of local anesthetic has been directly related to the serum concentration by many authors [113, 118–122]. Early signs of toxicity, usually occurring at serum levels of about 3–4 µg/ml for lidocaine, include circumoral numbness and lightheadedness, and tinnitus. As the serum concentration increases toward 8 µg/ml, tachycardia, tachypnea, confusion, disorientation, visual disturbance, muscular twitching, and cardiac depression may occur. At still higher serum levels above 8 µg/ml, unconsciousness and seizures may ensue. Complete cardiorespiratory arrest may occur between 10 and 20 µg/ml [113, 122]. However, the toxicity of lidocaine may not always correlate exactly with the plasma level of lidocaine, presumably because of the variable extent of protein binding in each patient and the presence of active metabolites [113] and other factors already discussed, including the age, ethnicity, health, and body habitus of the patient, and additional medications.

Ropivacaine, a long-lasting local anesthetic, has less cardiovascular toxicity than bupivacaine and may be a safer alternative to bupivacaine if a local anesthetic of longer duration is required [122, 123]. The cardiovascular toxicity of bupivicaine and etidocaine is much greater than that of lidocaine [122–124]. While bupivacaine toxicity has been associated with sustained ventricular tachycardia and sudden profound cardiovascular collapse [125, 126], the incidence of ventricular dysrhythmias has not been as widely acknowledged with lidocaine or mepivacaine toxicity. In fact, ventricular tachycardia of fibrillation was not observed despite the use of supraconvulsant doses of intravenously administered doses of lidocaine, etidocaine, or mepivacaine in the animal model [123].

Indeed, during administration of infiltrative lidocaine anesthesia, rapid anesthetic injection into a highly vascular area or accidental intravascular injection leading to sudden toxic levels of anesthetics resulting in sudden onset of seizures or even cardiac arrest or cardiovascular collapse has been documented [127, 128]. One particularly disconcerting case presented by Christie [129] confirms the fatal consequence of a lidocaine injection of 200 mg in a healthy patient. Seizure and death occurred following a relatively low dose of lidocaine and a serum level of only 4 µg/ml. A second patient suffered cardiac arrest with a blood level of 5.8 µg/ml [129]. Although continued postmortem metabolism may artificially reduce serum lidocaine levels, the reported serum levels associated with mortality in these patients were well below the 8–20 µg/ml considered necessary to cause seizures, myocardial depression, and cardiorespiratory arrest. The 4 µg/ml level reported by Christie is uncomfortably close to the maximum serum levels reported by Ostad et. al. [120] of 3.4 and 3.6 µg/ml following tumescent lidocaine doses of 51.3 and 76.7 mg/kg, respectively. Similar near-toxic levels were reported in individual patients receiving about 35 mg/kg of lidocaine by Samdal et. al. [130] Pitman [131] reported that toxic manifestations occurred 8 h postoperatively after a total dose of 48.8 mg/kg which resulted from a 12-h plasma lidocaine level of 3.7 µg/kg. Ostad et. al. [120] concluded that because of the poor correlation of lidocaine doses with the plasma lidocaine levels, an extrapolation of the maximum safe dose of lidocaine for liposuction cannot not be determined. Given the devastating consequences of toxicity due to local anesthetics, physicians must exercise extreme caution when administering these medications.

Patients who report previous allergies to anesthetics may present a challenge to surgeons performing liposuction. Although local anesthetics of the aminoester class such as procaine are associated with allergic reactions, true allergic reactions to local anesthetics of the aminoamide class, such as lidocaine, are extremely rare [132, 133]. Allergic reactions may occur to the preservative in the multidose vials. Tachycardia and generalized flushing may occur with rapid absorption of the epinephrine contained in some standard local anesthetic preparations. The development of vasovagal reactions after injections of any kind may cause hypotension, bradycardia, diaphoresis, pallor, nausea, and loss of consciousness. These adverse reactions may be misinterpreted by the patient and even the physician as allergic reactions [132]. A carefully taken history from the patient describing the apparent reaction usually clarifies the cause. If there is still concern about the possibility of true allergy to local anesthetic, then the patient should be referred to an allergist for skin testing.

In the event of a seizure following a toxic dose of local anesthetic, proper airway management and maintaining oxygenation is critical. Seizure activity may be aborted with intravenously administered diazepam (10–20 mg), midazolam (5–10 mg), or thiopental (100–200 mg). Although the ventricular arrhythmias associated with bupivacaine toxicity are notoriously intractable [125, 126], treatment is still possible using large doses of atropine, epinephrine, and bretylium [134, 135]. Some studies indicate that lidocaine should not be used during the resuscitation of a patient with bupivicaine toxicity [136]. Pain associated with local anesthetic administration is due to the pH of the solution and the may be reduced by the addition of 1 mEq of sodium bicarbonate to 10 ml of anesthetic [137].

Topical anesthetics in a phospholipid base have become more popular as a technique for administering local anesthetics. Application of these topical agents may provide limited anesthesia over specific areas such as the face for minor procedures, including limited laser resurfacing. (eutectic mixture of local anesthetics), a combination of lidocaine and prilocaine, was the first commercially available preparation. The topical anesthetic preparation must be applied under an occlusive dressing at least 60 min prior to the procedure to develop adequate local anesthesia [138]. Even after 60 min the anesthesia may not be complete and the patient may still experience significant discomfort. Many physicians prefer to use their own customized formula, which they obtain from a compounding pharmacy. However, these compounded formulas are not monitored by the FDA and compounding pharmacies may vary in the quality-control standards. Some of the formulas may contain up to 40% local anesthetics in various combinations. This type of preparation could deliver up to 400 mg per gram of ointment to the patient. The application of 30 g of a compounded formula containing a total of 20% local anesthetic over a wide area with subsequent occlusive dressing could expose the patient to 6,000 mg of local anesthetic. Studies have demonstrated that systemic absorption of local anesthetic after application of topical local anesthetic is limited to less than 5% [139, 140]. Even with limited systemic absorption, the development of toxic blood levels of local anesthetic, with the ensuing catastrophic results, would not be hard to envision if a large quantity of a concentrated compounded anesthetic ointment were applied under an occlusive dressing. There has been at least one case report of death after application of a compounded local anesthetic ointment while preparing for cosmetic surgery [141]. Physicians who prescribe compounded topical local anesthetics to patients prior to surgery should reevaluate the concentration of these medications as well as the total dose of medication that may be delivered to the patient. Frequently, the patient is given the topical anesthetic to be applied at home prior to arrival at the office or surgical center.

1.6.2
Sedative-Analgesic Medication

Most minimally invasive procedures may be performed with a combination of local anesthesia and supplemental sedative-analgesic medication (SAM) administered orally, intramuscularly, or intravenously. The goals of administering supplemental medications are to reduce anxiety (anxiolytics), the level of consciousness (sedation), unanticipated pain (analgesia), and, in some cases, to eliminate recall of the surgery (amnesia).

Sedation may be defined as the reduction of the level of consciousness usually resulting from pharmacological interventions. The level of sedation may be further divided into four broad categories, minimal sedation, moderate sedation, deep sedation (also referred to as conscious sedation), and general anesthesia. During minimal sedation patients may respond normally to verbal commands but have impaired cognitive function and coordination. Life-preserving protective reflexes (LPPRs), ventilatory function, and cardiovascular function are generally maintained during minimal sedation. During moderate sedation, while the level consciousness is depressed, the patient should respond in a purposeful manner to soft verbal commands. During deep sedation, the patient becomes difficult to arouse and may respond purposely only with loud verbal or painful tactile stimulation. During deep sedation the patient has a probability of loss of LPPRs and a depression of ventilatory function. Cardiovascular function is usually maintained. Finally, during general anesthesia there is complete loss of consciousness and the patient is not arousable by any means. There is a high likelihood of loss of LPPRs and suppression of ventilatory and cardiac function under general anesthesia [142].

LPPRs may be defined as the involuntary physical and physiological responses that maintain the patient's

Table 1.5 Clinical pharmacology of common local anesthetics for infiltrative

Agent	Without epinephrine		With epinephrine						
	Concentration (%)	Duration of action (min)	Maximum dose			Duration of action (min)	Maximum dose		
			(mg/kg)	(total mg)	(total ml)		(mg/kg)	(total mg)	(total ml)
Lidocaine	1.0	30–60	4	300	30	120	7	500	50
Mepivacaine	1.0	45–90	4	300	30	120	7	500	50
Etidocaine	0.5	120–180	4	300	60	180	5.5	400	80
Bupivacaine	0.25	120–240	2.5	185	75	180	3	225	90
Ropivacaine	0.2	120–360	2.7	200	80	120–360	2.7	200	80

Adapted from Covino and Wildsmith [111]

life which, if interrupted, result in inevitable and catastrophic physiological consequences. The most obvious examples of LPPRs are the ability to maintain an open airway, swallowing, coughing, gagging, and spontaneous breathing. Some involuntary physical movements such as head turning or attempts to assume an erect posture may be considered LPPRs if these reflex actions occur in an attempt to improve airway patency such as expelling oropharyngeal contents. The myriad of homeostatic mechanisms to maintain blood pressure, heart function, and body temperature may even be considered LPPRs. When a patient enters deep sedation, and the level of consciousness is depressed to the point that the patient is not able to respond purposefully to verbal commands or physical stimulation, there is a significant probability of loss of LPPRs. Ultimately, as total loss of consciousness occurs under general anesthesia and the patient no longer responds to verbal command or painful stimuli, the patient most likely loses the LPPRs [142].

In actual practice, the delineation between the levels of sedation becomes challenging at best. The loss of consciousness occurs as a continuum. With each incremental change in the level of consciousness, the likelihood of loss of LPPRs increases. The level of consciousness may vary from moment to moment, depending on the level of surgical stimulation. Since the definition of conscious sedation is vague, current ASA guidelines consider the term sedation-analgesia a more relevant term than conscious sedation [15]. The term "sedative-analgesic medication" (SAM) has been adopted by some facilities. Monitored anesthesia care has been generally defined as the medical management of patients receiving local anesthesia during surgery with or without the use of supplemental medications. Monitored anesthesia care usually refers to services provided by the anesthesiologist or the CRNA. The term "local standby" is no longer used because it mischaracterizes the purpose and activity of the anesthesiologist or CRNA.

Surgical procedures performed using a combination of local anesthetic and SAM usually have a shorter recovery time than similar procedures performed under regional or general anesthesia [143]. Using local anesthesia alone, without the benefit of supplemental medication, is associated with a greater risk of cardiovascular and hemodynamic perturbations such as tachycardia, arrhythmias, and hypertension particularly in patients with preexisting cardiac disease or hypertension [144]. Patients usually prefer sedation while undergoing surgery with local anesthetics [145]. While the addition of sedatives and analgesics during surgery using local anesthesia seems to have some advantages, use of SAM during local anesthesia is certainly not free of risk. A study by the Federated Ambulatory Surgical Association concluded that local anesthesia with supplemental medications was associated with more than twice the number of complications than local anesthesia alone. Furthermore, local anesthesia with SAM was associated with greater risks than general anesthesia [146]. Significant respiratory depression as determined by the development of hypoxemia, hypercarbia, and respiratory acidosis has been documented in patients after receiving even minimal doses of medications. This respiratory depression persists even in the recovery period [147, 148].

One explanation for the frequency of complications in patients receiving SAM is the wide variability of patients' responses to these medications. Up to 20-fold differences in the dose requirements for some medications such as diazepam and up to fivefold variations for some narcotics such as fentanyl have been documented in some patients [149, 150]. Even small doses of fentanyl as low as 2 µg/kg, considered by many physicians as subclinical, produce respiratory depression for more than 1 h in some patients [151]. Combinations of even small doses of sedatives, such as midazolam, and narcotics, such as fentanyl, may act synergistically (effects greater than an additive effect) in producing adverse side effects such as respiratory depression and hemodynamic instability [152]. The clearance of many medications may vary depending on the amount and duration of administration, a phenomenon known as context-sensitive half-life. The net result is increased sensitivity and duration of action to medication for longer surgical operations [153]. Because of these variations and interactions, predicting any given patient's dose-response is a daunting task. Patients appearing awake and responsive may, in an instant, slip into unintended levels of deep sedation with greater potential of loss of LPPRs. Careful titration of these medications to the desired effect combined with vigilant monitoring are the critical elements in avoiding complications associated with the use of SAM. Klein [154] acknowledges that most of the complications attributed to midazolam and narcotic combinations occur as result of inadequate monitoring. Supplemental medication may be administered via multiple routes including oral, nasal, transmucosal, transcutaneous, intravenous, intramuscular, and rectal. While intermittent bolus has been the traditional method to administer medication, continuous infusion and patient-controlled delivery result in comparable safety and patient satisfaction [155, 156].

Benzodiazepines such as diazepam, midazolam, and lorezepam remain popular for sedation and anxiolytics. Patients and physicians especially appreciate the potent amnestic effects of this class of medications, especially midazolam (using midazolam "means never having to say you're sorry"). The disadvantages of diazepam include the higher incidence of pain on intravenous administration, the possibility of phlebitis [157], and the prolonged half-life of up to 20–50 h. Moreover, diazepam has active metabolites, which may prolong the effects of the medication even into the postoperative recovery time [158]. Midazolam, however, is more rapidly metabolized, allowing for a quicker and more complete recovery for outpatient surgery [158]. Because the sedative, anxiolytic, and amnestic effects of midazolam are more profound than those of other benzodiazepines and the recovery is more rapid, patient acceptance is usually higher [159]. Since lorezepam is less affected by medications altering cytochrome P450 metabolisim [160], it has been recommended as the sedative of choice of liposuctions which require large-dose lidocaine tumescent anesthesia [121]. The disadvantage of lorezepam is the slower onset of action and the 11–22-h elimination half-life making titration cumbersome and postoperative recovery prolonged [158].

Generally, physicians who use SAM titrate a combination of medications from different classes to tailor the medications to the desired level of sedation and analgesia for each patient. Use of prepackaged or premixed combinations of medications defeats the purpose of the selective control of each medication. Typically, sedatives such as the benzodiazepines are combined with narcotic analgesics such as fentanyl, meperidine, or morphine during local anesthesia to decrease pain associated with local anesthetic injection or unanticipated breakthrough pain. Fentanyl has the advantage of rapid onset and duration of action of less than 60 min. However, because of synergistic action with sedative agents, even doses of 25–50 μg can result in respiratory depression [161]. Other medications with sedative and hypnotic effects such as a barbiturate, ketamine, or propofol are often added. Adjunctive analgesics such as ketorolac may be administered for additional analgesic activity. As long as the patient is carefully monitored, several medications may be titrated together to achieve the effects required for the patient characteristics and the complexity of the surgery. Fixed combinations of medications are not advised [15].

More-potent narcotic analgesics with rapid onset of action and even shorter duration of action than fentanyl include sufenanil, alfenanil, and remifenanil and may be administered using intermittent boluses or continuous infusion in combination with other sedative or hypnotic agents. However, extreme caution and scrupulous monitoring is required when these potent narcotics are used because of the risk of respiratory arrest [162, 163]. Use of these medications should be restricted to the anesthesiologist or the CRNA. A major disadvantage of narcotic medication is the perioperative nausea and vomiting [164].

Many surgeons feel comfortable administering SAM to patients. Others prefer to use the services of an anesthesiologist or a CNRA. Prudence dictates that for prolonged or complicated surgeries or for patients with significant risk factors, the participation of the anesthesiologist or CRNA during monitored anesthesia care is preferable. Regardless of who administers the anesthetic medications, the monitoring must have the same level of vigilance.

Propofol, a member of the alkylphenol family, has demonstrated its versatility as a supplemental sedative-hypnotic agent for local anesthesia and of regional anesthesia. Propofol may be used alone or in combination with a variety of other medications. Rapid metabolism and clearance results in faster and more complete recovery with less postoperative hangover than with other sedative-hypnotic medications such as midazolam and methohexital [165, 166]. The documented antiemetic properties of propofol yield added benefits of this medication [167]. The disadvantages of propofol include pain on intravenous injection and the lack of amnestic effect [168]. However, the addition of 3 ml of 2% lidocaine to 20 ml of propofol virtually eliminates the pain on injection with no added risk. If an amnestic response is desired, a small dose of a benzodiazepine, such as midazolam (5 mg i.v.), given in combination with propofol, provides the adequate amnesia. Rapid administration of propofol may be associated with significant hypotension, decreased cardiac output [169], and respiratory depression [170]. Continuous infusion with propofol results in a more rapid recovery than similar infusions with midazolam [171]. Patient-controlled sedation with propofol has also been shown to be safe and effective [172].

Barbiturate sedative-hypnotic agents such as thiopental and methohexital, while older, still play a role in many clinical settings. In particular, methohexital, with controlled boluses (10–20 mg i.v.) or limited infusions remains a safe and effective sedative-hypnotic alternative with rapid recovery. However, with prolonged administration recovery from methohexital may be delayed compared with recovery from propofol [173].

Ketamine, a phencyclidine derivative, is a unique agent because of its combined sedative and analgesic effects and the absence of cardiovascular depression in healthy patients [174]. Because the CNS effects of ketamine result in a state similar to catatonia, the resulting anesthesia is often described as dissociative anesthesia. Although gag and cough reflexes are more predictably maintained with ketamine, emesis and pulmonary aspiration of gastric contents are still possible [175]. Unfortunately, a significant number of patients suffer distressing postoperative psychomimetic reactions [176]. While concomitant administration of benzodiazepines attenuates these reactions, the postoperative psychological sequelae limit the usefulness of ketamine for most elective outpatient surgeries.

Droperidol, a butyrophenone and a derivative of haloperidol, acts as a sedative, hypnotic, and antiemetic medication. Rather than causing global CNS depression like barbiturates, droperidol causes more specific CNS changes similar to phenothiazines. For this reason, the cataleptic state caused by droperidol is referred to as neuroleptic anesthesia [177]. Droperidol has been used effectively in combination with various narcotic medications. While droperidol has minimal effect on respiratory function if used as a single agent, when combined with narcotic medication, a predictable dose-dependant respiratory depression may be anticipated [178]. Psychomimetic reactions such as dysphoria or hallucina-

Table 1.6 Common medications and doses used for sedative

Medication	Bolus dose	Average adult dose	Continuous infusion rate (μg/kg/min)
Narcotic analgesics			
Alfentanil	5–7 μg/kg	30 to 50 μg	0.2–0.5
Fentanyl	0.3–0.7 μg/kg	25 to 50 μg	0.01
Meperidine	0.2 mg	10–20 mg i.v., 50–100 mg i.m.	NA
Morphine	0.02 mg	1–2 mg i.v., 5–10 mg i.m.	NA
Remifentanil	0.5–1.0 μg/kg	10–25 μg	0.025–0.05
Sufentanil	0.1–0.2 μg/kg	10 μg	0.001–0.002
Opiate agonist–antagonist analgesics			
Buprenorphene	4–6 μg/kg	0.3 mg	NA
Butorphanol	2–7 μg/kg	0.1–0.2 mg	NA
Nalbupnine	0.03–0.1 mg/kg	10 mg	NA
Sedative-hypnotics			
Diazepam	0.05–0.1 mg/kg	5–7.5 mg	NA
Methohexital	0.2–0.5 mg/kg	10–20 mg	10–50
Midazolam	30–75 μg/kg	2.5–5.0 mg	0.25–0.5
Propofol	0.2–0.5 mg/kg	10–20 mg	10–50
Thiopental	0.5–1.0 mg/kg	25–50 mg	50–100
Dissociative anesthetics			
Ketamine	0.2–0.5 mg/kg	10–20 mg	10

Adapted from Philip [184], Sa Rego et al. [185] and Fragen [186]. The doses may vary depending on age, gender, underlying health status, and other concomitantly administered medications.
NA not available

tions are frequent, unpleasant side effects of droperidol. Benzodiazepines or narcotics reduce the incidence of these unpleasant side effects [179, 180]. Extrapyramidal reactions such as dyskinesias, torticollis, or oculogyric spasms may also occur, even with small doses of droperidol. Dimenhydrinate usually reverses these complications [180]. Hypotension may occur as consequence of droperidol's alpha-adrenergic receptor blocking characteristics. One rare complication of droperidol is the neurolept malignant syndrome [181], a condition very similar to malignant hyperthermia, characterized by extreme temperature elevations and rhabdomyolysis. The treatment of neurolept malignant syndrome and malignant hyperthermia is essentially the same. While droperidol has been used for years without appreciable myocardial depression [179], a surprising announcement from the FDA warned of sudden cardiac death

resulting after the administration of standard, clinically useful doses [182]. Unfortunately, this potential complication makes the routine use of this once very useful medication difficult to justify given the availability of alternative medications.

Butarphanol, buprenorphine, and nalbuphine are three synthetically derived opiates, which share the properties of being mixed agonist–antagonists at the opiate receptors. These medications are sometimes preferred as supplemental analgesics during local, regional, or general anesthesia, because they partially reverse the analgesic and respiratory depressant effects of other narcotics. While these medications result in respiratory depression at lower doses, a ceiling effect occurs at higher dose, thereby limiting the respiratory depression. Still, respiratory arrest is possible, especially if these medications are combined with other medications with respiratory depressant properties [183]. While the duration of action of nutarphanol is 2–3 h, nalbuphine has a duration of action of about 3–6 h and buprenorphan has one of up to 10 h, making these medications less suitable for surgeries of shorter duration. Table 1.6 summarizes the recommended doses for SAM.

1.6.3
Regional Anesthesia

Many limited cosmetic procedures may be performed using regional anesthesia, which is blockade of one or more sensory nerves with local anesthesia. Even though patients receive regional anesthesia, additional SAMs can be administered.

1.6.4
General Anesthesia

Although significant advances have been made in the administration of local anesthetics, SAMs, and regional anesthesia, the use of general anesthesia may still be the anesthesia technique of choice for many patients. General anesthesia is especially appropriate when working with patients suffering extreme anxiety, high tolerance to narcotic or sedative medications, or if the surgery is particularly complex. The goals of a general anesthetic are a smooth induction, a prompt recovery, and minimal side effects, such as nausea, vomiting, or sore throat. The inhalation anesthetic agents halothane, isoflurane, and enflurane have been widely popular because of the safety, reliability, and convenience of use. The newer inhalation agents sevoflurane and desflurane share similar properties with the added benefit of prompt emergence [187, 188]. Nitrous oxide, a long-time favorite anesthetic inhalation agent, may be associated with postoperative nausea and vomiting (PONV) [189]. Patients receiving nitrous oxide also have a greater risk of perioperative hypoxemia.

The development of potent, short-acting sedatives, opiates, analgesics, and muscle-relaxant medications has resulted in a newer medication regimen that permits the use of intravenous agents exclusively. The same medications that have been discussed for SAM can also be used during general anesthesia as sole agents or in combination with the inhalation agents [190]. The anesthesiologist or CRNA should preferentially be responsible for the administration and monitoring of general anesthesia.

Airway control is a key element in the management of the patient under general anesthesia. Maintaining a patent airway, ensuring adequate ventilation, and prevention of aspiration of gastric contents are the goals of successful airway management. For shorter operations, the airway may be supported by an oropharyngeal airway and gas mixtures delivered by an occlusive mask.

For longer or more complex operations, or if additional facial surgery is planned requiring surgical field avoidance, then the airway may be secured using laryngeal mask anesthesia or endotracheal intubation [191].

Orthognathic surgeries that require unrestricted access to the oral and lower facial regions often require nasotracheal intubation. Obviously, this procedure requires an anesthesiologist with extensive training and experience to avoid serious complications to the upper airway. Techniques that facilitate nasotracheal intubation are:

1. Pretreating of the nasopharynx with vasoconstrictor (0.05% oxymetolosine)
2. Nasotracheal tube one size smaller than the size normally used for oratracheal intubation
3. Prewarming the endotracheal tube to 45 °C
4. Progressively dilating the nasopharynx with lubricated rubber nasopharyngeal tubes after induction
5. Copious lubrication of the endotracheal tube with a dental anesthetic lubricant (with 10% benzocain)
6. Preflexing the tip of the endotracheal tube just prior to intubation to negotiate the nasopharynx
7. Using curved intubating forceps to direct the endotracheal tube through the larynx

Preflexing the tip of the endotracheal tube immediately prior to intubation that facilitates the passage of the tube around the nasopharyngeal junction is one helpful technique. When these precautions are followed, complications related to nasotracheal intubation, such as perioperative nasopharyngeal bleeding or nasopharyngeal trauma, are extremely rare (The Center for Oral and Facial Reconstruction and Reconstruction and Ambulatory Services, Irvine, CA, USA, unpublished data).

1.7
Preoperative Preparation

Generally, medications which may have been required to stabilize the patient's medical conditions should be continued up to the time of surgery. Notable exceptions include anticoagulant medications, monoamine oxidase (MAO) inhibitors [192, 193], and possibly ACE inhibitor medications [194, 195]. It is generally accepted that MAO inhibitors, carboxazial (Marplan), deprenyl (Eldepryl), paragyline (Eutonyl), phenelzine (Nardil), tranylcypromine (Parnate), should be discontinued 2–3 weeks prior to surgery, especially for elective operations, because of the interactions with narcotic medication, specifically, hyperpyrexia, and certain vasopressor agents, specifically, ephedrine [192, 193]. Patients taking ACE inhibitors (captopril, enalapril, and lisinopril) may have a greater risk for hypotension during general anesthesia [195]. As previously discussed, diabetics may require a reduction in the dose of their medication. However, if the risks of discontinuing any of these medications outweigh the benefits of the proposed elective surgery, the patient and physician may decide to postpone, modify, or cancel the proposed surgery.

Previous requirements of complete preoperative fasting for 10–16 h are considered unnecessary by many anethesiologists [196, 197]. More-recent investigations have demonstrated that gastric volume may be less 2 h after oral intake of 8 oz of clear liquid than after more-prolonged fasting [198]. Furthermore, prolonged fasting may increase the risk of hypoglycemia [199]. Many patients appreciate an 8-oz feeding of their favorite caffeinated elixir 2 h prior to surgery. Preoperative sedative medications may also be taken with a small amount of water or juice. Abstinence from solid food ingestion for 10–12 h prior to surgery is still recommended. Liquids taken prior to surgery must be clear [200], e.g., coffee without cream or juice without pulp.

Healthy outpatients are no longer considered higher risk for gastric acid aspiration and, therefore, routine use of antacids, histamine type-2 (H2) antagonists, or gastrokinetic medications is not indicated. However, patients with marked obesity, hiatal hernia, or diabetes mellitus have higher risks for aspiration. These patients may benefit form selected prophylactic treatment [201]. Sodium citrate, an orally administered, non-particulate antacid, rapidly increases gastric pH; however, its unpleasant taste and short duration of action limit its usefulness in elective surgery [202]. Gastric volume and pH may be effectively reduced by H2 receptor antagonists. Cimetidine (300 mg p.o., 1–2 h prior to surgery) reduces gastric volume and pH; however, it is also a potent cytochrome oxidase inhibitor and may increase the risk of reactions to lidocaine during tumescent anesthesia [203]. Ranitidine (150–300 mg, 90–120 min prior to surgery) [204] and famotidine (20 mg p.o., 60 min prior to surgery) are equally effective but have a better safety profile than cimetidine [205].

Omeprazole, which decreases gastric acid secretion by inhibiting the proton pump mechanism of the gastric mucosa, may prove to be a safe and effective alternative to the H2 receptor antagonists [205]. Metaclopramide (10–20 mg p.o. or i.v.), a gastrokinetic agent which increases gastric motility and lowers esophageal sphincter tone, may be effective in patients with reduced gastric motility, such as diabetics or patients receiving opiates. However, extrapyramidal side effects limit the routine use of the medication [164, 206].

Postoperative nausea and vomiting (PONV) remains one of the more vexing complications of anesthesia and surgery [207]. In fact, patients dread PONV more than any other complication, even postoperative pain [208]. PONV is the most common postoperative complication [209, 210], and the common cause of postoperative patient dissatisfaction [211]. Strategies to reduce PONV should be incorporated into the preoperative planning stages especially in patients with previous histories of PONV. Use of prophylactic antiemetic medication has been shown to reduce the incidence of PONV [212]. Even though many patients do not suffer PONV in the recovery period after ambulatory anesthesia, more than 35% of patients develop PONV after discharge [213].

Droperidol, 0.625–1.25 mg i.v., is an extremely cost-effective antiemetic [214]. However, troublesome side effects such as sedation, dysphoria, extrapyramidal reactions [215], and, more recently, cardiac arrest have been described [182]. These complications may preclude the widespread use of droperidol altogether. The serotonin antagonists ondansetron (4–8 mg i.v.), dolasetron (12.5 mg i.v.), and granisetron (1 mg i.v.) are among the most effective antiemetic medications available without sedative, dysphoric or extrapyramidal sequelae [216–218]. The antiemetic effects of ondansetron may reduce PONV for up to 24 h postoperatively [219]. The effects of ondansetron may be augmented by the addition of dexamethasone (4–8 mg) [220] or droperidol (1.25 mg i.v.) [221]. Despite the efficacy of the newer serotonin antagonists, cost remains a prohibitive factor in the routine prophylactic use of these medications, especially in the office setting.

Promethazine (12.5–25 mg p.o., p.r., or i.m.) and chlorpromazine (5–10 mg p.o. or i.m. and 25 mg p.r.) are two older phenothiazines which are still used by many physicians as prophylaxis, especially in combination with narcotic analgesics. Once again, sedation and extrapyramidal effects may complicate the routine prophylactic use of these medications [164].

Preoperative atropine (0.4 mg i.m.), glycopyrrolate (0.2 mg i.m.), and scopolamine (0.2 mg i.m.), anticholinergic agents, once considered standard preoperative medication because of their vagolytic and antisialogic effects, are no longer popular because of side effects such as dry mouth, dizziness, tachycardia, and disorientation [222]. Transdermal scopolamine, applied 90 min prior to surgery, effectively reduces PONV; however, the incidence of dry mouth and drowsiness is high [223], and toxic psychosis is a rare complication [225]. Antihistamines, such as dimenhydrinate (25–50 mg p.o., i.m., or i.v.) and hydroxyzine (50 mg p.o. or i.m.), may also be used to treat and prevent PONV with few side effects except for possible postoperative sedation [225].

The selection of anesthetic agents may also play a major role in PONV. The direct antiemetic actions of propofol have been clearly demonstrated [226]. Anesthetic regimens utilizing propofol, alone or in combination with other medications, are associated with significantly less PONV [227]. Although still controversial, nitrous oxide is considered by many authors a prime suspect among possible causes of PONV [189, 228, 229]. Opiates are also considered culprits in the development of PONV and the delay of discharge after outpatient surgery [164, 230–232]. Adequate fluid hydration has been shown to reduce PONV [233].

One goal of preoperative preparation is to reduce the anxiety of patients. Many simple, non-pharmacological techniques may be extremely effective in reassuring both patients and families, starting with a relaxed, friendly atmosphere and a professional, caring, and attentive office staff. With proper preoperative preparation, pharmacological interventions may not even be necessary. However, a variety of oral and parenteral anxiolytic-sedative medications are frequently called upon to provide a smooth transition to the operative room. Diazepam (5–10 mg p.o.), given 1–2 h preoperatively, is a very effective medication which usually does not prolong recovery time [234]. Parenteral diazepam (5–10 mg i.v. or i.m.) may also be given immediately preoperatively. However, because of a long elimination half-life of 24–48 h, and active metabolites with an elimination half-life of 50–120 h, caution must be exercised when using diazepam, especially in shorter operations, so that recovery is not delayed [235]. Pain and phlebitis with intravenous or intramuscular administration reduces the popularity of diazepam [157].

Lorezepam (1–2 mg p.o. or s.l., 1–2 h preoperatively) is also an effective choice for sedation or anxiolytics. However, the prolonged duration of action may prolong the recovery time after shorter operations [236]. Midazolam (5–7.5 mg i.m., 30 min preoperatively or 2 mg i.v. minutes prior to surgery) is a more potent anxiolytic-sedative medication with more rapid onset and shorter elimination half-life, compared with diazepam [237]. Unfortunately, orally administered midazolam has unpredictable results and is not considered a useful alternative for preoperative medication [238]. Oral narcotics, such as oxycodone (5–10 mg p.o.), may help relieve the patient's intraoperative breakthrough pain during operations involving more limited liposuction with minimal potential perioperative sequelae. Parenteral opioids, such as morphine (5–10 mg i.m. or 1–2 mg i.v.), demerol (50–100 mg i.m. or 10–20 mg i.v.), fentanyl (10–20 μg i.v.), or sufentanil (1–2 ug i.v.), may produce sedation and euphoria and may decrease the requirements for other sedative medication. The level of anxiolytics and sedation is still greater with the benzodiazepines than with the opioids. Premedication with narcotics has been shown to have minimal effects on postoperative recovery time. However, opioid premedication may increase PONV [239, 240].

Antihistamine medications, such as hydroxyzine (50–100 mg i.m. or 50–100 mg p.o.) and dimenhydrinate (50 mg p.o. or i.m. or 25 mg i.v.), are still used safely in combination with other premedications, especially the opioids, to add sedation and to reduce nausea and pruritis. However, the anxiolytic and amnestic effects are not as potent as for the benzodiazepines [241]. Barbiturates, such as secobarbital and pentobarbital, once a standard premedication have largely been replaced by the benzodiazepines.

Postoperative pulmonary embolism is an unpredictable and devastating complication with an estimated incidence of 0.1–5%, depending on the type of surgical case [242], and a mortality rate of about 15% [243]. Risk factors for thromboembolism include prior history or family history of DVT or pulmonary embolism, obesity, smoking, hypertension, use of oral contraceptives and hormone replacement therapy, and patients over 60 years of age [243]. Estimates for the incidence of postoperative DVT vary from 0.8% for outpatients undergoing herniorrhaphies [244] to up to 80% for patients undergoing total hip replacement [242]. Estimates of fatal pulmonary embolism also vary from 0.1% for patients undergoing general surgeries to up to 1–5% for patients undergoing major joint replacement [242]. The incidence of pulmonary embolism may be more common than reported. One study revealed that unsuspected pulmonary embolism may actually occur in up to 40% of patients who develop DVT [245].

Most minimally invasive cosmetic surgeries, especially of the head and neck, under local anesthesia, with or without sedation, are considered low risk for DVT or pulmonary embolism. Prevention of DVT and pulmonary embolism should be considered an essential component of the perioperative management, especially for operations which may last more than 2 h, when a general anesthetic is used or the patient has increased risk factors for DVT or pulmonary embolism. Although unfractionated heparin reduces the rate of fatal pulmonary embolism [246], many surgeons are reluctant to use this prophylaxis because of concerns of perioperative hemorrhage. The low molecular weight heparins enoxaparin, dalteparin, and ardeparin and danaparoid, a heparinoid, are available for prophylactic indications. Graduated compression stockings and intermittent pneumatic lower-extremity compression devices applied throughout the perioperative period, until the patient has become ambulatory, are considered very effective and safe alternatives in the prevention of postoperative DVT and pulmonary embolism [247, 248]. Even with prophylactic therapy, pulmonary embolism may still occur up to 30 days after surgery [249]. Physicians should be suspicious of pulmonary embolism if patients present postoperatively with dyspnea, chest pain, cough, hemoptysis, pleuritic pain, dizziness, syncope, tachycardia, cyanosis, shortness of breath, or wheezing [243].

1.8
Perioperative Monitoring

The adoption of a standardized perioperative monitoring protocol has resulted in a quantum leap in perioperative patient safety. The standards for basic perioperative monitoring were approved by the ASA in 1986 and amended in 1995 [7]. These monitoring standards are now considered applicable to all types of anesthetics, including local with or without sedation, regional, or general anesthesia, regardless of the duration or complexity of the surgical procedure and regardless of whether the surgeon or anesthesiologist is responsible for the anesthesia. Vigilant and continuous monitoring and compulsive documentation facilitates early recognition of deleterious physiological events and trends, which, if not recognized promptly, could lead to irreversible pathological spirals, ultimately endangering a patient's life.

During the course of action of any anesthetic, the patient's oxygenation, ventilation, circulation, and temperature should be continuously evaluated. The concentration of the inspired oxygen must be measured by an oxygen analyzer. Assessment of the perioperative oxygenation of the patient using pulse oximetry, now considered mandatory in every case, has been a significant advancement in monitoring. This monitoring is so critical to the safety of the patient that it has earned the nickname "the monitor of life." Evaluation of ventilation includes observation of skin color, chest wall motion, and frequent auscultation of breath sounds. During general anesthesia with or without mechanical ventilation, a disconnect alarm on the anesthesia circuit is crucial. Capnography, a measurement of respiratory end-tidal CO_2, is required, especially when the patient is under heavy sedation or general anesthesia. Capnography provides the first alert in the event of airway obstruction, hypoventilation, or accidental anesthesia circuit disconnect, even before the oxygen saturation has begun to fall. End-expiratory or inspiratory volatile gas monitoring is also extremely useful. All patients must have continuous monitoring of the ECG, and intermittent determination of blood pressure and heart rate at a minimum of 5-min intervals. Superficial or core body temperature should be monitored. Of course, all electronic monitors must have preset alarm limits to alert physicians prior to the development of critical changes.

While the availability of electronic monitoring equipment has improved perioperative safety, there is no substitute for visual monitoring by a qualified, experienced practitioner, usually a CRNA or an anesthesiologist. During surgeries using local anesthesia with SAM, if a surgeon elects not to use a CRNA or an anesthesiologist, a separate, designated, certified individual must perform these monitoring functions [15]. Visual observation of the patient's position is also important in order to avoid untoward outcomes such as peripheral nerve or ocular injuries.

Documentation of perioperative events, interventions, and observations must be contemporaneously performed and should include blood pressure and heart rate every 5 min and oximetry, capnography, ECG pattern, and temperature at 15-min intervals. Intravenous fluids, medication doses in milligrams, patient position, and other intraoperative events must also be recorded. Documentation may alert the physician to unrecognized physiological trends that may require treatment. Preparation for subsequent anesthetics may require information contained in the patient's prior records, especially if the patient suffered an unsatisfactory outcome due to the anesthetic regimen that was used. Treatment of subsequent complications by other physicians may require information contained in the records, such as the types of medications used, blood loss or fluid totals. Finally, compulsive documentation may help exonerate a physician in many medical-legal situations.

When local anesthesia with SAM is used, monitoring must include an assessment of the patient's level of consciousness as previously described. For patients under general anesthesia, the level of consciousness may be determined using the bispectral index (BIS), a measurement derived from computerized analysis of the electroencephalogram. When used with patients receiving general anesthesia, the BIS improves control of the level of consciousness, rate of emergence and recovery, and cost-control of medication usage. Moreover, BIS monitoring may reduce the risk of intraoperative recall [250].

1.9
Fluid Replacement

Management of perioperative fluids probably generates more controversy than any other anesthesia-related topic. For minimally invasive treatments in healthy patients, fluid replacement is not a critical part of the procedure. In this patient population, the intravenous access serves merely as a conduit for the administration of medications. Generally, the typical, healthy, 60-kg patient requires about 100 ml of water per hour to replace metabolic, sensible, and insensible water losses. After a 12-h period of fasting, a 60-kg patient may be expected to have a 1-l volume deficit on the morning of surgery. This deficit should be replaced over the first few hours of surgery. The patient's usual maintenance fluid needs may be met with a crystalloid solution such as lactated Ringer's solution.

Replacement fluids may be divided into crystalloid solutions, such as normal saline or balance salt solution, colloids, such as fresh frozen plasma, 5% albumin, plasma protein fraction, or hetastarch, and blood products containing red blood cells, such as packed red blood cells. Generally, balanced salt solutions may be used as standard fluid maintenance and to replace small amounts of blood loss. For every milliliter of blood loss, 3 ml of fluid replacement is usually required [251]. However, as larger volumes of blood are lost, attempts to replace these losses with crystalloid solution reduces the serum oncotic pressure, one of the main forces supporting intravascular volume. Subsequently, crystalloid solution rapidly moves into the extracellular space. Intravascular volume cannot be adequately sustained with further infusion of crystalloid solution [252]. At this point, many authors suggest that a colloid solution may be more effective in maintaining intravascular volume and hemodynamic stability [253, 254]. Given the ongoing crystalloid–colloid controversy in the literature, the most practical approach to fluid management is a compromise. Crystalloid replacement should be used for estimated blood losses (EBL) less than 500 ml, while colloids, such as hetastarch may be used for EBLs greater than 500 ml. One milliliter of colloid solution should be used to replace 1 ml of EBL [251]. However, not all authors agree on the benefits of colloid resuscitation. Moss and Gould [255] concluded that isotonic crystalloid replacement, even for large EBLs, restores plasma volume as well as colloid replacement.

Transfusion of red blood cells is rarely a consideration during minimally invasive cosmetic surgeries. Healthy, normovolemic patients, with hemodynamic and physiologic stability, should tolerate hemoglobin levels down to 7.5 g/dl [256]. The decision to transfuse must be made after careful consideration of the benefits and risks of transfusion and not rely on one transfusion trigger. Transfusion is generally indicated when hemoglobin concentrations fall below 6 g/dl [257]. The management of fluids during more invasive operations such as large-volume liposuction or abdominoplasty has been described in detail elsewhere [258].

1.10
Recovery and Discharge

The same intensive monitoring and treatment which occurs in the operating room must be continued in the recovery room under the care of a designated, licensed, and experienced person for as long as is necessary to ensure the stability and safety of the patient, regardless of whether the facility is a hospital, an outpatient surgical center, or a physicians office. During the initial stages of recovery, the patient should not be left alone while hospital or office personnel attend to other duties. Vigilant monitoring including visual observation, continuous oximetry, continuous ECG, and intermittent blood pressure and temperature determinations must be continued. Because the patient is still vulnerable to airway obstruction and respiratory arrest in the recovery period, continuous visual observation is still the best method of monitoring for this complication. Supplemental oxygenation should be continued during the initial stages of recovery and continued until the patient is able to maintain an oxygen saturation above 90% on room air.

The most common postoperative complication is nausea and vomiting. The antiemetic medications previously discussed, with the same consideration of potential risks, may be used in the postoperative period. Ondansetron (4–8 mg i.v. or s.l.) and other serotonin antagonists are probably the safest and most effective antiemetics [216–220]. However, the cost of such medication is often prohibitive, especially in an office setting [221]. Postoperative surgical pain may be managed with judiciously titrated intravenous narcotic medication such as demerol (10–20 mg i.v. every 5–10 min),

morphine (1–2 mg i.v. every 5–10 min), or butorphanol (0.1–0.2 mg i.v. every 10 min).

The number of complications that occur after discharge may be more than twice the number of complications occurring intraoperatively and during recovery combined [259]. Accredited ambulatory surgical centers generally have established discharge criteria. While these criteria may vary, the common goal is to ensure the patient's level of consciousness and physiological stability. The following is an example of discharge criteria which may be used [260]:

1. All life-preserving protective reflexes, i.e., airway, cough, gag, must be returned to normal.
2. The vital signs must be stable without orthostatic changes.
3. There must be no evidence of hypoxemia 20 min after the discontinuation of supplemental oxygen.
4. Patients must be oriented to person, place, time, and situation (times 4).
5. Nausea and vomiting must be controlled and patients should tolerate fluids per os.
6. There must be no evidence of postoperative hemorrhage or expanding ecchymosis.
7. Incisional pain should be reasonably controlled.
8. The patient should be able to sit up without support and walk with assistance.

Medication intended to reverse the effects of anesthesia should be used only in the event of suspected overdose of medications. Naloxone (0.1–0.2 mg i.v.), a pure opiate receptor antagonist, with a therapeutic half-life of less than 2 h, may be used to reverse the respiratory depressant effects of narcotic medications, such as morphine, demerol, fentanyl, and butorphanol. Because potential adverse effects of rapid opiate reversal of narcotics include severe pain, seizures, pulmonary edema, hypertension, congestive heart failure, and cardiac arrest [261], naloxone must be administered by careful titration. Naloxone has no effect on the actions of medications, such as the benzodiazepines, the barbiturates, propofol, or ketamine.

Flumazenil (0.1–0.2 mg i.v.), a specific competitive antagonist of the benzodiazepines, such as diazepam, midazolam, and lorezepam, may be used to reverse excessive or prolonged sedation and respiratory depression resulting from these medications [262]. The effective half-life of Flumazenil is one l h or less [263].

The effective half-lives of many narcotics exceed the half-life of naloxone. The benzodiazepines have effective half-lives greater than 2 h and, in the case of diazepam, up to 50 h. Many active metabolites unpredictably extend the putative effects of the narcotics and benzodiazepines. A major risk associated with the use of naloxone and Flumazenil is the recurrence of the effects of the narcotic or benzodiazepine after 1–2 h. If the patient has already been discharged home after these effects recur, the patient may be at risk for oversedation or respiratory arrest [261, 264]; therefore, routine use of reversal agents, without specific indication, prior to discharge is ill advised and should not be a routine practice of postoperative management. Patients should be monitored for at least 2 h prior to discharge if these reversal agents are administered [15].

Physostigmine (1.25 mg i.v.), a centrally acting anticholinesterase inhibitor, functions as a non-specific reversal agent which may be used to counteract the agitation, sedation, and psychomotor effects caused by a variety of sedative, analgesic, and inhalation anesthetic agents [265, 266]. The effects of neuromuscular blocking drugs, if required during general anesthesia, are usually reversed by the anesthesiologist or CRNA prior to emergence from the operating room with anticholinesterase inhibitors such as neostigmine or edrophonium. Occasionally, a second dose may be required when the patient is in the recovery room.

In the event patients fail to regain consciousness during recovery, reversal agents should be administered. If no response occurs, the patient should be evaluated for other possible causes of unconsciousness, including hypoglycemia, hyperglycemia, cerebral vascular accidents, or cerebral hypoxia. If hemodynamic instability occurs in the recovery period, causes such as occult hemorrhage, hypovolemia, pulmonary edema, congestive heart failure, or myocardial infarction must be considered. Access to laboratory analysis to assist with the evaluation of the patient is crucial. Unfortunately, stat laboratory analysis is usually not available if the surgery is performed in an office-based setting.

1.11
Summary

The preceding text is meant to serve as an overview of the extremely complex subject of anesthesia. It is the intent of this chapter to serve as an introduction to the physician who participates in the perioperative management of patients and should not be considered a comprehensive presentation. The physician is encouraged to seek additional information on this broad topic from [267–269]. At least one authoritative text on anesthesia should be considered a mandatory addition to the physician's resources.

References

1. Courtiss EH, Goldwyn RM, Joffe JM, Hannenberg AH: Anesthetic practices in ambulatory aesthetic surgery. Plast Reconstr Surg 1994;93(4):792–801
2. Bechtoldt AA: Committee on anesthesia study. Anesthetic-related death: 1969–1976. N C Med J 1981;42(4):253–259
3. White PF, Smith I: Ambulatory anesthesia: past present and future. Int Anesthesiol Clin 1994;32(3):1–16
4. Morello DC, Colon GA, Fredricks S, Iverson, RE, Singer R: Patient safety in accredited office surgical facilities. Plast Reconstr Surg 1997;99(6):1496–1500
5. West Group, West's Annotated California Codes, Business and Professions Code. 3A Article 11.5, Section 2216
6. West Group, West's Annotated Codes, Health and Safety Code. 38B, Chapter 1.3, Section 1248
7. American Society of Anesthesiologists: Standards for Basic Anesthetic Monitoring. Approved by the House of Delegates on October 21, 1986 and Last Amended on October 13, 1993. Directory of Members. American Society of Anesthesiologists, Park Ridge 1997:394
8. American Society of Anesthesiologists Guidelines for Ambulatory Surgical Facilities Last Amended 1988. Directory of Members. American Society of Anesthesiologists, Park Ridge 1995:386–387
9. American Academy of Cosmetic Surgery: 1995 Guidelines for Liposuction. 1995:2–6
10. West Group, West's Annotated California Codes, Health and Safety Code. 38B, Chapter 1.3, Section 1248.15
11. Press I: The last word. Hosp Health Netw 5 March, 1994:60
12. Anderson & Associates. Best Practices. Putting Insight into Practice. Anderson & Associates, Dallas 1992
13. Graham III DH, Duplechain G: Anesthesia in Facial Plastic Surgery. In Willett JM (ed), Facial Plastic Surgery. Appleton & Lange, Stamford 1997;5–26
14. The American Academy of Cosmetic Surgery: 2000 Guidelines for Liposuction Surgery. Am J Cosmet Surg 2000;25:31–37
15. American Society of Anesthesiologists Task Force on Sedation and Analgesia by Non-Anesthesiologists: Practice guidelines for sedation and analgesia by Non-Anesthesiologists. A report by the American Society of Anesthesiologists Task Force on Sedation and Analgesia by Non-Anesthesiologists. Anesthesiology 1996;84(2):459–471
16. Mannino MJ: Anesthesia for male aesthetic surgery. Clin Plast Surg, 1991;18(4):863–875
17. Jamison RN, Parris WC, Maxson WS: Psychological factors influencing recovery from outpatient surgery. Behav Res Ther 1987;25(1):31–37
18. Hampton JR, Harrison MJG, Mitchell JR, Pritchard JS, Seymour C: Relative contributions of history taking, physical examination, and laboratory investigation to diagnosis and management of medical outpatients. Br Med J 1975;2(5969):486–489
19. Delahunt B, Turnbull PRG: How cost-effective are routine preoperative investigations? NZ Med J 1980;92(673):431–432
20. Apfelbaum JL: Preoperative evaluation, laboratory screening, and selection of adult surgical outpatients in the 1990's. Anesthesiol Rev 1990;17:4–12

21. Gibby GL, Gravenstein JS, Layone AJ, Jackson KI How often does the preoperative interview change anesthetic management? (Abstract) Anesthesiology 1992;77:A1134

22. Sandler G: Costs of unnecessary tests. Br J Med 1979;2(6181):21–24

23. Rabkin SW, Horne JM: Preoperative electrocardiography effect of new abnormalities on clinical decisions. Can Med Assoc J 1983;128(2):146–147

24. Korvin CC, Pearce RH, Stanley J: Admissions screening: clinical benefits. Ann Intern Med 1975;83(2):197–203

25. Tape TG, Mushlin AI: The utility of routine chest radiographs. Ann Intern Med 1986;104(5):663–670

26. Turnbull JM, Buck C: The value of preoperative screening investigations in otherwise healthy individuals. Arch Intern Med 1987;147(6):1101–1105

27. Kaplan EB, Sheiner LB, Boeckman AJ, Roizen MF, Beal SL, Cohen SN, Nicoll CD: The usefulness of preoperative laboratory testing. J Am Med Assoc 1985;253(24):3576–3581

28. Bates DW, Boyle DL, Rittenberg E, Kuperman GJ, Ma'Luf N, Menkin V, Winkelman JW, Tanasijevic MJ: What proportion of common diagnostic test appear redundant? Am J Med 1998;104(4):361–368

29. Fowkes FGR, Lunn JN, Farrow SC, Robertson IB, Samuel P: Epidemiology in anesthesia. III. Mortality risk in patients with coexisting disease. Br J Anaesth 1982;54(8):819–825

30. American Society of Anesthesiologists: New classification of physical status. Anesthesiology 1963;24:111

31. Gold BS, Kitz DS, Lecky JH, Neuhaus JM: Unanticipated admission to the hospital following ambulatory surgery. J Am Med Assoc 1989;262(21):3008–3010

32. Tiret L, Desmonts JM, Hatton F, Vourc'h G: Complications associated with anesthesia—a prospective study in France. Can Anaesth Soc J 1986;33(3 Pt 1):336–344

33. Pedersen T, Eliasen K, Hendricksen E: A prospective study of mortality associated with anesthesia and surgery: Risk indicators of mortality in hospital. Acta Anaesthesiol Scan 1990;34:76

34. Vacanti CJ, VanHouten RJ, Hill RC: A statistical analysis of the relationship of physical status to postoperative mortality in 68,388 cases. Anesth Analg 1970;49(4):564–566

35. Goldman L, Caldera DL, Nussbaum SR, Southwick FS, Krogstad D, Murray B, Burke DS, O'Malley TA, Goroll AH, Caplan CH, Nolan J, Carbello B, Slater EE: Multifactorial index of cardiac risk in noncardiac surgical procedures: N Engl J Med. 1977;297(16):845–850

36. Goldman L, Caldera DL, Southwick FS, Nussbaum SR, Murray B, O'Malley TA, Goroll AH, Caplan CH, Nolan J, Burke DS, Krogstad D, Carabello B, Slater EE: Cardiac risk factors and complications in non-cardiac surgery. Medicine 1978;57(4):357–370

37. Mangano DT, Browner WS, Hollenberg M, London MJ, Tubau JF, Tateo IM: Association of perioperative myocardial ischemia with cardiac morbidity and mortality in men undergoing non-cardiac surgery. N Engl J Med. 1990;323(26):1781–1788

38. Krupski WC, Layug, EL, Reilly LM, Rapp JH, Mangano DT: Comparison of cardiac morbidity between aortic and infrainguinal operations. Study of Perioperative Ischemia (SPI) Research Group. J Vasc Surg 1992;15(2):354–363

39. L'Italien GJ, Cambria RP, Cutler BS, Leppo JA, Paul SD, Brewster DC, Hendel RC, Abbott WM, Eagle KA: Comparative early and late cardiac morbidity among patients requiring different vascular surgery procedures. J Vasc Surg 1995;21(6):935–944

40. Detsky AS, Abram HB, Mclaughlin JR, Drucker DJ, Sasson Z, Johnston N, Scott JG, Forbath N, Hilliard JR: Predicting cardiac complication in patients undergoing non-cardiac surgery. J Gen Intern Med 1986;1(4):211–219

41. Rose SD, Corman LC, Mason DT: Cardiac risk factors in patients undergoing noncardiac surgery. Med Clin N Am 1979;63(6):1271–1288

42. Pasternak LR: Screening patients: strategies and studies. In McGoldrick KE (ed), Ambulatory Anesthesiology, A Problem-Oriented Approach. Williams & Wilkins, Baltimore 1995:10

43. Buck N, Devlin HB, Lunn JN: Report of confidential inquiry into perioperative deaths: Nuffield Provincial Hospitals Trust. London King's Fund Publishing House 1987

44. Lunn JN, Devlin HB: Lessons from the confidential inquiry into perioperative death in three NHS regions. Lancet 1987;2(8572):1384–1386

45. Rabkin SW, Horne JM: Preoperative electrocardiography effect of new abnormalities on clinical decisions. Can Med Assoc J 1983;128(2):146–147

46. McCann RL, Clements FM: Silent myocardial ischemia in patients undergoing peripheral vascular surgery: incidence and association with preoperative cardiac morbidity and mortality. J Vasc Surg 1989;9(4):583–587

47. Deanfield JE, Maseri A, Selwyn AP, Ribeiro P, Chierchia S., Krikler S, Morgan M: Myocardial ischaemia during daily life in patients with stable angina: its relation to symptoms and heart rate changes. Lancet 1983;2(8353):753–758

48. Tarhan S, Moffitt EA, Taylor WF, Giuliani ER: Myocardial infarction after general anesthesia. J Am Med Assoc 1972;220(11):1451–1454

49. Sapala JA, Ponka JL, Duvernoy WF: Operative and non-operative risks in the cardiac patient. J Am Geriatr Soc 1975;23(12):529–534

50. Steen PA, Tinker JH, Tarhan S: Myocardial reinfarction after anesthesia and surgery. J Am Med Assoc 1978;239(24):2566

51. Rao TLK, Jacobs KH, El-Etr AA: Reinfarction following anesthesia in patients with myocardial infarction. Anesthesiology 1983;59(6):499–505

52. Shah KB, Kleinman BS, Sami H, Patel J, Rao TL: Reevaluation of perioperative myocardial infarction in patients with prior myocardial infarction undergoing noncardiac operations. Anesth Analg 1990;71(3):231–235

53. Mantha S, Roizen MF, Barnard J, Thisted RA, Ellis JE, Foss J: Relative effectiveness of preoperative noninvasive cardiac evaluation test on predicting adverse cardiac outcome following vascular surgery: a metaanalysis. Anesth Analg 1994;79(3):422–433

54. McPhail N, Calvin JE, Shariatmader A, Barber GG, Scobie TK: The use of preoperative exercise testing to predict cardiac complication after arterial reconstruction. J Vasc Surg 1988;7(1):60–68

55. Christopherson R, Beattie L, Frank SM, Norris EJ, Meinert CL, Gottlieb SO, Yates H, Rock P, Parker SD, Perler BA: Perioperative morbidity in patients randomized to epidural or general anesthesia for lower extremity vascular surgery. Perioperative Ischemia Randomized Anesthesia Trial Study Group. Anesthesiology 1993;79(3):422–434

56. Slogoff S, Keats AS: Randomized trial of primary anesthetic agents on outcome of coronary artery bypass operations. Anesthesiology 1989;70(2):179–188

57. Abraham S, Johnson CL: Prevalence of severe obesity in adults in the United States. Am J Clin Nutr 1980;33(2 Suppl):364–369

58. Anderson T, Gluud C: Liver morphology in morbid obesity: a literature study. Int J Obes 1984;8(2):97–106

59. Fauci AS, Braunwald E, Isselbacher KJ, Wilson JD, Martin JB, Kaspper DL, Hauser SL, Longo DL: Harrison's Principles of Internal Medicine, 14th Edition. McGraw-Hill, New York 1998:454–455

60. Lee JJ, Larson RH, Buckley JJ, Roberts RS: Airway maintenance in the morbidly obese. Anesth Rev 1980;71:33–36

61. Vaughan RW, Bauer S, Wise L: Volume and pH of gastric juice in obese patients. Anesthesiology 1975;43(6):686–689

62. Ray CS, Sue DY, Bray G, Hansen JE, Wasserman K: Effects of obesity on respiratory function. Am Rev Resp Dis 1983;128(3):501–506

63. Paul DR, Hoyt JL, Boutros AR: Cardiovascular and respiratory changes in response to change of posture in the very obese. Anesthesiology 1976;45(1):73–78

64. Drummond GB, Park GR: Arterial oxygen saturation before intubation of the trachea: An assessment of oxygenation techniques. Br J Anaesth 1984;56(9):987–993

65. Vaughn RW, Englehardt RC, Wise L: Postoperative hypoxemia in obese patients. Ann Surg 1974;180(6):877–882

66. Manchikanti L, Roush JR, Colliver JA: Effect of preanesthetic ranitidine and metaclopromide on gastric contents in morbidly obese patients. Anesth Analg 1986;65(2):195–199

67. Rakoczi I, Chamone D, Collen D, Verstraete M: Prediction of postoperative leg-vein thrombosis in gynaecological patients. Lancet 1978;1(8062):509–510

68. Snell AM: The relation of obesity to fatal post operative pulmonary embolism. Arch Surg 1927;15:237–244

69. Shiffman MA: Anesthesia risks in patients who have had antiobesity medication. Am J Cosmet Surg 1998;15:3–4

70. Smithwick RH, Thompson JE: Splanchnicectomy for essential hypertension; results in 1,266 cases. J Am Med Assoc 1953;152(6):1501–1504

71. Brown BR: Anesthesia and essential hypertension. In Hershey SG (ed), ASA Refresher Courses in Anesthesiology. Lippincott 1979;7:47

72. Veterans' Administration Cooperative Study Group on Antihypertensive Agents: Effects of treatment on morbidity in hypertension. II. Results in patients with diastolic blood pressure averaging 90 through 114 Hg. J Am Med Assoc 1970;213(7):1143–1152

73. Anonymous: The effect of treatment on mortality in "mild" hypertension: results of the hypertension detection and follow-up program. N Engl J Med 1982;307(16):976–980

74. Kannel WB: Blood pressure as a cardiovascular risk factor. Prevention and treatment. J Am Med Assoc 1996;275(20):1571–1576

75. Prys-Roberts C, Meloche R, Foex P: Studies of anesthesia in relation to hypertension. I. Cardiovascular responses of treated and untreated patients. Br J Anaesth 1971;43(2):122–137

76. Bedford RF, Feinstein B: Hospital admission blood pressure: a predictor for hypertension following endotracheal intubation. Anesth Analg 1980;59(5):367–370

77. Stone JG, Foex P, Sear JW, Johnson LL, Khambatta HJ, Triner L: Myocardial ischemia in untreated hypertension patients: effect of a single small oral dose of a beta-adrenergic blocking agent. Anesthesiology 1988;68(4):495–500

78. Katz JD, Cronau LH, Barash PG: Postoperative hypertension: a hazard of abrupt cessation on antihypertensive medication in preoperative period. Am Heart J 1976;92(1):79–80

79. Coriat P, Richer C, Douraki T, Gomez C, Hendricks K, Giudicelli JF, Viars P: Influence of chronic angiotensin-converting enzyme inhibition in anesthetic induction. Anesthesiology 1994;81(2):299–307

80. Leslie JB, Kalayjian RW, Sirgo MA, Plachetka JR, Watkins WD: Intravenous labetolol for treatment of postoperative hypertension. Anesthesiology 1987;67(3):413–416

81. O'Malley K, Segal JL, Israili ZH, Boles M, McNay JL, Dayton PG: Duration of hydralazine action in hypertension. Clin Pharmacol Ther 1975;18(5 Pt 1):581–586

82. Walsh DB, Eckhauser FE, Ramsburgh SR, Burney RB: Risk associated with diabetes mellitus in patients undergoing gall-bladder surgery. Surgery 1982;91(3):254–257

83. Fowkes FGR, Lunn JN, Farrow SC, Robertson IB, Samuel P: Epidemiology in anesthesia. III. Mortality risk in patients with coexisting physical disease. Br J Anaesth 1982;54(8):819–825

84. Hjortrup A, Rasmussen BF, Kehlet H: Morbidity in diabetic and non-diabetic patients after major vascular surgery. Br Med J 1983;287(6399):1107–1108

85. Burgos LG, Ebert TJ, Asiddao C, Turner LA, Pattison CZ, Wang-Cheng R, Kampine JP: Increased intraoperative cardiovascular morbidity in diabetics with autonomic neuropathy. Anesthesiology 1989;70(4):591–597

86. Hirsch IB, McGill JB, Cryer PE, White PF: Perioperative management of surgical patients with diabetes mellitus. Anesthesiology 1991;74(2):346–359

87. Roizen M: Anesthetic Implications of concurrent disease. In Miller RD (ed), Anesthesia, Fifth Edition. Churchill Livingstone, Philadelphia 2000:909

88. Walts LF, Miller J, Davidson MD, Brown J: Perioperative management of diabetes mellitus. Anesthesiology 1981;55(2):104–109

89. Malling B, Knudsen L, Christiansen BA, Schurzek BA, Hermansen K: Insulin treatment in non-insulin dependent diabetic patients undergoing minor surgery. Diabetes Nutr Metab 1989;2:125–131

90. Hirsch IB, White PF: Management of surgical patients with insulin dependent diabetes mellitus. Anesthesiology Rev 1994;21:53–59

91. Weiss KB, Wagner DK: Changing patterns of asthma mortality. Identifying target populations at high risk. J Amer Med Assoc 1990;264(13):1683–1687

92. Boushy SF, Billing DM, North LB, Helgason AH: Clinical course related to preoperative pulmonary function in patients with bronchogenic carcinoma. Chest 1971;59(4):383–391

93. Hall WJ, Douglas RG, Hyde RW, Roth FK, Cross AS, Speers DM: Pulmonary mechanics after uncomplicated influenza A infections. Am Rev Respir Dis 1976;113(2):141–148

94. Warner MA, Offord KP, Warner ME, Lennon RL, Conover MA, Jansson-Schumacher U: Role of preoperative cessation of smoking and other factors in postoperative pulmonary complication: A clinical prospective study of coronary artery bypass patients. Mayo Clin Proc 1989;64(6):609–614

95. Homer CJ: Asthma disease management. N Engl J Med 1997;337(20):1461–1463

96. Stein M, Cassara EL: Preoperative pulmonary evaluation and therapy for surgical patients. J Am Med Assoc 1970;211(5):787–790

97. Bartlett RH, Brennan ML, Gazzaniga AB, Hansen EL: Studies on the pathogenesis and prevention of postoperative pulmonary complication. Surg Gynecol Obstet 1973;137(6):925–933

98. National Commission on Sleep Disorders Research: Wake Up America. A National Sleep Alert. Government Printing Office, Washington 1993

99. Barsh CI: The origin of pharyngeal obstruction during sleep. Sleep Breath 1999;31:17–21

100. Shelton KE, Gay SB, Woodson H, Gay S, Suratt PM: Pharyngeal fat in obstructive sleep apnea. Am Rev Respir Dis 1993;148(2):462–466

101. Berman EJ, DiBenedetto RJ, Causey DE, Mims T, Conneff M, Goodman LS, Rollings RC: Right ventricular hypertrophy detected in echocardiography in newly diagnosed obstructive sleep apnea. Chest 1991;100(2):347–350

102. Orr WC: Sleep apnea, hypoxemia, and cardiac arrhythmias. Chest 1986;89(1):1–2

103. Chung F, Crago RR: Sleep apnea syndrome and analgesia. Can Anaesth Soc J 1982;29(5):439–445

104. Ostermeier AM, Roizen MF, Hautekappe M, Klock PA, Klafta JM: Three sudden postoperative respiratory arrests associated with epidural opioids in patients with sleep apnea. Anesth Analg 1997;85(2):452–460

105. Benumof JL: Obstructive sleep apnea in the adult obese patient: implications for airway management. J Clin Anesth 2001;13(2):144–156

106. Strollo PJ Jr, Rogers RM: Obstructive sleep apnea. N Engl J Med 1996;334(2):99–104

107. Wilson K, Stooks RA, Mulroony TF, Johnson IJ, Guilleminault C, Huang Z: The snoring spectrum: Acoustic assessment of snoring sound intensity in 1,139 individuals undergoing polysomnography. Chest 1999;115(3):762–770

108. Yentis SM, Levine MF, Hartley EJ: Should all children with suspected or confirmed malignant hyperthermia susceptibility be admitted after surgery? A 10-year review. Anesth Analg 1992;75(3):345–350

109. Gronert GA, Antognini JF, Pessah IN: Malignant Hyperthermia. In Miller RD (ed), Anesthesia, Fifth Edition. Churchill Livingstone, Philadelphia 2000:1047–1048

110. Kolb ME, Horne ML, Martz R: Dantrolene in human malignant hyperthermia: A multicenter study. Anesthesiology 1982;56(4):254–262

111. Covino BG, Wildsmith JAW: Clinical pharmacology of local anesthetics. In Cousins MJ, Bridenbaugh DL (eds), Neural Blockade in Clinical Anesthesia and Management of Pain, Third Edition. Lippincott Raven, Philadelphia 1998:98

112. Braid DP, Scott DB: The systemic absorption of local anesthetic drugs. Br J Anesth 1965;37:394–404

113. Moore DC, Bridenbaugh DL, Thompson GE, Balfour RI, Horton, WG: Factors determining doses of amide-type anesthetic drugs. Anesthesiology 1977;47(3):263–268

114. Nation R, Triggs F, Selig M: Lignocaine kinetics in cardiac and aged subjects. Br J Clin Pharmacol 1977;4(4):439–448

115. Meister F: Possible association between tumescent technique and life-threatening pulmonary edema. Clin Plast Surg 1996;23:642–645

116. Shiffman M: Medications potentially causing lidocaine toxicity. Am J Cosmet Surg 1998;15:227–228

117. Klein JA: The tumescent technique of liposuction surgery. Am J Cosmet Surg 1987;4:263–276

118. Klein JA: Tumescent technique for regional anesthesia permits lidocaine doses 35mg/kg for liposuction J Dermatol Surg Oncol 1990;16(3):248–263

119. Klein JA: Pharmacokinetic of tumescent lidocaine. In Klein JA (ed), Tumescent Technique: Tumescent Anesthesia and Microcannular Liposuction. Mosby, St Louis 2000:141–161

120. Ostad A, Kageyama N, Moy RL: Tumescent anesthesia with a lidocaine dose of 55mg/kg is safe for liposuction. Dermatol Surg 1996;22(11):921–927

121. Klein JA, Kassarjdian N: Lidocaine toxicity with tumescent liposuction. Dermatol Surg 1997;23(12):1169–1174

122. Corvino BG, Wildsmith JAW: Clinical pharmacology of local anesthetic agents. In Cousins MJ, Bridenbaugh DL (eds), Neural Blockade in Clinical Anesthesia and Management of Pain, Third Edition. Lippincott Raven, Philadelphia 1998:107–108

123. Feldman HS, Arthur GR, Covino BG: Comparative systemic toxicity of convulsant and supraconvulsant doses of intravenous ropivacaine, bupivacaine and lidocaine in the conscious dog. Anesth Analg 1989;69(6):794–801

124. Morishma HO, Peterson H, Finster M: Is bupivacaine more cardiotoxic than lidocaine? Anesthesiology 1983;59:A409

125. Albright GA: Cardiac arrest following regional anesthesia with etidocaine or bupivacaine. Anesthesiology 1979;51(4):285–287

126. Rosen M, Thigpen J, Shnider SM, Foutz SE, Levinson G, Koike M: Bupivacaine-induced cardiotoxicity in hypoxic and acidotic sheep. Anesth Analg 1985;64(11):1089–1096

127. Sunshine I, Fike WW: Value of thin-layer chromatography in two fatal cases of intoxication due to lidocaine and mepivacaine. N Engl J Med 1964;271:487–490

128. Yukioka H, Hayashi M, Fujimori M: Lidocaine intoxication during general anesthesia (letter). Anesth Analg 1990;71(2):207–208

129. Christie JL: Fatal consequences of local anesthesia: Report of five cases and a review of the literature. J Forensic Sci 1976;21:671–679

130. Samdal F, Amland PF, Bugge JF: Plasma lidocaine levels during suction-assisted lipectomy using large doses of dilute lidocaine with epinephrine. Plast Reconstr Surg. 1994;93(6):1217–1223

131. Pitman GH: Tumescent technique for local anesthesia improves safety in large-volume liposuction. (Discussion) Plast Reconstr Surg 1993;92:1099–1100

132. Fisher MM, Graham R: Adverse responses to local anesthetics. Anaesth Intens Care 1984;(4)12:325–327

133. Aldrete J, Johnson DA: Evaluation of intracutaneous testing for investigation of allergy to local anesthetic agents. Anesth Analg 1970;49(1):173–183

134. Kaster GW, Martin ST: Successful resuscitation after massive intravenous bupivacaine overdose in the hypoxic dog. Anesthesiology 1984;61:A206

135. Feldman H, Arthur G, Pitkanen M, Hudley R, Doucette AM, Covino BG: Treatment of acute systemic toxicity after the rapid intravenous injection of ropivacaine, bupivacaine, and lidocaine in the conscious dog. Anesth Analg 1991;73(4):373–384

136. Kasten GW, Martin ST: Bupivacaine cardiovascular toxicity: Comparison of treatment with bretylium and lidocaine. Anesth Analg 1985;64(9):911–916

137. McKay W, Morris R, Mushlin P: Sodium bicarbonate attenuates pain on skin infiltration with lidocaine, with or without epinephrine. Anesth Analg 1987;66(6):572–574

138. Buckley MM, Benfield P: Eutectic lidocaine/prilocaine cream: A review of the topical anesthetic/analgesic efficacy of a eutectic mixture of local anesthetics (EMLA). Drugs 1993;46(1):126–151

139. Gammaitoni AR, Davis MW: Pharmacokinetics and tolerabllity of lidocaine patch 5% with extended dosing. Ann Pharmacother 2002;36(2):236–240

140. Endo Pharmaceuticals: Lidoderm. In Physicians Desk Reference, 60th Edition, Thompson, Monyvale 2006:1107–1108

141. Young D: Student's death sparks concerns about compounded preparations. Am J Health-Syst Pharm 2005;62:450–454

142. Holzman RS, Cullen DJ, Eichhorn JH, Phillip JH: Guidelines for sedation by nonanesthesilogists during diagnostic and therapeutic procedures. J Clin Anesth 1994;6(4):265–276

143. White PF, Negus JB: Sedative infusions during local and regional anesthesia: A comparison of midazolam and propoful. J Clin Anesth 1991;3(1):32–39

144. Rothfusz ER, Kitz DS, Andrews RW: O2 sat, HR and MAP amoung patients receiving local anesthesia: how low/high do they go? Anesth Analg 1988;67:S189

145. Lundgren S, Rosenquist JB: Amnesia, pain experience, and patient satisfaction after sedation with intravenous diazepam. J Oral Maxiilofac Surg 1983;41(2):99–102

146. Federated Ambulatory Surgical Association: FASA Special Study I. Federated Ambulatory Surgical Association, Alexandria 1986

147. McNabb TG, Goldwyn RM: Blood gas and hemodynamic effects of sedatives and analgisics when used as as suppliment to local anesthesia in plastic surgery. Plastic Reconstr Surg 1976;58(1):37–43

148. Singer R, Thomas PE: Pulse oximeter in the ambulatory anesthetic surgical facility. Plast Reconstr Surg 1988;82(1):111–114

149. Giles HG, MacLeod SM, Wright JR, Sellers EM: Influence of age and previous use on diazepam dosing requirements for endoscopy. Can Med Assoc J 1978;118(5):513–514

150. Wynands JE, Wong P, Townsend G, Sprigge JS, Whalley DG: Narcotic requirements for intravenous ansthesia. Anesth Analg 1984;63(2):101–105

151. Kay B, Rolly G: Duration of action of analgesic suppliment to anesthesia. Acta Anaesthesiol Belg 1977;28(1):25–32

152. Bailey PL, Andriano KP, Pace NL: Small doses of fentanyl potentiate and prolong diazepam induced respiratory depression. Anesth Analg 1984;63:183

153. Reves JG: Benzodiazepines. In Prys-Roberts C, Hugg CC (eds), Pharmacokinetics of Anesthesia. Blackwell, Boston 1984

154. Klein JA: Tumescent technique for local anesthesia improves safety in large-volume liposuction. Plast Reconstr Surg 1993;92(6):1085–1098

155. Osborne GA, Rudkin GE, Curtis NJ, Vickers D, Craker AJ: Intraoperative patient-controlled sedation; comparison of patient-controlled propofol with anaesthetist-administered midazolam and fentanyl. Anesthesiology 1991;46(7):553–556

156. Zelcer J, White PF, Chester S, Paull JD, Molnar R: Intraoperative patient-controlled analgesia: An alternative to physician administration during outpatient monitored anesthesia care. Anesth Analg 1992;75(1):41–44

157. Hegarty JE, Dundee JW: Sequelae after intravenous injection of three benzodiazepines: Diazepam, lorezepam, and flunitrazepam. Br Med J 1977;2(6099):1384–1385

158. Greenblatt DJ, Shader RI, Dwoll M, Harmatz JS: Benzodiazepines: A summary of the pharmacokinetics. Br J Clin Pharmacol 1981;11(Suppl 1):11S–16S

159. White PF, Vasconez CO, Mathes SA, Way WL, Wender LA: Comparison of midazolam and diazepam for sedation during plastic surgery. Plast Reconstr Surg 1998;81(5):703–712

160. Blitt CD: Clinical pharmacology of lorezepam. In Brown BRJ (ed), New Pharmacologic Vista in Anesthesia. Davis, Philadelphia 1983:135

161. Rigg JR, Goldsmith CH: Recovery of ventilatory response to carbon dioxide after thiopentone, morphine and fentanyl in man. Can Anaesth Soc J 1976;23(4):370–382

162. White PF, Coe V, Shafer A, Sung ML: Comparison of alfentanil with fentanyl for outpatient anesthesia. Anesthesiology 1986;64(1):99–106

163. SaRego MM, Inagoki Y, White PF: Use of remifentanil during lithotripsy: Intermittant boluses vs continuous infusion [abstract]. Anesth Analg 1997;84:5541

164. Watcha MR, White PF: Postoperative nausea and vomiting: Its etiology, treatment and prevention. Anesthesiology 1992;77(1):162–184

165. Mackenzie N, Grant IS: Propofol (Diprovan) for continuous intravenous anaesthesia: A comparison with methohexitone. Postgrad Med J 1985;61(Suppl 3):70–75

166. White PF, Negus JB: Sedative infusions during local and regional anesthesia: A comparison of midazolam and propofol. J Clin Anesth 1991;3(1):32–39

167. McCollum JS, Milligan KR, Dundee JW: The antiemetic action of propofol. Anesthesia 1988;43(3):239–240

168. Smith I, Monk TG, White PF, Ding Y: Propofol infusion during regional anesthesia: Sedative, amnestic, anxiolytic properties. Anesth Analg 1994;79(2):313–319

169. Grounds RM, Twigley AJ, Carli F, Whitwam JG, Morgan M: The haemodynamic effects of thiopentone and propofol. Anaesthesiol 1985;40(8):735–740

170. Goodman NW, Black AM, Carter JA: Some ventilatory effects of propofol as sole anesthetic agent. Br J Anaesth 1987;59(12):1497–1503

171. Fanard L, Van Steenberge A, Demeire X, van der Puyl F: Comparison between propofol and midazolam as sedative agents for surgery under regional anesthesia 1988;43(Suppl):87–89

172. Rudkin GE, Osborne GA, Finn BP, Jarvis DA, Vickers D: Intraoperative patient-controlled sedation: Comparison of patient-controlled propofol with patient-controlled midazolam. Anesthesiology 1992;47(5):376–381

173. Meyers CJ, Eisig SB, Kraut RA: Comparison of propofol and methohexital for deep sedation. J Maxillofac Surg 1994;52(5):448–452

174. White PF, Way WL, Trevor AJ: Ketamine: Its pharmacology and therapeutic uses. Anesthesiology 1982;56(2):119–136

175. Taylor PA, Towey RM: Depression of laryngeal reflexes during ketamine anesthesia. Br Med J 1971;2(763):688–689

176. Garfield JM, Garfield FB, Stone JG, Hopkins D, Johns LA: A comparison of psychological responses to ketamine and thiopental, nitrous oxide, halothane anesthesia. Anesthesiology 1972;36(4):329–338

177. Corssen G, Reves JG, Stanley TH: Neuroleptanalgesia and neuroleptanesthesia. Intravenous Anesthesia and Analgesia.Lea & Febig, Philadelphia 1988:175

178. Prys-Roberts C, Kelman GR: The influence of drugs used in neurolept analgesia on cardiovascular and ventilatory function. Br J Anaesth 1967;39(2):134–145

179. Edmonds-Seal J, Prys-Roberts C: Pharmacology of drugs used in neurolept analgesia Anaesth Analg (Paris) 1959;16:1022

180. Melnick BM: Extrapyramidal reactions to low-dose droperidol. Anesthesiology 1988;69(3):424–426

181. Guze BH, Baxter LR Jr: Current concepts: Neuroletic malignant syndrome. N Engl J Med 1985;313(3):163–166

182. Food and Drug Administration: FDA Strenghtens Warnings for Droperidol. FDA Talk Paper, 12/5/01;T01–62

183. Bailey PL, Egan TD, Stanlet TE: Intravenous Opiod Anesthetics. In Miller RD (ed), Anesthesia, Fifth Edition. Churchill Livingsone, Philadelphia 2000:345–348

184. Philip BK: Supplemental medication for ambulatory procedures under regional anesthesia. Anesth Analg 1985;64(11):1117–1125

185. Sa Rego MM, Watcha MF, White PF: The changing role of monitored anesthesia care in the ambulatory setting. Anesthesiology 1997;85(5):1020–1036

186. Fragen RJ (ed): Drug Infusions in Anesthesiology. Raven, New York 1991

187. Naito Y, Tamai S, Shinguk, Fujimori R, Mori K: Comparison between sevoflurane and halothane for paediatric ambulatory anesthesia. Br J Anaesth 1991;67(4):387–389

188. Ghouri AF, Bodner M, White PF: Recovery profile following desflurane-nitrous oxide versus isoflurane-nitrous oxide in outpatients. Anesthesiology 1991;74(3):419–424

189. Bodman RI, Morton HJ, Thomas ET: Vomiting by outpatients after nitrous oxide anesthesia. Br Med J 1960;5182:1327–1330

190. Van Hemelrijck J, White PF: Intravenous anesthesia for day-care surgery. In Kay B (ed), Total Intravenous Anesthesia. Elsevier, Amsterdam 1991;323–350

191. Benumof JL: Laryngeal mask airway: Indication and contraindications. Anesthesiology 1992;77(5):843–846

192. Campbell GD: Dangers of monoamine oxidase inhibitors. Br Med J 1963;1:750

193. Sjoqvist F: Psychotropic drugs, 2. Interaction between monoamine oxidase (MAO) inhibitors and other substances. Proc R Soc Med 58(11 Part 2):967–978

194. Roizen M: Anesthetic implications of concurrent diseases. In Miller RD (ed), Anesthesia, Fifth Edition. Churchill Livingstone, Philadelphia 2000:998

195. Coriat P, Richer C, Douraki T, Gomez C, Hendricks K, Giudicelli JF, Viars P: Influence of chronic angiotensin converting enzyme inhibition in anesthetic induction. Anesthesiology 1994;81(2):299–307

196. Green CR, Pandit SK, Schork MA: Preoperative fasting time: Is the traditional policy changing? Results of a national survey. Anesth Analg 1996;83(1):123–128

197. Schreiner MS, Nicolson SC: Pediatric ambulatory anesthesia: NPO before or after surgery? J Clin Anesth 1995;7(7):589–596

198. Maltby JR, Sutherland AD, Sale JP, Schaffer EA: Preoperative oral fluids. Is a five-hour fast justified prior to elective surgery? Anesth Analg 1986;65(11):1112–1116

199. Doze VA, White PF: Effects of fluid therapy on serum glucose in fasted outpatients. Anesthesiology 1987;66(2):223–226

200. Kallar SK, Everett LL: Potential risks and preventative measures for pulmonary aspiration: New concepts in preoperative fasting guideline. Anesth Analg 1993;77(1):171–182

201. Manchikanti L, Canella MG, Hohlbein LJ, Colliver JA: Assessment of effects of various modes of premedication on acid aspiration risk factors in outpatient surgery. Anesth Analg 1987;66(1):81–84

202. Morgan M: Control of gastric pH and volume. Br J Anaesth 1984;56(1):47–57

203. Manchikanti L, Kraus JW, Edds SP: Cimetidine and related drugs in anesthesia. Anesth Analg 1982;61(7):595–608

204. Manchikanti L, Colliver JA, Roush JR, Canella MG: Evaluation of ranitidine as an oral antacid in outpatient anesthesia. South Med J 1985;78(7):818–822

205. Boulay K, Blanloeil Y, Bourveau M, Gray G: Comparison of oral ranitidine (R), famotidine (F), and omeprazole (O) effects on gastric pH and volume in elective general surgery (Abstract). Anesthesiology 1992;77:A431

206. Diamond MJ, Keeri-Szanto M: Reduction of postoperative vomiting by preoperative administration of oral metaclopromide. Can Anaesth Soc J 1980;27(1):36–39

207. Kapur PA: The big 'little' problem. (Editorial). Anesth Analg 1991;73(3):243–245

208. van Wijk MG, Smalhout B: Postoperative analysis of the patients' view of anesthesia in a Netherlands's teaching hospital. Anaesthesia 1990;45(8):679–682

209. Hines R, Barash PG, Watrous G, O'Connor T: Complications occurring in the post anesthesia care unit. Anesth Analg 1992;74(4):503–509

210. Green G, Jonsson L: Nausea: the most important factor determining length of stay after ambulatory anaesthesia. A comparison study of isoflurane and/or propofol techniques. Acta Anaesthesiol Scand 1993;37(8):742–746

211. Madej TH, Simpson KH: Comparison of the use of domperidone, droperidol, and metaclopramide on the prevention of nausea and vomiting following gynaecological surgery in day cases. Br J Anaesth 1986;58(8):879–883

212. White PF, Shafer A: Nausea and vomiting: causes and Prophylaxis. Semin Anesth 1987;6:300–308

213. Carroll NV, Miederhoff P, Cox FM, Hirsch JD: Postoperative nausea and vomiting after discharge from outpatient surgery centers. Anesth Analg 1995;80(5):903–909

214. Tang J, Watcha MF, White PF: A comparison of costs and efficacy of ondansetron and droperidol as prophylactic antiemetic therapy for elective outpatient gynecologic procedures. Anesth Analg 1996;83(2):304–313

215. Melnick BM: Extrapyramidal reactions to low-dose droperidol. Anesthesiology 1988;69(3):424–426

216. Alon E, Himmelseher S: Ondansetron in the treatment of postoperative vomiting: A randomized double-blind comparison with droperidol and metaclopromide. (Abstract), Anesth Analg 1993;79:A8

217. Wilson AJ, Diemunsch P, Lindeque BG, Scheinin H, Helbo-Hansen HS, Kroeks MV, Kong KL: Single-dose i.v. granisetron in the prevention of postoperative nausea and vomiting. Br J Anaesth 1996;76(4):515–518

218. Sung YF, Wetcher BV, Duncalf D, Joslyn AF: A double-blind placebo-controlled pilot study examining the effectiveness of intravenous ondansetron in the prevention of postoperative nausea and emesis. J Clin Anesth 1993;5(1):22–29

219. McKenzie R, Kovac A, O'Connor T, Duncalf D, Angel J, Gratz I, Tolpin E, McLeskey C, Joslyn A: Comparison of ondansetron versus placebo to prevent postoperative nausea and vomiting in women undergoing gynecological surgery. Anesthesiology 1993;78(1):21–28

220. McKenzie R, Tantisira B, Karambelkan DJ, Riley TJ, Abdelhady H: Comparison of ondansetron with ondansetron plus dexamethasone, 4 to 8 mg, in the prevention of postoperative nausea and vomiting. Anesth Analg 1994;79(5):961–964

221. McKenzie R, Uy NT, Riley TJ, Hamilton DL: Droperidol/ondansetron combination controls nausea and vomiting after tubal ligation. Anesth Analg 1996;83(6):1218–1222

222. Shafer A: Preoperative medication: Adults and children. In White PF (ed), Ambulatory Anesthesia and Surgery. Saunders, London 1997:173

223. Kotelko DM, Rottman RL, Wright WC, Stone JJ, Yamashiro AY, Rosenblatt RM: Transdermal scopolamine decreases nausea and vomiting following cesarean section in patients receiving epidural morphine. Anesthesiology 1989;71(5):675–678

224. Rodysill KJ, Warren JB: Transdermal scopolamine and toxic psychosis. Ann Intern Med 1983;98(4):561

225. Vener DF, Carr AS, Sikich N, Bissonette B, Lerman J: Dimenhydrinate decreases vomiting after stabizmus surgery in children. Anesth Analg 1996;82(4):728–731

226. Borgeat A, Wilder-Smith OH, Saiah M, Rifat K: Subhypnotic doses of propofol possess direct antiemetic properties. Anesth Analg 1992;74(4):539–541

227. Raftery S, Sherry E: Total intravenous anaesthesia with propofol and alfentanil protects against nausea and vomiting. Can J Anaesth 1992;39(1):37–40

228. Felts JA, Poler SM, Spitznagel EL: Nitrous oxide, nausea and vomiting after outpatient gynecological surgery. J Clin Anesth 1990;2(3):168–171

229. Melnick BM, Johnson LJ: Effects of eliminating nitrous oxide in outpatient anesthesia. Anesthesiology 1987;67(6):982–984

230. Shafer A, White PF, Urquhart ML, Doze UA: Outpatient premedication: Use of midazolam and opioid analgesics. Anesthesiology 1989;71(4):495–501

231. Meridy HW: Criteria for selection of ambulatory surgical patients and guidelines for anesthetic management: A retrospective study of 1553 cases. Anesth Analg 1982;61(11):921–926

232. Janhumen L, Tommisto T: Postoperative vomiting after different modes of general anesthesia. Ann Chir Gynaecol 1972;61:152

233. Yogendran S, Asokumar B, Chang DC, Chung F: A prospective randomized double-blind study of the effects of intravenous fluid therapy on adverse outcomes on outpatient surgery. Anesth Analg 1995;80(4):682–686

234. Jakobsen H, Hertz JB, Johansen JR, Hansen A, Kolliker K: Premedication before day surgery. Br J Anaesth 1985;57(3):300–305

235. Baird ES, Hailey DM: Delayed recovery from a sedative: correlation of the plasma levels of diazepam with clinical effects after oral and intravenous administration. Br J Anaesth 1972;44(8):803–808

236. Gale GD, Galloon S, Porter WR: Sublingual lorazepam: A better premedication? Br J Anaesth 1983;55(8):761–765

237. Reinhart K, Dallinger-Stiller G, Dennhardt R, Heinnemeyer G, Eyrich K: Comparison of midazolam and diazepam and placebo i.m. as premedication for regional anesthesia. Br J Anaesth 1985;57(3):294–299

238. Raybould D, Bradshaw EG: Premedication for day case surgery. Anesthesiology 1987;42(6):591–595

239. Conner JT, Bellville JW, Katz RL: Meperidine and morphine as intravenous surgical premedicants. Can Anaesth Soc J 1977;24(5):559–564

240. Pandit SK, Kothary SP: Intravenous narcotics for premedication in outpatient anaesthesia. Acta Anaesthesiol Scan 1989;33(5):353–358

241. Wender RH, Conner JT, Bellville JW, Schehl D, Dorey F, Katz RL: Comparison of i.v. diazepam and hydroxyzine as surgical premedicants. Br J Anaesth 1977;49(9):907–912

242. Roisen MF: Anesthetic implications of concurrent disease. In Miller R(ed), Anesthesia, Fifth Edition. Churchill Livingstone, Philadelphia 2000:959–960

243. Goldhaber SZ: Pulmonary embolism. N Engl J Med 1998;339(2):93–104

244. Sandison AJP, Jones SE, Jones PA: A daycare modified Shouldice hernia repair follow-up. J One-Day Surg 1994;3:16–17

245. Moser KM, Fedullo PF, LittleJohn JK, Crawford R: Frequent asymptomatic pulmonary embolism in patients with deep venous thrombosis. J Am Med Assoc 1994;271:223–225[erratum] J Am Med Assoc 1994;271(24):1908

246. Collins R, Scrimgeour A, Yusuf S, Peto R: Reduction in fatal pulmonary embolism and venous thrombosis by perioperative administration of subcutaneous heparin, an overview of results of randomized trials in general, orthopedic and urologic surgery. N Engl J Med 1988;318(18):1162–1173

247. Anonymous: Prevention of venous thrombosis and pulmonary embolism. NIH Consensus Development. J Am Med Assoc 1986;256(6):744–749

248. Gallus A, Raman K, Darby T: Venous thrombosis after elective hips replacement-the influence of preventative intermittent calf compression on surgical technique. Br J Surg 1983;70(1):17–19

249. Bergqvist D, Lindblad B: A 30-year survey of pulmonary embolism verified at autopsy: an analysis of 1274 surgical patients. Br J Surg 1985;72(2):105–108

250. Gan TJ, Glass PS, Windsor A, Payne F, Rosow C, Sebel P, Manberg P: Bispectral index monitoring allows faster emergence and improved recovery from propofol, fentanyl and nitrous oxide anesthesia. Anesthesiology 1997;87(4):808–815

251. Tonnesen AS: Crystalloids and colloids. In Miller R (ed), Anesthesia, Fourth Edition. New Churchill Livingstone, New York 1994;1595–1618

252. Linko K, Makelainen A: Cardiorespiratory function after replacement of blood loss with hydroxyethyl starch 120, Dextran-70, and Ringer's lactate in pigs. Crit Care Med 1989;17(10):1031–1035

253. Hankeln K, Radel C, Beez M, Laniewski P, Bohmert F: Comparison of hydroxyethyl starch and lactated Ringer's solution in hemodynamics and oxygen transport of critically ill patients in prospective cross over studies. Crit Care Med 1989;17(2):133–135

254. Dawidson I: Fluid resuscitation of shock: current controversies. Crit Care Med 1989;17(10):1078–1080

255. Moss GS, Gould SA: Plasma expanders: an update. Am J Surg 1988;155(3):425–434

256. Leone BJ, Spahn DR: Anemia, hemodilution, and oxygen delivery. Anesth Analg 1992;75(5):651–653

257. American Society of Anesthesiologists Task Force on Blood Component Therapy: Practice guidelines for blood component therapy. Anesthesiology 1996;84(3):732–747

258. Bennett GD: Anesthesia for liposuction and abdominoplasty. In Shiffman MA, Mirrafati S (eds), Aesthetic Surgery of the Abdominal Wall. Springer, Berlin 2005:29–54

259. Natof HE, Gold B, Kitz DS: Complications. In Wetcher BV (ed), Anesthesia of Ambulatory Surgery, Second Edition. Lippincott, Philadelphia 1991:374–474

260. Mecca RS: Postoperative recovery. In Borash PG, Cullen BF, Stoelting RK (eds), Lippincott, Philadelphia 1992:1517–1518

261. Bailey PL, Egar TD, Stanley TH: Intravenous opioid anesthetics. In Miller RD (ed), Anesthesia, Fifth Edition. Churchill Livingstone, Philadelphia 2000:273–376

262. Jensen S, Knudsen L, Kirkegaard L, Kruse A, Knudsen EB: Flumazenil used for antagonizing the central effects of midazolam and diazepam in outpatients. Acta Anesthesiol Scand 1989;33(1):26–28

263. Klotz U: Drug interactions and clinical pharmacokinetics of flumazenil. Eur J Anaesthesiol 1988;2:103–108

264. McCloy RF: Reversal of conscious sedation by flumazenil: current status and future prospects. Acta Anaesthsiol Scand Suppl 1995;108:35–42

265. Bourke DL, Rosenberg M, Allen PD: Physostigmine: Effectiveness as an antagonist of respiratory depression and psychomotor effects caused by morphine or diazepam. Anesthesiology 1984;61(5):523–528

266. Hill GE, Stanley TH, Slentker CR: Physostigmine reversal of postoperative somnolence. Can Anaesth Soc J 1977;24(6):707–711

267. McGoldrick K (ed): Ambulatory Anesthesiology. A Problem-Oriented Approach. Williams & Wilkins, Baltimore 1995

268. Miller RD (ed): Anesthesia, Fifth Edition. Churchill Livingstone, Philadelphia 2000

269. White PF (ed): Ambulatory Anesthesia & Surgery. Saunders, Philadelphia 1997

270. Roizen MF, Foss JF, Fischer SP: Preoperative evaluation. In Miller RD (ed), Anesthesia Fifth Edition. Churchill Livingstone, Philadelphia 2000:854–855

271. Roizen MF, Fischer SP: In White PF (ed), Ambulatory Anesthesia and Surgery. Saunders, London 1997:155–172

CHAPTER 2

Local Anesthetic Blocks of the Head and Neck

Joseph Niamtu III

2.1
Introduction

If there were an award for the most important advance of the last millennium it would be in the author's opinion, hands down, the discovery of local anesthesia. Although it is almost impossible for us in the civilized world to contemplate, it was a cruel world out there. Owing to the inability to obtund severe pain, medicine and dentistry stayed in the "dark ages" way past the renaissance. A simple tooth extraction or a laceration repair would be an extremely traumatic experience, and in fact just several generations ago.

In the head and neck there is some of the most intensely innervated real estate in the body. Our major sensory organs are located there and are well protected and endowed with sensory innervation. Innervation to the teeth conveys only a single stimulus: pain! The ability to master local anesthetic techniques of the head and neck is one of the most useful and appreciated skills a physician can master. Neuroanatomy of the head and neck can be boring and complex and it was not that fun to learn back in medical or dental school. Relearning it now may seem laborious but if you pay attention to the pictures of sensory dermatomes in this chapter, it is really not that hard and actually can be fun.

The ability to predictably administer successful facial nerve blocks can provide many benefits. Many of us become somewhat callous when performing procedures and even may admonish patients for "hurting" during a procedure. Remember how we would want our own family treated if they went somewhere. We would want treatment to be painless and we should all strive for this same level of excellence. The second advantage of adequate local anesthesia is the ability to perform better work. No physician can argue that they can do superior work on a patient who is numb. No patient will argue that they can appreciate better work when they are numb! A hidden and sometimes unappreciated benefit of "being good with the needle" is positive marketing. The absence of pain is a superior marketing strategy. Never forget this and if you have not been practicing like this, tomorrow is the first day of the rest of your practice!

Alcohol was widely used for pain control, but as we are well aware and the ancients were also aware, even the drunkest drunk still feels pain. Cocaine was the first local anesthetic to be widely used in surgical applications. In the nineteenth century it was reported that the Indians of the Peruvian highlands chewed the leaves of the coca leaf (*Erythroxylon coca*) for its stimulating and exhilarating effects [1–3]. It was also observed that these Indians observed numbness in the areas around the lips. In 1859, Albert Niemann, a German chemist, was given credit for being the first to extract the isolate cocaine from the coca shrub in a purified form [4]. When Niemann tasted the substance, his tongue became numb. This property led to one of the most humane discoveries in all of medicine and surgery. Over two decades later, Sigmund Freud began treating patients with cocaine for its physiologic and psychological effects. While he was treating a colleague for morphine dependence, the patient developed cocaine dependence [4].

Koller demonstrated the topical anesthetic activity of cocaine on the cornea in animal models and on himself. In an operation for glaucoma, Koller used cocaine for local anesthesia in 1894 [2–5].

William Halsted was a prominent American surgeon who investigated the principles of nerve block using cocaine. In November 1884, Halsted performed infraor-

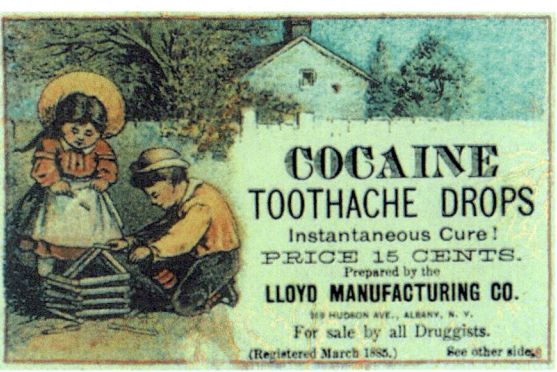

Fig. 2.1 Cocaine use in early dentistry

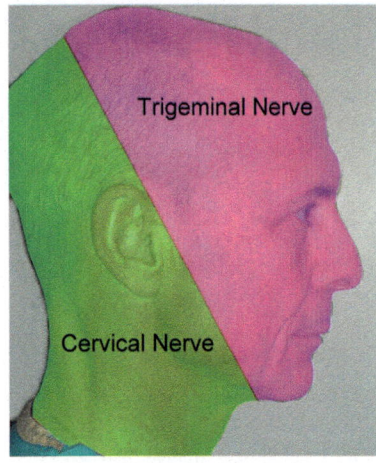

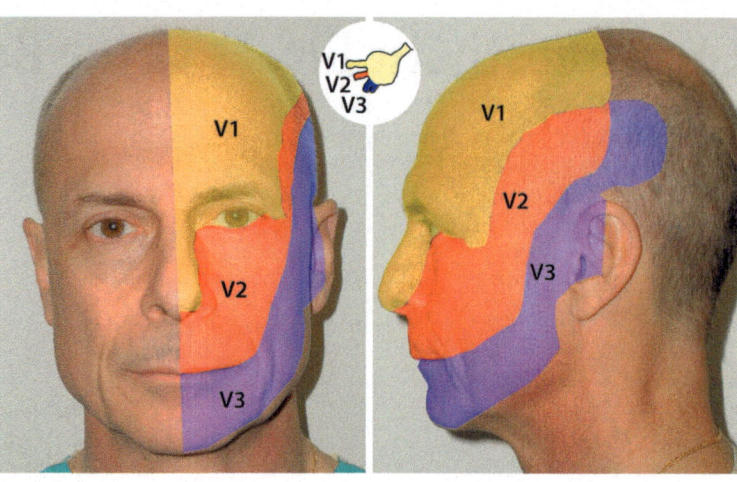

Fig. 2.2 The sensory innervation of the head and neck is derived from the trigeminal and upper cervical nerves

Fig. 2.3 The main branches of the trigeminal nerve supplying sensation to the respective facial areas. The *inset* shows the trigeminal ganglion with the three main nerve branches

bital and inferior alveolar (mandibular dental block) as well as demonstrated various other regional anesthetic techniques [4]. Halsted's self-experimentation with cocaine caused an addiction and it required 2 years to resolve and regain his eminent position in surgery and teaching [4].

Early dentists dissolved cocaine hydrochloride pills in water and drew this mixture into a syringe to perform nerve infiltrations and blocks. The extreme vasoconstrictive effects of cocaine often caused tissue necrosis, but nonetheless provided profound local anesthesia that revolutionized dentistry and medicine forever. Many proprietary preparations of that time period contained cocaine (Fig. 2.1).

By the early 1900s cocaine's adverse effects became well recognized. These deleterious effects included profound cardiac stimulation and vasoconstriction. Cocaine blocks the neuronal reuptake of norepinephrine in the peripheral nervous system, and myocardial stimulation in combination with coronary artery vasoconstriction has proven lethal in sensitive individuals, central nervous system stimulation and mood-altering euphoric effect [6, 7]. These effects coupled with the severe physical and psychological dependence proved to be significant drawbacks to cocaine use for local anesthesia.

In 1904 Einhorn, searching for a safer and less toxic local anesthetic, synthesized procaine (Novocain) [4, 8]. Novocain was the gold standard of topical anesthetics for almost 40 years until Lofgren synthesized lidocaine (Xylocaine), the first amide group of local anesthetics [4]. Lidocaine provided advantages over the ester group (procaine) in terms of greater potency, less allergic potential and a more rapid onset of anesthesia [1, 2, 9, 10].

2.2
Mechanism of Action of Local Anesthetics

Local anesthetics block the sensation of pain by interfering with the propagation of impulses along peripheral nerve fibers without significantly altering normal resting membrane potentials [11]. Local anesthetics depolarize the nerve membranes and prevent achievement of a threshold potential. A propagated action potential fails to develop and a conduction blockade is achieved. This occurs by the interference of nerve transmission by blocking the influx of sodium through the excitable nerve membrane [12].

2.3
Sensory Anatomy of the Head and Neck

The main sensory innervation of the face is derived from cranial nerve V (trigeminal nerve) and the upper cervical nerves (Fig. 2.2).

2.3.1
Trigeminal Nerve

The trigeminal nerve is the fifth of the 12 cranial nerves. Its branches originate at the semilunar ganglion (Gasserian ganglion) located in a cavity (Meckel's cave) near the apex of the petrous part of the temporal bone. Three large nerves, the ophthalmic, maxillary, and mandibular, proceed from the ganglion to supply sensory innervation to the face (Fig. 2.3).

Often referred to as "the great sensory nerve of the head and neck", the trigeminal nerve is named for its three major sensory branches. The ophthalmic nerve (V1), maxillary nerve (V2), and mandibular nerve (V3) are literally "three twins" (trigeminal) carrying sensory information of light touch, temperature, pain, and proprioception from the face and scalp to the brainstem. The commonly used terms "V1," "V2," and "V3" are shorthand notation for cranial nerve five, branches one, two, and three, respectively. In addition to nerves carrying incoming sensory information, certain branches of the trigeminal nerve also contain nerve motor components (the ophthalmic and maxillary nerves consist exclusively of sensory fibers; the mandibular nerve is joined outside the cranium by the motor root). These outgoing motor components include branchial motor nerves (nerves innervating muscles derived embryologically from the branchial arches) as well as "hitchhiking" visceral motor nerves (nerves innervating viscera, including smooth muscle and glands). The trigeminal nerve exits the trigeminal ganglion and courses "backward" to enter the mid-lateral aspect of the pons at the brainstem [13].

The ophthalmic nerve (V1) leaves the semilunar ganglion through the superior orbital fissure. The maxillary nerve (V2) leaves the semilunar ganglion through the foramen rotundum at the skull base and the mandibular nerve (V3) leaves the semilunar ganglion through the foramen ovale at the skull base (Fig. 2.3) [13]. The remainder of this chapter will only discuss the sensory components of this nerve system as they relate to local anesthetic blocking techniques for cosmetic facial procedures.

2.3.2
Ophthalmic Nerve (V1)

The ophthalmic nerve, or first division of the trigeminal nerve, is a sensory nerve. It supplies branches to the cornea, ciliary body, and iris; to the lacrimal gland and conjunctiva; to the part of the mucous membrane of the nasal cavity; and to the skin of the eyelids, eyebrow, forehead, and upper lateral nose (Fig 2.3). It is the smallest of the three divisions of the trigeminal nerve and divides into three branches, the frontal, nasociliary, and lacrimal [13]. The frontal nerve divides into the supraorbital and supratrochlear nerves providing sensation to the forehead and anterior scalp.

The nasociliary nerve divides into four branches, two of which supply sensory innervation to the face. These two branches are the infratrochlear nerve, which supplies sensation to the skin of the medial eyelids and side of the nose, and the ethmoidal nerve, which gives of a terminal branch called the external (or dorsal) nasal nerve and innervates the skin of the nasal dorsum and tip. The lacrimal nerve innervates the skin of the upper eyelid.

2.3.3
Maxillary Nerve (V2)

The maxillary nerve, or second division of the trigeminal nerve, is a sensory nerve that crosses the pterygopalatine fossa then traverses the orbit in the infraorbital groove and canal in the floor of the orbit, and appears upon the face at the infraorbital foramen as the infraorbital nerve [13]. At its termination, the nerve divides into branches which spread out upon the side of the nose, the lower eyelid, and the upper lip, joining with filaments of the facial nerve [13].

The zygomatic nerve arises in the pterygopalatine fossa, enters the orbit by the inferior orbital fissure, and divides at the back of that cavity into two terminal branches, the zygomaticotemporal and zygomaticofacial nerves.

The zygomaticotemporal branch runs along the lateral wall of the orbit in a groove in the zygomatic bone then passes through a foramen in the zygomatic bone and enters the temporal fossa. It ascends between the bone and substance of the temporalis muscle and pierces the temporal fascia about 2.5 cm above the zygomatic arch, where it is distributed to the skin of the side of the forehead (Fig. 2.3) [13].

The zygomaticofacial branch passes along the inferolateral angle of the orbit, emerges upon the face through a foramen in the zygomatic bone, and, perforates the orbicularis oculi and supplies the skin on the prominence of the cheek (Fig. 2.3).

As the maxillary nerve traverses the orbital floor and exits the infraorbital foramen, it branches into a plexus of nerves, which has the following terminal branches:
1. The inferior palpebral branches ascend behind the orbicularis oculi muscle and supply the skin and conjunctiva of the lower eyelid (Fig. 2.3).
2. The lateral nasal branches (rami nasales externi) supply the skin of the side of the nose (Fig. 2.3).
3. The superior labial branches are distributed to the skin of the upper lip, the mucous membrane of the mouth, and labial glands (Fig. 2.3) [13].

2.3.4
Mandibular Nerve (V3)

The mandibular nerve supplies the teeth and gums of the mandible, the skin of the temporal region, part of the auricle, the lower lip, and the lower part of the face (Fig. 2.3). The mandibular nerve also supplies the muscles of mastication and the mucous membrane of the anterior two thirds of the tongue. It is the largest of the three divisions of the fifth cranial nerve and is made up of a motor and sensory root [13].

Sensory branches of the mandibular nerve include:
1. The auriculotemporal nerve supplies sensation to the skin covering the front of the helix and tragus (Fig. 2.3).

2. The inferior alveolar nerve is the largest branch of the mandibular nerve. It descends with the inferior alveolar artery and exits the ramus of the mandible to the mandibular foramen. It then passes forward in the mandibular canal, beneath the teeth, as far as the mental foramen, where it divides into two terminal branches, incisive and mental nerves. The mental nerve emerges at the mental foramen, and divides into three branches: one descends to the skin of the chin, and two ascend to the skin and mucous membrane of the lower lip [13].

3. The buccal nerve which supplies sensation to the skin over the buccinator muscle.

2.4
Local Anesthetic Techniques

2.4.1
Infiltrative Peripheral Anesthesia Versus Regional Nerve Block Anesthesia

Local anesthesia can be effectively obtained by infiltrations and nerve blocks. Infiltrative local anesthesia applies to the injection of the local anesthesia solution in the area of the peripheral innervation distant from the site of the main nerve. An advantage of infiltrative anesthesia is that no specific skill is necessary, only the selected area of innervation is involved and vasoconstrictors can improve local hemostasis. A drawback of infiltrative local anesthesia is the distortion of the tissue at or around the site of injection that may obscure or hamper cosmetic procedures.

A nerve block involves placing the local anesthetic solution in a specific location at or around the main nerve trunk that will effectively depolarize that nerve and obtund sensation distal to that area. Advantages of nerve blocks include the fact that a single accurately placed injection can obtund large areas of sensation without tissue distortion at the operative site. Disadvantages of peripheral nerve block include the sensation of numbness in areas other than the operative site and the lack of hemostasis at the operative site from a vasoconstrictor.

Individual anatomic variances in patients are responsible for the sometimes unpredictable effect of peripheral nerve block. Foraminal position, nerves crossing the midline, accessory innervation, and nerve bifurcation are just some factors that affect the predictability and success of failure of local anesthetic nerve blocks. Nerves that innervate areas close to the midline may receive innervation from the contralateral side and require bilateral blocks. For the multiple, aforementioned reasons, some nerve blocks may require augmentative infiltrative local anesthesia to obtain adequate pain control.

Since many nerves are accompanied by corresponding veins and arteries, aspiration should always be performed to prevent intravascular injection.

2.4.2
The Use of Topical Preanesthesia

Any person who has pain-free dental treatment more than likely receives topical mucosal anesthesia prior to having a dental block. Although some of the effects of topical anesthesia may be psychological, all patients appreciate the extra pain control effort. Although topical anesthetic techniques are more effective and faster acting on mucosal surfaces, patients still appreciate the extra care for pain control. The use of a topical anesthetic agent on the lip mucosa will definitely augment injections in that area regardless of the blocking techniques used. In the author's practice, when a patient is seated for lip augmentation injections, the assistant immediately applies a thick coating of a topical anesthetic preparation to the lips, which will be in contact with the mucosa for at least 10 min before injection. This topical anesthetic is a custom mixture of benzocaine, lidocaine, and tetracaine (Bayview Pharmacy, Baltimore, MD, USA). This produces profound anesthesia in many patients and negates the need for further blocking techniques. Some patients will still require blocks, but topical anesthesia will assist by both psychological and physiological means. Many cosmetic surgeons also use topical agents for cutaneous anesthesia.

2.4.3
Local Anesthetic Techniques for Blocking the Main Sensory Nerves of the Head and Neck

A rudimentary knowledge of the neuroanatomy of the head and neck can enable the cosmetic surgeon to perform painless surgical procedures in this area. In addition, when used concomitantly with general anesthesia or intravenous sedation, local anesthetic blocks can decrease the amount of intravenous or inhalation agents needed. Finally, using local anesthetic blocks with intravenous or inhalation agents can provide excellent postanesthetic pain control.

2.4.3.1
Scalp and Forehead

The supraorbital nerve exits through a notch (in some cases a foramen) on the superior orbital rim approximately 27 mm lateral to the glabellar midline (Fig. 2.4). This supraorbital notch is readily palpable in most patients. After exiting the notch or foramen, the nerve traverses the corrugator supercilii muscles and branches into a medial and lateral portion. The lateral branches supply the lateral forehead and the medial branches supply the scalp. The supratrochlear nerve exits a foramen approximately 17 mm form the glabellar midline (Fig. 2.4) and supplies sensation to the middle portion of the forehead. The infratrochlear nerve exits a foramen

Fig. 2.4 The supraorbital nerve (*SO*) exits about 27 mm from the glabellar midline and the supratrochlear nerve (*ST*) is located approximately 17 mm from the glabellar midline. The infratrochlear nerve (*IT*) exits below the trochlea

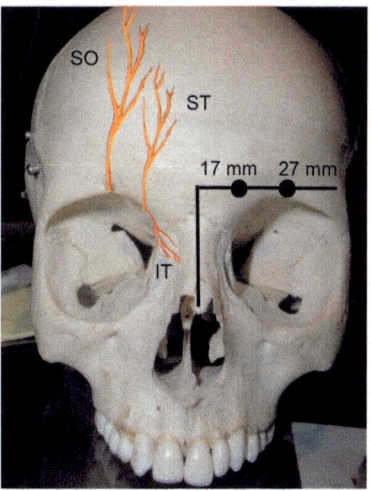

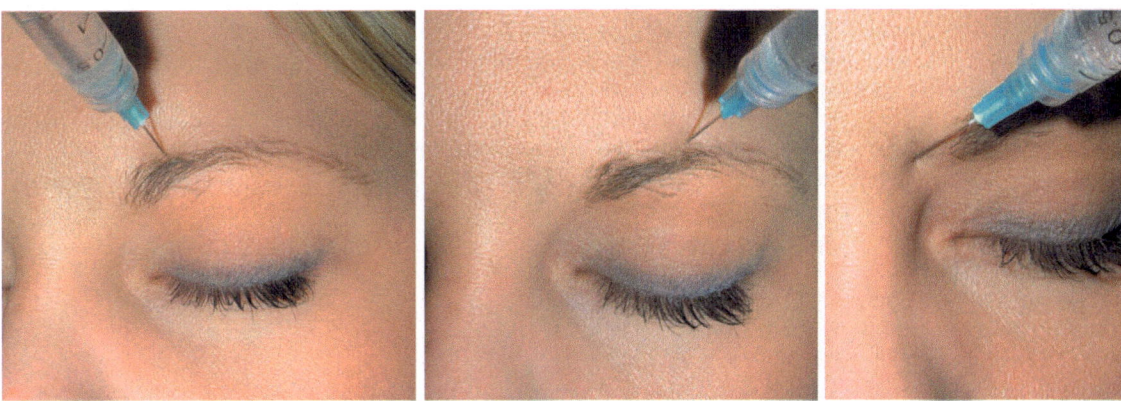

Fig. 2.5 The forehead and scalp are blocked by a series of injections form the central to the medial brow

below the trochlea and provides sensation to the medial upper eyelid, canthus, medial nasal skin, conjunctiva, and lacrimal apparatus (Fig. 2.4) [14].

When injecting this area it is prudent to always use the free hand to palpate the orbital rim to prevent inadvertent injection into the globe! To anesthetize this area, the supratrochlear nerve is measured 17 mm from the glabellar midline and 1–2 ml of 2% lidocaine with 1:100,000 epinephrine is injected (Fig. 2.5). The supraorbital nerve is blocked by palpating the notch (and or measuring 27 mm from the glabellar midline) and injecting 2 ml of local anesthetic solution (Fig. 2.6). The infratrochlear nerve is blocked by injecting 1–2 ml of local anesthetic solution at the junction of the orbit and the nasal bones (Fig. 2.6). In reality, one can block all three of these nerves by simply injecting 2–4 ml of local anesthetic solution from the central brow proceeding to the medial brow. Figure 2.6 shows the regions anesthetized by the aforementioned blocks.

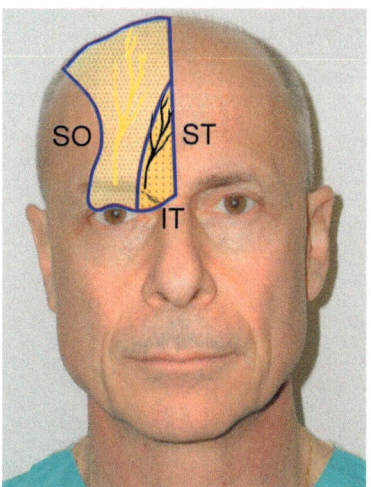

Fig. 2.6 The *shaded areas* indicate the anesthetized areas from supraorbital nerve (*SO*) and supratrochlear nerve (*ST*) and infratrochlear nerve (*IT*) blocks

2.4.3.2
Infraorbital Nerve Block

The infraorbital nerve exits the infraorbital foramen 4–7 mm below the orbital rim in an imaginary line dropped from the medial limbus of the iris [14] or the pupillary midline. The anterior-superior alveolar nerve branches from the infraorbital nerve before it exits the foramen and thus some patients will manifest anesthesia of the anterior teeth and gingiva if the branching is close to the foramen. Areas anesthetized include the lateral nose, anterior cheek, lower eyelid, and upper lip on the injected side. This nerve can be blocked by intraoral or extraoral routes. To perform an infraorbital nerve block from an intraoral approach, topical anesthetic is placed on the oral mucosa at the vestibular sulcus just under the canine fossa (between the canine and first premolar tooth) and left for several minutes. The lip is then elevated and a 1.5-in. 27-gauge needle is inserted in the sulcus and directed superiorly toward the infraorbital foramen (Fig. 2.7). The needle does not need to enter the foramen for a successful block. The anesthetic solution needs only to contact the vast branching around the foramen to be effective. It is imperative to use the other hand to palpate the inferior orbital rim to avoid injecting the orbit. Between 2 and 4 ml of 2% lidocaine with 1:100,000 epinephrine is injected in this area for the infraorbital block.

The infraorbital nerve can also be very easily blocked by a facial approach and this is the preferred route of the author. This may also be the preferred route in dental phobic patients. A 0.5-in. 27-gauge needle is used and is placed through the skin and aimed at the foramen in a perpendicular direction. Between 2 and 4 ml of local anesthetic solution is injected at or close to the foramen (Fig. 2.8). Again, the other hand must constantly palpate the inferior orbital rim to prevent inadvertent injection into the orbit.

A successful infraorbital nerve block will anesthetize the infraorbital cheek, the lower palpebral area, the lateral nasal area, and superior labial regions (Fig. 2.9).

The aforementioned techniques provide anesthesia to the lateral nasal skin but do not provide anesthesia to the central portion of the nose. A dorsal (external) nasal nerve block will supplement nasal anesthesia by providing anesthesia over the area of the cartilaginous nasal dorsum and tip. This supplementary nasal block is accomplished by palpating the inferior rim of the nasal bones at the osseous cartilaginous junction. The dorsal nerve (anterior ethmoid branch of the nasociliary nerve) emerges 5–10 mm from the nasal midline at the osseous junction of the inferior portion of the nasal bones (the distal edge of the nasal bones) (Fig. 2.10). The dotted line in Fig. 2.10 shows the course of this nerve under the nasal bones before emerging.

2.4.3.3
Augmentive Lip Anesthesia

Although in theory a bilateral infraorbital block should anesthetize the entire upper lip, some patients may still perceive pain for various anatomic (or sometimes psy-

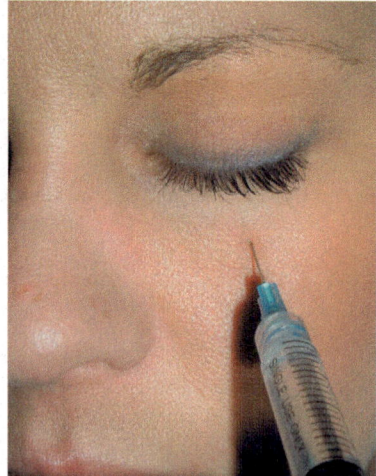
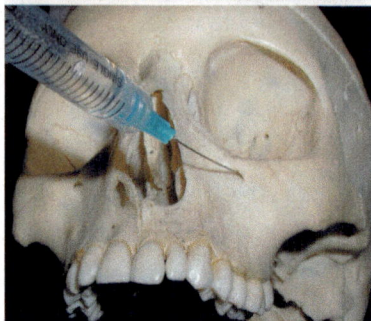

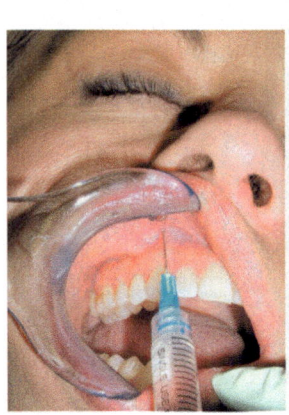
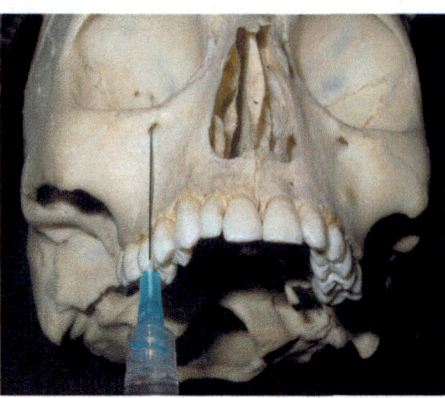

Fig. 2.7 The intraoral approach for local anesthetic block of the infraorbital nerve

Fig. 2.8 The facial approach for local anesthetic block of the infraorbital nerve

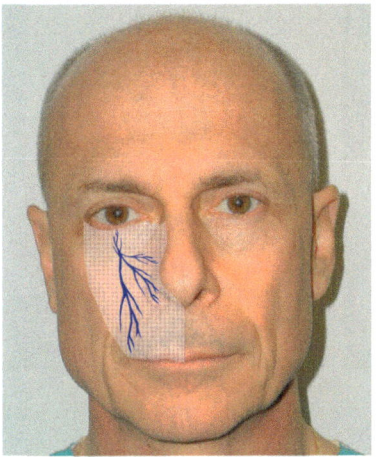
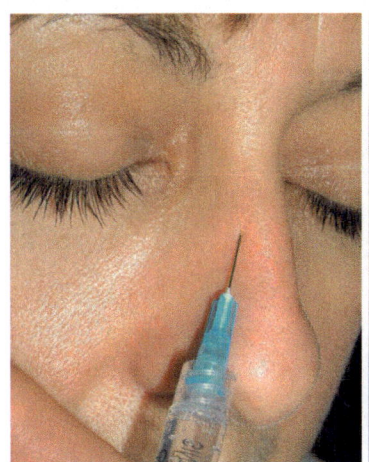
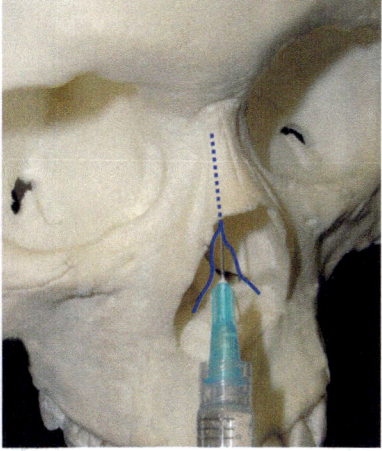

Fig. 2.9 Area of anesthesia from unilateral infraorbital nerve block

Fig. 2.10 The dorsal (external) nasal nerve is blocked subcutaneously at the osseous-cartilaginous junction of the distal nasal bones

chological) reasons detailed earlier in this chapter. Anecdotally, the author injects 0.5 ml of local anesthetic solution in the maxillary labial frenum (Fig. 2.11). Whether the effect is psychological or physiological, this seems to provide additional anesthesia. This can also be performed in the lower-lip labial frenum area to augment bilateral mental blocks as will be discussed later in this chapter. The combination of bilateral infraorbital and mental blocks and the just-described infiltrative augmentation (when necessary) is an ideal technique for anesthetizing the lips for filler injection or implant placement.

Two often overlooked nerves in facial local anesthetic blocks are the zygomaticotemporal and zygomaticofa-

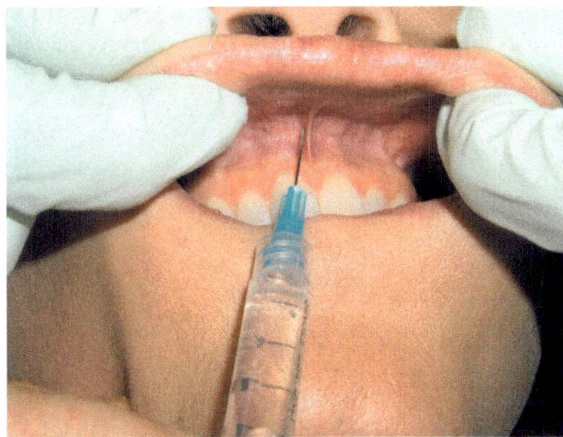

Fig. 2.11 An augmentative injection of local anesthetic in the maxillary frenum can assist subtotal anesthesia from infraorbital blocks when the upper lips are anesthetized

cial nerves. These nerves represent terminal branches of the zygomatic nerve. The zygomaticotemporal nerve emerges through a foramen located on the anterior wall of the temporal fossa. This foramen is actually behind the lateral orbital rim posterior to the zygoma at the approximate level of the lateral canthus (Fig. 2.12).

Injection technique involves sliding a 1.5-in. needle behind the concave portion of the lateral orbital rim. It is suggested that one closely examine this area on a model skull prior to attempting this injection as it will make the technique simpler. To orient for this injection, the physician needs to palpate the lateral orbital rim at the level of the frontozygomatic suture (which is frequently palpable). With the index finger in the depression of the posterior lateral aspect of the lateral orbital rim (inferior and posterior to the frontozygomatic suture), the operator places the needle just behind the palpating finger (which is about 1 cm poster to the frontozygomatic suture) (Fig. 2.12). The needle is then "walked" down the concave posterior wall of the lateral orbital rim to the approximate level of the lateral canthus. After aspirating, 1–2 ml of 2% lidocaine with 1:100,000 epinephrine is injected in this area with a slight pumping action to ensure deposition of the local anesthetic solution at or about the foramen. Again, it is important to hug the back concave wall of the lateral orbital rim with the needle when injecting.

Blocking the zygomaticotemporal nerve causes anesthesia in the area superior to the nerve, including the lateral orbital rim and the skin of the temple from above the zygomatic arch to the temporal fusion line (Fig. 2.13).

The zygomaticofacial nerve exits through a foramen (or foramina in some patients) in the inferior lateral portion of the orbital rim at the zygoma. If the surgeon

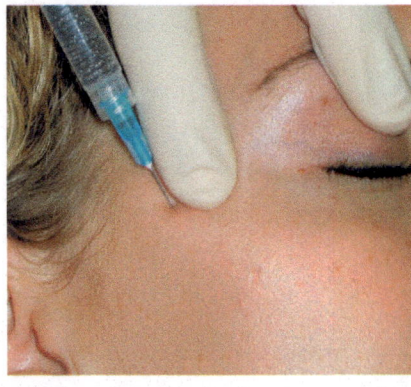
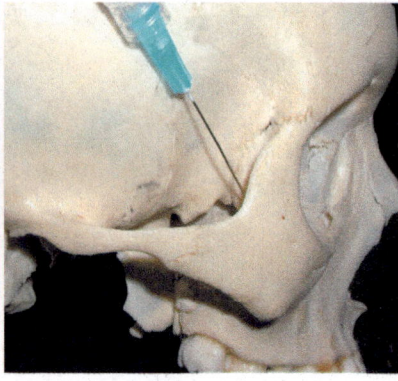
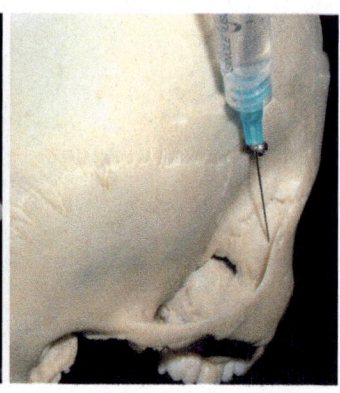

Fig. 2.12 The zygomaticotemporal nerve is blocked by placing the needle on the concave surface of the posterior lateral orbital rim

palpates the junction of the inferior lateral (the most southwest portion of the right orbit, if you will) portion of the lateral orbital rim, the nerve emerges several millimeters lateral to this point. By palpating this area and injecting just lateral to the finger, one successfully blocks this nerve with 1–2 ml of local anesthetic (Fig. 2.14). Blocking this nerve will result in anesthesia of a triangular area from the lateral canthus and the malar region along the zygomatic arch and some skin inferior to this area (Fig. 2.13) [14].

2.4.3.4
Total Second-Division Nerve Block

An efficient and simple technique to obtain hemi-midfacial local anesthesia is to block the entire second division or maxillary nerve. This will anesthetize the entire hemimaxilla and the unilateral maxillary sinus by blocking the pterygopalatine, infraorbital, and zygomatic nerves and their terminal branches. This is an easily learned technique and involves an intraoral approach at the posterior lateral palate (Fig. 2.15).

The maxillary nerve block via the greater palatine canal was first described in 1917 by Mendel [15]. The greater palatine foramen is located anterior to the junction of the hard palate and the soft palate medial to the second molar tooth (Fig. 2.15). The foramen is usually found about 7 mm anterior to the junction of the hard and soft palates. This junction is seen as a color change such that the tissue overlying the soft palate is darker pink than the tissue overlying the hard palate. The key to this block is to place a 1.5-in. needle through the greater palatine foramen. It sometimes takes multiple needle sticks to localize the foramen. Owing to the need for multiple sticks, the palatal mucosa in this area is first infiltrated with 0.5 ml of lidocaine to facilitate painless location of the greater palatine foramen. A 1.5-in. 25- or 27-gauge needle is bent to 45° and will usually easily negotiate the pterygopalatine canal, thereby placing the local anesthetic solution into the pterygopalatine fossa. The course of the maxillary division of the trigeminal nerve (V2) is as follows. The second division of the trigeminal nerve arises from the Gasserian ganglion in the medial cranial fossa and exits the skull via the foramen rotundum (Fig. 2.15). The nerve then traverses the superior aspect of the pterygopalatine fossa, where it divides into three major branches: the pterygopalatine

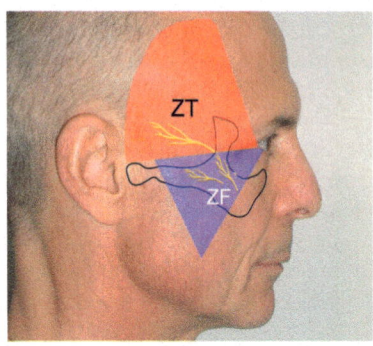
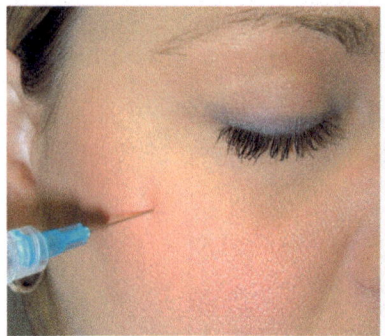
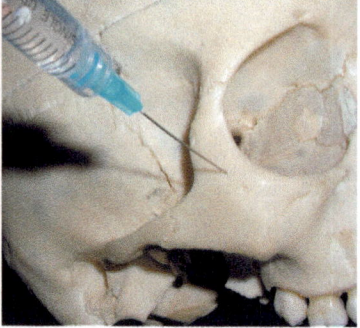

Fig. 2.13 The anesthetized areas from the zygomaticotemporal nerve (*ZT*) and the zygomaticofacial nerve (*ZF*)

Fig. 2.14 The zygomaticofacial nerve(s) are blocked by injecting the inferior lateral portion of the orbital rim

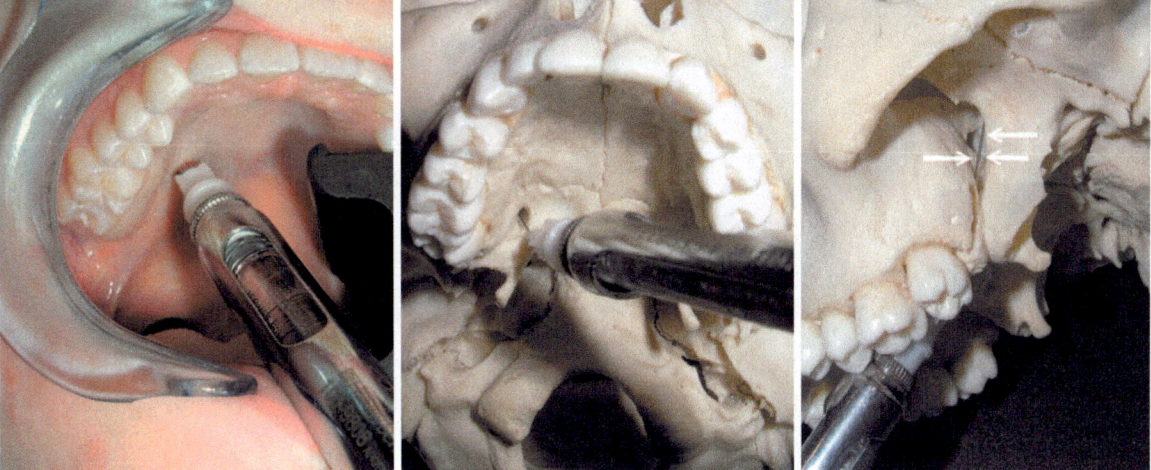

Fig. 2.15 The maxillary nerve block is performed by locating the greater palatine foramen (*left*) and inserting a bent needle up the pterygopalatine canal (*center*) to inject local anesthetic into the pterygopalatine fossa (*right*). Notice the needle tip in the pterygopalatine fossa in the *right* image. As the second division traverses this area it is blocked at the main trunk

nerve, the infraorbital nerve, and the zygomatic nerve [16]. It is these nerves that targeted in this block.

When the foramen is located, the needle should be gently advanced. If significant resistance is encountered, the needle should be withdrawn and redirected. Approximately 5% of the population has been shown to have tortuous canals that impede the needle tip and in some patients this technique is not possible [17]. It is also important to aspirate before injecting to prevent intravascular injection. When the needle is properly positioned (usually at a depth of 25–30 mm), the injection (2–4 ml) should proceed over 30–45 s.

Transient diplopia of the ipsilateral eye may occur [18]. This results from the local anesthetic diffusing superiorly and medially to anesthetize the orbital nerves. The patient must be assured that if this phenomenon occurs, it is transient.

Again, this technique will anesthetize all the terminal branches of the maxillary nerve with a single injection.

2.4.3.5
Mental Nerve Block

The mental nerve exits the mental foramen on the hemimandible at the base of the root of the second premolar (many patients may be missing a premolar owing to orthodontic extractions). The mental foramen is on average 11 mm inferior to the gum line (Fig. 2.16). There is variability with this foramen (like all foramina), but by injecting 2–4 ml of local anesthetic solution about 10 mm inferior to the gum line or 15 mm inferior to the top of the crown of the second premolar tooth the block is usually successful. In a patient without teeth, the foramen is often located much higher on the jaw and can sometimes be palpated. This block is performed more superiorly in the denture patient. As stated earlier, the foramen does not need to be entered as a sufficient volume of local anesthetic solution in the general area will be effective. By placing traction on the lip and pulling

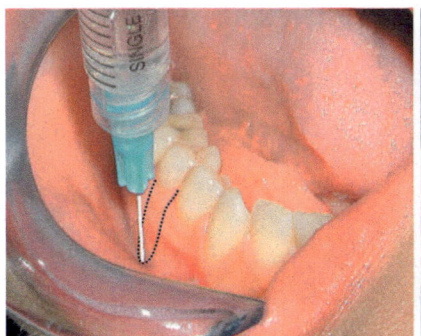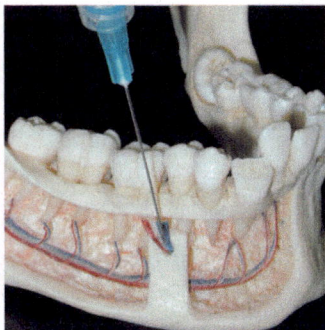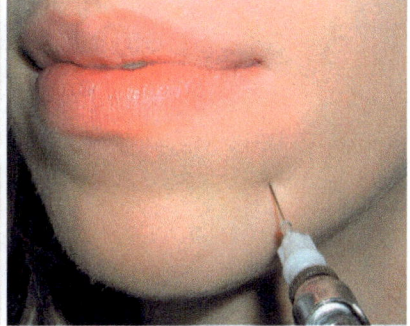

Fig. 2.16 The mental foramen is approached intraorally below the root tip of the lower second premolar (*left*) or from a facial approach (*right*)

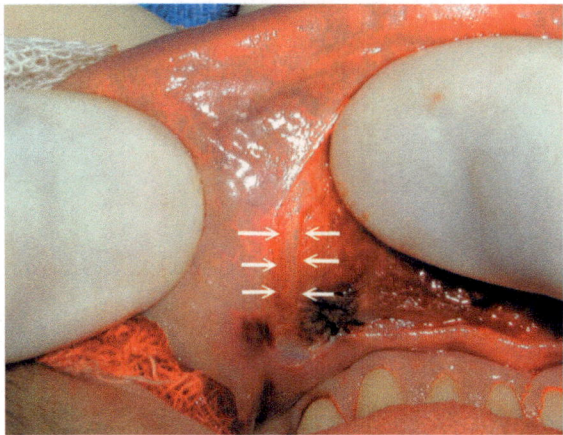

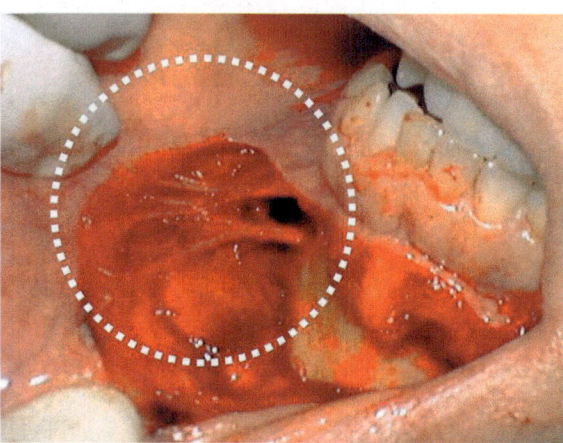

Fig. 2.17 By stretching the lower-lip mucosa, the underlying labial branches of the mental nerve are sometimes visible. This image shows the very superficial labial sensory nerve exposed with mucosal incision for a chin implant

Fig. 2.18 The vast arborization of the distal branches of the mental nerve (*circled*) is visualized intraoperatively in a genioplasty incision

it away from the jaw, one can sometimes see the labial branches of the mental nerve traversing through the thin mucosa (Fig. 2.17). The mental nerve gives off labial branches to the lip and chin (Fig. 2.18).

Alternatively, the mental nerve may be blocked with a facial approach aiming for the same target (Fig. 2.16).

When anesthetized, the distribution of numbness will be the unilateral lip down to the mentolabial fold but many times the anterior chin and cheek depending on the individual furcating anatomy of that patient's nerve (Fig. 2.19). The inferior alveolar nerve also supplies sensory innervation to the chin pad. The mylo-

hyoid nerve may also innervate this area. To augment or extend the area of local anesthesia on the chin, an inferior alveolar nerve (mandibular dental block) block can be performed instead of or with the mental nerve block. Additionally, local skin infiltration in that area may assist.

Sometimes patients may perceive pain despite bilateral nerve block in the upper or lower lips. When injecting fillers in the lower lip and bilateral mental nerve blocks are not totally effective, a supplemental infiltration of local anesthetic into the mandibular labial frenum can assist the blocks (Fig. 2.20).

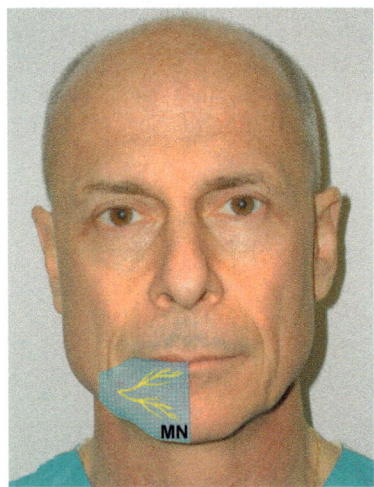

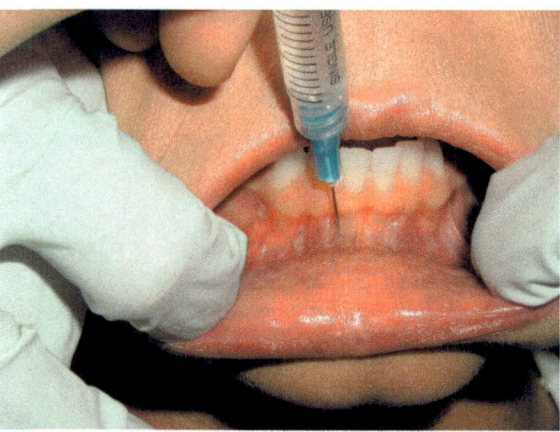

Fig. 2.19 The anesthetized areas from a unilateral mental nerve (*MN*) block. Owing to various anatomic factors, the area below the mentolabial fold or at the midline may share other innervation

Fig. 2.20 Supplemental anesthetic infiltration of the lower labial frenum area can be used to augment bilateral mental blocks when the patient still perceives pain

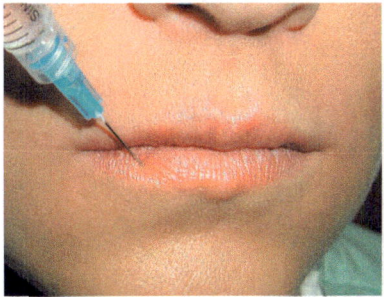
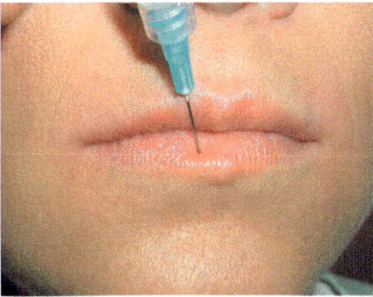
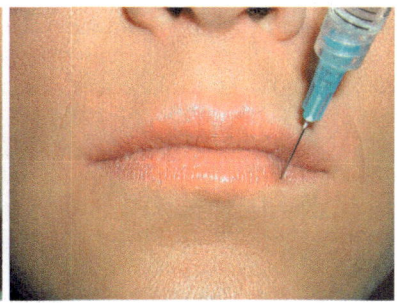

Fig. 2.21 Submucosal lip infiltration can be used to augment or in place of bilateral mental nerve block to treat the lower lip. Very small volumes will create adequate anesthesia. The solution is injected across the entire lip. The same technique can be used on the upper lip as well

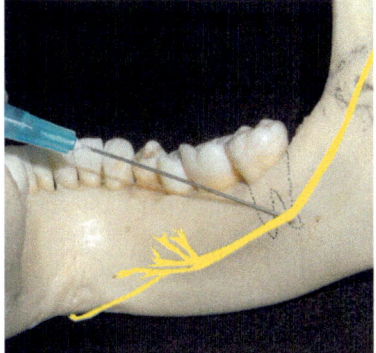
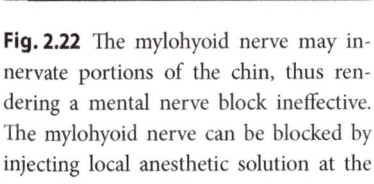
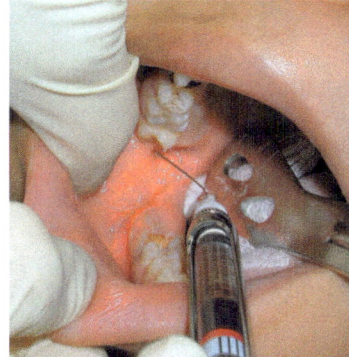
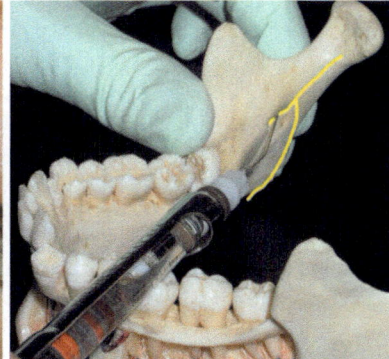

Fig. 2.22 The mylohyoid nerve may innervate portions of the chin, thus rendering a mental nerve block ineffective. The mylohyoid nerve can be blocked by injecting local anesthetic solution at the base of the roots of the second molar

Fig. 2.23 The target of the needle in the intraoral inferior alveolar nerve block is at the entrance of the nerve in the mandibular foramen on the medial ramus. The needle can be slightly bent with a medial angle to negotiate the flaring anatomy of the ramus. The mylohyoid nerve (inferior to needle) may or may not be blocked by this technique depending upon its level of branching

In the case of a "missed" or incomplete block, the lips may also be anesthetized by small amounts of submucosal local anesthetic infiltration (Fig. 2.21). This infiltration technique may be performed to assist or in place of mental nerve block, but a very small volume of local solution is used so as not to distort the lip. This is especially important when injecting fillers. Applying topical anesthesia prior to the injections will assist patient comfort.

The mental nerve block may fail to anesthetize the entire chin or area lateral to it owing to innervation from the mylohyoid nerve. Although infiltrative augmentation techniques may be used, complete anesthesia may be obtained by performing an inferior alveolar nerve block or blocking the mylohyoid nerve. The mylohyoid nerve branches off from the mandibular nerve and travels along the mylohyoid grove just below the apices of the mandibular second molars. This nerve is blocked by placing a 1.5-in. 27-gauge needle at the bottom of the roots of the lower second molar and depositing 2 ml of local anesthetic solution (Fig. 2.22).

2.4.3.6
Inferior Alveolar Nerve Block (Intraoral)

Almost every person who has ever been to a dentist has had this block and is aware of its effects, distribution, and duration. This block is technically more difficult to master, but is easily learned. The basis of this technique involves the deposition of local anesthetic solution at or about the mandibular foramen on the medial mandibular ramus where the inferior alveolar nerve enters the mandible (Fig. 2.23).

Detailed description of this technique is beyond the scope of this review but will be outlined as follows. The patient is seated upright and the surgeon places the index finger on the posterior ramus and the thumb in the coronoid notch on the anterior mandibular ramus (Fig. 2.23).

A 1.5-in. 27-gauge needle is then directed to the medial mandibular ramus at the level of the cusps of the upper second molar and the needle is advanced halfway between the thumb and index finger of the other hand that is grasping the mandible (Fig. 2.23). Two milliliters of 2% lidocaine with 1:100,000 epinephrine is then injected in a pumping motion to better the chances of anesthetic solution contacting the nerve and foramen. The needle can be slightly bent as shown in Fig. 2.23 to negotiate the sometimes outward curvature of the mandibular ramus. The surgeon should first aspirate to avoid intravascular injection. Anesthesia from this block sometimes takes 5–10 min to ensue. Proficiency in this blocking technique requires practice, but is very useful in cosmetic facial procedures. In addition, the ipsolateral tongue is usually anesthetized with this block. The area anesthetized includes the lower teeth and gums, the chin, and skin on the lateral chin. The inferior alveolar nerve block frequently includes the mylohyoid nerve. In some patients the mylohyoid nerve braches above the area of inferior alveolar injection and in this case needs a specific mylohyoid nerve block as outlined previously.

2.4.3.7
Mandibular Nerve (V3) Block (Facial Approach)

The mandibular nerve can also be blocked from a deep injection as the nerve exits the foramen ovale, posterior to the pterygoid plate (Fig. 2.24). This technique requires more experience and has more potential complications than the intraoral approach.

The technique for performing this block begins with the patient in supine position with the head and neck turned away from the side to be blocked. The patient is asked to open and close the mouth gently so that the operator can identify and palpate the sigmoid notch [19]. This is the area between the mandibular condyle and the coronoid process (Fig. 2.24). This notch is located about 25 mm anterior to the tragus. If one places a finger 25 mm anterior to the tragus and opens and closes the jaw, the mandibular condyle can be palpated with the jaw open. When the jaw is closed, the finger will be over the sigmoid notch. An 8-cm 22-gauge needle is inserted in the midpoint of the notch and directed at aslightly cephalic and medial angle through the notch until the lateral pterygoid plate is contacted (Fig. 2.24) [19]. This is usually at a depth of approximately 4.5–5.0 cm. Spinal needles frequently have measuring stops that can be adjusted to the position of original contact of the pterygoid plate. The needle is then withdrawn to a subcutaneous position and carefully "walked off" the posterior border of the pterygoid plate (Fig. 2.24) in

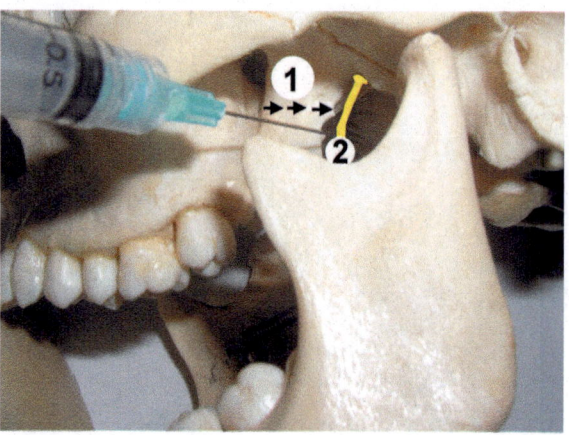

Fig. 2.24 The mandibular nerve (V3) block places the local anesthetic just posterior to the lateral pterygoid plate where the third division of the trigeminal nerve exits the foramen ovale. The needle is walked off the pterygoid plate (*1*) and the local anesthetic solution is deposited in the region of the third division of the trigeminal nerve (*2*)

a horizontal plane until the needle no longer touches the plate and is posterior to it. The needle depth should be the same as the distance on the needle stop marker when the pterygoid plate was originally contacted. The needle should not be advanced more than 0.5 cm past the depth of the pterygoid plate because the superior constrictor muscle of the pharynx can be pierced easily [19]. When the needle is in the appropriate position, 5 ml of local anesthetic solution can be administered. The area anesthetized is shown as "V3" in Fig. 2.3. Complications include hematoma formation and subarachnoid injection [20]. This block should be learned in a proctored situation and should not be attempted by novice injectors.

2.4.3.8   Blocking the Scalp

As outlined earlier in this chapter, the anterior scalp is anesthetized by injecting the branches of V1 (supraorbital and supratrochlear nerves) and V2 (the zygomaticotemporal nerve). The posterior scalp is innervated by the greater and lesser occipital nerves and the greater auricular nerve supplies the lateral scalp (Fig. 2.25).

By performing the "brow blocks" (Fig. 2.6), the cervical plexus block (Fig. 2.27), and the zygomaticotemporal block (Fig. 2.12), one anesthetizes most of the scalp, with the exception of the posterior area. This is anesthetized by blocking the greater occipital nerve. On can also perform a ring block where wheals of local anesthetic are injected every several centimeters around the entire scalp at about the level of the eyebrows. About 30 ml of local anesthetic is required to perform a scalp ring block.

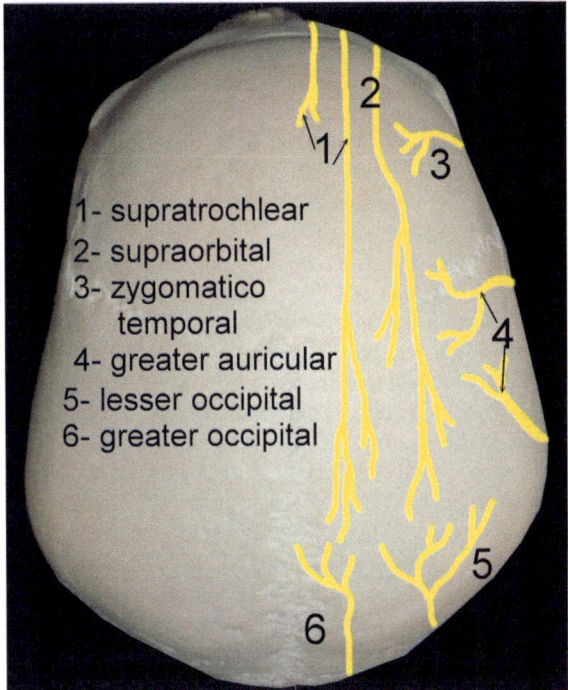

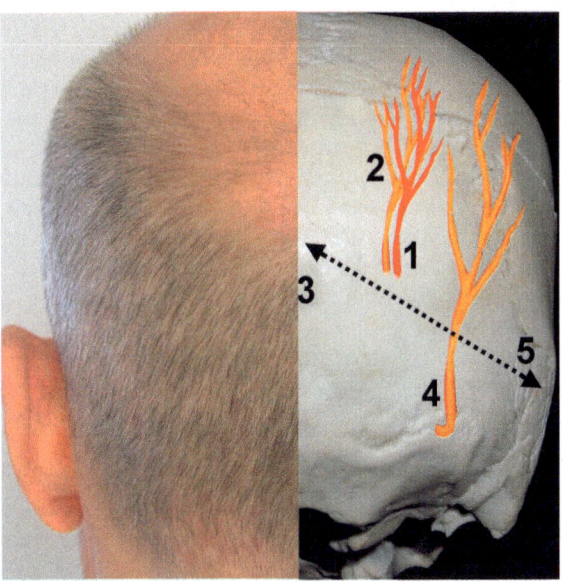

Fig. 2.25 Innervation of the scalp. *1* supratrochlear nerve, *2* supraorbital nerve(s), *3* zygomaticotemporal nerve, *4* greater auricular nerve, *5* lesser occipital nerve, *6* greater occipital nerve. (Innervation pattern adapted from Brown [19])

Fig. 2.26 The greater occipital nerve is in close approximation to the artery of the same name (*1*). The nerve can be located by palpating the artery and injecting just medial to it (*2*). Another landmark is injecting on the nuchal line, one third to half the distance between the mastoid prominence and occipital protuberance (*3, 5*). *4* the lesser occipital nerve

2.4.3.9
Greater Occipital Nerve Block Technique for Posterior Scalp Anesthesia

The greater occipital nerve arises from the dorsal rami of the second cervical nerve and travels deep to the cervical musculature until it becomes subcutaneous slightly inferior to the superior nuchal line [21]. It emerges on this line in association with the occipital artery, and the artery is the most useful landmark for locating the greater occipital nerve (Fig. 2.26). The most efficient patient position is sitting upright with the chin flexed to the sternum [20].

The nerve is identified at its point of entry to the scalp, along the superior nuchal line two thirds to half the distance between the mastoid process and the occipital protuberance in the midline (Fig. 2.26). Another measurement for locating the artery is 2.5–3.0 cm lateral to the occipital protrubence [22]. The patient will report pain upon compression of the nerve: the point at which maximal tenderness is elicited can be used as the injection site. A 0.625-in. 25-gauge needle is used for the block. The occipital artery is just lateral to the greater occipital nerve and can be used as a pulsitile landmark. Between 2 and 4 ml of local anesthetic solution can be infiltrated on either side of the artery to

ensure proximity to the nerve. Figure 2.29 shows the dermatomes anesthetized by blocking the greater occipital nerve.

2.4.3.10
Local Anesthesia of the Neck

Innervation of the Cervical Plexus

The cervical plexus is formed from the ventral rami of the upper four cervical nerves (Fig. 2.27). Their dorsal and ventral roots combine to form spinal nerves as they exit through the intervertebral foramen. The anterior rami of C2 through C4 form the cervical plexus [13]. The cervical plexus lies just behind the posterior border of the sternocleidomastoid muscle, giving off both superficial (superficial cervical plexus) and deep branches (deep cervical plexus). The branches of the superficial cervical plexus supply the skin and superficial structures of the head, neck, and shoulder. The deep branches of the cervical plexus innervate the deeper structures of the neck, including the muscles of the anterior neck and the diaphragm (phrenic nerve), and are not blocked for local anesthetic procedures.

Superficial Branches of the Cervical Plexus

The lesser occipital nerve arises from the second (and sometimes third) cervical nerve and emerges from the deep fascia on the posterior lateral portion of the head behind the auricle, supplying the skin and communicating with the greater occipital nerve, the greater auricular nerve, and the posterior auricular branch of the facial nerve [13].

The greater auricular nerve arises from the second and third cervical nerves and divides into an anterior and a posterior branch. The anterior branch is distributed to the skin of the face over the parotid gland, and communicates in the substance of the gland with the facial nerve.

The posterior branch supplies the skin over the mastoid process and on the back of the auricle, except at its upper part; a filament pierces the auricle to reach its lateral surface, where it is distributed to the lobule and lower part of the concha. The posterior branch communicates with the lesser occipital nerve, the auricular branch of the vagus, and the posterior auricular branch of the facial nerve [13].

The cutaneous cervical nerve (cutaneous colli nerve, anterior cervical nerve) arises from the second and third cervical nerves and provides sensation to the anterolateral parts of the neck (Fig. 2.25).

Cervical Plexus Block

This technique is used in cosmetic facial surgery to block the superficial branches of the cervical plexus to anesthetize skin of the lateral or anterior neck, the posterior lateral scalp, and portions of the periauricular area (Fig. 2.3).

The technique involves laying the patient back with the sternocleidomastoid flexed. The line from the mastoid process to the transverse process of C6 (Chassaignac's tubercle) (approximate level of the cricoid cartilage) (Fig. 2.27) is divided in half at the posterior border of the sternocleidomastoid to determine the injection point [19, 23]. Another technique is to simply bisect the distance from the origin and insertion of the sternocleidomastoid without osseous landmarks. The success of this block involves a larger volume of local anesthetic diffusing and spreading out over a larger area rather than absolute accuracy of the nerve position. Between 3 and 5 ml of local anesthetic solution is injected subcutaneously with the needle perpendicular to the skin. The needle is then redirected superiorly and another 3–5 ml is injected. Finally, the needle is then directed inferiorly and another 3–5 ml is injected. Figure 2.27 shows the areas anesthetized by a cervical plexus block.

Phrenic nerve involvement is rare with superficial cervical plexus block (it is more common with deep cervical blocks) but is technically possible as C3, C4, and C5 innervate the diaphragm. Healthy patients can tolerate a hemiparalysis of the diaphragm but caution must be used in patients with cardiopulmonary problems as assisted ventilation may be required. It must be kept in mind that a bilateral block could potentially denervate the entire diaphragm. To prevent unwanted spread of local anesthetic solution, this injection is just subcutaneous in placement and is never done bilaterally.

2.4.3.11
Ear Block

Four nerve branches supply sensory innervation to the ear. The anterior half of the ear is supplied by the

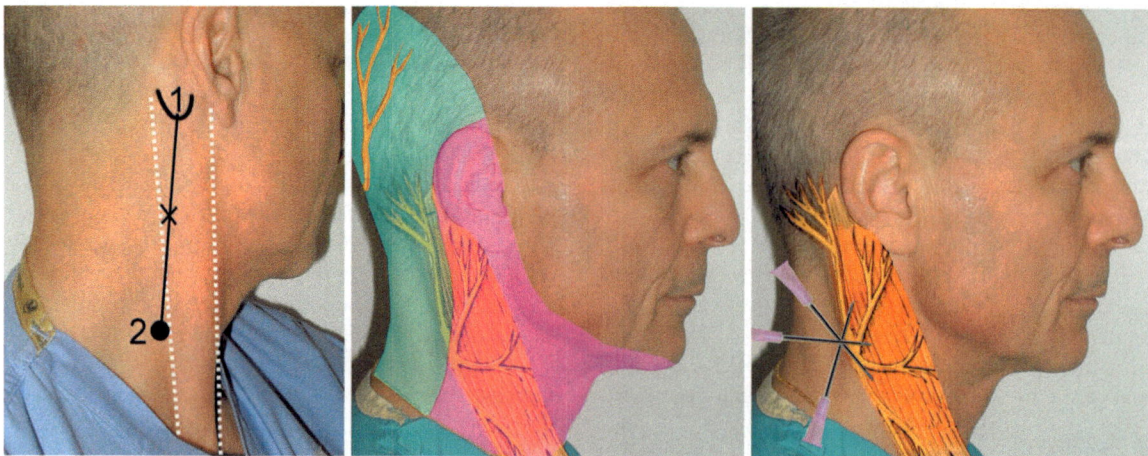

Fig. 2.27 The cervical plexus block is performed by making a line from the mastoid process (*1*) to the level of the transverse process of C6 (*2*) then finding the point halfway between these two marks (*X*) just posterior to the sternocleidomastoid (*dotted line*). Local anesthetic is then injected perpendicular, superiorly, and inferiorly in this region. The *middle picture* also shows the greater occipital nerve, which is not part of the cervical plexus

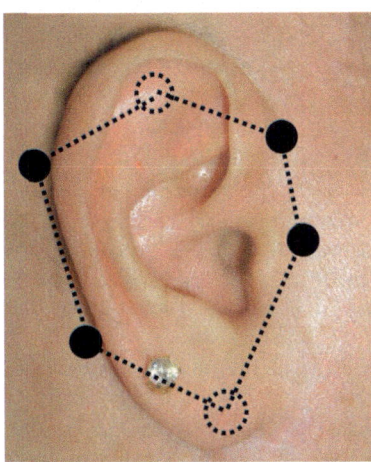

Fig. 2.28 Blocking the entire ear (with the exception of the area supplied by the vagus nerve) can be performed by inserting the needle at the *black dots* and infiltrating along the *dotted lines*. This will anesthetize the terminal branches of the auriculotemporal nerve, the lesser occipital nerve, and the anterior and posterior branches of the greater auricular nerve. The main trunks of these nerves could be blocked as detailed in the text, but this terminal infiltration technique may be more convenient

auriculotemporal nerve, which is a branch of the mandibular portion of the trigeminal nerve. The posterior half of the ear is innervated by two nerve branches derived from the cervical plexus: the great auricular nerve and the lesser occipital nerve (Fig. 2.27). The auditory branch of the vagus nerve innervates the concha and the external auditory canal.

Although these nerves can be individually targeted with blocks, a circumferential infiltration (ring block) will anesthetize the entire ear, except the concha and the external auditory canal, which are innervated by the vagus nerve. The needle is inserted into the skin at the junction where the earlobe attaches to the head. The anesthetic should be infiltrated while the needle is advanced to the subcutaneous plane. Infiltration is made in a hexagonal pattern around the entire periphery of the ear (Fig. 2.28). The chonal bowl and external auditory canal will need separate infiltration. One should aspirate (as with all injections) prior to injection to prevent intravascular injection.

2.5 Summary

A firm knowledge of the sensory neuroanatomy of the head and neck can benefit the practice of cosmetic facial surgery for both the surgeon and the patient. Although the pathways of sensation for the head and neck are complex, they can be easily and safely blocked by reviewing the basic innervation patterns.

The entire sensory apparatus of the face is supplied by the trigeminal nerve and several cervical branches. There exist many patterns of nerve distribution anomaly, cross-innervation, and individual patient variation; however, by following the basic techniques outlined in this chapter, the cosmetic surgeon should be able to achieve pain control of the major dermatomes of the head and neck. A basic dermatomal distribution is illustrated in Fig. 2.29 and can serve as road map to local anesthesia of the head and neck.

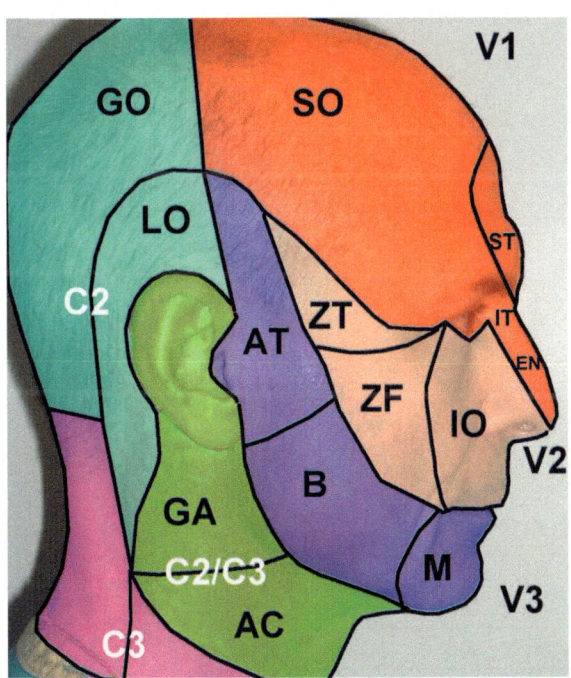

Fig. 2.29 The major sensory dermatomes of the head and neck. *AC* anterior cervical cutaneous colli, *AT* auriculotemporal nerve, *B* buccal nerve, *EN* external (dorsal) nasal nerve, *GA* greater auricular nerve, *GO* greater occipital nerve, *IO* infraorbital nerve, *IT* infratrochlear nerve, *LO* lesser occipital nerve, *M* mental nerve, *SO* supraorbital nerve, *ST* supratrochlear nerve, *ZF* zygomaticofacial nerve, *ZT* zygomaticotemporal nerve. (Adapted from Larrabee [24])

References

1. Hersh EV, Condouis GA: Local anesthetics: A review of their pharmacology and clinical use. Compend Contin Educ Dent 1987;8:374–382

2. Jastak JT, Yagiela JA, Donaldson D.: Local Anesthesia of the Oral Cavity. Philadelphia, Saunders 1995

3. Covino BG, Vassalo HG: Chemical aspects of local anesthetic agents. In Local Anesthetics: Mechanism of Action and Clinical Use, Kitz RJ, Laver MB (Eds), New York, Grune & Stratton, 1976:1–11

4. Hersh EV: Local Anesthetics. In Oral and Maxillofacial Surgery, Fonseca RJ (Ed), Philadelphia, Saunders 2000:58–78

5. Fink BR: History of neural blockade. In Neural Blockade in Clinical Anesthesia and Management of Pain, 2nd Edition, Cousins MJ, Bridenbaugh PO (Eds), Philadelphia, Lippincott 1988:3–21

6. Lathers CM, Tyau LSY, Spino MM, Agarwal I: Cocaine-induced seizures, arrhythmias, and sudden death. J Clin Pharmacol, 1988;28(7):584–593

7. Kosten TR, Hollister LE: Drugs of Abuse. In Basic and Clinical Pharmacology, 7th Edition, Katzung BG (Ed), Norwalk, Appleton & Lange 1998:516–531

8. Hadda SE: Procaine: Alfred Einhorn's ideal substitute for cocaine. J Am Dent Assoc 1962;64:841–845

9. Yagiela JA: Local Anesthetics. In Management of Pain and Anxiety in Dental Practice, Dionne RA, Phero JC (Eds), New York, Elsevier 1991:109–134

10. Malamed SF: Handbook of Local Anesthesia, 4th Edition, St. Louis, Mosby 1997

11. Aceves J, Machne X: The action of calcium and of local anesthetics on nerve cells and their interaction during excitation. J Pharmacol Exp Ther 1963;140:138–148

12. Stricharatz D: Molecular mechanisms of nerve block by local anesthetics. Anesthesiology 1976;45(4):421–441

13. Gray H: Anatomy of the Human Body, 13th Edition, Philadelphia, Lea & Febiger, 1918:1158–1169

14. Zide BM, Swift R: How to block and tackle the face. Plast Reconstr Surg 1998;101(3):840–851

15. Mendel N, Puterbaugh PG: Conduction, Infiltration and General Anesthesia in Dentistry, 4th Edition, New York, Dental Items of Interest Publishing Co 1938:140

16. Mercuri LG: Intraoral second division nerve block. Oral Surg 1979;47(2):9–13

17. Westmoreland EE, Blanton PL: An analysis of the variations in position of the greater palatine foramen in the adult human skull. Anat Rec 1982;204(4):383–388

18. Malamed SF, Trieger N: Intraoral maxillary nerve block: an anatomical and clinical study. Anesth Prog 1983;30(2):44–48

19. Brown DL: Atlas of Regional Anesthesia, Philadelphia, Saunders 999:170

20. Wheeler AH: Theraputic Injections for Pain Management, http://www.emedicine.com/neuro/topic514.htm#target10 2001

21. Bonica TT, Buckley FO: Regional anesthesia with local anesthetics. In: The Management of Pain, Bonica TT (Ed), Philadelphia, Lippincott Williams and Wilkins 1990:1883–1966

22. Gmyrek R: Local Anesthesia and Regional Nerve Block Anesthesia, http://www.emedicine.com/derm/topic824.htm 2002

23. http://www.nysora.com/techniques/basic/superficial_plexus/superficial_plexus.html

24. Larrabee W, Msakielski KH: Surgical Anatomy of the Face, New York, Raven Press, 1993:83

Part II
Classifications

CHAPTER 3

Universal Classification of Skin Type

Mitchel P. Goldman

Thomas Fitzpatrick [1] proposed a classification of skin type based on the efficiency of melanogenesis in response to ultraviolet exposure. This classification is based on a personal history of sunburning and/or sun-tanning following 45–60 min of exposure to midday sun. This "Fitzpatrick skin classification" (Table 3.1) has been universally adopted in all aspects of dermatology and cutaneous surgery to predict post-treatment pigmentary changes. My experience in treating hundreds of patients of both sexes of various races on various medications suggests that the Fitzpatrick classification is not an accurate predictor of pigmentary response to laser, surgical (dermabrasion) or chemical injury to the skin. In fact, I do not believe that the Fitzpatrick classification was ever meant to fulfill this purpose.

The Fitzpatrick classification is a good predictor of melanogenesis in response to ultraviolet exposure; however, other stimuli of melanocytic function have not been correlated to this classification. For example, other important stimuli of melanocytic function are inflammation [2, 3], hemosiderin [4] and free-radical formation [5]. Various hormones have also been associated with stimulation of melanocytic function [6, 7]. It is proposed that a more comprehensive classification of skin type regarding melanocytic function be based on its stimulation by these various factors in addition to ultraviolet light and surgical/chemical injury to the skin.

The approximately 3.5 billion nonwhite people in India, China, Northeast and Southeast Asia, the Middle East, Spain, Central and South America, and the black populations of African countries, the USA and elsewhere represent the majority of the world's human population. Racial differences in skin pathophysiology have been well documented [8, 9]. There is a high risk of pigmentary alteration and scarring following any procedure that produces inflammation of the skin in darkly pigmented races. Both genetic background and environmental factors are involved in these differences.

Melanosomes differ in their appearance and structure with regard to race [10]. Melanosomes from Caucasians are 0.6 μm × 0.2 μm in diameter and are oval-shaped. Melanosomes in Black races are denser on electron microscope images and measure 1.0 μm × 0.5 μm in diameter. Asian or Mongoloid melanosomes appear as single or aggregate forms on electron microscope images and measure 0.6 μm × 0.3 μm in diameter. In addition, although the density of melanocytes is similar with variations on different body parts, the melanocyte/epidermal cell interaction differs amongst the races.

The effects of light on skin (including laser light) begins with the absorption of incident light by chromophores [11]. Melanin, hemoglobin, oxyhemoglobin and water are the dominant natural chromophores in the skin [12]. The major determinant of differences in skin color between white and nonwhite skin is the amount of epidermal melanin. As described above, although there is no difference in the quantity of melanocytes between the two groups, the larger and more melanized melanosomes in nonwhite skin compared with white skin influence skin color. In addition, the degradation rate of melanosomes within the keratinocytes of dark skin is slower than that of white skin. The larger and more melanized melanosomes of Blacks absorb and scatter more energy, thus providing a higher photoprotection. Conversely, the melanocytes and mesenchyma in darker skin seem to be more vulnerable to trauma and inflammatory conditions than those in white skin [13].

Race as a determinate of skin color can be broadly broken down into five categories. These categories appear to be derived from geographic evolution of the *homo sapiens* species. There are obvious significant differences in skin color and thus melanocyte/melanosome/epidermal cell interaction even within geographic groups. Lancer [14] proposed a "Lancer ethnicity scale" to take race into consideration when treating patients with laser resurfacing. He also factored in additional patient genetic historical information to provide a method to presurgically correlate skin type to patient outcome (Table 3.2). However, his use of hair color as a factor in his skin type has been debated since light-skinned people can have dark hair, and vice versa [15].

The proposed world classification of skin type (Table 3.3) is the author's attempt at providing a useful classification to predict melanocyte response to multiple surgical and chemical stimuli (including laser resurfacing) in addition to ultraviolet radiation.

My experience and a review of the literature on laser resurfacing underlies the need for a new classification. All available studies on pigmentary response from laser resurfacing have used the Fitzpatrick classification. A

Table 3.1 Fitzpatrick classification of skin type

I	Always burns never tans
II	Burns easily, tans with difficulty
III	Rarely burns, tans easily
IV	Never burns, tans

review of these reports shows a wide variability in the incidence and extent of pigmentary alterations. It is my hypothesis that these variations are not merely secondary to the surgeon's expertise, technique or reporting accuracy, but are due to the variability within the Fitzpatrick skin type classification.

For example, our experience shows that hyperpigmentation occurs in 20–30% of patients with Fitzpatrick type III, and nearly 100% of patients with Fitzpatrick type IV skin at 3 months follow-up [16]. We have found that almost all episodes resolve in 2–4 months and usually respond faster to treatment. Other authors report hyperpigmentation in their Fitzpatrick type I–IV patients in 83% [17], 40% [18], 0% [19], 3% [20], 10% [21], and 25% [22] of their patients with Fitzpatrick types I–IV. Thus, many authors using similar laser resurfacing techniques in similar populations report vastly different pigmentation results. It is not possible to ask all the authors to recalculate their hyperpigmentation incidence based on a new classification scheme to prove its efficacy. This study is presently being performed in my office.

Decreasing the incidence of hyperpigmentation in Asian patients with laser resurfacing has been shown by pretreatment with hydroxyquinone. In one study, 100% of Asian patients developed hyperpigmentation after laser resurfacing without pretreatment vs. a 32% incidence in patients who were treated both preoperatively and postoperatively with hydroxyquinone solution [23]. Ho et al. [24] treated 30 Asian and Hispanic patients

Table 3.2 Lancer ethnicity scale (*LES*)

Geography	Fitzpatrick skin type	LES skin type
African background		
Central East, West African	V	5
Eritrean and Ethiopian	V	5
North African, Middle East	V	5
Arabian background		
Sephardic Jewish	III	4
Asian background		
Chinese, Korean, Japanese, Thai, Vietnamese	IV	4
Filipino, Polynesian	IV	4
European background		
Ashkenazi Jewish	II	3
Celtic	I	1
Central Eastern European	III	2
Nordic	I–II	1
Northern European (general)	I	1–2
Southern European, Mediterranean	III	3–4
Latin/Central/South American background		
Central/South American Indian	IV	4
North American background		
Native American (including Inuit)	II	3

and noted maximum pigmentation after 6 weeks which only persisted for 3–4 months following laser resurfacing. Our experience has been similar. However, when only using the Fitzpatrick classification, some of our type IV patients hyperpigment for 2–3 months, while other hyperpigment for 6–8 months. Thus, even in studies on Asian and/or type IV patients variability in pigmentation response occurs.

It is hoped that this chapter will stimulate a lively scientific discussion that will take surgical dermatology from "Caucasian-centric" to multiracial. The development of a new classification of skin type will allow physicians of all races to treat patients of all races with techniques specific for the particular race being treated. Equally important would be to more completely report adverse effects on the basis of a universal skin type classification that takes into account multiple factors and not merely the response to ultraviolet exposure.

References

1. Fitzpatrick TB: The validity and practicality of sun reactive skin type I through VI. Arch Dermatol 1988;124:869
2. Synder DS, Eaglestein WH: Intradermal antiprostaglandin agents and sunburn, J Invest Dermatol 1974;62:47
3. Black AK, et al: The effect of indomethacin on arachidonic acid and prostaglandins E2 and F2 levels in human skin 24 hours after UVB and UVC irradiation. Br J Clin Pharmacol 1987;6:261
4. Cawler EP, Hsu YT, Wood BT, Weary PE: Hemochromatosis and the skin. Arch Dermatol 1969;100:1–6

Table 3.3 World classification of skin type

1. European/Caucasian—white	(a) Pale, cannot tan, burns easily, no postinflammatory pigmentation
	(b) Tan, rarely burns, rarely develops postinflammatory pigmentation
	(c) Deep tan, never burns, develops postinflammatory pigmentation
2. Arabian/Mediterranean/Hispanic—light brown	(a) Pale, cannot tan, burns easily, no postinflammatory pigmentation
	(b) Tan, rarely burns, rarely develops postinflammatory pigmentation
	(c) Deep tan, never burns, develops postinflammatory pigmentation
3. Asian—yellow	(a) Pale, cannot tan, burns easily, no postinflammatory pigmentation
	(b) Tan, rarely burns, rarely develops postinflammatory pigmentation
	(c) Deep tan, never burns, develops postinflammatory pigmentation
4. Indian—brown	(a) Pale, cannot tan, burns easily, no postinflammatory pigmentation
	(b) Tan, rarely burns, rarely develops postinflammatory pigmentation
	(c) Deep tan, never burns, develops postinflammatory pigmentation
5. African—black	(a) Pale, cannot tan, burns easily, no postinflammatory pigmentation
	(b) Tan, rarely burns, rarely develops postinflammatory pigmentation
	(c) Deep tan, never burns, develops postinflammatory pigmentation

5. Kaidbey KH, Kurban AK: The influence of corticosteroids and indomethacin on sunburn erythema. J Invest Dermatol 1976;66:153

6. Esoda ECJ: Chloasma from progestational oral contraceptives. Arch Dermatol 1963;87:486

7. Mor A, Capsi E: Cutaneous complications of hormonal replacement therapy. Clin Dermatol 1997;15:147–154

8. Andersen KE, Maibach HI: Black and white human skin differences. J Am Acad Dermatol 1979;1:276–382

9. Berardesca E, Maibach HI: Racial differences in skin pathophysiology. J Am Acad Dermatol 1996;34:667–672

10. Szabo G, Gerald AB, Pathak MA, et al: The ultrastructure of racial color differences in man. In: Riley V, (Ed), Pigmentation: Its Genesis and Biologic Control. New York: Appleton-Century-Crofts 1972:23–41

11. Anderson RR: Laser-tissue interactions, 2nd ed. St. Louis: Mosby 1999

12. Anderson RR, Parrish JA: The optics of human skin. J Invest Dermatol 1981;77:13–19

13. Olson RL, Gaylor J, Everett MA: Skin color, melanin, and erythema. Arch Dermatol 1973;108:541–544

14. Lancer HA: Lancer ethnicity scale (LES) [letter]. Lasers Surg Med 1998;22:9

15. Wolbarsht ML, Urbach F: The Lancer ethnicity scale [letter]. Lasers Surg Med 1999;25:105–106

16. Fitzpatrick RE, Goldman MP, Satur NM, Tope WD: Pulsed carbon dioxide laser resurfacing of photoaged facial skin. Arch Dermatol 1996;132:395–402

17. Lowe NJ, Lask G, Griffin ME: Laser resurfacing: pre- and posttreatment guidelines. Dermatol Surg 1995;21:1017

18. Goodman GJ: Carbon dioxide laser resurfacing: preliminary observations on short-term follow-up: a subjective study on 100 patients' attitudes and outcomes. Dermatol Surg 1998;24:665

19. Weinstein C: Ultrapulse carbon dioxide laser removal of periocular wrinkles in association with laser blepharoplasty. J Clin Laser Med Surg 1994;12:205

20. Bernstein LJ, Kauvar ANB, Grossman MC, Geronemus RG: The short- and long-term side effects of carbon dioxide laser resurfacing. Dermatol Surg 1997;23:519–525

21. Ziering CL: Cutaneous laser resurfacing with the erbium: YAG laser and the char-free carbon dioxide laser. Int J Aesth Restor Surg 1998;5:29

22. Ruiz-Esparza J, Barba Gomez JM, Gomez de la Torre OL, Huerta Franco B, Parga Vazquez EG: Ultrapulse laser skin resurfacing in Hispanic patients. A prospective study of 36 individuals. Dermatol Surg 1998;24:59–62

23. Pham RT: Hyperpigmentation in Asians after carbon dioxide laser resurfacing. Dermatol Surg 1998;29:118–119

24. Ho C, Nguyen Q, Lowe NJ, et al: Laser resurfacing in pigmented skin. Dermatol Surg 1995;21:1035–1037

Chapter 4

Fasil Scale: Measurement of Facial Skin and Soft-Tissue Laxity

4

Hector Leal-Silva

4.1
Introduction

Human history is as recent or as ancient as 13,000 years [1] and for almost half that period evidence exists about efforts in widely diverse groups and times to enhance or modify physical attributes [2].

When efforts are made to enhance physical beauty, the attention frequently focuses on facial attributes. Facial skin, subcutaneous tissues and including bone experience constant structural modifications as time passes, modifications that together consist of growing and development in the earlier stages and later evidence the characteristic signs of aging and facial deterioration.

Several systems have been presented by some authors as an attempt to understand and explain the dynamics of the facial aging process.

Facial aging has been analyzed from the viewpoint of the presence or absence of wrinkles and photodamage [3], the persistency of wrinkles when manually pulling the skin [4], dynamic lines related to gestures and the effects of gravity and mechanical forces [5] or, furthermore, taking into account the degree of dermatoheliosis, considering pigmentary and textural changes [6].

The distinctive characteristics between a chronologically aged skin and a skin with actinic aging (photoaging), considering the various structures that define a young, healthy skin free from deterioration, have been described by Obagi [7].

Others, like Donofrio [8], have given profound relevance to the importance of facial volumetric distribution to reflect age and finding "antiaging" treatments for the correction or redistribution of the volume of specific "packs of soft tissue."

Recently Alam et al. [9] developed a numerical rating scale to assess the quality of cosmetic surgery procedures pertaining to clinical efficacy and patient satisfaction.

nonablative radiofrequency for skin and subdermal tissue contraction, or the diverse methods for volumetric redistribution of the face using fillers, the need for new methods to evaluate posttreatment outcomes became evident (Fig. 4.1).

The physical examination and photographic assessments of these cases reveled that there was no accurate method available to evaluate results with regard to facial skin and subdermal laxity/firmness (Fig. 4.2).

Not one of the classification systems presented before was accurate to evaluate the spectrum between laxity and firmness, and the only issue one was able to express in terms of results was whether the patient looked better, the same or worse on physical examination and in some cases on photographic evaluation before and after the procedure .

The approaches that have employed measurements and lines added by computer have failed, mainly due to the slightest degree of change in positioning the patient for photography also changes the measurement so greatly that they becomes useless for evaluation of facial laxity change as a result of treatments, time or events.

In my opinion the typical method for evaluating the percentage of improvement lacks precision in many ways. The most relevant reasons are the percentage of improvement in relation to what the appearance was before, other cases, personal experience or the degree of change that in the mind of the evaluator could constitute a 100% change. Even when evaluating half-face results, presented as the percentage of change when one compares the degree of change in the untreated half with the degree of change in the half treated, 100% change cannot be observed or determined by any method, and one can only guess from the data, becoming fully subjective again.

With the aim of giving some objectivity where subjectivity prevails, a method to measure facial laxity was developed by the author.

4.2
Justification

With the recent technological and procedural developments in cosmetic dermatology, like the several nonsurgical lifting techniques with autoanchorage threads or

4.3
Laxity Classification System

The following describes a quantitative method of accurate measurement of facial skin and deep tissue laxity. To classify a patient's laxity, two separate steps must be

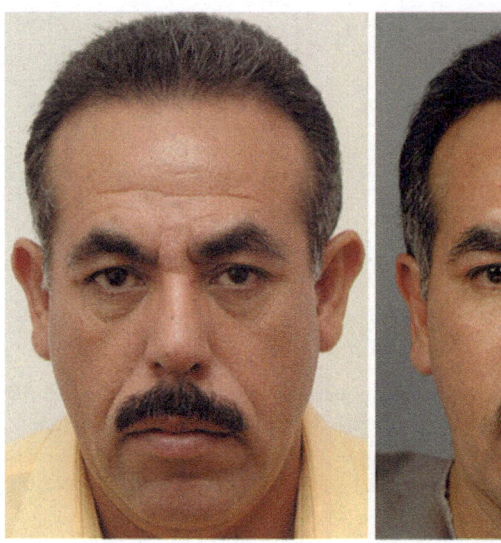

Fig. 4.1 Dermatologic cosmetic combined procedures

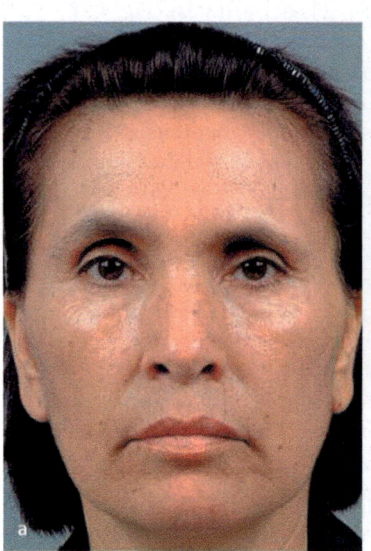 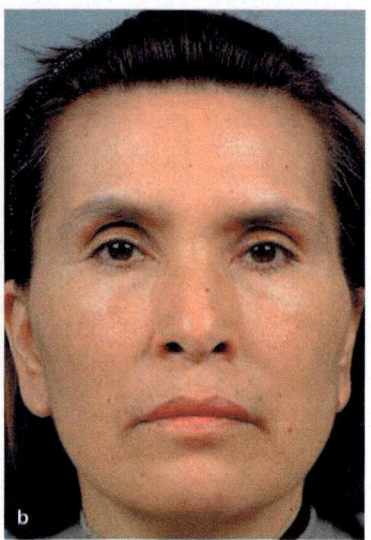

Fig. 4.2 Thermage™ patient. **a** Before and **b** 6 months after nonablative radiofrequency treatment

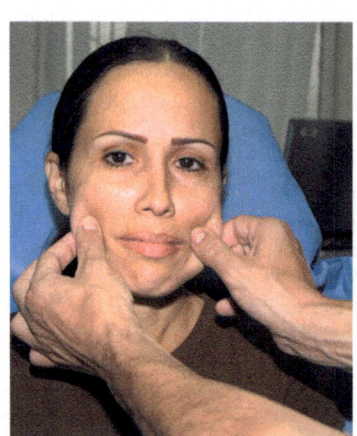 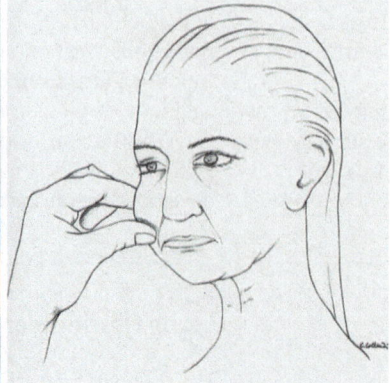

Fig. 4.3 Physical examination: pinch test

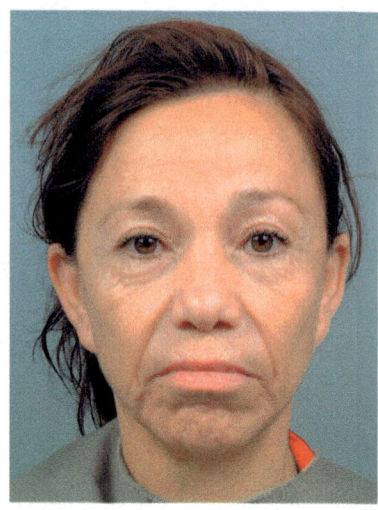

Fig. 4.4 Superficial laxity

performed: physical examination and photographic assessment.

4.3.1
Physical Examination

In the physical examination, the pinch test (Fig. 4.3) is critical to establish superficial (Fig. 4.4), deep (Fig. 4.5) or mixed (Fig. 4.6) laxity of facial skin and deep facial tissue (Table 4.1). The relevance of this differentiation resides in the fact that the physical expression of these variations in tissue laxity is structurally different and requires a specific approach.

Superficial laxity alone can be determined by positive slide displacement sign (skin easily performs shallow lateral movement). Since the expression of superficial laxity is mainly wrinkles, and since for the classification of rhytids, outstanding classification systems have already been developed as mentioned before, no attempt has been made by the author to classify this type of laxity.

The author's system focuses on deep or mixed tissue laxity assessed by photographic analysis. This initial physical examination is necessary mainly to avoid misinterpretation of data related to superficial expressions of age.

Table 4.1 Physical examination

Superficial	Deep	Superficial + deep

Table. 4.2 Signs

	Class					
	0	1	2	3	4	5
Upper face						
Eyelid	Eyelid fold slightly noticeable (thin line or absent)	Eyelid fold well defined (thick line)	Slight folding	Folding without reaching the eyelashes	Folding on the eyelashes	Eyelid fold interfering with the field of vision
Middle face						
Cheekbone roundness	Full	The central upper part of the cheekbone roundness is interrupted by an indentation	Nasojugal fold extends across the mid point of the cheekbone tissue	Nasojugal fold crosses the cheekbone tissue	The fold extend to form a flattened area	Completely flattened cheekbone tissue stretching the lower eyelid downward
Melolabial fold	Absent	Slightly noticeable	Defined	Prominent	Deeply marked crease	Line hidden by skin folding
Lower face						
Jowls	Absent	Slightly noticeable	Protruding forward	Protruding forward and downward	Forward protrusion with downward sagging	Forward sagging and lateral loss of definition in the neck
Upper neck						
Platysma bands	Absent	Absent	Slightly noticeable	Prominent	Sagging	Sagging to the point where bands or folds are no longer distinguishable
Horizontal folds	Absent	Absent	Absent	Slightly noticeable	Prominent	

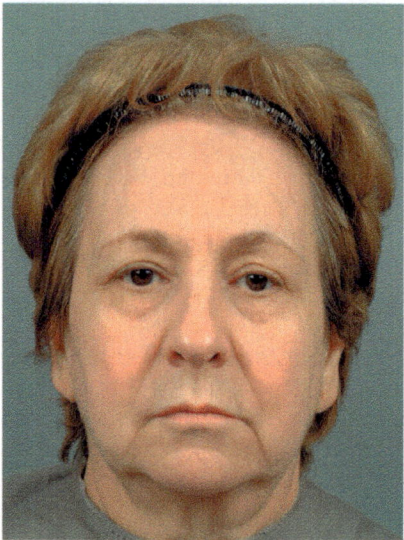

Fig. 4.5 Deep laxity

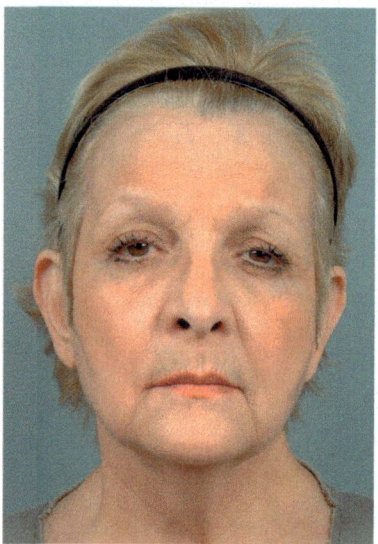

Fig. 4.6 Superficial plus deep laxity

4.3.2
Photographic Assessment

This part must be performed by observing the patient indirectly by using a set of five high-quality photographs (one frontal, two profiles and two intermediate) (Fig. 4.7).

In regards to the photographs we suggest a special area with indirect light, gray background, white lateral walls and a gray fabric on the chest. A static (on a tripod) digital camera with more than five megapixels should be used. The patient should be sitting and should only be rotated for positioning, using red dots in the lateral angles for sight standardization.

The photographic assessment includes two components: the division of the face into four regions and two sides (Figs. 4.8, 4.9); and classification of the observed laxity into one of six classes, each one with distinctive signs (Fig. 4.10) for each region and side (Figs. 4.11–4.34, Table 4.2).

The before mentioned regions mentioned before cover the area of study, including the zone around the sign that mainly or secondarily reflects the laxity of the whole region, like the eyelid fold in the upper region, the nasojugal and melolabial folds in the middle region, the jowls in the lower region and the platysma bands in the neck, this being the reason for not using the classic division by thirds in the anatomical approach to study the aging face [10].

Step 1: Divide the subject's face into regions and sides as follows:

1. Upper face: This region covers the area that begins at the hairline and extends to the horizontal line that crosses the pupils.
2. Middle face: This region covers the area that begins at a horizontal line that crosses the pupils and ex-

tends to a horizontal curved line that crosses the commissures of the mouth and the lower insertion of the ear.
3. Lower face: This region covers the area that begins at a horizontal curved line that crosses commissures of the mouth and the lower insertion of the ear, and extends downward up to the jaw line.
4. Upper neck: This region covers the area from the jaw line to the horizontal line that crosses the upper boundary of the thyroid cartilage.

Step 2: Classify the laxity in each region on each side of the face according to Table 4.2.

Step 3: Fill out the photographic assessment table (Table 4.3).

For statistical purposes, the mode can be observed and documented as 'the general facial grade'; the media can be used for more precise measurements and, of course, analyzing by region and side provides an abundance of data for specific purposes.

Some authors have used a half-grade (0.5) system in-between grades to express a degree of improvement that can be observed and recorded, but it does not meet the specified criteria to be considered as a 'full' change in grade (F. Mayoral 2005, personal communication).

Table 4.3 Photographic assessment

Region	Left	Right
Upper face		
Middle face		
Lower face		
Upper neck		

As a demonstration of the process of photographic assessment of patients, two cases have been classified by the author:

1. Case 1 (Fig. 4.35): The upper region corresponds to class 2 "eyelid slightly folding". The middle region also corresponds to class 2 "nasojugal fold extends across the mid point of the cheekbone and the melolabial fold is defined." The lower region of the face in this case presents an extensive laxity that corresponds to class 4 "forward protrusion with downward sagging." The neck presents changes corresponding also to class 4 "platysma bands sagging" even without the presence of horizontal folds. There are no significant differences between sides, so the table must be filled out as in Table 4.4.

2. Case 2 (Fig. 4.36): The upper region exhibits side to side differences: the right side corresponds to class 3 "eyelid folding without reaching the eyelashes," whereas the left side presents changes that correspond to class 4 "eyelid folding on the eyelashes." The middle region presents symmetrical changes that correspond to class 2 "nasojugal fold extends across the mid point of the cheekbone and melolabial fold is defined". The lower region is more or less symmetrical and corresponds to class 3 "jowls protruding forward and downward" (exhibits a mild asymmetry that fits within the same class). The neck presents changes in the horizontal folds (not in platysma bands) that correspond also to class 3 "slightly noticeable." The table must be filled out as in Table 4.5.

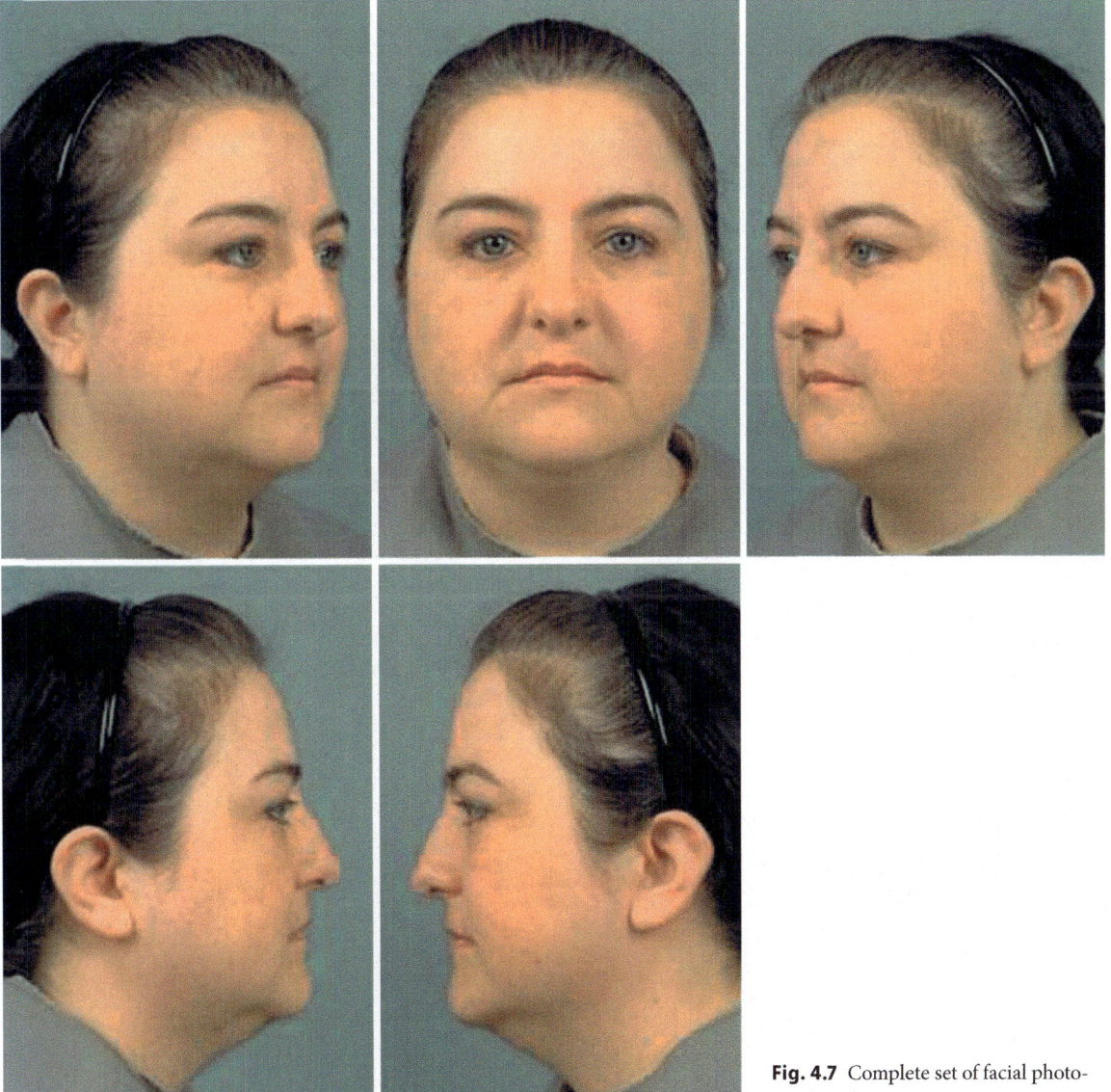

Fig. 4.7 Complete set of facial photographs

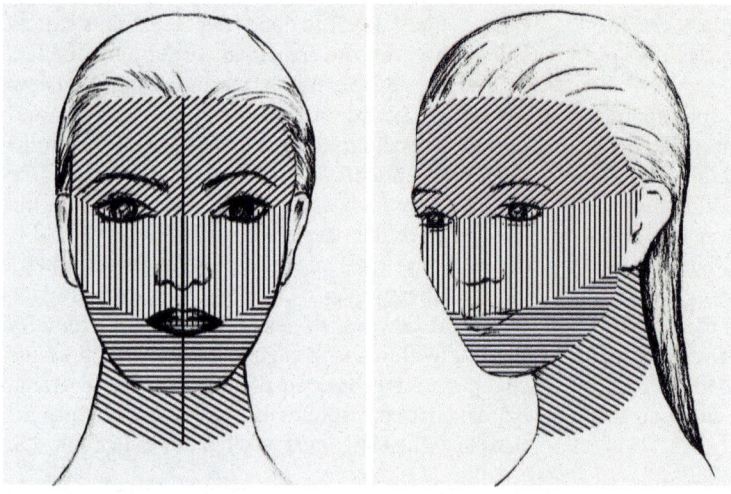

Fig. 4.8 Sections of face

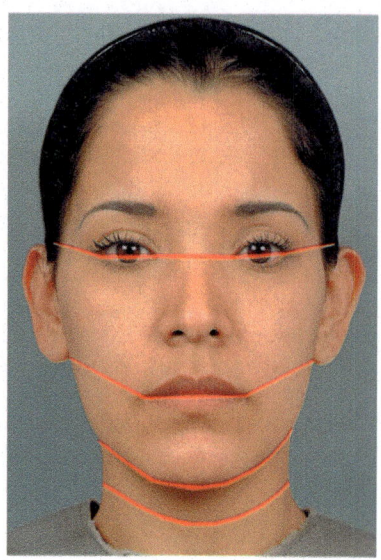

Fig. 4.9 Sections of face

Table 4.4 Photographic assessment of case 1

Region	Left	Right
Upper face	2	2
Middle face	2	2
Lower face	4	4
Upper neck	4	4

Table 4.5 Photographic assessment of case 2

Region	Left	Right
Upper face	4	3
Middle face	2	2
Lower face	3	3
Upper neck	3	3

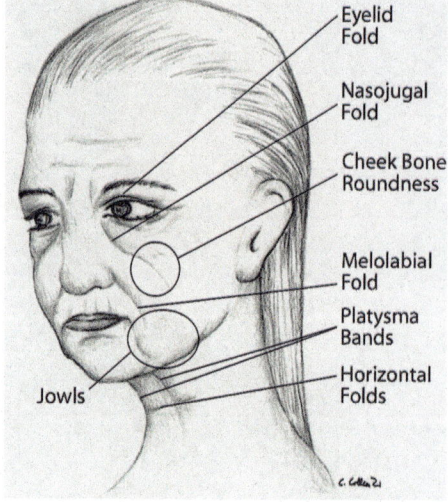

Fig. 4.10 Distinctive signs

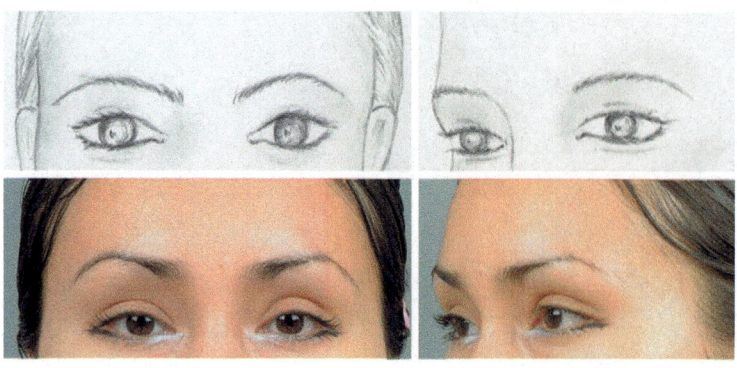

Fig. 4.11 Upper-face region, class 0. The eyelid fold slightly noticeable (thin line or absent)

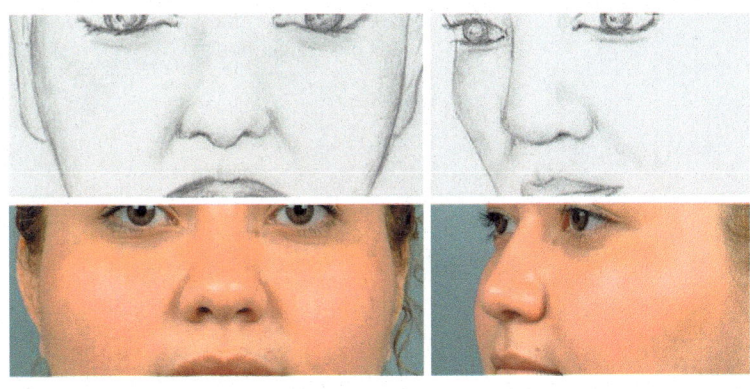

Fig. 4.12 Middle-face region, class 0. The cheekbone roundness is full and a melolabial fold is absent

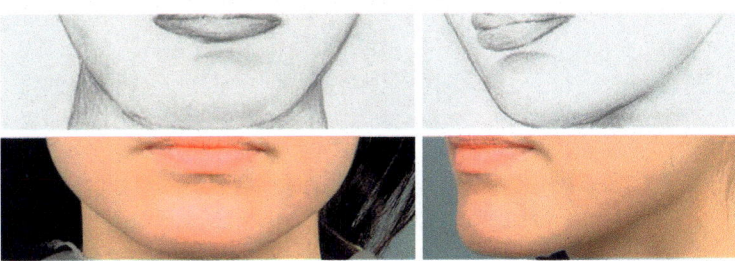

Fig. 4.13 Lower-face region, class 0. The jowls are absent

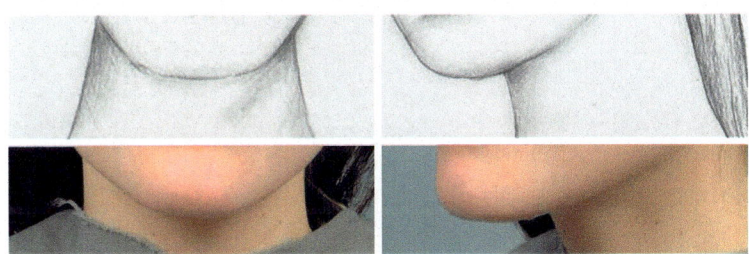

Fig. 4.14 Upper-neck region, class 0. Platysma bands and horizontal folds are absent

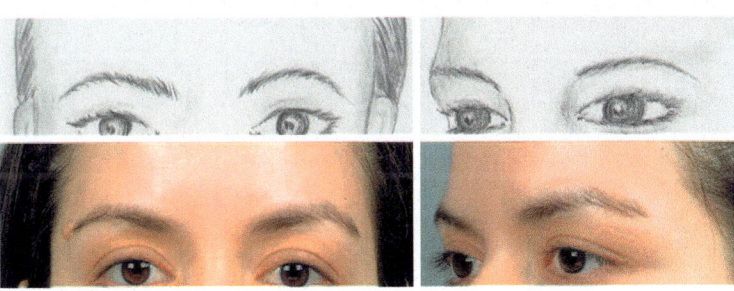

Fig. 4.15 Upper-face region, class 1. Eyelid fold is well defined (thick line)

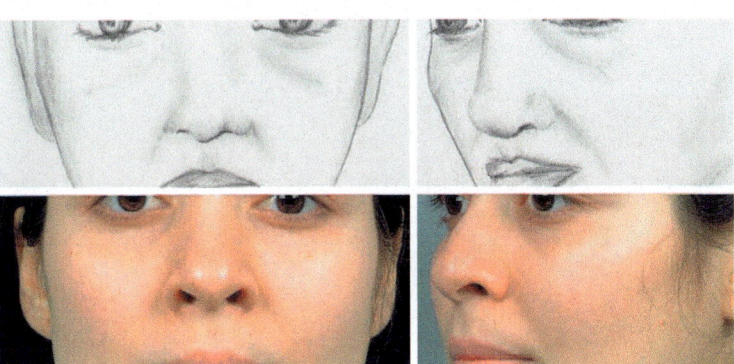

Fig. 4.16 Middle-face region, class 1. The central upper part of the cheekbone roundness is interrupted by an indentation and a melolabial fold is slightly noticeable

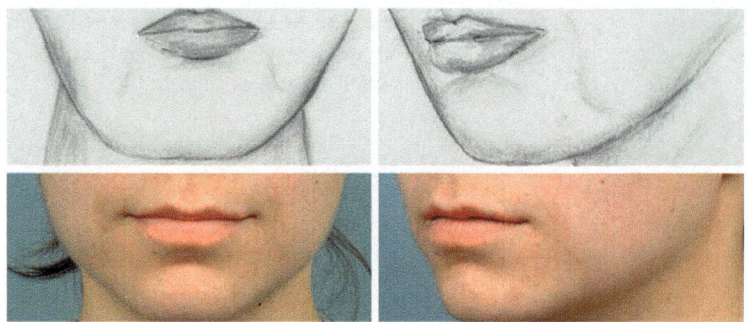

Fig. 4.17 Lower-face region, class 1. Jowls are slightly noticeable

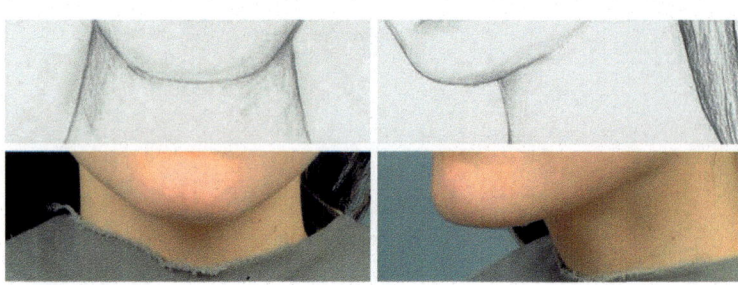

Fig. 4.18 Upper-neck region, class 1. Platysma bands and horizontal folds are absent

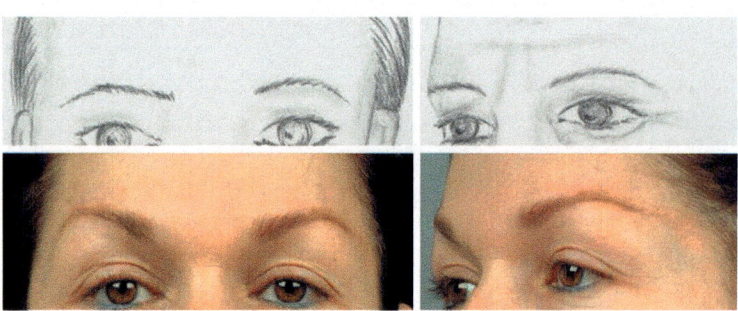

Fig. 4.19 Upper-face region, class 2. The eyelid is slightly folding

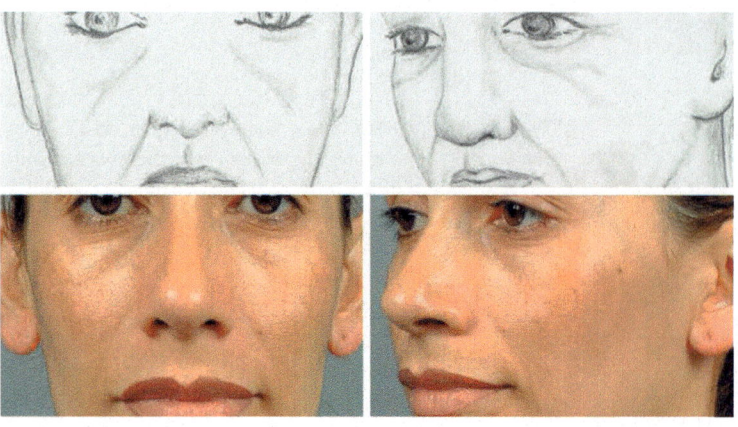

Fig. 4.20 Middle-face region, class 2. The nasojugal fold extends across the mid point of the cheekbone and the melolabial fold is defined

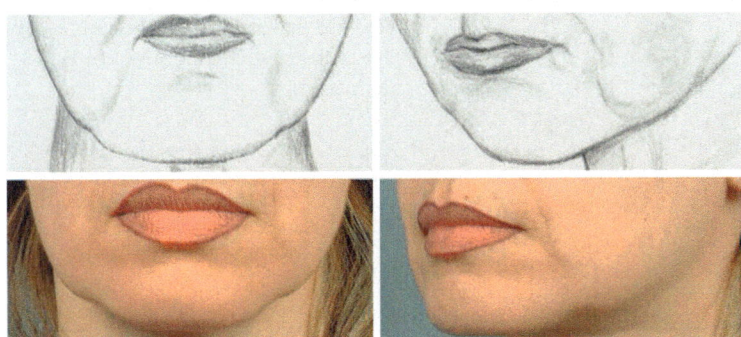

Fig. 4.21 Lower-face region, class 2. The jowls are protruding forward

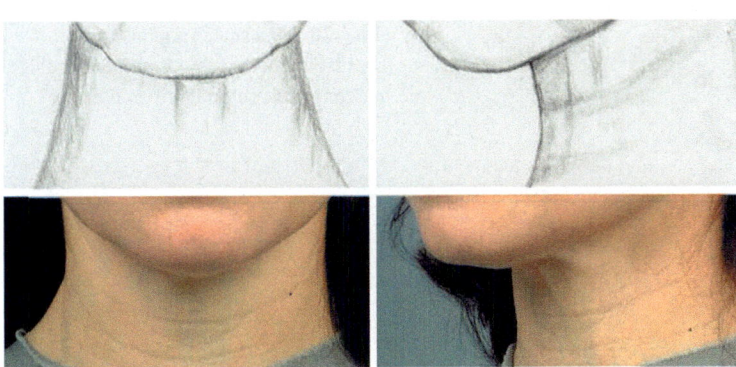

Fig. 4.22 Upper-neck region, class 2. The platysma bands are slightly noticeable and horizontal folds are absent

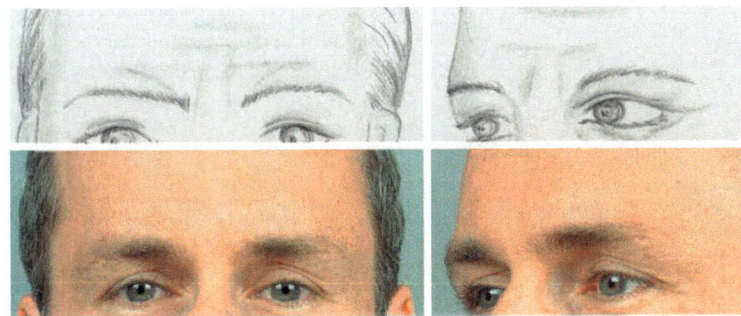

Fig. 4.23 Upper-face region, class 3. Eyelid folding without reaching the eyelashes

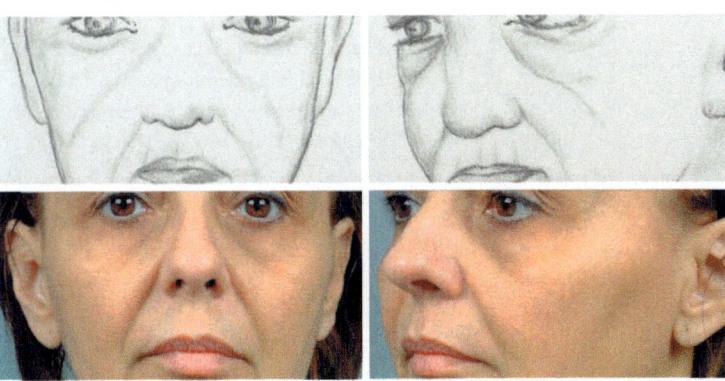

Fig. 4.24 Middle-face region, class 3. The nasojugal fold crosses the cheekbone and the melolabial fold is prominent

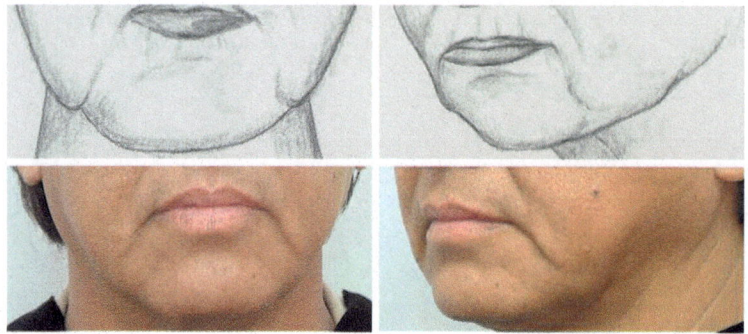

Fig. 4.25 Lower-face region, class 3. The jowls are protruding forward and downward

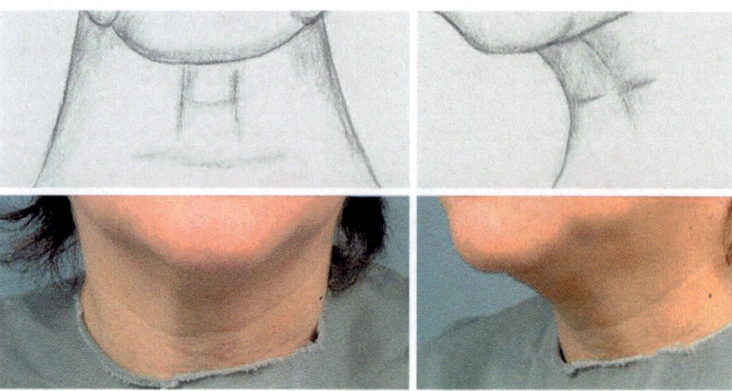

Fig. 4.26 Upper-neck region, class 3. The platysma bands are prominent and horizontal folds are slightly noticeable

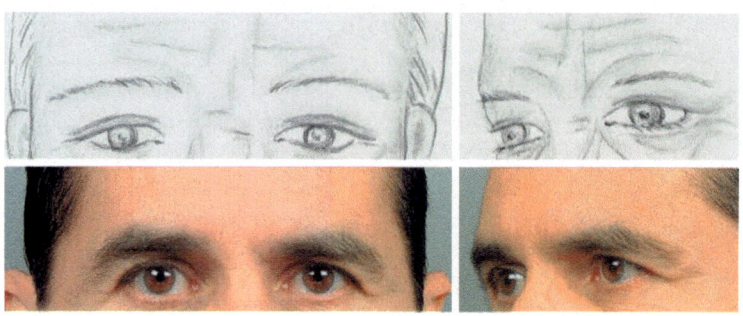

Fig. 4.27 Upper-face region, class 4. The eyelid is folding on the eyelashes

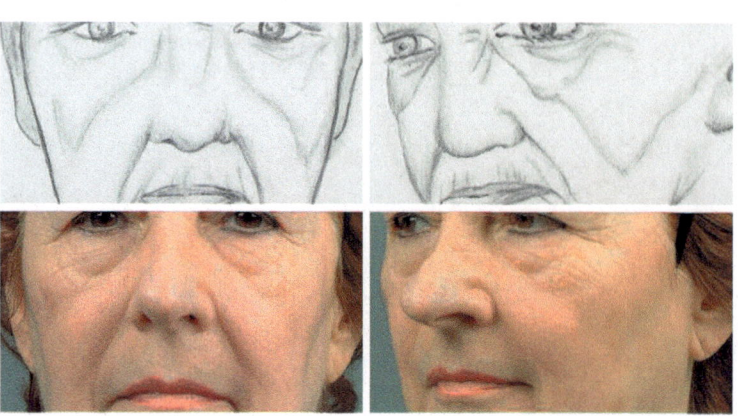

Fig. 4.28 Middle-face region, class 4. The nasojugal fold extends to form a flattened area and the melolabial fold forms a deeply marked crease

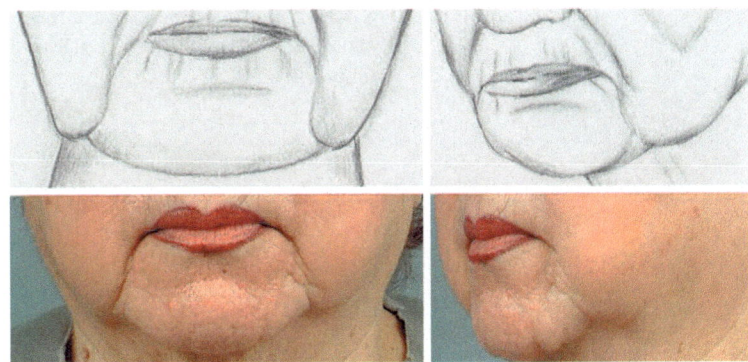

Fig. 4.29 Lower-face region, class 4. The jowls are protruding forward with downward sagging

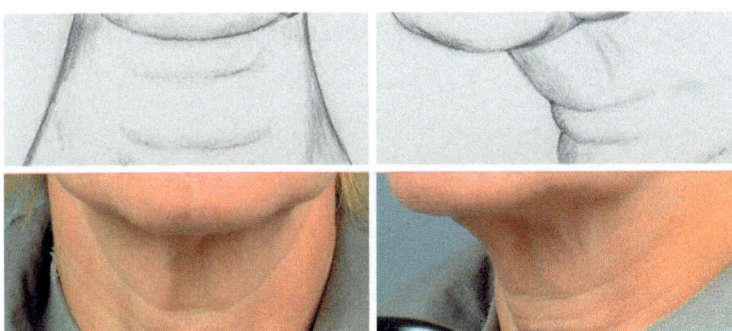

Fig. 4.30 Upper-neck region, class 4. The platysma bands are sagging and horizontal folds are prominent

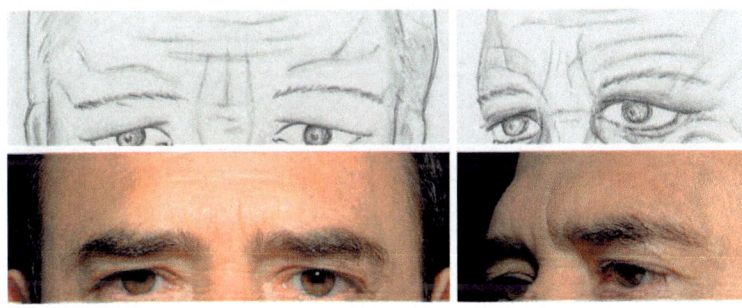

Fig. 4.31 Upper-face region, class 5. The eyelid fold interferes with the field of vision

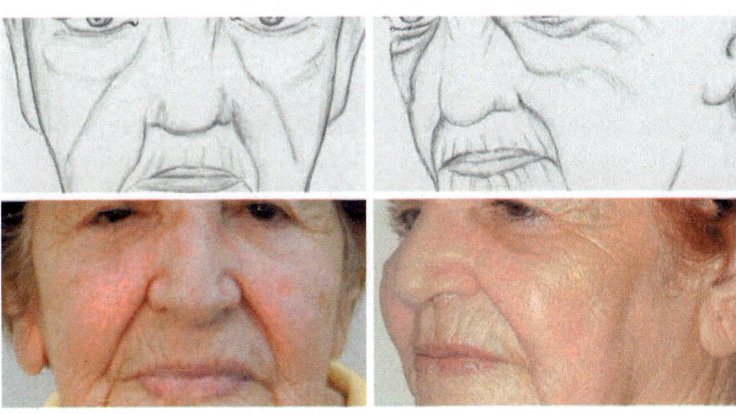

Fig. 4.32 Middle-face region, class 5. The completely flattened cheekbone stretches the lower eyelid downward and the line of melolabial fold is hidden by skin folding

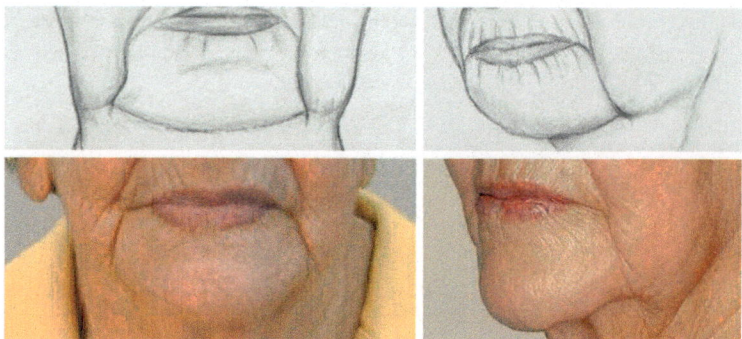

Fig. 4.33 Lower-face region, class 5. The jowls sag forward and there is lateral loss of definition in the neck

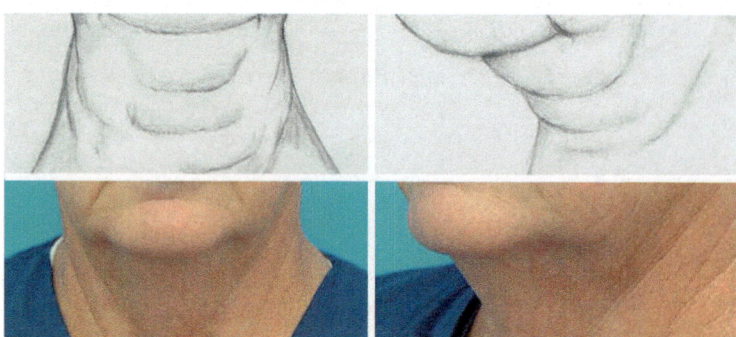

Fig. 4.34 Upper-neck Region, class 5. The platysma bands and horizontal folds are sagging to the point where bands or folds are no longer noticeable

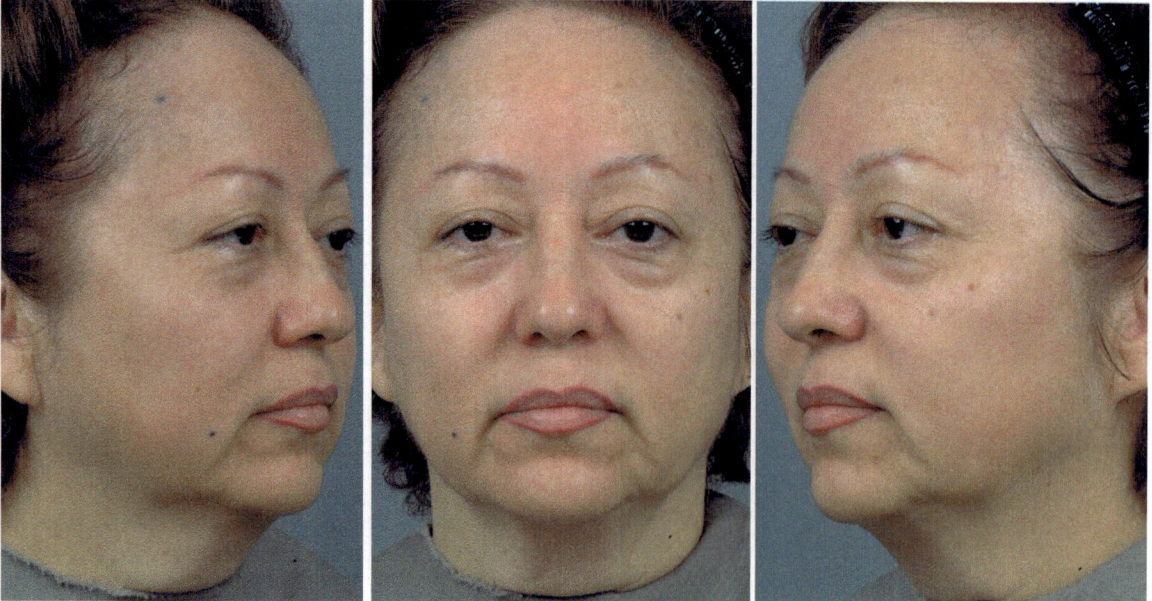

Fig. 4.35 Case 1

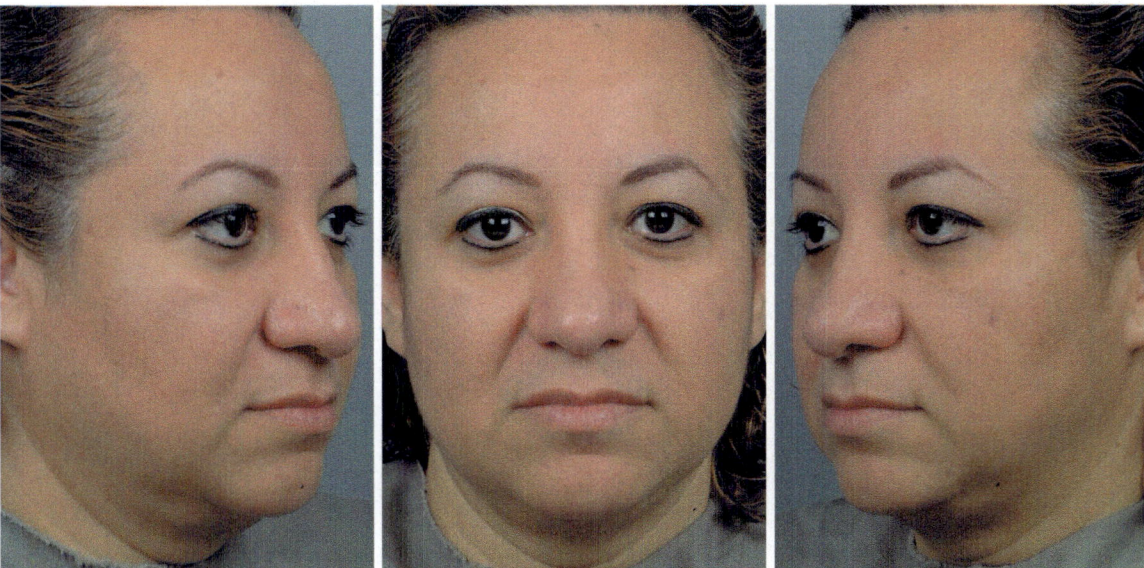

Fig. 4.36 Case 2

References

1. Diamond J.: Guns, Germs and Steel. The Fates of Human Societies. New York, Norton 1999

2. Bardinet T: Les Papyrus Medicaux del l'Egypte Pharonique. Paris, Fayard 1995

3. Matarasso SL, Brody H, Glogau RG: Chemical peels. In Atlas of Cutaneous Surgery, 1st Edition, Robinson, JK, Arndt KA, LeVoit PE et al. (Eds), Philadelphia, Saunders 1996:351–361

4. Tsuji T, Yorifuji T, Hayashi Y, Hamada T: Two types of wrinkles in aged persons. Arch Dermatol 1986;122(1):22–23

5. Lapiere C.M., Poerard GE: The mechanical forces a neglected factor in the age related changes of the skin. G Ital Chir Dermatol Oncol 1987;2:201–210

6. Fitzpatrick RE, Goldman MP, Satur NM, Tope WD: Pulsed carbon dioxide laser resurfacing of photoaged facial skin. Arch Dermatol 1996; 132(4):395–402

7. Obagi ZE: Obagi Skin Restoration and Rejuvenation. New York, Springer 2000

8. Donofrio LM, Augmentation with autologous fat. In: Soft Tissue Augmentation, Carruthers, J., Carruthers, A. (Eds), Philadelphia, Elsevier 2005:22

9. Alam M, DesJardin J, Arndt K, Dover JS, Hodapp RM, Baumann L, Brody HJ, Carruthers JB, Coleman EP 3rd, Garden JM, Geronemus RG, Glogau RG, Jacob CI, Katz BE, Klein AW, Krauss MC, Lawrence N, Moy RL, Narins RS, Sadick NS, Kaminer MS: A quality rating scale for aesthetic surgical procedures. J Am Acad Dermatol 2006;54(2):272–281

10. Tan SR, Glogau RG: Fillers esthetics. In: Soft Issue Augmentation, Carruthers J, Carruthers A (Eds), Philadelphia, Elsevier 2005:8

CHAPTER 5

Facial Aging: a Clinical Classification

5

Melvin A. Shiffman

5.1
Introduction

The purpose of this classification of facial aging is to have a simple clinical method to determine the severity of the aging process in the face. This allows a quick estimate as to the types of procedures that the patient would need to have the best results.

Procedures that are presently used for facial rejuvenation include laser, chemical peels, suture lifts, fillers, modified facelift, and full facelift. The physician is already using his or her best judgment to determine which procedure would be best for any particular patient. This classification may help to refine these decisions.

5.2
Clinical Classification

The classification utilizes four different areas of the face that are affected by the aging process (Table 5.1). The appearance of a tear-trough depression is one of the first manifestations of facial aging. This is followed by loss of cheek fat, prominence of the jowls, and then deepening of the various facial folds. The most prominent fold is the nasolabial fold, followed in time by the marionette lines.

The use of neck manifestations such as loose skin, platysmal bands, and transverse folds would be too variable since a heavy neck would hide these changes

and a thin neck would show the changes earlier. Rhytids (wrinkles) generally are a result of heredity, skin aging from sun damage, overuse of facial expression muscles, sleep pressure, and skin laxity. Laxity of eyelid skin and appearance of eyelid fat pads occur with aging, but the skin laxity may be associated with heredity and sun damage.

5.3
Use of the Classification

The first change of aging from stage 0 (no changes noted) to stage 1 is the appearance of a deepening in the tear trough and a very slight appearance of the nasolabial fold depth (Figs. 5.1, 5.2). This is followed by extension of the tear trough with slight loss of cheek fat medially, mild nasolabial fold deepening, and the appearance of the jowl prominence in stage 2 (Fig. 5.3). Stage 3 (Fig. 5.4) has a slightly more prominent tear-trough depth than stage 2, moderate loss of total cheek fat, moderate depth of the nasolabial fold, and mild to moderate prominence of the jowls. Stage 4 has severe changes in all of the areas being examined (Fig. 5.5). Not every patient presents with these changes at the same time or in the same order. The most prominent category of change is in the extent of the tear trough and loss of cheek fat. Classification should take this into account when deciding the type of procedure for any particular patient.

Table 5.1 Clinical classification of facial aging

Stage	Tear-trough depth	Cheek fat loss	Nasolabial fold depth	Jowl prominence
0	None	No loss	None	None
1	Slight: to cheek fat	No loss	Slight	None
2	Mild: into cheek fat	Slight loss medially	Mild	Slight
3	Moderate	Moderate	Moderate	Moderate
4	Severe	Severe	Severe	Severe

5.4
Treatment

Stage 0 ordinarily needs no treatment, whereas stage 1 would improve with a filler such as autologous fat to the tear trough. Stage 2 would be improved with fillers to the tear trough and cheeks, while suture lifts can be attempted to improve the jowl prominence (possibly with minimal liposuction) and nasolabial fold. Stage 3 would be treated with fillers in the defect areas, liposuction of the prominent jowls, as well as possibly a modified facelift if there were sufficient skin laxity. Stage 4 would benefit from fillers and possibly a full facelift.

As the skin gets more sun damage and more rhytids appear, consideration should be given to the use of chemical peels and laser. Suture lift of the neck for mild loose skin does not work very well. Neck lift surgery should be considered for moderate laxity of the neck skin.

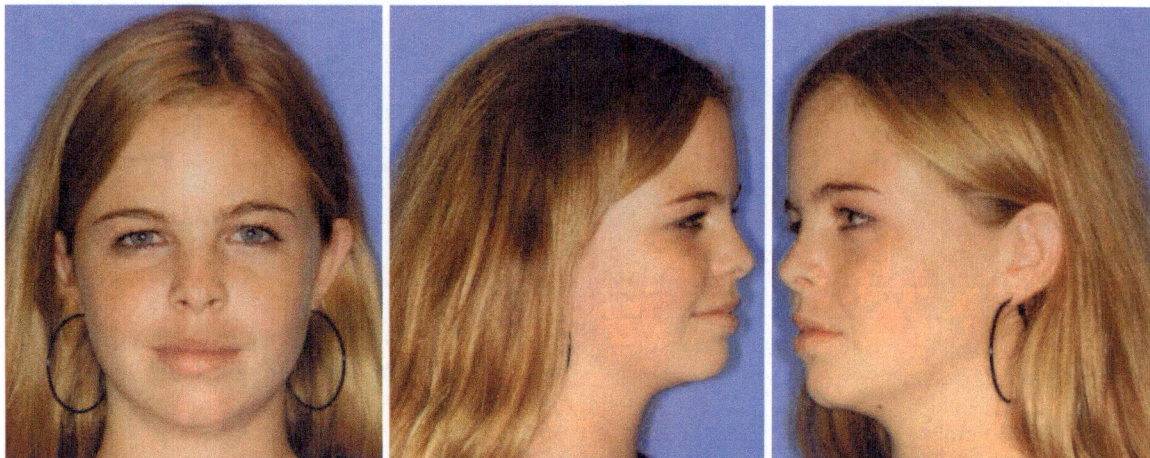

Fig. 5.1 Stage 0. No loss of fat in the cheeks or evidence of a nasolabial trough

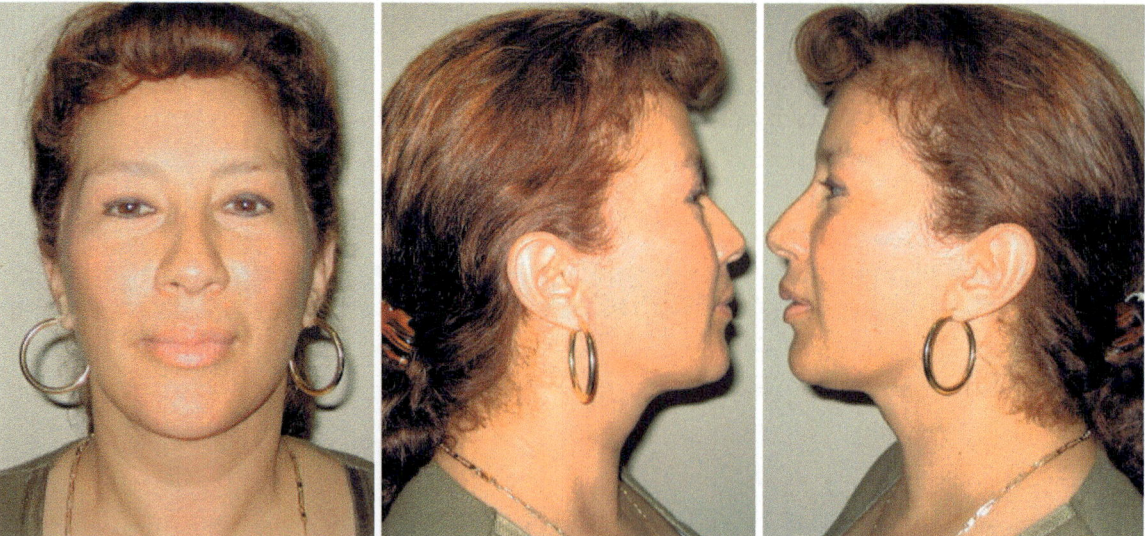

Fig. 5.2 Stage 1. No less of check fat but slight tear-trough depression

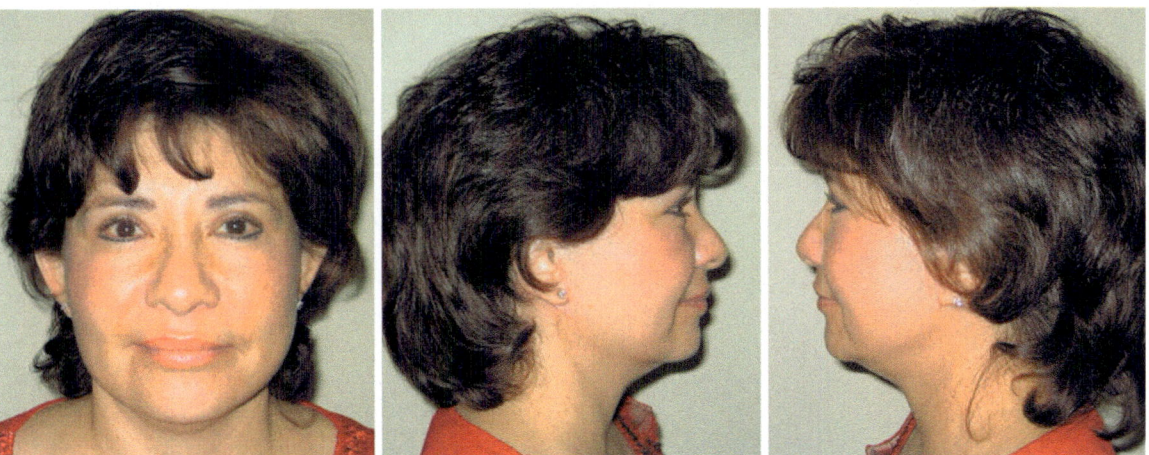

Fig. 5.3 Stage 2. Slight loss of cheek fat with mild tear-trough depression

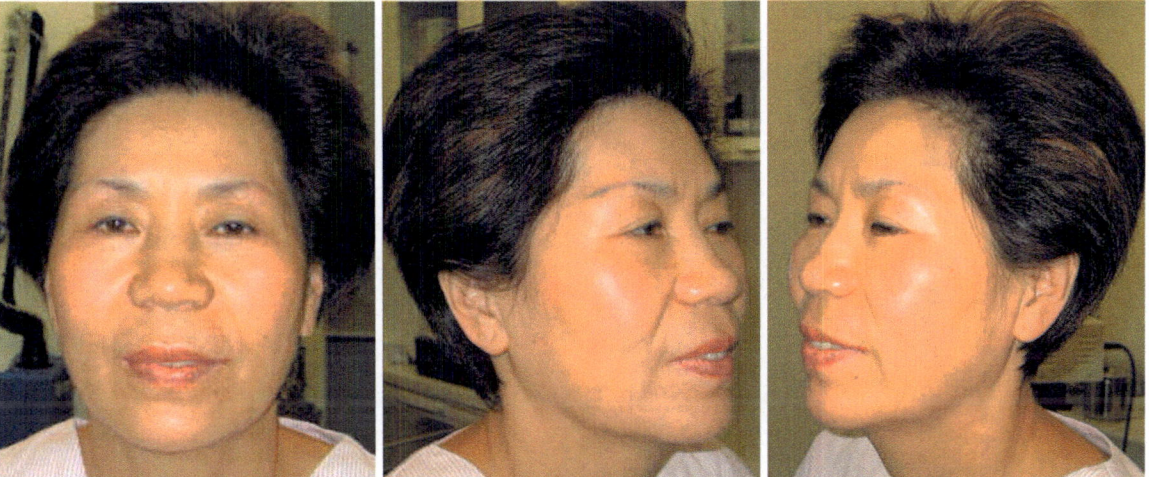

Fig. 5.4 Stage 3. Moderate loss of cheek fat with tear-trough depression into the cheek

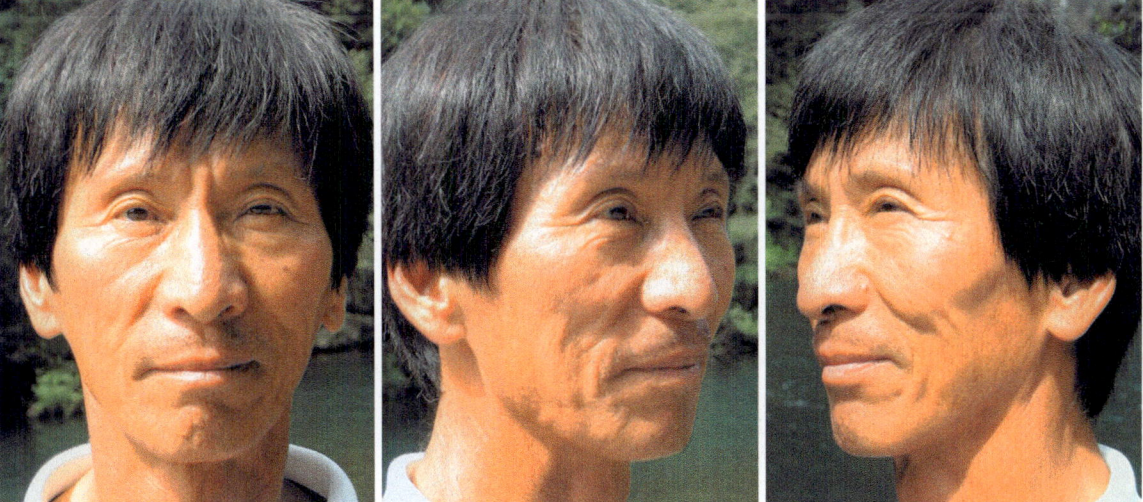

Fig. 5.5 Stage 4. Severe loss of cheek fat and tear trough extending into the cheek

CHAPTER 6

Facial Aging and its Mechanics

Ivo Pitanguy, Djenane Pamplona, Henrique N. Radwanski

6.1
Introduction

From prehistoric art to modern times, there has been clear evidence that humans have constantly attempted to improve and perpetuate physical beauty. Studies of the evolution of facial aesthetics over the centuries suggest that 35,000 years ago man possessed no less potential for facial attractiveness than today [1].

Aging has always been the greatest obstacle to eternal youthfulness, and mankind has had to content itself with myriad forms of camouflage and decoration of the body and face. A huge market has been created, offering different means to prolong signs of youth. These include biological methods (when the tissues lost owing to the aging process are replaced), beauty products, aesthetic surgery, and other newly discovered and promising rejuvenation strategies.

Although some cultures associate senescence with wisdom, most western cultures consider aging a sign of degeneration. In our modern society, the young face and athletic body are correlated with desirable traits, such as sexual vigor, power, wealth, and success. This can be attested by the ever-increasing number of men and women seeking rejuvenation procedures.

Since the original studies done by Leonardo da Vinci, generally accepted guidelines of facial aesthetics and measurements of proportions have been described, seeking to establish a well-defined concept of beauty [2].

When analyzing the external signs of the aging process, both the body and face suffer significant transformations, and the plastic surgeon should be familiar with the many processes involved. Facial aging affects anatomy and the body's physiology, and is characterized by visual changes in the skin and supporting tissues. Loss of the classic youthful contours occurs owing to factors such as atrophy of underlying tissues and thinning and loss of elasticity of the skin [3–5]. These alterations cause wrinkles, folds, and deepening furrows.

In simple biomechanical terms, the result is a gradually expanding outer envelope (i.e., the skin) that covers a progressively volumetrically decreased underlying tissue framework.

Mechanical factors, such as continuous muscle activity and gravity, accentuate the biology of aging. A theoretical model capable of studying the behavior of these variables in the face through time is fundamental for several reasons. These include finding ways to mechanically control the aging process, predicting the changes that may affect facial appearance, and improving face-lifting techniques. The final objective of this model is to supply surgeons with a quantitative tool capable of assessing aging parameters more accurately.

In this chapter, the authors analyze the mechanical processes of aging that occur specifically in the face. This has been the subject of a more extensive article, where mathematical equations were used to demonstrate the statistical findings of our research. We will here focus on the issues that are of more interest to the plastic surgeon.

An attempt is made to identify the physical signs of senescence, find the parameters that change throughout the years, and find ways to measure these alterations. Knowledge of the performance of some of the aging parameters, such as the upper lip and the ear lobe, in conjunction with a numerical model, designed as finite elements, can give helpful hints about the viscoelastic properties of tissues, including skin, muscles, and fat of the different regions of the face. Finally, designing a mathematical model that is capable of describing and predicting the behavior of these parameters over the years may prove to be useful for the surgeon to compare the facial aging process in both men and women.

6.2
The Aging Face

Careful analysis of the aging face reveals that much more than just wrinkling and/or skin flaccidity occur. Alterations in three-dimensional topography are responsible for the distinctive phenotypic presentations of the face throughout life [2]. Computer studies have attempted to model the aging face and its reconstruction. Although some qualitative criteria [3, 6] are available, quantitative information on the subject is still lacking. For example, Rowland and Perret [3] utilized composite images of different faces and manipulated factors such as shape and color (using computer graphics) to provide an empirical definition of the alterations that occur in the face. In 1999, Stack [7] summarized the latest digital and technological advances in facial plastic and reconstructive surgery.

In order to evaluate facial contour changes over time, Abramo and Oliveira [8] compared photographs taken before and 10 years after face-lifting procedures. The results demonstrated that neck contour after 10 years was similar to the presentation before the original procedure in a significant number of patients. One can conclude that 10 years is a reasonable time period after surgery to evaluate facial alterations due to aging.

Koury and Epker [9] outlined, in a very complete paper, the following specific features responsible for facial aging by discussing the basic anatomical units of the face: forehead, periorbital areas, cheek, nose, lips and perioral tissues, mandibular line, chin, and neck.

6.2.1
The Forehead

The youthful forehead possesses eyebrows that are positioned well above the superior orbital ridges, a softly curving ciliary arch that blends with the proximal tissues, and no wrinkles. Prominent signs of aging include horizontal and vertical forehead wrinkles and sagging of the eyebrows with loss of the youthful contour in the ciliary area. The horizontal forehead wrinkles begin as fine transverse lines resulting from contraction of the frontalis muscle. The vertical forehead wrinkles (or glabellar lines) occur owing to excessive corrugator muscle activity. With time, vertical forehead elongation occurs owing to hair loss and eyebrow descent (induced by factors such as gravity and winking). At first, lateral hooding of the eyes occurs; the eyebrows then descend as a unit to a position well below the superior orbital ridge, giving the face a tired or even angry look. The concomitant eyebrow thickening, which occurs particularly in men, accentuates this phenomenon.

6.2.2
Periorbital Areas

A youthful periorbital contour consists of a well-shaped and correctly positioned eyebrow, a well-defined upper-eyelid platform and supratarsal crease, and absence of excess fat pads, loose skin, and wrinkles in the upper and lower eyelids. Ptosis commonly accompanies these signs and lateral rhytids (i.e., crow's-feet) accentuate aging of the eyes during facial expression.

6.2.3
Cheeks

The youthful cheek consists of a well-defined prominence located approximately 10 mm lateral and 15 mm inferior to the lateral canthus. The overlying skin is smooth and a slight depression exists below the cheek and slightly above the nasolabial fold, separating it from the upper lip. The common signs of aging in this area are loss of the normally positioned cheek prominence and a skeleton-like hollow defect. The latter occurs in the temporal and buccal regions owing to the gravitational displacement of soft tissue and atrophy of skin, muscle, and fat. The skin may appear "sucked-in" around the bony prominences, which produces the gaunt, aged look.

6.2.4
The Nose

The appearance of the youthful nose varies among different ethnic groups and between men and women. However, a straight dorsum, a well-defined tip with good projection and rotation, a normal nasolabial angle (90–110°), and almond-shaped nostrils should be present. The principal changes that occur with aging are an increase in vertical length and a decrease in tip projection. The drooping tip is characteristic of the older patient. These conditions may exist even in young individuals, creating an illusion of advanced age.

6.2.5
Lips and Perioral Tissue

In young individuals, the perioral area has no wrinkles and minimal nasolabial folds; the interlabial line lies above the incisal line. Signs of aging include nasolabial fold prominence, fine vertical wrinkles, altered display of the teeth, and loss of exposed vermillion.

A line at the lip–cheek junction represents the junction of the lip skin, tightly bound to muscle, and the cheek skin, which is loosely bound to fat. With time, the nasolabial folds tend to span obliquely downwards.

The appearance of fine vertical rhytids around the mouth is greatly affected by exposure to ultraviolet light and tobacco smoking. Gravitational soft-tissue displacement alters the youthful display of teeth. Visibility of the upper teeth is decreased and the lower anterior teeth become more apparent. Particularly in the upper lip, the amount of exposed vermilion decreases. This occurs because thinning of the lip reduces the circumference of the edges and causes inward rotation of the vermillion.

6.2.6
The Mandibular Line

The mandible is important because it defines the face with a lower border, separating the neck into an independent aesthetic unit. A youthful contour is smooth and well-defined; an aged appearance is created by poor bony definition, accumulation of fat, and soft-tissue sagging may produce this effect. Loss of teeth may accentuate a poorly defined jaw line.

With aging, ptosis of elements such as the skin, superficial musculoaponeurotic system, muscles, and submandibular glands (as well as the accumulation of subcutaneous fat) may produce jowls. This deformity appears as a bulging mass of tissue that hangs lateral and inferior to the mandibular body.

6.2.7
The Chin

Viewed frontally in young individuals, the apex of the chin is normally located high above the mandibular line and fullness is provided by alveolar support. In profile, the chin should be well projected relative to the nose and lips and should blend smoothly with the neck. An aged appearance is produced by descent of the chin, lack of submental definition, and prominence of "marionette lines" that run from the nasolabial folds to underneath the mandible.

Sagging of the soft tissues and resorption of the alveolar ridge, in the inferior and posterior directions, create a "witch's" chin in the inferior and posterior directions (due to atrophy caused by the loss of teeth).

6.2.8
The Neck

A youthful neck is composed of a thin tissue lining over the underlying structures, a cervical-mental angle of 90°, and the absence of clinically visible accumulations of fat, sagging of soft tissues, and rhytids.

6.3
Aging Parameters

Face-lifting procedures can be enhanced with the knowledge of the facial aging parameters. When considering the aging process, each area of the face will change at different rates. For example, individuals who constantly smile may develop nasolabial wrinkles more rapidly. Also, the accumulation of cervical-facial fat in an overweight individual will result in loss of the youthful neck and mandibular contours. The upper eyelids may present fat pad bulging and excessive skin even in the young individual.

Changes in three-dimensional topography are responsible for the distinctive phenotypic presentations of the face throughout life [10]. Therefore, engineers and plastic surgeons have worked together to define ag-

ing patterns and this cooperation has resulted in the selection of characteristic anatomical points that may be observed and measured during the aging process.

A first study by the authors defined various aging parameters of the female face [11]. Here we will present the improvements of our technique by studying aging in male patients. Although trying to find general behavior patterns in facial aging is difficult because each face possesses individual characteristics (such as size and shape), the objective is to find a general model that can serve as a reference for patient analysis.

The aging parameters chosen to be measured and analyzed were:

1. Height of the forehead (only in women because many men have the genetic tendency to be bald)
2. Aging of the eyelids, which was measured from the eyebrow and folds
3. The height of the eyebrow
4. Palpebral pouch

In our original paper, facial modeling and the aging process were evaluated in women photographically. The mechanical alteration of the nasolabial fold as well as the height and width of the nose were analyzed.

6.4
Measurement of Aging Parameters

After defining the aging parameters, the second objective was to measure the behavior of these variables in people who were photographed throughout their lives. An attempt was made to find a pattern of change for each facial parameter in the same person after years of aging. Photographs of the person's face at a younger age were used as a reference for analysis.

All images had to be standardized. The photographs were scanned using a 600-dpi Hewlett-Packard scanner or taken with a digital camera, digitally processed, and rotated until the line that connects the center of the two pupils was horizontal. The photographs were then normalized in terms of size, with all linear measurements of each person divided by the horizontal distance between the pupils. (The images were enhanced and lines were drawn using Adobe® software.) Coordinates of the points in pixels were obtained using Microsoft Photo Editor® software according to the following procedure.

The two pupils (A and B) and their midpoint (C) were marked and the line AB was rotated (with the entire image) until it became a horizontal line. Vertical lines were drawn passing through points A, B, and C and through the external limiting points of the eyes and mouth. These lines define the points G, G′, H, H′, I, I′, J, J′ on the eyebrow and on the upper-eyelid fold; K, L on the palpebral pouch; O, P, Q, R, S, T, U on the contour of the face; and M, M′, N, N′ on the lips. The remaining points V^1, V^2, V^3 and X^1, X^2, X^3 were located

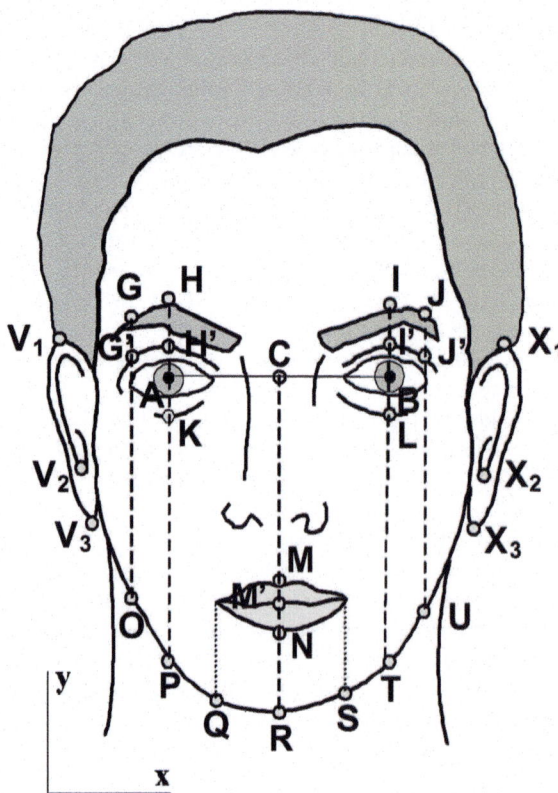

Fig. 6.1 Characteristic points defining the aging parameters

The 27 aging parameters studied were (Fig. 6.1):

- Eyebrows $(AG)_y$, $(AH)_y$, $(BI)_y$, $(BJ)_y$
- Eyelids $(AG')_y$, $(AH')_y$, $(BI')_y$, $(BJ')_y$
- Eyelid fat pads $(AK)_y$, $(BL)_y$
- Central midface tissues $(CR)_y$
- Height of the lips $(MN)_y$, $(MM')_y$, $(NN')_y$
- Length of the upper lip $(CM)_y$
- Lateral pouches of the midface $(AO)_y$, $(AP)_y$, $(AQ)_y$, $(BS)_y$ $(BT)_y$, $(BU)_y$
- Ears $(AV^1)_y$, $(V^1V^3)_y$, $(AV^3)_y$, $(BX^1)_y$ $(X^1X^3)_y$, $(BX^3)_y$

The research model can only be considered meaningful if a time-dependent general aging curve $U_k(t)$ is determined for each of the defined and measured parameters k.

A complete presentation of our mathematical findings can be found in our previous work [14, 15].

6.5
Materials and Methods

Our first work [14, 15] was conducted in a group of 40 women, photographed at two different ages (at least 5 years apart). Not every parameter could be measured in every person owing to the presence of earrings, hair over the forehead, or a slight smile on one of the photographs. Histogram results showed seven to ten measurements in every 5-year range of the selected interval (i.e., from 25 to 65 years of age). The reason for choosing this sample was the availability of frontal pattern photographs at different ages. The parameters for each person were measured at two different ages and a strong correlation was found between age and behavior of these variables.

on the left and right ears. The vertical distance between two points, $()_y$, defined the following 27 Cartesian linear measurements y^k. Each measurement done for each person i, at ages t_1 and t_2 defined the size of an aging parameter k.

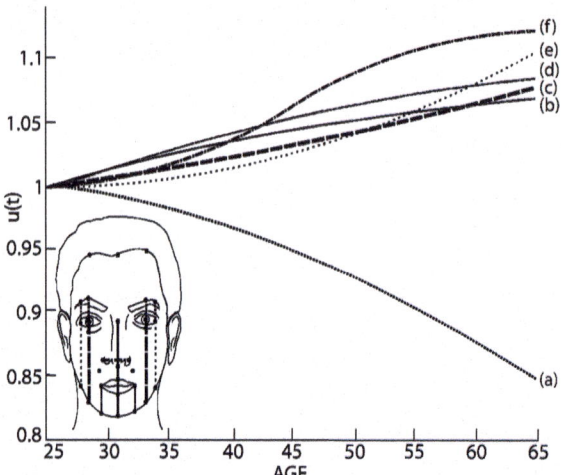

Fig. 6.2 General curves for *a* eyelids, *b* central pouch of the face, *c–e* lateral pouches of the face, and *f* width of the nose

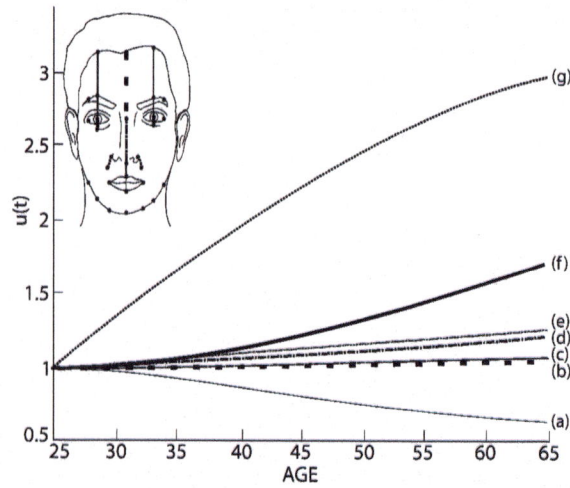

Fig. 6.3 General curves for *a* height of the lips, *b*, *c* central and lateral height of the forehead, *d* height of the nose, *e* height of the upper lip, *f* palpebral pouches, and *g* nasolabial fold

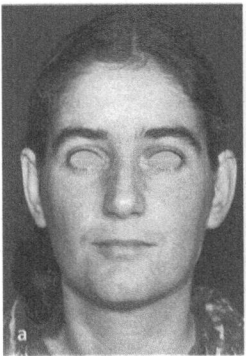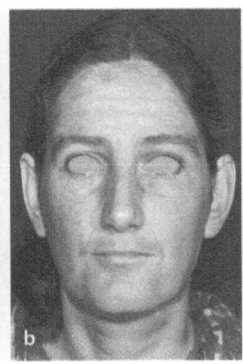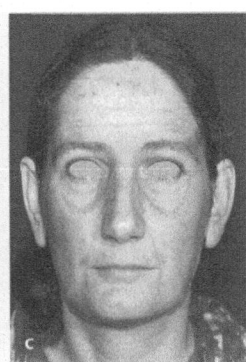

Fig. 6.4 Patient photographed at age 30 (**a**) and manipulated to ages 45 (**b**) and 65 (**c**)

6.6
Results in Women

The curves $U_k(t)$ in Figs. 6.2 and 6.3 represent the results of the method employed in our previous research in women. These curves, together with their respective mathematical equations, can be used to predict the magnitude of the aging parameters at certain ages.

From Figs. 6.2 and 6.3, it is interesting to observe that in women the vertical dimension of the lateral forehead increases more than the central region; the central and external areas of the eyelids behave in the same manner. Nose length increases significantly and almost linearly and the width of the nostrils changes slightly according to an S-shaped curve. The rate of increase in the length of the nasolabial fold decreases after 50 years of age. The height of the upper lip shows an astonishing increase, although its width narrows. Descent of the central and lateral pouches of the face demonstrates the action of gravity on the relatively loose facial tissues, resulting in loss of facial contour.

Computer simulations (Fig. 6.4) were carried out us-

ing Corel 5.0 software and grids containing coordinates of the calculated points at ages 45 and 65. The photograph of a patient at age 30 (Fig. 6.4a) was manipulated in each region so that the defined points would fit the new coordinates on the grid at ages 45 (Fig. 6.4b) and 65 (Fig. 6.4c).

6.7
Results in Men

Analysis of Fig. 6.5 showing the descent of the central and lateral pouches of the face indicates the action of gravity on relatively loose facial tissues, resulting in loss of facial contour. This is similar to the alterations observed in women. Tissue descent was most significant and almost linear in the area under the pupil (Fig. 6.5c) and the corner of the mouth (Fig. 6.5d). On the other hand, the central facial tissue (Fig. 6.5a) was the least affected. Peripheral tissues such as the external corner of the eye (Fig. 6.5b) showed intermediate results.

The mouth is an area in which the aging process is

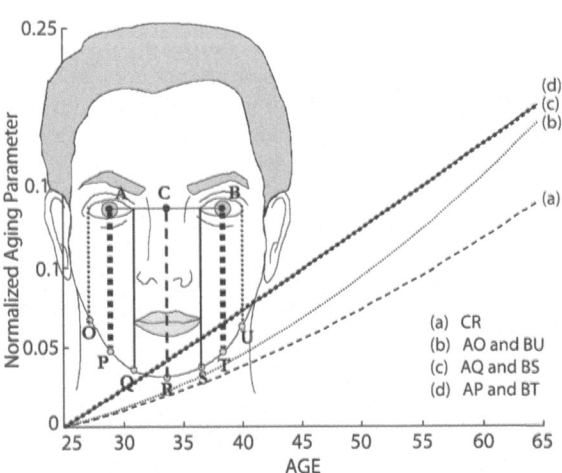
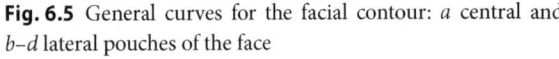

Fig. 6.5 General curves for the facial contour: *a* central and *b–d* lateral pouches of the face

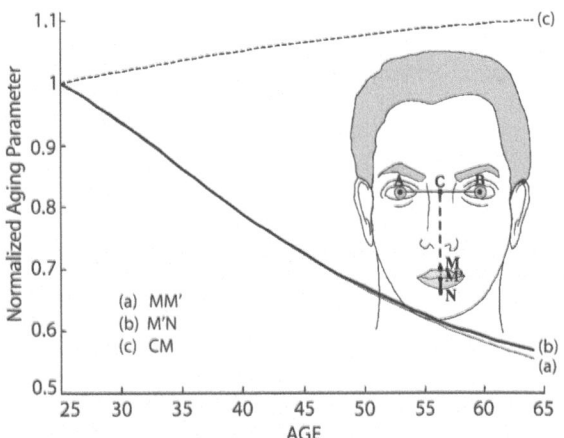

Fig. 6.6 General curves for height of the superior (*a*) and inferior (*b*) lips and for height of the upper lip (*c*)

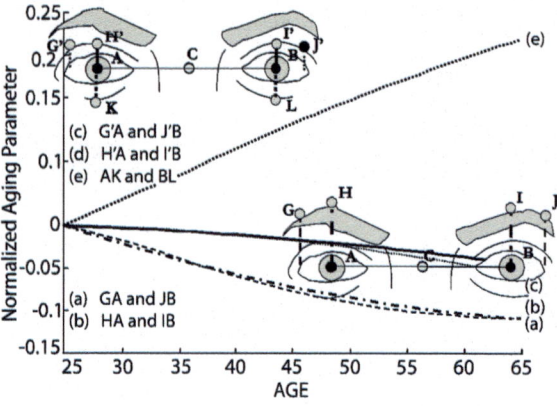

Fig. 6.7 General curves for external (a) and central (b) eyebrow, external (c) and central (d) eyelid fold, and fat pads (e)

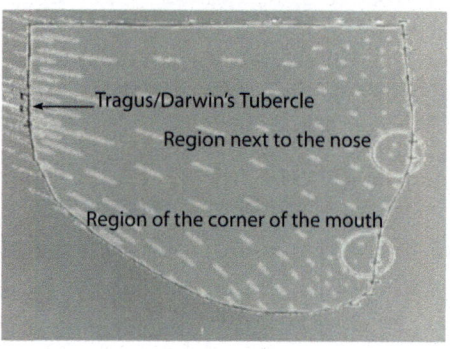

Fig. 6.8 Computer model shows the physical effects of traction following the vectors described in Sect. 6.8

especially noticeable. Alterations such as narrowing of the lip lines (Fig. 6.6) and an increase in the height of the upper lip (Fig. 6.6c) are characteristic as were also observed in women.

The appearance of the eyes throughout life is fundamental. Finer details such as brightness of the iris and whiteness of the conjunctiva could not be measured in the old photographs used in our study. The measurable factors are the ones chosen and depicted in Fig. 6.7. The central and external aspects of the fold between the eyelid and eyebrow (Fig. 6.7c, d) descended less than the eyebrow (Fig. 6.7a, b). The eyelid fold was not considered in our previous investigation in women. In some men this variable could not be considered owing to the growth of hair in the eyebrow. This is because thicker, bushy hair creates an illusion of descent and ascent of the lower and upper borders of the eyebrow, respectively. The eyelid fat pads (Fig. 6.7e) showed an astonishing increase with age.

6.8
The Round-Lifting Technique and Facial Aging

The surgical procedure known as the round-lifting technique was originally proposed by Pitanguy as the most efficient means to surgically correct the signs of facial aging.

The effects of the "round-lifting" technique have been studied by analyzing the mechanical forces applied and the displacements produced [14]. The method of finite elements was employed and, by means of computers, the relevant equations were defined. Human skin was modeled as a pseudoelastic, isotropic, non-compressible, and homogeneous membrane, and a computational study of the fields of displacement and the forces applied to the flaps during a rhytidoplasty demonstrated that the di-

rection of traction creates areas of tension that can be either negative or positive (Fig. 6.8). These forces ultimately result in the correction of signs of aging.

Interestingly, the vectors described in the round-lifting technique address both the main features that suffer distortion with aging as well as maintaining anatomical parameters. There were limits owing to the variety of factors involved because of the complexities of human skin (basic properties and individual variations) yet the study holds a close parallel to a real surgical procedure.

6.9
Discussion

Biological data are generally quite difficult to represent mathematically. This investigation attempted to describe the aging process of the face by assessing the behavior of various aging parameters over the years. In this way, it would be possible to predict a person's appearance in the future, with a known amount of error, by measuring and normalizing a present photograph of that same person. The study was successful in its purpose and a representative fraction of the patient's data behaved sufficiently similarly to each parameter's general aging curve. The scientifically supported computer graphic manipulation was performed with excellent results [14].

The project's main objective was to establish general curves by defining an increase (or decrease) in the aging parameters at a proportional or displaced rate of change. A strong correlation was found between age and the behavior of the parameters. The model's quantitative verification was performed by comparing the measured and predicted parameters.

Finally, comparison of the aging curves for some of the parameters in the investigations in men and women indicates a strong equivalence between the behavior of some parameters in both sexes. For example, lip length (or thickness) in both sexes decreased almost equivalently. On the other hand, some parameters did not have this equivalence. We observe that in men, eyelid fat pads increased twice as much as in women (Figs. 6.9, 6.10).

6.10
Conclusions

The expectations and demands in facial aesthetic surgery have grown with the evolution of surgical techniques. Treatment of the aging face should be individualized to each patient's structural characteristics. The objective of any surgical procedure should be to offer a harmonious result without distorting anatomical landmarks and causing undesirable surgical stigmas. It is the opinion of the senior author that the round-lifting technique, as originally described by him and which is extensively covered in Chap. 47, is the one that ensures maintenance of facial anatomy while optimally correcting the signs of aging.

Biological data are generally quite difficult to represent mathematically. This investigation attempted to describe the aging process of the face by assessing various aging parameters and their behavior over the years. The study was successful in its purpose and a representative fraction of the patient's data behaved sufficiently similarly to each parameter's general aging curve. The development of an automatic computer graphic manipulation (i.e., warping) system for the female face [15] has been an important spin-off of this study.

The identification of the mechanical forces involved in the process of facial aging is one of the main contributions of this study. A review of the literature reveals that a complete study in this field is still lacking. We consider that a better understanding of this process may lead to important improvements in the numerous currently employed treatment strategies. On the other hand, it might also be possible to predict a person's appearance in the future, with a known amount of error, by measuring and normalizing a present photograph of that same person. Finally, one might even imagine that, in understanding the mechanics of the aging process, sometime in the future, it may be possible to control this progressive and unavoidable process.

Acknowledgments

The authors thank Hilde Zemann for providing the data from the photographs that were used in the research in men, and for giving permission to print some of these photographs. We also thank Hans Ingo Weber, who co-authored a significant part of this project. Finally, we express our gratitude to the Brazilian National Council for Research (CNPq) for financially supporting this project.

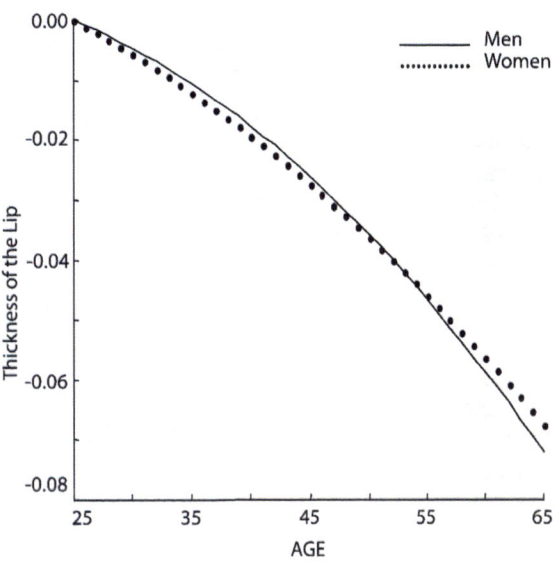

Fig. 6.9 Male and female general aging curves for the parameter "length of the lip"

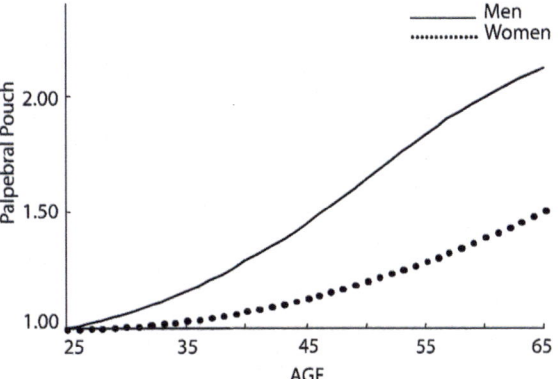

Fig. 6.10 Male and female general aging curves for the parameter "eyelid fat pads"

References

1. Peck H, Peck S: A concept of facial esthetics. Esthetics 1970;40(4):284–318
2. Nassif PS, Nowadays MSK: Aesthetic facial analysis. Facial Plast Surg 1999;7(1):1–15
3. Rowland DA, Perrett DI: Manipulating facial appearance through shape and color. IEEE Comput Graph Appl 1995:70–76
4. Erol OO: Facial autologous soft-tissue contouring by adjunction of tissues cocktail injection. Plast Reconstr Surg 2000;106(6):1375–1387
5. Guyuron B: Forehead rejuvenation. Ann Int Symp Rec Adv Plast Surg 1992;III(10):56–66
6. Leta F, Conci A, Pamplona D, Pitanguy I: A Model for Facial Aging. In: ISWC3D'97 International Workshop on Synthetic Natural Hybrid Coding and Three Dimensional Imaging, 1997, Rhodes City, Rhodes. International Symposium on Wearable Computers—3D 1997;1:204–207
7. Stack BC: Computer modeling. Update and applications on facial imaging, contouring and reconstruction. Facial Plast Surg 1999;7(1):115–124
8. Abramo AC, Oliveira VR: The lazy S shaped plication of the SMAS–platysma musculoaponeurotic system: A 10-year review. Aesthet Plast Surg 2000;24(6):433–439
9. Koury ME, Epker BN: The aged face: the facial manifestations of aging. Int J Adult Orthodont Orthog Surg 1991;6(2):81–95
10. Pellacani G, Seidenari S: Variations in facial skin thickness and echogenicity with site and age. Acta Dermatol Venereol 1999;79(5):366–369
11. Pitanguy I, Quintaes G, Cavalcanti M, Leite L: Anatomia do envelhecimento da face (Anatomy of facial aging). Rev Bras Cir 1977;67:79–84
12. Pitanguy I: Facial cosmetic surgery: A 30-year perspective. Plast Reconstr Surg 2000;105(4):1517–1529
13. Pitanguy I: The face. In: Pitanguy I (Ed), Aesthetic Surgery of Head and Body. Berlin, Springer 1984:165–200
14. Pitanguy I, Pamplona DC, Giuntini ME, Salgado F, Radwanski HN: Computational simulation of rhytidectomy by the "round-lifting" technique. Rev Bras Cir 1995;85:213–218
15. Pitanguy I, Pamplona D, Weber HI: Defining and measuring aging parameters. Appl Math Comp 1996;78:217–227
16. Pitanguy I, Pamplona D, Weber H, Leta F, Salgado F, Radwanski H: Numerical modeling of facial aging. Plast Reconstr Surg 1998;102:200–204.

Part III
Dermatologic

CHAPTER 7

Peptides for Facial Skin Aging

Mary P. Lupo

7.1
Introduction

Proteins have been an important category in cosmetics since the inception of the beauty product industry. Cosmetics were originally designed and categorized as formulations that temporarily enhance the appearance of the skin, hair, or nails. In contrast to drugs, which are strictly tested, controlled, and distributed, cosmetics are meant to adorn rather than alter biological structure or function of the skin. Kligman suggested a hybrid category to better classify formulations that have not been tested as drugs, but clearly exhibit clinical effects beyond that of mere skin hydration or temporary adornment. The resulting cosmeceutical industry has grown at an astonishing rate.

Protein peptide fragments, as cosmeceutical formulation ingredients, have become one of the most popular in the recent marketplace. Cosmeceutical proteins have evolved from the large molecular weight hydrolyzed proteins such as collagen in moisturizers and keratin in hair-repair formulas to the smaller oligopeptide chains of amino acids that may function in skin repair. Proteins of old were mere humectants in moisturizers; large molecules that would soften the stratum corneum and epidermal skin layer. In addition to use as skin moisturizers, proteins are also added to hair conditioners. The hair shaft's cuticle layer becomes fractured and raised from normal wear and tear, as well as chemical treatments and certain grooming practices. Hydrolyzed proteins such as keratin can be applied and absorbed through the damaged cuticle to restore tensile strength as well as cationically bind anions on the hair shaft that give damaged hair its dull and frizzy appearance.

Quite commonly, the appearance of an ingredient in a cosmeceutical formula is preceded by the intake of that, or a similar ingredient, in oral supplements. Amino acid extracts have been reported to increase collagen deposition. Amino acids are the building blocks of peptides. A recent published study on healthy individuals over the age of 70 demonstrated significant results after oral intake of amino acids such as arginine and leucine [1]. These data may translate into a safe nutritional supplement to enhance wound healing, and add further credence to incorporation of peptides into cosmeceuticals.

Short-chain amino acid sequences form these peptides that are the new, popular ingredient in antiaging skin cosmeceuticals. Peptides are used by cells to trigger cellular actions. Cosmeceutical peptides are theorized to mimic these actions. The main benefit is, as with oral supplementation with amino acids, collagen stimulation. Other cosmeceutical peptides act as carriers for copper, an important cofactor in wound healing. A third category is the neurotransmitter-inhibiting peptides.

7.2
"Signal" Peptides

Short chains of amino acids have been studied that may trigger the production of large proteins in the dermis of the skin. There has been a good deal of basic science research in the response of dermal fibroblasts to skin injury. After injury, dermal proteins are damaged and healing reactions of the skin result in skin repair. Cosmeceutical peptides are the result of in vitro studies of wound healing and growth stimulation of human skin fibroblasts. Elastin-derived peptides have been described that stimulate human dermal fibroblast proliferation [2]. Peptides have also been identified that have effects that potentially decrease collagen breakdown [3]. The six-chain hexapeptide valine–glycine–valine–alanine–proline–glycine stimulates human fibroblasts while downregulating elastin expression [4]. Peptide sequences can result in a feedback stimulation of dermal fibroblasts in vitro. This feedback or "signal" to repair could be used in a cosmeceutical formula to stimulate new collagen production in photodamaged skin. One specific peptide sequence, lysine–therine–therine–lysine–serine (KTTPS), is found on type I collagen. It has been found to stimulate production of extracellular matrix proteins such as collagen and glycosaminoglycans [5]. In topical formulas, the peptide must be linked to a lipophilic tail to enhance penetration. This pentapeptide sequence, KTTPS–palmitic acid, has been clinically tested and found to improve the appearance of aging skin [6]. Other proprietary palmitoyl dipeptide and oligopeptide complexes are also very popular in the cosmeceutical armamentarium. All of these products claim to improve skin appearance by stimulating new collagen production.

7.3
Carrier Peptides

The stimulation of collagen production and other important healing mechanisms are also achieved by other factors. Copper is an important trace element that has been found to be important in wound healing and enzymatic processes. There are several mechanisms whereby copper may have beneficial effects in the skin. Lysyl oxidase is an important enzyme in collagen and elastin production. It is dependant upon the action of copper. Tyrosinase and cytochrome c oxidase require copper as well. The detrimental effects of free radicals on the skin have been elucidated in basic science research into skin photoaging. Superoxide dismutase acts as an important antioxidant and requires copper as a cofactor.

The tripeptide complex glycyl–l–histidyl–l–lysine (GHK) spontaneously complexes with copper and facilitates the uptake of copper by cells [7]. This peptide sequence is found in proteins of the extracellular matrix such as the α chain of collagen, and it is believed to be released during wounding and inflammation. A feedback stimulation of collagen repair has also been proposed for this peptide [8], but the main benefit to photoaged skin is believed to be the enhanced delivery of copper. Both the tripeptide alone as well as the copper–tripeptide complex have been found to have beneficial effects on collagen stimulation. This carrier peptide–copper combination has also been found to increase levels of MMP-2 and MMP-2 messenger RNA, as well as tissue inhibitors of metalloproteinase (TIMP) 1 and 2. As such, it could function in collagen remodeling [9]. Experiments using GHK–Cu have demonstrated stimulation of both type I collagen and the glycosaminoglycans dermatan sulfate and chondroitin sulfate in rat wounds as well as cultured rat fibroblasts [10]. Human fibroblast cultures showed increased synthesis of dermatan sulfate and heparin sulfate after addition of the GHK–Cu complex [11]. Limited clinical trials with patients using a facial cosmeceutical product containing the complex as the active ingredient demonstrated an improvement in the appearance of fine lines as well as an increase in skin density and thickness [12].

7.4
Neurotransmitter-Inhibiting Peptides

Clinical benefit from peptides may also occur because of other cellular actions. A very popular peptide is a hexapeptide sequence known as argireline. It is a sequence of acetyl–glutamyl–glutamyl–methyoxyl–glutaminyl–ar-

ginyl–arginyl–arginylamide and its action is inhibition of lines from facial muscle movement. Argireline interferes in vitro with the formation or stabilization of the protein complex in the muscle cell that is responsible for calcium-dependent exocytosis [13]. The clinical effect of this peptide could be the result of elevation of the minimum threshold for muscle movement, relaxing the action of the muscle over time and smoothing movement-induced wrinkling. Other peptide sequences have been engineered that mimic the peptide fragment that binds proteins of the exocytic complex and inhibit secretory vesicle docking [14, 15]. If a cosmeceutical peptide of this class is added to a cosmeceutical formula that penetrates to the level of the targeted muscle, clinical reduction of visible lines may result.

7.5
How to Incorporate Peptides in a Facial Anti-skin-aging Protocol

Practicing dermatologists, as well as their patients, may be confused as to the real benefit of peptide cosmeceuticals and if and when to utilize them. The clinical benefit of improved skin hydration and resulting clinical improvement of the skin's appearance can be very important. Remember the original benefit of proteins was indeed moisturization. In my practice, I use these products in a complementary manner to retinoids, which, though proven to improve photoaged skin by the United States Food and Drug Administration, often cause dryness and irritation. When compliance with retinoids is improved, clinical results improve. In a comprehensive skin care program for photoaged skin, the daily use of sunscreens in the daytime and retinoids at night is the gold standard. The addition of cosmeceuticals such as peptides may speed visible results by enhancing collagen production, relaxing mimetic wrinkling, by improving hydration and barrier function, or by a combination of these benefits. Unless intolerance to retinoids exists, cosmeceuticals should never be used instead of retinoids, but rather in addition to them. Peptides are just one option. Antioxidants, α-hydroxy acids, growth factors, and bleaching agents are other possible options. These cosmeceuticals can be used in daytime in addition to sunscreens, alternated with retinoids at night, or in addition to the retinoids in the evening. Often the only way to assess individual response is by trial and error, since the only real goal of any cosmeceutical is to improve the appearance of aging skin.

7.6
Conclusions

Peptides in cosmeceuticals are one of the new, popular options to treat aging skin. Most studies used to justify the incorporation of these ingredients into skin care products have been in vitro. As dermatologists well know, these results do not always translate into in vivo actions. For any active ingredient to work, it must be absorbed in a stable form into the viable dermis. It is not an easy task to penetrate the barrier of the skin. Double-blinded, placebo-controlled drug study data are lacking, as it is with all cosmeceuticals owing to regulatory concerns by industry. There are, however, soft clinical data and anecdotal evidence to suggest that they are beneficial, and may have a place in a comprehensive skin care protocol for aging skin.

References

1. Williams JZ, Abumrad N, Barbul A: Effect of a specialized amino acid mixture on human collagen deposition. Ann Surg 2002;236:369–375

2. Kamoun A, Landeau JM, Godeau G, Wallach J, Duchesnay A: Growth stimulation of human skin fibroblasts by elastin-derived peptides. Cell Adhes Commun 1995;3(4):273–281

3. Njieha FK, Morikava T, Tuderman L, Prockop DJ: Partial purification of a procollagen C-protenase. Inhibition by synthetic peptides and sequential cleavage of type I procollagen. Biochemistry 1982;21:757–764

4. Tajima S, Wachi H, Uemura Y, Okamoto K: Modulation by elastin peptide VGVAPG of cell proliferation and elastin expression in human skin fibroblasts. Arch Dermatol Res 1997;289:489–492

5. Katayama K, Armendariz-Borunda J, Raghow R, Kang AH, Seyer JM: A pentapeptide from type I collagen promotes extracellular matrix production. J Biol Chem 1993;268(14):9941–9944

6. Lintner K: Promoting production in the extracellular matrix without compromising barrier. Cutis 2002(Suppl);70(6S):13–16

7. Pickart L, Freedman JH, Loker WJ, Peisach J, Perkins CM, Stenkamp RE, Weinstein B: Growth-modulating plasma tripeptide may function by facilitating copper uptake into cells. Nature 1980;288(5792):715–717

8. Maquart FX, Pickart L, Laurent M, Gillery P, Monboisse JC, Borel JP: Stimulation of collagen synthesis in fibroblast cultures by the tripeptide complex glycyl-L-histidyl-L-lysine-Cu²+. FEBS Lett 1988;238(2):343–346

9. Simeon A, Emonard H, Hornebeck W, Maquart FX: The tripeptide-copper complex glycyl-L-histidyl-L-lysine-Cu²+ stimulates matrix metalloproteinase-II expression by fibroblast cultures. Life Sci 2000;67(18):2257–65

10. Simeon A, Wegrowski Y, Bontemps J, Maquart FX: Expression of glycosaminoglycan and small Proteoglycans in wounds: modulation by the tripeptide-copper complex glycyl-L-histidyl-L-lysine-Cu²+. J Invest Dermatol 2000;115(6):962–968

11. Wegrowski Y, Maquart FX, Borel JP: Stimulation of sulfated glycosaminoglycan synthesis by the tripeptide-copper complex glycyl-L-histidyl-L-lysine-Cu²+. Life Sci 1992;51:1049–1056

12. Leyden JJ: Skin care benefits of copper peptide containing facial cream. Presented at the American Academy of Dermatology 60th Annual Meeting; New Orleans, February

13. Blanes-Mira C, Merino JM, Valera E, Fernandez-Ballester G, Gutierrez LM, Viniegra S, Perez-Paya E, Ferrer-Monteil A: Small peptides patterned after the SNARE complex assembly and regulated exocytosis. J Neurochem 2004;88(1):124–135

14. Gutierrez LM, Cannes JM, Ferrer-Monteil AV, Reig JA, Montal M, Viniegra S: A peptide that mimics the carboxyl-terminal domain of SNAP-25 blocks Ca²+-dependant exocytosis in chromaffin cells. FEBS Lett 1995;372(1):39–43

15. Gutierrez LM, Viniegra S, Rueda J, Ferrer-Monteil AV, Canaves JM, Montal M: A peptide that mimics the C-terminal sequence of SNAP-25 inhibits secretory vesicle docking in chromaffin cells. J Biol Chem 1997;272(5):2634–2639

Treatment of Hyperpigmented Photodamaged Skin

8

Zoe Diana Draelos

8.1
Introduction

Photodamaged skin is one of the most common problems addressed by the dermatologist. It can be simplistically characterized by the visual changes of dyspigmentation, fine wrinkles, and tactile roughness [1, 2]. The hyperpigmentation aspect of photodamage is probably one of the most disconcerting to patients as healthy skin is perceived to be even-colored. The discoloration results from stimulation of the melanocytes by UV-A radiation that causes excess pigment production. While the pigment produced by the skin is photoprotective, the inability of the melanocytes to evenly generate melanin causes localized pigmented spots, known as lentigenes, and a reticulated dyspigmentation, known as melasma. This chapter will focus on the topical treatments available for hyperpigmented photodamaged skin.

The most effective topical agent for treating hyperpigmentation is hydroquinone. Hydroquinone, a phenolic compound chemically known as 1,4-dihydroxybenzene, functions by inhibiting the enzymatic oxidation of tyrosine and phenol oxidases, which suppresses melanocyte pigment production; thus, hydroquinone induces gradual lightening of the dyspigmentation through decreased melanocyte pigment production, but does nothing for photodamage. As a matter of fact, hydroquinone is an unstable radical that may indeed perpetuate the inflammation of photodamage if used alone; thus, it might seem prudent to combine hydroquinone with other agents to assist in the treatment of photodamage.

One group of substances that could be utilized in combination with hydroquinone are the retinoids. The use of prescription tretinoin (all-*trans*-retinoic acid) for repairing photodamaged skin and improving dyspigmentation was first elaborated in the latter half of the 1980s [3, 4]; however, more recently the use of topical forms of naturally occurring over-the-counter (OTC) vitamin A in skin care products has been popularized. Vitamin A can perform several different functions when topically applied. It is a known humectant, meaning that it can attract water from the dermis and viable epidermis to the stratum corneum. This aids in skin hydration when the humectant vitamin A is combined with an occlusive agent, such as petrolatum or mineral oil, to prevent water evaporation. OTC forms of vitamin A, such as retinol, can function as topical antioxidants, enhancing functioning of the skin. Retinol can be converted to retinoic acid, also known as tretinoin, in the dermis, which is responsible for the biologic activity of OTC retinoid forms [5].

Retinoids are some of the most important cosmeceuticals for purposes of decreasing and reversing the signs of cutaneous aging [6–9]. The initial effect observed following the first few weeks of topical treatment with tretinoin is improvement in tactile smoothness. This is felt to be due to a stratum corneum with a more compact pattern with increased epidermal thickness due to spongiosis [10]. Increased hyaluronic acid is also produced, allowing the water-holding capacity of the skin to increase, also contributing to the early improvement in skin smoothness [11]. Thickening also occurs in the epidermal granular cell layer [12]. The effects of topically applied tretinoin following 4 months of use are improvement in fine wrinkles, representing a dermal effect. This improvement is due to an increase in collagen production [13]. Furthermore, it has been demonstrated that tretinoin decreases UV-B-induced collagenase activity, thus preventing photoaging [14]. Side effects are consistent with hypervitaminosis A of the skin and include mild skin irritation, such as erythema, peeling, and burning [15].

Topically applied tretinoin also appears to have an effect on skin pigmentation as seen by a decrease in cutaneous freckling and lentigenes [16]. It is the irregular grouping and activation of melanocytes that accounts for the dyspigmentation associated with photoaging [17], but normalization of this change has been histologically demonstrated through the use of retinoids [18]. While this effect is more dramatic with topically applied tretinoin, topically applied retinol has been thought to provide similar effects as a cosmeceutical.

While a 0.05% tretinoin emollient cream was approved for the treatment of photodamaged skin in the mid-1990s and has been used successfully since that time [19], it can cause a number of irritant responses, including erythema, dryness, and/or scaling, in some patients depending on the skin type and age of the patient [20–22]. Recent studies have demonstrated that retinol induces changes in the skin similar to those produced by tretinoin but without the irritation caused by retinoic acid [23]. Retinol has been shown to convert to retinoic acid in a two-step oxidation process in the skin. Although retinol has a lower potency than retinoic acid and requires tenfold higher concentrations to produce similar epidermal effects, it can be effective in improving the appearance of photodamage [24]. The main challenge to retinol formulations has been the successful development of high-concentration stabilized formulas.

Thus, one technique for improving the appearance of hyperpigmented photodamaged skin is the combination use of hydroquinone and retinoids, either prescription or OTC varieties, to optimize the efficacy of both actives. This technique and the results of a study demonstrating its utility are discussed next.

8.2
Technique

In order to study the effect of retinoids alone and in combination with hydroquinone, a study was performed comparing the efficacy and tolerance of a topically applied 4% hydroquinone plus high-concentration stabilized 0.3% retinol cream compared with those of topically applied 0.05% tretinoin emollient cream over a 16-week period in the treatment of hyperpigmentation, fine lines, and tactile roughness associated with photodamage. Subjects were instructed to apply a green-pea-sized amount of their assigned study product to create a thin layer over the entire face, since excess product application might cause undue irritation. Because some irritation during the first weeks of usage is common with both of the research medications, the study was designed as a step-up usage trial. For the first 2 weeks of the study, subjects used their test medication at half the usual recommended dose. Beginning with week 3, usage was increased to the recommended dose for each of the test agents.

Subjects in the 4% hydroquinone/0.3% retinol cream group were instructed to apply their medication once daily in the evening for the first 2 weeks. Beginning with week 3, usage was increased to twice daily application, morning and evening. Subjects in the 0.05% tretinoin emollient cream group applied their medication every other evening for the first 2 weeks and then every evening until the completion of the study. Subjects were instructed to wash their face morning and evening with a foaming face wash followed by application of a broad-spectrum zinc oxide containing SPF 15 facial moisturizer to prevent further UV-A pigmentation and to minimize retinoid-induced photosensitivity.

To evaluate the 4% hydroquinone/0.3% retinol cream versus the 0.05% tretinoin emollient cream 44 nonpregnant, non-lactating Caucasian (38 subjects), Asian (two subjects), and Hispanic women (four subjects), between 30 and 50 years of age, in good general health, with Fitzpatrick skin color classifications of types I–IV,

modified Glogau classification of I or II, and mild to moderate fine lines in the periocular area were followed for 16 weeks. The subjects demonstrated baseline pigmentation with a score of 5 or greater on a 10-point visual analog scale with 0 indicating no dyspigmentation, 5 indicating moderate dyspigmentation, and 10 indicating severe dyspigmentation. The subject panel was constructed to mimic the diversity of pigmentation disorders present in photoaged skin. Systemic retinoids, topically applied retinoids, skin-lightening products, and hydroxy acid products were not allowed within 1 year, 3 months, and 1 month, respectively, of enrollment. Daily sun exposure on the treatment areas and use of tanning beds were contraindicated during study participation.

8.3
Complications

Thirty-two of 44 women completed the entire 16-week protocol, 19 in the hydroquinone/retinol group and 13 in the tretinoin emollient cream treatment group. Those women that did not continue were released from the study owing to facial irritation. More women in the tretinoin emollient cream treatment group than in the hydroquinone/retinol treatment group did not continue. More dryness, scaling, and erythema occurred in women in the tretinoin emollient cream group than in women in the hydroquinone/retinol group. The differences between treatments were significant ($P<0.02$) at weeks 4, 8, and 16 for irritation.

8.4
Results

In general, the 4% hydroquinone/0.3% retinol cream performed better than the tretinoin emollient cream in the evaluated measures of photodamage. Within the hydroquinone/retinol treatment, the change from the baseline in tactile roughness was significant at all treatment visits starting with week 4, while in the tretinoin emollient cream group, tactile roughness worsened during the 16-week study (Fig. 8.1). This may be due to cosmeceutical effect of the study product emollient vehicle.

Similarly, for the appearance of fine lines, the change from the baseline was significant for the hydroquinone/retinol treatment at all visits after 4 weeks, while the tretinoin emollient cream treatment did not show statistically significant improvement. Between-treatment differences were statistically significant at weeks 12 and 16, showing greater response to 4% hydroquinone/0.3% retinol than to 0.05% tretinoin emollient cream (Fig. 8.2). Some of this improvement is probably due to the cosmeceutical moisturization effect of the study product vehicle.

Clinical evaluations of mottled hyperpigmentation, overall melasma severity, and the melasma area and severity index (MASI) score were analyzed to determine the effectiveness of the two treatments on hyperpigmentation. Consistently, the 4% hydroquinone/0.3% retinol cream was statistically more effective than the tretinoin emollient cream at improving each of these three pigmentation measures.

Both treatments caused significant changes from the baseline in mottled hyperpigmentation; however, these differences were apparent for the hydroquinone/retinol group at week 4 but not until week 8 for the tretinoin emollient cream group. Statistically significant between-treatment differences showed greater reduction in mottled hyperpigmentation with hydroquinone/retinol cream than with tretinoin emollient cream at each study visit (Fig. 8.3).

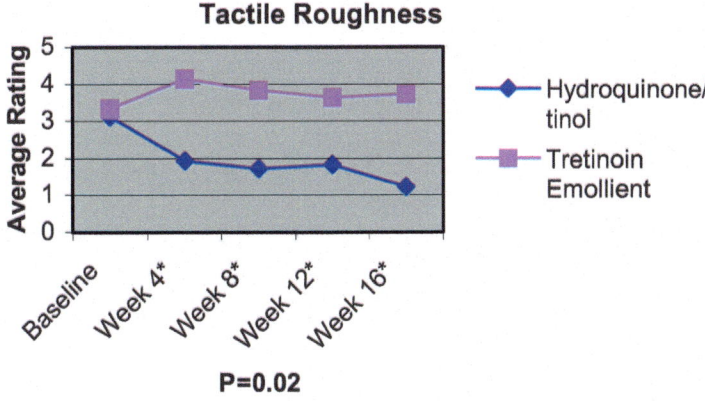

Fig. 8.1 Hydroquinone/retinol compared with tretinoin emollient cream for tactile roughness

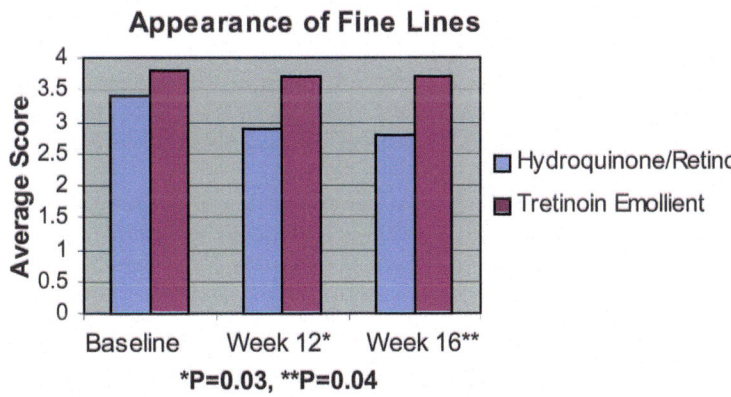

Fig. 8.2 Hydroquinone/retinol compared with tretinoin emollient cream for the appearance of fine lines

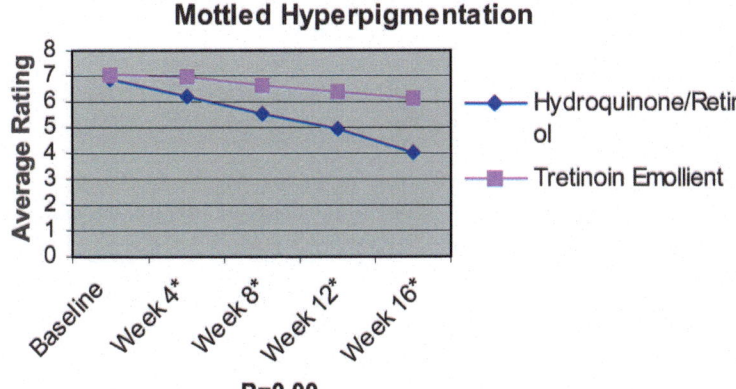

Fig. 8.3 Hydroquinone/retinol compared with tretinoin emollient cream for mottled hyperpigmentation

8.5
Discussion

The optimal treatment of hyperpigmented photodamaged skin is a combination of actives that address both pigmentation and wrinkling. Photodamage is a condition that is not characterized by one physical finding. This research demonstrated that 4% hydroquinone with stabilized 0.3% retinol in an emollient cream may be a viable treatment for hyperpigmented photodamaged skin. The hydroquinone/retinol cream provided more improvement in tactile roughness and fine lines than the 0.05% tretinoin emollient cream. This is probably due to the enhanced cosmeceutical moisturization properties of the hydroquinone/retinol vehicle and the lower irritancy of the cosmeceutical retinol active versus the prescription tretinoin active. Tretinoin can rapidly destroy the skin barrier upon application, which has led to interest in less irritating OTC retinoid forms, such as retinol. Hydroquinone too can produce skin irritation, since it can function as a cutaneous oxidant. The addition of a moisturizing vehicle and a less irritating retinoid can decrease skin roughness in formulations for dyspigmentation. The findings of this study point to the importance of the vehicle in prescription medications for photodamage. This is a concept that has been well recognized in the cosmetics industry.

The hydroquinone/retinol cream also resulted in a more rapid and greater reduction in the pigmentation associated with photodamage. This is probably due to the increased ability of the hydroquinone to decrease melanocyte pigment production, while the tretinoin primarily decreased melanosome transfer. It is possible that tretinoin might have functioned better if the study period had been lengthened. Nevertheless, one possible treatment for hyperpigmented photodamaged skin is the use of a retinol moisturizer in combination with hydroquinone.

8.6
Conclusions

It may be worthwhile to consider the use of a retinol moisturizer in combination with hydroquinone for patients with hyperpigmented photoaged skin. Even though prescription tretinoin has been considered the gold standard topical therapy, this research demonstrated the efficacy of a retinol moisturizer combined with hydroquinone to be efficacious. Rapid improvement in fine lines may be facilitated by an efficacious moisturizer with slower long-term non-irritating photodamage improvement induced by a stabilized retinol. Immediate and sustained improvement in dyspigmentation can be achieved with hydroquinone. This chapter has elucidated some of the clinical benefits of using a combination approach to the treatment of hyperpigmented photoaged skin by combining cosmeceutical and pharmaceutical attributes.

References

1. Kligman LH, Gans EH: Re-emergence of topical retinol in dermatology. J Dermatol Treat 2000;11:47–52
2. Draelos ZD: Hydroquinone: Optimizing therapeutic outcomes in the clinical setting of melanin-related hyperpigmentation. J New Devel Clin Med 2001;19(3):191–201
3. Kligman AM, Grove GL, Hirose R, Leyden JJ: Topical tretinoin for photoaged skin. J Amer Acad Dermatol 1986;15(4):836–859
4. Kligman AM: The treatment of photoaged human skin by topical tretinoin. Drugs 1989;38(1):1–8
5. Duell EA, Derguini F, Kang S, Elder JT, Voorhees JJ: Extraction of human epidermis treated with retinol yields retro-retinoids in addition to free retinol and retinyl esters. J Invest Dermatol 1996;107:178–182
6. Kligman LH, Do CH, Kligman AM: Topical retinoic acid enhances the repair of ultraviolet damaged dermal connective tissue. Connect Tissue Res 1984;12:139–150
7. Kligman AM, Grove GL, Hirose R, Leyden JJ: Topical tretinoin for photoaged skin. J Am Acad Dermatol 1986;15:836–859
8. Goodman DS: Vitamin A and retinoids in health and disease. N Eng J Med 1984;310(16):1023–1031
9. Noy N: Interactions of retinoids with lipid bilayers and with membranes. In Retinoids, MA Livrea, L Packer (eds), Dekker, New York 1993:17–27
10. Weiss JS, Ellis CN, Headington JT, Tincoff, T, Hamilton TA, Voorhees JJ: Topical tretinoin improves photoaged skin: a double-blind, vehicle controlled study. J Am Med Assoc 1988;259(4):527–532
11. Fisher GJ, Tavakkol A, Griffiths CE, Elder JT, Zhang OY, Finkel L, Danielpour D, Glick AB, Higley H, Ellingsworth L, et al: Differential modulation of transforming growth factor-beta one expression and mucin deposition by retinoic acid and sodium lauryl sulfate in human skin. J Invest Dermatol 1992;98(1):102–108
12. Olsen EA, Katz I, Levine N, Shupack J, Billys MM, Prawer S, Gold J, Stiller M, Lufrano L, Thorne EG: Tretinoin emollient cream: a new therapy for photodamaged skin. J Am Acad Dermatol 1992;26(2 Pt 1):215–224
13. Woodley DT, Zelickson AS, Briggaman RA, Hamilton TA, Weiss JS, Ellis CN, Voorhees JJ: Treatment of photoaged skin with topical tretinoin increases epidermal-dermal anchoring fibrils: a preliminary report. J Am Med Assoc 1990;263(22):3057–3059
14. Fisher GJ, Datta SC, Talwar HS, Wang ZO, Varani J, Kang S, Voorhees JJ: Molecular basis of sun-induced premature skin ageing and retinoid antagonism. Nature 1996;379(6563):335–339
15. Weiss JS, Ellis CE, Headington JT, Voorhees JJ: Topical tretinoin in the treatment of aging skin. J Am Acad Dermatol 1988;19:169–175

16. Weinstein GD, Nigra TP, Pochi PE, Savin RC, Allan A, Benik K, Jeffes E, Lufrano L, Thorne EG: Topical tretinoin for treatment of photodamaged skin. Arch Dermatol 1991;127:659–665

17. Gilchrest BA, Blog FB, Szabo G: Effects of aging and chronic sun exposure on melanocytes in human skin. J Invest Dermatol 1979;73:141–143

18. Bhawan J, Gonzalez-Serva A, Nehal K, Labadie R, Lufrano L, Thorne EG, Gilchrest BA: Effects of tretinoin on photodamaged skin a histologic study. Arch Dermatol 1991;127(5):666–672

19. Olsen EA, Katz I, Levine N, Shupack J, Billys MM, Prawer S, Gold J, Stiller M, Lufrano L, Thorne EG: Tretinoin emollient cream: a new therapy for photodamaged skin. J Am Acad Dermatol 1992;26:215–224

20. Weinstein GD, Nigra TP, Pochi PE, Savin RC, Allan A, Benik K, Jeffes E, Lufrano L, Thorne EG: Topical tretinoin for treatment of photodamaged skin. Arch Dermatol 1991;127(5):659–665

21. Kimbrough-Green CK, Griffiths CE, Finkel LJ, Hamilton TA, Bulengo-Ransby SM, Ellis CN, Voorhees JJ: Topical retinoic acid (tretinoin) for melasma in Black patients. Arch Dermatol 1994;130(6):727–733

22. Griffiths CE, Goldfarb MT, Finkel LJ, Roulia V, Bonawitz M, Hamilton TA, Ellis CN, Voorhees JJ: Topical tretinoin (retinoic acid) treatment of hyperpigmented lesions associated with photoaging in Chinese and Japanese patients. J Am Acad Dermatol 1994;30(1):76–84

23. Kang S, Duell EA, Fisher GJ, Datta SC, Wang ZO, Reddy AP, Tavakkol A, Yi JY, Griffiths CE, Elder JT, et al: Application of retinol to human skin in vivo induces epidermal hyperplasia and cellular retinoid binding proteins characteristic of retinoic acid but without measurable retinoic acid levels of irritation. J Invest Dermatol 1995;105(4):549–556

24. Duell EA, Kang S, Voorhees JJ: Unoccluded retinol penetrates human skin in vivo more effectively than unoccluded retinyl palmitate or retinoic acid. J Invest Dermatol 1997;109(3):301–305

CHAPTER 9

Chemical Peels and Other Rejuvenation Methods for the Face

9

Yang-Che Kim

9.1
Introduction

A chemical peel leads to regeneration of new cells at a faster rate than they would regenerate naturally. The treatment causes the surface of the skin to exfoliate or flake, which leaves the skin with a fresher and smoother appearance and texture. This freshens the skin, removes some sunspots and rough scaly patches, and reduces freckles and irregular pigmentation. It also reduces fine wrinkles. A chemical peel may be used prior to facelifts to maintain or preserve facial skin tone. It is safest and most effective on the face. Hands can be peeled but the risk of scarring is higher and the results are less predictable. Sometimes the results are dramatic and satisfying and a facelift can be avoided altogether. There are several types of peels in use today, and each has its own area of clinical use.

9.2
Types of Peels

9.2.1
Phenol Peel

Phenol, also known under the old name carbolic acid, is a colorless crystalline solid with a typical sweet tarry odor. Its chemical formula is C_6H_5OH and its structure is that of a hydroxyl group (–OH) bonded to a phenyl ring; it is thus an aromatic compound. The Baker–Gordon formula is 3 ml 88% phenol USP, 2 ml tap water, three drops of croton oil, and three drops of hexachlorophene soap (Septisol).

9.2.1.1
Technique

A full-face deep chemical peel takes 1–2 h to perform. A more limited procedure (such as treatment of wrinkling above the lip) will generally take less than 0.5 h. A solution is applied to the area to be treated (avoiding the eyes, brows, and lips). There is a slight burning sensation, but it is minimal since the solution also acts as an anesthetic. After the peel solution has worked on

the skin, it is neutralized with water. Approximately 1 h later, a thick coating of petroleum jelly is layered over the patient's face, covering the protective crust which develops rapidly over the area. This stays in place for 1–2 days. In an alternative technique, the patient's face is covered by a "mask," composed of strips of adhesive tape, with openings for the eyes and mouth (this is particularly effective in cases of severe wrinkling).

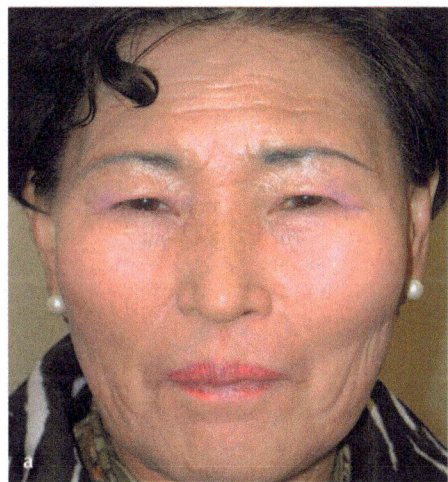

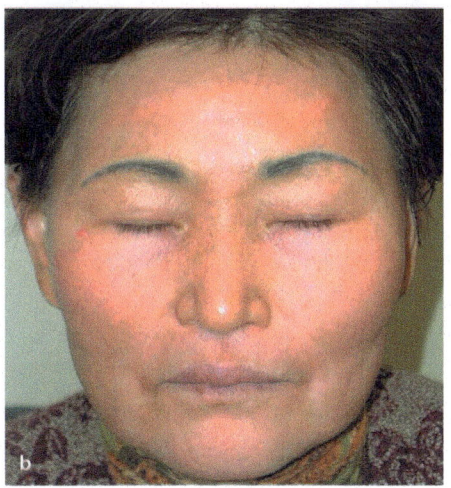

Fig. 9.1 a Before phenol peel. **b** After phenol peel

9.2.1.2
Complications

The toxic oral dose of phenol for adults is 8–15 g, which is usually fatal within 24 h. Blood levels of phenol resulting from a total facial peel are well below the toxic range. Although reports of systemic toxicity are rare, myocardial changes such as premature ventricular contractions are not uncommon; therefore, all phenol peels are monitored by ECG with slow application of the phenol and an intravenous line in place to treat any cardiac arrhythmias.

9.2.1.3
Results

Since peeling with phenol results in a peel at a deep dermal level, it may be anticipated that the end result is skin lightening. However, since the deeper rhytids of the face (perioral and orbital) respond well to this technique, judicious use of phenol in these areas is often combined with dermabrasion and or trichloroacetic acid (TCA) without the use of taping. The bleaching effect is therefore minimized and healing time is shortened (Fig. 9.1).

9.2.2
Trichloroacetic Acid Peel

TCA is the other commonly used peeling agent that was reintroduced as a skin rejuvenator. The present formulation for phenol peels was published in 1961 [1]. TCA also denatures protein and is used in concentrations ranging from 20 to 50%. Although the depth of peeling that may be achieved with 50% TCA is comparable to that with 50% phenol, the risk of scarring is greater with TCA in this higher concentration.

9.2.2.1
Dilution

For a 12% solution, mix 1 part 25% TCA with 1 part water (equal amounts). For variations between 25 and 12%, just add a little more or less water. A 25% solution will result in a medium peel, whereas a 12% solution will give a lighter "lunchtime" peel, comparable to that from a 30% glycolic acid treatment.

9.2.2.2
Technique

Pretreatment cream (Retin-A or other desquamating agents) must be applied 4–6 weeks prior to treatment.

This provides a more uniform skin peel. The face is cleansed thoroughly and degreased with acetone. As with phenol, degreasing the skin with acetone or absolute alcohol enhances penetration of the peel chemical. Jessner's solution is then be applied to one area of the face at a time. The solution is left on the skin for several minutes. The skin will burn and tingle. Next, 35% TCA

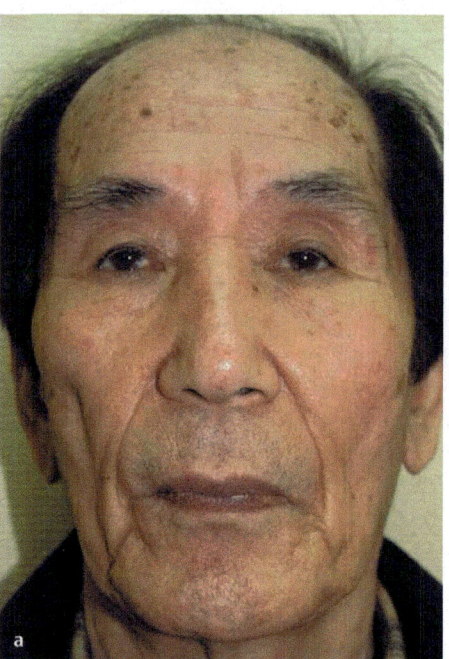
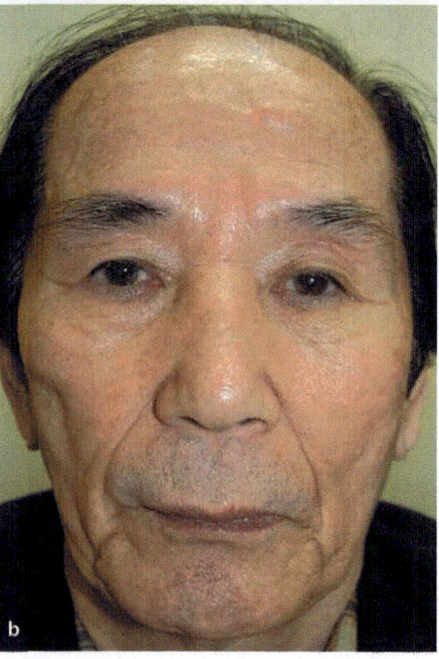

Fig. 9.2 a Before trichloroacetic acid peel. **b** After trichloroacetic acid

is applied. During this time the burning will be very intense. The TCA is neutralized at the appropriate time with water or rubbing alcohol. Cool compresses are applied followed by Polysporin. During this time the skin will begin to feel better. The peeled areas are then covered with A&D ointment or Vaseline and rinsed daily.

9.2.2.3
Complications

Because there is no systemic toxicity to TCA when used in the proper concentrations, it is considered safer for older patients. There is no evidence that allergic reactions to TCA or to phenol occur, but the TCA peel also requires monitoring for cardiac arrhythmias.

9.2.2.4
Results

TCA peeling lasts for 2 weeks after the treatment with significant redness (Fig. 9.2). Sunscreen must be applied 4–6 weeks prior to treatment and 6 months after treatment and repeat treatment may be needed to maintain results.

9.2.3
Glycolic Acid Peel

Glycolic acid (or hydroxyacetic acid) is the smallest α-hydroxy acid (AHA). Glycolic acid is isolated from sugar cane, sugar beet, and unripe grapes. Its polymerization yields polyglycolide, although the most common route to synthesize this polymer uses glycolide, the cyclic dimer of glycolic acid as starting material. Glycolic acids (AHAs) rejuvenate the skin by encouraging the shedding of old, sun-damaged surface skin cells. Glycolic acid that is derived from sugar cane is the AHA most frequently used for facial treatments but lactic acid and citric acid are also useful. Lactic acid comes from milk.

9.2.3.1
Technique

Two weeks before the peel, begin the pretreatment regimen. At least 3–4 weeks before the first peel, Retin-A and exfoliating sponges should stop being used. All forms of hair removal should be stopped at least 3–4 weeks before the peel. The face is cleansed thoroughly with cleanser. Petroleum jelly is applied to the corners of the eyes, nose, and mouth. Glycolic acid is then applied to one area of the face at a time. The glycolic acid is be left on the skin for several minutes. The skin will burn and tingle. When the skin becomes uncomfortable, the

peel is neutralized. After the peel has been neutralized, the face is rinsed and sunscreen is then applied.

9.2.3.2
Complications

The most common side effect after a glycolic acid peel is brown discoloration of the skin. This is usually reversible but can rarely be permanent. This side effect usually occurs only in those who have had sun exposure after a peel. Peels can cause persistent redness of the skin. If the patient gets cold sores, a peel can cause them to flare. This can be prevented by taking the prescription drug Acyclovir.

9.2.3.3
Results

Glycolic acid peel smoothes rough and dry skin and improves the texture of sun-damaged skin and aids in acne control. Bleaching agent can be mixed with the glycolic acid to correct pigment problems. Glycolic acid peel can usually be used as TCA pretreatment. A series of peels (a monthly treatment) may be needed. As with most peel treatments, sunblock use is recommended.

9.2.4
Conclusions

Skin resurfacing with chemical peeling has been practiced in some form for hundreds of years. Dramatic improvements in skin texture and appearance can be achieved with proper peels and techniques. Experience and training are necessary to prevent untoward sequelae of chemical peeling. For the physician and patient alike, this can be a valuable tool in the arsenal of choices for facial rejuvenation.

9.3
Treatment of Wrinkles with Intense Pulsed Light

9.3.1
Introduction

The treatment of facial rhytids has traditionally centered on methods that destroy the epidermis and cause a dermal wound, with resultant dermal collagen remodeling. Theses methods have included dermabrasion, chemical peels and, more recently, the use of the pulsed CO_2 laser and Er:YAG lasers. These procedures are effective enough to improve photoaging; however, they have not been widely accepted because of postoperative complications such as persistent hyperemia, hyperpigmentation, and even hypertrophic scar formation. The complication or downtime sometimes will last more than 1 year.

Nonablative full-face rejuvenation is in many ways an ideal treatment modality in the sense that it provides many of the benefits that patients seek to restore skin color and texture without significant complications and posttreatment downtime associated with more invasive options. Recently, intense pulsed light (IPL) photorejuvenation has been indicated and is effective for cosmetic disorders including fine wrinkles and large pores.

9.3.2
Technique

IPL systems are high-intensity pulsed sources which emit polychromatic light in a broad wavelength spectrum from 515 to 1,200 nm. The mechanism of action of such light systems corresponds to selective photothermolysis. Because of the varying absorption maximum of the respective target structures, appropriate wavelengths can be selected to deliberately heat (above 80°C) and destroy them. Hemoglobin primarily absorbs at 580 nm; melanin absorbs over the entire visible spectral range (400–750 nm).

The wavelength determines not only the absorption behavior but also the penetration depth of the light. With the aid of different cutoff filters (515–755 nm), which only allow a defined wavelength to pass through them, the spectrum can be filtered out that corresponds to the depth of the target structure (vessels of different depth and sizes, hair follicles, pigmented structures).

The pulse duration of IPL systems can be set to ranges between 0.5 and 88.5 ms and should be lower than the thermal relaxation time of the target structure so that the surrounding tissue is not damaged. The use of single pulses is possible, and high fluences can be split into multiple pulses as well; the intervals between the individual pulses can be set at values between 1 and 300 ms. This delay allows the epidermis cells and smaller vessels to cool down between pulses, while the heat is retained in the larger (target) vessels, hair follicles, resulting in selective thermal damage.

9.3.3
Beginning the Procedure

1. Determine the Fitzpatrick skin type.
2. Apply anesthetic if needed. Wait 20–30 min.
3. Use safety eyewear for the patient and the operator.
4. Select parameters; pulse type, pw1, delay, pw2, filter, fluence.
5. Apply 2–3 mm cold gel to the skin for the light guide.
6. Test the pulse to the periauricular area.
7. Await clinical response; slight erythema (3 min).
8. Confirm settings or make adjustments.
9. Begin the full-face procedure.

9.3.4
Complications

There are many factors that have major effects on the prevalence of side effects: skin type, skin tone, thickness of dermis, the degree of sensitivity, and relative number of sebaceous glands on various parts of the body Transient erythema lasts for 2–48 h and is occasionally accompanied by edema. Transient purpura, crusting, and hyperpigmentation and hypopigmentation can occur, most often observed in patients with dark skin or tanned skin. To protect the epidermis from being burned, the cooling can be performed using cooling gels, ice gels, contact spray cooling, or special cooling handpieces.

9.3.5
Discussion

The reason why IPL is effective in improving skin texture is that microthermal damage causes an increase in collagen production during the wound-healing process. The activation of intracellular fibroblast activity and resultant collagen proliferation is stimulated by three mechanisms: first, from thermal damage to collagen fibers caused by ducted heat from light selectively absorbed by structures containing melanin or oxyhemoglobin; second, from thermal damage to collagen fibers caused by light absorbed in the fibers themselves; third, from thermal damage to collagen fibers through the nonselective heating of the dermis. Since light between 400 and 600 nm is highly absorbed by collagen fibers, we can conclude that IPL in the 560–1,200-nm range is partially absorbed and may therefore mildly damage dermal collagen fibers.

The piled-up collagen influences the smoothness of the epithelial layer and acceleration of epithelial turnover. The shrinkage of collagen and increased superficial collagen proliferation following thermal generation will greatly accelerate the improvement ratio in wrinkle treatment.

9.3.6
Conclusions

IPL simultaneously improves both skin texture and superficial degeneration, including pigmentation and telangiectasia (Fig. 9.3). Unlike conventional procedures, photorejuvenation is a nonablative procedure, requiring almost no downtime. Because of these advantages it will be easily accepted be socially active people.

9.4
Treatment of Wrinkles with Radiofrequency Devices: ThermaCool, Polaris, and Internal Radiofrequency

9.4.1
Introduction

Over the past several years, lasers have replaced chemical peels and dermabrasion as the treatment to improve photodamaged skin. Although the ablative laser techniques are associated with impressive efficacy in reducing facial wrinkles and tightening sagging skin, dermabrasion-type side effects following laser surgery are common. Nonablative technologies have been developed in an effort to reduce complications, minimize perioperative pain, and shorten the healing time by creating a dermal wound without ablating the epidermis. While the incidence of adverse effects is unquestionably lower with nonablative techniques, the cosmetic improvement is subtle, and often requires serial treatment over a 6–12-month period.

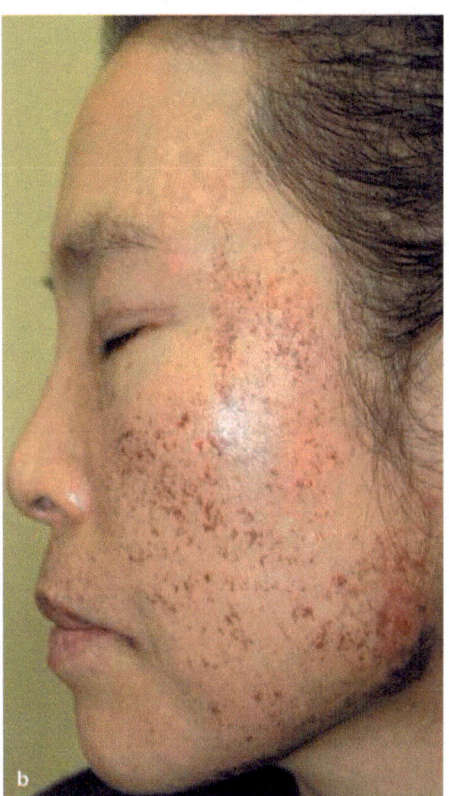

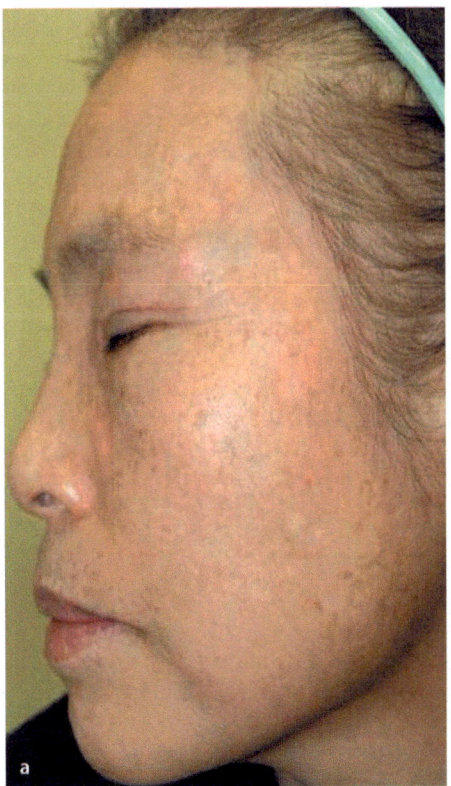

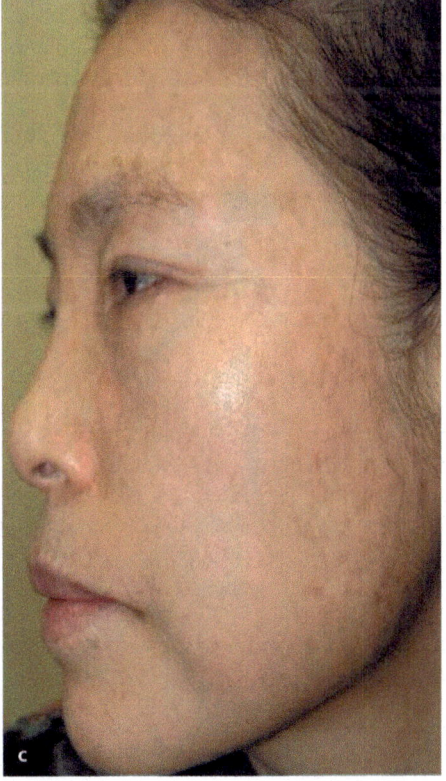

Fig. 9.3 a Before intense pulsed light (IPL) treatment. **b** Three weeks after IPL treatment. **c** Much improved pigmentation without scar 6 weeks after IPL treatmentv

In contrast to light-based nonablative resurfacing, radiofrequency (RF) treatment applies RF energy to the skin with concomitant cryogen cooling of the epidermis. Tissue resistance to RF energy generates heat, which causes a controlled thermal dermal injury.

Internal RF treatment is a new technique which applies RF energy to the dissected forehead to treat wrinkles on the forehead, glabella, and nasal root.

9.4.2
Techniques and Complications

RF technology produces an electric current that generates heat through resistance in the dermis and subcutaneous tissue. The depth and the degree of thermal injury are dependent on the geometry and the size of the treatment tip and the conductive properties of the tissue being treated.

The thermal effect is determined by the formula
Energy $(J) = I^2 RT$,
where I is the current, R is the impedance of the tissue, and T is the time of application.

9.4.2.1
ThermaCool Radiofrequency Device

The ThermaCool (Thermage, Hayward, CA, USA) system heats tissue using a proprietary method of coupling RF to skin by a thin capacitive membrane that distributes RF energy over a volume of tissue beneath the membrane surface. A cryogen system simultaneously cools the epidermal surface for protection. This combination of deep volumetric tissue heating and surface cooling allows sustained delivery of high energy fluences in a single treatment.

Device

1. RF generator producing a 6-MHz alternating-current RF signal.
2. Handpiece for directing the RF energy to the skin, delivering cooling cryogen spray, monitoring temperature, pressure, RF feedback.
3. A treatment-electrode tip, for transferring RF energy to skin and serving as a membrane for contact cooling.
4. A cooling module that feeds a cryogen through a controlled valve on the handpiece to the tip's contact cooling membrane.

Procedure

1. Topical anesthetic (5% lidocaine) is applied to the designated treatment area under occlusion for 60

min and then completely removed with water-soaked gauze before the RF procedure.
2. The treatment area is marked in ink with a grid pattern of contiguous squares, each square slightly larger than the selected RF treatment (0.25 or 1 cm²).
3. A RF return pad is adhered to the subject's back to create a return path for RF travel.
4. A proprietary coupling fluid iss spread over the treatment area to enhance thermal and electrical contact with the treatment-electrode tip.
5. Each application consists of three continuous and automatic phases of cryogen precooling/simultaneous RF heating and cryogen cooling/cryogen postcooling.
6. Treatment is delivered in a single, nonoverlapping pass over the treatment area through an applied conductive fluid.

Complications

The most frequently noted treatment-related events were erythema and edema. Scabbing was the next most frequent procedure-related adverse event. Burning pain and altered sensation can occur related to use of nerve block.

9.4.2.2
Polaris

The Polaris (ELOS) laser consists of a bipolar RF generator and flashlamp pulsed light delivered through a contact sapphire light guide with the bipolar RF energy delivered through electrodes embedded in the system applicator and brought into contact with skin surface. The RF component of the ELOS system is a bipolar configuration for both electrodes. The two electrodes are laterally affixed on opposing sides of the rectangular sapphire guide. Electrical current is passed between the two electrodes and is limited by the area between the electrodes. The penetration depth of the electrical current can be calculated as half of the distance between the electrodes.

The device also includes an active dermal monitoring system that measures changes in the skin impedance, which can be adjusted by the user to provide an integrated safety mechanism to prevent overheating of the dermis. A thermoelectric cooling handpiece provides contact cooling at approximately 5 C before, during, and after energy delivery.

Procedure

1. Hydrate and cool the epidermis.
2. Apply optical energy to selectively heat the target and bipolar RF energy to provide additional ther-

mal energy to the heated target. The applied energy should be at the level at which the temperature of the epidermis does not exceed the target temperature.

3. Discontinue the optical pulse and continue with the RF pulse for additional selective heating of the target.
4. Each treatment consists of one to three passes over the face using a fluence of 28–34 J/cm² and a RF current of 20 J/cm².

Complications

Transient blistering and erythema may occur that can be minimized by proper technique.

9.4.2.3
Internal Radiofrequency

ThermaCool treatment protects the epidermis with a cryogen cooling spray while delivering RF energy to dermis and heating the dermis. But, the effect on upper dermis will be insufficient because of short dermal heating time and continuing application of the cooling device. A new technique to treat the wrinkles on the forehead, glabella, and nasal root by using RF internally and evaluating the efficacy and safety of the new technique was introduced and named internal RF (Fig. 9.4).

Anatomically, it is easy to dissect the forehead in the subperiosteal level. In delivering the RF internally after dissection, there are several benefits:

1. There is no need for a cooling device.
2. RF energy can transfer to the dermis directly.
3. Subcutaneous fat tissue prevents heat loss and continuous dermal heating is possible.

In addition, subperiosteal dissection provides a path to access the corrugator muscle, procerus muscle, and depressor supercilii muscle.

Device

The Timed TD 50A micropulse™ (Korpo, Genoa, Italy) produces a 920-kHz alternating-current RF signal, the energy level of which is set by the operator. A RF transmitter delivers the RF energy to the skin. Dermal heat is generated based on the tissue's natural resistance to the movement of electrons within RF fields. Dermal heat energy output can be stated in terms of joules as calculated by the following formula:

Energy density (J/cm²)=PT/S,

where P is the power of the RF generator (watts), T is the time to deliver the RF (seconds), and S is the surface area (square centimeters).

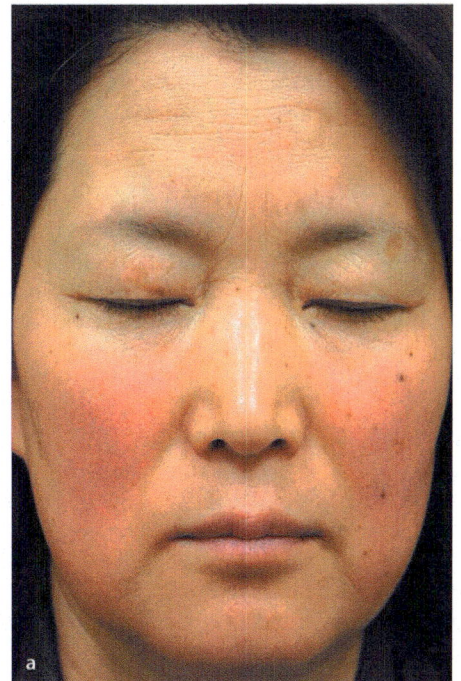

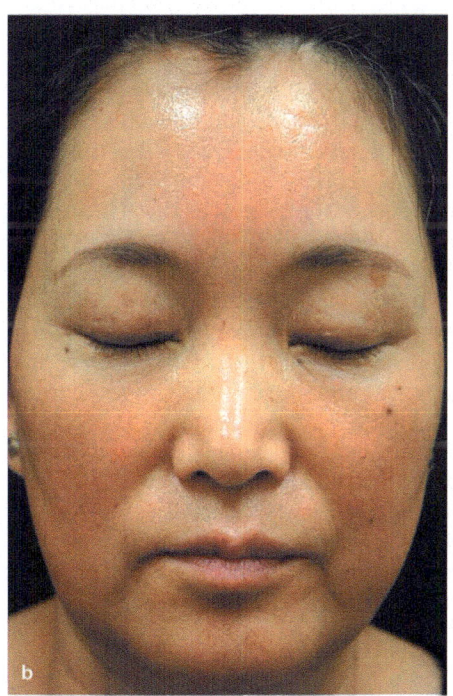

Fig. 9.4 a Before internal radiofrequency (IRF) treatment. **b** After IRF treatment with much improvement in forehead and frown wrinkles

Procedure

1. Before the treatment, the medical histories of all the subjects should be checked and a routine laboratory test should be performed.
2. Calculate the surface area of the forehead of each subject using section paper and the time to deliver the RF to skin for 90–110 J/cm^2 of heat energy.
3. To relieve pain, 50 µg fentanyl citrate is injected about 30–60 min before the treatment and a 25 µg Fentanyl patch (Duragesic patch) is applied on the chest. Blood pressure, oxygen saturation, and electrocardiogram are monitored before and during the treatment.
4. The scalp and forehead are disinfected with povidone and alcohol. Right before the treatment, the parts of forehead are marked to incise in the midline about 2 cm from the frontal hair line. The forehead is marked into four areas to apply a fixed amount of RF energy to the each area.
5. Lidocaine (2%) with 1:100,000 epinephrine is used for the regional blockade of the supraorbital nerve and the supratrochlear nerve, and iss injected in the marked incision site.
6. A transverse incision of 1 cm on the midline about 2 cm from the frontal hair line is made using a no. 15 scalpel blade, and the forehead is dissected up to the superolateral edge of the orbital rim on a subperiosteal level with a blunt dissector. After dissection of the forehead, the nasal root area is dissected using the same method. After dissection of the forehead and the nasal root, RF energy is applied all over the dissected forehead using a RF transmitter. When applying the RF energy, we timed the duration of so that the same amount of RF radiation was applied on the four areas marked before the treatment. After delivering the RF energy, the frontalis muscle, the procerus muscle, and the corrugator supercilii muscle were destroyed selectively using the hook.
7. When the treatment was completed, the dissected forehead skin was fixed on the upper-level frontal bone tightly with a 4-in. elastic bandage.
8. The subject had to take antibiotics and analgesics for 1 week after the treatment. The incision site in the frontal scalp was sutured with nylon 4.0. Then, dressing and changing of the elastic bandage on the treatment area were performed every 3 days for 2 weeks.

Complications

Erythema and edema are most common. Other complications are ecchymosis, erosion on the treatment site and transient paresthesia on the forehead and scalp, transient hair loss, itching sensation, and brow malposition.

9.4.3
Discussion

9.4.3.1
ThermaCool Radiofrequency Device

This RF method of heating tissue-with controlled volumetric heating of deeper cutaneous tissues resulting in tissue tightening differs radically from traditional laser methods. The mechanism of action after RF treatment is hypothesized to be that of immediate collagen contraction, followed by secondary collagen synthesis and remodeling.

This system is thought to improve skin texture and remove fine lines not via tissue tightening but by induction of minor superficial dermal wounding and subsequent regeneration of new collagen in the papillary dermis Thus, clinical findings suggesting that the RF device can induce skin tightening via controlled volumetric heating of the deeper cutaneous tissues are noteworthy.

9.4.3.2
Polaris

A new technology that integrates bipolar RF and optical energies, ELOS, is based on the premise of synergistic activity between the two forms of energy. The bipolar RF component enables the use of a lower-power optical component, reducing the risk from optical energy and potentially improving its use across different skin types. The optical component is believed to help the bipolar RF energy to concentrate where the optical component has selectively heated the target.

9.4.3.3
Internal Radiofrequency

The basic principle of internal RF treatment is similar to that of the nonablative RF device ThermaCool system. The RF current created by the generator transforms into thermal energy and heats the dermis. The collagen fibril, with a thermal injury of appropriate temperature, denatures as the intermolecular hydrogen bond is interrupted. As a result, the tissue contracts and skin is tightened. The mechanism of this treatment not only brings the RF effect to the collagen, but also achieves an additional therapy effect. The vertical fixing fibril, from the skin towards the periosteum, is destroyed by dissecting the forehead, and the RF on the tendon, periosteum, and muscle sheath causes them to contract. In addition, tissue repositioning, partial destruction of the depressor muscle group on the forehead, and frontalis muscle contraction can contribute to the treatment effect.

9.4.4
Conclusions

As demand grows for minimally invasive techniques to treat the signs of aging and photodamaged skin, cosmetic surgeons are challenged to develop procedures that provide clinical improvement while minimizing side effects.

Noninvasive RF is a new and very promising tool for the nonsurgical tightening of sagging skin. In its current configuration, most patients will see at least a mild improvement, with minimal downtime and minimal risk. This technology offers a very attractive alternative to invasive facelift surgery.

A single treatment with internal RF produces objective and subjective reductions in wrinkles on the forehead, glabella, and nasal root. The benefits of this treatment include no need for an additional cooling device, rapid treatment time, no secondary hyperpigmentation, long-lasting effect, and a safe and simple technique.

9.5
Treatment of Wrinkles with an Infrared Laser

9.5.1
Introduction

Near-infrared lasers, primarily at 1,064, 1,320, and 1,450 nm, produce light that is absorbed by primarily by water and heat both the epidermis and the dermis. These lasers use aggressive skin cooling to limit thermal damage to the epidermis, creating a controlled injury to the dermal collagen, with subsequent remodeling and tightening. There is generally little effect on pigmentation or blood vessels, making them less useful for pigmented lesions, and because of the deeper penetration and heating effect on the skin, these laser wavelengths tend to cause more discomfort during treatment.

9.5.2
Techniques

The Titan skin tightening system consists of handheld infrared light source and an attached cooling system that protects the skin. The infrared light penetrates the deep, inner layer of the skin, uniformly heating the existing collagen and subsequently causing it to shrink and firm up. This shrinkage promotes long-term collagen production, which lifts the targeted areas and gives patients a smoother, more toned appearance (Fig. 9.5). While the infrared light source heats the collagen, the cooling attachment continuously cools the surface of the skin in order to protect the epidermis and prevent any heat-related damage.

No anesthesia is required for this virtually painless procedure, and postoperative pain is practically nonexistent.

9.5.3
Complications

Mild blistering, erythema, and edema, immediately afterward, resolve within a few days.

9.5.4
Discussion

Titan lasers stimulate new collagen formation by heating collagen in the upper layers of the skin. The infrared light from these longer-wavelength lasers is absorbed by water in the upper dermis, heating the tissue and thereby inducing a wound-repair response. In order to avoid damaging the epidermis, various strategies are employed to cool the epidermis and avoid a visible epidermal wound.

Absorption by melanin and hemoglobin is minimal at these wavelengths, so these devices are not useful for treating discoloration as a "photofacial". Typically a series of three to six treatments performed about 1 month apart are recommended for best results.

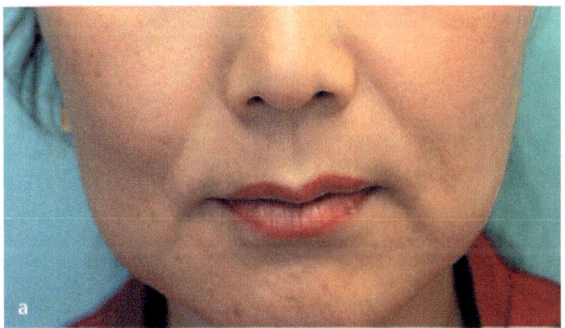

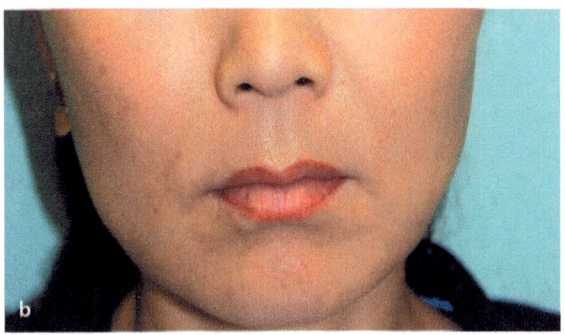

Fig. 9.5 a Before Titan. **b** After Titan

9.5.5
Conclusions

Titan technology, which uses carefully modulated, infrared light to improve skin quality, is safer and more effective than traditional nonsurgical skin rejuvenation treatments. Other heat treatments use RF, which can burn the skin and may require a significant recovery period.

Titan technology is an effective alternative to surgery with minimal side effects and virtually no recovery time.

Reference

1. Baker TJ: The ablation of rhytids by chemical means, a preliminary report. J Fla Med Assoc 1961;48:451–454

CHAPTER 10

Superficial and Medium-Depth Chemical Peels   10

Benjamin A. Bassichis

10.1
Introduction

Chemical peeling of facial skin has become an integral part of the armamentarium for resurfacing aging, sun-damaged, and diseased skin. The desire to reverse the aging process has generated tremendous interest throughout history. Ancient texts describe the application of substances to the skin in an attempt to rejuvenate the appearance. More recently, many factors have contributed to the explosion of popularity of skin resurfacing procedures, including excess ultraviolet exposure both naturally and via tanning booths, the aging baby boomer cohort, youth-centric culture, smoking, ozone layer depletion, and the prevalence of both hot and cold weather outdoor recreations, and all have had a significant effect on people's skin health and premature wrinkling.

The modern body of knowledge regarding chemical agents began with the description of a variety of agents still in use today by Unna [1], including salicylic acid, resorcinol, phenol, and trichloroacetic acid (TCA). Over the ensuing century, peeling became popularized by non-medical practitioners and cosmeticians who attracted increasing attention because of the rejuvenating results they achieved. Subsequent scientific studies of chemical peels by the medical community have further delineated the indications and limitations of these procedures and improved safety and efficacy. We are currently in an era of rapid development of new techniques for skin enhancement and rehabilitation, some of which offer the possibilities of dramatic results, with minimized discomfort and diminished downtime [2].

There are many products currently available for chemical resurfacing of the skin, from over-the-counter superficial peeling agents to deep-peeling chemicals that should only be applied by a physician in a controlled setting [3]. Many of these products and procedures have proven very successful in improving the quality and appearance of facial skin. The goal of chemical peeling is to remove a controlled uniform thickness of damaged skin to improve and smooth the texture of the facial skin by removing the superficial layers and stimulate a wound-healing response. In response to the chemical injury, fibroblasts in the papillary dermis in-crease production of collagen and growth factors. The collagen increase in turn thickens the dermis, which enhances the tensile strength of the skin and yields the clinical appearance of rejuvenation.

10.2
Skin Anatomy

The approach to chemical resurfacing of the skin necessitates a thorough knowledge of skin anatomy and normal wound healing. The skin is composed of two mutually dependent layers, the epidermis and the dermis, which reside on a layer of subcutaneous adipose tissue. The epidermis is the most superficial layer of the skin and provides a critical barrier of protection. The epidermis is composed of keratinocytes in four layers: the stratum corneum, stratum granulosum, stratum spinosum, and stratum basale.

The stratum corneum is the outermost layer of the epidermis and is shed about every 2 weeks. Providing significant protection to the skin, it is formed from flattened, anucleate keratinocytes filled with mature keratin. Depending on the area of the body, the stratum corneum varies in thickness, with the eyelid being the thinnest and the palms and soles the thickest. The cells of the stratum granulosum contain dense basophilic keratohyalin granules, hence the granular layer. These granules are composed of lipids, which along with the desmosomal connections help form a waterproof barrier that functions to prevent fluid loss from the body. The stratum spinosum keratinocytes contain numerous desmosomes on their outer surface that provides the characteristic spiny or prickled appearance of the cells in this layer. The stratum basale or basal layer, the deepest layer of the epidermis, contains basal cells whose replicative effort replaces the cells of the superficial layers every 2 weeks. The basal layer also contains melanocytes, which provide pigmentation in the skin.

The epidermis is avascular and thus dependent on the underlying dermis for nutrient delivery and waste disposal by diffusion through the dermoepidermal junction. In addition to thermoregulation, the dermis functions to sustain and support the overlying epidermis. The dermis is divided into two zones, the upper papillary dermis and the deeper reticular dermis. The dermis contains numerous fibroblasts that are responsible for secreting collagen, elastin, and ground matrix that provide the support and elasticity of the skin. Also, present in the dermis are a variety immune cells that are involved in defense against foreign invaders passing through the epidermis.

As we mature, the skin undergoes changes over time. The epidermal layer tends to thin and atrophy. The stratum corneum becomes disorganized and less effective as a protective barrier to the external environment. The dermoepidermal junction flattens and exhibits fewer papillae. However, the most significant changes occur in the dermis as it thins with age. The amount of ground substance and collagen fibers decreases, and elastic fibers degenerate and become irregular, making the skin less resistant to deformational forces. As the relatively inelastic epidermis loses dermal volume and support beneath it, fine wrinkles form.

After a chemical peel has removed the superficial skin, the epidermis regenerates from the epidermal appendages located in the remaining dermis. This process begins within 24 h of wounding and is usually complete in 7–10 days. The new epidermis shows greater organization and vertical polarity, with the disappearance of actinic keratoses and lentigines. Dermal regeneration is a slower process but is usually complete within several months. Chemical peeling has been shown to improve the quality of the dermis with the formation of a dense, homogenous 2–3-mm band of parallel collagen fibers [4].

Histological sections of skin after a chemical peel procedure reveal a layer of new, denser connective tissue above the older, degenerated elastotic tissue. Clinically this results in the effective ablation of the fine wrinkles and a diminution of pigmentation. Dermal ground substance is decreased, and telangiectasias are absent. Increased angiogenesis occurs in the dermis, which is thought to aid the appearance of the skin by adding a warm glow. The overall result is soft supple skin that appears more youthful with fewer rhytids and dyschromias. These clinical and histological changes are long-lasting (15–20 years) and may be permanent in some patients.

10.3 Technique

10.3.1 Patient Selection

Indications for more superficial chemical peels include dyschromias, comedonal acne, and for skin refreshing. Indications for medium and deep peels are treatment of actinic changes, fine rhytids, pigmentary dyschromias, selected superficial scars, and acne vulgaris and rosacea.

Thorough evaluation and photographic documentation prior to chemical peeling is vital for a successful outcome. This includes consideration of the severity of actinic damage, depth and number of rhytids, and need for additional or alternative procedures. Patients with deep rhytids and excess or lax facial skin are likely best served by traditional rhytidectomy. However, patients with severe sun damage and fine to medium rhytids are optimal candidates for chemical peeling. Some patients may benefit from both procedures as rhytidectomy addresses skin quantity, whereas peeling treats skin quality. The procedures are not recommended for simultaneous application. A minimum of 3 months between chemical peel and other surgical procedures is advised to permit complete wound healing.

Skin type, quality, color, ethnic background, and age are important factors that should be considered prior to chemical peel. Patients should be evaluated using Fitzpatrick's scale of sun-reactive skin types (Table 10.1), which denotes a patient's sensitivity to ultraviolet radiation and existing degree of pigmentation. Fitzpatrick type I patients always burn and never tan. Type II describes patients who only tan with difficulty and usually burn. Type III patients usually tan, but sometimes burn. Type IV patients tan with ease but rarely burn. Fitzpatrick type V patients tan very easily and very rarely burn, and type VI patients tan very easily and never burn [5]. Patients with lighter skin types often tolerate chemical peeling with minimal pigmentary alterations, whereas individuals with darker skin are at a higher risk for either hyperpigmentation or hypopigmentation problems after chemoexfoliation.

Another useful grading system for pretreatment classification is the Glogau system describing four types of photoaging (Table 10.2). According to the individual patient's classifications, skin type, and problems, the

Table 10.1 Fitzpatrick skin types

Skin type	Skin color	Tanning response
I	Very white or freckled	Always burns, never tans
II	White	Usually burns, tans with difficulty
III	White to olive	Mild burn, average tan
IV	Brown	Rarely burns, tans easily
V	Dark brown	Very rarely burns, tans very easily
VI	Black	Does not burn, tans very easily

Table 10.2 Glogau classification of photoaging

Group I mild	Group II moderate	Group III advanced	Group IV severe
Age 28–35	Age 35–50	Age 50–60	Age 65–70
No keratoses	Early actinic keratoses	Obvious actinic keratoses	Actinic keratoses/skin cancer
Little wrinkling	Early wrinkling-smile lines	Wrinkling at rest	Wrinkling/laxity
No scarring	Mild scarring	Moderate acne scarring	Severe acne scarring
Little makeup	Small amount of makeup	Always wear makeup	Makeup cakes on

type and depth of the peels can be customized to suit the patient's needs [6].

Patients must have realistic expectations and the physician must understand what can be accomplished with chemical peeling. A successful peel procedure is a result of good communication between patient and surgeon. Superficial skin resurfacing cannot achieve flawless skin. Rather the goal of chemical peeling is to improve the appearance of the skin as much as possible.

In addition to the physical examination, a thorough medical history and review of systems should be obtained in patients considering chemical peel. Preexisting cardiac, hepatic, and renal disease may influence treatment decisions and choice of peeling agents. A history of melasma, recent pregnancy, exogenous estrogens, oral contraceptives, other photosensitizing medications, or an unwillingness to avoid the sun may portend postpeel hyperpigmentation problems. The patient's medication use, skin sensitivities, and allergy history must also be documented.

In patients with a history of herpes simplex virus (HSV) infections, prophylactic antiviral therapy should be initiated at least 1 day before the peel procedure and continued until reepithelialization is complete. With the ubiquity of HSV, some authors advocate prophylaxis for all patients undergoing chemical peels beyond the superficial dermis. Any existing lesions should be allowed to heal completely prior to proceeding with a chemical peel [7].

A history of prior recent resurfacing by any modality or other facial surgical procedures is another important possible contraindication. Caution is warranted when resurfacing an area with vascular compromise secondary to a recent procedure.

Patients with collagen vascular disease, history of hypertrophic scarring or keloid development, advanced HIV disease, and general poor mental and physical well-being may be poor candidates for chemical peeling.

Compliance with the postpeel regimen is necessary to ensure normal wound healing and to avoid complications. Patients likely to be non-compliant or unable to avoid sun exposure because of occupation are unsuit-

able candidates. Men are less optimal candidates for chemical peels as their thicker, oilier skin promotes uneven penetration of the chemical agents. Patients with decreased numbers of epithelial appendages from radiation therapy or isotretinoin (Accutane) use are also poor candidates because of slower healing and an increased likelihood of scarring. Recent use of Accutane is considered a contraindication to medium or deep peels. It is recommended to wait at least 1 year after stopping using Accutane prior to embarking on chemical peel procedures. This allows for regrowth of epithelial appendages, which are essential for postpeel reepithelialization. While the technique of chemical peeling is relatively simple, the real challenge lies in appropriate patient and peeling agent selection.

10.3.2
Pretreatment

Once a patient has been appropriately selected to undergo a chemical peel, informed consent, including a detailed discussion of possible complications, is obtained. The patient should have the procedure and the recovery process explained in detail before the peel is performed. Especially for medium and deeper peels, patients should receive postoperative instructions in advance so they may prepare for the recovery period. Some physicians also routinely prescribe oral antibiotics in advance for the postoperative period [8].

Some authors recommend preconditioning the skin in order to maximize results from a chemical peel. The exfoliative agent transretinoic acid (tretinoin, Retin-A, Renova) may be helpful to facilitate uniform penetration of the peeling agent and promote more rapid reepithelialization. Retin-A promotes thinning of the stratum corneum with shedding of keratinocytes, disperses melanin throughout the epidermis, and induces activation of dermal fibroblasts.

Pretreatment with 4–8% hydroquinone blocks can be useful when treating dyschromias or Fitzpatrick types III–VI. Hydroquinone functions by blocking tyrosinase from forming precursors for melanin.

Many patients tolerate the chemical peels without any sedation or analgesia. If needed, patients can be offered diazepam or celecoxib (Celebrex) orally 1 h before the peel. Both EMLA and ELA-Max have been shown to decrease the discomfort felt during medium-depth combination chemical peeling without influencing either the clinical or the histopathologic result [9]. Reassurance and a cooling fan are always helpful for patient comfort throughout the procedure.

Patients are instructed to avoid using makeup for 24 h before the peel. Prior to the peel, the patient should thoroughly clean the face with non-residue soap the evening before and the morning of the procedure. The patient is instructed not to apply makeup or moisturizers. The skin is cleansed in the physician's office immediately prior to the procedure with acetone, ether, Freon, or isopropyl alcohol to remove any residual cosmetics, oil, or debris. Although a vigorous degreasing is important, care must be taken not to abrade the skin as this may cause increased uptake of the chemical and thus an uneven peel. Some authors have also suggested the use of povidone–iodine or Septisol prior to the alcohol or acetone wash. This cleansing step is important to ensure uniform penetration of the peeling agent.

10.3.3
Chemical Peels

A variety of chemical agents can be used to accomplish chemoexfoliation for facial rejuvenation. The effect of the peel is secondary to the depth of epidermal–dermal injury incurred. Thus, in selecting a peel one must factor in the depth of injury needed for the desired result, the pigmentary changes associated with each agent, the toxicities, and the individual physician's experience and comfort with the various agents.

Chemical peeling is generally classified by the depth of penetration into superficial, medium, and deep peels. Superficial peels typically have a depth of penetration of 0.06 mm, removing the most superficial stratum corneum and stratum granulosum. Medium-depth peels penetrate to a clinical depth into the papillary and upper reticular dermis, approximately 0.45 mm. Deep peels target the mid reticular dermis with a depth of penetration of 0.6 mm [10]. The process of healing after a chemical peel primarily involves coagulation and inflammation, followed by reepithelialization, granulation tissue formation, angiogenesis, and a prolonged period of collagen remodeling. It is this prolonged process of remodeling that accounts for the continuing clinical improvement in the months after the procedure.

Application of most peeling agents is similar. Before application, the skin to be treated is first cleansed with acetone or alcohol. Because most chemical peels are lipophobic, this facilitates greater depth and promotes even distribution of the peel. The peel is carefully applied to the subunits of the face with gauze or a cotton-tipped applicator. To ensure a consistent effect, it is important to apply the chemical evenly and avoid pooling of the agent on the face. The peel should be delicately blended with the neighboring untreated skin by feathering the edges to prevent a discrete line of demarcation.

10.3.3.1
Superficial Peels

Superficial chemical peeling is an exfoliation of the stratum corneum or entire epidermis to promote epidermal regrowth with a more rejuvenated appearance. Superficial chemical peeling is a treatment with many benefits and few risks or side effects. It is can be performed on individuals of all ages, as early as ages 25–30, when the first effects of photoaging become evident. Superficial chemical peels can minimize fine lines resulting from sun damage, acne, and rosacea. Repeat superficial peels may be required to achieve optimal effects. Patients must be counseled that multiple superficial peels do not produce results equivalent to those of a medium or deep chemical peel. Superficial peeling agents include α-hydroxy acids (AHAs) such as 20–50% glycolic acid, salicylic acid, Jessner's solution, and 10–30% TCA.

α-Hydroxy Acids

AHAs have been used for thousands of years to improve the appearance of the face. Cleopatra herself is rumored to have used the debris from the bottom of wine barrels for facial rejuvenation. AHAs function by promoting keratinocyte discohesion in the granular cell layer, causing increased cell turnover. Commonly used AHAs are derived from fruit and dairy products, such as glycolic acid from sugar cane, lactic acid from fermented milk, citric acid from fruits, tartaric acid from grapes, and malic acid from apples. Glycolic acid is currently the most commonly used AHA.

The efficacy and penetrating depths of AHAs are dependent on their concentration, the vehicle, and the pH. Over-the-counter AHA products containing 3–10% glycolic acid or other naturally occurring organic acids cause exfoliation over several weeks and may be used as a prepeel primer to potentiate the effects of higher-concentration peel procedures or other resurfacing modalities.

Professional-grade AHA peels usually contain 50% or higher AHA. Unlike other peeling agents, penetration of AHAs is time-dependent. The time to peel is dependent on both the concentration and the pH of the acid. Higher concentrations and lower pHs require shorter peeling periods. The AHA peel is applied with a sponge or gauze, systematically proceeding from one facial region to another. After placement of an AHA preparation, the skin becomes erythematous. The mild stinging and redness typically disappears 1 h after treatment. Development of a white frost is not a desirable outcome of an AHA peel as it denotes penetration depth into the dermis. Removal of the agent is achieved by rinsing with water or neutralization with an alkaline solution such as sodium bicarbonate. Deeper than intended peeling may occur if neutralization is not performed within the correct time. The subsequent exfoliation takes place over a few days and reepithelialization is usually complete within 7–10 days. Multiple treatments may be required to achieve the desired results and should be spaced several weeks apart to allow epidermal recuperation. AHA peels produce the least profound results of the chemical peeling agents; however, they are associated with the lowest frequency of complications.

AHAs, such as glycolic acid, can also be mixed with facial cleaners or creams in lesser concentrations as part of a daily skin-care regimen to improve the skin's texture or to maintain results following a resurfacing procedure.

Salicylic acid

β-Hydroxy acids, also known as salicylic acids, provide a safe, mild rejuvenation to skin. Salicylic acid functions via keratolysis, is lipid-soluble, and has a predilection for sebum-containing cells, making it an excellent peel for comedonal acne. In addition to acne, salicylic acid is helpful in treatment of oily skin, textural changes, melasma, and postinflammatory pigmentation with minimal side effects. Another benefit of salicylic acid is that it does not need to be neutralized. After applying salicylic acid to the skin, salt formation on the skin is seen.

Jessner's peel

Jessner's solution is a combination of salicylic acid, lactic acid, and resorcinol in alcohol [11]:
- 14 g resorcinol
- 14 g salicylic acid
- 14 ml 85% lactic acid
- 100 ml 95% ethanol (qs)

Considered a mild-medium peeling agent, this formulation was designed to minimize the toxicities inherent to each individual agent. This solution must be stored in a dark bottle as light will discolor the solution and cause staining. Repetitive layers of Jessner's solution may be applied to effect a slightly deeper peel. Jessner's solution peeling action is through intense keratolysis. Its ability to disrupt the barrier function of the epidermis makes it an ideal primer for TCA peels, allowing the TCA to penetrate effectively and evenly [11]. Independently, Jessner's solution is an easy-to-use peeling agent with-

out timing restriction. Skin sloughing occurs within 2–4 days after application with subsequent epidermal regrowth.

10.3.1.2
Medium-Depth Peels

Medium-depth chemical peeling is defined as controlled damage to the papillary dermis, and can be performed in a single procedure [12]. Indications for medium-depth peel include destruction of epidermal lesions and actinic keratoses, resurfacing moderately photoaged skin, correction of dyschromias, and repair of mild acne scars. Although agents such as pyruvic acid or full-strength phenol can be used to achieve a medium-depth peel, the classic agent is TCA.

10.3.1.3
Trichloroacetic Acid

TCA is a versatile chemoexfoliative agent in that it can be used as a superficial-intermediate to deep peeling agent in varying concentrations (Figs. 10.1–10.3). The depth of penetration of a TCA peel corresponds to increasing concentrations of TCA. At lower concentrations of 10–35% TCA, only a superficial peel is rendered. The results of superficial-depth TCA peels include mild reversal of fine wrinkles and improvement in dyspigmentation with less recovery period and risk than deeper TCA peels or peel combinations.

At higher concentrations, such as 50% and above, TCA behaves comparably to a phenol peel; however, the depth of the wound to the reticular dermis with 50%+ TCA increases concurrently with the rate of scarring and dyschromias. Many authors feel that 35% is the highest concentration of TCA which can be reliably used. Therefore, to safely improve epidermal penetration to the desired medium-depth peel, 35% TCA is usually preceded by a superficial keratolytic agent such as solid CO_2, Jessner's solution, or 70% glycolic acid. Two proprietary TCA-based agents, the TCA Masque (ICN Pharmaceuticals, Costa Mesa, CA, USA) and the TCA Blue Peel (Obagi), are also commonly used.

TCA's peeling mechanism of action at lower concentrations is via protein precipitation. TCA is a keratocoagulant that produces a frosting or whitening of the skin, which is dependent on the concentration used. Level I frosting, which is defined as erythema with streaky whitening of the face, is the end point for superficial resurfacing. Level II frosting is described as even white-coated frosting with patches of erythema showing through. Level III frosting, clinically signifying penetration through the papillary dermis, is a solid white enamel frost with minimal visible erythema. Level III frosting should be reserved for regions exhibiting severe actinic damage.

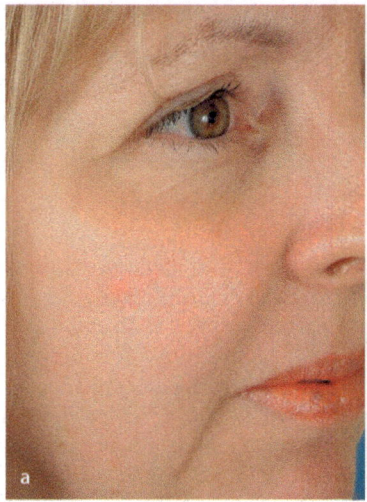 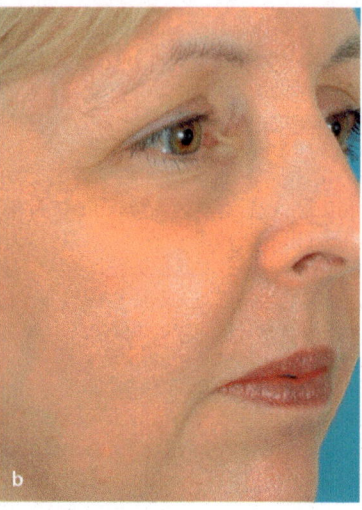

Fig. 10.1 Forty-eight year-old woman. **a** Prior to treatment. **b** Three months after 35% trichloroacetic acid medium-depth chemical peel

The dose of TCA applied is dependent on the amount of agent used, the concentration, and the physician's technique. For example, vigorous rubbing of the agent, as compared with blotting, yields a deeper penetration. The systematic application of TCA with a sponge or brush involves treating the face in a sequence of subunits. During the procedure, if frosting is not uniform, reapplication may be performed until the desired level is reached. To achieve effective treatment of the whole face, certain areas and lesions require specialized care. Thicker keratotic areas may necessitate additional or more vigorous application of the TCA for deeper penetration. Eyelid skin is treated with the patient's head elevated and the eyes closed. The TCA is carefully applied with a semidry applicator extending to within 2–3 mm of the lid margin. With many variables involved, which can be specifically adjusted according the patient's skin type and the areas being treated, the medium-depth TCA peel can be individualized for each patient.

Appropriate analgesia is necessary as TCA application is associated with an intense burning sensation that resolves within 30 min. Patient comfort may also be improved by cooling the face with a fan and by applying iced saline-soaked sponges prior to moving from one facial region to another. Once the procedure is completed, skin sloughing proceeds for several days, and reepithelialization occurs within 7–10 days. Patient discomfort can be controlled with oral pain medications. An advantage of the TCA peels is that the solution is neutralized by the body's serum, and there is no other associated toxicity.

10.4
Adjunctive Measures

In patients susceptible to hyperpigmentation, pretreatment with a bleaching agent may be preventive. Hydroquinone, an isomer of resorcinol and phenol, is commonly used. Other bleaching agents include kojic acid and azelaic acid.

Individuals with more significant laxity of deeper skin structures may benefit from other facial rejuvenative procedures, including rhytidectomy, browlift, and/or blepharoplasty in appropriately selected patients. Simultaneous facelift and chemical peel are generally approached with caution as there is a higher likelihood of full-thickness flap loss when peeling over elevated flaps.

Other adjunctive cosmetic procedures include treatment of dynamic wrinkles with Botox and filling very deep furrows or scars with facial fillers.

10.5
Postoperative Care

Postoperative care is designed to provide an ideal environment for moist wound healing. Initially, a generous amount of bland ointment, such as Aquaphor, petroleum jelly, or A&D ointment, is applied to the entire treatment area. This serves as an occlusive ointment, which protects and hydrates the skin. The use of more heavily formulated products can irritate the delicate, healing skin and interfere with the peeling process. Crisco vegetable shortening historically was used quite successfully, but has since been reformulated and now may actually be irritating. Patients are instructed to reapply the ointment throughout the day or night, whenever the face feels tight or dry. The initial inflammatory response is an erythematous and edematous reaction lasting from 12 to 36 h. During this period, patients may experience marked edema of the periocular region as well as the entire face. As the outer layers begin to shed, the patient is allowed to shower and gently wash the face with a mild cleanser. After showering, the face should be patted dry and a new coating of ointment applied.

Patients are instructed not to pick at the face during the recovery period. For the best results, the patient should allow the skin to peel independently and resist the temptation to assist the peeling process. The use of loofahs, natural facial sponges, skin brushes, or any skin exfoliants is forbidden as manipulation of the skin prior to complete reepithelialization can result in prolonged erythema, bacterial infection, and scarring. Cool clean compresses and elevation of the head of the bed can provide symptomatic relief of discomfort. The skin is generally reepithelialized by 7–10 days after the peel, at which point makeup can be applied. A formal consultation with an aesthetician is valuable in educating patients on how to camouflage resolving erythema. Skin-care services such as superficial peels and microdermabrasion are not to be resumed until 3 months af-

ter a medium-deep peel. Medium-depth chemical peels need not be repeated for at least 1 year. Sunscreen is crucial to prevent further actinic damage and to prevent hyperpigmentation. The patients should be meticulous in avoiding sun exposure during this period, as any sun damage during this delicate recovery time could prolong postprocedure erythema and the wound-healing process.

Following, some practitioners prescribe topical agents containing platelet products or growth factors. Although these products have been reported to improve wound healing, no randomized controlled clinical trials

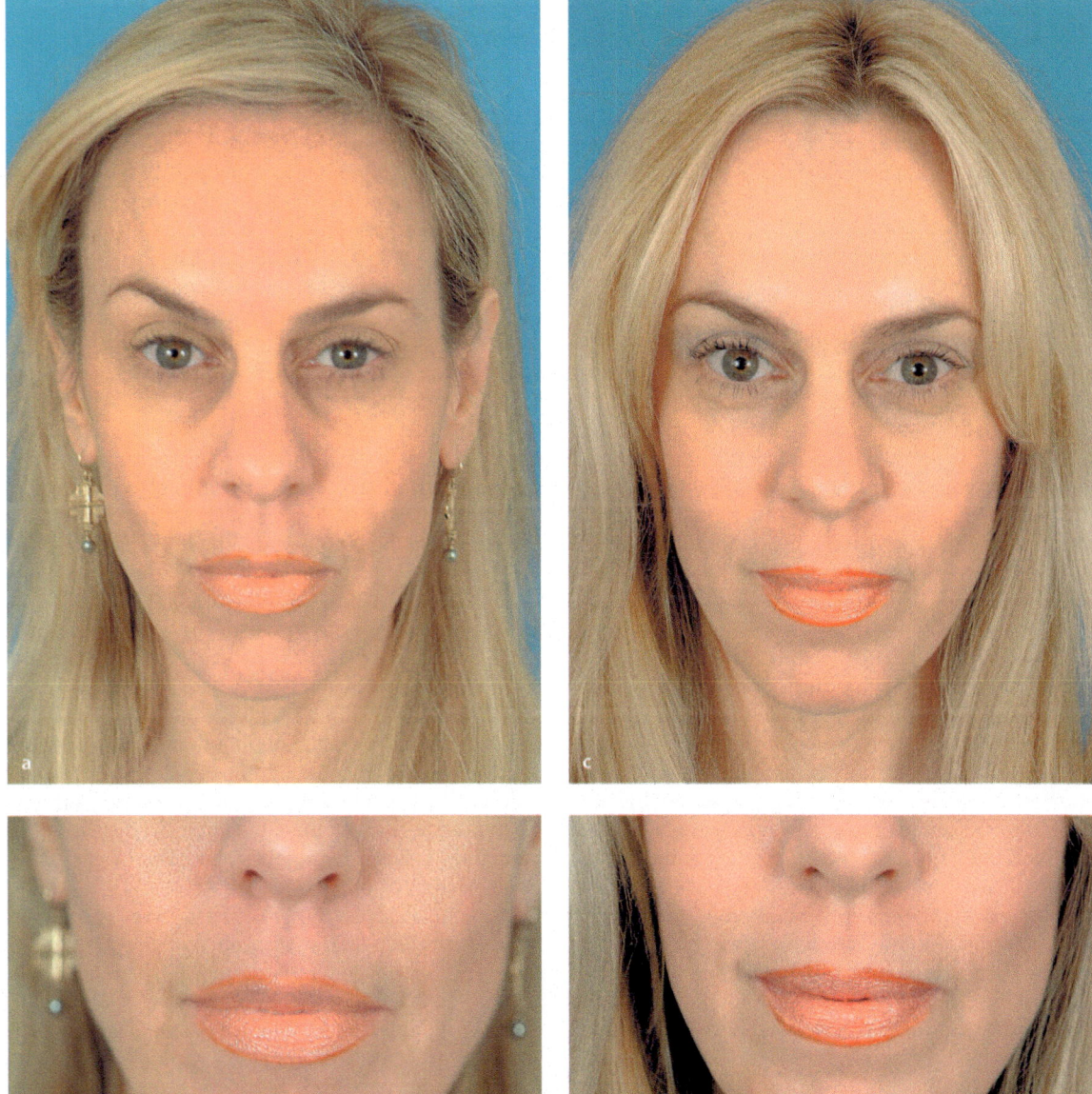

Fig. 10.2 Forty-nine year-old woman. **a**, **b** Prior to treatment. **c**, **d** After 35% trichloroacetic acid medium-depth peel

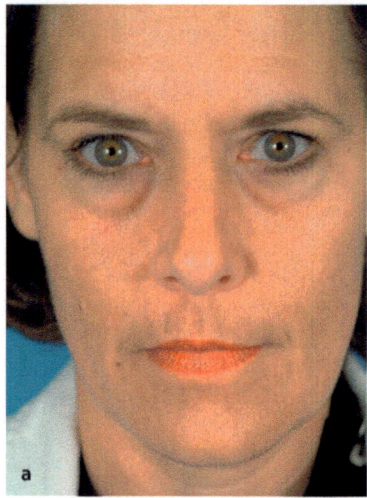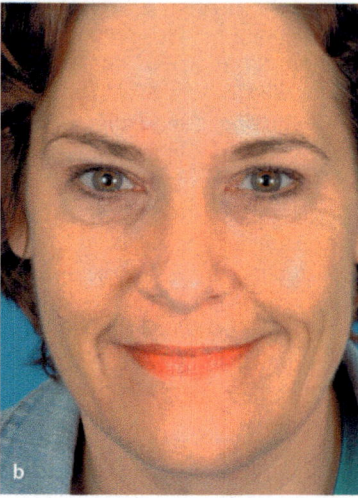

Fig. 10.3 Forty-seven year-old woman. **a** Prior to treatment. **b** After superficial chemical peel

presently support their use in this specific setting. Further research is necessary to determine the clinical utility of these agents in the chemical peel process.

10.6 Complications

Chemical peeling may result in a profound rejuvenation of facial skin; however, this treatment is not without potential complications. Results and complications are generally related to the depth of wounding, with deeper-penetration peels providing more marked results and a concomitant higher incidence of complications.

When the resurfacing agent removes the epidermis and a portion of the dermis, an important immunologic barrier between the patient and the environment no longer exists. An occlusive dressing, a topical ointment, or the body's own exudate provides some protection; however, the healing wound is more susceptible to both bacterial and fungal infections than the undisturbed skin. Delayed healing can be seen secondary to viral, bacterial, and fungal infections. Although bacterial infections are relatively rare, these infections can be avoided with the use of perioperative antiviral and antibiotic medications and good wound care. Infectious complications demand vigilance and aggressive therapy with oral and topical antibiotics. *Staphylococcus* and *streptococcus* are the most common culprits when bacterial infections occur. Pseudomonas infections occasionally occur and may be recognized by Woods-lamp examination. Treatment of pseudomonas infections includes cleansing with 0.25% acetic acid and appropriate antibiotics. The trauma of the resurfacing procedure may reactivate a viral infection (e.g., HSV). Persistent pain after the peel may be an indication of secondary herpetic infection. Preoperative prophylaxis for HSV is prudent as herpes infections have been documented in patients with no prior history of outbreaks. Herpes

exacerbations are treated with oral and topical antivirals until resolution. The physician must be vigilant for signs of infection to prevent scarring.

Cicatricial complications may be cosmetic failures alone or they may complicate a case by imposing a functional deficit on a patient, particularly in the periorbital area. Scarring is one of the most significant complications following chemical peel. Care must be taken to properly screen patients. The use of Accutane in the last 1–2 years, history of keloid formation, radiation therapy, and collagen vascular disease all may predispose the patient to scarring and may make the patient a poor candidate for chemical peel. Scarring is unusual when the chemical agent is properly mixed and when the skin is effectively cleansed of all surface debris. Nevertheless, scarring may occur if multiple passes of the peeling agent are applied to a single area during the same session. An initial pass weakens the barrier and can permit a subsequent pass of the chemical to penetrate to a deeper level in the skin. Patiently waiting for frosting to occur can prevent this technical error. Delay in wound healing may lead to scarring, a severe complication requiring close follow-up and aggressive early treatment. Steroids administered topically or intralesionally, silicone sheeting, pressure dressing, and scar massage may improve outcome. Scar excision or dermabrasion may be necessary in cases of persistent unsatisfactory results.

Pigment changes after resurfacing are among the most frustrating to the surgeon and the patient because they can occur despite proper patient selection and excellent technique. They also are among the most common complications. Pigment complications after chemical peels may involve either hyperpigmentary or hypopigmentary changes. Erythema generally subsides within 90 days, but may persist as hyperpigmentation. Patients at increased risk are those taking oral contraceptive pills, exogenous estrogens, or other photosensitizing medications or patients with a history of posttraumatic hyperpigmentation. Hyperpigmentation after a chemical peel is best avoided by careful patient selection. Test spots may be performed on darker-skinned patients before the peel. The application of hydrocortisone topically or a short course of systemic steroids may lead to earlier resolution. Other treatments, including transretinoic acid, glycolic acid, or hydroquinone, can be useful in reducing pigmentary changes after the peel. Accompanying pruritus may be treated with oral antihistamines. Following chemical peeling, the skin is typically hypersensitive to the sun, which may be a source of additional hyperpigmentation. Sun avoidance and daily sunscreen application following the peel should be strongly endorsed to minimize pigmentary alterations. Pretreatment and posttreatment with a bleaching agent, such as hydroquinone, may minimize this problem in the susceptible patient.

Hypopigmentation is a late sequela of resurfacing and is extremely difficult to treat. Hypopigmentation is the result of melanocyte destruction or inhibition. Melanocytes are not capable of regeneration or division. It is encountered most frequently following phenol peeling, which has caused many clinicians to abandon phenol in favor of other peeling agents. Most noticeable in darker-skinned patients, hypopigmentation may be difficult to assess until postprocedure erythema has subsided, at which point the condition may have unfortunately become permanent. Care must be taken upon initial application of the peel agent to feather the margins to avoid a sharp border between the treated and untreated areas. This may be accomplished either by using a less concentrated formulation or by applying less of the peeling agent in these regions. Camouflage makeup may conceal this and other pigmentary disturbances. When a line of demarcation is apparent between peeled and unpeeled areas of the face, the untreated skin may be resurfaced. Feathering a chemical peel into the neck can help blur the demarcation between the jaw and the neck.

Milia commonly develop after a chemical peel. Their appearance 2–3 weeks after a peel may be secondary to the use of occlusive ointments used during the healing period. They may spontaneously resolve or require removal by mild exfoliation or lancing.

Although uncommon, marked conjunctivitis and corneal abrasions have been reported after seepage of 35% TCA into the eye of a patient undergoing peel application. Chemical peel solutions must be applied extremely carefully in the periorbital regions to avoid ocular complications, which can be quite grave if not addressed in a timely manner [13].

Systemic complications from chemical peel resurfacing are quite uncommon, yet potentially disastrous. Toxic shock syndrome (secondary to *Staphylococcus aureus infection*) has been rarely reported, and can occur in association with any infected wound. Most often, toxic shock syndrome begins on the second or third day after treatment, with the patient often presenting with fever, a desquamating rash, and hypotension. Treatment includes hospital admission, supportive care, aggressive cleansing of the wound, and antibiotics.

10.7
Discussion

The art of facial chemical peels encompasses a wide variety of chemical agents and application techniques. When a standardized technique is used, it is possible to quantify the therapeutic effects and to predict the outcome reliably. Variations of chemical peels will be used as clinicians try to achieve better results. If possible, variations from standard techniques should be scientifically studied and quantified to establish their safety and efficacy. Using careful clinical assessment and technique, one can safely and reliably undertake facial chemical peeling to combat photoaging.

10.8
Conclusions

Expertly performed chemical peels with healthy wound healing can achieve a significant reduction in facial rhytids, dyschromias, solar changes, acne, and superficial scarring. The best results for a chemical peel rest both with the cosmetic surgeon as well as with the patient. The need for explicit pretreatment education and stringent posttreatment care cannot be overemphasized. Ultimately it is a combination of the surgeon's technique and the patient's compliance with the wound-care instructions that determines the overall result. Setting realistic expectations for patients is imperative to the success of the chemical peeling process and will serve to maximize patient satisfaction.

References

1. Unna PG: Die Histopathologie der Hautkrankheiten. Berlin, Hirschfeld 1894:816–820
2. Hirsch RJ, Dayan SH, Shah AR: Superficial skin resurfacing. Facial Plast Surg Clin North Am 2004;12(3):311–321
3. Fulton JE, Porumb S: Chemical peels: their place within the range of resurfacing techniques. Am J Clin Dermatol 2004;5(3):179–187
4. Rubin M: Manual of chemical peels. Philadelphia, Lippincott 1995
5. Fitzpatrick TB: The validity and practicality of sun-reactive skin types I through VI. Arch Dermatol 1988;124:869–871
6. Glogau RG: Aesthetic and anatomic analysis of the aging skin. Semin Cutan Med Surg 1996;15(3):134–138

7. Sabini P: Classifying, diagnosing, and treating the complications of resurfacing the facial skin. Facial Plast Surg Clin North Am. 2004;12(3):357–361

8. Manuskiatti W, Fitzpatrick RE, Goldman MP, Krejci-Papa N: Prophylactic antibiotics in patients undergoing laser resurfacing of the skin. J Am Acad Dermatol 1999;40:77–84

9. Koppel RA, Coleman KM, Coleman WP: The efficacy of EMLA versus ELA-Max for pain relief in medium-depth chemical peeling: a clinical and histopathologic evaluation. Dermatol Surg 2000;26(1):61–64

10. Matarasso SL, Glogau RG: Chemical face peels. Dermatol Clin 1991;9(1):131–150

11. Monheit GD: The Jessner's-trichloroacetic acid peel. An enhanced medium-depth chemical peel. Dermatol Clin 1995;13(2):277–283

12. Halaas YP: Medium depth peels. Facial Plast Surg Clin North Am 2004;12(3):297–303

13. Fung F, Sengelmann RD, Kenneally CZ: Chemical injury to the eye from trichloroacetic acid. Dermatol Surg 2002;28:609–610

Chapter 11

Chemical Peeling Rejuvenation of the Neck

11

Samuel M. Lam, Ross A. Clevens

11.1
Introduction

Skin rejuvenation of the neck is a subject that has received little attention owing mainly to the fear that ablative resurfacing in this area was simply thought to be unsafe and risky. However, the authors' clinical experience with ablative chemical resurfacing in this area has borne out a remarkable aesthetic benefit without concomitant morbidity profile. Understanding how to approach the neck area can be an important adjunct in the armamentarium of global facial rejuvenation.

Rejuvenation of facial skin alone can lead to a marked and glaring disparity between the treated face and untreated neck that can be unsatisfying for the patient and also appear generally unnatural, especially in those individuals with advanced cervical skin aging. The major reward in treating the extended décolletage area is the ability to achieve rejuvenation that blends more seamlessly with a rejuvenated face. The major treatment modality that has been used for neck-skin rejuvenation is a combination of Jessner's solution pretreatment followed by 25–35% trichloroacetic acid (TCA) application. Traditionally, most practitioners have advocated a more conservative policy of a TCA concentration not exceeding 20% in the cervical region, as the pilosebaceous glands, the primary skin regenerative unit, are sparser in the entire body compared with the face proper. However, this low concentration can oftentimes fail to achieve the desired aesthetic improvement. Even Jessner's solution-35% TCA may require an additional treatment session after several months to arrive at the intended cosmetic result. Nevertheless, chemical rejuvenation of the neck with Jessner's solution and TCA has led to notable and satisfactory improvements when combined with similar (TCA) or deeper treatment modalities for the face (plasma or CO_2 laser resurfacing).

11.2
Patient Selection

The patient who is typically a candidate for ablative chemical rejuvenation of the neck region falls within the Fitzpatrick I–III range (Table 11.1) [1] and has sufficient solar damage to render facial ablative therapy appear mismatched with the untreated neck area.

Certain predisposing factors may make an individual unsuitable for ablative neck-skin rejuvenation, including use of isotretinoin (Accutane) over the recent preceding 1–2 years, a history of radiation exposure to the intended treatment area or a history of hypertrophic scarring in general. If the patient reports marked sensitivity to various topical agents, like fragrances or skin-care products, he or she may not be an ideal candidate either. Recent tanning may predispose toward a more exuberant postinflammatory hyperpigmentation response and may benefit from both delays in treatment as well as pretreatment with 4% hydroquinone. Obviously, the physician should proceed with caution in any smoker or past smoker owing to the higher risk of poor wound healing. Although the majority of treated

Table 11.1 Fitzpatrick's sun-reactive skin types

Skin type	Skin color	Tanning response
I	White	Always burn, never tan
II	White	Usually burn, tan with difficulty
III	White	Sometimes mild burn, tan average
IV	Brown	Rarely burn, tan with ease
V	Dark brown	Very rarely burn, tan very easily
VI	Black	No burn, tan very easily

patients have fallen within the Fitzpatrick I–III range, it can be safe to treat sun-damaged Fitzpatrick type IV individuals with lower concentrations (20–25% TCA) and with possibly repeat treatments as necessary.

During the preoperative phase, it is important also to evaluate the patient carefully for any suspicious skin lesions that would indicate dermatologic referral or confirmatory biopsy. For actinic keratoses and other non-frankly malignant cutaneous lesions, chemical peeling may also lead to a reduction or elimination of these entities. Unlike topical treatments like 5-flouro-uracil (Effudex) that may leave the patient unsightly for 3–4 weeks, chemical rejuvenation not only reduces the incidence of actinic keratoses but also yields wonderful aesthetic improvement to the entire treated area at the same time.

The Glogau scale (Table 11.2) [2] for skin wrinkles can also be a useful guide in determining the strength of TCA to be used. For a patient with only Glogau type II aging, 25% TCA may be sufficient; whereas for more advanced Glogau type IV aging, 35% TCA could be warranted. Although ablative chemical rejuvenation can have a quite impressive aesthetic benefit, the patient should not anticipate the profound rejuvenation that is possible following deeper ablative treatment options in the facial area. The prospective patient should expect that the principal reason for treatment of the neck is to achieve a more blended result in which the neck area more closely matches the rejuvenated state of the face. Secondarily, TCA treatment can offer the hope of some reduction in texture, tone, and color of the skin with more modest improvements in wrinkles and skin laxity. For true skin laxity, however, face and neck lifting should really be the treatment of choice to correct this condition. Like any cosmetic endeavor, preparing the patient for what to expect afterwards can be the difference between a realistic expectation and what is perceived as a feeble excuse.

As part of the preoperative regimen, use of a daily glycolic acid regimen for 4–6 weeks preceding the date of treatment can help reduce the overall thickness of the stratum corneum so that a deeper and more uniform peel can be achieved. Patients need only cease usage of the glycolic-acid regimen the day prior to resurfacing. In addition, a sunblock containing physical blocking agents like zinc oxide or titanium dioxide with a protective SPF value that equals or exceeds 30 can also reduce the incidence of postinflammatory hyperpigmentation. Those individuals who exhibit a tan or who are at greater risk for postinflammatory hyperpigmentation can also be pretreated for 4–6 weeks with 4% hydroquinone to be stopped 1 day prior to intervention.

11.3 Technique

On the day of the procedure, the patient takes a combination of an oral sedative and a narcotic, specifically 10–20 mg diazepam orally and one to two Percocet or Vicodin tablets 1 h prior to the procedure. Alternatively, Mepergan forte, which includes 50 mg Demerol, 25 mg phenergan, and 10 mg diazepam, can be administered 1 h prior to the procedure. If the patient still appears awake or anxious, an additional 5–10 mg diazepam can be given sublingually prior to the procedure as needed. The patient should also routinely take an antibiotic like Levaquin prior to the chemical peel and for the duration of reepithelialization, which lasts typically 1 week.

Prior to arriving at the clinic, the patient is advised to shampoo the hair with a baby-shampoo formulation and cleanse the face, neck, and chest with a mild skin cleanser like Eucerin or Cetaphil that morning. The patient is also instructed to avoid any kind of makeup or camouflage application that morning and should come in with a loose-fitting, button-up style shirt that he or she does not mind soiling and perhaps jettisoning if needed.

Table 11.2 Glogau's classification of skin aging

Type I: no wrinkles	Type II: wrinkles in motion	Type III: wrinkles at rest	Type IV: only wrinkles
Early photoaging: mild pigmentary changes; no keratoses; minimal wrinkles	Early to moderate photoaging: early senile lentigines visible; keratoses palpable but not visible; parallel smile lines beginning to appear	Advanced photoaging: obvious dyschromias, telangiectasia; visible keratoses; wrinkles even when not moving	Severe photoaging: yellow-gray color of skin; prior skin malignancies; wrinkled throughout, no normal skin
Patient age: 20s or 30s	Patient age: late 30s or 40s	Patient age: 50s or older	Patient age: 6th or 7th decade
Minimal or no makeup	Usually wears some foundations	Always wears heavy foundation	Cannot wear makeup— "cakes and cracks"

The entire area for treatment should then be thoroughly cleansed again with Septisol or Dial soap using a folded 4 × 4 gauze. Typically, the neck area to be included covers the entire neck including the occipital region up until where the tan-line demarcation is observed. Acetone (100%) is then used to vigorously cleanse and degrease the area, again with a folded 4×4 gauze. If the nurse or medical assistant completes these tasks, it is wise for the physician to pass over the area one more time with acetone to ensure that the entire area is thoroughly and adequately prepared.

The next step is to apply a single-pass coating of standard, unmodified Jessner's solution to the entire area using a folded 4 × 4 gauze that is moderately damp but not soaking wet (Fig. 11.1). The patient is cooled with a rotating fan as needed during this application. The physician then waits approximately 10–15 min for the Jessner's solution to accomplish the task of further reduction of the stratum corneum that will permit a deeper and more uniform TCA peel. A light and uniform frost should appear at the end of this treatment time. If an adequate frost is not observed and the patient does not complain of any notable discomfort, the physician should apply an additional coat of Jessner's solution and wait an additional 10–15 min. In the majority of cases, a single pass of Jessner's solution is adequate prior to starting chemical peeling with TCA. If the patient begins to complain of marked discomfort and a more exuberant erythema is noted, the physician may decide to modify the strength of TCA from the standard 35% concentration down to a more conservative 25% concentration.

At this point, TCA administration can be undertaken. Again, a folded 4 × 4 gauze that is moderately damp but not soaked is used to apply a single uniform pass over the entire treatment area. The patient is carefully observed for discomfort or signs of advancing depth of penetration. If the patient experiences too much discomfort, the process can be aborted with the liberal application of petrolatum ointment. Typically, mild discomfort passes after 4–10 min. The desired color end point is a relatively uniform white with a light-pink hue. A deeper opaque white or white-gray color would indicate possibly overtreatment. As the desired color end

Fig. 11.1 a Appearance of the neck and chest 3 min following the application of Jessner's solution. Note the early faint frost of the treated region. **b** Appearance of the neck and chest 7 min following the application of Jessner's solution. The frost is more uniform with greater accentuation in regions of actinic damage. **c** Appearance of the neck and chest 2 min following the application of 35% trichloroacetic acid (TCA) solution. The frost is faint with a pink hue suggesting a medium-depth peel. **d** Appearance of the neck and chest 5 min following the application of 35% TCA solution. The frost is increasingly dense and uniform, but a pink hue remains apparent confirming a medium-depth peel

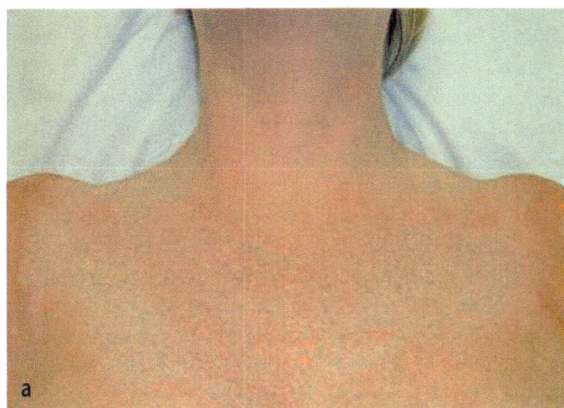
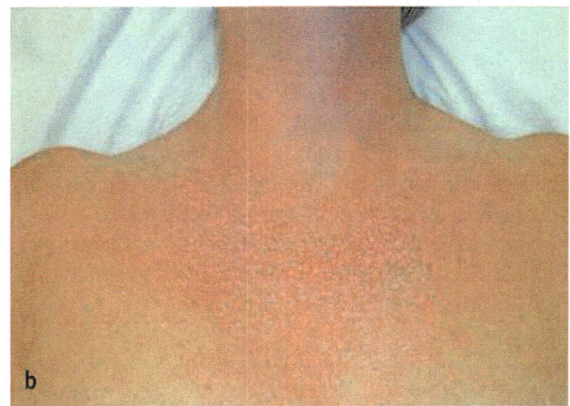
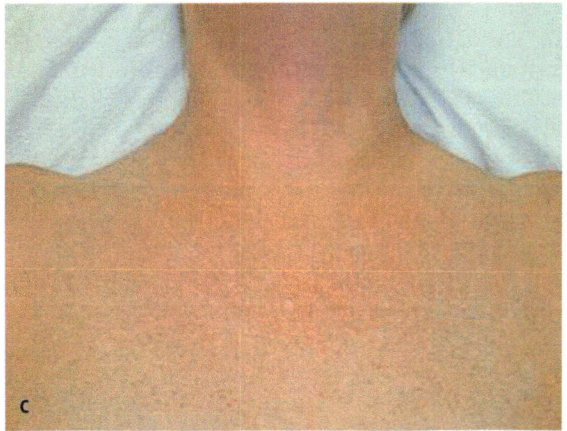
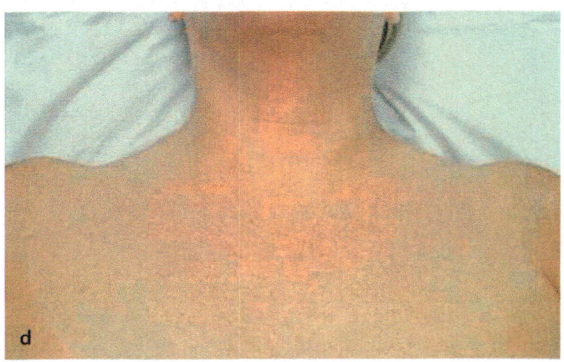

point is approached, the process can be aborted with application of petrolatum ointment. After 10–15 min, the process should be arrested with petrolatum ointment. If there is not a good response during this time, an additional single coat of 20% TCA can be applied, and the tissue reaction observed.

If the patient is under deeper sedation, then obviously patient response will be blunted or entirely muted; therefore, the physician must use appropriate judgment based only on the color changes that occur. It is advisable for a physician who has never undertaken TCA peeling of any kind to start with the face, which is a more forgiving area, when judging skin color changes that occur during the peeling process. When undertaking undermining in the submental and cervical regions, it is advisable to wait a minimum 2–3 days before initiating peeling over the undermined areas to allow time for the flaps to properly sit down. Clearly, if there is robust edema or ecchymosis, chemical peeling in the neck should be deferred for a longer time until bruising and swelling begin to subside. Generally, many patients are not inclined to undergo chemical peeling 2–3 days following a face lift owing to some fatigue and discomfort, and it may be advisable to defer treatment until the fifth to seventh postoperative day as needed.

11.4
Postoperative Care

The postoperative care for the peeled patient is straightforward. The patient should wait approximately 24 h before bathing and showering to minimize irritation to the recently treated area. In addition, only mild cleansers like Eucerin and Cetaphil should be used to cleanse the skin to reduce the risk of contact dermatitis. All treated areas need to be coated with a thick application of petrolatum ointment, like Vaseline or Aquaphor. Unlike the epithelial peeling and shedding that is typically observed in the face, the neck tends not to peel in sheets

but simply turns a bright red and may flake occasionally. These differences in the peeling process between the neck and the face should be remarked and explained to the patient, especially when concurrent face and body peeling is undertaken. The erythema may linger for typically a period of 5–12 days following the peel session.

11.5
Complications

The authors have had no cases of observed hypertrophic scarring, keloid scarring, or infection. The standard risks following chemical peeling or other resurfacing are always possible and should be kept in mind. The most common sequela that has been encountered is prolonged erythema that can linger for 7–14 days and is accompanied by the sensations of tightness, pruritus, and discomfort. A topical steroid cream, 0.05% fluocinonide, delivered two or three times daily until resolution, is the treatment of choice. Supportive care with antihistamines can ameliorate the pruritus and avoid the temptation to excoriate the peeled areas.

11.6
Discussion

Although more advanced technologies exist today for neck rejuvenation, like plasma resurfacing (Portrait PSR[3], Rhytec), chemical peeling of the neck has remained a reliable, fast, and cost-effective modality to treat the neck. Oftentimes, plasma resurfacing is used to treat the face to provide a result that is comparatively superior to that achieved by TCA chemical peeling, and is then combined with TCA of the neck. Although plasma resurfacing can be used safely and effectively over the neck, it can be a tedious, time-consuming, and expensive venture. Other ablative modalities like CO_2 laser resurfacing and phenol peels are too aggressive to

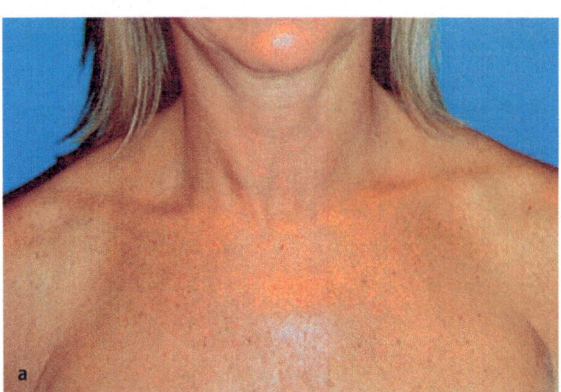
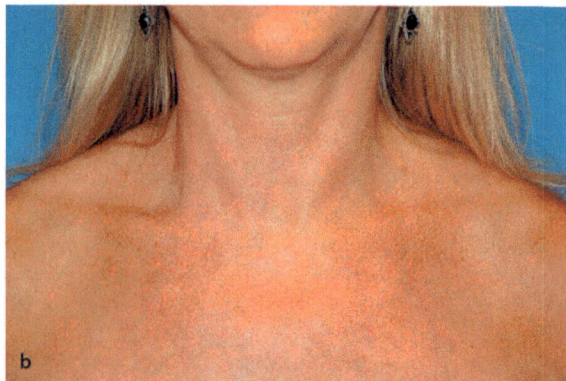

Fig. 11.2 A 44-year-old woman. **a** Before treatment. **b** Four months after a single combined Jessner's solution–35% TCA chemical peel of the neck and chest in conjunction with nitrogen plasma resurfacing of the full face

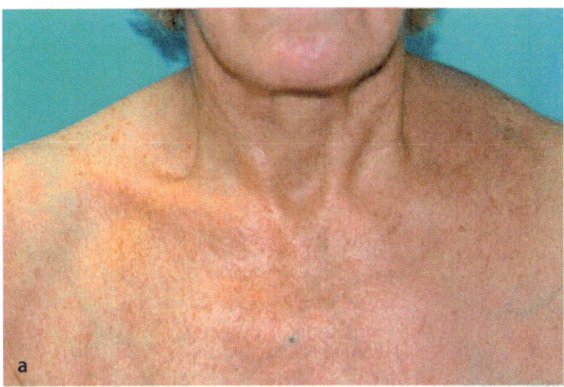 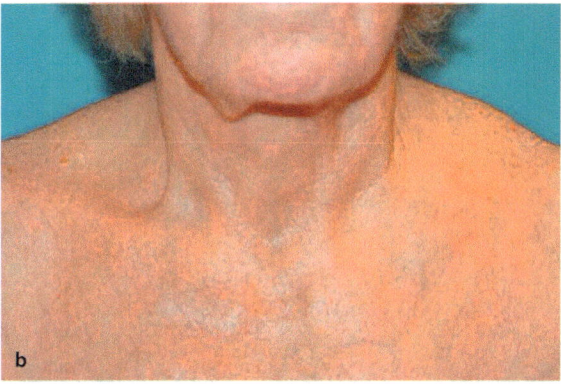

Fig. 11.3 A 51-year-old woman. **a** Before treatment. **b** Six months after a single combined Jessner's solution–30% TCA chemical peel of the neck and chest in conjunction with combined Jessner's solution–35% TCA chemical peel of the full face

be used on the neck and should be avoided for the risk of prolonged healing and ultimately scarring. When using plasma resurfacing on the sensitive neck area, caution should be adhered to in using only low settings of 1–1.9 J/cm² and to repeat treatment every 3–4 weeks as necessary.

damaged individual (Figs. 11.2, 11.3). This stepwise approach has enjoyed a limited morbidity profile with good aesthetic outcome, with the occasional need for a secondary session several months afterward to attain the desired results. Patient satisfaction has been high and complications low for this valuable ancillary treatment modality.

11.7
Conclusions

Ablative TCA peeling with Jessner's solution and 35% TCA has become a useful adjunct in global skin rejuvenation to provide an expedient, safe, cost-effective solution that helps to achieve a more seamless result with concurrent facial skin resurfacing in the very sun

References

1. Fitzpatrick TB: The validity and practicality of sun-reactive skin types I through VI. Arch Dermatol 1988;124:869–871
2. Glogau RG: Chemical peeling and aging skin. J Geriatr Dermatol 1994;2:30–35

CHAPTER 12

Deep Phenol Chemical Peels

12

Michel Siegel, Benjamin A. Bassichis

12.1
Introduction

In the early 1960s, Baker and Gordon [1, 2] reported their experience with phenol chemical face peeling. Their initial technique involved "taping," or occluding the skin after phenol application, to prevent evaporation and increase the penetration of phenol. In 1985 Beeson and McCollough [3] reported their technique without taping, which eliminated the inability to monitor the wound after the procedure, but still achieved excellent results. Regardless of the technique used [4], phenol chemical peeling continues to offer a method of achieving spectacular results for skin rejuvenation [5]. When performed properly and with appropriate patient selection, the complication rate remains low. As with any method of skin resurfacing, the goal involves the production of a controlled and predictable, partial thickness chemical injury. In the case of phenol, penetration is to the superficial dermis, without ablation of the pilo-sebaceous unit.

12.2
Patient Selection

The most important factor in achieving a good result with phenol chemical peeling is the selection of the proper patient. Because of the depth of penetration with phenol, some degree of injury to the pigment-producing cells will occur, resulting in hypopigmentation or depigmentation of the skin. In order to camouflage this appearance, patients with lighter skin will have a better result. It is not who is a good candidate but who should not undergo phenol chemical peeling. Patients with Fitzpatrick skin types V and VI are very poor candidates, as any hypopigmentation will be obvious. Also red-haired freckled Fitzpatrick type I patients are poor candidates. Owing to the freckling, hypopigmentation in this category of patients will be more obvious as a freckled and "non-freckled" zone is created. Asian patients, notorious for pigmentary problems, are poor candidates for phenol resurfacing. Male patients with their thicker and oilier skin are less than ideal candidates. Patients with a long history of sun exposure will make poor candidates, as a line of demarcation may

be obvious after peeling owing to the mottled skin appearance of the non-peeled areas. Having excluded these categories of patients, the more ideal patients are non-freckled Fitzpatrick types I and II. Type III and IV patients can be cautiously treated as long as the patient understands the possible risks of depigmentation [6].

12.3
Technique

Phenol chemical peeling can be done as a regional peel, a periorbital and/or perioral peel, or as a full-face peel. Regional peels are done in the office after the patient's medical history has been reviewed and the patient is deemed a good candidates for phenol peeling. Either topical anesthetic cream placed 30 min prior to the procedure to the region to be peeled or a local block with 1% Xylocaine with 1:100,000 epinephrine is satisfactory for performing the procedure in the office.

Full-face peeling must be performed in an accredited facility where intravenous access is available, the patient can be sedated, the cardiac status of the patient can be continuously monitored, and immediate intervention is accessible if needed.

Skin preparation is the most important step regardless of the area to be treated. The skin must be thoroughly washed with soap to remove any traces of makeup and dirt. This is followed by skin degreasing with 100% medical grade acetone soaked gauze. It is extremely important to remove all skin oils to ensure even penetration during the peel. Once the skin has been degreased, the peeling is performed with a freshly made phenol solution. The traditional Baker–Gordon mixture (3 ml USP liquid phenol, 2 ml tap water, eight drops of Septisol liquid soap, three drops of croton oil) yields an 88% phenol solution. The solution is made by the physician in the office prior to each procedure to prevent changes in concentration from evaporation and is mixed multiple times during the procedure to prevent settling.

The mixture is applied with dampened cotton-tip applicators using a rolling motion into the skin, ensuring that the area is painted evenly and that each applicator is used only once. One pass per area is performed, allowing the skin to become frosty white, a sign of mid-dermal penetration. After waiting approximately 30 s, any areas with signs of poor penetration will be self-evident, and a limited second pass to these areas is undertaken.

The limits of perioral peeling are as follows: laterally to the nasolabial folds, inferiorly feathering 2 cm below the border of the mentum, and feathering at the vermillion border of the lips.

For periorbital peeling, the orbital subunits are marked and the patient is placed at 45°. Cotton-tip applicators are placed at the medial and lateral canthus to prevent tears from running down and possibly mixing with the phenol to produce a stronger concentration. Along the upper lid no phenol is placed along the tarsus. When the lower lids are peeled, the patient is instructed to fix the eyes on a superior point at the ceiling to increase the taughtness of the skin. The lid border is marked to 3 mm. Whenever a periorbital peel is performed the sedation is kept to a minimum so the patient is cooperative and awake enough to complain of pain in case phenol contacts the cornea. Cool saline is kept on hand in case ocular irrigation becomes necessary. Because of the anesthetic properties of phenol, discomfort during the initial application is self-limited and no further medication is given to the patient.

To avoid the possibility of cardiac arrhythmias from full-face peeling the patient's cardiac status is continuously monitored and the procedure is lengthened approximately 2 h by peeling the face as subunits. Each subunit is peeled separately, with a 20-min interval between subunits, to prevent rapid absorption of the phenol solution. Because of the renal clearance of phenol, normal renal function is essential; thus, blood urea nitrogen and creatinine levels are obtained prior to the procedure. The patient also receives about 2 l of intravenous fluids to enhance renal excretion of phenol during the peel procedure. Full-face peeling is recommended in the following order: forehead, periorbital, cheeks, perioral area, and nose. Because the action of this peel is of coagulation, no neutralization of the acid is required. At the conclusion of the procedure, Vaseline is placed along the peeled areas, providing a "semiocclusive" dressing. However, non-occlusive phenol peeling can be achieved by avoiding any petroleum-based ointments after the procedure.

Patients undergoing full-face phenol peeling are started on antiherpetic medication 3 days prior to the peel and are given antibiotics after the procedure. Patients undergoing regional peeling will be given antiviral drugs only if they have a history of cold sores.

Some patients will experience a severe burning sensation after the procedure, lasting 6–7 hours. For regional peeled patients pain and antianxiety medications will give some relief. For full-face peeled patients intravenous pain management is preferred. The pain and burning associated with this procedure usually subsides after 8 h.

During the first 7–10 days after the peel the patient is instructed to wash the face three to four times a day with vinegar, followed by application of a petroleum-based ointment. The vinegar mixture decreases the risk of fungal infection. After reepithelialization, usually after the seventh to tenth day, the patient is permitted to wash the face with a non-comedogenic, non-perfumed soap followed by application of a skin moisturizer and sunscreen. It is imperative that patients are counseled on avoiding sun exposure to prevent developing dyschromias. Any itching may be controlled with antihistamines.

Patients are followed very closely for erythema persisting after 12 weeks. Any signs of prolonged erythema are treated with a 3-week course of 2.5% hydrocortisone applied to the face twice per day.

12.4
Complications

With proper patient selection and diligent technique, the complication rate with phenol chemical peeling should be low. It is important to differentiate between true complications and transient postpeel reactions. Because of the depth of penetration of phenol there will, invariably, be injury to the pigment-producing cells. Because recovery of these cells is unpredictable, proper patient selection is imperative.

Poor feathering of the peel will result in a suboptimal cosmetic result owing to an obvious demarcation line. Feathering too low in the neck will not only cause this, but will also increase the risk of scarring because of the paucity of adnexal structures below the jaw line.

It is important to counsel patients before a phenol peel about the length of erythema associated with this procedure. It is not uncommon for patients to experience erythema from 4–12 weeks after the peel. Makeup may be applied after 2 weeks to conceal redness, but patients should be followed closely to treat persistent erythema with topically applied steroids.

The use of sunscreen for a minimum of 6 months after a peel is vital to prevent hyperpigmentation from sun exposure. Patients need to be educated that their postpeel skin is highly sun sensitive; thus, suntanning and excess sun exposure after a phenol peel are not advised.

The most common problem after a phenol peel is transient hyperpigmentation. The darker the patient, the more likely this may occur. Hyperpigmentation is usually seen around the third to fourth week after the peel. The most important step in preventing this is avoiding sun exposure. The first signs will be marked by erythema followed by the appearance of blotchy skin spots. A treatment regimen of Retin-A and hydroquinone is started and patients are seen at intervals of

2 weeks. Patients not responding to this regimen are offered a trichloroacetic acid peel.

The most feared complication of a phenol peel is postpeel hypertrophic scarring. Hypertrophic scarring results from violation of tissues deep to the reticular dermis. It may be the result of a treated herpes simplex virus (HSV) infection, peeling of tissues with poor adnexal structures, like the neck, or performing multiple passes on the face with phenol solution. Fortunately, HSV leading to hypertrophic scarring is rare as this infection responds well to antiviral therapy. The best treatment though is prevention. Patients with a history of cold sores or patients undergoing full-face phenol chemical peeling should be treated prophylactically with antiviral therapy. Hypertrophic scarring, once diagnosed, should be aggressively treated with intralesionally and topically applied steroids.

Patients should be monitored for signs of infection in the postpeel period. Bacterial infections are usually a result of poor facial hygiene. Antistaphylococcal oral antibiotics will usually resolve this problem. Fungal infections are rare as the patient keeps the pH of the skin in the acidic range using daily vinegar treatments.

Patients with a history of cold sores or undergoing full-face peeling should be started on prophylactic therapy to prevent HSV breakouts. If the patient develops an HSV outbreak after the peel, the oral dose of antiviral medication is doubled.

Milia formation is a sequela rather than a complication. Milia represent small superficial inclusion cysts, usually lasting days to weeks. Most will spontaneously resolve, but the larger ones can be "unroofed" with an 18-gauge needle.

One should be careful to perform this type of peel on patients with previous history of blepharoplasty or on patients with lower-lid laxity as these patients may develop an ectropion. Most of them will resolve, but corrective surgery may be needed in some instances.

12.5 Conclusions

Phenol chemical peeling has been safely performed for almost half a century. Phenol chemical peeling is a means of providing a controlled and predictable chemical injury to the skin (Fig. 12.1). Microscopically, phenol induces new collagen and elastin formation as well as the reorganization of melanocytes within the basement membrane. Clinically, the results of phenol chemical peeling are significant and long-lasting.

Proper patient selection and counseling regarding the length of recovery is the key to excellent results and happy patients. Because of the properties of phenol it is imperative that the patient be in good health prior to the procedure. Phenol is absorbed through the skin, detoxified in the liver, and excreted by the kidneys. Poor renal or hepatic function will result in toxic levels of phenol producing cardiac arrhythmias. Thus, patients with poor renal function, liver problems, or heart conditions may not be the best candidates for this resurfacing modality. The safety of the patient remains the number one priority. Healthy patients undergoing full-face chemical peeling should have their cardiac function continuously monitored, and application of phenol should be performed in increments of facial subunits with rest in-between applications to prevent cardiac problems.

There are certain conditions that phenol chemical peeling produces poor to minimal results, and patients with these conditions are not offered phenol peeling as an option. These include capillary hemangiomas, facial telangiectasia, port-wine stains, thermal burns, deep-pitted acne scars, and hypertrophic scars. Phenol peeling is not performed on Fitzpatrick types V and VI, or type I with freckles, owing to the abnormal hypopigmentation with severe demarcation changes. Phenol should not be applied to areas with minimal to no adnexal structures, like the neck, chest, and hands, owing to the high risk of hypertrophic scarring.

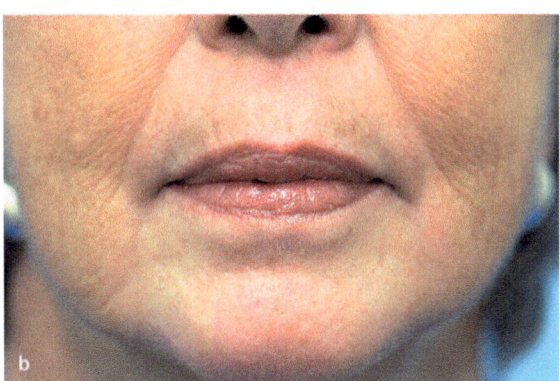

Fig. 12.1 **a** Before and **b** after deep phenol chemical peel

With the proper technique, patient selection, and counseling about the recovery time, phenol chemical peeling remains a safe and effective means of skin resurfacing.

References

1.   Baker TJ, Gordon HL: The ablation of rhytids by chemical means. A preliminary report. J Fla Med Assoc 1961;48:451–454

2.   Baker TJ, Gordon HL, Seckinger DL: A second look at chemical face peeling. Plast Reconstr Surg 1966;37(6):487–493

3.   Beeson WH, McCollough EG: Chemical face peeling without taping. J Dermatol Surg Oncol 1985;11(10):985–990

4.   Baker TJ, Stuzin JM, Baker TM: Facial Skin Resurfacing. St. Louis, Quality Medical Publishing 1998:117–143

5.   Cortez EA: Phenol chemical face peeling. Facial Plast Clin North Am 1994;2:29–41

6.   Kligman AM, Baker TJ, Gordon HL: Long term histologic follow up of phenol face peels. Plast Reconstr Surgery 1985;75(5):652–659

CHAPTER 13

The Golden Peel

13

Enrique Hernández-Pérez, Hassan Abbas Khawaja

13.1
Introduction

The two drugs most commonly used in chemical peels as an office cosmetic surgical procedure are trichloroacetic acid (TCA) and phenol. The authors use special combinations of resorcinol in different formulations that are called Golden Peel. Their formulations are shown in Tables 13.1 and 13.2. These formulations are simple, effective, inexpensive, and safe chemical peels.

The physician's skill and experience determines the technique classification for the depth of peel. The classification of Golden Peel (resorcinol) is [1, 2]:

- Superficial Golden Peel: 24% resorcinol
- Medium Golden Peel: 53% resorcinol
- Golden Peel Plus: Jessner solution plus 53% resorcinol

Table 13.1 Formulation for superficial Golden Peel

Raw materials	Percentage
Sulfur	24.0
Resorcinol	24.0
Carboxymethyl cellulose (7 mf)	0.5
Aluminum magnesium silicate	1.0
Veegum HV	
Sorbitol	2.5
Glycerin	2.5
Deionized water	45.5

Table 13.2 Formulation for medium Golden Peel

Raw materials	Percentage
Resorcinol	53.0
Glycerin monostearate	5.0
Cetyl alcohol	5.0
Deionized water	37.0

The depth of peeling agents depends on various factors, including type of skin (dry or oily), age of the patient, anatomical region, presence of previous dermatosis, preparation and defatting of the skin, strength and amount of the chosen agent, intensity of previous scrubbing, number of applications of the drug [3–5], and contact time of the peel with the skin.

13.2
Active Principle

Resorcinol, or 1,3-dihydroxybenzene, is a phenol derivative with keratolytic properties and precipitates cutaneous proteins [2]. It is soluble in water, alcohol, ether, and oil, has great affinity for oxygen, and acts as an effective reducing agent [3, 4]. The mechanism of its action is by inducing keratolysis and protein precipitation [5, 6].

When topically applied, it separates stratum corneum and the most superficial layers of the epidermis from the deeper ones; such a split seems to occur in the stratum granulosum [7]. A deep inflammatory reaction, histologically noticeable, is associated with vasodilatation, visible 6 h following its application. Findings 1 week later consist of increased mitosis in the stratum germinativum, prolonged vasodilatation of dermal vessels, proliferation of fibroblasts, a thickened papillary dermal band, and a higher concentration of elastic fibers in the deep dermis. With the exception of vasodilatation, dermal changes are still visible 4 months later [7]. The nature and intensity of these changes depend on the concentration of resorcinol applied.

In clinical terms, a resorcinol peel improves skin texture and homogenizes pigmentation, reducing senile pigmentary changes and actinic keratosis and smoothing fine perioral wrinkles [8–10]. Serious complications are rare and should not be seen when the peel is used carefully [11–13].

If deeper penetration is needed, 53% Golden Peel may be combined with Jessner solution (Golden Peel Plus) [14]. This combination provokes a reduction in solar lentigines, fine wrinkles, seborrheic keratoses, and freckles. Progressive improvement in the general appearance, skin lightening, wrinkle depth, and skin oiliness is observed after each peel [14]. Histopathologic examination shows improvement in the epidermal thickness, as well as reduction in atrophy, keratinous plugs, loss of polarity, and basal cell degeneration. Decreases in elastosis, edema, and telangiectasias are also observed. According to the depth of the biological changes (wounding) induced by this combination of peeling agents (papillary dermis and upper part of reticular dermis), it must be considered as a medium-depth peel [14].

13.3
Indications for Golden Peels

The more common indications are superficial wrinkles mostly located on the cheeks and around the eyelids and mouth. In cases of deeper wrinkles, the patients should understand the convenience of combining these peelings with the injection of filler substances. This method is not a substitute for other specific surgical procedures, such as face-lifting, which can improve the skin in a very different way. These facts must be carefully explained to the patient [1].

The procedure is also very effective in cases of oily and thick skin, in actinically damaged skin, in some patients with postinflammatory pigmentations (for instance, brown or dark-brown pigmentations secondary to acne), or to improve some superficial scars (mostly as a consequence of dermatoses such as acne, chicken pox, or neurotic excoriations). This method is also convenient for patients with busy daily schedules or those with a "tired-looking" appearance who wish a change toward a new younger look, but who are not able to take time off from their jobs [1]. They are useful, in combination with other therapeutic modalities, in the treatment of active acne, even in patients undergoing treatment with orally administered isotretinoin (Table 13.3).

A careful explanation is given to patients. Golden Peels permit only a temporary improvement of the skin, but require no convalescence period or special postoperative care. Nevertheless, with the idea in mind of maintaining an improved appearance, it is necessary to perform these interventions periodically.

These peelings can also be used in combination with other surgical procedures in order to obtain the maximum benefit; we frequently perform them along with (before or after) face-lifts, blepharoplasties, injections or filler substances, or in preparation for deep chemical peeling, according to the schedule and wishes of the patient.

Golden Peel Plus can be used for the improvement of photodamage affecting face, V-line of the neck, and dorsum of the hands and forearms. It permits a pleasing easy improvement of fine wrinkles, atrophy, yellowish discolorations, and brown spots due to age- and sun-related damage in these anatomical regions. If the surface in these areas seems to be too large, it is preferable to divide them by zones, recalling that resorcin is a phenol derivative (focal Golden Peel). In this way, no more than one area should be done per session, so as to avoid the possibility of significant absorption. Improvement may also be found in pigmentations and scars affecting the face and back. In the latter case, focal use (by sections) of Golden Peel Plus is recommended. These combinations of agents act together well to improve breast flaccidity, and in striae distensae, as well as the treatment of cellulite and lifting of the gluteus; the rational for such an effect is microscopic improvement in collagen and elastic fibers (Table 13.4). [13, 14] Treatment should be repeated every 2–4 weeks, depending upon the degree of improvement observed and the availability of the patient. Such improvement may be accentuated by combining the treatment with sunscreens, topically applied

Table 13.3 Indications for Golden Peel

Superficial wrinkles
Actinically damaged skin
Oily and thick skin
Active acne[a]
Postinflammatory pigmentations
Superficial scars
Convenience: patients with busy daily schedules
"Tired-looking" appearance
In combination with other surgical procedures

By increasing the contact time on the skin, the penetration (wound) can be made deeper.
[a]Even in patients taking isotretinoin per os

Table 13.4 Indications for Golden Peel Plus

Photodamage
Facial
V-line of the neck
Dorsum of the hands and forearms
Pigmentation and scars
Facial
Back
Breast flaccidity
Striae distensae
Lifting of the gluteus
Cellulite

tretinoin, or low doses of orally administered isotretinoin.

13.4
Technique

Patients are permitted to come to the office wearing their own cosmetics. No sedation or special preoperative preparation is required. After putting the patient in a comfortable decubitus dorsalis position, the nurse assistant removes all cosmetics or oils from the face using a cotton ball or gauze impregnated with rose water or other mild astringent.

This procedure is carried out in a very casual manner, talking continuously to the patient, with pleasant music playing in the background so that the patient remembers the procedure as a gratifying one.

A scrubbing of the face is performed, up to tolerance, using a cream containing granules of poly(ethylene glycol). Immediately after this preparation the superficial Golden Peel is begun. Paste is applied with an art brush over all the facial skin surface, sparing the eyelids (Fig. 13.1). With the patient in this position and the eyes covered with cotton balls impregnated with a cool, mild astringent, we leave the paste on the skin for 10 min the first time according to the tolerance of the patient's skin. We try to increase the time of each subsequent application progressively. Increases of 5 min each time are often very well tolerated. The applications are repeated once a week or once every 2 weeks at the beginning; after two or three treatment sessions and depending upon the availability of the patient, the patients are ready to progress to medium peeling [1]. The patients wishes must be carefully respected, however; if they feel comfortable with the same number of minutes, application is repeated for this length of time in the subsequent sessions.

Paste for performing medium Golden Peel treatment is applied in the same way (the skin is prepared by cleansing with alcohol–acetone or a mild astringent, and scrubbing with polyethylene granules). This time, however, it is left in place for 1–2 min the first time. It is necessary to have cotton balls impregnated with rose water to remove the medication as rapidly as necessary.

Depending on the tolerance of the patient's skin, we perform a new application 1 or 2 weeks later. The time is then increased by 1 min each session. However, frequently it is not necessary to apply the paste for more than 30 s to 1 min per session to achieve the desired results.

According to the patient's wishes and the time available a treatment is performed in a series of six to ten sessions on average. However, the time is never increased or nor is a different grade of peeling used until the patient's skin tolerance has been well established. Frequently patients ask for increases. The patient returns to the office once a month or once every 2–3 months.

Immediately after the removal of these pastes, the patient will notice some numbness in the area of the skin treated as well as a tingling and a mild burning. Mild to more severe burning, as well as pain, is observed only

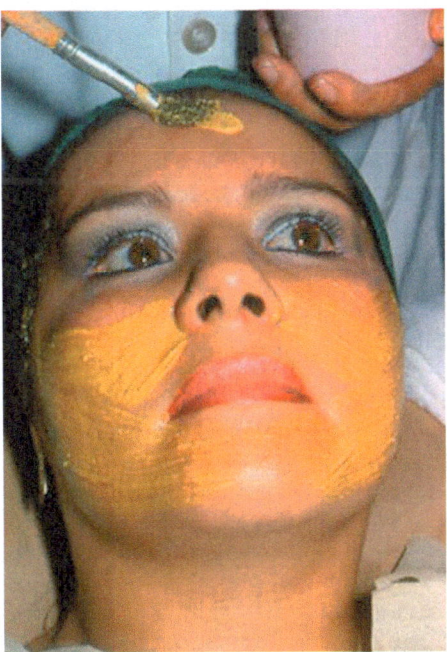

Fig. 13.1 Application of superficial and medium Golden Peel

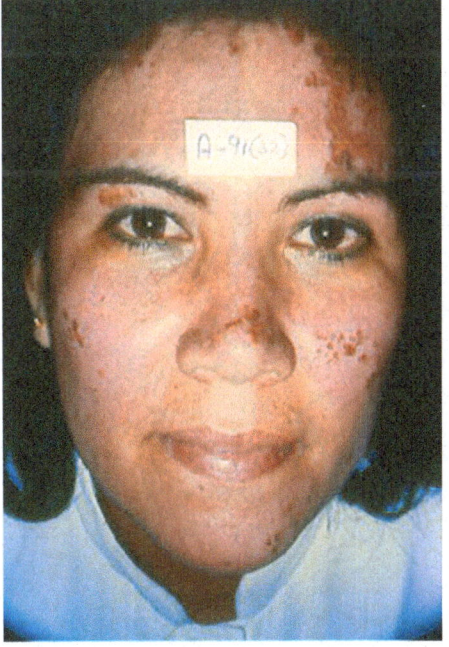

Fig. 13.2 Golden Peel Plus. Scales are thicker, but the end result is nicer (eighth day)

with application of medium Golden Peel. Sometimes acetaminophen orally or topical low-potency corticoid cream (hydrocortisone) may be necessary. These symptoms are common in periods of no more than 30 min after application.

When the patient leaves the office, most often after the medium Golden Peel treatment, the skin is slightly swollen and erythematous, showing variable grades of edema; this is more noticeable in the bony prominences (malar areas) and around the mouth. This remains for at least 2 days. It is not of sufficient magnitude to require the patient to stay at home [1].

Throughout the process, the patient is permitted to wear her own cosmetics and is asked only to avoid excessive sun exposure and to use sunscreens of SPF 15 or more.

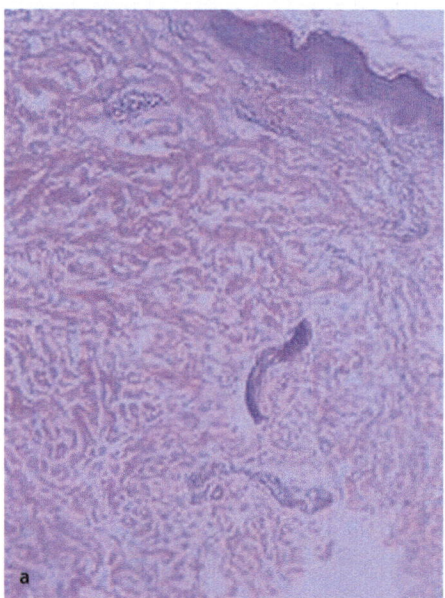

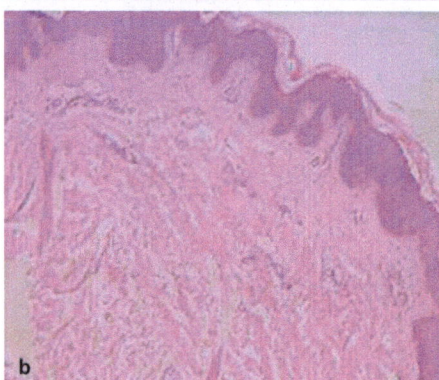

Fig. 13.3 Changes are clearly noted in epidermis and dermis, **a** before and **b** after (hematoxylin and eosin stain, ×10)

For the application of Golden Peel Plus, the skin is prepared in the same way: cleansing with astringents, scrubbing with polyethylene granules [14]. Then the Jessner solution is applied in several passes up to the point of frosting, on average 1–3 min. The medium Golden Peel paste (53% resorcinol) is then applied and left on the skin for 1 min in the first session. This time may subsequently be increased according to the patient's skin tolerance, with a burning sensation indicating termination. On average the paste is left for 2–5 min. The skin where the paste is removed becomes white in the center and edematous and congestive at the periphery. During the next 2–3 days the skin changes from congestive, red, and swollen to brown and sometimes deep brown. After 4–5 days desquamation occurs (Fig. 13.2) [14].

The effects of Golden Peel are highly selective. That can to be observed on the top of inflamed acne nodules as well as when it is used in striae distensae. Microscopic improvement in the epidermis and the dermis is also easily noted (Fig. 13.3).

Other indications for Golden Peel include striae distensae, lifting of the gluteus, breast flaccidity, and cellulite.

13.5
Complications

With the use of these formulations, the authors have not seen any case of hypopigmentation, milia, or unsightly scars as is commonly observed after deeper peelings [1, 14]. Serious complications related to resorcinol absorption [11–13] can be avoided if the appropriate precautions are taken concerning the time of contact on the skin and application of the formulations over several anatomical regions (or large areas) in the same session is avoided. On the back, for instance, the procedure must be performed focally.

In only four cases have there been mild and transitory dizziness when the patient stood up immediately after Golden Peel Plus treatment. In all of these cases, resorcinol paste had been applied at the same time on the dorsum of the hands, forearms, and V-line of the neck. No changes in blood pressure or cardiac rhythm were noted, and patients recovered after drinking a cup of coffee and reclining for 10 min in the Trendelenburg position.

There were two cases that seemed to be an authentic allergic contact dermatitis to resorcinol. The patients experienced the rapid onset of pruritus and burning, and the skin became erythematous, edematous, and showed multiple small vesicles. The condition was treated with orally administered antihistamines and topically applied corticoids, and improved rapidly.

The most common complication has been mild to moderate grades of hyperpigmentation. This occurs in less than 1% of patients, even though most are of Hispanic origin. This pigmentation does not need anything more than time in most cases to effect healing, since it is usually self-limited. However, sometimes treatment with sunscreens and 3% pure hydroquinone at night is necessary and unnecessary sun exposure as long as the skin remains erythematous should be avoided.

13.6
Discussion

Golden Peel has been successfully used for more than 30 years. Resorcinol is a phenol derivative that precipitates cutaneous proteins [8, 11]. Biopsies and microscopic analysis of women using 53% gel once a week for 10 weeks demonstrated an increase in epidermal thickness, formation of small rete pegs, decreased liquefaction of the basal layer, and formation of a subepidermal band of neocollagen [2, 11, 13]. Clinical improvement following resorcinol peel has been highly satisfactory.

The main indications for resorcinol peels in facial cosmetic surgery are [1, 14–20] acne and acne scars, superficial wrinkles, actinically damaged skin that is thick and oily, postinflammatory pigmentation (secondary to acne, neurotic excoriations or smallpox), superficial scars, and "tired" skin.

Resorcinol peels are safe, effective, inexpensive, and easy to apply. The time dedicated to each patient is very short and the peel can be applied by the assistants, not necessarily by the physician [1, 14–21]. There is no risk to patients undergoing simultaneous treatment with isotretinoin. A special period of convalescence or special care before or after the peel is not required. The patient should be told that the improvement in the skin is transitory in nature, and treatment should be repeated every 6–12 months. This period of time can be increased or the improvement can be more evident when the peel is combined with other elements of a facial rejuvenation program.

One of the hazards of phenol peel is the cardiotoxicity of phenol [16]. At high concentrations, TCA peel can produce chemical burning with unacceptable scars [17, 22, 23]. New protocols of treatment with phenol are being developed in order to avoid its inherent toxicity [16, 17]. Golden Peel, even though made of resorcinol, a phenol derivative, is free of its toxic effects.

13.7
Conclusions

Different grades of Golden Peel are simple and effective procedures can be performed in the office. Combination of Golden Peel with Jessner solution allows the physician to increase the depth of penetration. Good results are observed not only on a clinical basis but also under the microscope. Golden Peel is worth recommending.

References

1. Hernandez-Perez E: Different grades of chemical peels. Am J Cosmet Surg 1990;7:67–70
2. Hernandez-Perez E, Carpio E: Resorcinol peels: gross and microscopic study. Am J Cosmet Surg 1995;12:337–340
3. Brody HJ: Chemical Peeling. St. Louis, Mosby Year Book 1992:53–73
4. McCollough EG, Langsdon PR: Dermabrasion and Chemical Peel. A Guide for Facial Plastic Surgeons. New York, Thieme; 1988:VII
5. Rubin MG: Manual of Chemical Peels. Superficial and Medium Depth. Philadelphia, Lippincott, 1995:7–25
6. Harvey SC: Antisépticos y desinfectantes; fungicidas y ectoparasiticidas. In: A Goodman Gilman, LS Goodman, and A Gilman (eds): Las Bases Farmacológicas de la Terapéutica, 6th ed. Mexico, Panamericana, 1982:953–954
7. Drake L, Dinehart SM, Goltz RW, Graham GF, Hordinsky MK, Lewis CW, Pariser DM, Salasche SJ, Skouge JW, Turner ML, et al: Guidelines of care for chemical peeling. J Am Acad Dermatol 1995;33(3):497–503
8. Caldeira A, Lucas A: Chemical face peeling: eight years' experience. Int J Aesthet Restor Surg 1991;4:117–114
9. Chiarello SE, Resnik BI, Resnik SS: The TCA masque: a new cream formulation used alone and in combination with Jessner's solution. Dermatol Surg 1996;22(8):687–692
10. Lawrence N, Cox SE, Brody HJ: Treatment of melasma with Jessner's solution versus glycolic acid: a comparison of clinical efficacy and evaluation of the predictive ability of Wood's light examination. J Am Acad Dermatol 1997;36(4):589–593
11. Letessier SM: Chemical Peel with resorcinol. In: RK Roegnik, and HH Roegnik (eds): Dermatologic Surgery: Principles and Practice. New York, Dekker 1989:1017–1024
12. Nelson BR, Fader DJ, Gillard M, Majmudar G, Johnson TM: Pilot histologic and ultrastructural study of the effects of medium depth chemical facial peels and dermal collagen in patients with actinically damaged skin. J Am Acad Dermatol 1995;32(3):472–478
13. Hernández-Pérez E, Carpio E: Resorcinol peels: gross and microscopic study. Am J Cosmet Surg 1997;12:337–340
14. Hernández-Pérez E: Resorcinol peel as a part of facial rejuvenation program. Am J Cosmet Surg 1997;14:35–40
15. Hopping SB: Chemical peeling in 1996: what have we learned? Int J Aesth Restor Surg 1996;4:73–80
16. Coleman WP 3rd, Alt TH: Dermatologic cosmetic surgery. J Dermatol Surg Oncol 1990;16(2):170–176
17. Brandy DA: Medium-deep chemical peel utilizing Jessner's solution, 20% TCA, and Baker's phenol solution. Am J Cosmet Surg 1997;14:4–48

18. Hernández-Pérez E, Jáurez-Arce V: Gross and microscopic findings with a combination of Jessner's solution plus 53% resorcinol paste in chemical peels. Am J Cosmet Surg 2000;17:85–89

19. Hernández-Pérez E: El versátil "Golden Peel". Act Terap Dermatol 2002;25:90–97

20. Hernández-Pérez E, Jáurez-Arce V: Cutaneous aging: a review. Am J Cosmet Surg 1999;16:59–61

21. Hernández-Pérez E, Khawaja HA, Alvarez TY: Oral isotretinoin as part of the treatment of cutaneous aging. Dermatol Surg 2000;26(7):649–652

22. Rullan PP, Lemon J, Rullan J: The 2-day light phenol chemabrasion for deep wrinkles and acne scars: A presentation of face and neck peels. Am J Cosmet Surg 2004;21:199–210

23. Peters W: Full-thickness facial chemical burn from a 50% TCA peel. Plast Reconstr Surg 1995;95(3):602–603

Combined Techniques of Ablative Skin Resurfacing: Phenol, Trichloroacetic Acid, and Mechanical Dermabrasion

14

Samuel M. Lam, Thomas L. Tzikas

14.1
Introduction

Skin resurfacing is a vital component to an overall, global strategy for comprehensive facial rejuvenation that would include facial lifting procedures to counteract gravity, volume restoration to combat soft-tissue depletion associated with aging, and other ancillary modalities, like botulinum toxin and dermal fillers. Skin resurfacing can be divided into two principal categories: ablative and non-ablative. Non-ablative therapies include laser, light, and radiofrequency treatments in which the epidermis is not violated, thereby limiting recovery time but which would also potentially be less effective compared with ablative therapies. Ablative skin resurfacing entails a treatment modality (chemical, laser, and/or mechanical) that removes the overlying epidermis and partial thickness of the dermal layer in order to elicit the desired rejuvenation. By their very nature, ablative therapies require a convalescence of varying duration when the individual will not look socially acceptable. The myriad ablative skin options carry with them unique profiles that include the extent of rejuvenation, viz., the capacity to eliminate rhytids, improve dyschromias and other skin abnormalities, and a proportionate degree of recovery time depending on the depth of imparted injury. Accordingly, a combination of ablative skin therapies can effect the optimal aesthetic changes while minimizing recovery time and the likelihood of related adverse events.

This chapter will outline a strategy of how to combine different ablative skin therapies for optimal advantage for the patient and discuss the technical details of how to execute these treatment methods in a concurrent, combined fashion.

14.2
Strategy

Although many patients may benefit from only one type of ablative skin therapy, a judicious selection of different modalities can oftentimes provide the most aesthetic gain without undue morbidity. This chapter is not intended to recount every possible type of ablative skin intervention but instead to outline a strategy of combining various therapies that have worked effectively in the authors' clinical practices.

The three major types of ablative skin therapies that will be discussed herein include phenol-based peels (both straight 88% phenol and various strengths of more potent Baker–Gordon mixtures), 35% trichloracetic acid (TCA) peels, and mechanical dermabrasion. By combining these three major skin treatments, the physician can attain remarkable skin improvement with or without concurrent surgical therapies. By understanding the advantages and limitations of each modality, the physician can act like an artist with many brushes to create the desired artistic rendering.

Being aware of the salient attributes of each treatment modality will allow an understanding of the basic differences between these resurfacing methods. TCA peels can be applied lightly, as by an aesthetician, to effect mild to no epidermal ablation, typically in the range of 10–20% concentrations. Alternatively, TCA peels can be used as an ablative instrument in concentrations of 30–35% in order to provide more definitive improvement but concomitant downtime of about 1 week in duration. This higher-strength TCA treatment will be the focus of discussion herein. TCA peels work well to improve unwanted skin pigmentation and undesirable dyschromias but only effect limited improvement in rhytids. Phenol peels can provide more dramatic improvement in both rhytids and dyschromias but can result in a prolonged recovery time and the risk of hypopigmentation that is proportionate to the type of phenol mixture administered. Phenol peels work well to address the more recalcitrant lower-eyelid/periorbital and perioral rhytids and can be combined with 35% TCA in the remainder of the face to achieve the desired effect. For younger patients who only exhibit primarily uneven skin coloration, a straight 35% TCA peel may be sufficient. For older patients with pan facial rhytids, a full-face phenol peel may be preferable so long as the patient understands the recovery and risk involved. As an alternative strategy to phenol peel, mechanical dermabrasion can yield equivalent or at times even superior results in the perioral region for recalcitrant circumoral rhytids compared with phenol peel. Also, mechanical dermabrasion can be used to address various contour deformities such as acne scarring, scarring, or other uneven skin textures. For patients with undesirable pigmentation, a full-face TCA peel can be undertaken along with dermabrasion in order to feather and blend the areas untreated by dermabrasion.

Besides a general health history, the physician must diligently confirm that the patient has not been on isotretinoin over the past year, which can reduce the pilosebaceous units and thereby lead to potentially disastrous scarring. Also, recent or current outbreaks of perioral herpes should caution a physician from entertaining any thought of resurfacing until the patient has been vesicle-free for a minimum of several weeks. Antiviral prophylaxis should also be a mainstay in any ablative resurfacing protocol that involves the perioral region even in those individuals without a frank history of herpetic outbreaks. Valcyclovir or famcyclovir 500 mg orally twice daily should be instituted 2 days prior to the treatment session and continued for a total of 7 days. Any outbreaks that arise in the postresurfacing period must be immediately reported to the physician and carefully followed. In addition, the dose should be doubled until complete resolution of the outbreak.

14.3
Technique

14.3.1
Phenol

Many practitioners consider CO_2 laser resurfacing an equivalent to phenol peel as a deep ablative therapy. We have found that oftentimes CO_2 laser resurfacing is initially very effective but over time may not sustain the durability of the aesthetic result. Moreover, the thermal damage imparted by the CO_2 laser can frequently be associated with progressive and irreversible hypopigmentation that greatly exceeds that of phenol. The recovery time can also be protracted, as the erythema with 88% phenol typically resolves after a couple of weeks and with a traditional Baker–Gordon phenol formulation tends not to be as profoundly beefy red as that resulting from a CO_2 laser over the ensuing weeks of convalescence. For these enumerated reasons, we have almost altogether abandoned the CO_2 laser as a treatment modality.

Phenol peels are most effective to address the recalcitrant rhytids in the periorbital and perioral regions with or without concurrent TCA in the remainder of the face. For more extensive rhytids and facial skin aging, a full-face phenol peel may be required to attain the desired level of aesthetic change. For any patient contemplating a full-face phenol treatment (whether 88% plain phenol or a Baker–Gordon modification), it is imperative that the patient undergoes complete preoperative medical clearance, considering the risk of cardiac toxicity with the product. In addition, cardiac monitoring and sequential treatment of each facial subunit with a delay of 10–15 min between each subunit must be undertaken to ensure safety. For an individual who will undergo treatment in the periorbital and/or perioral regions alone with phenol, cardiac monitoring and slow therapy need not in general be a concern.

As with any chemical peel, thorough degreasing with an acetone scrub is the essential first step to ensure an even and effective peel. In particular, streaking of phenol can occur when the patient is insufficiently prepared with an acetone scrub. After the patient has removed all makeup and washed the face thoroughly, the physician applies 100% acetone to the entire face using a 4×4 gauze in a deliberate and abrasive manner to degrease the skin and to remove the outer stratum corneum. The patient will usually not appreciate the physician's abrasive manner in scrubbing the skin with acetone nor the noxious odors that emanate forth. Reassurances that this critical step will ensure a safe and consistent result can help the patient comprehend the necessity of this action and thereby better tolerate it.

Plain phenol, 88%, is not as effective as a Baker–Gordon phenol peel but also carries with it a lower morbidity profile. The recovery time for 88% phenol peel approximates that of a 35% TCA peel, i.e., about 1 week or slightly more. Further, older patients with lower-eyelid laxity or already poor lower-eyelid position are at significant risk of ectropion with a Baker–Gordon peel and should be approached cautiously using this higher concentration. Eighty-eight percent phenol, in contrast, can be used more safely in these individuals. Another very important preoperative consideration for a prospective candidate is limiting a phenol-based peel only to individuals of a Fitzpatrick 1 or 2 skin type in order to minimize the potential for noticeable and deforming hypopigmentation. Even individuals with a Fitzpatrick 1 or 2 skin type should be warned that some degree of hypopigmentation might occur. Typically, isolated treatment of the lower-eyelid region with phenol should not be a concern in these lighter-skinned individuals as many people have either a slightly darker skin tone in this region already owing to the visible orbicularis oculi muscle through the attenuated eyelid skin or a lighter skin tone owing to the use of sunglasses or it is just naturally so.

Phenol, 88%, comes prepared from the compounding pharmacist and is ready for use. However, we recommend freshly preparing a Baker–Gordon mixture for several reasons. First, the contents of the Baker–Gordon peel separate out and it is difficult to ensure that they remain uniform when mixed beforehand. Second, effectiveness of the mixture may be compromised when it is prepared in advance. Third, the strength of the Baker–Gordon peel can be adjusted by reducing the amount of croton oil in the mixture to titrate to optimal effect and to reduce morbidity, like the risk of hypopigmentation and the extent of the recovery time.

A Baker–Gordon mixture consists of the following: 3 ml of 88% plain phenol, 2 ml of distilled water, eight drops of septisol, and three drops of croton oil. Each of these constituent ingredients can be placed into a plastic medicine cup in preparation for use. When only treating a smaller area, like the periorbital region, the amounts can be reduced to minimize waste, e.g., 1 ml of 88% phenol, 2–3 ml of distilled water, three drops of septisol, and one drop of croton oil. Croton oil is the most important determinant of the strength of the Baker–Gordon mixture. In order to titrate down the depth of penetration of the mixture, the croton oil can be proportionately reduced. For example, a weaker mixture (but still more potent than straight 88% phenol) would be as follows: 3 ml of 88% plain phenol, 2 ml of distilled water, eight drops of septisol, and one drop of croton oil.

Phenol, especially the Baker–Gordon modification, is quite uncomfortable for the patient to endure. Whereas a TCA peel can be undertaken with an oral sedative and a topically applied betacaine preparation, these adjunctive techniques will fail to provide sufficient comfort for the patient during and after the procedure. With the Baker–Gordon peel, the patient may experience discomfort for even several hours after the treatment. When undertaking a limited phenol peel, e.g., in the periorbital region, infiltration of a long-acting local anesthetic like bupivicaine is very helpful. Phenol applied periorally should be supported by nerve blocks with bupivicaine to provide adequate duration of anesthesia. For a full-face phenol peel, the patient should also receive intravenous sedation in addition to the aforementioned nerve blocks and local infiltration in order to achieve an adequate comfort level.

After appropriate anesthesia is established and the patient is well hydrated, the phenol peel can be undertaken. If a Baker–Gordon mixture is used, the contents must be swirled vigorously to ensure a uniform suspension. A cotton-tipped applicator is dipped in the phenol solution, and then ringed around the lip of the container to remove any excessive solution before applying it onto the face. Starting at the lower-eyelid ciliary margin, the applicator is applied at a deliberate, even speed over the entire lower-eyelid subunit, which can be feathered gently beyond the orbital rim to encompass some crow's-feet rhytids. As the applicator approaches the orbital rim inferiorly, there is less product on the applicator, so the surrounding skin can be feathered easily. Generally speaking, phenol immediately keratocoagulates the skin and does not need to be constantly reapplied to achieve a uniform frost. A single pass should suffice in most instances. A gentle second pass can be made in undertreated areas. Frosting should occur generally within 10–15 s of application. However, the speed of application should not be too slow, which can translate into overtreatment. The medial inferior orbital rim along the nasojugal groove is particularly susceptible to overtreatment, which in turn can lead to prolonged healing and risk of scarring. Accordingly, less aggressive application of phenol should be undertaken in this

area and no product should pool there (or anywhere for that matter). At the end of treatment, no water should be applied to the treated areas because the more dilute the phenol is, the deeper the penetration. After a few minutes, the chemical reaction should be entirely arrested and should not be deepened should any water contact the area, as would be needed to stop reaction in TCA-treated areas.

If the perioral area is the only additional facial zone to be treated with phenol, the physician need not wait the prescribed 10–15 min as would be indicated when performing a full-face phenol peel. Oftentimes, only the upper-lip subunit need be addressed with phenol to manage the deeper rhytids that are present in this area. The wooden, backside of the applicator or a broken toothpick can be used to first apply the phenol into the perioral rhytids themselves with the non-dominant hand spreading open the skin to facilitate placement of phenol into the depth of the rhytid. The remaining subunit is then completed as described above.

The forehead, right cheek, left cheek, and nose constitute the remaining subunits, which should be completed with a 10–15 min delay between each subunit. The nasal subunit can be combined with the lower-eyelid or perioral subunit, as it is a smaller treatment zone. If any cardiac changes become evident, e.g., bigeminy, they will usually reverse given sufficient time. Obviously, no further treatment should be initiated until complete cessation of any evidence of cardiac toxicity.

14.3.2
Trichloroacetic Acid

A TCA peel should always follow a phenol peel, since the former is keratolytic and the latter is keratocoagulant, i.e., the phenol peel is self-limiting and will not be affected by the subsequent application of TCA. Unlike phenol, which rapidly frosts to a uniform color, TCA may need to be applied with several passes until the desired color end point is achieved. In addition, if a simultaneous facelift is entertained, it is generally safer to undertake a rhytidectomy concurrent with full-face TCA peel than with the more deeply penetrated full-face phenol peel. Phenol treatments around the eyes and mouth, however, are far away from the elevated flaps of a facelift and thereby pose no risk to flap viability.

Ablative treatments with 30–35% TCA are uncomfortable for the patient but not as unbearable or for as long a time as with treatment with phenol. Nevertheless, oral sedation with topically applied betacaine or intravenous sedation is preferable when treating a patient with higher concentrations of TCA.

If a full-face TCA or a combined phenol–TCA peel is planned, then the patient should always receive full-face acetone treatment prior to initiating any portion of the peeling to ensure a consistently, uniform result. After the patient has undergone selective phenol peeling in the periorbital area with or without perioral areas, the patient can be treated with TCA. Pretreatment with Jessner's solution may help achieve a deeper and more uniform TCA peel by removing the remaining stratum corneum. Jessner's solution is applied several minutes after the phenol peel to ensure that the phenol reaction is complete and it can be liberally applied to the entire remainder of the face where TCA will then be applied. Generally speaking, 90 s is sufficient for Jessner's solution to afford adequate pretreatment prior to starting the TCA peel.

TCA is applied to the face by subunit like phenol but no waiting time is necessary between treating subunits. The reason the subunit principle is followed when applying TCA is that after a few minutes a previously treated area will change from a uniform frost back to a faded or almost non-existent frost. The physician may then interpret this area as undertreated and reapply a coat of TCA, which will most likely lead to overtreatment, prolonged healing, and potential scarring. A cotton-tipped applicator or ringed-out cotton ball can be used to apply 30–35% TCA to the face in broad, even strokes. Generally, it takes about 30–60 s to witness changes of the skin color to the desired frost. The initial color change is a light erythema, then a speckled gray-white, finally a more uniform white color. Additional passes can be applied to achieve the desired uniform white color. Oftentimes about three to five passes with 35% TCA will attain the level of color change desired. The higher the concentration of TCA, the faster the result will occur. Accordingly, it takes longer and is more difficult to control 10–20% TCA when trying to achieve ablative levels of rejuvenation; whereas 50% and beyond has a higher likelihood of leading to overcorrection. A TCA range of 30–35% is ideal for attaining a safe and effective ablative skin intervention. As the color of the skin begins to become more uniform, the physician can apply a cold water soaked or saline-soaked 4×4 gauze (rung out dry first so that it does not drip onto not yet treated areas). If the color of the skin becomes more of a uniform grayish white, then the area may have been overtreated. The use of a water-impregnated 4×4 gauze is intended to slow down and arrest the chemical reaction of the TCA. Of note, water dilution of phenol only serves to deepen the reaction (in an uncontrolled fashion), whereas it helps slow down and stop the reaction of the TCA peel. As phenol is a keratocoagulant, by the time the physician starts the TCA peel portion of the procedure, it is safe to apply the cold, soaked gauze even in areas that were previously treated with phenol. In order to maintain a consistent result, the physician should apply the cold, soaked gauze after each subunit is completed before continuing on to the next subunit. This cycle of treating a subunit with TCA until the desired color change is observed followed by application of water-soaked gauze onto the subunit should be followed until the entire face is completed in this fashion.

14.3.3
Dermabrasion

Mechanical dermabrasion with either a diamond fraise or a wire brush is an effective tool in correction of deeper skin abnormalities, like deep rhytids or acne scarring. It can be used as an alternative strategy for perioral rhytid reduction in combination with periorbital phenol and full-facial TCA treatments. It is safe and effective to dermabrade over TCA-treated areas but this may be less than ideal over phenol-treated areas. Fundamentally, it may be an obvious point but one worth stating explicitly: always peel a patient first before performing dermabrasion. It is absolutely unsafe to peel in an area of denuded skin where the patient was just dermabraded. Therefore, when performing a combination of phenol, TCA, and dermabrasion, the appropriate chronologic sequence would always be phenol, then TCA, then dermabrasion. Mechanical dermabrasion, if performed well, can rival if not exceed the therapeutic benefits of phenol peel for rhytids in the perioral region and is the first choice for acne scarring or other scarring abnormalities (except hypertrophic, keloid, or raised scars that would be worsened with dermabrasion).

Diamond-fraise dermabrasion is more easily and safely undertaken in a physician's hands, especially a neophyte, when compared with the more aggressive wire-brush kind of dermabrader. Nevertheless, the technique for treatment remains essentially the same. The target end point is just beyond the punctate bleeding that is encountered in the papillary dermis. By the time the physician reaches this depth, the dermabrader should have passed in perpendicular directions to facilitate maximal and even laceration of the collagen. Rephrased another way, the physician should initiate treatment with the dermabrader in one direction until just before punctate bleeding is encountered, then rotate the instrument in a perpendicular orientation to the first pass in order to complete the treatment. It is imperative that a 4×4 gauze not get too close to the dermabrader head during treatment, as it will invariably get caught in the instrument. Also, protective eyewear should be donned, e.g., a visor mask, in order to protect against the aerosol plume of particulate matter that arises during dermabrasion. If the physician is just starting out with dermabrasion, he or she should practice the art of dermabrading on an orange before approaching a patient for the first time.

14.4
Postoperative Care and Management of Complications

After any kind of ablative resurfacing, the major goal is to maintain adequate moisture to all treated areas in order to avoid desiccation, crusting, and scarring. A thick, long-lasting emollient, e.g., Aquaphor (Beiersdorf), that is also hypoallergenic should be applied liberally to all treated areas until complete epithelialization occurs. After 1–2 weeks when complete reepithelialization has been observed, a lighter hypoallergenic moisturizer can be substituted for a petroleum-based product, e.g., Cetaphil or Eucerin. It is important that the patient abstain from usage of standard skin-care products that can be very irritating if not outright harmful in the immediate postresurfacing period of 30 days. In addition, perfumes and other fragrances should not make contact with the resurfaced areas to minimize the likelihood of dermatitis. Any dermatitis that arises should be immediately reported to the physician, evaluated, and treated.

Characteristically, dermatitis presents clinically as a pruritic, raised, and erythematous area, which should be treated by discovering and removing the offending product that elicited the problem and treating the condition with topically applied 1% hydrocortisone cream twice daily until resolution. Smoldering dermatitis can eventually lead to scarring if left untreated in the postresurfacing patient so early detection and intervention is mandatory. Similarly makeup application early on can engender dermatitis and should be withheld until at least full epithelialization. Further, mineral-based products may be less prone to inciting an unfavorable dermatologic response.

Hyperpigmentation is a common sequela following TCA peel and can be exacerbated by early sun exposure. A sunblock with a minimum sun protection factor rating of 25 should be used on the skin after complete epithelialization to minimize the likelihood and severity of hyperpigmentation. At times, chemical blocking agents (octyl methoxycinnamate) in sunblocks can more likely give rise to dermatitis, which should be avoided, compared with physical blocking agents (zinc oxide, titanium dioxide), which are preferable. Fortunately, postinflammatory pigmentary changes are only temporary in nature and gradually subside over a period of weeks to months. Typically, hyperpigmentation is encountered after the third week and remains for a few months. Use of 4% hydroquinone, or an alternative bleaching product, should not be initiated during the first postoperative month in order to minimize the chance of inducing dermatitis. As phenol does not typically cause hyperpigmentation, it is not uncommon to see a demarcated border of hyperpigmentation on the TCA side where the TCA-treated area abuts the phenol-treated area.

Whereas hyperpigmentation is uncommon with phenol, hypopigmentation is not only the norm but should be expected. Varying levels of hypopigmentation occur with phenol depending on the patient's skin type and the strength of phenol used. At times when hypopigmentation occurs, it can be reversible over time. Patients must fully understand the reality that some hypopigmentation may or will occur after phenol peel. There really is no practical treatment for hypopigmentation, although a repeated series of Psoralen and UV-A (PUVA) therapy has been shown to ameliorate the condition. Hypopigmentation is generally much less noticeable if TCA is used in adjoining areas to minimize any overt dyschromias that may lessen the disparity between phenol-treated and non-phenol-treated areas. Furthermore, staying within subunit boundaries for each type of peel/resurfacing modality can also help minimize the visibility of the treatment.

Erythema is relatively short lived with TCA, typically lasting 1–2 weeks after treatment but could be somewhat extended beyond that time period. Phenol (88%) follows a similar time period in The extent of erythema following 88% phenol peel is similar to that following TCA peel, but the duration may exceed that of TCA peel by 1–2 weeks. Erythema following a Baker–Gordon peel can be more prominent and linger for even several weeks to months, which should not raise alarm. Accordingly, women who wear makeup for cosmetic camouflage may be more accepting of this condition than men, who may decline this option. Nevertheless, the erythema is generally less beefy red and prolonged than following CO_2 laser treatment.

Herpetic outbreaks can occur following any kind of resurfacing, especially in the perioral region. A prophylactic regimen and management routine were already thoroughly discussed earlier on and will not be repeated here.

Scarring can occur after any resurfacing treatment owing to overtreatment, prolonged healing, or dermatitis, to name the major etiologic inciting factors. If any area does not appear to have been completely epithelialized by the tenth posttreatment day, the risk of potential scarring increases proportionately. For a denuded area that remains, it is advisable to place a tailored Duoderm patch until resolution to minimize the chance of scarring. Injection of 10 mg/ml triamcinolone acetonide diluted down to half strength can be used in the area to minimize the risk of scarring as well.

14.5
Conclusions

Although one single modality for ablative resurfacing can at times suffice, oftentimes a combination of skin therapies can be more effective to attain the optimal aesthetic result and to minimize the morbidity profile (Figs. 14.1, 14.2). This chapter should have elucidated the principles and properties of various ablative skin therapies and how to implement them in an effective strategy for combined and concurrent intervention. Like an artist with many brushes, the physician can exercise creativity and control when approaching a prospective patient with combined resurfacing tools.

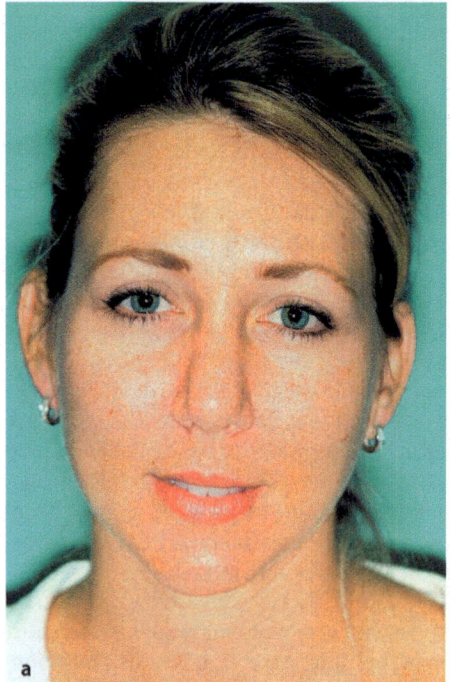
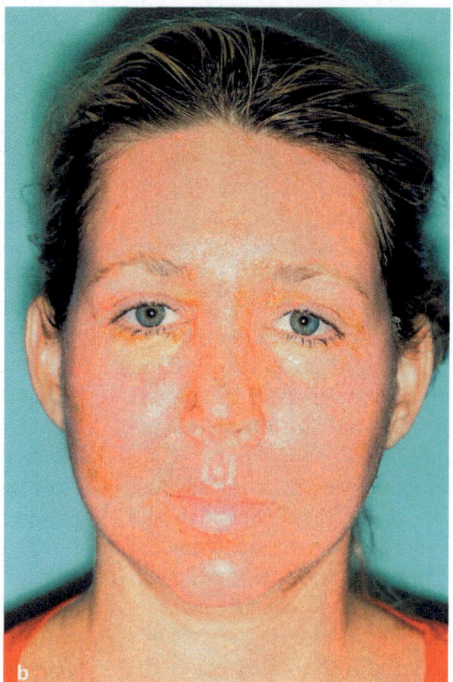
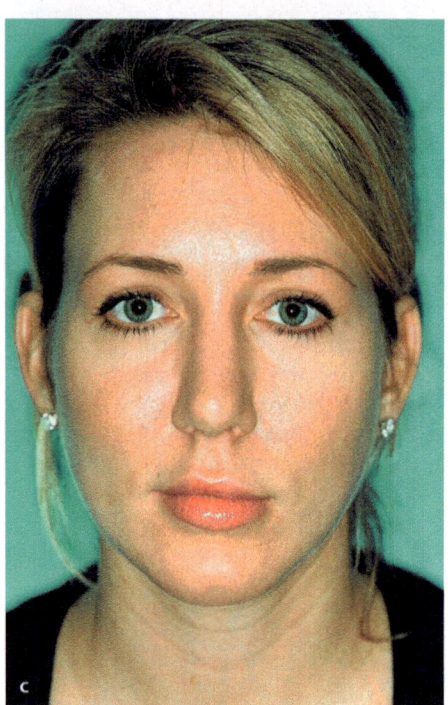

Fig. 14.1 a Thirty-year-old woman wanted a dramatic improvement in her skin appearance. **b** Three days after a full-face Baker–Gordon phenol peel. **c** Aesthetic improvement 8 months after the peel

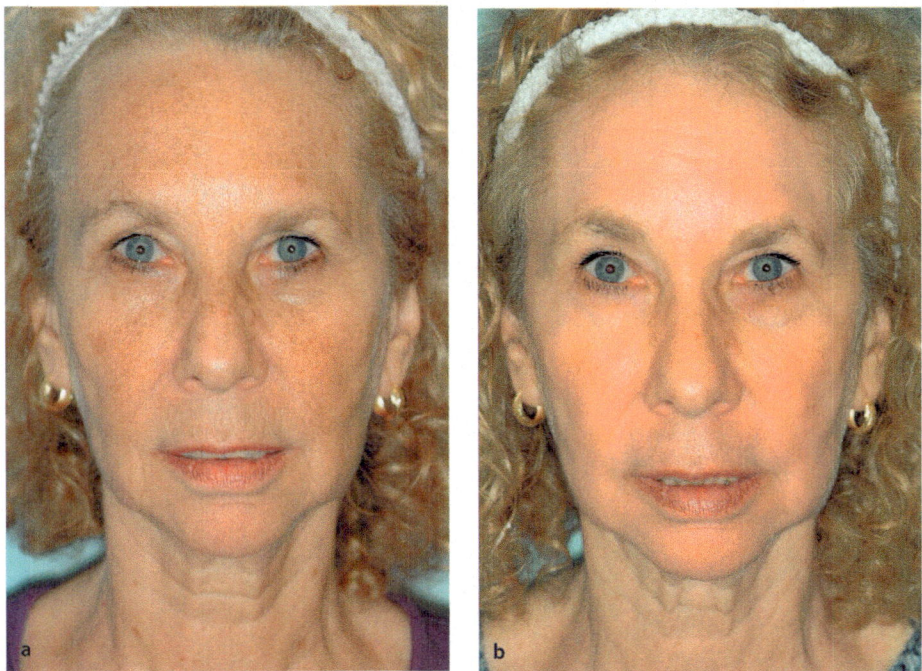

Fig. 14.2 **a** Fifty-five year-old woman prior to treatment. **b** Six months after full-face Baker–Gordon phenol peel

CHAPTER 15

Comparison of Laser and Phenol Chemical Peel   **15**

Phillip R. Langsdon, David Armstrong

15.1
Introduction

Photodamaged skin and wrinkled skin are signs of aging that humans have, for centuries, sought to diminish. The innate desire to look as youthful as possible for as long as possible is not new. The ancient Egyptians used acidic substances from wine in an attempt to improve aging skin. Milk, wine, as well as various fruits and vegetables have been applied to the skin by various cultures over the centuries.

Today, the billions of dollars of over-the-counter cosmetic products purchased represent the continued human drive for improved appearance. But, over-the-counter products have limited benefit. New medical-grade exfoliation products have improved possible results, and the public demand has come into the physician's office. However, even the medical-grade self-application products cannot always do enough to improve the condition of very aged/damaged skin. For those requiring more advanced intervention, surgical exfoliation is required.

For years dermabrasion and phenol chemical peeling were the mainstay procedures used to improve facial rhytids. These techniques were used very successfully by surgeons experienced with these procedures.

Each procedure had and still has its limits. Dermabrasion, for instance, must be used with extra caution in the perioral and periorbital regions because of the risk of snagging the soft tissue around the eyes or mouth. The thin skin of the eyelids cannot be dermabraded in the same manner as thicker-skinned areas of the face. Chemical peeling, on the other hand, works well on the thin eyelid skin and lateral cheeks, but may not improve deep rhytids of the lips or middle third of the face to the extent as that which can be obtained with dermabrasion. But, no matter the limitations, these techniques work and have provided satisfying results for many decades.

In the 1990s use of the CO_2 laser became a popular method to reduce facial wrinkling. The rapid growth in use by both experienced as well as new resurfacing physicians can be attributed to aggressive promotion by the manufactures of the lasers. This occurred in spite of the fact that up until October 2000 [1] no prospective clinical trials comparing the results of the use of lasers with those of using chemical peels had compared postoperative course, histologic examination, patient satisfaction, or long-term outcome. Therefore a study was undertaken at this institution to compare methods.

15.2
Aging Skin

Through the normal aging process human skin loses volume and elasticity. On a microscopic level the skin demonstrates flattening of the rete pegs in the dermis–epidermis junction. Collagen fibers become course and disorganized, vascular supply recedes, and the dermis thins. Sun damage causes acanthotic changes, cellular atypia, and disorganization of elastin fibers. Normal aging changes plus sun damage results in keratosis, telangiectatias, wrinkling, and sagging.

15.3
Surgical Treatment Methods

Whatever treatment method chosen, laser, chemical peeling, or dermabrasion, the depth of insult or stimulation is related to the level of improvement sought as well as the capacity to heal. Insult, or tissue removal, that does not penetrate the reticular dermis usually results in reasonable healing, and hopefully an improvement in the condition under treatment.

15.4
Chemical Peeling

LaGasse, during World War I, noted the use of phenol and an occlusive dressing improved the appearance of skin after a period of healing. Later his daughter Antoinette began a "lay" peeling center for the improvement of wrinkles and scars. By the mid-1950s Gillies [2] began using phenol to treat wrinkled eyelid skin. Then in the early 1960s Litton began using Antionette's technique to treat wrinkled skin for his patients seeking improvement otherwise not obtainable with aging face surgery. In 1966 Baker [3] reported on the use of phenol, plus croton oil. His report help broaden awareness of phenol peeling with the cosmetic surgery community.

Chemical peeling involves the application of a chemical that reacts with the skin, resulting in a sloughing of the tissues. The resultant healed skin usually provides a smoother tone and texture. Phenol peeling, usually used for medium to deep peeling, is best used to treat fair-complexion, thin-skinned patients with fine rhytids. Other agents have been used to chemexfoliate skin. Trichloroacetic acid, resorcinol, salicylic acid, and glycolic acid can also produce medium to deep peeling. Chemical peeling has been used to improve wrinkles, superficial acne scarring, keratosis, pigmentation abnormalities, and solar elastosis.

15.5
Dermabrasion

In 1905, Kromayer [4] reported cylindrical knives for treating scars, tattoos, pigmentation abnormalities, and other conditions. This evolved into the use of rotating burrs attached to dental drills. Eventually rotating wire-brush instruments were used to smooth damaged skin; only the obscuring impact of the resulting bleeding limited treatment. Kurtin's [5] 1953 description of the use of refrigeration anesthesia, which impeded surgical bleeding, aided the surgical popularity of the wire-brush motor-driven method of surgical abrasion.

Dermabrasion involves the mechanical removal of tissues, usually with either a rotating wire brush or a diamond fraise. Tissue depth can be observed by the surgeon and advanced as necessary.

Dermabrasion may be used to improve acne scarring, wrinkles, keratosis, rhinophyma, pigmentation abnormalities, tattoos, as well as many other skin abnormalities.

15.6
Laser Abrasion

Lasers were developed in the 1950s and began being used in medicine in the 1960s. The CO_2 laser gained popularity in medicine because of the ability to precisely vaporize tissue, with little carbonization, edema, or inflammation. It has the added advantage of its hemostatic impact on the vaporized tissue bed.

CO_2 lasers have many uses, but considering abrasive surgery the main use is to vaporize the layers of skin involved with wrinkles, scaring, keratosis, etc. In 1989, David et al. [6] demonstrated improvement in the stratum corneum, improvement in solar elastosis, and the creation of a new subepidermal band of collagen; results similar to those obtained with phenol peeling or dermabrasion.

The development of computer-controlled hand pieces capable of generating preprogrammed patterns of skin injury, allowing a large area of the face to be treated in a short period of time, with minimal surrounding tissue injury, brought CO_2 laser use into the realm of practical skin resurfacing. Unfortunately, the rapid growth of laser skin resurfacing in the 1990s was promoted more by the aggressive marketing of the laser manufactures than by traditional medical examination processes.

In 2000 the senior author published a study evaluating the comparison of phenol peeling and laser resurfacing. A prospective study was performed comparing the two methods. Postoperative course, patient satisfaction, histologic examination, and long-term outcome were evaluated.

15.7
The Study

Four patients were studied. Each received two passes of the CO_2 laser to the right side of the face. The Sharplan Silktouch Flashscanner CO_2 laser was used at 3-mm spot size, 6-W power, and 0.2-s exposure time for the periorbital region and 3-mm spot size 16-W power, and 0.2-s exposure time for the remainder of the right side of the face.

The left side of the face was peeled with a chemical peel formula consisting of 3 ml of 88% phenol, three drops of croton oil, eight drops of Septisol soap, and 2 ml of distilled water. The peel procedure was performed according to the standard procedure described in [7]. Postoperative care included showering the face, followed by the application of a moisturizing cream, six times per day until there was no skin flaking and all areas were healed. The results and postoperative course were examined for 1 year following treatment.

There was more postoperative erythema on the laser-treated side, early in the healing process. The laser-treated side also exhibited more prolonged stinging and discomfort. By the first 24-h after treatment there was significantly more swelling on the chemically peeled side of the face. The greater amount of swelling did not resolve and equal out until about 7 days postoperatively.

Erythema was more patchy and less intense on the peeled side of the face, and it resolved earlier than on the laser-treated side. The early stinging of the peeled area resolved in 6–8 h, while that of the laser-treated side persisted for several days.

One patient developed spotty hyperpigmentation on the laser-treated side at 2 months postoperatively. This was successfully treated with 2.5% hydrocortisone and 4% hydroquinone cream.

The patients and evaluating surgeons felt there was overall improvement on both sides of each patient's face; with a reduction in wrinkles. However, the patients and surgeons appreciated some differences between the two sides. Greater improvement was noted on the laser-treated side in the thicker, more glandular areas of the nasolabial fold and chin regions. The surgeons felt that there was near-uniform improvement of the two sides in the thinner skin areas of the lateral cheek and eyelids. They also noted a slight advantage on the laser-treated side of the upper lip and forehead areas. However, the early advantage in smoothness had diminished somewhat by the 6 month evaluation.

Additionally, the treatment response of improved skin texture was initially patchy on the chemical peel treated side of the face; the laser-treated side demonstrated a more uniform response. This was not unexpected since the laser treatment involves a mechanical removal of cutaneous tissue while the chemexfoliated skin can be limited in tissue response by the varying amount of sebaceous glandular concentration throughout the face; even aggressive preoperative degreasing did not prevent the patchy response.

This lack of postoperative uniformity in skin appearance of the peeled side diminished over the course of the first 12 months postoperatively, and it was not as apparent in the drier skin areas of the upper lip, forehead, lateral cheek, and periorbital areas.

One year after treatment hypopigmentation was more significant on the laser-treated side in all four patients. One patient required repeeling at 3 years postoperatively because of the worsening significance in disparity of the intense hypopigmentation of the laser-treated side compared with the peeled side.

Another patient underwent rhytidectomy 44 days after the laser/peeling. Histologic evaluation, by a blinded pathologist, of the excised facial skin (not treated, laser treated, and peeled) revealed that there was deeper injury on the peeled side; down into the reticular dermis. The laser-treated side demonstrated tissue injury into the papillary dermis. Considering that the skin was only 44 days after treatment, it was discovered that sun-damaged elastic connective tissue was significantly reduced in the laser-treated skin and totally obliterated in the peeled skin. If later tissue samples can be obtained the long-term impact on elastin fibers can be determined.

15.8 Discussion

It is understood that one difficulty with this type of comparison is the inherent differences in depth of tissue injury between laser treatment and peeling, as well as the impact of operator control in depth of injury. Previous studies have consistently demonstrated the CO_2 laser produces a depth of injury approximating that of a medium-depth chemical peel (0.14–0.25 mm) [8] while deep phenol peeling created an injury depth of 0.6–0.8 mm [9]. In spite of these understood differences in depths of injury, as well as the deeper insult of deep peeling, in our study the laser produced slightly better results in the thicker and more glandular areas of the facial skin; but the advantage was only more significantly pronounced in the early phases of the healing process. The laser-treated side demonstrated more

significant hypopigmentation that became ever more apparent, the longer the patients were observed postoperatively. There was more prolonged erythema and discomfort with this method. The chemical peel was as effective in the thinner skin areas of the face, such as the eyelids, lateral cheeks, and the nonglabellar portions of the forehead. The discomfort resolved within the first few hours after treatment and the erythema was not as prolonged.

15.9 Conclusions

Phenol chemical peeling remains a good technique to use when attempting to improve aged, wrinkled, sun-damaged facial skin. It is certainly less costly than lasers, which may cost close to $100,000 in many instances. For the deeper wrinkled and/or more sebaceous areas of the face, dermabrasion may be combined with chemical peeling or the area of concern may simply be repeeled at a later date. Therefore, phenol chemical peeling of the face remains an effective technique to reverse the signs of facial aging in selected patients. New technologies will certainly continue to become available, but they must have proven significant advantages in order to supplant phenol chemical peeling and justify the costs of laser treatment or other technologies.

References

1. Langsdon PR, Milburn M, Yarber R. Comparison of the laser and phenol chemical peel in facial skin resurfacing. Arch Otolaryngol Head Neck Surg 2000;126(10):1195–1199
2. Gillies HD, Millard DR Jr: Principles and Art of Plastic Surgery. Boston, Little Brown, 1957
3. Baker TJ, Gordon HL, Seckinger DL: A second look at chemical face peeling. Plast Reconstr Surg 1966;37(6):487–493
4. Kromayer E: Die Heilung der Akne durch in neves norbenlases Operations Verfahren. Das Stanzen. Illus Monatsschr Aerztl Polytech 1905;27:101
5. Kurtin A: Corrective surgical planing of skin: new technique for treatment of acne scars and other skin defects. Arch Dermatol Syphilol 1953;68(4):389–397
6. David LM, Lask GP, Glassberg E, Jacoby R, Abergel RP. Laser abrasion for cosmetic and medical treatment of facial actinic damage. Cutis 1989;43(6):583–587
7. McCollough EG, Langsdon PR: Dermabrasion and Chemical Peel; A Guide for Facial Plastic Surgeons. New York, Thieme, 1988
8. Cotton J, Hood AF, Gonin R, Beesen WH, Hanke CW: Histological evaluation of preauricular and postauricular human skin after high-energy, short-pulse carbon dioxide laser. Arch Dermatol 1996;132(4):425–428
9. Body HJ (ed): Chemical Peeling. St. Louis, Mosby Year Book, 1991:1–5

CHAPTER 16

Face and Neck Remodeling with Ultrasound-Assisted (VASER) Lipoplasty

Alberto Di Giuseppe, George Commons

This chapter is dedicated to my dear friend Franco Antognini M.D. (1945–2006) who was the anesthesiologist in my clinic for over 13 years. His great talent and humanity should be remembered as an example for young physicians. He will be missed by all, especially his wife, daughter, and son (who is just starting his medical career).

16.1
Introduction

The first published reported use of ultrasound-assisted liposculpture (SMEI, Italy) was in 2000 [1]. A solid probe 25 mm in diameter and 17-cm long was utilized on 115 patients operated on to defat heavy faces or to undermine lax neck skin and to possibly achieve skin retraction. When utilizing the solid probe in the face, the power administrated was 30% of the total potential of the ultrasound tool in order to reduce undesired side effects of ultrasound energy (heat essentially). The aim of the technique was:

1. To reduce the numbers and extension of scars of the face for remodeling procedures of the face and neck.
2. To perform under local tumescent anesthesia essentially the majority of facial contouring surgeries.
3. To induce skin retraction in the face and neck, even with lax skin, avoiding major open surgery operations such as standard face-lift.
4. To undermine and induce skin retraction with minimal trauma by utilizing a solid probe and the ultrasound energy instead of an open approach and a scalpel.
5. To debulk heavy faces, neck, and jowls, with a smooth device able to emulsify fat in specific targets with minimal trauma, low energy, and safe surgical planes.
6. To contour difficult areas, such as the mandible border, the neck line, and the chin.
7. To make facial surgery accessible even to patients who refused major open surgery operations, which normally lead to a longer recovery time.

Under those circumstances the authors did not substitute the standard rhytidectomy, but offered an alternative technique in facial contouring surgery called "the harmonic lift."

16.2
Material and Methods

In total 150 patients were included in the study, consisting of 112 women and 38 men with an age range from 28 to 76 (mean age 45). From 1996 ultrasonically assisted skin remodeling was the sole procedure in 79 patients and was used concomitantly with a mini lift in 71 patients, blepharoplasty in 48 patients, rhinoplasty in seven patients, chin augmentation in ten patients, breast augmentation in one patient, breast reduction in two patients, and mastopexy in six patients. Abdominoplasty was performed in five patients, and gynecomastia was treated in two patients. All patients were followed for at least 1 year.

16.3
Patient Selection

The harmonic lift can be used in young patients with fatty necks and cheeks as well as in older patients with loose skin and wrinkles. Each patient was evaluated as to the aims of surgery such as treatment of crow's-feet, nasolabial and commissural folds, jowls, and waddle neck.

The procedure is appropriate in the following cases:

1. Face-lift and neck-lift in Fitzpatrick skin types 4–6, thus avoiding keloid formation and postinflammatory hyperpigmentation that may occur with skin rejuvenation with laser or peel techniques.
2. Young patients who require only treatment of chubby cheeks and double chin.
3. To enhance neck definition with chin augmentation.
4. To substitute for endoscopic forehead-lift in balding scalps.
5. To achieve dermal stimulation and retraction in the neck beyond areas amenable to laser resurfacing.
6. To reduce acne scarring of the cheeks.
7. In secondary and tertiary face-lifts when partial removal of the skin is a questionable procedure but the central face needs further tightening.

Other indications include rhytids in the malar area, crow's-feet, frontal, nasolabial, glabella (horizontal and vertical), and neck folds as well as descent of the cheek fat, ptosis of the lateral eyebrows, laxity of the upper lids, jowls, and diffuse acne scarring of the cheeks and neck.

16.4
Technique

Lines are drawn on the face to show the full area of undermining, the vectors of muscle tension, relaxation creases and folds, crisscrossing lines of tunneling, and dermal stimulation.

Incisions are placed at different sites to allow ease of access depending on the target areas (Fig. 16.1). In the forehead, incisions are vertical to avoid nerve damage and are at the hairline, midline, or frontal recess. Temporal incisions are parallel to the hairline, while submental incisions are at the submental crease. Preauricular incisions are made at the earlobe and upper-eyelid and lower-eyelid incisions are at blepharoplasty sites.

The use of the tumescent technique reduces bleeding, bruising, and surgery time. Analgesia used for the full face is 1,000 ml Ringer's lactate, 1 ml adrenaline, and 1–1.5 g lidocaine.

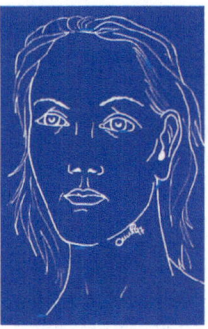

Incision Lines:

- frontal
- temporal
- retroauricola
- submental
- laterocervical
- eyelid

Fig. 16.1 Incision lines

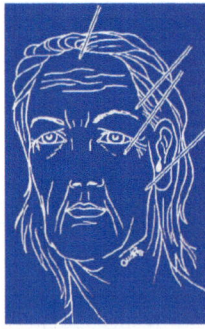

Tension lines of action with Vaser UAL solid probe: 50% of total power, 5–12 minutes of full face undermining

Fig. 16.2 Tension lines of action with a VASER ultrasound-assisted liposuction (*UAL*) solid probe

Klein's solution [2] contains 1,000 ml normal saline with 1.5 ml epinephrine (15 mg), 1,500 mg lidocaine, and 12.5 mEq sodium bicarbonate.

Intravenous sedation is generally utilized, but when general anesthesia is used the amount of lidocaine is reduced to 200 mg and sodium bicarbonate is eliminated. Approximately 350–500 ml of solution is utilized on each side. A blunt-tipped, 14-gauge cannula is used to infiltrate the subcutaneous tissues of the neck, jowls, cheeks, temple, and brow. Digital pressure aids in directing and expanding the fluid evenly.

16.5
Ultrasound-Assisted Dissection

Ultrasonic dissection was performed with a titanium solid probe (VASER, from SST Denver CO, USA) which is 2,2 mm diameter [3, 4]. The areas include frontal from the hairline to the brow, glabella, dorsum of the nose, temple, lateral canthal region (crow's-feet), cheeks to nasolabial grooves, chin, jowls, and anterior neck from the chin to the sternal notch (anterior triangles). The probe is advanced subdermally and the tip of the probe tents the skin while it is withdrawn. Blanching of the skin occurs with treatment and is more noticeable in the patient with ruddy complexion. The skin softens and smoothes following use of the probe.

The sequence of dissection starts with the submental area and the neck from the submental and earlobe incisions. The probe is then used over the mandible, cheek, and temple, reaching the nasolabial fold, the side of the nose, and the crow's-feet in a radiating fashion through the earlobe incision. An upper-eyelid incision allows access to the glabella and the central portion of the forehead, releasing the cutaneous insertion of the corrugator and procerus muscles without altering skin

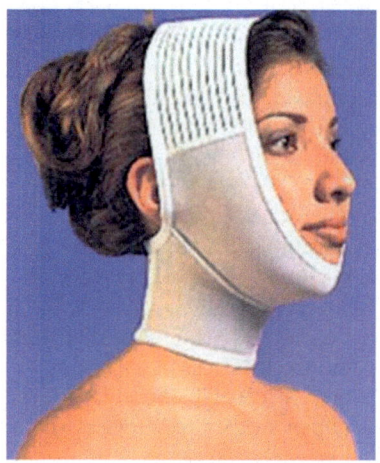

Fig. 16.3 Face-supporting garment

sensation. The rest of the forehead is dissected through a separate hairline incision (Fig. 16.2).

The fat emulsion and tumescent fluid are evacuated by gentle massage of the areas. When the harmonic face-lift (ultrasonic skin rejuvenation) is used alone, the skin incisions are closed with skin sutures and Epifoam is applied to the skin and a chin strap is applied. Ice packs are used on the face and orbital regions not covered by the foam. A supporting garment is applied for 1 week, and then for 2 weeks more, at night (Fig. 16.3).

16.5.1
Concomitant Procedures

The superficial musculoaponeurotic system (SMAS) can be tightened by dissection and resection or imbrication for face-lift and neck-lift. Skin excisions are usually minimal, if required at all (Fig. 16.4).

Any other cosmetic procedure can be performed at the same time, including upper and lower blepharoplasty, platysmaplasty, face-lift, neck-lift, chin or cheek implants, temporal-lift, forehead-lift, and skin rejuvenation with laser treatment or chemical peel. The authors have utilized VASER face remodeling with autologous fat transfer.

16.5.2
Complications

Two patients developed postoperative hematomas, which required aspiration; however, both were hypertensive and noncompliant with their medications. Contour deformities of the neck were noted in three patients, with two of them improving over 2 months. One patient required surgical release of the subdermal scar and asked for a more extensive surgery, a standard open face-lift with the SMAS [5, 6].

There were no instances of nerve injury, alopecia, or a vascular necrosis. The ultrasound-assisted facial rejuvenation was safe, effective, and reproducible. The results were comparable to those of more extensive, difficult surgeries with higher morbidity, risks, and costs.

16.6
Discussion

There has been a lot of interest in the use of ultrasonic liposuction for body contouring. Skin retraction has been reported as a result of the concomitant use of internal ultrasound from the large amount of fat removed, removal of subdermal fat, skeletonization of the super-

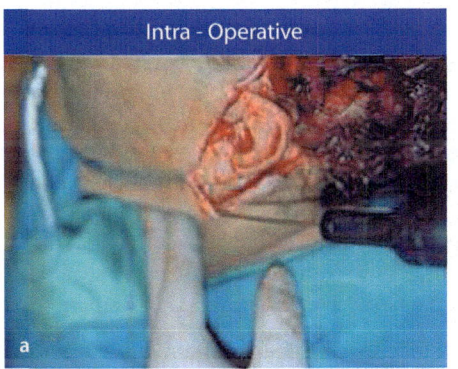
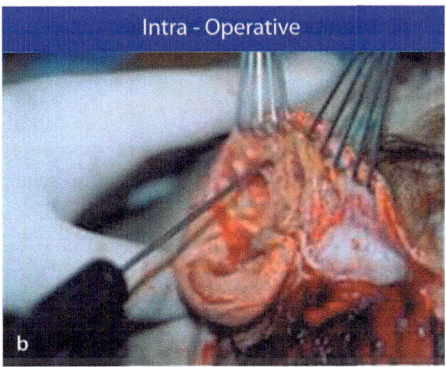
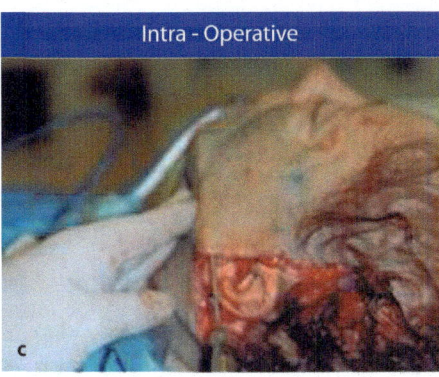
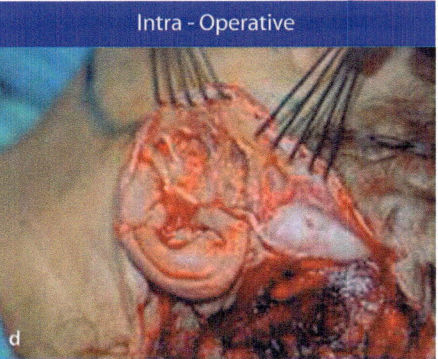

Fig. 16.4 a Flap harvesting. **b** VASER undermining. **c** Emulsion cleaning **d** Verifying tunnels made by the probe. Note untouched supporting structures of the skin

ficial fascial system, and thermal effects on the subdermal surface and collagenous structures of the superficial facial system [7–10]. There are three theories of skin contracture:

1. Collagen contraction due to injury (thermal? Original proposition).
2. Defatting the superficial layer-retained structures minus fat allows the skin to retract.
3. Gentle stimulation to cause contraction through controlled damage.

Facial aging is due to fat and skin ptosis and is not due to muscle or facial ptosis; therefore, the supra-SMAS plane is ideal for the harmonic lift with ultrasonic rejuvenation of the face. The osteofacial dermal ligaments can be released or attenuated in this plane allowing direct contouring of the malar, nasolabial, jowl, and submental fat collections. Fat removed close to the under surface of intact skin results in skin retraction with permanent contour changes.

Postoperative care requires careful nursing assistance, punctilious wound protection, and prolonged avoidance of elaborate makeup. The recovery time varies from 4 to 14 days. The postoperative care is limited to the use of Reston foam and elastic compression bandages that are changed by the patient. Although there were no histology examinations in this study, there have been previous reports on the results of subdermal ultrasound and liposuction [11, 12]. The long-term results have not been evaluated and are probably related to the type of skin, patient age and sex, and the long-term effect of ultrasound energy.

Disadvantages are the cost of the ultrasound machine, increased hassle factor in the operating room, and machine dependency, but after achieving proficiency in using the machine there is no turning back because it is addictive. The conclusion, at that time, was that the harmonic lift is a safe, effective, and reproducible form of skin remodeling. It can be performed under local, regional, or general anesthesia and can be repeated with no increase in surgical difficulty or cumulative effect. Advantages include negligible blood loss and pain, short and uncomplicated recovery, and simple postoperative care. The results are comparable to those obtained with more extensive surgery that frequently involves overnight stay, higher risks, increased morbidity, and higher costs.

There is some skepticism concerning the utilization of ultrasound energy in the face, mainly related to the potential risks of burns. In the USA, from 1995 to 2000, a series of articles published in the medical literature pointed out the increasing number of complications related to body-contouring procedures when ultrasound energy was involved [13].

The analysis of all these complications, even with the difficulty of assembling all clinical data, produced the following results:

- Seroma (30% of body-contouring cases)
- Delayed wound healing (18% of clinical cases)
- Prolonged edema (15% of clinical cases)
- Dysesthesia (12% of clinical cases)
- Fibrosis (8% of clinical cases)
- Asymmetries (4% of clinical cases)
- Skin necrosis (0.3% of clinical cases)
- Burn (0.2% of clinical cases)

Despite the fact that burns and skin necrosis were largely the least common related complications and represented really a rare issue, the potential risks of these two complications were overemphasized.

A major issue was introduced by many authors in the literature, probably because burns and skin necrosis related to procedure complications were not seen with the other technique of liposuction (superficial, traditional, power-assisted).

A task force was established by the Educational Foundation of the American Society of Aesthetic Plastic Surgery (ASAPS) and by the American Society of Plastic and Reconstructive Surgery (ASPRS), and met many times in order to establish safety criteria for utilization of ultrasound energy in body-contouring surgery. The first safety indication, to prevent complications such as burns and skin necrosis, was to avoid using the ultrasound probe close to the underlying dermis, which was the most important step of the "harmonic lift." However, only working "superficially" with a solid ultrasound probe, the surgeon can undermine the cutaneous and subcutaneous layers, assembling a skinny but vascularized flap, more prone to retract and adapt to a reduced body volume. The great misunderstanding in those years which led to and created confusion and mixing of clinical data was due to the fact that all the complications-related data came through the utilization of the two most diffuse ultrasound tools, in the US market: The Contour Genesis, from Mentor (Santa Barbara, CA, USA), and the Lysonics (from Inamed Corporation). These two ultrasound tools have similar technical characteristics:

- High energy
- Hollow probes, with simultaneous ultrasound energy administration; thus there is emulsification and simultaneous, subsequent aspiration
- A 5.0-mm-diameter probe

The vaser system has smaller diameter probes, in solid titanium, with no aspiration at the time of emulsification (which were, and are, two different clinical phases).

Adopting a finer probe for the face and neck has not led to such kinds of complications. However, the number of ultrasound tools sold by SMEI (probably 700) was far less than the number sold by Mentor and Lysonics (probably more than 2,500 units). The American market was far superior to all the remaining worldwide market; thus the published literature included only the experience (and complications) of American technology in internal ultrasound energy. In 2001, Cimino [14] reported on quantification and efficiency of ultrasound energy. This article was of capital importance to understand all the mistakes made by the two main American manufacturers in assembling the two most common ultrasound tools:

- Too much energy, which produced unnecessary overheating, which increased the side effects of ultrasound (seroma, mainly) without enhancing the results and the clinical outcomes.
- Too large probes, with low efficacy in transmitting energy to the tip, and thus reducing the emulsification rate.
- Poor design of the tip of the probe due to lack of technological research, with a reduced efficacy of the system. In order to raise the rate of emulsification, the manufacturer increased the power of the tools.

The two main ultrasound devices were far from a good technical standard, technologically were not well-developed machines, and the majority of complications came from these limitations. Performing liposculpture with the SMEI machine, the authors have never had the complications pointed out in the literature in those years which progressively destroyed the "name" of the ultrasound technique for fat emulsification. Fortunately in 2001 a new ultrasound device, called VASER (SST-Denver, CO, USA), was introduced to the US market.

This new tool has new features such as:

- New designed probes, of different caliber and shape.
- The tip is designed (with one, two, or three rings) to increase the efficiency of the emulsification, which now affects not only the tip, but also the sides of the last part of the shaft (Fig. 16.5).
- The number of rings is related to the efficacy of the emulsion depending on the type of tissue encountered (more or less fibrotic, type of fat, more or less dense).
- A new generator of ultrasound energy, with less power, but optimization of the distribution of energy at the different frequencies and wavelengths. High efficiency with less energy, which means fewer related complications due to overheating of the system. So far, in the last 5 years of the "VASER ultrasound generation," no report of burns or skin necrosis was published. An insignificant percentage of seroma was reported.
- A new aspiration system, the so-called Ventex, with a new pathway expressly designed for increasing the rate of aspiration, without damaging the tissue, thus aspirating "noble" structures, such as vessels, nerves, and elastic tissue, and impossible to block by undue aspiration of the wrong tissue.
- Skin protector, expressly designed to prevent tissue damage from friction injuries, related to the consecutive passages of the probe from the same entrance point (Fig. 16.6).

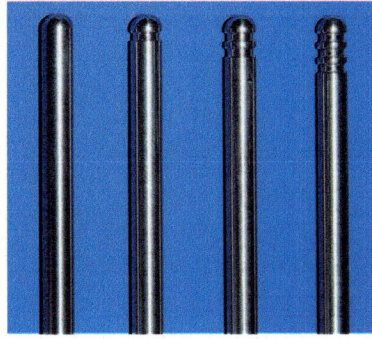

Fig. 16.5 Different probes with one , two, and three rings at the top of the shaft

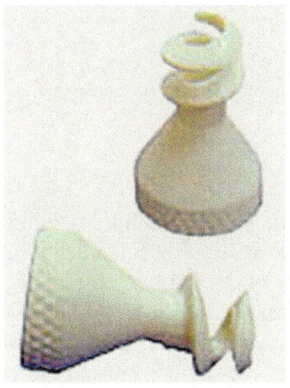

Fig. 16.6 Skin ports

- Reduced extension entrance scar of the skin, to allow the introduction of the solid titanium probes, which are smaller in diameter (standard probe varies from 2.2 to 3.7 mm). The facial probe is 2.2 mm in diameter.

Even the entrance sites are now compatible with the typical diameter of the standard liposuction cannulas (between 2 and 4 mm in diameter). The author began using the VASER system in 2001 for body-contouring surgery, breast reduction, face-contouring reduction of breast tissue in men and women, in treatment of Buffalo hump lipodystrophies, in face and neck contouring, and in axillary hyperhidrosis treatment. This is a new, excellent ultrasound tool that is safe and efficient for fat emulsification, which, commercially, has led to the term "liposelection." VASER emulsifies body fat sparing important structures of the skin and subcutaneous tissues such as vessels, nerves, and elastic fibers. Tissue trauma is minimal, edema is largely reduced, bleeding is virtually absent, and the time of recovery of tissues is consistently reduced [15, 16].

The role of the dermis in the subcutaneous anatomical structure has been undervalued in the past. The dermal layer is important for skin retraction [17]. A split skin graft (no dermis left, in this case) is not really indicated to cover joint areas (such as the elbow)

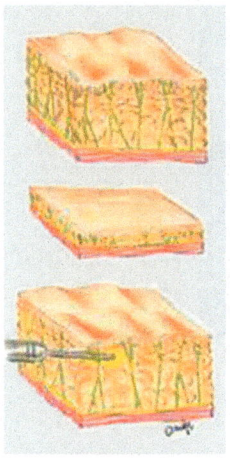

The thinner the subcutaneous fat, the greater retraction is achieved.

UAL solid titanium probe works close to the dermis, to thin the subcutaneous fat, and achieves contraction.

Fig. 16.7 The thinner the subcutaneous fat, the more the contraction

Layers of subcutaneous emulsification with Vaser UAL

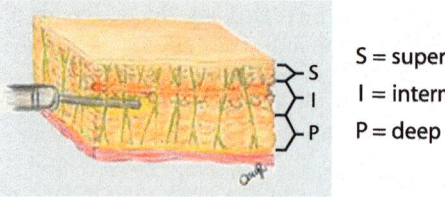

S = superficial
I = intermediate
P = deep

Fig. 16.8 Layers of emulsification of subcutaneous fat by VASER UAL

because of the possibility of skin retraction causing functional problems to the area. If a full-thickness graft is utilized (with a layer of dermis but no fat) the same area is less prone to contraction, and to functional problems (Fig. 16.7). This aspect has never been considered in skin contraction after ultrasound-assisted body contouring [18, 19]. Emulsifying the body fat, and thus conserving the connective, supporting structure of the subcutaneous tissue (Fig. 16.8), causes skin retraction much more than in standard conditions. If the surgeon can harvest a well vascularized skin dermal flap with the help of an instrument that helps prepare such a surgical plane, the potential of skin retraction is minimized and is a safe procedure (Fig. 16.9). This is the VASER technique for face and neck contouring (Figs. 16.10, 16.11). The surgeon can emulsify fat areas (chin, jowls) or just extensively undermine the areas of interest, counting on a deep, severe, intense, skin retraction, simulating the effect of a subcutaneous rhythidectomy but without cutaneous scars [20].

16.7
Commons's Technique

Facial liposuction has long been recognized as a valid procedure in the treatment of facial lipodisproportion.

Areas that can be treated include the submental area, the mandibular border, the jowls, the mid cheek, the preparotid area, and at times even the mid to the lower neck The posterior and lateral cervical areas can be included where fat deposition can disproportionately occur, especially as a sequela of protease inhibitor use in HIV patients. As far as liposuction modalities are concerned, many modes work; simple suction-assisted liposuction (SAL), ultrasound-assisted liposuction (UAL), power-assisted liposuction, and more recently UAL via the VASER (Sound Surgical) system. Laser-assisted liposuction has been generally deemed of no value.

General principles of small cannula use in all modalities, SAL, UAL, and VASER UAL, have been agreed upon (1.8–2.7-mm diameter). Procedures of head and neck liposuction can be done with local anesthesia or general anesthesia. Head and neck liposuction can be done as component maneuvers in face-lift surgery (primary or secondary) to help achieve the best possible results.

The concept of applying ultrasonic energy to face-lift relapsed lack skin to tighten this skin is useful but not always effective. For the past 4 years the VASER UAL system (Sound Surgical) has been used in 178 cases in the head and neck and has been safe and productive. The breakdown of cases includes 121 primary virgin UAL procedures. Twelve secondary facial procedures

Fat thickness varies in different body areas.

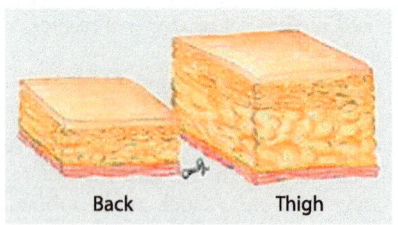

Back   Thigh

☐ Thigh and abdomen are the thickest areas

☐ Back and face are the thinnest

Fig. 16.9 Fat thickness varies in different body areas

were performed for weight gain in underdone or new (cheek) areas. The VASER UAL system has been used to assist dissection in 45 face-lift procedures (six virgin) and (31 secondary face-lift procedures) and to improve face-lift submental relapse in eight cases. In all 178 cases, safety has prevailed. There have been no nerve injuries, no burns, no seromas, and no deformity.

The VASER ultrasound times, cannula modes, cannula choice, and intensities are important. In head and neck procedures the mode is always the pulsed mode, the intensity is the lowest that is effective, 30–50. The cannulas used are 9 cm × 2.2 mm or 14 cm × 2.2 mm. Suction is done with either the Mercedes 2.4- or 1.8-mm cannula or the smallest Ventex cannula available (2.7 mm or less). Any small-aspiration cannula works but avoid cannulas over 2.7 mm.

The times of ultrasonic energy application vary, but in general use only what is needed to get the loose feeling sought in other areas of ultrasonic treatment. The times range from 30 s to 5 min in each cheek–jowl area, from 30 s to 5 min in each lateral neck area, and from 30 s to 5 min in each submental area. The nondominant "thinking hand" is always on the cannula tip and feeling location, movement, and heat.

Use only what is needed and not more. Regarding cannulas, smaller is better (ultrasonic probe or aspiration cannula). The mode is always pulsed VASER, intensity 30–50. The time is as short as is needed. Just like in eyelid surgery, or rhinoplasty, this is a thinking, planned procedure.

A wetting solution is used with a mixture of 1 l of lactated Ringer's solution with 50 ml of 1% lidocaine and 50 ml of 0.25% Marcaine (bupivacaine). To this mixture is added 1 ml of 1:1,000 epinephrine and 20 mg Kenalog (triamcinolone). Since 500 ml is adequate (almost always) one could make half of this and add the same ingredients, but it is nice to have a little extra if needed. If 500 ml is chosen of course all ingredients should be halved, or not, as is desired. Calculate all doses by the size of the patients, age, other areas done, total doses (lidocaine), etc. Safety always, perfection always.

It takes about 150–250 ml of wetting solution for the

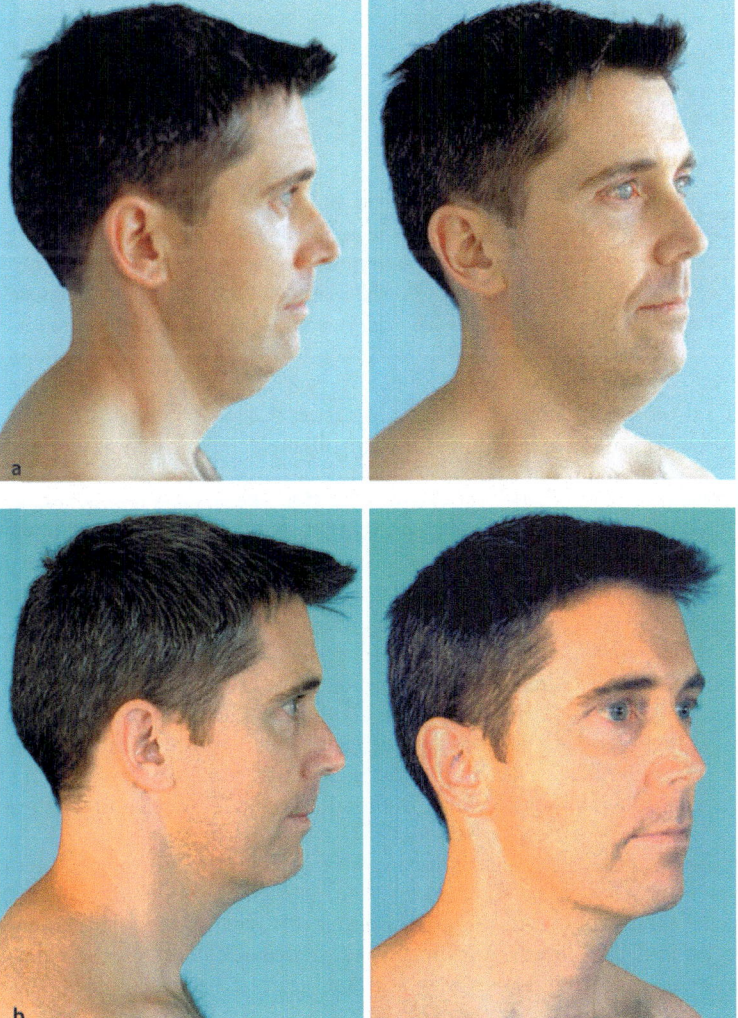

Fig. 16.10 A 38-year-old patient. **a** Preoperatively. **b** Postoperatively following jowl, chin, and neck contouring

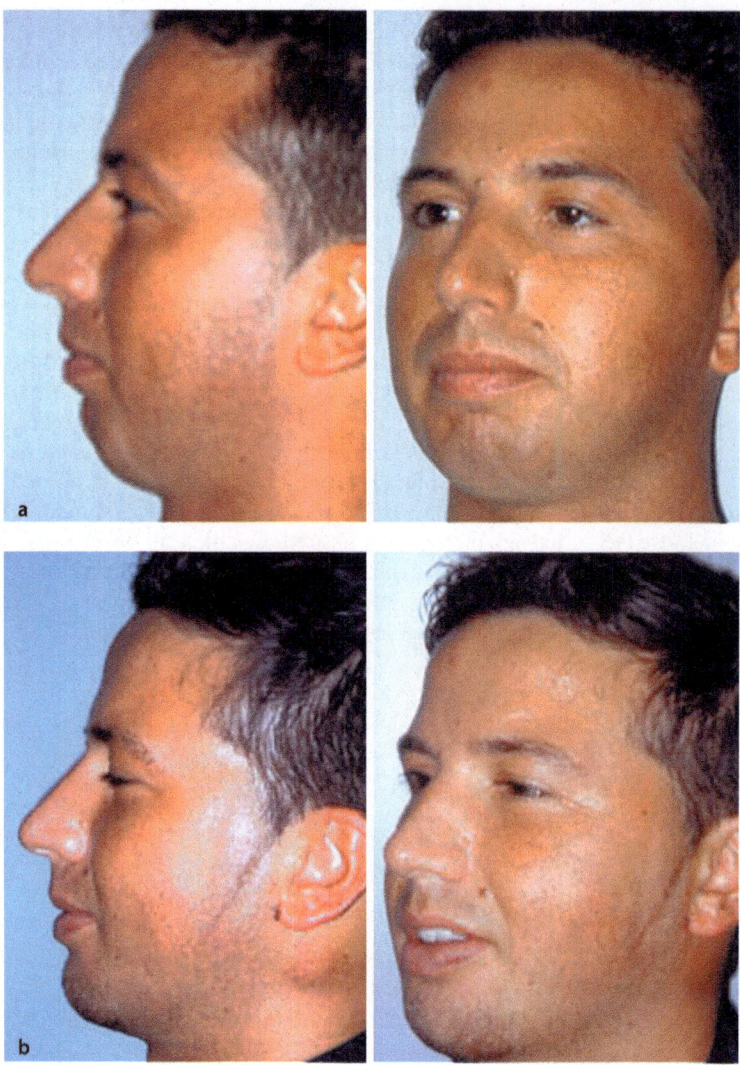

Fig. 16.11 a Preoperative 28-year-old male patient with heavy cheeks and chin retrusion. **b** One month postoperatively following VASER UAL of cheeks and neck for contouring and intraoral chin implant

full neck and submental area and 50–100 ml for each cheek area. After injection, a waiting period of 10 min allows good epinephrine effect.

The procedure is accomplished via incisions (2–3 mm) behind each earlobe and under the chin (submental) area. Skin protectors are not used but do have the assistant drop cold saline at the entrance site during UAL, and protect with wet saline gauze during the entire ultrasonic application. Again start with the 2.2-mm titanium, three-ring probe, use pulse mode, intensity 30, and time the application for each area. If desired, skin protectors can be used but slightly larger incisions are needed. After appropriate looseness is felt, stop ultrasonic energy applications and go to the next area and so on.

If the right neck or cheek is larger than the left, plan to use more time on the larger side. Do this both for UAL and the suction phases. After all areas have treated with ultrasonic energy, liposuction is begun and the emulsified fat removed with a small Ventex or other small cannulas (Mercedes 1.8 or 2.4 mm). Cannulas greater than 2.7-mm diameter are not indicated and can cause overcommitment, inaccuracy, and deformity.

The larger cheek or side of the neck almost always requires a little extra UAL and aspiration time and then the surgeon must judge the volumes, evaluate the volumes, look, feel, check preoperative pictures, and fine-tune the result with whatever final finesse is needed.

When completed, apply a circumferential light head dressing similar to a face-lift dressing and remove this the next day. Light compression head supports can then be used as well as cold compresses to assist in reducing swelling. Sutures are removed in 4–5 days or subcuticular Vicryl, Monocril, or PDS II is used and does not need to be removed.

There is usually little bruising in the low neck area near the clavicles. A turtle neck may hide this bruising.

All the usual precautions regarding aspirin, nonsteroidal anti-inflammatory drugs, etc, are given 10 days preoperatively and antibiotics are generally not used.

Pain is very minimal, but all patients are given some pain medication (Vicodin, Tylenol with codeine) in case of need.

Recovery is rapid and return to comfortable normal activity takes 4–7 days. Ultimate recovery takes longer. If confidence is not an issue, the patient can often return to work in 1–2 days. Turning the neck while driving may be restricted postoperatively so patients need to be cautioned.

16.8
Discussion

VASER UAL is useful in the head and neck area. Is it better than SAL? In some cases, yes. In others, the results may be similar. Is it easier for patient and surgeon when the VASER is used? Yes. Some necks and cheeks (especially secondary) are fibrous and the VASER ultrasonic procedure allows delicate accurate sculpting. There is less pain with VASER ultrasonic procedures than with earlier techniques. This is a mystery. Possibly the procedures are more delicately done via the VASER ultrasonic device. This lower thermal unit does not produce the burning feeling experienced by some patients with earlier UAL devices. In fibrous cases, simply less mechanical force is used via the VASER compared with traditional SAL. The VASER ultrasonic device can be used in the manner of delicately playing a violin as opposed to the somewhat sword-fighting technique of traditional SAL. Power-assisted liposuction is more traumatic to tissue, resulting in more bleeding, in all areas of the body and especially in the head and neck. Power-assisted liposuction has no place in head and neck liposuction in my opinion. It is very tissue unfriendly.

So why use this VASER UAL system as opposed to simple SAL? Certainly both work. Both may be at times equal. Overall, however, the authors feel that the influence of the ultrasonic energy on the deep dermis causes some enhanced skin shrinkage. While at times the results are similar, as operation after operation is done the results are often just a little better to considerably better in many patients. The larger the neck, the fuller the cheeks, the more excess skin there is, the better the VASER ultrasonic device proves itself.

Application of ultrasonic energy to the deep dermis is safe enough via the VASER but of course the procedure must be done safely to be safe. The Stanford plastic surgical residents working with the authors seem to quite rapidly adapt to the VASER UAL system and although there is a learning curve to this procedure, it is not difficult to achieve safe performance. Fine points, perfection of use, and maximal benefits come with experience as in most procedures.

When do the authors use ultrasonic energy? All of the time and in all cases and in all areas. It is simply easier, allows more delicate sculpting, patients are more comfortable, it is faster and more accurate, and the results are better. Defining better means better skin adaptation, a smoother surface results, there is less pain, and this in all areas of the body, including the head and neck.

What about the application of VASER ultrasonic techniques in face-lift surgery? As a liposuction tool it is useful. As a pure dissection enhancement it is very useful. In addition, dissection can be done in primary or secondary face-lift procedures and it allows a rapid, safe, dissection-assistance tool. For secondary procedures it is quick and easy and safe but is it any better? No. It works. It may speed up the procedure. Are the results better? No, they are the same, but it is an interesting consideration. In the case of face-lift relapses with some submental skin laxity, the application of VASER ultrasonic energy shows promise. In all cases there is some benefit and in some cases the results can be pleasing, but do not have 100% satisfaction.

Local anesthesia without sedation using 50 ml or so of 0.25% lidocaine with 1:400,000 epinephrine is used in the submental area or the jowl or both. Ultrasonic energy (pulsed, intensity 30, 2.2-mm cannula, 4 or 5 min or a little more) and a dressing with support are used, and there is hope for maximal skin contraction with this procedure. Some will occur. The ultrasonic energy can be applied directly subdermally and the thinking hand is used to constantly feel the tip of the cannula and to monitor the temperature. A little warmth is okay, but warmer is not okay. There have been no skin losses, burns, or nerve-damage issues.

This ultrasonic energy technique has been attempted in the nasolabial areas (no liposuction) but the improvements were minimal. Note that this ultrasonic energy technique is not liposuction. This is purely an attempt to shrink the skin or influence the skin favorably by subdermal ultrasonic energy application. The mechanism here is likely related to heating the deep dermis. It works sometimes, as occasionally does Thermage or Titan treatments, but certainly far from 100% of the time.

Liposuction works in the head and neck area. It has multiple arenas of application. The VASER ultrasonic system is a favorable, satisfying method of accomplishing liposuction. This system is safe when used in a safe manner. There likely is some useful application of this ultrasonic energy system in an attempt to shrink skin and in face-lift dissection procedures. Improvement in face-lift submental skin relapse is possible. Work, research, time, and assessment of many surgeons will better define the full parameter of use and usefulness.

Fat grafting to the head and neck area is a very valuable technique. Certainly fat removal and replacement go hand in hand. If harvested fat is to be transplanted, the removal of graft fat is done with gentle SAL initially. Final detailing is accomplished with the VASER UAL technique fully employed. Harvested fat is then appropriately grafted.

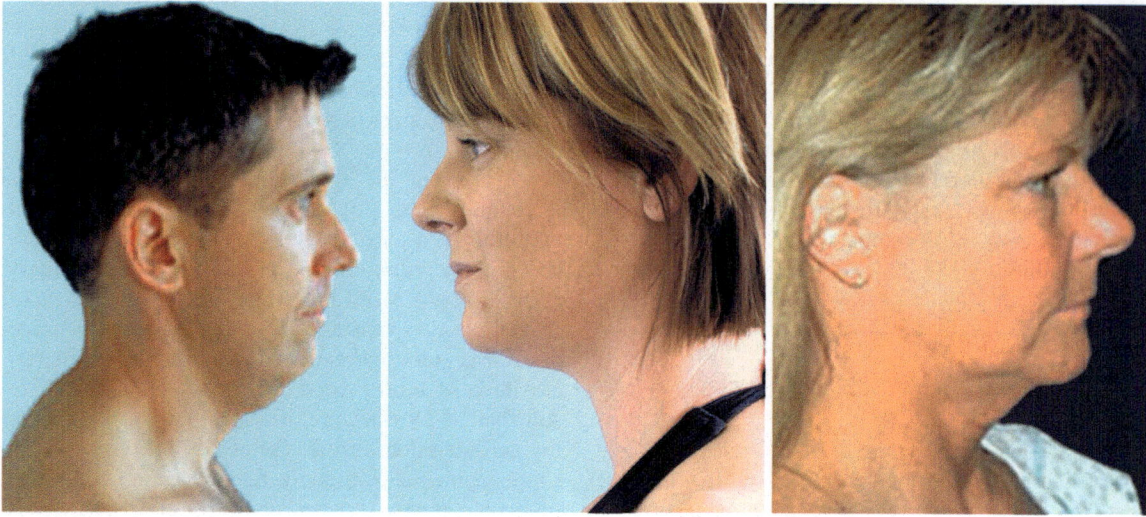

Fig. 16.12 Patients with good indications for VASER treatment

16.9
Technique of VASER

16.9.1
Indications

Patients with heavy neck and/or chin with moderate to good skin tone and where extra volume is expected to be excess fatty tissue can have VASER treatment if the neck.

16.9.2
What Patients Are Seeking?

Patients are seeking a good predictable aesthetic outcome (contouring of the neck/jowls) with maximum safety and fast recovery, with the minimum downtime.

The protocol establishes that VASER-assisted neck contouring should only be performed by surgeons already experienced with the VASER system for fatty tissue emulsification, which means at least 20 cases of standard liposelection are recommended before moving to application to the face and neck. Indicated patients (Fig. 16.12) are those who are seeking contouring of the neck and jowl areas, who have heavy neck and/or chins with moderate to good skin tone, and where extra volume is expected to be excess fatty tissue.

16.9.3
Markings

1. Plan the strategy for volume removal and associated marking.
2. Landmarks are the lower border of the mandible, corticoid, and thyroid cartilage.

3. Divide the neck into thirds infiltrating about 100 ml in each.

16.9.4
Incisions

Placement of incisions under the chin, neck, and in front or behind the ears (bilaterally). Incisions may be placed bilaterally in the neck at the lowest anticipated level of treatment.

16.9.5
Infusion

The face and the neck are more vascular and have more innervations that typical fat layers in the body. The concentration of epinephrine should be increased to

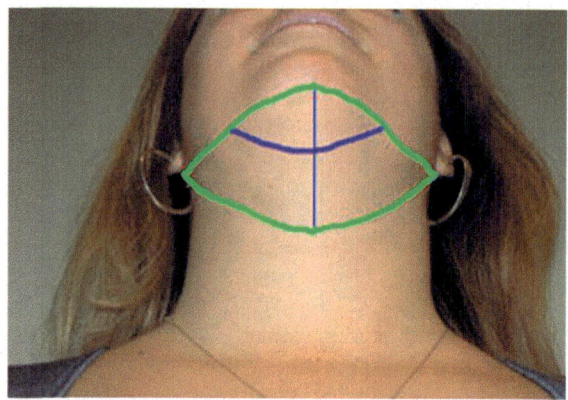

Fig. 16.13 Area of tumescent infusion. Make sure the area targeted for infusion is beyond the *upper green line*

1:500.000 and the concentration of lidocaine to 0.3–0.5%, in order to guarantee enough analgesia and vaso-constriction of the area.

The surgeon must wait between 8 and 10 min before starting surgery, until the effects of lidocaine and epinephrine begin. It is advisable to infuse with a small-diameter blunt infusion cannula (2.0 mm or smaller 14 gauge or smaller). Never use a needle. The infusion should be uniform and into all locations where the VASER or the suction cannula may be used (Fig. 16.13). The infusion should be slow, 100 ml/min, with gentle action.

16.9.6
Skin Protection

Skin protection should be used in all incisions, utilizing the black skin parts with the orange silicone discs. The discs should be sutured into place (three anchor sutures are necessary) using 3/0 or 4/0 nylon. The surgeon must make sure the knots are tight as the silicone disc tends to cause the knots to unwind. The skin ports protect the incision edges and reduce visible incision scarring. The incisions and tissues below the incision should be stretched with a hemostat to ease insertion.

16.9.7
Emulsification

Utilize the 2.2-mm diameter (18-cm- or 11-cm-long) probes, initially with the VASER mode at 20 or 40% of the maximum power of the system. The 20% amplitude in the face and neck works well when the tissues encountered are soft. The 30% amplitude is better for moderate/average fat. The 40% amplitude is indicated if the face is fibrous. Never exceed 40% with the 2.2-mm diameter probes, they may break. Apply the VASER until the targeted fat has emulsified, likely 2–3 min in total per side depending on the volumes, with an additional 2–3 min under the chin depending on how the VASER was applied on the sides. The total VASER time is 6–10 min depending on the patients and the volumes infused. The surgeon must try to achieve the targeted 6–10 min of VASER time to minimize aspiration trauma.

16.9.8
Aspiration/Cleaning

Two small stab incisions are sometimes placed in the lateral aspects of the neck at the lowest point of treatment and are left open for drainage purposes. A small suction cannula with no vacuum applied is passed through the stab incisions to open channels into the treated areas. At the end, it is advisable to massage and press tissues to force emulsified fat and fluids out of the incisions. The emulsified fat and fluids can be massaged out or will drain out of the incisions on their own.

16.9.9
Postoperative Taping/Dressing

The recommended dressing will make a gentle compression to help the skin redrape and settle into position and will aid in preventing ripples or folds in the skin. The options include cotton pads with elastic wraps, cold compresses, silicone foam padding, and elastic face garments typically applied for 2–4 days, then overnight for 1–2 weeks, depending on preference. The head should be kept elevated overnight for 4 weeks to help reduce any edema more quickly. The typical follow-up schedule is 1 day, 1 week, 6 weeks, 6 months, and as needed.

16.9.10
Protocol for External Ultrasound and for Light Massage

Endermologie-LPG or just lymphatic massage may be beneficial. External ultrasound, 10 W for 5 min with a small head twice a week for 3–4 weeks, is recommended as an alternative to Endermologie to soften tissues.

16.9.11
Results

The patients have been satisfied with the liposuction procedure using VASER technology. The results have been excellent.

References

1. Di Giuseppe A, Menna G: The harmonic lift: ultrasonic assisted skin remodelling. Int J Cosmet Surg Aesthet Dermatol 2000;2(2):125–131
2. Klein J: Tumescent technique: Tumescent Anesthesia & Microcannular Liposuction, St. Louis, Mosby 2000
3. Grotting JC, Beckestein MS: The solid probe technique in ultrasound-assisted lipoplasty. Clin Plast Surg 1999;26(2):245–254
4. Rohrich RJ, Beran SJ, Kenkel JM: Ultrasound Assisted Liposuction. St. Louis, Quality Medical Publishing 1998
5. Gingrass MK: Lipoplasty complications and their prevention. Clin Plast Surg 1999;26(3):341–354
6. Tebbetts JB: Minimizing complications of ultrasound-assisted lipoplasty: an initial experience with no related complications. Plast Reconstr Surg 1998;102(5):1690–1697
7. Illouz YG: Study of subcutaneous fat. Aesthet Plast Surg 1990;14(3):165–177
8. Gibson T: Physical properties of skin. In McCarthy Plastic Surgery, Philadelphia, Saunders 1990

9. Gibson T, Kenedi RM: The structural components of the dermis. In Montagna W, Bentley JP, Dobson L, (Eds.), The Dermis. New York, Appleton—Century Crofts 1970

10. Southwood WF: The thickness of the skin. Plast Reconstr Surg 1955;15(5):423–429

11. Pitman GH: Liposuction and Aesthetic Surgery. St. Louis, Quality Medical Publishing 1993

12. Fodor PB, Watson J: Personal experience with ultrasound-assisted lipoplasty: a pilot study comparing ultrasound-assisted lipoplasty with traditional lipoplasty. Plast Reconstr Surg 1998;101(4):1103–1116

13. Scheflan M, Tazi H: Ultrasonically assisted body contouring. Aesthet Surg J 1996;16:117–122

14. Cimino WW: Ultrasonic surgery: Power quantification and efficiency optimization. Aesthet Plast Surg J 2001; 21:233

15. Jewell ML, Souza Pinto E.B., Fodor P.B., Shamarri M.A.: Clinical application of Vaser assisted lipoplasty: a pilot clinical study. Aesthet Plast Surg J 2002; 22:131

16. Di Giuseppe A: Ultrasonically assisted liposculpture: Physical and technical principles and clinical application. Am J Cosmet Surg 1997:14(3) 317–327

17. Rudolph R, Guber S, Suzuki M, Woodward M: The life cycle of the myofibroblast. Surg Gynecol Obstet 1977;145(3):389–400

18. Becker H: Subdermal liposuction to enhance skin contraction: a preliminary report. Ann Plast Surg 1992:28(5):479–484

19. Gasparotti A: Superficial liposuction: a new application of the technique for aged and flaccid skin. Aesthet Plast Surg 1992:16:141–153

20. Shiffman MA, Di Giuseppe A: Liposuction: Principles and Techniques. Springer, Berlin 2006

CHAPTER 17

Complications of Laser

Melvin A. Shiffman

17.1
Introduction

Laser facial skin resurfacing requires an understanding of the laser capability, such as extent of burn, as well as the safety requirements for the use of the laser. Early diagnosis and treatment of complications may be necessary to prevent serious injury.

17.2
Complications

17.2.1
Hyperpigmentation

Hyperpigmentation tends to occur more often in the Asian or Hispanic. Sun avoidance in the postoperative period is most important. Postinflammatory hyperpigmentation is treated with hydroquinone followed by kojic acid, azelaic acid, and glycolic acid if necessary.

17.2.2
Hypopigmentation

If the hypopigmentation is from destruction of the melanocytes, the loss of pigmentation is usually permanent. If the hypopigmentation is postinflammatory, then steroids or nonsteroidal anti-inflammatory drugs may be helpful. Light peels may help to blunt the contrasting skin.

17.2.3
Infection

If infection is suspected the area should be cleansed with mild soap and/or Burrow's solution. Smears should be taken for culture to distinguish between bacterial and fungal infection and to determine antibiotic treatment.

Herpes simplex infection should be avoided with the use of perioperative antivirals. If infection occurs the dose should be increased and intravenously administered acyclovir should be considered for disseminated herpes.

17.2.4
Milia

Treatment consists of needle insertion to open the skin and then the white material can be squeezed out with a comedone extractor.

17.2.5
Prolonged Erythema

Erythema is a side effect of laser resurfacing, but if it is prolonged or increased in intensity steroids should be used either topically or orally (Medrol Dosepak) [1]. Thickening of the skin with erythema requires more-intensive treatment for impending hypertrophic scar (steroid ointment, silicone patches and gel, and Kenalog injections). A flashlamp-pumped pulsed dye laser may be considered [1].

17.2.6
Pain

Pain is usually temporary during the period of healing. Persistent pain may indicate infection or inflammation.

17.2.7
Scar

Prolonged inflammation is the precursor of scarring and should be treated with steroid creams 1 week at a time with stopping for 2 weeks in-between treatments.

Hypertrophic or keloid scars can occur and may be treated with the usual method of steroid injection, 5-fluorouracil injection, silicone sheeting, surgery, or a combination of these. Keloids recur in 80% of cases.

17.2.8
Telangiectasia

Telangiectasias may be present preoperatively and become more prominent after laser treatment. Telangiectatic lesions may increase in number as well. Treatment may require an appropriate vascular laser (1,064-nm laser) or intense pulsed light.

Reference

1. Keller GS, Lacombe VG: Laser resurfacing: An overview. In Lasers in Aesthetic Surgery, Keller GS, Lacombe VG, Lee PK, Watson JP (Eds), New York, Thieme 2001:41–66

Chapter 18

Thermage Radiofrequency

18

Rhoda S. Narins, Kenneth Beer, David J. Narins

18.1
Introduction

The ideal device for skin tightening would be able to accomplish a nonsurgical facelift with minimal downtime, risk and discomfort. Various devices have been introduced with the promise of delivering this miracle, but perhaps none has so captivated the attention of consumers (and physicians driven by their patients) as ThermaCool TC™ by Thermage®. This device employs a radiofrequency energy source to heat and subsequently tighten dermal connective tissue.

Rather than using light to heat the skin, ThermaCool TC™ utilizes an elegant application of electrical engineering to deliver uniform heating to an area of dermis without burning the intervening epidermis. A 6-MHz current is generated by the radiofrequency generator within the main part of the device [1]. This current is delivered to the skin via a disposable tip. The disposable tip and software that govern it are the truly novel aspects of the system. The tip contains a contact surface of a known area and software constantly measures skin temperature, resistance and other key parameters. This information is evaluated in real time by a computer and if any monitored data fall out of predetermined parameters, energy delivery is aborted to avoid tissue injury. For instance, with the newer treatment tips if all four corners of the tip are not in contact with the patient's skin, the device will not deliver a pulse since doing so would most likely result in the delivery of current to a smaller area of skin than was intended and likely result in a burn. Cryogen spray is delivered by the hand piece to cool the inner surface of the treatment tip membrane. Unlike lasers and light sources, which produce heating in tissue depending on the differential absorption of optical energy by the target (selective photothermolysis), the ThermaCool TC™ uses radiofrequency energy to deliver a uniform volumetric heating effect into the deep dermis and underlying tissue. Heat is generated by the tissue's natural resistance to the flow of current within an electric field, rather than from photon absorption. The ThermaCool TC™ has a unique capacitive coupled electrode design that disperses energy uniformly across the surface area of the treatment tip membrane. This creates a uniform electric field (zone of heating) in tissue at controlled depths. The electric field changes polarity six million times per second. Charged particles within the electric field change orientation at that same frequency, and the tissue's natural resistance to this electron movement generates heat (resistive heating). Utilization of a unique method of contact cooling prior to, during and after application of the energy produces a reverse thermal gradient with the greatest heating in the deep dermis while protecting the epidermis from thermal injury. It tightens deep tissue while sparing the epidermis. The depth of heating is treatment tip dependent not wavelength-dependent. Depths of heating and cooling are controlled by treatment tip geometry and/or cooling parameter adjustments within the tip. In the future new treatment tips may enable different levels of the dermis and subcutaneous tissue to be targeted. The complete mechanism of action of the tissue tightening is unclear. It has been hypothesized that the ThermaCool TC™ delivers enough heat into a large volume of tissue to cause immediate collagen contraction followed by a significant wound-healing response, resulting in gradual tissue tightening over time. The heat produced by the radiofrequency energy changes the molecular structure of the triple-helix collagen molecule by heating it to a point where it breaks the hydrogen bonds, resulting in collagen contraction. Unpublished transmission electron microscopy research performed immediately after treatment reinforces this hypothesis. This research demonstrated an immediate morphological change in individual collagen fibrils and confirmed the presence of partial denatured (contracted) collagen in the mid and deep dermis.

The elegance and efficacy of the ThermaCool TC™ system lies in what is referred to as volumetric heating. To picture this, it is useful to first banish traditional perceptions of heating in which a continuous front of heat is delivered to a surface and subsequently penetrates whatever lies beneath. Traditional heating implies that heat diminishes as the radiation travels through a target as energy is absorbed by the material it interacts with. Radiofrequency waves, as utilized by ThermaCool TC™, are more akin to microwaves, which heat deeply rather than superficially. A homogenous wave of heat is pro-

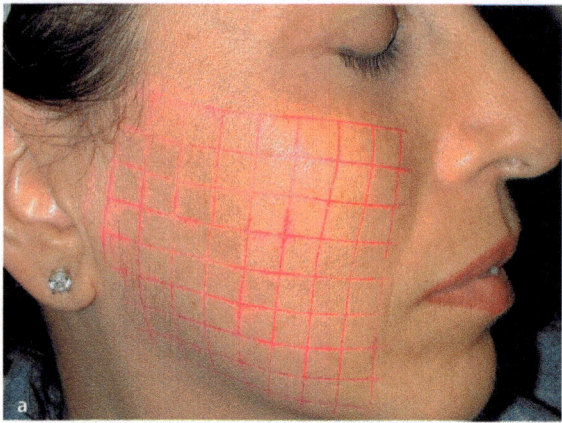

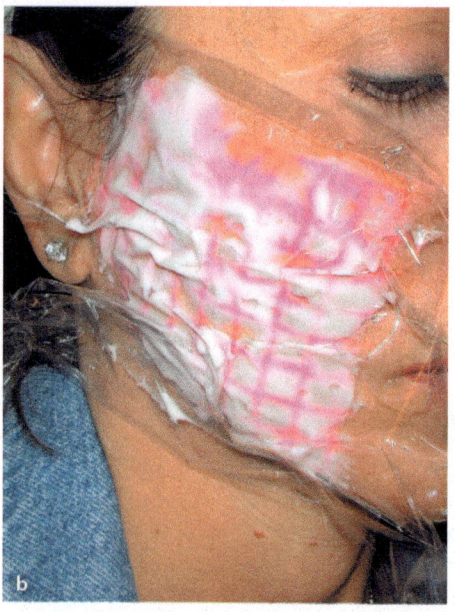

Fig. 18.1 a Grid used for area to be treated. **b** Occlusion for 1 h

duced at a precise level of the dermis. The depth, size and energy delivered are governed by the impedance of the tissue, size of the tip applied and current generated [1]. ThermaCool TC™ links the amount of heat generated with cooling provided to govern where and how much heat is applied to different levels of the skin. Thus, by controlling the variables of heating and cooling, energy is efficiently applied at a level deeper than is possible with most light-based nonablative technologies.

Histology studies demonstrate several changes following treatment with this device [2]. Collagen fibers become tighter immediately after the treatment and, on a longer term, become thicker and more youthful in histologic appearance.

18.2
Technique

As with other nonablative technologies, results with ThermaCool TC™ are technique-dependent. One critical component of the technique for this procedure is patient selection and education. Although the procedure is capable of tightening the skin, it is not adequate for patients who absolutely require rhytidectomy (nor was it intended for these people). It is important to select patients who have a realistic understanding of the procedure, its limitations, its benefits and the possible requirement for several treatment sessions. Treating patients who expect to have a facelift result from one session will be counterproductive for physician and patient alike.

Additional patient selection criteria have been published by Fisher et al. [3], who indicate that treating obese patients with ThermaCool TC™ will not produce satisfactory results. They also report that the device should not be used in patients with pacemakers.

Patients who will benefit from treatment include those with mild to moderate skin laxity in areas that are amenable to treatment. These areas include the forehead and brow regions, the regions of the neck and jaw and the cheeks.

Kaminer and Hsu [4] treated 16 patients with ThermaCool TC™ and reported an improvement of skin laxity of the cheeks after a single pass. In addition, their findings illustrate several technical considerations that improve the likelihood of having good outcomes. These include the use of higher energy settings, treating larger surface areas and treating patients who are younger. Using settings of 134 J/cm² to the left side of the forehead, 115 J/cm² to the left temple and cheeks and 97 J/cm² to the left jaw, Nahm et al. [5] demonstrated objective improvements of skin laxity using a single pass. Thus, these parameters are a good baseline for beginning patient treatments. A larger series that specifically evaluated neck and cheek laxity following a single treatment demonstrated significant improvement that lasted for at least 6 months [6]. The parameters used in this study were between 97 and 144 J/cm² (Fig. 18.1). Approximately 80% of those patients treated in this study had moderate improvement with the single treatment (Figs. 18.2, 18.3). Kaminer and Jacob [1] recommend parameters as follows: for the temple and crow's-feet 13–13.5; for the forehead 72.5–74.5; for the temples 73 or less; and 14.5–15.5 for the first pass of the lower face with slightly lower settings for subsequent passes.

Recent improvements in technique have enhanced patient outcomes. One significant advance has been the addition of additional passes during a treatment session. After one pass, a second and sometimes a third pass may be performed. Many practitioners recommend that ThermaCool TC™ treatments be repeated approximately 1 month apart. How many treatments are optimal and what additional passes do for the longevity of correction remain to be defined.

Fisher et al. [3] have found greater improvements in patient outcomes as they have evolved to more treatment sessions (should this be "multiple passes and several treatment sessions") conducted at lower energy settings. They report that they typically treat the face with two passes at 107 J using the 1.5-cm tip. Following two passes at this setting, they use an energy setting of 83 J for an additional three passes for a total of five passes. This is significantly different from initial reports which recommended higher settings for fewer passes and is consistent with recommendations by other experienced operators of this device, including Kaminer.

One additional technical consideration for treat-ment with ThermaCool TC™ is pain management. The treatment is uncomfortable and although some patients can tolerate it with topical anesthetic such as lidocaine or compounded topical anesthetics, most patients require additional anesthesia. Since the device measures tissue impedance and injections of large volumes of liquid reduce impedance, it is presently not suggested that infiltration with lidocaine or tumescent anesthesia be utilized. The manufacturer recommends avoiding local anesthesia or anesthetic block injections as pain feedback is believed to be an important parameter for treatment end points. Nerve blocks are helpful for regions amenable to them, but in many areas of Therma-Cool TC™ treatment, the sites undergoing treatment are innervated by small cutaneous branches not easily treated by regional blocks. Exceptions to this include the glabella and forehead areas. Physicians performing the procedure with any degree of frequency will most

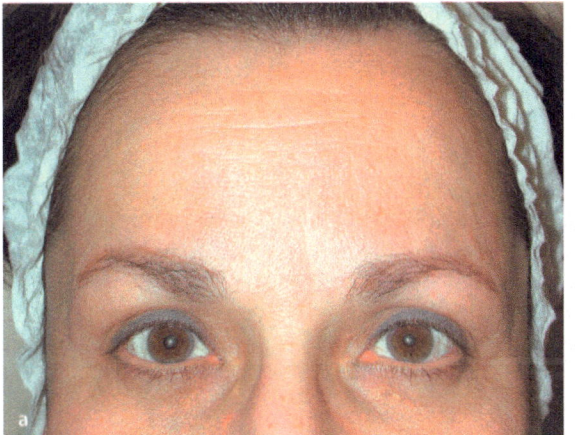
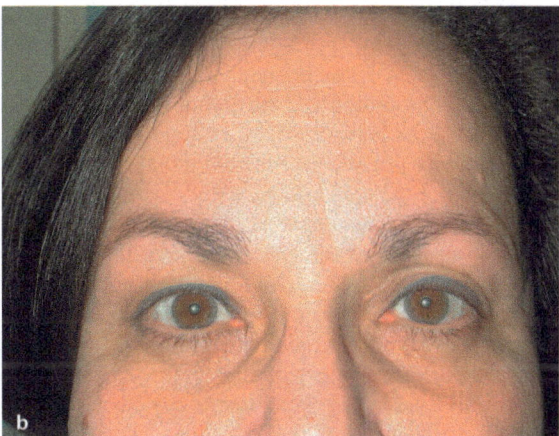

Fig. 18.2 **a** Before treatment. **b** Six weeks after treatment of the brow

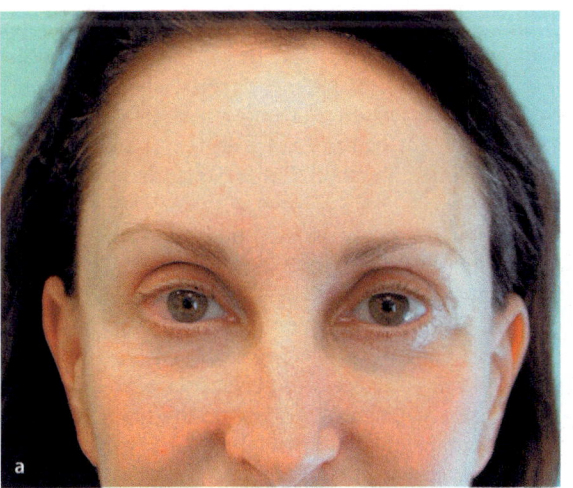
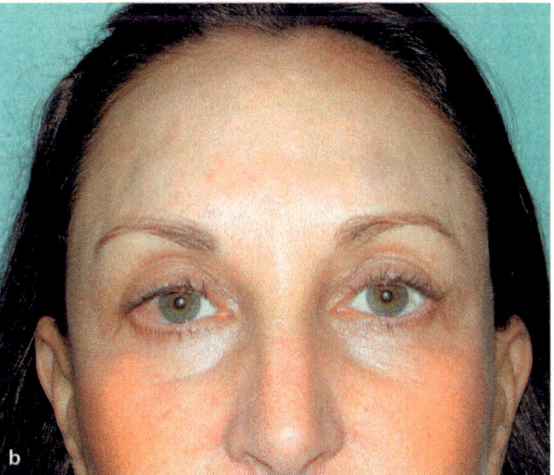

Fig. 18.3 **a** Before treatment. **b** Six weeks after treatment of the brow

likely find it useful to administer some form of amnestic, sedative or opioid derivative alone or in combinations. Among the medications that may be utilized are Demerol, Atarax, Valium, Versed and other drugs from each of these families. Obviously, when administering any of these medications, the physician should be well versed in the doses, side effects and potential complications that may result. Many physicians who administer sedatives find it helpful to have monitoring equipment readily available.

18.3
Complications

The overall rate of complications with ThermaCool TC™ procedures has been low and it is likely that if it were possible to parse the data for nonspecialist and nonphysician providers of the procedure, it would be lower still. In one study, the most common complications were mild erythema and edema, consistent with other noninvasive rejuvenation procedures [3]. Alster and Tanzi [6] reported mild erythema in all patients treated with this device. They noted that the erythema was mild and that it lasted for between 2 and 12 h. Other complications that were initially noted with increased frequency in early use of the device include vesiculation, crusting and erosions [3]. These have become less frequent with increased experience with the device, but may be seen as new operators, particularly those with no dermatology or plastic surgery training, adopt the procedure.

More serious complications reported have included formation of granuloma, scarring, fat atrophy and neuralgia. The incidence of granulomas has been variable and seems to depend on the area treated as well as the energy parameters used. Erythematous papules that spontaneously resolved were noted in 6% of patients treated on the neck in one study [6]. It has been noted that the incidence of subcutaneous papule has diminished with the adoption of lower-energy, multiple-pass protocols [3]. Perhaps the lower energy settings do not disrupt the adipocytes and therefore do not induce the same degree of phagocytosis induced with higher settings. One interesting question that should be evaluated clinically and histologically is whether intentional use of higher energy settings may be useful in treating areas of unwanted fat and cellulite. It would be worthwhile to conduct this trial and determine whether ThermaCool TC™ or the reaction it stimulates can be helpful in treating these conditions. Fat atrophy has been noted to occur following treatments with higher energies and was reported to spontaneously resolve over the span of 2 years [3].

Alster and Tanzi [6] noted that 56% of their patients reported some mild discomfort in the areas treated. It should be noted that post-treatment discomfort appears to be increased when the neck is treated. In this same study, one of 50 patients treated developed a dysesthesia that resolved spontaneously several days after treatment. Again, this seems to be consistent with other reports that have documented increased sensitivity following treatments to the neck and jaw. Fisher et al. [3] have reported a single patient with temporary anesthesia of the earlobe after treatment of the posterior neck and another patient with trigeminal neuralgia.

More recently, treatment of "delayed contour irregularities" by using subcision and autologous fat transfer has been reported by Narins et al. [7]. These authors suggest that long-term contour irregularities may be avoided by staying within recommended treatment parameters, waiting 2 min before a second pass and paying attention to patient "feedback" especially when treating the malar, temple and forehead areas. If contour irregularities occur, they report that they are correctable provided that certain steps are taken.

Fortunately, the majority of complications reported with this device have been mild and self-limited. Most of the complications appear to be related to higher energy parameters and the incidence of these complications has fallen with experience and adoption of lower energy guidelines. One cautionary note that should be addressed is the frequent use of this technology by those least capable of understanding its method of action or comprehending the complications that may ensue. As with other devices, this machine continues to be marketed and utilized by physicians who have no training in dermatology or plastic surgery and by nonphysicians who are entering the cosmetic marketplace spurred by the lack of regulation and aggressive marketing by several corporations.

18.4
Discussion

The advent of a nonsurgical radiofrequency skin tightening device is a significant milestone for dermatologic and plastic surgeons. The ThermaCool TC™ device is FDA-approved to treat periorbital skin laxity and rhytids. Several studies have demonstrated its efficacy albeit it has not had the same degree of consistent results in clinical practice that these studies would suggest.

Efficacy was first evaluated by Fitzpatrick et al. [8], who evaluated 86 patients treated with a single pass for treatment of periorbital rhytids. They found that 83% of those treated had an improvement of their rhytids at 6 months. Other investigators have reported efficacy of the device in other areas of the face. Jacobson et al. [9] have treated patients with laxity on the lower face and neck. Significantly, they treated patients with multiple passes at each session and repeated sessions at intervals of 4 weeks. Patients were allowed to have up to three sessions in this study. In this study 17 of the 24 patients studied had visible improvement of their skin laxity. Similar findings have been reported by other investigators [6].Given the outcomes reported with these studies, it seems reasonable to use the treatment parameters and outcomes reported to guide patient expectations and physician treatment protocols. Treatment parameters reported in these latter two studies are more consistent with the clinical parameters that are presently in widespread usage.

Radiofrequency skin tightening is one of the most interesting advances in aesthetic surgery in several years. The initial device approved by the FDA has undergone several refinements with software upgrades and improvements to the tip. Additional improvements in technique have improved patient outcomes and reduced complications. It is anticipated that radiofrequency skin tightening will continue to advance as newer devices and adjunctive treatments become widely utilized.

18.5
Conclusions

Until recently, surgical rhytidectomy was the only option available for patients with skin laxity. The advent of radiofrequency skin tightening brings a new option for patient care to the expanding horizon of noninvasive skin rejuvenation. Combinations of fillers and volumizers, photorejuvenation, botulinum toxins, cosmeceuticals, prescription medications and thread lifting procedures are now available, and when used in individualized combinations can now bring comprehensive noninvasive rejuvenation to an increasing number of patients. There is no doubt that future iterations of radiofrequency devices will improve upon the technology presently available. As this occurs, advances in technique and patient outcomes will follow.

References

1. Kaminer M, Jacob C: In Laser and Lights, Procedures in Cosmetic Dermatology, Goldberg D. Elsevier, Philadelphia. 43–60
2. Zelickson BD, Kist D, Bernstein E, Brown DB, Ksenzenko S, Burns J, Kilmer S, Mehregan D, Pope K: Histologic and ultrastructural evaluation of the effects of a radiofrequency based non ablative dermal remodeling device: A Pilot Study. Arch Dermatol. 2004;140(2):204–209
3. Fisher GH, Jacobson LG, Bernstein LJ, Kim KH, Geronemus RG: Nonablative Radiofrequency Treatment of Facial Laxity. Dermatol Surg. 2005;31(9 Pt 2):1237–1241
4. Hsu TS, Kaminer MS: The use of nonablative radiofrequency technology to tighten the lower face and neck. Semin Cutan Med Surg. 2003;22(2);115–123
5. Nahm WK, Su TT, Rotunda AM, Moy RL: Objective changes in brow position, superior palpebral crease, peak angle of the eyebrow, and jowl surface area after volumetric radiofrequency treatments to half of the face. Dermatol Surg. 2004;30(6);922–928
6. Alster TS, Tanzi E: Improvement of neck and cheek laxity with a nonablative radiofrequency device: A lifting experience. Dermatol Surg. 2004; 30(4 Pt 1):503–507
7. Narins RS, Tope WD, Pope K, Ross EV: Overtreatment effects associated with a radiofrequency tissue tightening device: rare, preventable, and correctable with subcision and autologous fat transfer. Dermatol Surg. 2006;32(1):115–124
8. Fitzpatrick R, Geronemus R, Goldberg D, Kaminer M, Kilmer S, Ruiz-Esparza J: Multicenter study of noninvasive radiofrequency for periorbital tissue tightening. Lasers Surg Med. 2003;33(4):232–242
9. Jacobson LG, Alexiades-Armenakas M, Bernstein L, Geronemus RG: Treatment of nasolabial folds and jowls with a noninvasive radiofrequency device. Arch Dermatol. 2003;139(10):1371–1372

CHAPTER 19

Capacitive Radiofrequency Skin Rejuvenation

19

Manoj T. Abraham

19.1
Introduction

Radiofrequency (RF) energy is part of the electromagnetic spectrum. RF energy has been used extensively in medicine over the past century as electrocautery to generate focused heat to cut and to coagulate tissue during surgery. There have been some recent reports of electrocautery being used directly for aesthetic skin resurfacing [1–6]. In a process called coblation, RF current is applied to the skin surface via a conductive medium such as saline, creating a superficial zone of injury [7]. As with other modalities of ablative skin resurfacing (dermabrasion, deep chemical peels, lasers), controlled destruction of the epidermis and dermis down to the reticular layer, followed by the expected 7–14-day healing response, results in rejuvenation of the skin. Ablative resurfacing must be confined to facial skin, where adequate hair density allows for safe reepithelialization. Proper technique and meticulous aftercare to maintain a moist environment conducive to healing are essential to avoid potential scarring. Areas that are resurfaced may remain erythematous and sensitive for several months after treatment, and may be prone to long-term alteration in pigment.

Techniques to use RF energy in a non-ablative fashion have been developed over the past several years. This less-invasive approach has been used successfully to tighten joint capsules, alter corneal contour, enhance esophageal tone, and shrink obstructive palate and turbinate tissue contributing to snoring and sleep apnea.

Non-ablative RF tightening and rejuvenation of the skin has also recently gained popularity. Thermage, based in Hayward, CA, USA has pioneered the aesthetic application of non-ablative RF skin tightening. The ThermaCool™ system utilizes the company's proprietary technology incorporating large capacitive electrodes to deliver RF energy into the skin while simultaneously protecting the skin surface with a cryogen cooling spray. Thermage was initially granted FDA regulatory clearance for treatment of periorbital wrinkles and rhytids in November 2002. This was followed by clearance for full-face treatment in June 2004. In January 2006, the FDA expanded its clearance to treatment of all skin surface wrinkles and rhytids. Although there are currently other non-ablative RF and non-RF devices available for skin tightening (Table 19.1), these devices and technologies do not have the same accumulation of studies reporting efficacy in the scientific literature [8–34].

19.2
Technique

The ThermaCool™ system delivers RF energy via a monopolar capacitive electrode while concurrently cooling the epidermis with a cryogen spray. This creates a reverse thermal gradient (Fig. 19.1), which causes partial collagen denaturation within the dermis without injury to the skin surface [8, 26]. Initial contraction of the skin collagen network in the dermis occurs immediately as the collagen fibrils reanneal. Tightening continues as a healing response is triggered within the dermis, leading to an overall increase in skin collagen content (Fig. 19.2).

Non-ablative capacitive RF treatment is most ap-

Table 19.1 Devices for non-ablative skin tightening

RF devices	Non-RF devices
Capacitive monopolar RF (Thermage, Hayward, CA, USA)	Intense pulsed light sources
Bipolar RF and optical energy (Syneron, Yokneam, Israel)	Long-pulse 1,064-nm Nd:YAG lasers
	Infrared energy (Titan) (Cutera, Brisbane, CA, USA)
	Fraxel laser (Reliant Technologies, Palo Alto, CA, USA)

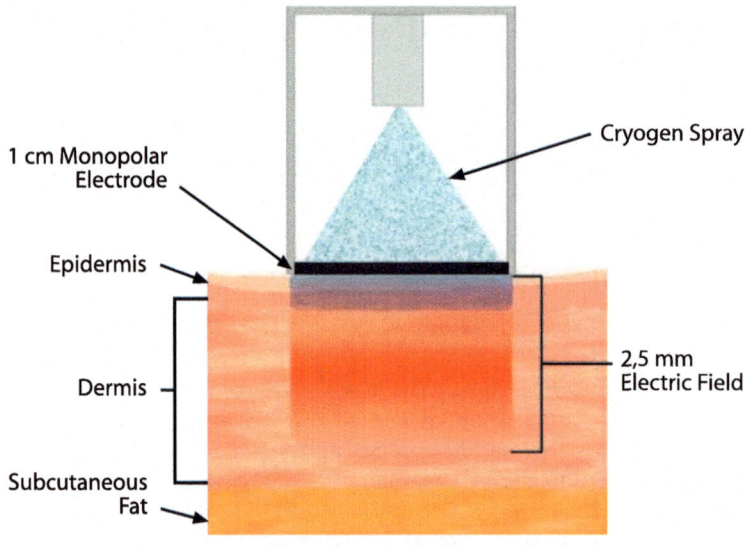

Fig. 19.1 The reverse thermal gradient created within the skin during Therma Cool™ capacitive RF treatment. The cryogen spray cools and protects the epidermis, while RF energy is delivered volumetrically to the dermis

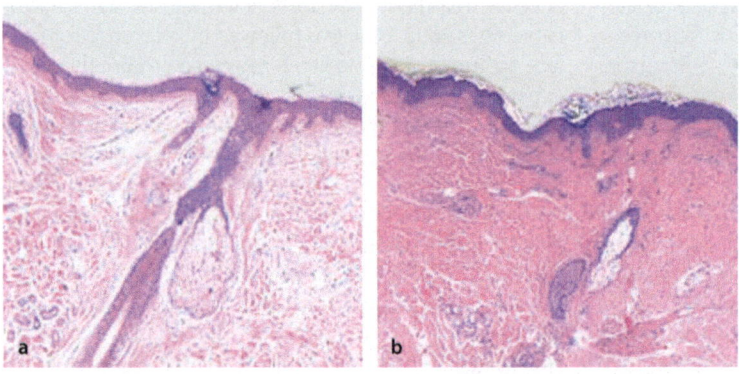

Fig. 19.2 Biopsy of aging human skin stained with hematoxylin and eosin **a** before and **b** 4 months after capacitive RF treatment. There is increased density of collagen in the dermis, sebaceous gland atrophy and thickening of the epidermis. (Histology courtesy of Thermage, Hayward, CA, USA; Julio Barba Gomez and Javier Ruiz-Esparza)

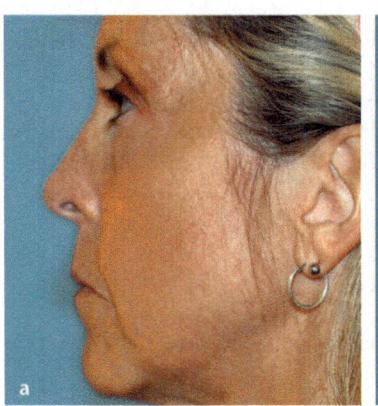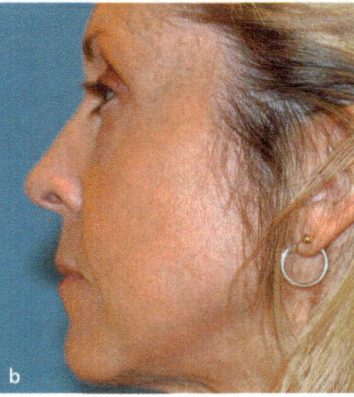

Fig. 19.3 a Before treatment. **b** Patient 2 months after non-ablative capacitive RF treatment of the face and upper neck. Brow elevation and improvement in jaw line and midface profile are evident

propriate for patients with mild to moderate aging and wrinkling of the skin. Patients with significant skin laxity or those with noticeable underlying structural ptosis, who are not interested in surgical options for rejuvenation, may still obtain a theoretical antiaging benefit from collagen stimulation in the skin. Patients must be cautioned to have realistic expectations. It is the author's experience that those with thinner skin typically achieve a more dramatic result. Patients with thicker, more sebaceous skin may require more then one treatment session. ThermaCool™ treatment can be combined with other minimally invasive office-based or surgical procedures to obtain a cumulative result (Table 19.2) [9–11, 27, 28]. When performed alone, there are few contraindications to ThermaCool™ treatment (Table 19.3).

Table 19.2 Minimally invasive procedures that can be combined effectively with capacitive RF skin rejuvenation

Surgical procedures	Non-surgical treatments
Facial and neck liposuction	Chemodenervation
Blepharoplasty	Tissue fillers
Percutaneous suture techniques	Intense pulsed light and non-ablative lasers
	Microdermabrasion and superficial chemical peels

Table 19.3 Contraindications to capacitive RF skin rejuvenation

Absolute contraindications	Relative contraindications
Implanted medical device (pacemaker, defibrillator, etc.)	Dermatologic conditions
Pregnancy	Collagen-vascular or autoimmune diseases
	Impaired collagen production (radiation, metabolic, etc.)

Despite newer multiple-pass treatment algorithms that require less energy to be delivered at one time, capacitive RF treatment is uncomfortable. There is an initial cooling sensation as the cryogen cooling spray is applied, overcome by a burst of heat as RF energy is delivered, followed by cooling again. Since a typical full-face and upper-neck treatment with the 1.5-cm² tip involves 600 RF pulses and can take 1 h or more to perform, some form of anesthesia is recommended to optimize patient comfort. Most patients with appropriate temperament are able to tolerate treatment using oral narcotic analgesics (oxycodone, hydrocodone) and short-acting anxiolytics (lorazepam, alprazolam). Topical anesthetics are counterproductive as they numb the epidermis and the cooling sensation, but are not effective in alleviating the discomfort of penetrating RF heat [30]. Local injection anesthetics can alter skin resistance and interfere with proper RF energy delivery [9, 12, 32]. Sedation or general anesthesia should only be utilized by experienced providers, since the additional safety measure of patient feedback is removed.

Typically, all non-hair-bearing areas of the face and upper neck are treated. Upper-lid skin is distracted onto the orbital rim and away from the globe prior to treatment. The skin over the nose is densely adherent and does not require treatment. Areas to be treated are first cleansed with mild soap and water. All metal accoutrements are removed, and the grounding pad is applied to an area distant from the treatment site. The manufacturer-supplied ink grid is used to guide treatment topography, and coupling fluid is used to ensure uniform delivery of energy. An initial test pulse is performed on each patient to allow the machine to calibrate skin resistance. Complete, even contact of the electrode with the skin surface is necessary to initiate cooling and RF delivery.

The patient is asked to provide feedback using a 0–4 point scale (0 nothing, 1 warm, 2 hot, 3 very hot, 4 burning), with treatment settings calibrated to a 2–2.5 level. With the 1.5-cm² tip, this usually translates to a setting of 61–96 J/cm² in most areas. Energy levels are reduced (44–61 J/cm²) in areas of thinner skin (around the orbital rim), over vulnerable superficial fat pads (temporal, malar), over sensory nerve trunks (greater auricular, supraorbital, infraorbital, mental) and over the platysma in the neck.

One or two initial passes are performed to cover the entire treatment area to achieve uniform contraction of the collagen skin scaffold. Where more skin tightening is desired, additional passes are performed along vectors perpendicular to the relaxed skin tension lines of the face. For instance, contiguous treatment around the mouth is avoided since circumferential tightening would accentuate perioral rhytids. Instead, superior and lateral vectors are targeted to lift, tighten and stretch the skin around the lips, nasolabial folds and marionette creases.

RF energy is known to conduct through collagen-based fibrous septae that surround fat lobules in the subcutaneous tissue [11]. Additional shrinkage and definition can be accomplished by targeting these fibrous septae. This strategy works well in areas of fullness such as the submental and jowl regions. Stacking of treatment pulses on top of each other without time in-between pulses is generally not recommended owing to concerns of excessive heat buildup, but can be used effectively in experienced hands to achieve further tissue sculpting [25].

Visible tightening, erythema of the skin and patient discomfort are all subjective clinical end points of treatment. If other complementary procedures are to be done concurrently (Table 19.2), they should be performed after ThermaCool™ treatment has been completed [9, 11, 18, 27].

If capacitive RF treatment is performed alone, aftercare is minimal. Most patients can resume normal activities immediately after the procedure. Patients are instructed to avoid using ice or anti-inflammatory medications that may blunt the healing response and impede collagen stimulation.

In patients with thin skin and moderate laxity, initial improvement is seen immediately owing to thermally mediated collagen tightening. Thickening, toning and lifting of the skin peaks a few weeks after treatment and continues for 4 months or longer, as a result of increased collagen production in the skin [9–17]. Contour changes seen in the face typically include 2–4 mm of brow elevation, smoothing of the nasolabial folds and marionette creases, and better definition of the jaw line and cervicomental angle (Fig. 19.3) [9–22, 24, 25, 31–34]. Intrinsic characteristics of the skin such as pore size, acne and tone are also improved [9, 23, 24].

19.3
Complications

Compared with the incidence of complications following invasive surgical procedures and ablative methods of skin rejuvenation, the incidence of complications following capacitive RF treatment is extremely low [9, 11–17, 20, 25–29, 33, 34]. Clinically noticeable asymmetry is unlikely if the face is treated uniformly and treatment guidelines are followed. A mild amount of transient erythema and edema is common after the procedure, and resolves within a few days. On rare occasion, low-dose oral steroid therapy may be useful, but is avoided unless it is necessary since the inflammatory and healing response is what is believed to trigger new collagen formation.

There can be some numbness of the skin, most often in the distribution of the greater auricular nerve, possibly as a result of perineural inflammation. Numbness may take a few weeks to recover, but permanent nerve injury has not been reported [9–11]. Localized inflammation of the platysma can cause temporary ridging or lumping in the neck which may take 1–2 months to dissipate. Anecdotally, patients who have the greatest evidence of inflammation appear to get the most amount of skin tightening.

If the treatment tip is not kept completely flat against the skin surface, arcing of RF energy can occasionally cause a small less than 5 mm superficial burn [11, 13]. In the author's experience, these are self-limited and can be treated with topical antibiotic ointment. The treatment tip has built-in sensors, which continuously monitor temperature and surface pressure. RF-energy delivery is aborted if measurements are outside a safe threshold, making significant skin burns unlikely.

The complication of greatest concern with capacitive RF treatment is localized overtightening of subcutaneous collagen-based fibrous septae or possible fat atrophy resulting in skin surface irregularity [29]. This complication was more common initially when single-pass high-energy regimens were being followed, often with the patient under profound anesthesia [11, 29]. The author has found in two patients with this complication the indentations improved over the course of a few months without any additional intervention, most likely as a result of new collagen formation. Other treatments including autologous fat transfer have been advocated [29]. With current lower-energy multiple-pass treatment algorithms and in experienced hands, complications in general are rare.

19.4
Discussion

The ThermaCool™ system represents the current generation of capacitive RF skin rejuvenation devices, and has been show to stimulate dermal collagen change [8, 26]. As the process is non-ablative and depends on energy delivery based on tissue resistance rather than absorption of laser light energy, it can be used with all Fitzpatrick sun-reactive skin types.

Gradual, modest tightening and lifting of the skin is expected over the course of several months, with softening of facial rhytids and definition of facial contours. Skin tone, thickness and pore size may also improve [9]. The patient is spared the incisions, complications and recovery time associated with traditional aging face procedures. Collagen stimulation in the skin may also provide a theoretical antiaging benefit by replenishing collagen lost during aging. Setting realistic patient expectations is crucial to achieving patient satisfaction [11].

ThermaCool™ treatment is better suited to address deeper rhytids such as the nasolabial folds and marionette creases, rather then fine, superficial crepe-paper-type wrinkles along the skin surface. This relates to the currently available medium-depth treatment tip that targets RF energy to the mid and deep layers of the dermis, rather then the skin surface. The manufacturer has recently released a superficial-depth treatment tip for eyelid treatment that may be more effective in treatment of superficial rhytids. The current gold standard for treatment of fine skin surface wrinkles is ablative resurfacing (carbon dioxide and erbium lasers, deep chemical peels and dermabrasion).

As RF energy is not visible-light-based, pigmentary dyschromias, hair, and capillary and vascular ectasias are all relatively unaffected by capacitive RF treatment—there may be some reduction in capillary dilation with increased skin collagen content. Non-ablative lasers and intense pulsed light systems are more effective for these applications, and these treatments can be performed in conjunction with capacitive RF skin rejuvenation.

The manufacturer is continuing to develop the technology for non-ablative capacitive RF rejuvenation. With the release of larger and faster treatment tips, FDA approval has been granted for treatment of wrinkles outside the face. Evolving treatment algorithms have helped achieve more consistent results. Treatment tips that allow for deeper penetration of the RF field and allow targeted lipolysis are being investigated.

19.5
Conclusions

Capacitive RF skin treatment provides an additional avenue of rejuvenation of the aging face, especially for patients not interested in invasive surgical options. Candidates for treatment must be made aware of the limitations of the procedure and the gradual nature of the changes seen. Patients with significant skin laxity or underlying structural ptosis should be counseled that capacitive RF treatment does not currently achieve the dramatic changes provided by traditional surgery, although there is a theoretical antiaging benefit to stimulating collagen formation in the skin. Combining RF treatment with other non-surgical or minimally invasive procedures can achieve a more significant result. Future developments and refinement of RF technology will undoubtedly expand the role of capacitive RF treatments for facial and body rejuvenation.

References

1. Sarradet MD, Hussain M, Goldberg DJ: Electrosurgical resurfacing: a clinical, histologic, and electron microscopic evaluation. Lasers Surg Med 2003;32:111–114

2. Alster TS: Electrosurgical ablation: a new mode of cutaneous resurfacing. Plast Reconstr Surg 2001;107:1890–1894

3. Acland KM, Calonje E, Seed PT, Stat C, Barlow RJ: A clinical and histologic comparison of electrosurgical and carbon dioxide laser peels. J Am Acad Dermatol 2001;44:492–496

4. Grekin RC, Tope WD, Yarborough JM Jr, Olhoffer IH, Lee PK, Leffell DJ, Zachary CB: Electrosurgical facial resurfacing: a prospective multicenter study of efficacy and safety. Arch Dermatol 2000;136:1309–1316

5. Burns RL, Carruthers A, Langiry JA, Trotter MJ: Electrosurgical skin resurfacing: a new bipolar instrument. Dermatol Surg 1999;25:582–586

6. Tope WD: Multi-electrode radio frequency resurfacing of ex vivo human skin. Dermatol Surg 1999;25:348–352

7. Mancini PF: Coblation: a new technology and technique for skin resurfacing and other aesthetic surgical procedures. Aesthet Plast Surg 2001;25:372–377

8. Zelickson BD, Kist D, Bernstein E, et al.: Histological and ultrastructural evaluation of the effects of a radiofrequency-based non-ablative dermal remodeling device: a pilot study. Arch Dermatol 2004;140:204–209

9. Abraham M, Chiang S, Keller G, Rawnsley J, Blackwell K, Elashoff D: Clinical evaluation of non-ablative radiofrequency facial rejuvenation. J Cosmet Laser Ther 2004;6:136–144

10. Koch RJ: Radiofrequency non-ablative tissue tightening. Facial Plast Surg Clin North Am 2004;12:339–346

11. Abraham MT, Ross EV: Current concepts in non-ablative radiofrequency rejuvenation of the lower face and neck. Facial Plast Surg 2005;21:65–73

12. Narins DJ, Narins RS: Non-surgical radiofrequency facelift. J Drugs Dermatol 2003;2:495–500

13. Fitzpatrick R, Geronemus R, Goldberg D, Kaminer M, Kilmer S, Ruiz-Esparza J: Multicenter study of noninvasive radiofrequency for peri-orbital tissue tightening. Lasers Surg Med 2003;33:232–242

14. Nahm WK, Su TT, Rotunda AM, Moy RL: Objective changes in brow position, superior palpebral crease, peak angle of the eyebrow, and jowl surface area after volumetric radiofrequency treatments to half of the face. Dermatol Surg 2004;30:922–928

15. Fritz M, Counters JT, Zelickson BD: Radiofrequency treatment for middle and lower face laxity. Arch Facial Plast Surg 2004;6:370–373

16. Alster TS, Tanzi E: Improvement of neck and cheek laxity with a non-ablative radiofrequency device: a lifting experience. Dermatol Surg 2004;30:503–507

17. Bassichis BA, Dayan S, Thomas JR: Use of a non-ablative radiofrequency device to rejuvenate the upper one-third of the face. Otolaryngol Head Neck Surg 2004;130:397–406

18. Jacobson LG, Alexiades-Armenakas M, Bernstein L, Geronemus RG: Treatment of nasolabial fold and jowls with a noninvasive radiofrequency device. Arch Dermatol 2003;139:1371–1372

19. Ruiz-Esparza J: Noninvasive lower eyelid blepharoplasty: a new technique using nonablative radiofrequency on periorbital skin. Dermatol Surg 2004;30:125–129

20. Ruiz-Esparza J, Gomez JB: The medical face lift: a noninvasive, nonsurgical approach to tissue tightening in facial skin using nonablative radiofrequency. Dermatol Surg 2003;29:325–332

21. Hsu TS, Kaminer MS: The use of non-ablative radiofrequency technology to tighten the lower face and neck. Semin Cutan Med Surg 2003;22:115–123

22. Iyer S, Suthamjariya K, Fitzpatrick RE: Using a radiofrequency energy device to treat the lower face: a treatment paradigm for a nonsurgical facelift. Cosmet Dermatol 2003;16:37–40

23. Ruiz-Esparza J, Gomez JB: Non-ablative radiofrequency for active acne vulgaris: the use of deep dermal heat in the treatment of moderate to severe active acne vulgaris (thermotherapy): a report of 22 patients. Dermatol Surg 2003;29:333–339

24. Fisher GH, Jacobson LG, Bernstein LJ, Kim KH, Geronemus RG: Non-ablative radiofrequency treatment of facial laxity. Dermatol Surg 2005;31:1237–1241

25. Finzi E, Spangler A: Multipass vector (mpave) technique with non-ablative radiofrequency to treat facial and neck laxity. Dermatol Surg 2005;31:916–922

26. Meshkinpour A, Ghasri P, Pope K, Lyubovitsky JG, Risteli J, Krasieva TB, Kelly KM: Treatment of hypertrophic scars and keloids with a radiofrequency device: a study of collagen effects. Lasers Surg Med 2005;37:343–349

27. England LJ, Tan MH, Shumaker PR, Egbert BM, Pittelko K, Orentreich D, Pope K: Effect of mono-polar radiofrequency treatment over soft-tissue fillers in an animal model. Lasers Surg Med 2005;37:356–365

28. Shumaker PR, England LJ, Dover JS, Ross EV, Harford R, Derienzo D, Bogle M, Uebelhoer N, Jacoby M, Pope K: Effect of mono-polar radiofrequency treatment over soft-tissue fillers in an animal model: part 2. Lasers Surg Med 2006;38:211–217

29. Narins RS, Tope WD, Pope K, Ross CE: Over treatment effects associated with a radiofrequency tissue-tightening device: rare, preventable, and correctable with subcision and autologous fat transfer. Dermatol Surg 2006;32:115–124

30. Kushikata N, Negishi K, Tezuka Y, Takeuchi K, Wakamatsu S: Is topical anesthesia useful in noninvasive tightening using radiofrequency? Dermatol Surg 2005;31:526–533

31. Kushikata N, Negishi K, Tezuka Y, Takeuchi K, Wakamatsu S: Non-ablative skin tightening with radiofrequency in Asian skin. Lasers Surg Med 2005;36:92–97

32. Lack EB, Rachel JD, D'Andrea L, Corres J: Relationship of energy settings and impedance in different anatomic areas using a radiofrequency device. Dermatol Surg 2005;31:1668–1670

33. Sadick N, Sorhaindo L: The radiofrequency frontier: a review of radiofrequency and combined radiofrequency pulsed-light technology in aesthetic medicine. Facial Plast Surg 2005;21:131–138

34. Sadick NS, Makino Y: Selective electro-thermolysis in aesthetic medicine: a review. Lasers Surg Med 2004;34:91–97

CHAPTER 20

Photorejuvenation

Kenneth Beer, Rhoda S. Narins

20.1
Introduction

The concept for rejuvenation of the face by using light sources has been present since the advent of laser technologies. Lasers used to accomplish this goal include the ablative (CO_2 and erbium) and nonablative lasers. However, the sequelae associated with ablative lasers and the lack of compelling efficacy associated with nonablative lasers created a realization that a nonlaser light source might be the best means of accomplishing facial photorejuvenation. These pulsed light sources began to become popular in the cosmetic surgery community in 2004 and have since undergone various refinements.

The benefits of photorejuvenation are numerous and include improvements of the tone and texture of the skin, diminished pigment irregularity, reduction of vascular lesions and improvement in the appearance of fine lines and wrinkles.

Intense pulsed light (IPL) differs from laser light in a number of theoretical and clinical aspects. Whereas laser emissions are coherent beams of the same wavelength and frequency, IPL contains light with a variety of wavelengths. Intense IPL used for photorejuvenation is light between 500 and 1,200 nm [1]. As such, it targets numerous chromophores within the epidermis and dermis, including melanin, vascular structures, collagen and other structures. The use of filters to limit the spectra of light emitted enables one to focus on one particular aspect of the skin when using this device. Since the process of photoaging (and thus of photorejuvenation) affects each of these aspects, it is worthwhile to consider the interaction of IPL with each one.

The actual IPL device consists of a flashlamp light source that produces polychromatic light [2]. Depending on the desired wavelength, filters may be introduced to remove light of a specific wavelength. It is this capability that enables IPL to provide diverse types of treatments with one device and is partially responsible for the popularity of IPL with physician and nonphysician practitioners alike.

One hallmark of aging skin is the pigmentary irregularity frequently seen after photodamage has occurred. The degree of pigment present is a function of the skin type of the individual in question, the amount of ultraviolet exposure they have sustained, mitigating treatments such as the use of topically applied retinoids, bleaching creams, chemical peels or cosmeceuticals and the capacity for intrinsic rejuvenation that a given individual possesses.

Hypopigmentation associated with photodamage is, at present, not treated with IPL with any degree of success. To date, attempts to stimulate melanocytes to produce pigment once they have undergone apoptosis have not resulted in restoration of a normal complement of pigment-producing cells within the basal layer of the epidermis.

Hyperpigmentation associated with a variety of conditions, including photodamage, pregnancy and postinflammatory hyperpigmentation, has been more effectively treated with photorejuvenation. The absorption spectrum for melanin is continuous and thus IPL is well suited for this indication. Actinic lentigines, melasma and postinflammatory hyperpigmentation may be treated with IPL. When treating hyperpigmentation, it is critical to ensure that patients have not had any significant ultraviolet exposure for the preceding several weeks (2–4), have used either broad-spectrum sunscreen or physical-barrier sunblocks and that they have no planned sun exposure for a few weeks after the procedure. Prior sun exposure will prime the melanocytes to respond to the IPL by making more pigment as does sun exposure following the treatment.

Skin types I, II and III tend to develop telangectasias with increased sun exposure and aging. In addition, these types of skin are prone to rosacea as the skin ages. IPL can address many of the vascular proliferations seen with both of these problems. Since hemoglobin has a series of absorption peaks, including 585 nm, IPL is readily absorbed. One study evaluating the use of IPL for rosacea-associated telangectasias found significant improvement after five treatments each 3 weeks apart [3].

The addition of porphyrins to the skin may increase the efficacy of this treatment [4]. This treatment is known as photodynamic therapy, or PDT. The addition of this photosensitizer has increased the energy absorption for IPL, rendering it more effective at treating the various stigmata of photoaging. Various protocols may be utilized, each involving cleansing of the skin prior to application of aminolevulinic acid for an amount of time that may vary between 15 and 60 min. Energy levels and filters for IPL depend on the skin type, degree of damage present, degree of erythema present, tolerance for downtime by the patient and goals of the treatment. The marriage of IPL with aminolevulinic acid may provide for highly effective photorejuvenation.

Under the microscope, photoaging is associated with disorganization and atrophy of the epidermis, degeneration of the papillary and reticular dermis as the collagen and elastic fibers diminish and a host of other subtle and overt changes [5]. At a subcellular level, IPL treatments stimulate production of type I collagen transcripts [6]. Devices that optimize this collagen production stimulate elastin production, and remodeling will enhance the ability of IPL machines to perform photorejuvenation. The addition of medications such as low-dose antibiotics, including doxycycline, may inhibit collagenase and addition of this medication may improve patient outcomes.

IPL has been useful in reversing several of these signs of aging and it is in this category of photorejuvenation that the potential may be the greatest. After observations that nonablative lasers in the 585-nm region of the spectrum were able to cause collagen remodeling, other methods of accomplishing the same goals were investigated. Goldberg and Cutler [7] demonstrated the efficacy of IPL for the treatment of rhytids and since that time various devices and protocols have been utilized for this goal. It is anticipated that this indication will most likely remain extremely popular.

20.2
Technique

The techniques for using IPL for photorejuvenation are as varied and diverse as the number of machines and operators using them and the goals of a treatment regimen for a given patient. Perhaps the most important part of the technique for photorejuvenation is the one that is sometimes overlooked—the consultation and consent process. During the consultation, it is important to listen to what the potential patient is saying about his or her expectations and tolerance for risk and downtime. One signal that the nonablative photorejuvenation might be the wrong procedure for a particular patient is statements indicating that the patient wants to "get rid" of wrinkles or the patient wants a nonsurgical facelift. Many of the patients that have these types of expectations are fed by the reports of various procedures in the popular media. Since these types of reports tend to present only the best cases, patients who demand these results are most likely going to be disappointed and thus are not good candidates unless one can educate them about the realities of the procedure. Other

signs that a patient might not be a good candidate for photorejuvenation are similar to warning signs to heed for any cosmetic surgery patient: patients who speak poorly of other physicians, patients who are financially stretched for the procedure and cannot financially afford adjunct treatments such as botulinum toxins or fillers that might be needed for optimal outcomes and interactions with ancillary staff that simply give reliable staff a sense of dread towards the individual.

Consent for photorejuvenation should include discussions of the risks, need for multiple treatments, the fact that each session has a cost, confirmation that the patient is required to avoid the sun, informing the physician if the patient is pregnant or has certain types of photosensitive diseases and other relevant considerations for the type of procedure being performed. Many physicians recommend photographic documentation of the patient's baseline and this should be seriously considered for each patient.

For a particular device, the initial technical considerations are the parameters for the treatment. The first parameter to consider is the reason the patient is undergoing the treatment. Since many devices are capable of emitting light from 400–1,200 nm, filters that limit the wavelengths emitted are used to emit light most appropriate for each indication. For instance, when treating vascular or red lesions, filters are used to limit the light emitted to wavelengths that will be efficacious. Other filters may be used when melanin is the target.

Once the proper handpiece has been selected, energy settings must be considered. When beginning a treatment with a type I or II skin type that has not been exposed to recent ultraviolet light, settings can be at the upper end of recommended parameters. Darker skin types will need to be treated at the lower end of these settings.

The fluence, pulse duration and size of the spot are technical considerations whose parameters change with each device. The presence and type of skin cooling available also help to determine the settings for each treatment. Depending on the manufacturer, fluences from 15 to 90 J/cm^2 may be used. Spot size must be selected to best suit the area being treated and these may be as large as several centimeters or small as a few millimeters. Prior to using any IPL device, it is imperative to familiarize oneself with the particular recommendations and literature that are specific for it.

At each treatment, makeup and sunscreen should be removed before the treatment begins. A topical anesthetic cream may be applied for 30 min and removed before treatment begins. Once the treatment is completed, chemical-free sunscreen should be applied if the patient will have any outdoor exposure. The patient should be positioned comfortably and the operator should be able to readily access the area undergoing treatment. Eye protection must be worn during the procedure.

Using a double-stacked IPL pulse instead of a single

pulse may result in improvements in erythema, skin roughness and hyperpigmentation [8]. This protocol, using the Lux G handpiece from Palomar, suggests that operator variables may strongly influence outcomes when treating the visible signs of aging and suggests that using two stacked pulses is better than a single pulse when treating photoaging. Future devices or techniques will likely expand on this finding. Other devices, including the IPL Quantum system (Lumenis, Santa Clara, CA, USA), the Ellipse system (Candela, Wayland, MA, USA) and several other systems offer a variety of light filters that are suitable for treating multiple skin issues, including photorejuvenation, hyperpigmentation, telangectasias, rosacea and a host of other skin conditions. It is anticipated that advances in skin cooling, power delivery and light filters will continue to make these products more effective and more versatile.

Prior to treatment, a chilled gel is applied to the skin. Following a few pulses of the treated area, inspection of the skin must be performed to ensure that no blisters or incipient burns are occurring. At the completion of the treatment, ice or cool gel packs may be applied to reduce the swelling. Post-treatment care instructions are provided and documentation that this was completed should be in the patient record.

Treatments for photorejuvenation are usually separated by 2–4 weeks. For most devices it is recommended that a series of between four and six sessions be scheduled for maximum benefit.

Combining photorejuvenation with other types of cosmetic procedures may enhance the outcomes from each procedure and this is one technical consideration that only recently has begun to be explored. Carruthers and Carruthers [9] reported improvement of pore size, dyspigmentation, telangectasias and skin texture when botulinum toxin A was used concomitantly with IPL.

20.3
Complications

Complications that may occur with IPL for photorejuvenation include common ones such as swelling, bruising and transient erythema and less common ones including hyperpigmentation, infection, burns and scarring. The incidence of transient crusting is reported as 2% and Goldman et al. [2] note that this superficial crusting is self-limited, lasting approximately 1 week. The same authors report a 4% rate of purpura and a rate of swelling of 25% and these are consistent with the experience of the authors [2]. Both purpura and swelling occur at a much higher rate in areas such as the eyelids and care should be taken when treating the upper-cheek/lower-eyelid area.

The incidence of scarring is rare and it usually is the result of using excessive energy or from using the IPL device on someone who has been exposed to the sun. Infections from herpes simplex virus may occur after treatment of an area prone to outbreaks and prophylaxis with antiviral medication is recommended for patients with a history of herpes. Bacterial infections are extremely rare with nonablative photorejuvenation and they may be the result of patients who excoriate the skin following treatment. Any infection in a treated patient should be treated with appropriate antibiotic or antiviral medication. A single case of a vesiculobullous eruption following IPL performed by a nonphysician has been reported [10]. In this instance, the patient sustained significant vesicles and bulla that were thought to be a function of poor technique, although other causes were also entertained.

In order to minimize the risks of complications, patient education and screening are important. Patients with increased ultraviolet exposure should not be treated as they are at significant risk for transient hyperpigmentation as well as for scarring owing to the increased epidermal melanin with increased absorption of energy.

20.4
Discussion

The popularity of nonablative photorejuvenation with physicians, nonphysician providers and patients attests to the excellent results, thereby increasing the demand for these types of treatments. Users of each of these devices, in conjunction with industry, are searching for better outcomes with less downtime. Recent IPL devices are now approaching the goal of improving photoaging with minimal risk and downtime.

Since IPL is a broad spectrum of light that can be administered with varied levels of fluence, its potential for treating telangectasias, fine lines, hyperpigmentation, skin surface roughness and other signs of aging continues to be realized (Fig. 20.1).

Results for the treatment of small blood vessels as well as the erythema associated with rosacea have approached those obtained with a pulsed dye laser with significantly less post-treatment purpura. IPL is also useful for maintenance after using other lasers, such as the Vbeam or Nd:YAG. While not as dramatic as the outcomes that follow ablative skin resurfacing, the marked reduction of risk when compared with that for the latter procedure has made IPL extremely popular for the treatment of fine lines and skin surface roughness. The improvements of collagen fibers have been documented and modifications of both devices and protocols (including the adjunctive use of medications to foster collagen production) will continue to enhance outcomes. One likely scenario that will enhance nonablative photorejuvenation will be the combination of various types of light for synergistic outcomes. Fractional ablation, infrared light and radiofrequency are among

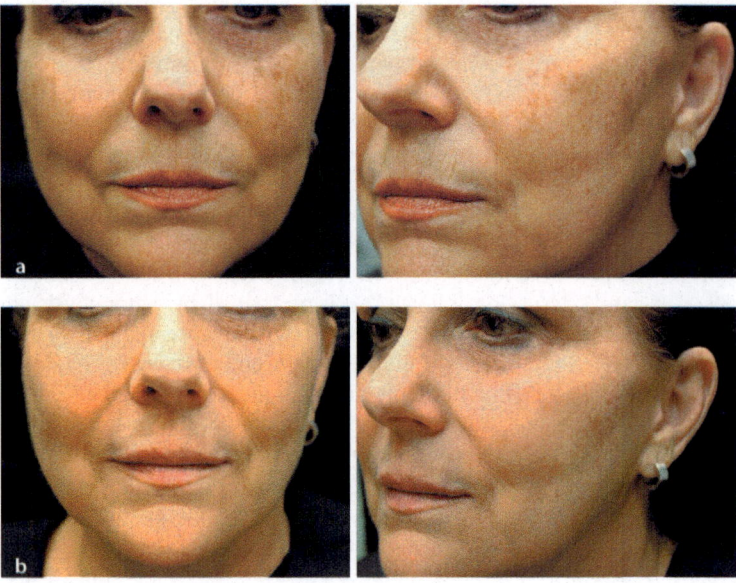

Fig. 20.1 a Before treatment. **b** After treatment following photorejuvenation

the possible candidates for this. Results from one study have suggested that combing IPL with Botox will yield dramatically better results than the sum of their parts would suggest likely. Undoubtedly, other combinations, including the use of other types of type A toxin and the use of fillers to stimulate collagen remodeling and to fill deep rhytids, will also be explored.

Photoaging may stigmatize the skin with production of pigment on the face, neck and dorsal hands. Poikilodermatous changes on the neck as well as the chest, arms, legs and other parts of the body are amenable to treatment with IPL and handpieces that can treat these are presently in use. The lentigines on the dorsal hands and face that serve notice of a life spent in the sun are also effectively treated with IPL and the use of this device in combination with prescription bleaching creams (including those with combinations of hydrocortisone, tretinoin and hydroquinone) and sunblocks has dramatically improved the appearance of both. Skin surface irregularity and roughness are similarly restored to a more youthful appearance following treatment with IPL and it remains to be considered whether advance treatment with topically applied vitamin C, tretinoin, green tea or oral medications may enhance the outcomes obtained, and if so what the optimal parameters are.

One problem with the use of IPL for the treatment of photoaging involves not the actual devices but the regulations governing them. In many states, the use of these devices is not regulated to any large extent. This, in conjunction with what can graciously be termed "overly enthusiastic" marketing to the masses of nonspecialists that comprise the larger market for several of the manufacturers, has led to a proliferation of devices placed in the hands of those least educated about the potential for harm that may ensue from their use. Scarring, hyper-

pigmentation, hypopigmentation and a host of other complications that may occur under the best of circumstances have become more frequent as the treatment of photoaging has been moved (to a large degree) from the dermatologist's office to the mall. Regulations to govern the use of these devices, including the need for supervision, will, at some point, catch up with the technology and marketing and this will hopefully bring the situation back into a balance that favors patient safety. Likewise, providers of seminars that train nonspecialists may eventually become liable for the damages that these practitioners cause. This may have a chilling effect on the seminars that exchange official-looking certificates designed to confer credibility for the price of the course.

20.5 Conclusions

Nonablative photorejuvenation is here to stay because it is safe and effective. Enhancements to the technology will continue to improve the ability of the devices to treat the signs of aging. Improvements in technique, including the use of double-stacked pulses and the adjunctive uses of other procedures and medications will increase the efficacy of the devices used. Regulations and public awareness campaigns will serve to decrease the complications associated with usage by nonphysicians and nonspecialists.

The use of these devices has transformed cosmetic dermatology by providing a safe and effective means to renovate the surface of the skin. Outcomes associated with these devices will continue to improve with refinements in training, techniques and technology.

References

1. Marmur E, Goldberg D: Nonablative Skin Resurfacing. Procedures in Cosmetic Dermatology. Lasers and Lights, Volume 2. Elsevier. Philadelphia. 2005:29–30

2. Goldman M, Weiss, R, Weiss M: Intense pulsed light as a nonablative approach to photoaging. Dermatol Surg. 2005;31:1179–1187

3. Mark K, Sparacia R, Voight A, Marenus K, Sarnoff D: Objective and quantitative improvement of rosacea associated erythema after intense pulsed light treatment. Dermatol Surg. 2003;29:600–604

4. Gold MH: The evolving role of aminolevulinic acid hydrochloride with photodynamic therapy in photoaging. Cutis 2002;69(6 Suppl):8–13

5. Hernandez-Perez F, Ibiett EV: Gross and microscopic findings in patients submitted to nonablative full face resurfacing using intense pulsed light. Dermatol Surg. 2002;28:651–655

6. Zelickson B, Kist D: Pulsed dye laser and photoderm treatment stimulate production of type I collagen and collagenase transcripts in papillary dermis fibroblasts, (abstract). Lasers Surg Med Suppl. 2001;13:33

7. Goldberg DJ, Cutler KB: Nonablative treatment of rhytids with intense pulsed light. Lasers Surg Med. 2000;26:196–200

8. Kligman D, Zhen Y: Intense pulsed light treatment of photoaged skin. Dermatol Surg. 2004;30(8);1085–1090

9. Carruthers J, Carruthers A: The effect of full face broadband light treatments alone and in combination with bilateral crow's feet botulinum toxin type A chemodenervation. J Dermatol Surg. 2004;30:355–366

10. Sperber B, Walling H, Arpey C, Whitaker D: Vesiculobullous eruption from intense pulsed light treatment. Dermatol Surg. 2005;31:345–349

CHAPTER 21

Coblation Skin Resurfacing Technique

21

Pier Francesco Mancini

21.1
Introduction

Skin resurfacing is a very common technique in aesthetic surgery and can be performed in very different ways. Acids, dermabrasion, lasers and radiofrequency can be used [1].

Two main results should be achieved:

1. Renewal of the epidermis surface to correct the fine lines, age spots, etc.
2. Dermal shrinkage in order to improve deep lines and get a lifting effect.

Removal of the epidermis and damage to the dermis to stimulate new collagen deposition have to be achieved. The most important problem during the process is to control the dermal damage because too much damage will result in a long and uncomfortable postoperative period and increase complications such as scarring, long lasting erythema, and hypopigmentation.

Dermal damage from the use of lasers or radiofrequency occurs from heating the dermis, so there is a need to control the temperature, because if it is too low the proper result will not be obtained, but if it is too high unwanted damage in the surrounding tissues will occur [2, 3]. The temperature has to be higher then 60°C to stimulate collagen shrinkage, but with higher temperatures undesired damage occurs in the deep dermis.

Visage Coblation (Arthrocare, Sunnyvale, CA, USA) is a device that is based on the modification of a bipolar surgical unit. This radiofrequency device is able to achieve tissue removal using a range of temperature between 40 and 70°C, so it can exfoliate the epidermis causing collagen contraction and stimulating new collagen deposition without causing too much damage in the deep dermis. Coblation can coagulate small vessels, controlling intraoperative bleeding [4–7].

Clinically this will result in good aesthetic improvement of lines and rhytids, improvement of age spots and the quality of the skin, and the achievement of a lifting effect with a short and comfortable postoperative period and very few complications.

21.2
Coblation: Technology and Device

Coblation is a registered technology based on two main modifications of a bipolar surgical unit. The first is that the two poles are set very close to each other so that the electrical arch that is formed between them is very short. The second modification is that the gap existing between the electrodes and the target tissue is filled with an electrically conductive solution (saline, lactated Ringer's solution).

Under this condition if a sufficiently high voltage is applied to the electrodes, the solution is transformed into an ionized vapor layer that is called "plasma" [8]. In the plasma the ions have high energy and are accelerated towards the target tissue, causing disruption of the intercellular bonds and so achieving exfoliation. Meanwhile, the ions lose their energy very quickly and are unable to overheat the surrounding tissues.

The range of temperatures during this process is always between 40 and 70°C, so it is high enough to cause the shrinkage of collagen and superficial necrosis in the dermis, but it is not enough to damage the surrounding tissues [4–6, 8]. This limited damage in the surrounding tissues is responsible for rapid reepithelialization and minimal postoperative inflammation that reduce the erythema, pain, and swelling.

Coblation technology fits what can be assumed are the main goals in a good skin-resurfacing procedure:

1. It exfoliates the epidermis.
2. It causes shrinkage of collagen.
3. It causes dermal damage promoting the postoperative regeneration of collagen.
4. The dermis is only superficially damaged and this allows a fast recover with minimal complications.

21.3
Coblation Device

Coblation is a bipolar electrosurgical unit so it is able to coagulate the small vessels and achieve a bloodless surgical field [4, 5].

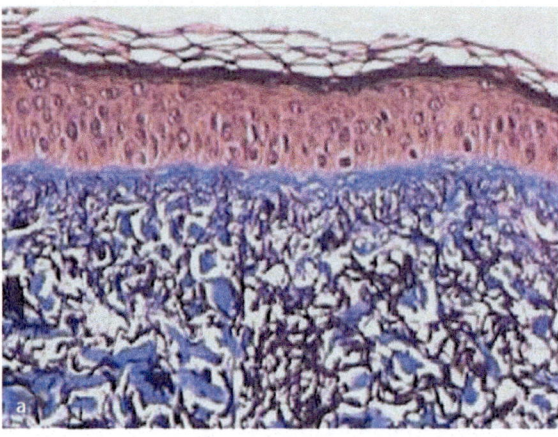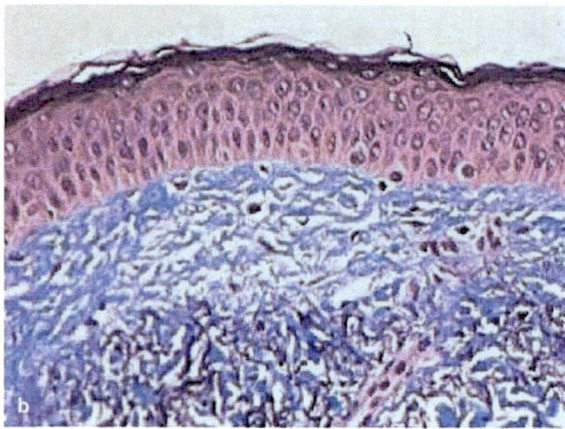

Fig. 21.1 Skin biopsy. **a** Before treatment. **b** Six months after treatment. Note collagen deposition

The Coblation device has different parts: (1) the controller is a modified bipolar surgical unit; (2) the footswitch allows the power setting to be adjusted and activates the system and the coagulation mode; (3) the hand piece is sterilizable and allows the connection between the controller and the stiletto; (4) the stiletto is disposable and represents the "heart" of the system.

The resurfacing model has three lines of gold-plated microelectrodes and a connection to the saline solution flow system that allows a continuous saline flow over the surgical field.

21.4
Histology Results

Coblation was tested on mammary skin of a patient who was undergoing a reduction mammoplasty. The following results were obtained using different power settings and different numbers of passes:

1. Two passes at 75 V exfoliate the epidermis without any kind of damage in the dermis.
2. Passes at 125 V achieve similar results.
3. Two passes at 175 V cause thermal damage in the dermis up to 0.23 mm.

4. Four passes at 175 V produce dermal damage up to 0.31 mm.

The damage that is caused with four passes at 175 V represents the maximum depth that can be achieved and dermal necrosis is limited. Injury to sweat glands and hair follicles is minimal and reepithelialization more rapid. Histologic evidence shows an increased amount of collagen 6 months after treatment and this explains the lifting effect that can be achieved in the postoperative period (Fig. 21.1).

21.5
Basic Technique

Treatment of the skin starts with 2 weeks of using creams with glycolic acid (12%) and hydroquinone (2%). Two days before Coblation treatment, the patient has to start wide-spectrum antibiotics and Aciclovir. Antibiotics and Aciclovir are used orally until complete reepithelization is achieved (about 3–7 days).

The procedure can be performed using nerve block anesthesia for a single aesthetic area but treatment of the whole face will probably need intravenous sedation.

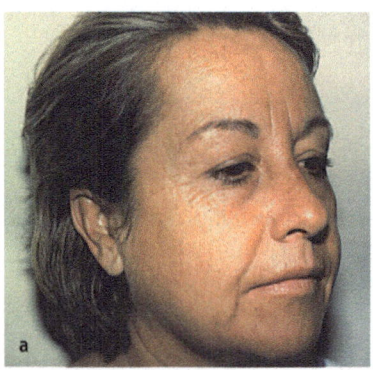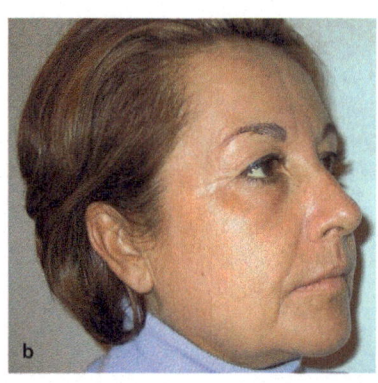

Fig. 21.2 Full-face skin resurfacing. **a** Before treatment. **b** Six months after treatment

Coblation resurfacing is performed on an outpatient basis.

Treatment begins by cleaning the face with a chlorhexidine solution. The preparation of the device begins by connecting the chosen stiletto to the hand piece and to the saline solution. The power is turned on and the power setting is selected (125–175 V). Saline solution flow is one drop per second. Prior to using the footswitch, it is important to be sure that the surgical field is wet, that the stiletto is in contact with the skin, and that it is perpendicular to the surface.

The assistant has to stretch the skin while the surgeon, holding the hand piece like a pencil, starts moving the stiletto over the surface, with an approximate speed of 1–2 cm/s. Parallel overlapping lines are drawn (about one third) to avoid non-treated strips and when more then one pass is planned it is better to criss-cross them forming a net.

During the first pass it is important to clean all the epidermal debris from the electrodes and from the skin surface using wet gauze. Cleaning is not as important in the following passes since Coblation causes minimal tissue ablation and only the upper dermis is heated.

The number of passes and the power setting are chosen depending on the skin type, the skin lesions (fine lines, deep rhytids, age spots, etc.), the aesthetic area, and the desired amount of postoperative skin retraction (Fig. 21.2). Usually, two to three passes at maximum power (175 V) are used in the forehead and the perioral area, one to two passes at 125 V in the periorbital area, and one to two passes at 175 V over the cheeks. These settings can achieve very good results without causing any special problems.

21.6
Advanced Techniques

Coblation can be safely used in combination with other aesthetic surgical procedures like facelifts and blepharoplasty.

21.6.1
Facelifting

If Coblation is combined with a facelift, the skin resurfacing can be used in order to improve the quality of the skin, erase the fine lines, and treat age spots.

Coblation resurfacing is safe and effective but, when combined with other surgical techniques, the number of passes has to be reduced and the power settings have to be reduced for the areas where a superficial flap has been elevated (cheeks). It can be used normally in the forehead, if the undermining was subperiosteal, and in the perioral area where any undermining does not exist. Over the cheek area it can be used with a low power setting (125 W) performing only one pass. In these cases

the resurfacing does not increase the postoperative recovery time and complications but the final result can be improved.

21.6.2
Blepharoplasty

Transconjuntival blepharoplasty is easily performed using a special Coblation stiletto that is called a microdissector. The microdissector is a needle that works with Coblation technology and that can cut tissues without causing large thermal damage but still coagulate small vessels. With use of this stiletto it is possible to remove eye bags. Then, changing to a normal resurfacing piece, the device can exfoliate the epidermis and stimulate postoperative shrinkage of the lid skin [4–7].

21.6.3
Lip Border

Coblation can be used to define and design the lip border to achieving an aesthetic result (Paris lip) similar to that from the use of dermal fillers. In order to achieve this result, the stiletto has to be moved vertically and stopped exactly on the lip border (vermillion) (Fig. 21.3). A second pass is performed parallel to the border and stops at the point where the lip filtrum is to be defined (Fig. 21.3). Postoperative collagen contraction will define the lip border and the nasolabial fold, giving the aesthetic result (Fig. 21.4).

21.7
Postoperative Period and Treatment

During the first 48 h mild edema and serous exudation are common.

A special dressing is used that contains epidermal growth factor that helps to absorb the exudation and

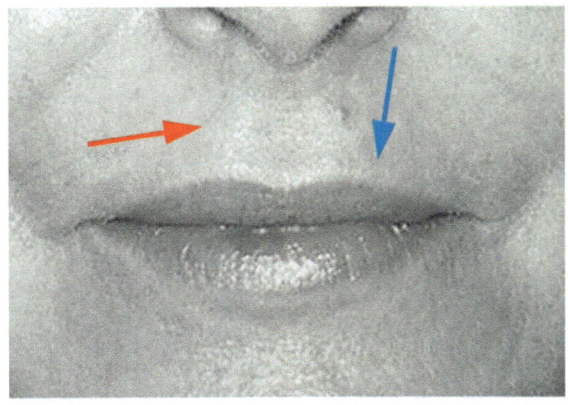

Fig. 21.3 Lip design technique

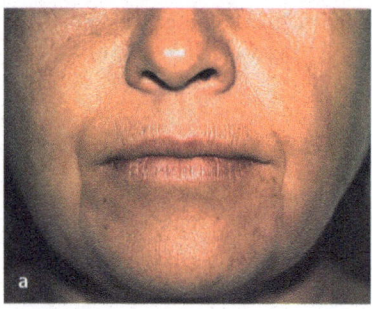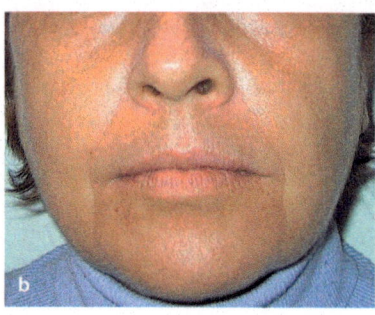

Fig. 21.4 Lip border design. **a** Before treatment. **b** Six months after treatment

accelerate the recovery. On the second postoperative day the dressings are removed and the patient starts washing the treated areas, with a cold chamomile solution that has to be applied over in a thin layer of cold epidermal growth factor gel.

Reepithelization is normally complete in 3–7 days. At this time extreme dryness of the skin has to be controlled with moisturizing creams and inflammatory hyperpigmentation prevented with the use of local corticoids. Antibiotics and Acyclovir can be discontinued at this time.

During the next 4–6 weeks mild erythema (light pink) persists that can be easily covered by makeup. Postoperative pain is uncommon, but itching can be frequent during the second postoperative week and can be controlled with cold chamomile applications.

21.8
Complications

There were no cases of scars, hypopigmentation, infection, or long-lasting erythema. The only complication that can be considered common (about 30%) is the postinflammatory hyperpigmentation that starts during the second or third postoperative week and at the beginning looks like areas of erythema with a darker (purple) color. It then turns to a light brown color, giving the appearance of leopard skin.

This kind of erythema can be treated and resolves in about 1 month, using bleaching creams and local corticoids.

21.9
Results

The aesthetic results can be considered complete in about 3 months. The results can be compared with those that can be achieved with CO_2 laser resurfacing, but the difference is the better postoperative period [3, 9]. Patients suffer less inflammation, less erythema (which disappears in about 1 month), and fewer complications. Improvement of deep rhytids can be achieved and fine lines and age spots disappear completely. The skin texture changes and it looks younger and healthier.

In all patients the results improve over several months and, clinically, confirm the postoperative regeneration of collagen. When Coblation skin resurfacing is combined with other aesthetic surgical procedures the final result can be improved further with complete rejuvenation in treating ptosis of the deep structures and the skin appearance improves with complete rejuvenation. Using the proper technique, the combination of surgical procedures and Coblation resurfacing will improve the aesthetic results without increasing the complications.

The lip border design technique gives a very nice and natural appearance and it can be performed by driving the skin contraction in the direction desired.

21.10
Conclusions

Coblation is a technology that allows the performance of skin resurfacing in a safe and effective way. Good aesthetic results can be achieved with a fast and comfortable recovery. This device can erase fine lines and age spots and deep rhytids can be improved. A lifting effect can be achieved by stimulating regeneration of collagen. The results are similar to those with the CO_2 laser, but reepithelialization is faster with less edema, no pain, less erythema, and fewer complications.

The technique is very easy to learn and with a little experience it is possible to perform changes like lip design and combine the resurfacing with facelift or blepharoplasty. It is an easy and safe technique that can improve many of the skin-aging signs.

References

1. Sperli AE: Electrosurgical peeling (peeling by high frequency cellular volatilization) Rev Soc Bras Cir Plast Estet Reconstr 1996;11:21–34

2. Ross VE, Domankevitz Y, Skrobal M, Anderson RR: Effects of CO2 laser pulse duration and residual thermal damage: implications for skin resurfacing. Laser Surg Med 199;19(2):123–129

3. Weinstein C: Why I abandoned CO2 laser resurfacing: the dilemma o evolving technologies Aesthet Surg J 1999;19:67–69

4. Mancini PF: La nuova tecnología per lo skin resurfacing. Conference at Fondazione Sanvenero Rosselli, Milan, Italy, 2000

5. Mancini PF: A new system for skin resurfacing: preliminary clinical and histologic reports. Aesthet Surg J 1999;19:459–464

6. Mancini PF: Coblation: A new technology and technique for skin resurfacing and other aesthetic surgical procedures. Aesthet Plast Surg 2001;25:372–377

7. Olhoffer IH, Leffel R: What's new in electrosurgery? Coblation: a new method for facial resurfacing. Aesthet Dermatol Cosmet Surg 1999;1:31–33

8. Grekin RC, Tope WD, Phil M, Yarborough J, Olhoffer I, Lee PK, Leffel DJ, Zachary CB: Electrosurgical facial resurfacing: a prospective multicenter study of efficacy and safety. Arch Dermatol 2000;136(11):1309–1316

9. Burkhardt BR, Maw R: Are more passes better? Safety versus efficacy with the pulsed CO2 laser. Plast Reconstr Surg 1997;100(6):1531–1546

CHAPTER 22

Removal of Rhytids with Electrocoagulation

22

Susanna Nikitina

Published posthumously

22.1
Introduction

Use of electrocoagulation (EC) in surgery is not new [1] but in many countries it has unfortunately fallen into ill-deserved oblivion. Since 1932 tens of thousands of patients with various disorders have been treated with EC at the Cosmetic and Plastic Surgery Center in Leningrad (CPSCL) (now renamed St. Petersburg).

Widely used EC for treating postleishmaniasis scarring allowed the doctors at CPSCL to gain much practical experience and to develop and update it for facial rejuvenation and for treating facial rhytids. More than 60 years of experience has shown that superficial EC is a perfect complementary procedure to surgical facial rejuvenation, sometimes postponing a facelift for years.

EC, as a thermal injury, causes contraction of the skin's natural collagen, which results in a significant lifting effect. While the other methods of facial rejuvenation, such as laser resurfacing, dermabrasion, or various peelings, are effective in removing fine lines and fine wrinkles, EC resurfacing (ECRS) has proven to be an excellent method for treating the most problematic cases such as deep rhytids and atrophic scarring. The long-lasting results of 5–10 or even 20 years are impressive.

ECRS more often than not is performed on an outpatient basis. Simple equipment is needed for the procedure. It is a "thermocauter" connected to an ordinary AC/DC apparatus (transformer regulating the amount of electricity). A special thermocauter convenient for quick full-face resurfacing was designed by leading dermatological surgeons at CPSCL.

The author was trained to perform ECRS in 1978 while was working at CPSCL. Since then 11,060 skin rejuvenation procedures have been performed. Of these patients none had any serious complications such as scarring or infection. There were occasional patients with temporary hyperpigmentation. Very few patients had reactivation of herpes labialis after EC of the upper lips. One patient had telangiectasia.

22.2
Technique

Although ECRS may be performed on practically all healthy people, the possibilities for the procedure must be thoroughly evaluated. Preoperative selection is very important.

Direct contraindications are acute inflammatory disorders, HIV, severe psychosomatic diseases, and contagious skin diseases. The patient's medical history, current medications, and relaxation technique should be noted. The last of these is important as some of techniques prolong postoperative redness significantly.

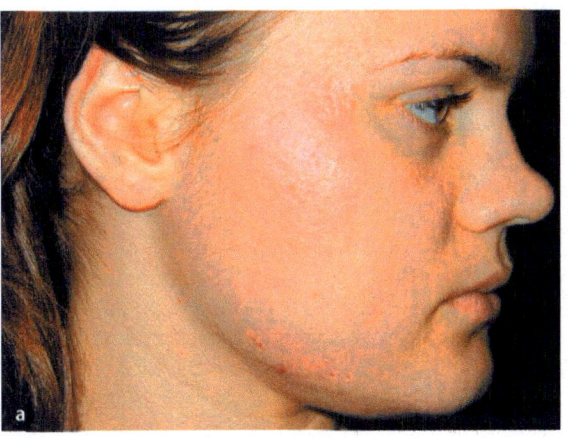 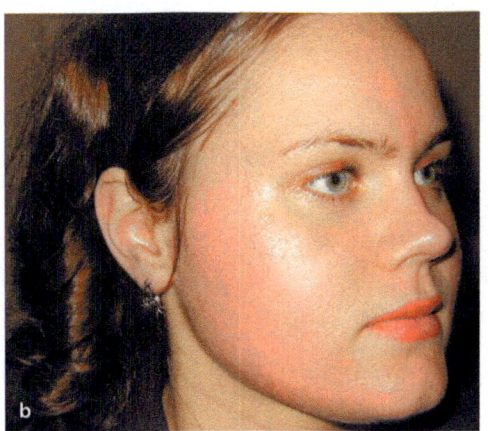

Fig. 22.1 a Acne scarring before treatment. **b** Seven days after treatment

The following groups of patients may be treated with EC:

- Young women and men with severe acne scars and premature skin aging.
- Patients with crow's-feet around the eyes.
- Patients with sun-damaged skin.
- Elderly women with severe wrinkling and skin laxity.
- Patients after surgical facelifts with remaining wrinkles and bad skin quality.
- Patients who had previously undergone other treatments, such as laser, chemical peels, and filling methods.

ECRS is performed with an ordinary transformer regulating the amount of electricity—AC/DC apparatus—to which the thermocauter is connected. Thermocauters of various shapes are used during the procedure.

The operative area should be marked. Then a numbing cream is applied to the surgical areas. Rejuvenation of a small portion of a face (e.g., eyelids, upper lips, or forehead) needs local anesthesia. Usually this is a numbing EMLA cream. Nevertheless, it is not a totally pain-free experience. The patients experience a burning and pinching sensation.

In the case of full-face resurfacing the patient needs intravenous anesthesia (Fig. 22.1) and the procedure

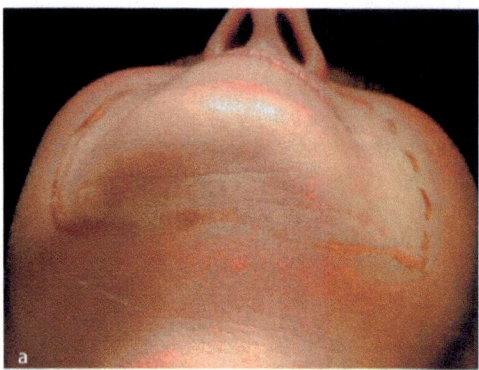
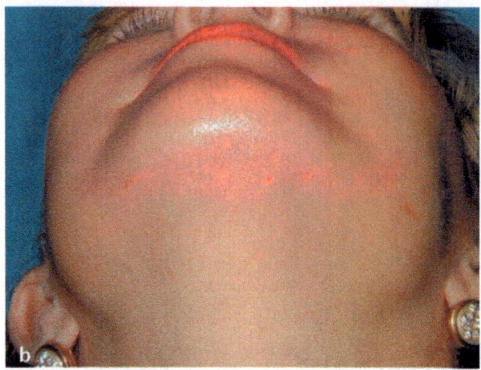

Fig. 22.2 a Rhytids under chin before treatment. **b** One week after treatment

should be performed in a surgical room with the assistance of an anesthesiologist.

After anesthesia the surface layer of the skin is removed to the reticular layer by a very quick, superficial, light, gliding touch of a thermocauter held parallel to the skin. Fine scars and fine wrinkles are completely removed with this method. For deeper scars and rhytids, after the first superficial coagulation, the coagulated tissue is removed, and the outer edges of the scar are flattened out almost to the bottom of the scar to make it as flat as possible. Therefore, the deeper the scar, the larger the skin area around the scar that has to be coagulated. The depth of skin resurfacing depends on the nature of the defects and skin types. Patients with thin, sensitive skin and with personal or family history of keloid formation should be approached with caution. Overaggressive EC can cause permanent damage, such as depigmentation, hypertrophic scars, or keloid.

In some cases, when there are atrophic and hypertrophic scars on the same area of a face or scarring along suture lines, a combination of ECRS and cryotherapy gives better cosmetic results.

The procedure of ECRS itself is performed over a period of 5–10 or 20 min, depending on the area involved. The coagulated area is covered by a gauze compress (such as Fucidin or fibrin cover) that is left on the wound for 1 day. The author has tried many types of dressings and found that the best is perforated fibrin film. It is permeable to air and water and significantly reduced healing time and postoperative redness. Fibrin film is left on the wound for 5–7 days (while healing) and there is no need to change the dressing.

After the procedure the patient is discharged home and seen in a 7–10 days. Some of the patients may experience edema of the face on 2–3 days, especially when the skin around the eyes and forehead is resurfaced. Usually it takes about 24 h for swelling to dissolve. The patients must be warned about all temporary changes that may occur after the procedure. A PowerPoint presentation during the preoperative consultation with all the pictures including "before" and "after" photographs would be very helpful.

If full facial rejuvenation is to be performed, the patient is treated in two sessions with an interval of 7 days, which is needed for healing. Therefore, it takes from 14 to 20 days for a full-face resurfacing, and 7–10 days for resurfacing of a small part of a face.

After ECRS the skin remains red for 7–10 days, then fades to a pink color that is easily camouflaged with makeup. The pink color disappears in 1–3 months. New skin regenerates, providing a fresher, smoother appearance with total resolution of rhytids (Fig. 22.2).

With full-face resurfacing there is significant skin retraction, giving the patient a real lifting effect accompanied by quite a rejuvenation of the face, without changing its natural expression.

The author has refined the technique making possible treating rhytids and scarring of a small portion of a face without a visible demarcation line. Patients used to undergo full-face EC in order to avoid a permanent demarcation line even if they had small problems (e.g., wrinkles on forehead, eyelids, upper lips). That was time-consuming and expensive. Now patients are happy to be able to get rid of unwelcome wrinkles for 7 days. Some of the patients somehow managed to continue working just wearing a facial mask.

Special care must be taken for 2–3 months after the ECRS. The use of potentially irritating topical products, abrasive soaps, cleansers, and cosmetics that have a strong drying effect, and products with a high concentration of alcohol, astringents, spices, or lime should be avoid. Particular caution should be exercised in using preparations containing sulfur, resorcinol, or salicylic acid.

Exposure to sunlight should be minimized. Use of sunscreen products and protective clothing over treated areas is recommended when exposure cannot be avoided.

patients with a pigmentary problems may have temporary hyperpigmentation (Fig. 22.3) These temporary changes can be avoided or reduced to a minimum by taking orally an antiviral medications at least 2 days before and 7 days after the procedure, and methionine with vitamin C.

An overzealous coagulation may cause permanent damage, such as depigmentation, edge pigmentation hypertrophic scars, and even keloid. To avoid scarring it is very important to make a proper assessment to ensure that coagulation is at the right strength. Attention must be paid to the individual characteristics of the skin in each and every case, for the patients' skin responds individually.

Nowadays, with an incredible growth in popularity of herbal medicines and supplements such as *Ginkgo biloba*, garlic, ginger ginsing, and vitamin E dermatologists have to be on the lookout. It is advisable to stop taking them prior to ECRS, for some of the herbal preparations can cause postoperative telangiectasia.

22.3
Complications

Occasionally, patients with a history of recurrent herpes simplex may have reactivation of the virus. Some

22.4
Discussion

ECRS is a perfect procedure for treating facial rejuvenation, rhytids, and scarring.

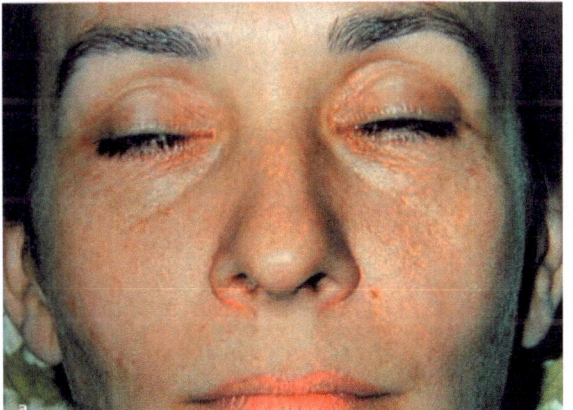

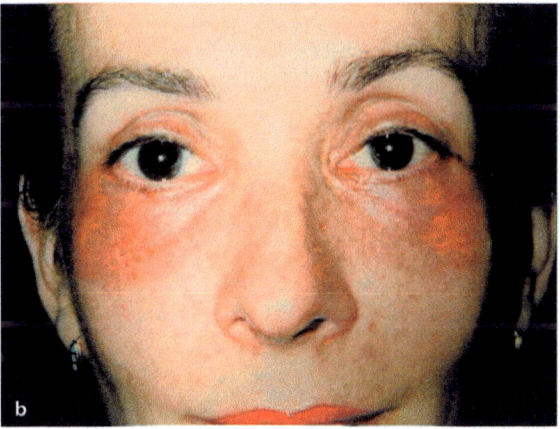

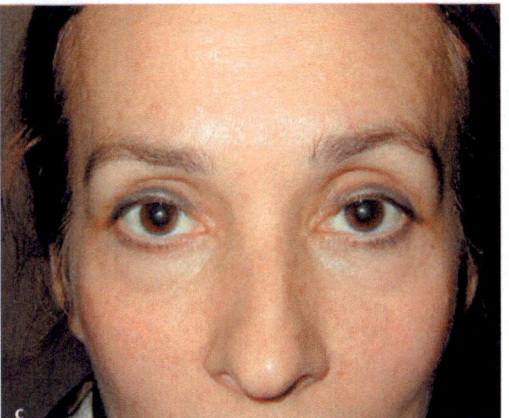

Fig. 22.3 a Patient prior to treatment. **b** Posttreatment hyperpigmentation under eyes. c Six months after treatment with resolution of the hyperpigmentation

The advantages of the technique are obvious:

- The equipment is portable and simple: transformer and a thermocauter.
- There is no bleeding during the procedure.
- There is no need for patients to take antibiotics because any kind of infection is excluded since the electrode is heated to 200–300°C.
- The procedure can be performed easily at any place as no surgical room and no assistance are required.
- It is simple and quick with long-lasting effects.

Altogether it has particular advantages. The procedure can be performed easily at any place. It appeals to those patients who prefer to have the treatment in the privacy of their own home. Simplicity, a high degree of effectiveness, as well as low incidences of complications make this method very attractive. The long-lasting results are impressive and result in a high degree of patient satisfaction.

Nevertheless, despite of the popularity of ECRS among patients, the method is not popular among dermatological surgeons because of the subtlety of the technique.

The skill of an experienced dermatological surgeon is essential to obtain superb results. That is why only very few dermatologists—six physicians remain from those 18 practitioners who were trained in the Soviet era—can perform this procedure.

22.5
Conclusions

EC is an effective conservative treatment for rhytids and scarring, as well as for facial rejuvenation. More often than not, no anesthesia is used. Instead, a numbing cream is applied to the areas to be work on. No assistance and no surgical room are required. The equipment is portable and easy to use at any place. The procedure is safe and does not cause any systematic side effects, or permanent damage if performed correctly.

Overall, this method can be widely used in cosmetic dermatology.

Reference

1. Nikitina S: Removal of fine wrinkles and correction of atrophic scars with electrocoagulation. Int J Cosmet Surg Aesthet Dermatol 2000;2(4):223–225

CHAPTER 23

Plasma Skin Resurfacing

23

Samuel M. Lam, Thomas L. Tzikas

23.1
Introduction

Traditional ablative techniques, including CO_2 laser resurfacing, medium-to-deep chemical peeling, and mechanical dermabrasion, have provided excellent and durable skin rejuvenation results. However, each treatment modality carries with it a potential morbidity profile and/or aesthetic limitations. Lighter treatment therapies like 35% trichloroacetic acid (TCA) peeling can rejuvenate mildly sun-damaged skin including dyschromias and fine rhytids, but may fail to correct deeper rhytids and more profound skin textural problems. Deeper treatments like CO_2 laser resurfacing and phenol can correct deeper rhytids but are associated with a more significantly protracted recovery period and risk of hypopigmentation. Mechanical dermabrasion works well to correct discrete contour problems like acne scarring and perioral rhytids but is technically more difficult to achieve consistency across the entire face when used as a standalone treatment modality. Obviously, a combination approach toward skin rejuvenation using various modalities can optimize aesthetic improvement while minimizing the side-effect profile.

A new technology has arisen in the past few years that offers the prospect of replacing many of these traditional techniques by optimizing aesthetic benefit without the untoward side-effect profile and prolonged recovery period associated with deeper treatments. Plasma skin resurfacing (PSR; Portrait PSR[3] from Rhytec, Waltham, MA, USA) relies on a technology in which ultra-high-frequency energy stimulates pulses of inert, nitrogen gas into a physical state known as plasma. Plasma, or ionized gas, is considered the fourth state of matter, along with solid, liquid, and gas. PSR achieves the intended skin rejuvenation via blind heat, i.e., the energy imparted is not chromophore-specific, unlike with lasers, so the thermal injury imparted to the skin is more controlled and uniform. Also unlike traditional ablative laser technology, PSR does not immediately remove the skin surface, but maintains the outer layer of skin as a biologic dressing akin to chemical peels that sloughs off after several days. The recovery time is generally 1 week with almost complete epithelialization by that time and with very little lingering erythema. The risk of hypopigmentation has also not been evident with PSR, which stands in contradistinction to the CO_2 laser and phenol. The recovery time is analogous to a medium-depth therapy like 35% TCA. By altering the settings of the device, one can also adjust the degree of rejuvenation to provide medium-depth rejuvenation where needed and deeper rejuvenation where indicated, thereby obviating the need for multiple combined resurfacing techniques. At very low settings, the patient can even undergo multiple sessions over monthly intervals to achieve a comparable result with only 2–3 days of downtime per treatment. The Portrait PSR[3] device is FDA-approved to treat multiple skin abnormalities, including facial rhytids, superficial skin lesions, actinic keratoses, viral papillomata, and seborrheic keratoses for Fitzpatrick skin types I–IV. It has also been used off-label to improve the skin tone and texture of the neck, chest, and hands using the lower-energy settings (1–1.5 J/cm^2) over repeated monthly sessions.

23.2
Technique

23.2.1
Anesthesia Considerations

Although the discomfort engendered by PSR is not as severe as that from CO_2 laser resurfacing, the pain scale is significant and adjunctive anesthetic measures are mandatory to achieve adequate pain control. Ideally, the patient is treated under intravenous sedation, moderate sedation to twilight, with concurrent regional anesthetic blocks. However, preoperative oral sedation and oral narcotic usage combined with topical anesthesia along with regional and tumescent anesthetic blocks can be adequate in most cases. With the latter type of anesthesia, the patient is given the oral sedative and narcotic (e.g., valium and vicodin, respectively) 1–2 h prior to the start of the procedure and a topical anesthetic (e.g., topically applied lidocaine preparation) 30–45 min beforehand. The patient can also receive supplemental intramuscular anesthesia that consists of 50 mg Demerol and 50 mg phenergan to enhance overall patient comfort.

Immediately prior to starting the procedure, the patient should receive regional anesthetic nerve blocks that include the infraorbital, mental, supraorbital, zygomatico-temporal, and zygomatico-maxillary nerves. The buccal and preauricular areas are more difficult areas to fully anesthetize with regional blockade so tumescent anesthesia can be carried out (i.e., direct local infiltration) in these areas and any area that is not adequately anesthetized despite a regional nerve block. The authors have found that the fine blunt infiltration cannulas used for autologous fat grafting can provide a convenient delivery system for tumescent anesthesia while minimizing the risk of ecchymosis that may arise with sharp-needle placement. Although lidocaine alone is adequate to achieve appropriate anesthesia levels during the procedure, we supplement our anesthesia with bupivicaine, as patients oftentimes have an intense burning sensation that can linger for 2–3 h after completion of the treatment.

As the plasma delivered is flammable, only moistened 4 × 4 gauze and fabrics should be present in the proximal field. Further, the oxygen supply should be completely turned off during PSR. It is also important to reiterate that perioperative herpetic prophylaxis is important for anyone receiving perioral PSR treatments, and current or recent isotretinoin usage is a contraindication like for all ablative therapies.

23.2.2
Protocols and Procedure

After adequate anesthesia levels have been verified, treatment can begin. Although the Portrait PSR[3] device can be dialed to any setting of fluence, there are only certain recommended fluences based on clinical experience. For lower-energy resurfacing, 1.5 J/cm² is preferred. This energy level reduces the recovery time to only 2–3 days but does not truly achieve the remarkable benefit that follows high-energy settings. The lower-energy setting can be used for individuals who desire a shorter recovery time and who are willing to undergo multiple, typically three, treatments spaced at monthly intervals to achieve comparable results. With lower-energy settings, the discomfort level is commensurately reduced. Lower-energy settings can also be used for areas where a concurrent facelift flap will be raised in order to minimize the chance of a problem with flap viability.

Generally, it is recommended to undertake PSR after all other facial surgical procedures have been completed. Higher-energy settings include 3.0 J/cm² for periocular resurfacing and 3.5 J/cm² for the remainder of the face. When approaching deeper cheek and perioral rhytids, the physician can elect to undertake a second pass at the same 3.5-J/cm² setting over the linear distance of the rhytid itself to improve the clinical result but at the expense of several more days of potential erythema. Settings between 1.6 and 2.9 J/cm² are not advisable,

as they can elicit the same degree of recovery time as the higher recommended settings without the clinical benefits.

In order to deliver the appropriate energy to the skin, the correct protocol that will be described must be followed. The Portrait PSR[3] device is intended not to contact the skin. Instead, the hand piece should be held perpendicular to the skin surface so that approximately a 5-mm distance is maintained between the nozzle and the skin surface (Fig. 23.1). In the past, a physical distance gauge was used to ensure maintenance of proper nozzle-to-skin distance but the marker melted under the heat of the plasma or caused undue skin damage as it was dragged across the skin surface. Therefore, the physician must be mindful of maintaining the appropriate nozzle-to-skin distance throughout the procedure. At a 5-mm distance, an illuminated ring that is projected onto the skin should appear in focus and approximately 5 mm in diameter. If feathering is desired, the nozzle can be pulled back to a distance of 2–3 cm so that the illuminated ring is enlarged and defocused. Changing the angle of the hand piece vis-à-vis the skin is not advisable owing to the risk of non-uniform delivery of energy.

The physician should move the hand piece in a smooth linear direction so that there is minimal overlap between rows. Slight overlap of each row is permitted given the Gaussian distribution of the imparted energy, i.e., most of the energy delivered is focused in the center of the beam with radial drop off from that central point of maximal cellular vacuolation. In addition, owing to the increased thermal injury that can be imparted when a physician passes from lateral to medial then turns around and goes from medial to lateral in the adjacent following row and continuing in this serpentine fashion, it is advised to go only in one direction for the entire face, i.e., lateral to medial, lateral to medial, and so forth. When delivering the energy, moving the hand

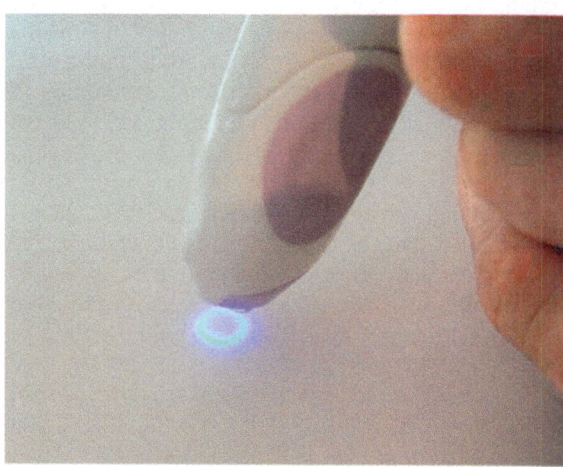

Fig. 23.1 The illuminated ring that appears on the skin to guide plasma skin resurfacing

piece at about 1.5 Hz can help deliver energy to the skin without skipped or stacked areas.

When passing the beam near any hair-bearing areas like the eyebrows and eyelashes, a tongue blade should be used to protect the singeing and vaporization of any hair. Although a corneal shield may not be necessary, lacrilube ointment and care to avoid corneal contact should always be undertaken. As mentioned, only moistened gauze should be used and the oxygen supply should be turned off during PSR to minimize the risk of an inadvertent flame and consequent burn.

When performing facial skin resurfacing, the physician can elect either to complete the full face or only regional areas like the perioral and periorbital regions. The Portrait PSR[3] device can be fitted with two different nozzles that are designed either for full-face or regional PSR and which must be replaced after the allotted pulses have been fired or the allotted time has elapsed. For a full-face PSR, a nozzle that permits 1,200 high-energy (3.0 or 3.5 J/cm^2) or 2,400 low-energy (1.5 J/cm^2) pulses is used. For a regional PSR treatment, a specific nozzle that yields 300 high-energy (3.0 or 3.5 J/cm^2) or 600 low-energy (1.5 J/cm^2) pulses is generally sufficient.

23.3
Postoperative Care and Management of Complications

As mentioned, the recovery after a standard high-energy treatment is approximately 7 days (Fig. 23.2). For the first 3–4 days, the charred debris of the outer skin remains intact, serving as a biologic dressing and making the patient look quite socially unacceptable. The skin can appear ashened and mottled until the old skin begins to fall away in a piecemeal fashion over the first 3–4 days. Typically, by the fifth postoperative day, most if not all of the old skin has fallen away and the new skin is in the process of regeneration. The patient will appear variably erythematous from a medium shade of pink to a bright red depending on the degree of epithelialization that has occurred by that point. By the seventh day, the patient should appear by most standards socially acceptable with near-complete or complete epithelialization and a very light pink color remains. This light pink color may persist for an additional 7 days, especially if a second high-energy pass was performed in the areas of deeper rhytids. However, the pinkness that remains is far less noticeable than the conspicuous erythema that lingers for weeks to months after CO_2 laser resurfacing.

As the old skin remains intact unlike with ablative CO_2 laser resurfacing, the patient does not feel the intense discomfort and occasional pruritus that follows CO_2 laser therapy. Nevertheless, the first 2 days that follow PSR can oftentimes still be somewhat uncomfortable so as to require relief by oral narcotic medication. This initial discomfort should pass within 2–3 days. As mentioned, the first few hours that follow immediately after PSR can be quite uncomfortable for the patient so bupivicaine regional and tumescent blocks are recommended as a preventative measure.

Postoperative care follows the exact same prescribed formula as for any kind of ablative resurfacing, i.e., application of thick petrolatum-based emollients over all treated areas until full epithelialization occurs. Aquaphor ointment (Beiersdorf) has proven to be a convenient, inexpensive product to serve as the ointment of choice until epithelialization is complete. Thereafter, a lighter

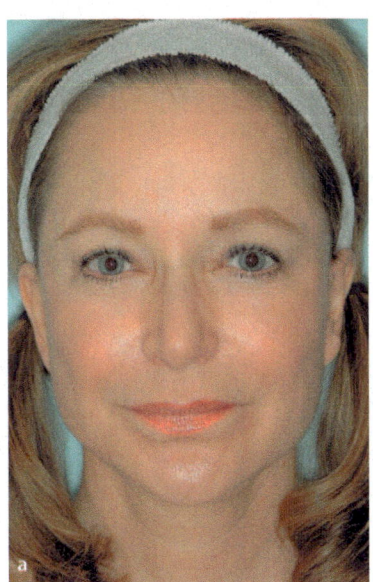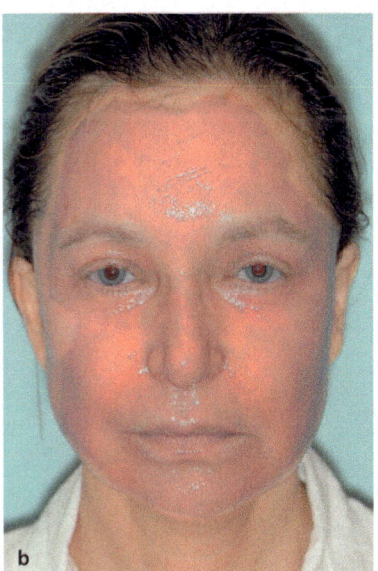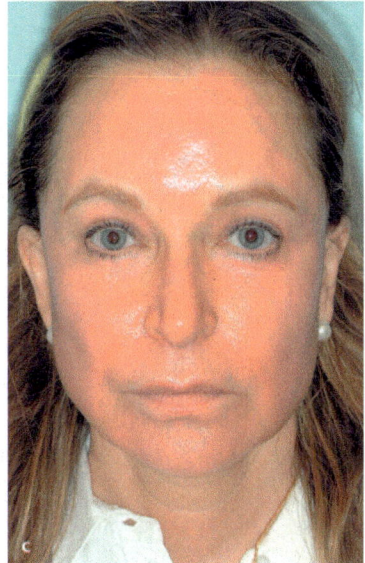

Fig. 23.2 A 53-year-old woman. **a** Preoperatively. **b** Five days following full-face plasma skin resurfacing at a high-energy level. **c** Seven days postoperatively

moisturizer can be used like Eucerin or Cetaphil for the first 30 days following resurfacing to maintain proper conditioning to otherwise partially desiccated skin during the healing phase. For the first few days while epithelialization occurs, the patient may experience some discomfort and mild pruritus. Cold, moistened compresses soaked in saline or water can be helpful in soothing the inflamed skin. A tablespoon of white vinegar in a cup of distilled water can be used to clean the skin and to remove the Aquaphor before reapplication of the ointment. The vinegar/water combination can also be used as a soaked compress to soothe the face.

Complications that occur after PSR are the same as those that arise after traditional ablative resurfacing, which include herpetic outbreak, dermatitis, hyperpigmentation, scarring, and limited aesthetic improvement. Hypopigmentation has not been reported to date after 2 years of clinical experience. Sun avoidance and sunscreen usage are important to minimize the onset and severity of hyperpigmentation. A detailed review of identification and management of complications that follow ablative resurfacing can be found in Chap. 14.

Generally speaking, with proper skin care and sun avoidance, PSR is only intended for a single, one-time treatment; however, a repeat treatment can be undertaken with a recommended minimum interval of 18 months between sessions. Although some rhytids will persist after treatment, ongoing improvement will be evident several months following PSR, a fact of which the patient should be aware. Explaining to patients that rhytids should continue to dissipate over time will help prepare them for the apparent return of some rhytids when the edema subsides after 1 week or so (Fig. 23.3).

23.4
Conclusions

With the advent of new technology, ongoing improvement in our capacity to achieve desired aesthetic objectives while minimizing downtime and the adverse side-effect profile continues to take place. Plasma resurfacing offers the hope of replacing the need to combine medium and deep skin therapies, as explained in Chap. 14, or at least an alternative treatment modality. However, any new technology must be borne out with long-term clinical evidence and the reality that newer technology stands always on the horizon.

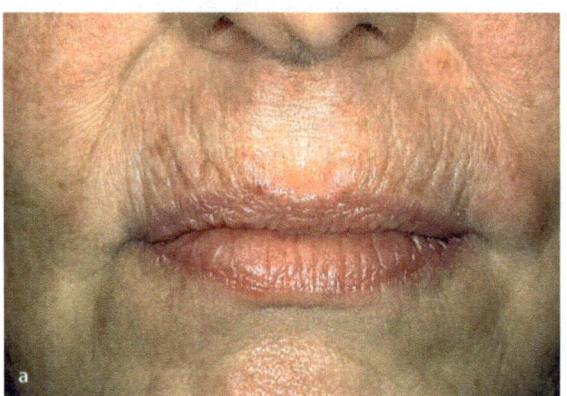
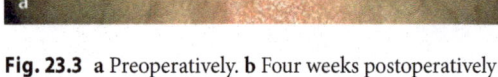
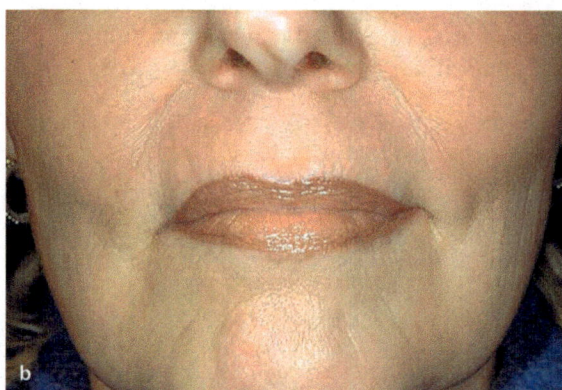

Fig. 23.3 **a** Preoperatively. **b** Four weeks postoperatively

CHAPTER 24

Botulinum Toxin: Products, Techniques, Complications

24

Melvin A. Shiffman, Sid J. Mirrafati

24.1
History

Justinus Kerner, in 1793 [1], discovered a substance he called *Wurstgift* found in spoiled sausage that caused gastrointestinal and muscular disorders that could result in death. The disease was called "Kerner's disease" and ultimately named by Muller, in 1870, botulism from the Latin term *botulus* meaning "sausage" [1]. In 1895, Emile van Ermengem first isolated the bacterium *Clostridium botulinum* [1]. Edward Schantz, in 1994 [1], first isolated the toxin and in 1973 Alan B. Scott [2] used BTX-A for the first time to treat strabismus.

BTX-A (Botox) was approved by the US Food and Drug Administration for the treatment of strabismus, blepharospasm, and hemifacial spasm in patients younger than age 12 years [1].

24.2
Introduction

The bacterium *Clostridium botulinum* produces eight serotypes (subspecies), of which there are seven serologically distinct exotoxins [3]. The toxin inhibits acetylcholine (a neurotransmitter) release at the neuromuscular junction, resulting in temporary muscle paralysis. Serologic types include A, B, C, D, E, F, and G. Type E is also produced by *Clostridium butyricum* and type F is also produced by *Clostridium baratii*. Only types A, B, E, and F cause illness in humans. Botulinum toxin is colorless, odorless, and tasteless. The toxin is inactivated by heat, 85°C (185°F) or greater for 5 min.

The standard measurement of the potency of the toxin is that one international unit (IU) of botulinum toxin kills 50% of a group of 18–20 female Swiss-Webster mice (LD_{50}) [4]. The LD_{50} in humans is estimated to be approximately 2,730 IU [5].

24.3
Products

Botox (Allergan Corporation, Irvine, CA, USA; Table 24.1) is a dry, protein crystalline complex of botulinum toxin A that contains 100 mouse units (MU) per bottle. "One unit of BOTOX® COSMETIC corresponds to the calculated median intraperitoneal lethal dose (LD_{50}) in mice" [6]. The product is unstable unless kept frozen. The instructions are to dilute the contents of bottle with 2 ml of sterile saline without preservative, leaving 25 MU for each 0.5 ml of solution (Fig. 24.1). The onset of paralysis takes 24–48 h and the effect usually lasts 4–6 months. Repeat injections may delay the onset of paralysis but sometimes a more protracted paralysis will occur [3]. One nanogram contains 2.5 IU [7].

Dysport (Ipsen, Slough, UK; Table 24.1) is botulinum type A. Four units of Dysport is approximately equal to one unit of Botox [8, 9]. Mybloc (Neurobloc) (Elan Pharmaceuticals, San Francisco, CA, USA; Table 24.1) is type B. When reconstituted, Mybloc has a shelf life of more than 12 months; however, larger volumes than

Table 24.1 Botulinum toxin

BTXA	Botulinum toxin type A	Lanzhou Institute of Biological Products, China
Botox	Botulinum toxin type A	Allergan, USA
Dysport	Botulinum toxin type A	Ipsen, UK
Mybloc	Botulinum toxin type B	Elan, Ireland
Neurobloc	Botulinum toxin type B	Elan, Ireland

Modified from [18]

Botulinum Toxin

Name: _____   Date: _____

Muscle   Number of Units

A. Frontal   _____

B. Corrugator   _____

C. Procerus   _____

D. Orbicularis Oculi   _____

E. Other _____   _____

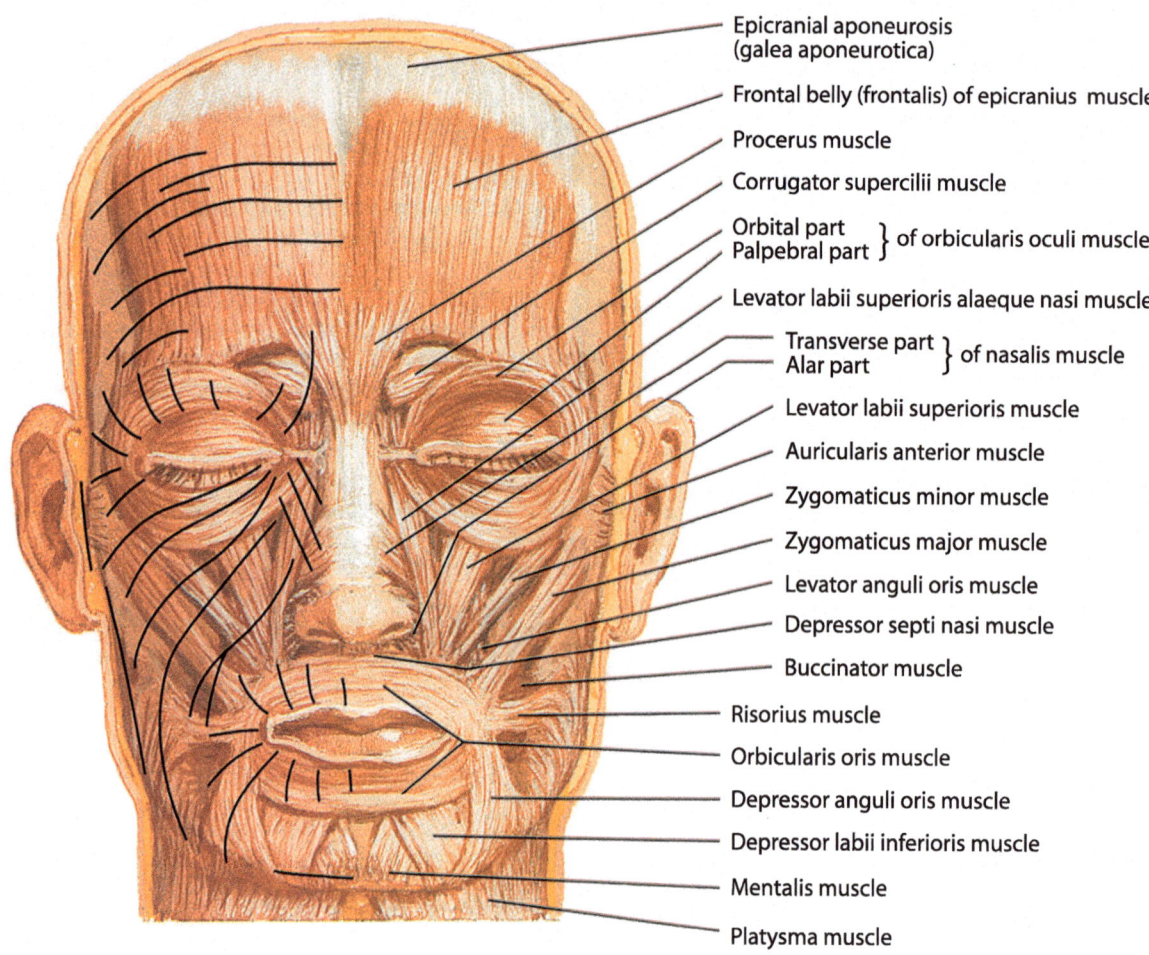

Epicranial aponeurosis
(galea aponeurotica)

Frontal belly (frontalis) of epicranius muscle

Procerus muscle

Corrugator supercilii muscle

Orbital part
Palpebral part } of orbicularis oculi muscle

Levator labii superioris alaeque nasi muscle

Transverse part
Alar part } of nasalis muscle

Levator labii superioris muscle

Auricularis anterior muscle

Zygomaticus minor muscle

Zygomaticus major muscle

Levator anguli oris muscle

Depressor septi nasi muscle

Buccinator muscle

Risorius muscle

Orbicularis oris muscle

Depressor anguli oris muscle

Depressor labii inferioris muscle

Mentalis muscle

Platysma muscle

Fig. 24.1 Medical record form for botulinum toxin injection

with Botox may be needed. Antibody formation against Myobloc may occur more often, because of its higher protein content, than with Botox [9]. One nanogram contains 40 IU [4].

Each company has its own test protocol.

24.4
Indications for Cosmetic Purposes

Wrinkles may be caused by muscular action or solar damage. Botulinum toxin is only indicated for wrinkles caused by muscular action (Figs. 24.2–24.5). Common indications include treatment of glabellar frown lines [10, 11], transverse forehead lines, lateral canthal fold wrinkle (crow's-feet) [12], and medial and lateral brow lifts. Other indications may include wrinkle on the upper lip, nasal scrunching and flaring, marionette lines, neck lines and platysmal bands, mental creases, and dimpling of the chin (these indications can lead to complications that interfere with physiologic functions). Off-

label uses include palmar [13] and plantar hyperhidrosis, focal dystonias, spasticity, hemifacial spasm, axillary hyperhidrosis [13, 14], tics, tremors, tension headaches [15], and migraine headaches (these are experimental in nature).

24.5
Cautions and Contraindications

24.5.1
Cautions

Caution is required for patients on the following medications:

1. Aminoglycoside antibiotic may increase the effect of botulinum toxin.
2. Chloroquine and hydroxychloroquine may reduce effect of botulinum toxin.
3. Blood-thinning agents such as aspirin or warfarin may result in bruising.

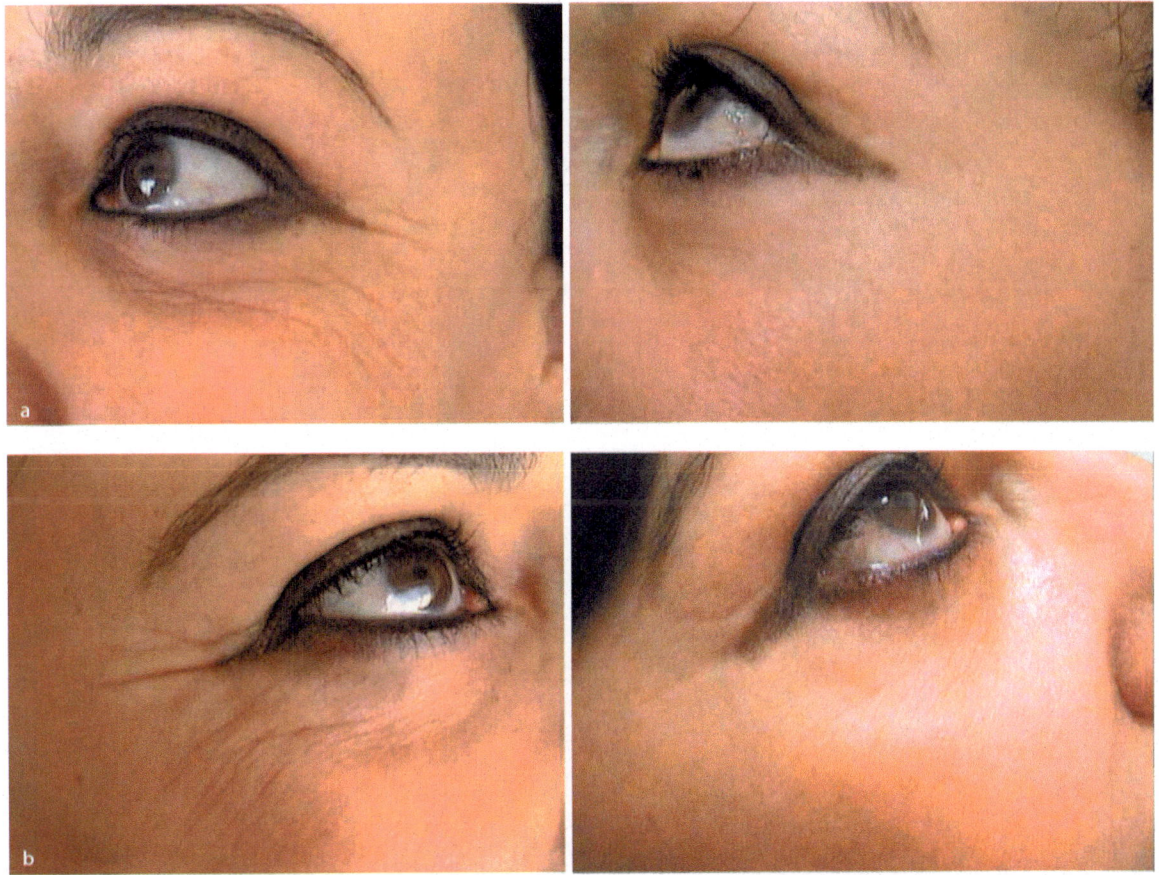

Fig. 24.2 a Preoperatively. **b** Two weeks after botulinum toxin injection into the orbicularis oculi muscle

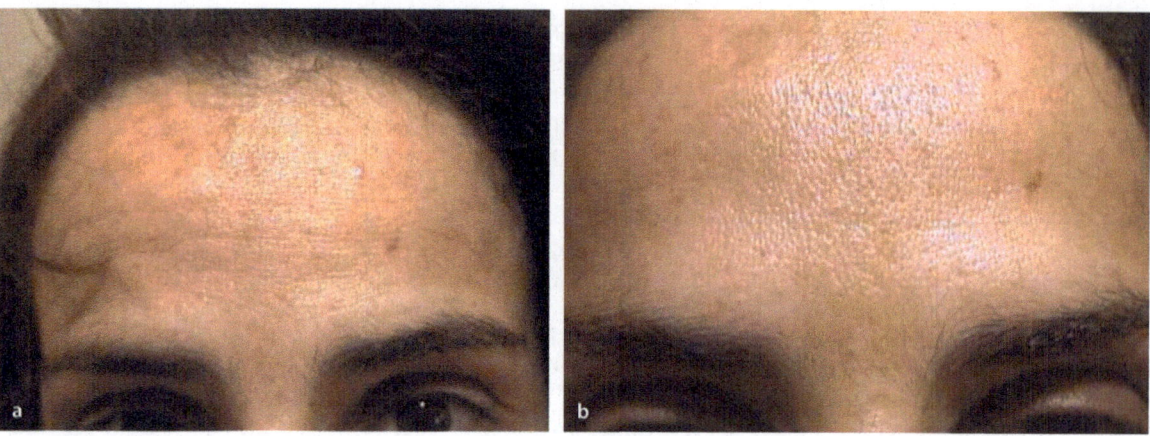

Fig. 24.3 a Preoperatively with forehead muscles at rest. Note persistent wrinkle. **b** Two weeks after botulinum toxin injection into the frontalis muscles

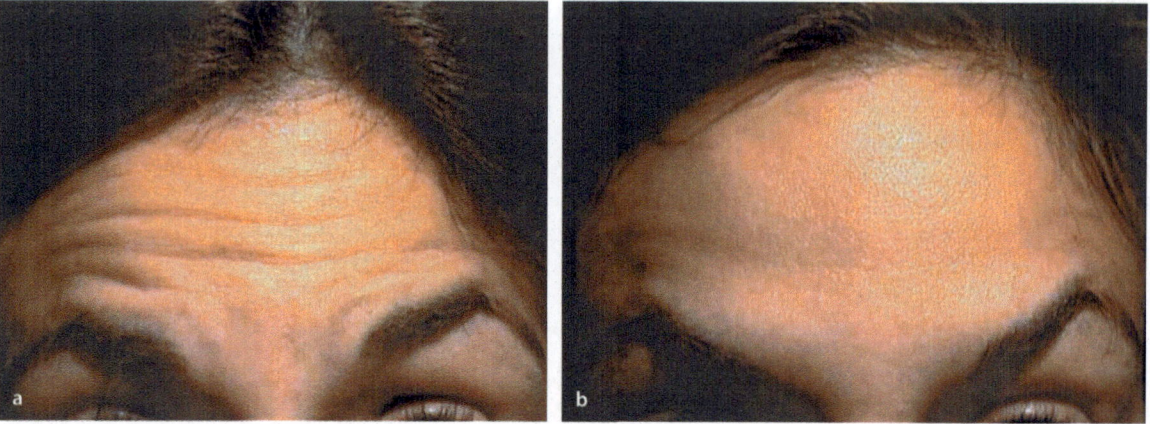

Fig. 24.4 a Preoperatively with frontalis muscles contracted. **b** Two weeks postoperatively following injection into frontalis muscles, with frontalis muscles contracted

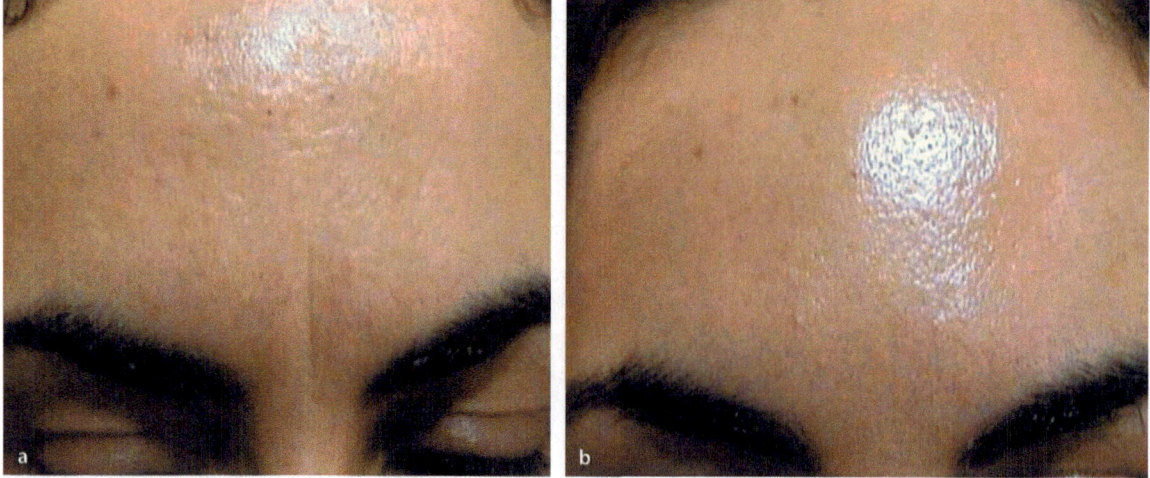

Fig. 24.5 a Preoperatively showing glabellar line. **b** Two weeks postoperatively following injection of botulinum toxin into corrugator muscles

24.5.2
Contraindications

Contraindications include neuromuscular disorders, known hypersensitivity to any ingredient of the formulation, pregnancy or breast feeding, unrealistic patient expectations, or infection at the proposed injection site(s).

24.6
Technique

24.6.1
Corrugator Muscle

The origin of the muscle is at the junction of the nasal and frontal bones close to the supramedial orbital rim. A transverse line drawn coronally through the middle of the eyebrow identifies the horizontal position of the bulk of the muscle. Do not inject lateral to the midpupillary line.

24.6.2
Procerus Muscle

The procerus muscle in located in the midline of the nose. The optimal injection site is the midline just caudal to the nasal root.

24.6.3
Frontalis Muscle

Inject the thickest portions of the muscle at points 1.5–2.0 cm apart. Laterally raise the line of the injections away from the brow to prevent lateral brow droop.

24.6.4
Orbicularis Oculi Muscle

Mark the lateral canthal line 1 cm lateral to the canthus. Inject along this line. Do not inject too close to the lids.

24.6.5
Orbicularis Oris Muscle

Inject at the point halfway between the vermillion border of the lower lip and the inferior edge of the mentum, approximately 0.5–1.0 cm medial to the oral commissure. Use only small amounts of toxin.

24.6.6
Platysma Muscle and Bands

The needle should be inserted perpendicular to the muscle fibers [16].

24.7
Postoperative Instructions

Do not massage the areas of the injections. Use the facial expression muscles to help block more of the acetylcholine every 15 min for the first hour after injection. Use ice packs for discomfort or pain.

24.8
Possible Risks and Complications

These are:
1. Delayed eyelid closure
2. Ptosis
3. Decreased blink response
4. Excessive tearing
5. Blurred vision
6. Asymmetry of face
7. Drooling
8. Headache
9. Infection
10. Bruising

Necrotizing fasciitis has been reported as a complication of botulinum toxin injection [17].

24.9
Conclusions

Botulinum toxin injected into muscles is a good temporary fix for rhytids. Very deep rhytids would need treatment with other modalities such as fillers or sugary.

References

1. Kedlaya D: Botulinum toxin: overview. In: eMedicine Word Medical Library, 2006, http://www.emedicine.com/pmr/topic216.htm
2. Scott AB: Botulinum toxin injection of eye muscles to correct strabismus. Trans Am Ophth 1981;79:734–770
3. Guyuron B: Forehead rejuvenation. In Plastic Surgery: Indications, Operations, and Outcomes. St. Louis, Mosby, 2000:2563–2582
4. Keen MS, Khosh M..: The role of botulinum toxin A in facial plastic surgery. In Facial Plastic Surgery, Willett JM (ed), Stanford, Appleton & Lange 1997:323–329

5. Jancovic J, Brin M: Therapeutic use of botulinum toxin. N Engl J Med 1991;324:1186–1194

6. Allergan (2005) BOTOX® COSMETIC (botulinum toxin type A) purified neurotoxin complex. http://www.botox-cosmetic.com/resources/pi.aspx. Cited 11 April 2007

7. Quinn N, Hallett M: Dose standardization of botulinum toxin. Lancet 1989;1:964

8. Odergren T, Hjaltason H, Kaakkola S, Solder S, Hanko J, Fehling C, Marttila RJ, Lundh H, Gedin S, Westergren, I., Richardson A, Dott C: A double blind, randomized, parallel group study to investigate the dose equivalence of Dysport and Botox in the treatment of cervical dystonia. J Neurol Neurosurg Psychiatry 1998;64(1):6–12

9. Trizna Z: Botulinum toxin. In: eMedicine Word Medical Library, 2006, http://www.emedicine/derm/topic779.htm. Cited 9 Sept 2004

10. Carruthers JD, Carruthers JA: Treatment of glabellar frown lines with C. botulinum-A exotoxin. J Dermatol Surg Oncol 1992;18(1):17–21

11. MacDonald MR, Spiegel JH, Raven RB, Kabaker SS, Maas CS: An anatomical approach to glabellar rhytids. Arch Otolaryngol Head Neck Surg 1998;124(2):1315–1320

12. Matarasso SL, Matarasso A: Treatment guidelines for botulinum toxin type A for the periocular region and a report on partial upper lip ptosis following injections to the lateral canthal rhytids. Plast Reconstr Surg 2001;108(1):208–214

13. Naver H, Swartling C, Aquilonius SM: Palmar and axillary hyperhidrosis treated with botulinum toxin: one-year clinical follow-up. Eur J Neurol 2000;7(1):55–62

14. Heckmann M, Ceballos-Baumann AO, Plewig G, Hyperhidrosis Study Group: Botulinum toxin A for axillary hyperhidrosis (excessive sweating). N Engl J Med 2001;344(7):488–493

15. Schulte-Mattler WJ, Wieser T, Zierz S: Treatment of tension-type headache with botulinum toxin: a pilot study. Eur J Med Res 1999;4(5):183–186

16. Matarasso A, Matarasso SL, Brandt FS, Bellman B: Botulinum A exotoxin for the management of platysmal bands. Plast Reconstr Surg 1999;103(2):645–652

17. Latimer PR, Hodgkins PR, Vakalis AN, Butler RE, Evans AR, Zaki GA: Necrotizing fasciitis as a complication of botulinum toxin injection. Eye 1998;12(Pt 1):51–53

18. Ichikawa K: Soft-tissue implantable materials A to Z. Plast Reconstr Surg 2005;115(3):966–968

CHAPTER 25

Laser Facial Hair Removal

25

Benjamin A. Bassichis

25.1
Introduction

As governed by cultural norms, excess hair, especially on the face, is a very common and often embarrassing issue for many patients. In the past century, unwanted hair was traditionally treated with many different modalities that were slow, tedious, painful, impractical, and resulted in poor long-term efficacy. Consequently, there has been a public demand for novel, rapid, reliable, safe, and affordable hair-removal techniques. In the last couple of decades, a number of laser and light-based technologies have been developed for hair removal that specifically target hair follicles and allow for the potential treatment of large areas with long-lasting results. The quest for truly permanent photoepilation and the ability to treat white hairs and darker-skinned patients are the current goals for improvement in this evolving field.

Laser hair removal works by sending a beam of laser light to a group of hair follicles. The light energy causes thermal injury to the follicles. This occurs because laser light is converted into heat as it passes through the skin and is absorbed in the target pigment melanin found in the hair follicle. This process is called selective photothermolysis [1]. It is selective because it targets only the hair and not the skin. The surrounding skin is usually cooled via several methods, including gels, cryogenic sprays, or a cooling tip.

Hair grows in cycles. Anagen is the active growth phase; catagen is the transition phase; and telogen is the resting phase. The laser is effective only in the active growth or anagen phase, during which time the hair has an abundance of melanin and the hair follicles are easily targeted. When the temperature in a hair follicle reaches a high enough level during its active growth phase, the treated hair structures are disabled, thus inhibiting hair regrowth.

The laser beam finds the hair follicles by targeting the melanin pigment that gives skin and hair dark coloration. Therefore, the ideal candidate for laser hair removal has dark hair and light skin. These patients will have more significant photoepilation results in fewer treatments than patients with red, white, gray, or true blond hair. The laser light is also attracted to the melanin in the skin, so individuals with suntans

or dark skin types have an increased risk for discoloration of pigment and other side effects with most types of lasers, making this category of patients a treatment challenge. However, new laser technologies, especially YAG lasers, have made it possible for people with many skin color and hair color combinations to enjoy the benefits of laser hair removal. These newer lasers have been designed to safely treat patients of all skin types [2].

Excess and unwanted facial hair is a common problem in both men and women. Women frequently experience this condition on the face, especially the upper lip, chin, or eyebrow area. Men often wish to rid themselves of unwanted hair between their eyebrows or on other parts of their face.

There are several laser and laserlike devices currently used for hair removal. These include, but are not limited to:

- Ruby laser—including the EpiTouch or the Epilaser
- Alexandrite laser—such as the Candela GentleLase Plus
- Light-based or intense pulsed light (IPL) devices—for example, the Palomar Starlux
- Diode laser—such as the Light Sheer
- Long-pulse Nd:YAG laser—for example, the Candela GentleYAG

These are all effective, fast, comfortable and safe for permanent hair removal. Each hair-removal system has a specific set of advantages and disadvantages depending on the skin color and hair color for the particular laser hair removal candidate. A good laser practitioner can achieve excellent results with a wide range of skin types, hair types, and colors.

A general paradigm (Table 25.1) to follow for selecting the best laser for your patients would be to treat clients with light hair or thin hair, and Fitzpatrick skin types I and II with radiofrequency technology, 694-nm ruby lasers, or 755-nm alexandrite lasers. Patients with brown and medium-thickness hair, who are Fitzpatrick types II–IV are best treated with the 755-nm alexandrite laser or with broad wavelength spectrum 515–1,200-nm IPL devices. The black hair, coarse hair texture patients with Fitzpatrick skin types IV–VI are optimally treated with the 800-nm diode laser or the 1,064-nm Nd:YAG laser [3, 4].

There are also several factors that a laser technician can control to customize treatments for efficacy, safety, and comfort:

- Pulse length—long-pulse lasers are considered safest.
- Fluence—selection of energy levels can be varied for skin type.
- Delay—the time in-between pulses of light affects how much the skin and hair follicle are allowed to cool off.
- Spot size—affects the speed and penetration of the laser. A larger spot penetrates deeper. A good selection of spot sizes helps the technician reach the hair at the depth at which it grows.
- Cooling—the surrounding skin may be protected by a cooling gel, spray, or cooled tip pressed against the skin.

Patients who are not ideal candidates for laser hair removal are those with red, white, gray, or very light blond hair, those who presently or have recently used Accutane or Bactrim, those taking photosensitizing medications, those who are tanned or very dark skinned (except when using a Nd:YAG laser), and those who are pregnant. Anabolic steroids should certainly not be taken unless medically necessary, as these can increase male-pattern hair growth in some cases. Medicines which inhibit hair growth (for example, spironolactone, Diane-35 birth control pills, Euflex, Androcur, and Vaniqua cream) might slightly reduce the pigment in hair roots and make laser treatments less efficient, but this seldom interferes with the overall effectiveness of the treatment. Laser hair removal can take place while the patient is on these medications, at the patient's request.

Even if a patient is not an "ideal candidate" he or she may still enjoy some of benefits of laser hair removal.

Early in the evolution of the procedure, patients with Fitzpatrick skin types V and VI were not candidates for laser hair removal, and even patients with skin types III and IV were considered high risk. However, innovations in laser technology have permitted more effective hair removal in a broader spectrum of patients, including the more challenging suntanned and Fitzpatrick skin types IV–VI. Long-pulse Nd:YAG lasers have been shown to effectively treat darker skin types, including patients of Afro-American, Asian, Hispanic, Mediterranean, European, and Middle Eastern heritages. The design of this laser, with deeper penetration and minimal scattering of laser energy, allows treatment of most skin types up to and including Afro-American skin types and people with tanned skin. If a traditional laser hair removal device is used on darker skin types, it can result in serious burning or loss of skin pigment (hypopigmentation). However, by utilizing a long pulse Nd:YAG, we can treat these patients with confidence. Fitzpatrick skin type VI can be treated with Nd:YAG lasers; however, there must be a differentiation between the hair and skin colors to proceed safely. The hair color must be darker than the skin color for effective photoepilation. Additionally, caution should be exercised when treating Asian skin, as excess precooling of the skin may cause hyperpigmentation. Because hair that is naturally blond, light red, grey, or white does not have enough pigment in the roots, it cannot be reliably treated with any type of laser at this time [3, 5].

25.2 Technique

25.2.1 Pretreatment Recommendations

1. Patients should avoid the sun, tanning creams, and tanning salon for 4–6 weeks before and after the

Table 25.1 Fitzpatrick skin types and recommended hair-removal devices

Skin type	Skin color	Tanning response	Recommended hair-removal device
I	White, freckled	Always burns, never tans	Radiofrequency, ruby laser (694 nm), alexandrite laser (755 nm)
II	White	Usually burns, tans with difficulty	IPL, radiofrequency, ruby laser (694 nm), alexandrite laser (755 nm)
III	White to olive	Mild burn, average tan	IPL, alexandrite laser (755 nm)
IV	Brown	Rarely buns, tans easily	IPL, diode laser (800 nm), Nd:YAG laser (1,064 nm)
V	Dark brown	Very rarely burns, tans very easily	Diode laser (800nm), Nd:YAG laser (1,064nm)
VI	Black	Does not burn, tans very easily	Diode laser (800nm), Nd:YAG laser (1,064nm)

IPL intense pulsed light

treatment regimen. A tan can interfere with the effectiveness of the treatment and possibly even cause complications. Patients should wear broad-spectrum (UV-A and UV-B) sunblock with an sun-protection factor (SPF) of 25 or higher before, between, and after treatments.

2. When patients with darker skin tones are treated, a bleaching cream may be started 4–6 weeks before treatment to optimize results.

3. The area to be treated should be shaved or trimmed the day before or the morning of treatment. Shaving prior to treatment also allows the patient to shape the exact area desired for treatment—this is sometimes very useful in areas such as the hairline and sideburns, and the bikini line. Excess hair above the surface of the skin absorbs and wastes laser energy, and reduces the amount of energy that reaches the hair root, where it is most effective. Excess hair above the surface of the skin also increases the chance of burning or irritating the skin.

4. Electrolysis, tweezing, plucking, threading, sugaring, or waxing hair must be stopped for at least 2–3 weeks prior to treatment. Hair follicles which do not have hair shafts in them to absorb laser energy will not be treated by the laser energy.

5. If a patient has a history of perioral cold sores or genital herpes in the treatment zone, prophylactic pretreatment with antiviral therapy (Acyclovir, Valtrex, or Famvir) should be prescribed.

6. The skin should be thoroughly cleaned and dried, removing any makeup, creams, oils, or topical anesthetics before laser treatments.

7. It may helpful for the patient to take Tylenol and/or Advil a couple hours prior to treatment. Some women find they are less sensitive after their menses and should schedule their treatment sessions accordingly.

8. The physician should engage in a detailed and honest discussion of desired results and expected improvements with each patient. Together the physician and patient can decide if laser treatment is the best option.

9. The most important step in laser hair removal is the skin patch test. The results of skin patch testing determine the settings for the laser and the safety profile. Testing should be performed in a low-visibility area with the same skin type as the area intended for treatment. If possible, at least 3 days should be allowed before the site is reexamined to assess for efficacy and for a reaction. If sufficient energy is delivered and absorbed, a generalized hyperemia reaction with mild focal swelling is visible after 3–5 min. The fluence should be increased for the particular skin type, and the patient's pain reaction should be noted until the hyperemia reaction is observed. For light or thin hair, the reaction may be minimal even at high settings. The laser setting for each type of treated area should be noted.

Patients have described the sensation from laser hair removal as discomfort rather than pain. After the laser hair removal treatment, patients can expect the treated area to be red and feel similar to a sunburn. For some patients, a topical anesthetic may be used prior to treatment, although it should be mentioned that some research has shown that topical anesthetics may decrease the effectiveness of treatment by decreasing blood flow to the follicles [3].

The number of treatments required depends upon the patient's skin color and coarseness of the hair. At minimum, two or three treatments are required as the process is only effective on hair during the hair growth cycle. Repeat sessions will be necessary to treat these follicles as they reenter the anagen phase. Most laser practitioners report treatments at 4–8-week intervals or at the first signs of hairs regrowth [6].

25.2.2
Posttreatment Recommendations

1. After the treatment, the patient may have redness or bumps in the treatment area. Cold compresses will alleviate this.

2. The skin should be kept moisturized. It is not be uncommon for the treated skin to be slightly drier after treatment and to require more moisturizer.

3. The sun and tanning salon should be avoided. Tanning creams should not be used between treatments.

4. Sunblock of SPF 25 or higher should be used.

5. The only other acceptable hair-removal method during the treatment series is shaving, if needed.

6. Tweezing, plucking, threading, waxing, and sugaring should be avoided because they can reduce the effectiveness of subsequent treatments.

7. Hair shafts will be released from hair follicles in the treated area for 1–2 weeks after the treatment. Gentle exfoliation or shaving the areas is fine.

8. Blistering or scaling after laser hair removal is uncommon, but usually resolves over a few days with Polysporin cream or hydrocortisone several times a day.

9. Makeup may be used if needed [7].

25.3
Complications

Most complications of laser hair removal are generally temporary. Special considerations are important when lasers are used on darker skin tones to allow for safe and effective therapy.

Hyperpigmentation and hypopigmentation are the most common side effects, occurring in 10–20% of treated individuals, and usually resolves within 6 months without any intervention. Mild edema lasting for 12–36 h is common after treatment. Bland emollients and medium-strength topical corticosteroid lotions can be applied in this setting. Blistering is usually superficial and resolves without scarring. The following complications are also possible: pruritis, pain, tingling, or a feeling of numbness, crusting or scab formation on ingrown hairs, bruising, redness, swelling, infection, and temporary hyperpigmentation or hypopigmentation. Scarring may also occur, but this is usually only a consequence when the patient is treated with improper fluences and inappropriate skin cooling [8].

Caution is advised when treating around the eye as ocular injury can occur even when light is delivered through the intact eyelid and sclera combined. Even the insertion of laser-protective eye shields over the cornea does not provide complete safety because they cover only the anterior surface of the globe. IPL sources do not carry this risk because of the biologic nature this technology.

Laser hair removal has not been studied long enough to permit a full assessment of its long-term health effects. However, short-term data indicate that laser hair removal is a safe procedure when the appropriate precautions are taken.

25.4
Discussion

One of the greatest advantages of laser hair removal is speed of treatment in conjunction with long-lasting results. For example, treating the back with laser hair removal only takes about 1 h, while treating a full back with electrolysis usually takes 125 h. Another advantage of laser hair removal is that for hairs that do grow back they are typically finer in texture.

Photoepilation, when properly used, offers clear ad-

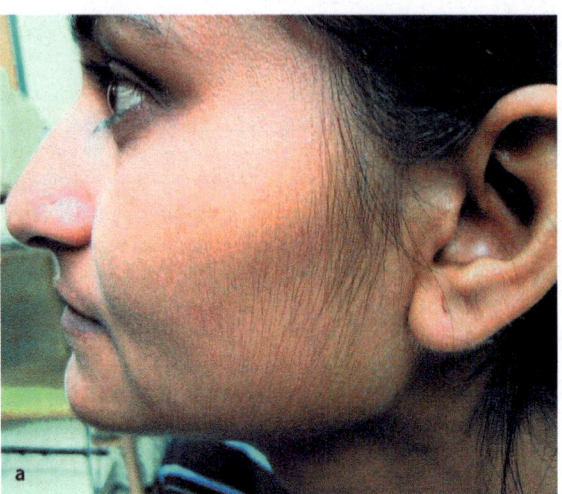 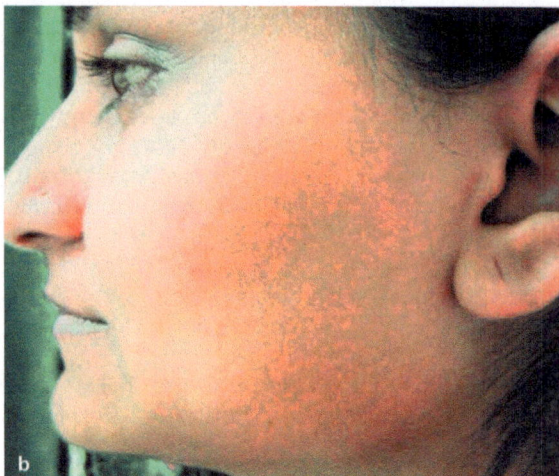

Fig. 25.1 **a** A 28-year-old Indian woman before treatment. **b** After six treatments with a Nd:YAG laser

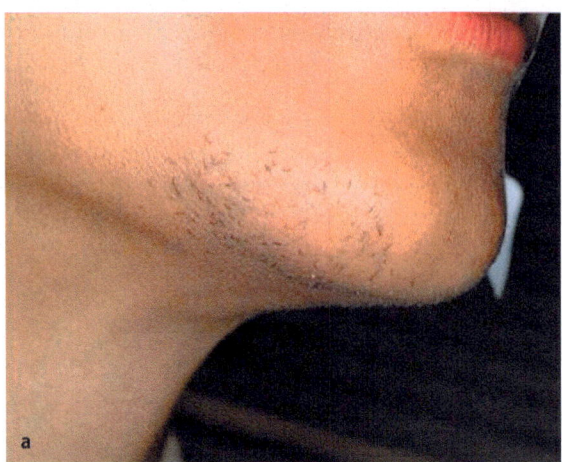 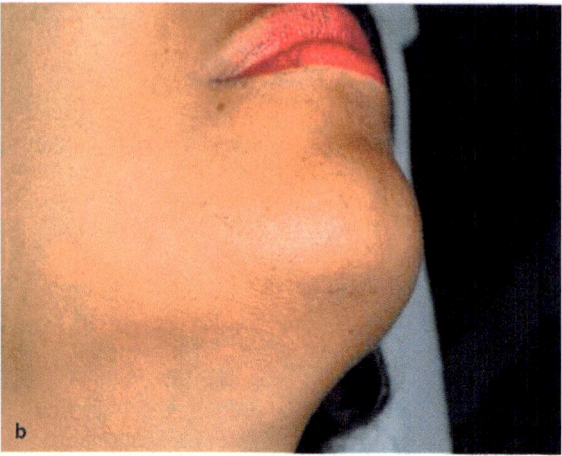

Fig. 25.2 **a** A 33-year-old Mediterranean woman before treatment. **b** After six treatments with a Nd:YAG laser

vantages when compared with older, traditional techniques. Although an ever-increasing number of published studies have confirmed the safety and short- and long-term efficacy of laser hair removal, the technology still has limits and risks.

While permanent hair removal is the goal of therapy, some patients may experience hair regrowth that is usually finer and lighter in color. In addition, long-lasting laser hair removal typically requires multiple treatments, which can make it more costly. Possible adverse side effects, though uncommon, include damage to the surrounding healthy tissue in the form of scars, burns, redness, pigment changes, and swelling. Most complications are generally temporary. Special considerations are important when lasers are used on darker skin tones to allow for safe and effective therapy.

25.5
Conclusions

The evolution of new technologies has improved the clinical efficacy of laser hair removal (Figs. 25.1, 25.2) and increased understanding of hair biology. With the recent FDA approval of lasers for tanned and darker skin types, long-term hair removal is now a realistic goal in the majority of individuals. Newer radiofrequency technologies might address the difficult issue of white and light blond hair phenotypes; however, their exact role

in the laser hair removal armamentarium remains to be further determined. Until then, current laser treatments provide gratifying and effective results.

References

1. Anderson RR, Parrish JA: Selective photothermolysis: precise microsurgery by selective absorption of pulsed radiation. Science 1983;220(4596):524–527

2. Goldberg DJ, Silapunt S: Histologic evaluation of a millisecond Nd:YAG laser for hair removal. Lasers Surg Med 2001;28(2):159–161

3. Sadick NS: Laser hair removal. Facial Plast Surg Clin North Am 2004;12(2):191–200

4. Fitzpatrick TB: The validity and practicality of sun-reactive skin types I through VI. Arch Dermatol 1988;124:869–871

5. Dierickx C, Alora MB, Dover JS: A clinical overview of hair removal using lasers and light sources. Dermatol Clin 1999;17(2):357–366

6. Wanner M: Laser hair removal. Dermatol Ther 2005;18(3):209–216

7. Dierickx CC: Hair removal by lasers and intense pulsed light sources. Dermatol Clin 2002;20(1):135–146

8. Nanni CA, Alster TS: Laser-assisted hair removal: side effects of Q-switched Nd:YAG, long-pulsed ruby, and alexandrite lasers. J Am Acad Dermatol 1999;41:165–171

CHAPTER 26

Mesotherapy for Facial Rejuvenation

26

Oh Sook Kwon

26.1
Introduction

There are many ways to treat skin aging. No matter what type of aging, the truth of skin aging is the combination of intrinsic skin aging and photoaging. The signs of aging are wrinkles (fine wrinkles, furrows), reduction of skin elasticity, pigmentation, dryness, and so on.

The formation of fine wrinkles is caused by transformation of epidermis and dermis, especially papillary dermis, and also this phenomenon is fairly relevant to the reduction, transformation, and dryness of elastic fiber and collagen fiber. Furrows have many causes, such as expression muscles, gravity, and sunlight. Particularly, expression muscles take part in the formation of furrows. During this process, the amount of elastic fiber decreases and transforms so that the formation of furrows is accelerated. Skin elasticity reduces because of the reduction of skin thickness, tension elasticity, and subcutaneous fat thickness. Skin elasticity reduces because of gravity.

Another sign of aging is pigmentation. Freckles, lentigines, irregular pigmentations, and dark spots are important signs of aging. Also, dryness, rough skin, and itchiness can be major signs of aging. These aging signs can be treated by laser resurfacing, chemical peeling, laser rejuvenation, microdermabrasion, and mesotherapy.

The author prefers mesotherapy for treating skin aging. There are many different kinds of mesotherapy techniques, for example, symptomatic technique, intradermal technique, and regional technique. To maximize the result, four units must be considered: (1) microcirculation unit, (2) autonomic nerve and sensory nerve unit, (3) immunologic unit, and (4) nutritional unit.

The basic concept of mesotherapy is needle therapy and other means of drug delivery. In needle therapy, the needles make small pores in the epidermis and dermal layers. Bleeding is intended by the needle stimulation, this causes growth factors (such as transforming growth factor, platelet-derived growth factor, connective tissue activating peptide, connective tissue growth factor, insulin-like growth factor, and fibroblast growth factor) for regeneration of skin to accumulate around the wounded area. Epidermal rejuvenation factors as well as dermal regeneration factors are gathered rapidly by thousands of cytokines to recover injured tissues.

Drug delivery is the main intent in mesotherapy. Drugs can be applied according to a variety of indications, such as hyperpigmentation, wrinkle, and scar. This makes it possible to treat skin elasticity, skin tone, roughness, and dryness. To treat skin aging, holistic care of pigmentation, wrinkles, and elasticity must be considered. Face rejuvenation should be approached by the combination of dermal substances such as hyaluronic acid, cytokine, which is a growth factor, vitamins, minerals, amino acids, DNA and RNA, antioxidants, etc.

26.2
Instrument

With the DermaRoller (Fig. 26.1) nearly 200 stainless steel micropoints are painlessly driven into the skin and dermis (Fig. 26.2).

26.3
Clinical Uses

The DermaRoller was developed for the less invasive collagen-induction-therapy (CIT). This device is designed to induce the body's own production of collagen. Its needles have a length of 1.5 mm and according to the applied pressure they penetrate the skin from 0.1 to 1.3 mm. The needles induce the production of collagen (CIT) in deeper skin layers to strengthen the connective tissue and to minimize the typical "orange-peel skin appearance." The device is equipped with 192 stainless steel needles in eight rows. The needle diameter is 0.25 mm and the penetration of the skin is 0.5 mm in depth. This model has a width of 20 mm and can be used on the face, neck, and body.

26.4
Techniques

The pretreatment procedure is necessary to maximize the treatment result. This includes steaming and scaling. Steaming is the step that removes keratin and moisturizer and scaling is the process of removing the corneum layer to clean pores and to make drug delivery better.

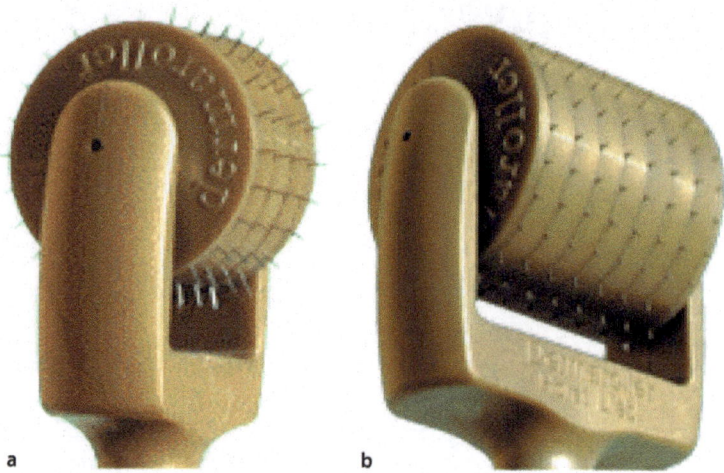

Fig. 26.1 DermaRoller

a   b

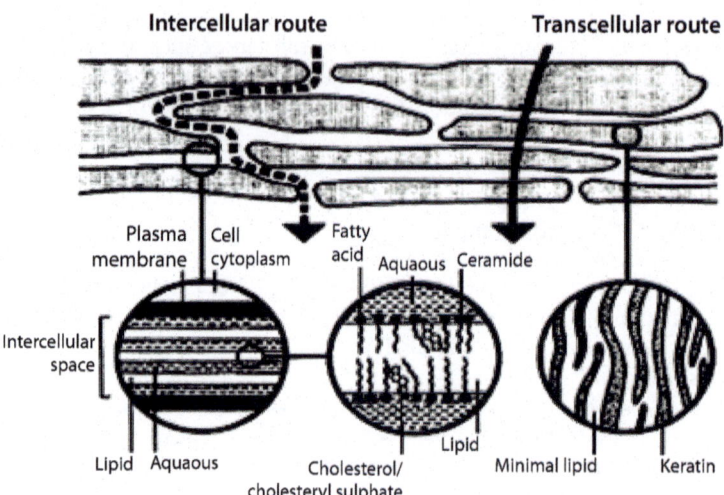

Fig. 26.2 The molecular size is smaller than the intercellular size in order to reach the target layer of skin. On the other hand, no matter how big the molecular size is, drugs can be delivered through the channels made by needles. This is the advantage of mesotherapy. The skin can be improved with the correct drug for the skin type

The patient is given intravenous injection of 0.3 ml ketamine (0.005 ml/kg).

Mesorolling is then performed. There should be careful selection of the roller because the key to this treatment depends on the length of the needle. The needles should reach the dermal layer so bleeding can occur. That is why the length of the roller should be 1.5 mm.

The drug mixture should be prepared in a 10-ml syringe for the mesogun technique. The combination of drugs is:

1. 2.5 ml of 25 mg/2.5ml hyaluronic acid (sodium hyaluronate)
2. 2 ml of 250 mg/5 ml tranexamic acid
3. 2 ml of 50 mg/5 ml buflomedil
4. One vial (100 mg) of Tathion
5. 2 ml placenta extract

Injections are made at 1-cm intervals on the skin. The injection should be more intense around the eyes where there are more wrinkle lines (perioral, nasolabial). The injection depth should be controlled so that the injection is in the upper dermal layer. Vessels should be avoided to reduce bruising.

The second procedure is with the mesoroller technique. The roller should be selected very carefully. To cause proper bleeding so that collagen formation is induced, the needle should pierce the correct layer. A 1.5-mm or longer needle is the best. The drug mixture should be applied with rolling. The contents of the drug mixture are:

1. One vial (100 mg) of DNA and RNA diluted with 1 ml normal saline
2. 10,000 IU (2 ml) vitamin A
3. 2 ml collagen peptide
4. 2 ml ascorbic acid

The technique involves starlike movements, back and forth, pierce-and-go technique. Caution must be taken with rolling, so as not to roll on the same area too many times. The roll should be even over all the area using many different directions. It is better to roll around the

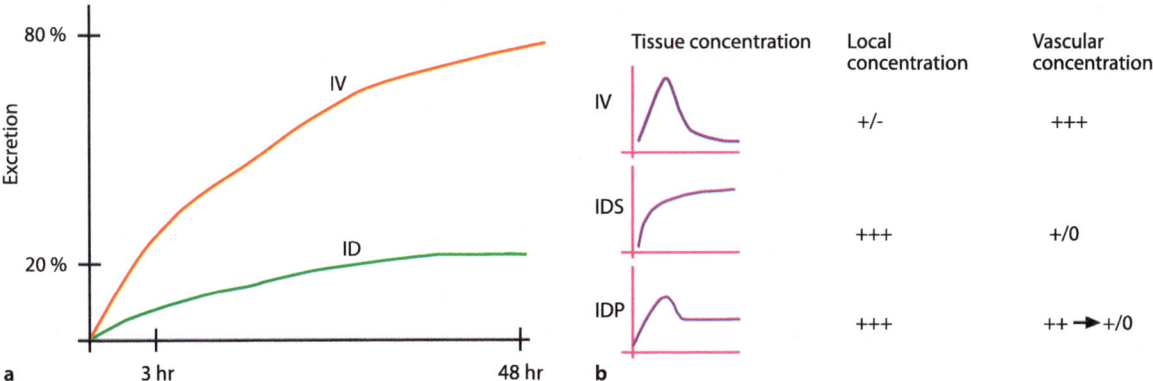

Fig. 26.3 a Intradermal (*ID*) and intravenous (*IV*). After 48 h 80% of intravenously injected drugs are excreted. The drugs are not kept in the body for a long time. On the other hand, when injected intradermally, only 20% of the drugs are excreted. The rest (80%) remain inside the skin, and the effect is maintained. **b** Intravenous, intradermal superficial (*IDS*), and intradermal profound (*IDP*). When the injection is intravenously, the concentration of the drugs in the tissue goes rapidly up and down. This is why the local concentration of the drug cannot be maintained for a long time. On the other hand, for intradermal superficial injection, the drug does not take a long time to get to the specific point and the peak concentration is maintained for a long time. For intradermal profound injection, the concentration of the drugs in the tissue goes up to its peak value rapidly, then it goes down a little bit and stays at the same level. As shown in the graph, intradermal superficial injection is most effective with regard to the concentration of the drugs in the tissue

eye area, nasolabial fold, and forehead where there are a lot of wrinkle lines but rolling should not be repeated on the same spot. After rolling, the blood on the face should be removed with normal saline and then the drug mixture should be applied quickly with a clean brush so that the drug mixture can be delivered through the pores. The drug should be allowed to penetrate enough (Fig. 26.3). The patient may experience edema and heat on the face, but this is normal. Hydrocortisone cream (0.5%) can be helpful for the discomfort. Cooling should follow immediately to suppress the discomfort. An ice-cold gauze can be used for 10 min. After that, strong moisturizer containing ceramide should be applied. The patient does not need to take an analgesic or antibiotic but will need to apply 0.5% hydrocortisone cream with moisturizer for 3 days.

26.5
Possible Complications

Possible complications are:
1. From the needle itself and too much stimulus
   (a) Needle tattoo
   (b) Postinflammatory hyperpigmentation by too much stimulus
   (c) Facial flush
   (d) Facial edema
   (e) Facial heating
   (f) Dryness
   (g) Too much scaling
   (h) Pain
   (i) Bleeding

2. From anesthesia
   (a) Dizziness
   (b) Hallucination (visual), including nightmare
   (c) Drug side effect
3. From the drug mixture
   (a) Drug allergy

26.6
Conclusions

After wounding, the correlation between cellular components, extracellular components, and cytokine is very important for recovery. This concept can be applied to cosmetics as well as the wound healing process. By the stimulation from "needling," growth factors gather around the wounded area and secrete cytokine, which correlate with the ability of cellular and extracellular structures to restore collagen, new vessels, the dermal layer, and the epidermal layer. Through this process aging can be treated. Mesorolling therapy gives the needling stimulation intended for treatment spontaneously and not artificially. The tiny holes close in 5–6 h and the drug can be delivered effectively and easily to the targeted layer of the skin. The limitation of transdermal delivery and patch is that if the molecular size is bigger than the intercellular space, the molecules will not be able to reach the targeted skin layer. But with needling treatment, the drugs can be delivered to the targeted layer of skin directly through hundreds of tiny holes. If the correct drugs that improve skin problems and conditions are used on the correct place that needs to be treated, the result should be very satisfactory. After 1 month, about 70% of collagen regeneration can be found and collagen regeneration reaches its peak in 2 months after needling (Fig. 26.4). Treatment can be repeated at 1–2 months. There is improvement in patients using mesotherapy with the DermaRoller in the treatment of acne scar, wrinkle, pigmentation, elasticity, rough skin tone, and dried and keratinous skin (Figs. 26.5–26.7).

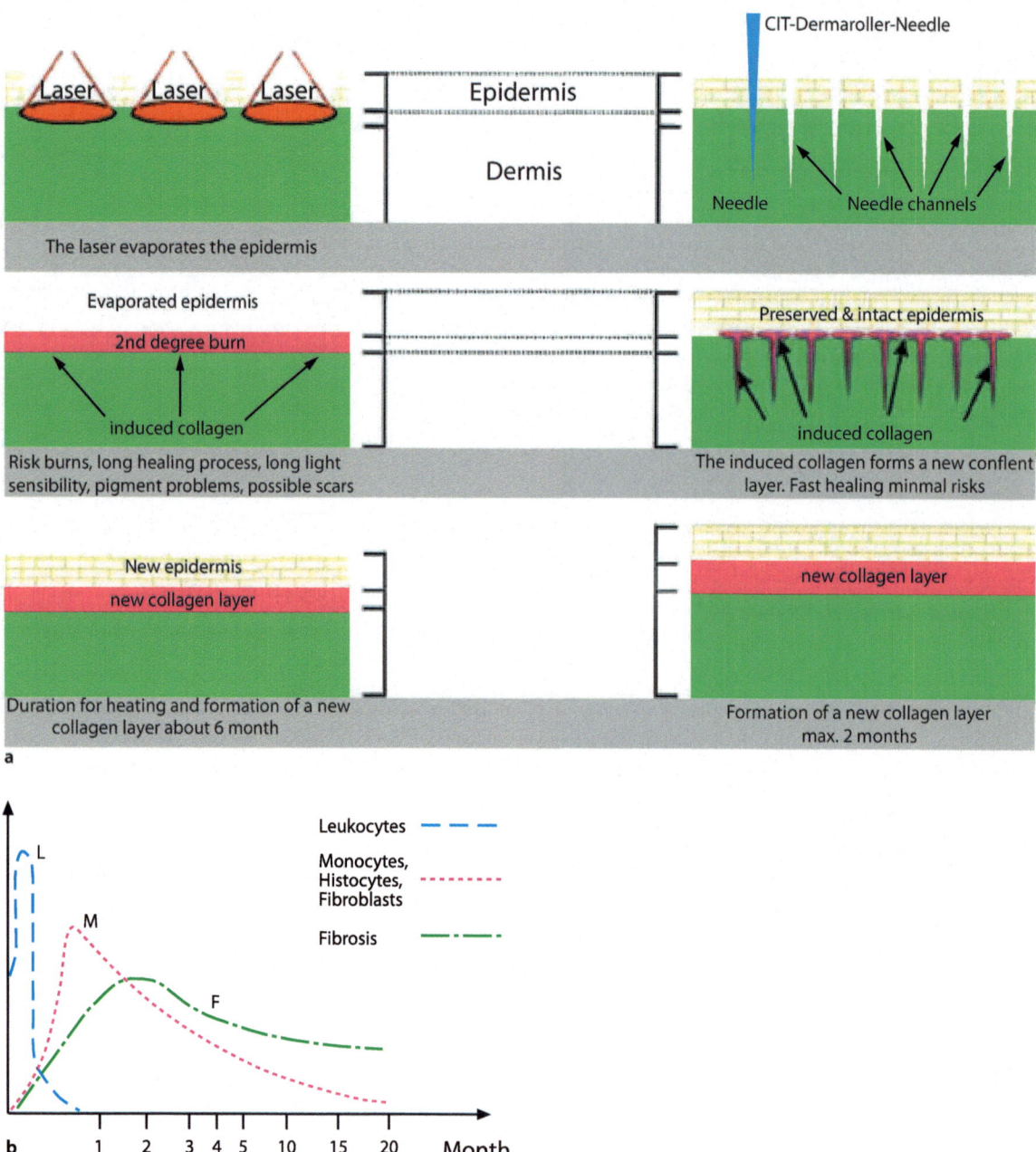

Fig. 26.4 a Skin rejuvenation by laser treatment has possible side effects, such as burning, long healing process, long light sensitivity, pigment problem, and scar, because there is the possibility of damaging the epidermal layer. On the other hand, needle rejuvenation does not damage the epidermis much because it does not have side effects such as those from laser treatment and the pores are closed within hours. Between those stimulated pores, because collagen is restored, tissues are elastic and harden, so wrinkles are treated and also the pores become smaller. This treatment does not have side effects like burning, pigmentation, and scar. The collagen restoration time is much shorter than with laser treatment. It only takes 2 months to reach its peak, but with laser treatment requires about 6 months. **b** Collagen restoration after needle treatment. After needle stimulation, leukocytes gather in the wounded area first of all, and then monocytes are found. After 2 months fibrosis reaches its peak. *c see next page*

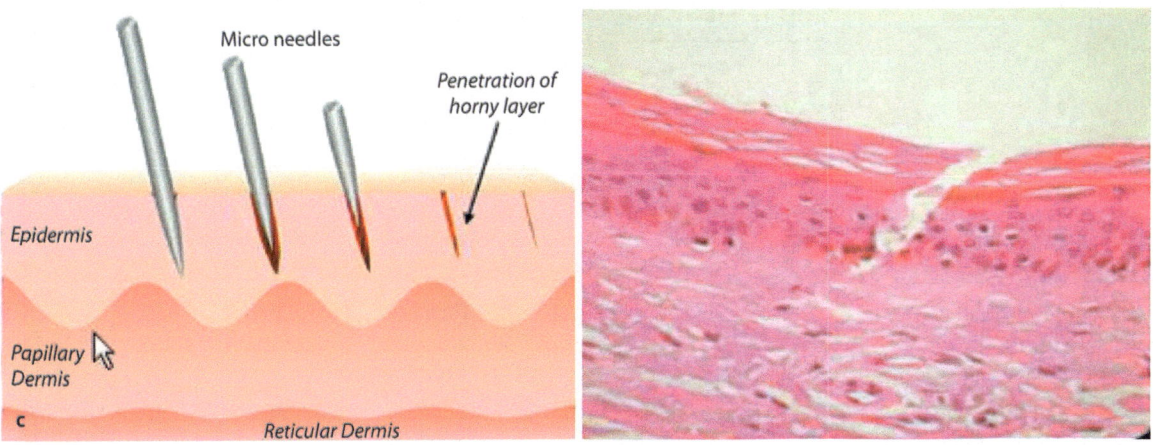

Fig. 26.4 *(Continued)* **c** This is what happens when needles stimulate the skin. Needles do not pierce the dermal layer but only the epidermis. Notice the open channels on the epidermis. The open pores close within hours and drugs are delivered though them

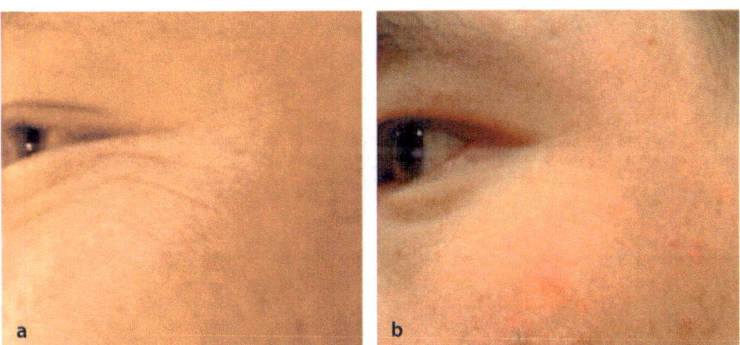

Fig. 26.5 Wrinkles. **a** Before treatment. **b** After treatment

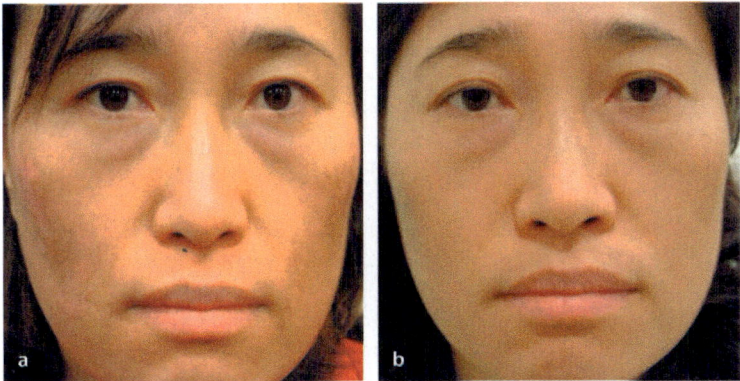

Fig. 26.6 Pigmentation. **a** Before treatment. **b** After treatment

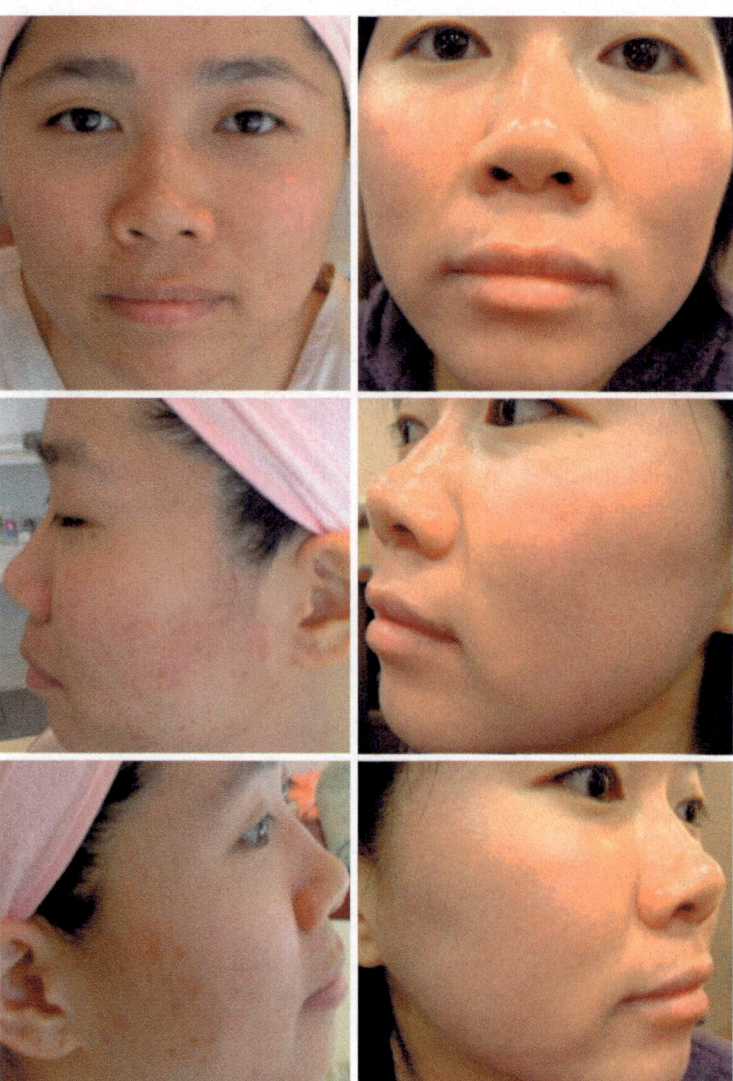

Fig. 26.7 Acne and acne scars. Before and after treatment

Suggested Reading

1. Ahn SK, Hwang SM, Jiang SJ, Choi EH, Lee SH: The changes of epidermal calcium gradient and transitional cells after prolonged occlusion following tape stripping in the murine epidermis. J Invest Dermatol 1999;113(2):189–195
2. Ahn SK, Jiang SJ, Hwang SM, Choi EH, Lee JS, Lee SH: Functional and structural changes of the epidermal barrier induced by various types of insults in hairless mice. Arch Dermatol Res 2001;293(6):308–318
3. Choi EH, Kim MJ, Ahn SK, Park WS, Son ED, Nam GW, Chang I, Lee SH: The skin barrier state of aged hairless mice in a dry environment. Br J Dermatol 2002;147(2):244–249
4. Choi EH, Kim MJ, Yeh BI, Ahn SK, Lee SH: Iontophoresis and sonophoresis stimulate epidermal cytokine expression at energies that do not provoke a barrier abnormality: lamellar body secretion and cytokine expression are linked to altered epidermal calcium levels. J Invest Dermatol 2003;121(5):1138–1144
5. Elias PM, Ahn SK, Denda M, Brown BE, Crumrien D, Kimutai LK, Komuves L, Lee SH, Feingold KR: Modulations in epidermal calcium regulate the expression of differentiation-specific markers. J Invest Dermatol 2002;119(5):1128–1136
6. Jiang SJ, Hwang SM, Choi EH, Elias PM, Ahn SK, Lee SH: Structural and functional effects of oleic acid and iontophoresis on hairless mouse stratum corneum. J Invest Dermatol 2000;114(1):64–70
7. Kalia YN, Nonato LB, Lund CH, Guy RH: Development of skin barrier function in premature infants. J Invest Dermatol 1998;111:320–326
8. Parienti IJ: Mésothérapie. 2nd Ed. Masson, Paris 1995
9. Pistor M: Mésothérapie Pratique. Masson, Paris 1998
10. Le Coz J: Traité de Mésothérapie. Masson, Paris 2004

Part IV
Facial Fillers and Implants

CHAPTER 27

Fat Transfer to the Face

Melvin A. Shiffman, Mitchell V. Kaminski

27.1
Introduction

The minimally invasive technique using autologous fat transplantation has become a standard procedure in facial rejuvenation. It is simple, inexpensive, permanent, and effective.

Injectable fillers, such as collagen and hyaluronic acid, are only temporary and, therefore, have minimal indication. Goretex, which is a permanent material, may extrude or be palpable. Since 1994, when Adatasil (silicone) was approved by the Federal Drug Administration for use in ophthalmic problems, the use of silicone injected into other areas of the body has been called an "off-label use" and is considered legal if it is used for a specific patient with a specific product and there is no advertising.

Autologous fat can be used to augment facial structures, rejuvenate rhytids, or fill depressed scars or defects of the face. Since the introduction of liposuction in 1975 [1] for body contouring, there has been an easy way to obtain fat for transplantation through very small incisions. The use of the tumescent technique for retrieving large amounts of fat for transfer has reduced the amount of blood loss and made the technique safer [2]. Although some reports have shown that fat transfer had disappointing results in some cases, the success of fat transfer is operator-dependent and can be quite successful if attention is paid to the details of the techniques of the procedure. The transfer of fat to the face, where vascularity is excellent, has an excellent chance for fat survival.

The only relative drawback has been the resorption of some of the fat graft. With proper technique, approximately 30–70% of the fat is retained. Low-speed, short-time centrifugation of the fat decreases the fluid in the transplant and reduces the apparent loss of graft by compacting the fat and separating out the excess liquid. Since some of the apparent graft loss is the resorption of fluid from the transplanted fat, there is less fluid in centrifuged fat and, therefore, more mass is retained.

A newer concept to facilitate graft retention is the use of albumin during the harvesting and transfer phases. Albumin reduces the colloid osmotic pressure disparity between the low colloid osmotic pressure of the fat graft with saline, epinephrine, lidocaine, and sodium bicarbonate and the interior of the fat cells. The higher the difference in colloid osmotic pressure between the cells and the surrounding fluids, the more fluid that will enter the cells and the more the likelihood of cell destruction. If the colloid osmotic pressure between the fat cells and that of the surrounding fluid with albumin are almost equal, the more likely there will be improved fat survival and retention.

27.2
History of Fat Transfer

Since Neuber [3], in 1893, reported that transplanted fat can be used to fill in a depressed area of the face, there have been many reports [4–14] that have shown fat, in pieces, can be transplanted and survive in various areas of the body. Since liposuction was conceived by Fischer and Fischer [15] in 1974 and put into practice in 1975 [1], the aspirate has been used to fill defects and for contouring [16–22]. Aspirated fat should be atraumatically washed in physiologic solution to remove blood, which would allow better fat survival [23].

Certain principles of fat transfer have evolved [24–69] over the years, which include aspiration at lower vacuum rather than at atmospheric pressure (Fig. 27.1). It is essential to avoid desiccation of the fat during transfer. Fat that is present for over 60 days after transfer will survive and grow, and fat grafts survive when there is vascular ingrowth. The survival of free fat used as an autograft is operator-dependent and requires delicate handling of the graft tissue, careful washing of the fat to minimize extraneous blood cells, and installation into a site with adequate vascularity. There is evidence that fat cells will survive and that filling of defects is not from the residual collagen following cell destruction. There is some loss of fat after transplantation and most surgeons will overfill the recipient site.

27.2.1
Insulin

Some physicians have added insulin to the fat in preparation for transplantation [19, 70, 71]. The theory is that insulin inhibits lipolysis. Sidman [72] found that

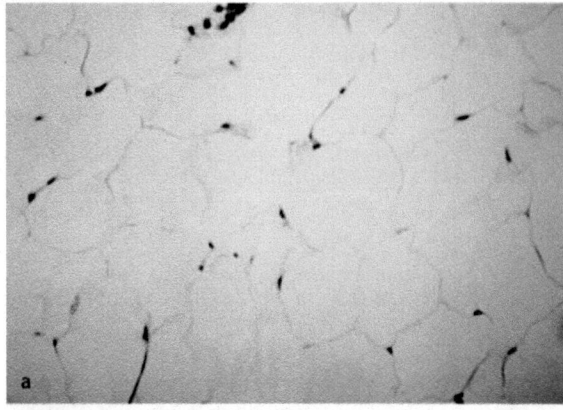

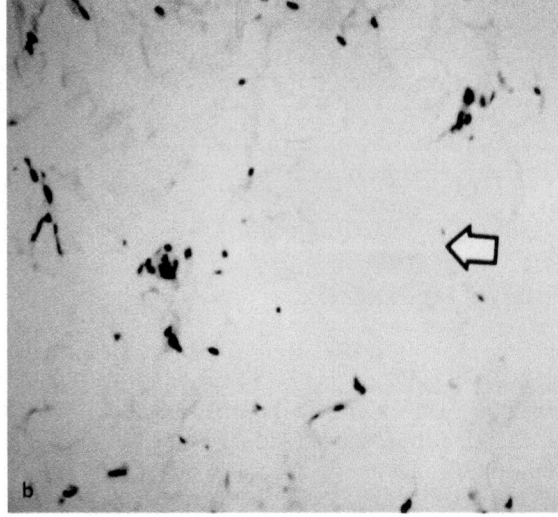

Fig. 27.1 Hematoxylin and eosin stain × 200. **a** Central core of fat with 95–100% intact fat cells that was harvested with a 3-mm cannula at –500-mmHg vacuum. **b** Periphery of core with more than 10% fat cell disruption (arrow) when harvested with a 3-mm cannula at –700-mmHg vacuum

insulin decreases lipolysis. Hiragun et al. [73] stated that theoretically insulin may induce fibroblasts to pick up the lipid lost and become adipocytes. Chajchir et al. [74] found that the use of insulin did not show any positive effect on adipocyte survival during transplantation compared with fat not prepared with insulin.

27.2.2
Centrifugation

Some physicians centrifuge the adipose tissue to remove blood products and free lipids to improve the quality of the fat to be injected [70–72]. Asken [42] stated that his "method of reducing the material to be injected to practically pure fat is to place the fat-filled syringe with a rubber cap (the plunger having been previously removed and kept in a sterile environment) into a centrifuge. The syringe is then spun for a few seconds at

the desired rpm and the serum, blood, and liquefied fat collects in the dependent part of the syringe...." Toledo [75] reported that "for facial injection we spin the full syringes for 1 minute...in a manual centrifuge (about 2000 rpm), eject the unwanted solution, and transfer the fat..."

Chajchir et al. [73] centrifuged 1 ml of bladder fat pad from mice (both at 1,000 rpm for 5 min and at 5,000 rpm for 5 min) and injected this into the subdermis of the malar area. Microscopically, after 1–2 months there were macrophages filled with lipid droplets, giant cells, focal necrosis of adipocytes, and cystlike cavities of irregular size and shapes. After 12 months following injection, no recognized adipocytes could be found. Total cellular damage was present in both groups.

Brandow and Newman [76] found that centrifugation of harvested fat did not after the microscopic structured integrity of cells. Spun and unspun samples were examined and were found to be similar. Fulton et al. [69] noted that centrifuged fat, 3 min at 3,400 rpm, works well for small-volume transfers, but not for large-volume transfers into breasts, biceps, or buttocks. Centrifugation at low speeds for a short time will compact the fat cells and not destroy them (Fig. 27.2).

27.2.3
Ratchet Gun for Injection

Newman and Levin [23] designed a lipo-injector with a gear-driven plunger to inject fat tissue evenly into desired sites. Fat injected with excessive pressure in the

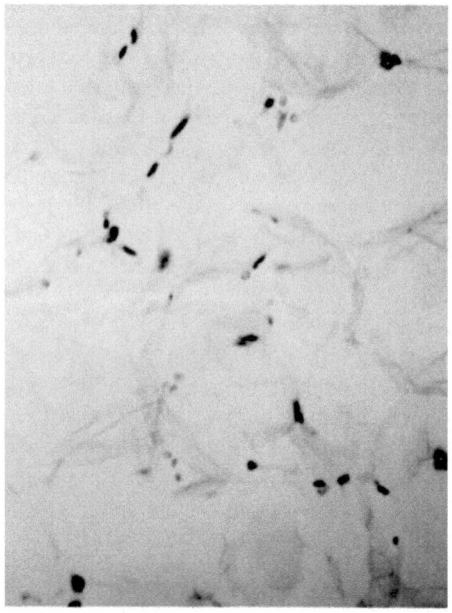

Fig. 27.2 Hematoxylin and eosin stain × 200. Centrifugation at 3,600 rpm for 1 min showing cell compaction

barrel of a syringe can cause sudden injections of un-desired quantities of fat, which will pour into recipient sites. Agris [45] stated that a ratchet-type gun allows controlled, accurate deposition of autologous fat. Each time the trigger is pulled, 0.1 ml is deposited. Asaadi and Haramis [56] described the use of a gun with a dis-posable 10-ml syringe for fat injection. Niechajev and Sevcuk [61] utilized a special pistol and a blunt-type cannula, with 2.3-mm internal diameter, to inject the fat.

Berdeguer [77] used a lipo transplant gun to inject fat into areas to be enhanced. Fulton et al. [69] stated that it is beneficial for a beginning surgeon to use a ratcheted pistol for injection as this gives a more uni-form injection volume.

27.3
Albumin in Improving Fat Cell Survival

27.3.1
Oncotic Pressure

When a molecule with molecular mass greater than 10,000 Da (the dalton is an arbitrary unit of mass equal to the mass of the nuclide of carbon-12, or 1.657×10^{-24} g), it is called a colloid and is capable of generating an oncotic pressure if it is restricted to one side of a semi-permeable membrane. Colloid restricted to one side of a semipermeable membrane creates an osmotic gradient measured in millimeters of mercury. Very small mole-cules and ions such as sodium, potassium, glucose, and urea easily cross a capillary membrane and can increase osmolarity toward isotonicity to prevent red blood cells from taking up water and bursting. Osmolarity is mea-sured by freezing-point depression and the greater the number of particles in solution, the colder the solution must be before it will freeze.

27.3.2
Colloid Osmotic Pressure

In determining the colloid osmotic pressure, the Lan-dis–Pappenheimer equation [78] takes into account that soluble proteins, whether albumin, globulin, or fi-brinogen, are highly negatively charged:

$$COP = 2.1TP + 0.16TP^2 + 0.009TP^3,$$

where COP is the colloid osmotic pressure and TP is the total amount of protein.

Positively charged sodium ions surrounding the core protein attract and hold water; thus, more fluid is accu-mulated on one side of the semipermeable membrane. The combination of the oncotic pressure of the protein and the osmotic pressure of the sodium ions resulting in an increased pressure gradient is called the colloid osmotic pressure.

Albumin has a molecular mass of 69,000 Da,

whereas globulin and fibrinogen have molecular masses of 150,000 and 400,000 Da, respectively. Since it is the number of molecules that are held on one side of the semipermeable membrane that creates colloid osmotic pressure, albumin will create the most pressure because 1 g of albumin has twice as many molecules as 1 g of globulin and 5 times the number of molecules as 1 g of fibrinogen. Starch molecules, found in hetastarch and dextran, should not be used for fat transfer since such molecules are too large to be evacuated through the lymphatics and will cause localized edema in the inter-stitial space.

27.3.3
Starling's Equation

Starling's equation [79, 80] represents the hydrostatic pressure pushing fluid through the capillary pore (P_c through δ) versus the colloid osmotic pressure forces holding fluid in circulation, and the rate of fluid flow across the gel–sol matrix (k_f is inversely proportional to π_i) and back into circulation via lymphatic channels (Qlymph). When all of these factors are combined, the entire equation is written as

$$Jv = k_f[(P_c - P_i) - \delta(\pi c - \pi_i)] - Q_{lymph},$$

where Jv is the interstitial fluid flow, k_f is the filtra-tion coefficient, P_c is the central venous pressure and P_c through δ is the hydrostatic pressure pushing fluid through a capillary pore, P_i is the interstitial space pres-sure, π_c is the total amount of protein in circulation, π_i is the amount of interstitial protein, and Q_{lymph} is the rate of lymph flow.

The pressure in the capillary minus the opposing pressure in the interstitial space is known as the hy-drostatic pressure. Central venous pressure (P_c) is the pressure pushing fluid across the endothelial mem-brane through the body. The total protein in circulation creates colloid osmotic pressure (π_c). At any given time at any given pore in the vascular endothelium, there is more protein concentrated in circulation than there is at that site in the interstitial space. The colloid osmotic pressure creates a constant negative force holding the fluid in circulation and keeping interstitial fluid flow to a minimum, packing cells together, and preventing edema.

27.3.4
Avoiding Hypo-oncotic Trauma in Fat Transfer

When Klein's solution or any modification is used in harvesting fat, the infranatant of the harvested fat con-tains 1.1–1.2 g% protein. The normal level is 2.0–4.0 g%. When one ampule of concentrated human albumin (12.5 g in 50 ml) is added to 1 l of tumescent solution or 8.3 ml is added to a 60-ml harvesting syringe, the har-vested fat contains 2.6 g% protein. Three washes of harvested fat also increase the difference in colloid osmotic pressure and, therefore, it is necessary to add 18.75 g of albumin to each liter of washing solution. Adequate time must be allowed between each wash to allow the fat cells to pack above the infranatant layer. The process can be accelerated by centrifugation. The supranatant oil must be removed before insertion of the fat into the recipient site.

27.4
Indications for Fat Transfer

There are a variety of indications for fat transfer, which can be distilled down to the following:
1. Fill Defects
   (a) Congenital
   (b) Traumatic
   (c) Disease (acne)
   (d) Iatrogenic
2. Cosmetic
   (a) Furrows (rhytids, wrinkles)
   (b) Refill of lost supportive tissue (aging)
   (c) Enhancement

27.5
Preoperative Consultation

The patient is carefully examined in relation to the specific complaint for which the patient has come in for consultation. A description of the physical problem needs to be recorded with appropriate measurements. Photographs should be taken before any procedure is undertaken and postoperative photographs should be taken at an appropriate interval of time when healing is completed.

If other problems are detected by the physician, other than that of which the patient complains, these must be recorded and possible treatment explained to the patient so that steps may be taken to correct other deficits not previously identified by the patient or so that the patient understands that adequate correction may require other procedures. At the same time the patient must not be talked into procedures that are not really wanted by the patient. An interval of time may be needed for the patient to think about what surgery may be necessary and to seek other consultations.

The patient must understand the need for using autologous fat as a filler substance in comparison with other fillers presently available. To conform to the standard of care for informed consent, the patient must have sufficient information to be knowledgeable about the procedure, the possible material risks and complications, and the alternatives and their possible material risks. Someone in the office must take time to explain this information and the physician must at least make sure the patient understands the procedure, risks, and alternatives and answer any questions about the procedure. It is suggested that the physician include in the record the statement that "the surgical procedure was discussed as well as viable alternatives and all material risks and complications."

27.6
Technique

Fat survival depends upon the careful handling of fat during harvesting, cleansing, and injecting. Harvesting is performed by liposuction in areas of fat with alpha-2 receptors where the fat responds poorly to diet such as the abdominal or lateral thigh areas (genetic fat) [42]. The fat can be retrieved with liposuction using a 2.0–3.0-mm cannula or needle (14–16 gauge) with a syringe (10–50 ml).

The fat should be cleansed with a physiologic solution of normal saline or lactated Ringer's solution by gently mixing and decanting the infranatant liquid consisting of tumescent fluid, serum, and blood (Fig. 27.3). Fat can be concentrated with the use of centrifugation at 3,600 rpm for 2 min. This allows less need for as much overfilling (30–50%) as is usually used. Kaminski et al. [81] have proposed the addition of 12.5 g of concentrated human albumin for each 1,000 ml of Klein's solution used for harvesting and 18.5 g for each 1,000 ml washing fluid in order to maintain the normal extracellular oncotic pressure necessary to prevent the influx of solution into the cells with possible rupture. Alternatively,

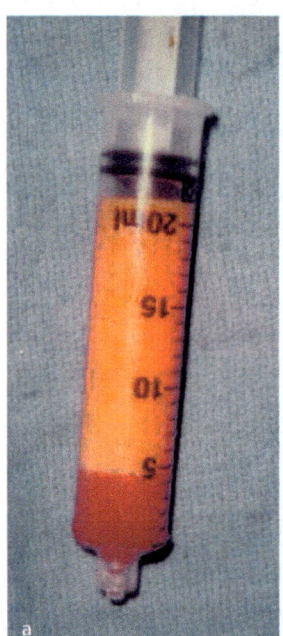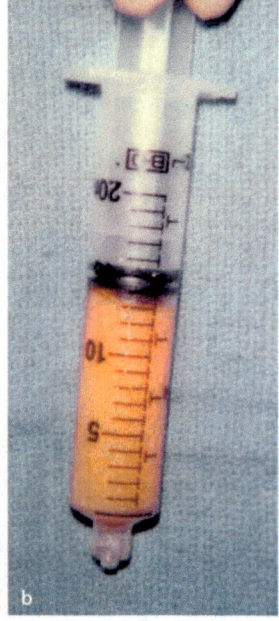

Fig. 27.3 a Fat retrieval with supranatant fat and infranatant fluid of blood and local tumescent fluid. **b** Fat following washing with sterile saline

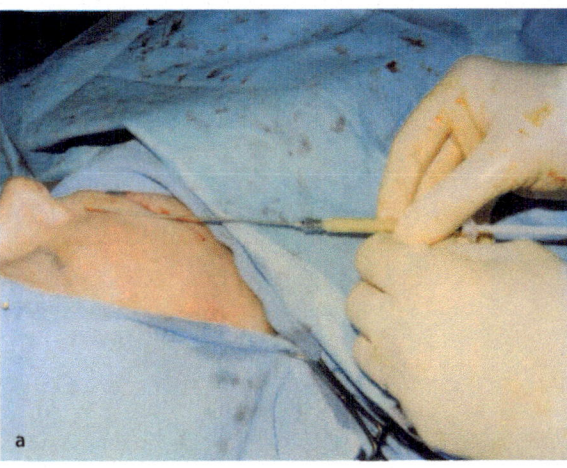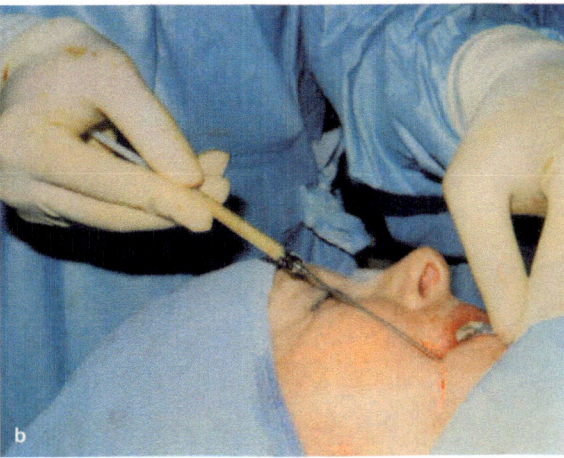

Fig. 27.4 a Fat transferred to 1-ml syringe with small cannula attached. **b** Injecting fat into face with palm of hand pressing on the plunger

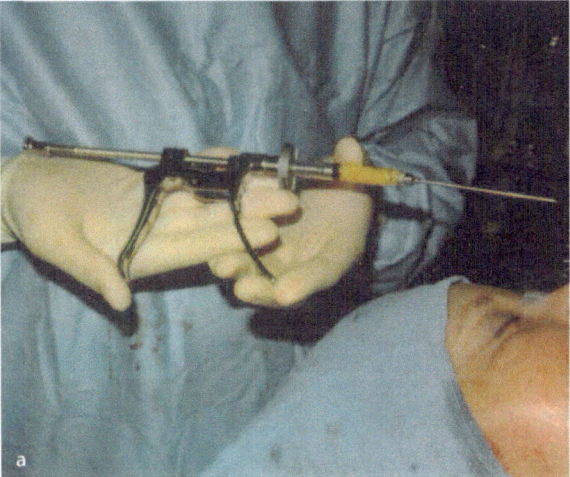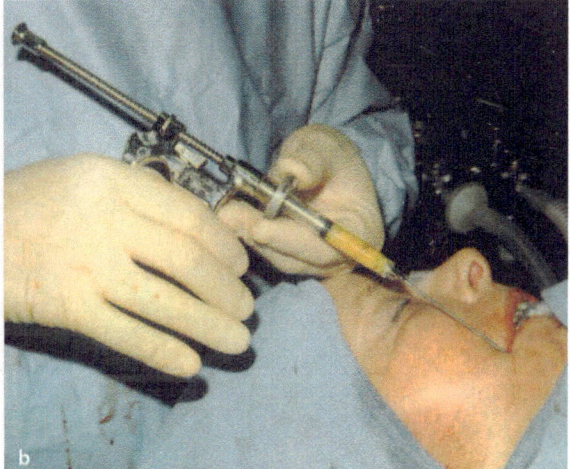

Fig. 27.5 a Ratchet gun with 1-ml syringe and cannula. **b** Fat being injected with a ratchet gun

8.3 ml of human serum albumin can be added to a 60-ml harvesting syringe.

Injection of the fat is with a needle (18 gauge) or cannula (1.5–2.0 mm) uniformly distributed into tunnels in multiple layers to fill the defect (Figs. 27.4, 27.5). With depressed scars, the attachments to the skin should be subcised before fat injection. The use of the ratchet gun for injection does not damage fat cells [82].

The areas of the face that can be enhanced include the cheeks (malar, submalar), lips, and chin (mentum) (Fig. 27.6). The brows may be lifted with fat transfer to the forehead and indentations can be improved in almost any area of the face. Rhytids in the glabella, nasolabial fold, and marionette lines can be improved. If the glabella is to be injected, the patient should be informed of the rare possibility of blindness. Any area of the face can have a depressed scar elevated by subcision and fat transfer.

27.7
Complications

There are very few serious complications of autologous fat transfer. Since it is the patient's own tissue, there is no rejection phenomenon or allergic reaction. The harvesting of large amounts of fat using liposuction is prone to the complications of liposuction in the donor area but facial fat transfer is usually with small amounts of fat. If small amounts of fat (under 50 ml) are retrieved, then one may expect the possibility of bruising or infection in the donor site.

The injection of autologous fat may be associated with the following risks:

1. Loss of fat volume (the most frequent problem)
2. Possible need for repeat injection(s) of fat
3. Bruising, hematoma
4. Swelling (especially with over injection)

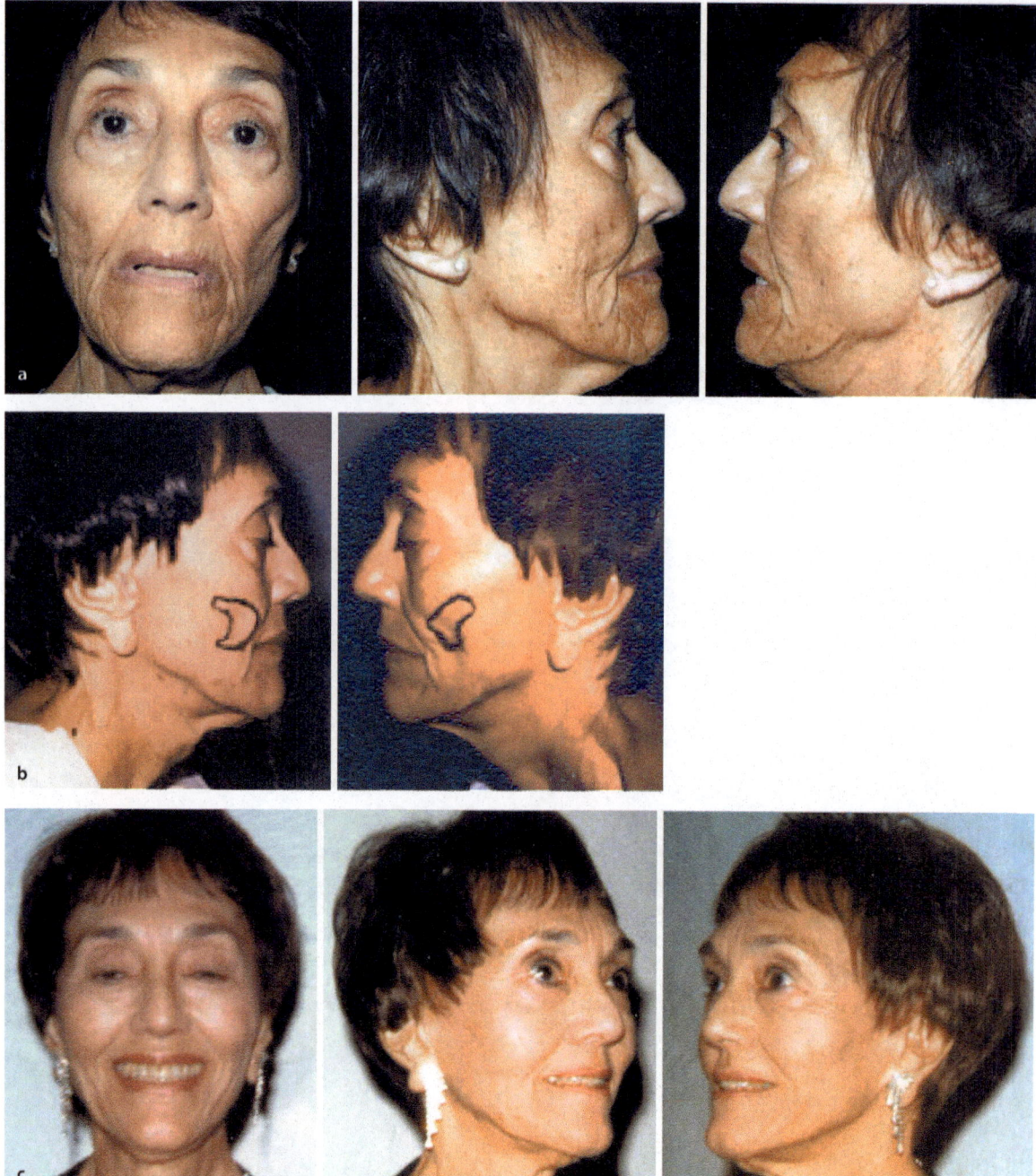

Fig. 27.6 A 60-year-old woman with atrophy of facial fat. **a** Preoperatively. **b** Fat transfer markings in submalar area. **c** Four years postoperatively

5. Asymmetry
6. Prolonged erythema (usually temporary over a short period of time)
7. Scar that is depressed or thickened (rare except in the area of liposuction)
8. Tenderness, pain
9. Fibrous capsule around fat accumulation (from too much fat injected into one area)
10. Fat cyst (mass)
11. Infection (rare)
12. Microcalcifications (has not been reported in the face)
13. Central nervous system damage or loss of sight from retinal artery occlusion (can occur with injection in the glabellar area)
14. All of the problems following liposuction if a large amount of fat is removed

27.8
Conclusions

Autologous fat transfer has been a very successful filler in the facial area. If care is taken in the transfer process and postoperatively, there will be 40–60% fat survival on the first transfer. At times a second or even a third fat transfer (using the patient's frozen fat) may be necessary to reach the volume best for the patient.

References

1. Fischer, G.: Surgical treatment of cellulitis. 3rd Congress International Academy of Cosmestic Surgery, Rome, Italy, 31 May 1975
2. Klein, J.A.: The tumescent technique for liposuction surgery. Amer J Cosmet Surg 1987;4:263–267
3. Neuber, F.: Fettransplantation. Chir Kongr Verhandl Dtsch Ges Chir 1893;22:66
4. Czerny, M.: Plastischer Ersatz der brusterlruse durch ein lipom Verh Dtsch Ges Chir
5. Verderame, P.: Ueber fettransplantation bei adharenten knochennarben am orbitalrand. Klin Monatsbl Augenheilkd 1909;47:433–442
6. Lexer, E.: Freie Fettransplantation. Dtsch Med Wochenschr 1910;36:640
7. Bruning, P.: Cited by Broeckaert, T.J., Steinhaus, J.: Contribution e l'etude des greffes adipueses. Bull Acad R Med Belg 1914;28:440
8. Tuffier, T.: Abces gangreneux du pouman ouvert dans les bronches: hemoptysies repetee operation par decollement pleuro-parietal; guerison. Bull Mem Soc Chir Paris 1911;37:134
9. Willi, C.H.: The Face and Its Improvement by Aesthetic Plastic Surgery. London, MacDonald & Evans, 1926:15–41
10. Straatsma, C.R., Peer, L.A.: Repair of postauricular fistula by means of a free fat graft. Arch Otolaryngol 1932;15:620–621
11. Cotton, F.J.: Contribution to technique of fat grafts. N Engl J Med 1934;211:1051–1053
12. Peer, L.A.: The neglected free fat graft. Plast Reconstr Surg 1956;18:233
13. Peer, L.A.: Loss of weight and volume in human fat grafts. Plast Reconstr Surg 1950;5:217
14. Peer, L.A.: Transplantation of Tissues, Transplantation of Fat. Baltimore, Williams and Wilkins, 1959
15. Fischer, G.: The evolution of liposculpture. Am J Cosmet Surg 1997; 14(3):231–239
16. Fischer, G.: First surgical treatment for modeling body's cellulite with three 5 mm incisions. Bull Int Acad Cosmet Surg 1976;2:35–37
17. Fischer, A., Fischer, G.: Revised technique for cellulitis fat reduction in riding breeches deformity. Bull Int Acad Cosmet Surg 1977;2(4):40–43
18. Bircoll, M.: Autologous fat transplantation. The Asian Congress of Plastic Surgery, February, 1982
19. Illouz, Y.G.: The fat cell "graft": A new technique to fill depressions. Plast Reconstr. Surg 1986;78(1):122–123
20. Johnson, G.W.: Body contouring by macroinjection of autologous fat. Am J Cosmet Surg 1987;4(2):103–109
21. Bircoll, M.J.: New frontiers in suction lipectomy. In: Second Asian Congress of Plastic Surgery, Pattiyua, Thailand, February, 1984
22. Krulig, E.: Lipo-injection. Am J Cosmet Surg 1987;4(2):123–129
23. Newman, J., Levin, J.: Facial lipo-transplant surgery. Am J Cosmet Surg 1987;4(2):131–140
24. Verderame, P.: Ueber fettranslantation bei adharenten knochennarben am orbitalran. Klin Montsbl Augenheilkd 1909,7:433
25. Lexer, E.: Ueber freie fettransplantation. Klin Ther Wehnschr 1911;18:53
26. Kanavel, A.R.: The transplantation of free flaps of fat. Surg Gynecol Obstet 1916;23:163–176
27. Davis, C.B: Free transplantation of the omentum, subcutaneously and within the abdomen. J Am Med Assoc 1917;68:705–706
28. Lexer, E.: Fatty tissue transplantation. In: Die Transplantation, Part I, Stuttgart, Ferdinand Enke, 1919:265–302
29. Mann, F.C.: The transplantation of fat in the peritoneal cavity. Surg Clin N Am 1921;1:1465–1471
30. Neuhof, H.: The Transplantation of Tissues. New York, Appleton & Co., 1923:74
31. Guerney, C.E.: Experimental study of the behavior of free fat transplants. Surgery 1938;3:679–692
32. Hilse, A.: Histologische Ergebnisse der experimentellen freien Fettgewebstronsplantation. Beitr 2 Path Anal U Z Allg Path 1928;79:592–624
33. Green, J.R.: Repairing bone defects in cranium and tibia. South Med J 1947;40:289
34. Wertheimer, E., Shapiro, B.: The physiology of adipose tissue. Physiol Rev 1948;28:451
35. Bames, H.O.: Augmentation mammoplasty by lipotransplant. Plast Reconstr Surg 1953;11:404
36. Hansberger, F.X.: Quantitative studies on the development of autotransplants of immature adipose tissue of rats. Anat Rec 1995;122:507
37. Schorcher, F.: Fettgewebsverpflanzung bei zu kleiner. Brust Munch Med Wochenschr 1957;99(14):489
38. Van, R.L.R., Roncari, D.A.K.: Complete differentiation of adipocyte precursors: a culture system for studying the cellular nature of adipose tissue. Cell Tissue Res 1978;195:317
39. Van, R.L.R., Roncari, D.A.K.: Complete differentiation in vivo of implanted cultured adipocyte precursors from adult rats. Cell Tissue Res 1982;225:557
40. Saunders, M.C., Keller, J.T., Dunsker, S.B., Mayfield, F.H.: Survival of autologous fat grafts in humans and mice. Connect Tissue Res 1981;8:85

41. Illouz, Y.-G.: New applications of liposuction. In: Illouz, Y.-G. (ed), Liposuction: The Franco-American Experience Beverly Hills, California, Medical Aesthetics, 1985:365–414

42. Asken, S.: Autologous fat transplantation: Micro and Macro techniques. Am J Cosmet Surg 1987;4:111–121

43. Campbell, G.L.M., Laudenslager, N., Newman, J.: The effect of mechanical stress on adipocyte morphology and metabolism. Am J Cosmet Surg 1987;4:89–94

44. Johnson, G.W.: Body contouring by macroinjection of autogenous fat. Am J Cosmet Surg 1987;4(2):103–109

45. Agris, J.: Autologous fat transplantation: A 3-year study. Am J Cosmet Surg 1987;4(2):95–102

46. Bircoll, M.: Autologous fat transplantation: An evaluation of microcalcification and fat cell survivability following (AFT) cosmetic breast augmentation. Am J Cosmet Surg 1988;5(4)283–288

47. ASPRS Ad-Hoc Committee on New Procedures: Report on autologous fat transplantation. 30 September 1987

48. Billings, E., Jr., May, J.W.: Historical review and present status of free fat graft autotransplantation in plastic and reconstructive surgery. Plast Reconstr Surg 1989;83(2):368–381

49. Markman, B.: Anatomy and physiology of adipose tissue. Clin Plast Surg 1989;16:235

50. Illouz, Y.-G.: Fat injection: A four year clinical trial. In: Hetter, G.P. (ed), Lipoplasty: The Theory and Practice of Blunt Suction Lipectomy, Second edition, Boston, Little, Brown and Company, 1990:239–246

51. Hudson, D.A., Lambert, E.V., Block, C.E.: Site selection for fat autotransplantation: some observations. Aesthet Plast Surg 1990;14:195–197

52. Nguyen, A., Pasyk, K.A., Bouvier, T.N. et al: Comparative study of survival of autologous adipose tissue taken and transplanted by different techniques. Plast Reconstr Surg 1990;85:378–386

53. Kononas, T.C., Bucky, L.P., Hurley, C., May, J.W., Jr.: The fate of suctioned and surgically removed fat after reimplantation for soft-tissue augmentation. A volume and histologic study in the rabbit. Plast Reconstr Surg 1993;91:763–768

54. Ersek, R.A.: Transplantation of purified autologous fat: A 3-year follow-up is disappointing. Plast Reconstr Surg 1991;87:219–227

55. Courtiss, E.H., Choucair, R.J., Donelan, M.B.: Large-volume suction lipectomy: An analysis of 108 patients. Plast Reconstr Surg 1992;89:1068–1079

56. Asaadi, M., Haramis, H.T.: Successful autologous fat injection at 5-year follow-up. Plast Reconstr Surg 1993;91(4):755–756

57. Samdal, F., Skolleborg, K.C., Berthelsen, N.: The effect of preoperative needle abrasion of the recipient on survival of autologous free fat grafts in rats. Scand J Reconstr Hand Surg 1992;26:33–36

58. Eppley, B.L., Sidner, R.A., Plastis, J.M., Sadove, A.M.: Bioactivation of free-fat transfers: a potential new approach to improving graft survival. Plast Reconstr Surg 1992;90:1022–1030

59. Carpaneda, C.A., Ribeiro, M.T.: Study of the histologic alterations and viability of the adipose graft in humans. Aesthet Plast Surg, 1993;17:43–47

60. Carpaneda, C.A., Ribeiro, M.T.: Percentage of graft viability versus injected volume in adipose autotransplants. Aesthet Plast Surg 1994;18(1):17–19

61. Niechajev, I., Sevchuk, O.: Long-term results of fat transplantation: clinical and histologic studies. Plast Reconstr Surg, 1994;94:496–506

62. Courtiss, E.H.: Surgical correction of postliposuction contour irregularities. Plast Reconstr Surg 1994;94:137–138

63. Fagrell, D., Enerstrom, S., Berggren, A., Kniola, B.: Fat cylinder transplantation: An experimental comparative study of three different kinds of fat transplants, Plast Reconstr Surg 1996;98(1):90–96

64. Jones, J.K., Lyles, M.E.: The viability of human adipocytes after closed-syringe liposuction harvest. Am J Cosmet Surg 1997;14:275–279

65. Coleman, S.: Long-term survival of fat transplants: Controlled demonstrations. Aesthet Plast Surg 1995;19:421–425

66. Sattler, G., Sommer, B.: Liporecycling: immediate and delayed. Am J Cosmet Surg 1997;14:311–316

67. Ullmann, Y., Hyams, M., Ramon, Y., Peled, I.J., Linderbaum, E.S.: Enhancing the survival of aspirated human fat injected into mice. Plast Reconstr Surg 1998;101:1940–1944

68. Fulton, J.E., Jr.: Breast contouring by autologous fat transfer. Am J Cosmet Surg 1992;9(3):273–279

69. Fulton, J.E., Suarez, M., Silverton, K., Barnes, T.: Small volume fat transfer. Dermatol Surg 1998;24(8):857–865

70. Ellenbogen, R.: Free autogenous pearl fat grafts in the face—a preliminary report of a rediscovered technique. Ann Plast Surg 1986;16:179–194

71. Newman, J.: Preliminary report on "fat recycling"—liposuction fat transfer for facial defects. Am J Cosmet Surg 1986;3:67–69

72. Sidman, R.L.: The direct effect of insulin on organ cultures of brown fat. Anat Rec 1956;124:723

73. Hiragun, A., Sato, M., Mitsui, H.: Establishment of a clonal line that differentiated into adipose cells in vitro. In Vitro 1980;16:685

74. Chajchir, A., Benzaquen, I., Moretti, E.: Comparative experimental study of autologous adipose tissue processed by different techniques. Aesthet Plast Surg 1993;17:113–115

75. Toledo, L.: Syringe liposculpture: a two-year experience. Aesthet Plast Surg 1991;15:321–326

76. Brandow, K., Newman, J.: Facial multilayered micro lipoaugmentation. Int J Aesthet Restor Surg 1996;4(2):95–110

77. Berdeguer, P.: Five years of experience using fat for leg contouring. Am J Cosmet Surg 1995;12(3):221–229

78. Guyton, A.C.: Capillary dynamics and exchange of fluid between the blood and interstitial fluid. In: Guyton, A.C. (Ed), Textbook of Medical Physiology, 7th edition, Philadelphia, Saunders, 1986:348

79. Kaminski, M., Haase, T.: Use of albumin in total parenteral nutrition solutions: Understanding Starling's law and the resolution of hypo-oncotic edema. In: Van Way, C. (Ed), Handbook of Surgical Nutrition, Philadelphia, Lippincott, 1992:272–282

80. Civetta, J.: A new look at the Starling equation. Crit Care Med 1979;7:84–91

81. Kaminski, M.V., Jr., Fulton, J.E., Wolosewick, J.J.: New consideration in fat transfer: A possible role for maintaining interstitial protein to reduce shrinkage of transferred volume. In: Shiffman, M.A. (ed), Autologous Fat Transplantation. New York, Dekker, 2001: 299–309

82. Shiffman, M.A.: Effect of various methods of fat harvesting and reinjection. J Aesthet Dermatol Cosmet Surg 2000;1(4):231–235

CHAPTER 28

Face Rejuvenation with Rice-Grain-Sized Fat Implants: Fischer's Technique

28

Giorgio Fischer

The Plastic Surgeon is undoubtedly the greatest of all contemporary artists. He paints on living canvas and sculpts in human flesh.

C. H. Willi

28.1
Introduction

Augmentation and restoration of different parts of the body has been for centuries the cosmetic surgeons' primary goal. Various alloplastic, allogenic and xenograft materials have been used with this intent. The perfect filler has not been invented yet but I believe that fat is the best material we can use. No allergic reaction has ever been reported in the literature with the use of autologous fat. Facial enhancement for young women or rejuvenation for elder women with rice-grain-sized fat parcels is, according to me, one of the greatest inventions of the century. Along with the aging process goes the loss of fat and consequently the texture of face skin itself. It is only in this way that we are able to restore vitality and new skin texture to an elderly looking face.

28.2
History

After the invention of liposuction together with my father, Arpad, in 1974, I started being confronted with the problem of having to correct depressed areas where too much fat had been taken out. The corrections were made by filling the depressions with the adipose tissue taken with the cannula from the patient. The areas were frequently overfilled. More than 50% of the graft was lost. For many years I did not realize the mistakes I was making. Today the technique I use differs very much from these first attempts.

It is only about 12 years ago that my interest in facial rejuvenation with the use of autologous fat returned. Fournier and I were in London and we came across a book that have changed my career. The book was entitled "*The Face and Its Improvement by Aesthetic Plastic Surgery*" by Charles H. Willi, written in 1926 (Fig. 28.1).

Almost 100 years ago Willi described the use of autologous fat delivered with a syringe for the correction of face lines and the loss of tissue. This technique employed by Willi represents the method that is most similar to our current approach.

Around 1985 I began to augment the zygomatic and malar regions with autologous fat and to fill deep nasolabial folds. At that time I was overfilling the areas, trying to compensate early graft loss. As a result more than 50% of the graft was lost.

By 1992, with better understanding of grafting techniques and the physiology of adipose tissue, I began to harvest the adipose tissue with small syringes and a sharp needle. I abandoned the processing technique. I started to notice that since less fat was transferred, there was a great increase in long-term survival and a decrease in early graft loss.

The larger the graft, the less chance it has to survive and this is because the implants survive by imbibitions. If the graft is too big, the central part of it undergoes the phenomenon of necrosis.

In 1997 I developed a technique that consisted of the transfer of rice-grain-sized fat parcels for total facial rejuvenation. The technique focuses on multiple transfers to the subdermal, intradermal, muscular and fat layers using a microcannula to deposit tiny parcels of adipose tissue. The size of the graft is fundamental to ensure early and reliable neovascularization. This is why any implant whose size is bigger than that of a rice grain has less possibility for survival.

Different authors describe different techniques of the procedure with regard to instrumentation, harvesting processes, processing and transfer techniques. The data for survival rates are inconsistent. I have 80–90% survival of the rice-grain-sized implant if the face is not overfilled. The procedure has to be repeated at least two times.

The procedure is ideal for relatively young patients, or in older patients when it is associated with other procedures. The implants stimulate new vessel formation and give the skin an improved color, consistency and texture.

The next step in the evolution of this grafting technique focuses on the lines of gravity and other factors that determine the vector of placement of the fat parcels. Fat is placed in an oblique manner, perpendicular to the

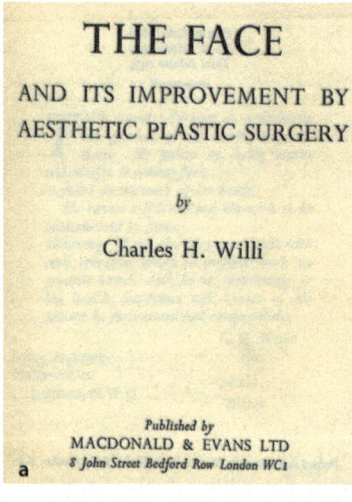

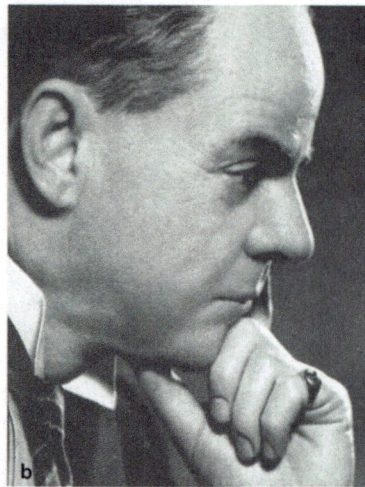

Fig. 28.1 **a** The cover of Willi's book. His book has never been cited in any plastic surgeon's work. **b** Willi's portrait. **c** Willi correcting facial lines and loss of tissue. **d** Willi transferring fat to face. **e** Willi's results with peeling and restoration of with fat implantation around the mouth. *Left*: Before. *Right*: After

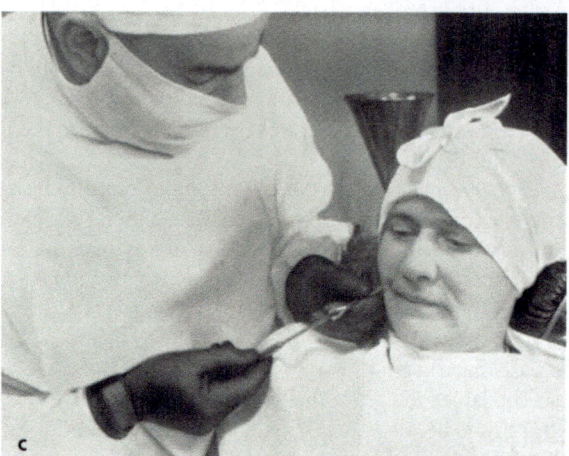

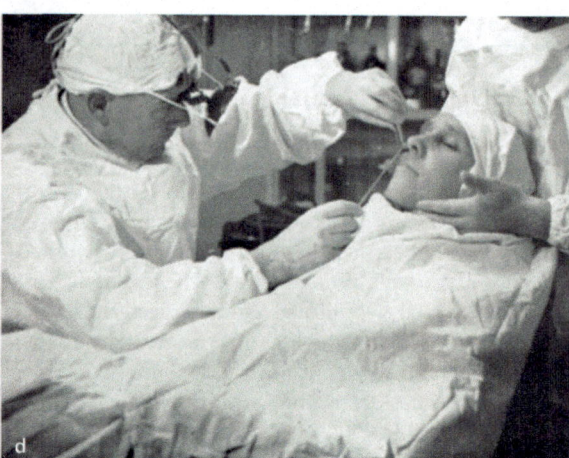

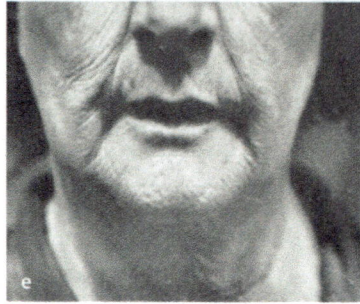

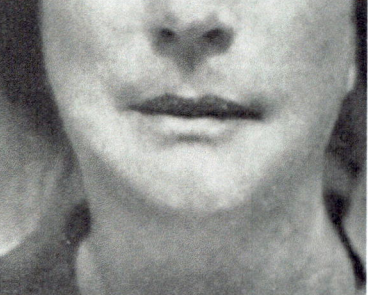

nasolabial, marionette, orbicularis and crow-feet's folds. Before we used to work parallel to these folds. The great innovation of this technique is the fact that we now work perpendicular to them. Inserting the grafts in this way, we create strength lines that contrast these same folds. Fat is deposited from the chin to the forehead in a herringbone manner; the head of the herringbone at the chin and the tail towards the forehead (Fig. 28.2). Much still has to be learned and proved with this technique but I believe this will be our future.

28.3
Preoperative Evaluation

As in any other cosmetic procedure, preoperative evaluation is very important both for the surgeon and for the patient. It is only by observing the patient in his/her normal expressions that we are able to note the harmonies or disharmonies of a face. We must also try to understand what type of objective the patient wants to achieve.

The patient must be informed that he/she will need at least another procedure, in 3 months time. The patient must also be informed that smoking is forbidden in the month prior to and following the procedure. Initial consultation is also important because filling might represent only an adjunct procedure. Donor sites must be recognized and marked. Photographs are taken.

28.4
Harvesting

All harvesting procedures are performed using intravenous sedation and modified tumescent anesthesia for harvesting. The donor site is selected on the basis of the availability of fat. Preferred areas are the flanks, the lower abdomen, the medial part of the thighs and knees, with the middle plane of fat being harvested from these anatomical sites. The donor site is prepared and draped in the usual sterile fashion as for liposuction.

Modified tumescent technique is used for the infiltration: lactated Ringer's solution, 10% Xylocaine and epinephrine. Approximately 25% of the normal amount usually administered for liposculpture is used. This quantity allows a more concentrated aspirate. An 18-G needle attached to a 1-ml Luer-Lok syringe is used. The 1-ml syringe is optimal since use of a larger one would end up with too much strength being used to aspirate the fat; what we want instead is lobulated rice-grain-sized fat. The cannula used to transfer the fat is attached to the same syringe. The cannula is 1.6 mm wide. This avoids manipulation of the fat and contamination of it by air, decreasing the rate of graft death.

The harvest needle is directed in a spoke-wheel fashion in order to prevent depressions of the skin overlying the donor site.

Harvesting should be carried out in a slow and constant manner. It should be a constant and delicate movement. Excessive pressure on the donor site will end up with too much oil in the graft as a result of the rupture of the adipose cells. The syringe is then placed on the server in an upright position.

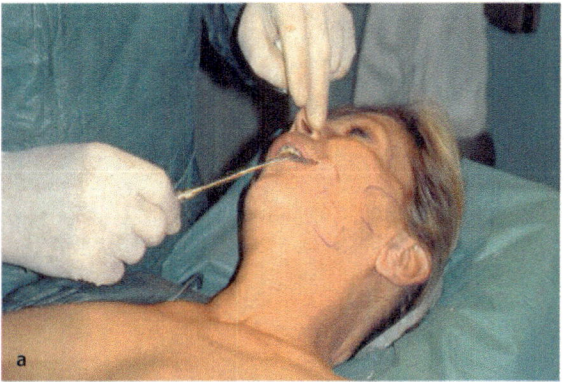
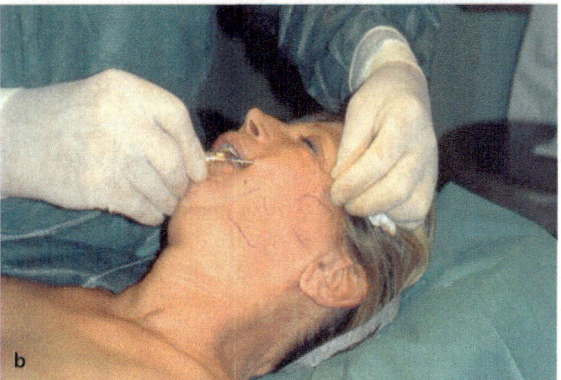
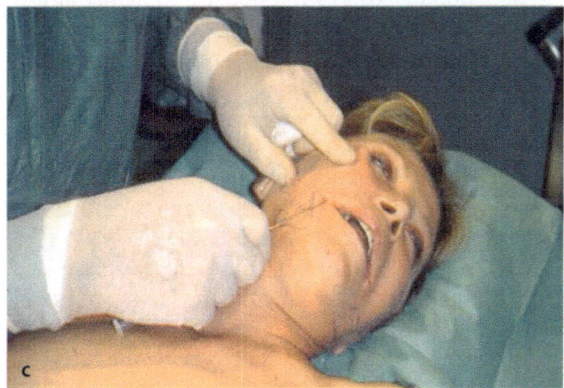

Fig. 28.2 Entry site at the angle of the mouth allows transfer of fat. **a** Cheek. **b** Posterior zygomatic area. **c** Anterior zygomatic area

28.5
Fat Processing

Fat can be processed in three ways. It can be centrifuged. Centrifuging will allow the graft to be isolated and separated quickly. The author believes this has a high risk of damaging the fat cells. The fat can also be washed with saline solution.

I believe that the less we manipulate the fat, the less we risk damaging it. This is why I allow the aspirate to settle for 5–6 min into two distinct layers. The bottom and denser layer contains Xylocaine and lactated Ringer's solution, and the top layer will contain only vi-

able fat cells. If the fat is harvested in the correct way, the two layers will not be present and only fat will be present in the syringe. I do not manipulate or touch the graft in any way.

28.6
Fat Transfer

Face rejuvenation with my technique should be a sculpture, a contouring of the anatomical variations that can be present in every patient. The face should be studied in each aesthetic unit; not even an inch should remain unstudied. As already said, the transfer cannula is attached to the Luer-Lok syringe. The entry site for the cannula is anesthetized and a small stab incision is made with a no. 11 blade. The entrance incisions are placed on the margin of the hairline in the temple, at the angle of the mouth and under the chin (Fig. 28.2).

From these entry sites we are able to transfer fat throughout the entire face. The fat parcels are transferred in a herringbone manner and the microcannula moves in a fanwise direction following the lines of the herringbone. The fat is deposited slowly and the fat lobules are transferred on insertion and withdrawal of the cannula. The cannulas are 1.6 mm wide and 10–13 cm long. The tip of the cannula is blunt, flattened and resembles a duck's beak. The cannulas can be straight or curved, depending on the different necessities of the anatomical region.

Total face rejuvenation with rice-grain-sized fat parcels placed in a herringbone manner is able to give thickness to those areas of the face that have defattened with time.

I do not use more than seven or eight syringes of fat for each side of the face, and this means that no more than 14 or 16 ml of fat is used for the entire face. Anything more than this will not survive. Only in this way the lobules of fat will have the maximum capacity of receiving blood and rapid neovascularization will occur.

The face can be divided into a third superior, a third medial and a third inferior part. Each of these parts contains critical key points in which fat has to be placed. For the superior part of the face, the frontal and temporal areas are very important. The slight ptosis of the eyebrows that occurs with time is due to increased skin laxity and loss of the fatty layer overlying the galea. Deposits of fat over the forehead will give a lifting effect of the eyebrows. The fat deposits on the forehead act against the force of gravity, lifting the forehead and brow in an upward direction. Fat should not de deposited at more than 2-cm distance from the superior margin of the eyebrow, otherwise a ptosis of the brow might occur.

The eyebrow lift should be finished with filling of the shadows under the eyes. These are a frequent sign of aging but are often seen in young patients as well. Eye shadows are caused by the orbicularis oculi muscle that shines through the delicate transluscent infraorbital skin. This can be corrected by infiltrating a couple of milliliters of fat. Fat inserted in this area must be massaged by the patient. The implantation must be carried out in a very delicate way. Single deposits are needed otherwise lumps might be visible after the operation.

The temporal area is another important key point that should not be forgotten. Frequently with age, this area loses the normal quantity of fat present. The absence of fat here gives the patient a "skeleton look." The roundness of this area is one of the criteria for a young-looking face. Fat transfer in this area is, however, only for expert surgeons. This is a very delicate area where superficial vessels are very well represented.

For the third inferior part of the face, an important area is certainly the nasolabial fold. Today I do not place the grafts in the same way I did in the past. Fat is always deposited perpendicular to the fold. Attention should be paid to the triangle placed under the ala of the nose. This triangle has its apex facing the chin. If this triangle is filled, the immediate effect will be that disappearance of the nasolabial fold. The perioral area can be thickened with this technique.

Insertion of grafts in the chin and along the whole mandibular region enhances and rejuvenates the whole face.

28.7
Postoperative Care

No sutures are needed on the temporal and perioral areas. Reston foam is applied on the donor site. Patients remove the Reston foam after 2 days. After a further 7 days they come for a first check, and then after 3 months. Photographs are taken on both occasions. After 3 months, the restored area is evaluated further and additional augmentation is performed.

28.8
Conclusion

Face rejuvenation with rice-grain-sized fat implants is a versatile procedure. If carried out in the correct manner it has an effective and long-lasting result. The technique avoids excessive and unnecessary manipulation of the graft. Processing of the fat is eliminated. Recontouring using autologous rice-grain-sized fat parcels involves precise layering of the graft in order to ensure a natural result. Overfilling the face should be avoided.

Chapter 29

Complementary Fat Grafting

29

Samuel M. Lam, Mark J. Glasgold, Robert A. Glasgold

29.1
Introduction

Autologous fat transfer has become an increasingly important method of facial rejuvenation both as a standalone procedure as well as in combination with traditional rejuvenative methods, like facelifting, browlifting, and blepharoplasty. In certain respects, fat grafting stands in contradistinction to previous efforts at rejuvenation in that the face is augmented with tissue rather than subtracted by lifting, pulling, and excising. A simple analogy to understand the benefits of fat grafting is looking at a full and ripe grape that becomes prunelike (wrinkled, puckered) over time like a convex, youthful face that undergoes contraction and involution with aging. Rather than remove what appears to be redundant tissue and transform that raisin into a pea, perhaps it would be better to reinflate that tiny raisin back into a grape.

Obviously, any analogy can suffer from the obvious problem of being overly reductionistic. Although many surgeons have approached fat grafting as the only correct method to rejuvenate the face (and have demonstrated wonderful results by doing so), the authors contend that fat grafting can serve more effectively as a complement to other rejuvenative techniques. For example, if a patient has significant neck descent and platysmal

dehiscence, a cervicofacial rhytidectomy would provide a more assured method of rejuvenation than copious fat grafting into the neck to mask the unfavorable contours. Fat grafting could then be combined simultaneously with facelifting to enhance the midfacial, periorbital, and prejowl depression to attain an overall improved aesthetic result (Fig. 29.1). A conservative transconjunctival blepharoplasty or skin-only upper blepharoplasty combined with fat grafting can provide reliable rejuvenation and limit morbidity associated with higher volumes of fat grafting that would otherwise be necessary without concomitant excisional-based surgery.

This focused and cogent chapter will elucidate the method that has proven effective for autologous fat grafting over a 10-year experience. Details of lifting procedures (like facelift, blepharoplasty, etc.) are assumed and not described herein.

29.2
Technique

The operative technique is outlined as a surgeon would approach a patient on the day of the procedure: marking the recipient sites, selection of donor site, donor-site harvesting, processing the fat, injection techniques, and immediate postoperative care.

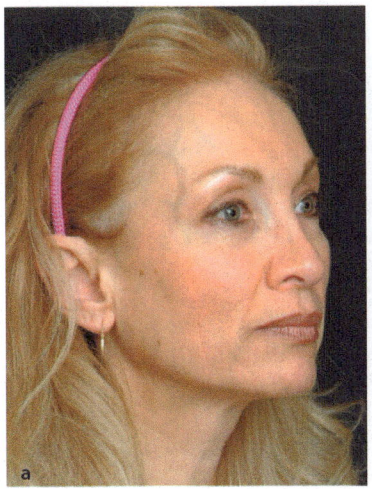 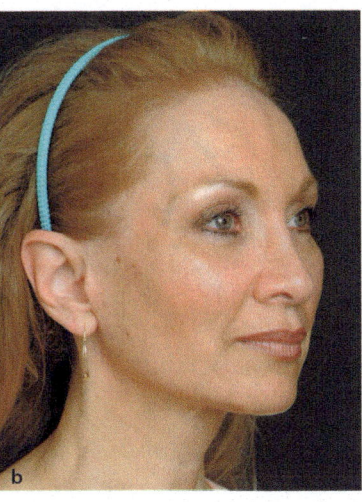

Fig. 29.1 a Preoperatively. **b** Postoperatively following facelift autologous fat transfer to the midface. (Reprinted with permission from Lam SM, Glasgold MJ, Glasgold RA: *Complementary Fat Grafting*. Philadelphia: Lippincott Williams & Wilkins; 2007)

29.2.1
Marking the Recipient Sites

On the day of surgery the surgeon should establish or reestablish with the patient the areas for facial augmentation with fat grafting. A permanent marker, e.g., a Sharpie (gentian violet is too tenacious and will remain on the patient's face for several days, which can be a nuisance; eyebrow crayons/pencils are wiped off too quickly to be useful) is the most effective tool to outline the targeted areas with the patient in the sitting position when the effects of gravity are the most apparent. The anatomic zones that are typically enhanced are as follows: the lateral brow, the inferior orbital rim, the nasojugal groove, the anterior cheek, especially the depression along the malar septum, the lateral cheek, the buccal recess, and the prejowl region (Fig. 29.1). Other areas that can be enhanced as well are the precanine fossa, the lateral mandible (The lateral mandible can only be addressed if a concurrent facelift is not performed, as a facelift typically undermines the soft tissue overlying the lateral aspect of the mandible), and the temple. The patient should confirm with the surgeon the areas for augmentation in a mirror before the surgeon proceeds. Another useful resource is a patient's old photograph that can help the surgeon and the patient achieve mutually agreed upon objectives in terms of volume and distribution of that volume.

29.2.2
Selection of Donor Site

The easiest method to determine the most favorable donor site for fat harvesting is to ask the patient where he or she has the greatest difficulty losing fat or where the patient thinks the most adipose reserve resides. Whereas most men are predominantly truncal-dominant, women can be either truncal-dominant or extremity-dominant (or both) in regard to fat distribution. If the patient has had prior liposuctioning, the surgeon should know where, as the quality of fat harvested from areas of previous liposuctioning can be less than desirable. Prior abdominal surgery does not usually prevent harvesting of the abdomen. As most fat is harvested from the lower lateral quadrants, midline and "bikini" incisions are generally not in the field of harvesting and should not pose a hindrance. Even lower lateral quadrant incisions are not a contraindication as long as the surgeon carefully palpates for any signs of herniation in these areas during valsalva. In general, the lower abdomen and inner thigh are the easiest sites for harvesting as the patient does not require full-body repositioning. However, the hip, the waist roll that descends along the lower back, the outer thigh, the anterior thigh, and rarely the inner knee are alternative sites that are excellent, but require patient repositioning. The area of the triceps is another source for fat harvesting that is easy

to undertake but requires the assistant to hold the arm extended during harvesting. Although fat harvesting from only one side should very rarely cause any noticeable asymmetry between the two sides of the body, it is always wiser to extract fat symmetrically in order to allay patient anxiety about this unlikely occurrence.

29.2.3
Donor-Site Harvesting

The donor site is anesthetized with a mixture of 0.25% lidocaine with 1:400,000 epinephrine by mixing 5 ml of 1% lidocaine/1:100,000 epinephrine with 15 ml saline in a 20-ml syringe fitted with a 22-gauge spinal needle for infiltration. The donor site is anesthetized by placing the anesthesia above (in the superficial subcutaneous plane below the dermis) the fat pad and in the deeper aspect of the fat pad, leaving the central portion of the fat pad itself relatively free of anesthetic. A total of 20 ml of anesthetic is delivered to each site, except for the abdomen, which receives 10 ml per lower lateral quadrant. For optimal patient comfort, the procedure should be performed under intravenous sedation (or general anesthesia if so desired, but which is typically unnecessary). If the patient is under lighter anesthesia or surgery is being performed with just local anesthetic, a mixture of 10 ml of 1% lidocaine with 1:100,000 epinephrine and 10 ml saline should be used in order to lessen discomfort.

The key to successful harvesting is atraumatic extraction of donor fat. Several principles should be elaborated to achieve this objective. First, only hand suctioning should be undertaken, i.e., not liposuctioning with wall or machine suction. Second, only 1–3 ml of negative pressure on the syringe plunger should be manually applied to minimize traumatic injury to the fat cells. Third, proper centrifugation, not overspinning or underspinning the fat, should be performed so as to preserve the fat cells while still purifying the fat from other non-fat-constituent elements, respectively.

Entry sites to pass the harvesting cannula are made with a 16-gauge Nokor needle or an abbreviated stab incision with a no. 11 Bard-Parker blade in an anatomically discreet location. For example, the lower abdomen can be easily accessed bilaterally from a simple stab incision along the inferior aspect of the umbilicus. The inner thigh can be approached from a stab incision along the inguinal line, and the lateral thigh accessed from the lateral infragluteal fold.

Harvesting is undertaken with a blunt harvesting cannula from any number of reputable manufacturers of fat harvesting equipment (Tulip Medical, San Diego, CA, USA; Miller Medical, Mesa, AZ, USA; Byron Medical, Tucson, AZ, USA). A 10-ml Luer-Lok syringe is ideal for harvesting. During harvesting, the surgeon should focus on the middle of the fat pad layer. If the harvesting is too superficial, tethering of the skin will be noted as the cannula approaches the dermis, which can in turn lead to potential contour deformities as well as elicit patient discomfort. Similarly, harvesting more deeply near the fascial layer can also provoke patient pain and under lighter anesthesia will not be easily tolerated. As the surgeon harvests fat, he or she should be cognizant of the cannula passage in the following ways. First, the cannula tip is where fat enters the cannula and thereby the syringe for collection. Accordingly, the surgeon should always be mindful of where the cannula tip is situated in the fat pad. The neophyte surgeon may unwittingly pass the cannula tip too far beyond the fat pad, which would limit potential harvest and also increase patient discomfort as the tip abrades unanesthetized structures (e.g., fascia, muscle, dermis). Second, after passage of the cannula several times in a specified area of the fat pad, the surgeon should consciously withdraw the cannula all the way back almost to the entry site before reorienting the cannula to pass into another part of the fat pad. Simply turning the cannula direction without first withdrawing the cannula back to the entry site can lead to overharvesting in one place since the cannula oftentimes remains exactly in the same place as it was previously.

Use of the non-dominant hand to stabilize the fat pad can be helpful to increase harvesting ease and efficiency; however, the surgeon should resist the temptation to squeeze the fat pad with the non-dominant hand, as this maneuver can lead to the potential for uneven contours. Another tip that is useful concerns harvesting from the inner thigh. The patient should have the contralateral side frog-legged to facilitate harvesting from the straightened leg. It is important not to harvest from the frog-legged side, as doing so can lead to possible contour irregularities. Also, the cannula must first pass through an initial fascial layer before harvesting commences. If the harvesting remains superficial, the cannula can be easily seen to tent and deform the overlying skin, which is too superficial a passage. The surgeon will feel an initial pop or release of tension when entering the correct fascial layer for the inner thigh.

29.2.4
Processing the Fat

The entire procedure, including fat processing, should be completed in a sterile fashion to minimize risk of infection. The donor and recipient sites are prepared with povidone–iodine, or an equivalent solution, and draped sterilely. Similarly, centrifugation of the fat should be done sterilely as well. There are many models of centrifuges that permit sterility to be maintained. For instance, the entire centrifuge hub into which the syringes are inserted can be removed and sterilized. Alternatively, the authors use a model in which the syringes are placed into individual sterilized sleeves (Miller Medi-

cal), which are in turn placed into the circular centrifuge hub, which remains non-sterile.

The 10-ml syringe containing harvested fat is prepared by removing the syringe plunger and affixing a cap and the Luer-Lok side, a Luer-Lok-style plug—both of which can be purchased from the aforementioned manufacturers. It is important to emphasize that the small plastic cap that comes packaged with the syringe should never be used for centrifugation, as it is not secure enough to hold the contents. The fat is then spun in the centrifuge in a balanced manner (i.e., the syringes are spaced equally around the centrifuge to avoid damage to the machine and poor centrifugation). Generally speaking, the fat is spun at around 3,000 rpm for 3 min give or take 1 min or about 1,000 rpm either way.

The syringes are then removed, and the supranatant (from the plunger side) is poured off into a waste basin on the sterile field to remove the free fatty oils released from lysed fat cells. The bloody infranatant is then allowed to drain off the bottom of the syringe into the waste basin. Any remaining supranatant is then wicked away with uncut 4 × 4 gauze tucked into the exposed plunger side to make contact with the fat. Five to ten minutes is allowed to transpire for complete wicking of the supranatant to occur. Then, the contents of the syringe are poured from the exposed plunger side into the back end (exposed plunger side) of a 20-ml Luer-Lok transfer syringe. Doing so expedites transfer into the 1-ml Luer-Lok infiltration syringes and also allows removal of any remaining bloody infranatant in the original 10-ml syringe. The 20-ml transfer syringe is filled to the 15 ml mark, and air is gently removed through the Luer-Lok side, taking care not to spill any of the fat contents through the aperture prematurely. A Luer-Lok transfer hub is then affixed on one side to the 20-ml syringe and on the other side to the 1-ml Luer-Lok syringe and the fat contents are transferred in a slow deliberate fashion. It is important to push the fat all the way to the back of the 1-ml syringe so that the plunger is actually removed from the back of the 1-ml syringe and reinserted to the 1.0 ml mark. There is always a tiny air bubble that remains at the base of the syringe, and this maneuver removes the bubble. The assistant then continues to refill each 1-ml syringe, as the surgeon continues to infiltrate the face systematically. Generally, four 1-ml syringes are sufficient for continual refilling without a wait time between fills.

29.3
Injection Techniques

29.3.1
General Principles

Use of blunt cannulas throughout the infiltration procedure can minimize hematoma formation and thereby aid fat-cell viability. In addition, blunt infiltration cannulas limit the potential for nerve damage, as tissue planes are followed more naturally and are less traumatically disturbed. Besides direct injection of the three proposed entry sites with local anesthesia, almost all of the anesthetic should be delivered with the same blunt infiltration cannula used for fat infiltration to minimize hematoma and swelling prior to starting injection of fat. The three ports of entry are as follows (Fig. 29.2):

1. The base of the malar septal depression in the mid-cheek of the face (port A)
2. Lateral to the lateral canthus (port B)
3. Posterior to the prejowl sulcus (port C)

Each of these ports of entry is made with a stab incision using a standard 18-gauge needle through which the blunt cannula can be inserted for both anesthetic delivery and fat infiltration.

Placing only tiny parcels of fat—either three to five passes per 0.1 ml (in unforgiving areas) or 0.1 ml per pass (in more forgiving areas)–is the key to successful fat transfer. In the past, larger boluses of fat were used that led to potential visible contour irregularities and could compromise fat viability. It is important for the surgeon to visualize the depth of infiltration basically into the following three zones:

1. Deep (immediately supraperiosteal)
2. Intermediate (in the musculofascial layer)
3. Superficial (in the subcutaneous plane)

For the supraperiosteal plane, the non-dominant hand can be used to provide tactile feedback during infiltration and to guide supraperiosteal placement. In addition, the dominant hand can feel that the cannula tip is gently abutting the bony surface. For the intermediate and superficial planes, the cannula passage is less precise and the surgeon must simply visualize that the cannula is passing through the central thickness of the soft tissue or more superficially.

29.3.2
Systematic Site-Specific Infiltration

29.3.2.1
Inferior Orbital Rim (from Port A)

The most difficult area to inject safely and accurately is the inferior orbital rim, and this is where most complications can arise; therefore, only small amounts (a total of 2–3 ml for the entire inferior orbital rim) should be placed per session when beginning. As comfort with the technique is gained, maximal infiltration in this area should still not exceed 4–5 ml per session. Moreover, only small quantities of fat per pass (three to five passes per 0.1 ml) should be delivered into the deep supraperiosteal plane. Injection of the inferior orbital rim from the inferiorly positioned entry site (port A)

at a perpendicular angle greatly reduces the incidence of complications. The non-dominant hand should be used to protect the globe and to provide tactile feedback that the cannula tip is dancing gently across the inferior orbital rim. It is very important that if the cannula tip feels plugged that the cannula be entirely withdrawn and cleared external to the body before continuing to avoid an inadvertent large bolus of fat in an unforgiving area like the inferior orbital rim. It is easier to divide the inferior orbital rim into a medial and a lateral half and place 1 ml of fat into each side as a way of being systematic and precise.

29.3.2.2
Nasojugal Groove (from Port A)

The nasojugal groove can be more recessed in some individuals than in others. Nevertheless, it is almost always of empiric benefit to place some fat along this bony triangular recession that resides between the medial inferior orbital rim and the nasal sidewall, as youthful individuals tend to exhibit some degree of favorable convexity here. Placement of 1 ml of fat into the supraperiosteal plane can be undertaken a bit more aggressively by delivering 0.1 ml per pass without significant risk of contour irregularity.

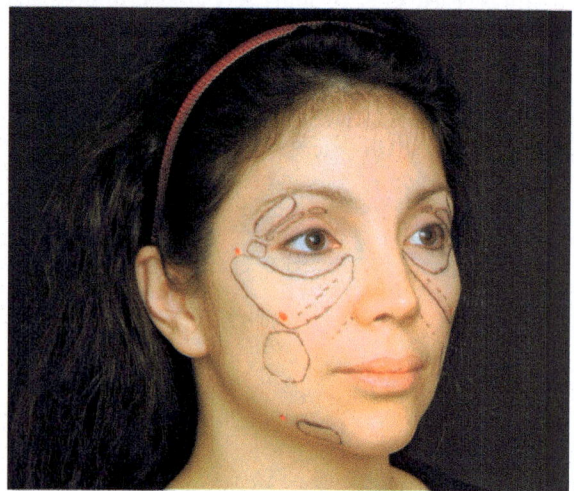

Fig. 29.2 Preoperative markings on a patient undergoing autologous fat transfer. The three planned entry sites for fat infiltration are marked in *red* and are referred to as ports B, A, and C, respectively, from superior to inferior. (Reprinted with permission from Lam SM, Glasgold MJ, Glasgold RA: *Complementary Fat Grafting*. Philadelphia: Lippincott Williams & Wilkins; 2007)

29.3.2.3
Lateral Canthus (from Port B)

If the patient exhibits some lateral-canthal hollowing, the surgeon can place 0.5 ml into the supraperiosteal plane from the laterally positioned entry port B. There tends to be considerable fibrous attachments that must be broken to insert the fat in this area. These fibers must be gently and gradually severed with the cannula tip, as a hematoma can arise from the traumatic disruption.

29.3.2.4
Lateral Brow (from Port B)

The lateral brow tends to be an excellent area for fat infiltration to achieve a balanced frame around the eye with fat. The lateral brow is approached from lateral entry port B and placement is undertaken in either a deep or an intermediate plane (Fig. 29.3). More realistically, the cannula should simply be passed in the plane of least resistance. As this area is more forgiving, placement of 0.1 ml per pass can be undertaken to place a total of 1 ml of fat in most cases. If a cigar roll appears at the end of infiltration, this deformity should not raise concern as it typically dissipates over time.

29.3.2.5
Anterior Cheek/Malar Septum (from Port B)

The anterior cheek, which often exhibits a linear depression that runs superomedially down inferolaterally and that corresponds with the ligamentous malar septum, should be addressed next. The cannula is passed from port B that is superolateral to the malar septum so that the cannula can break through the malar septum in a perpendicular orientation to it. Individuals exhibit varying degrees of resistance when the cannula passes through the malar septum. The goal is to place fat in the malar septal depression and on either side of it to raise the anterior cheek along with the unsightly depression. Generally, 2–3 ml of fat can be placed into the intermediate and superficial planes. The deep plane can also be addressed, but the surgeon need not hug the bony contour. Placement of a generous 0.1 ml per pass can be undertaken with impunity. The surgeon should be careful in aggressively enhancing the anterior cheek in men, as this characteristic can be somewhat feminizing.

29.3.2.6
Lateral Cheek (from Port A)

The lateral cheek is more easily elevated in continuity with the anterior cheek from an inferomedial position of entry port A. The bony zygomatic arch can serve as a helpful guide over which the fat can be placed. The

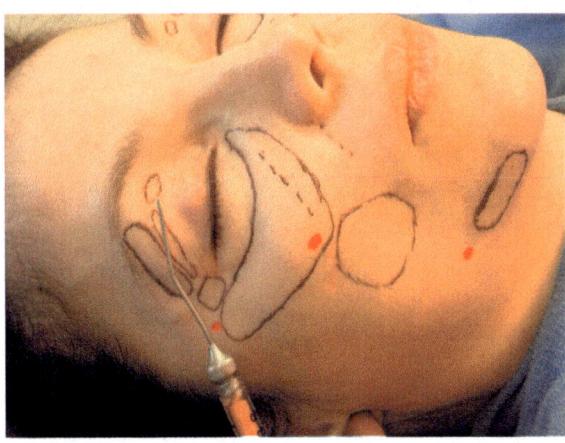

Fig. 29.3 Fat placed along the inferior orbital rim. (Reprinted with permission from Lam SM, Glasgold MJ, Glasgold RA: *Complementary Fat Grafting*. Philadelphia: Lippincott Williams & Wilkins; 2007)

placement of 2–3 ml of fat into the lateral cheek can be undertaken with a generous 0.10 ml per pass into all tissue depths, but again the cannula need not pass immediately in the supraperiosteal plane.

29.3.2.7
Buccal Recess (from Port A)

The buccal recess can be quite hollow with aging and can be even more exacerbated by augmenting the cheek above. The buccal hollow can accommodate a generous amount of fat on the order of 5–8 ml without difficulty. Placement of fat is into the intermediate and superficial tissue planes from entry site A. If the entry site is too proximal to the buccal region, the more distally situated port B can be used as an alternative or together with port A in a cross-hatching fashion.

29.3.2.8
Prejowl Sulcus (from Port C)

The prejowl sulcus is an important area to augment to achieve a more youthful facial contour but also to enhance a facelift result by straightening the jawline further with fat enhancement. Fat should be infiltrated into all three tissue planes described previously with a generous 0.1 ml per pass without difficulty. We generally start with 3 ml. It is important to conceptualize the prejowl sulcus three-dimensionally with fat placed along the anterior border of the mandible, the inferior border of the mandible, and the transition between these two borders. Doing so will provide a more even and complete fill of the prejowl depression. Additional fat can be feathered into the mental sulcus and anterior chin as aesthetically mandated.

29.4
Immediate Postoperative Care

As no actual incisions are made, there is no need for any suturing of the entry sites. Also, no dressings for the body or face are required either. Simply, head elevation and icing are sufficient to expedite the recovery process. The patients are discharged after adequate postoperative observation.

29.5
Complications

Obviously, the best situation is to avoid a complication altogether, as complications can be difficult to correct. It is important to be more conservative when starting out with autologous fat transfer, especially in the periorbital region, as it is a relatively simple task to add more fat but an arduous one to remove an excess. The first order of business when approaching a complication is to identify the nature of the complication to permit an accurate treatment protocol. For simplicity, we have divided the complications that can arise into the following four categories: lumps, bulges, overcorrection, and undercorrection. Each type of complication mandates a different, unique treatment strategy.

29.5.1
Lumps

A lump refers to a discrete, contour deformity that arises from either placement of too much fat into a specific locus or placement of fat too superficially near the skin in an unforgiving anatomic region, like the periorbital region. Although steroid injections may help, we have found that removal of the offending lump through a direct, cutaneous incision is the most effective method of resolving the problem.

29.5.2
Bulges

A bulge refers to a wider zone of fibrotic fat that can arise like a cigar-roll deformity along the inferior orbital rim owing to imprecise placement of a large quantity of fat in an unforgiving area. Since we have migrated away from injecting the inferior orbital rim from a lateral entry site now to exclusively an inferior-based entry site (i.e., perpendicular to the rim itself), we have encountered significantly fewer such complications. A bulge can also arise when a patient gains a considerable amount of weight after fat transplant, making the areas of fat grafted literally bulge owing to fat hypertrophy.

In these cases, we have found microliposuction and direct excision to be less favorable when compared with repeated, intralesional steroid injections. The authors typically inject the area with low-dose triamcinolone acetonide (10 mg/ml) and gradually increase the dose on a monthly basis if needed to a full 40 mg/ml until resolution. Conservative aliquots of steroid using only 0.05–0.1 ml per problem area help to minimize the risk of dermal atrophy and unfavorable divots that arise from steroid use.

29.5.3
Overcorrection

Overcorrection can be most apparent in the lateral cheek, and manifests itself as a roll that appears when the patient smiles. It is always wiser to start with a more conservative policy of enhancement, especially for the inexperienced surgeon. Overcorrection is best handled with an 18-gauge Klein-Capistrano microliposuction cannula (HK Surgical, San Clemente, CA, USA).

29.5.4
Undercorrection

Undercorrection is the most favorable situation, as additional fat can be easily harvested and infiltrated into the deficient areas. Unlike in facelift surgery, "hitting a double" and not trying for a "homerun" should be the goal in fat grafting. This conservative policy should be a useful guiding philosophy, especially for the starting surgeon. Some patients also tend to absorb fat more quickly, and an additional session 6 months after fat infiltration may be required to restore an optimal result.

29.6
Discussion

Autologous fat transfer has come to be recognized as an important, if not indispensable, tool in the facial aesthetic surgeon's armamentarium. The question arises whether traditional blepharoplasty has yielded the optimal rejuvenation for the patient. Removal of skin and fat around the eye alone during blepharoplasty can actually hollow the eye and thereby age the patient even more dramatically rather than serve to rejuvenate the appearance. If one studies the hallmarks of a youthful face, the periorbital region can be seen richly padded rather than hollow and that aging only serves to deplete the volume around the eye further. Conservative removal of some prolapsed fat in the lower eyelid should in most cases be combined with periorbital fat transfer to achieve the best aesthetic results. At times, fat transfer alone to the periorbital region will suffice. As hair restoration provides a frame for the face, autologous fat transfer should be thought of as a way to frame the eye and thereby bring back the luster of youth (Fig. 29.4).

A youthful face is heart-shaped, with a prominent cheek which tapers down to the chin area, which forms the apices of the heart. As aging occurs, the face becomes more deflated and gravity accentuates the heaviness of the jowls and lateral mandible. Accordingly, the face becomes not only more aged but also more masculinized with a rectangular/square shape. The goal of autologous fat transfer is to return the face back to a more ideal heart shape that is both youthful and feminine (Fig. 29.5). When dealing with male patients the anterior cheek augmentation is done to a lesser degree so as to avoid the risk of feminizing the male face.

Another feature of the aging face that is observed is the rise of depressions, concavities, and shadows, e.g., along the inferior orbital rim, the malar septum, the lateral brow, and the prejowl sulcus. The objective in autologous fat transfer is to return the face toward a more youthful convexity free of these shadowed concavities.

Although fat transfer is an excellent method to restore facial contour, it is not ideal for addressing the perioral lines like the nasolabial and labiomandibular folds or the lips. The authors prefer the use of soft-tissue fillers, other than fat, to achieve restoration of these areas, as correction of these kinds of lines with fat tends to be shorter-lived in our hands and also less than ideal. The lips are also an area that is more difficult to correct with any degree of longevity and the recovery time for lip enhancement with fat transfer can be considerable.

Fat transfer, when combined with other traditional rejuvenative procedures like blepharoplasty and/or face-lifting, can more effectively restore the aging face than any procedure alone in many cases. The authors advocate using the appropriate combination of procedures to arrive at the most targeted solution to the problem at hand. Using fat grafting as a complement to traditional rejuvenative procedures can possibly enhance patient satisfaction and reduce morbidity associated with aggressive fat grafting alone.

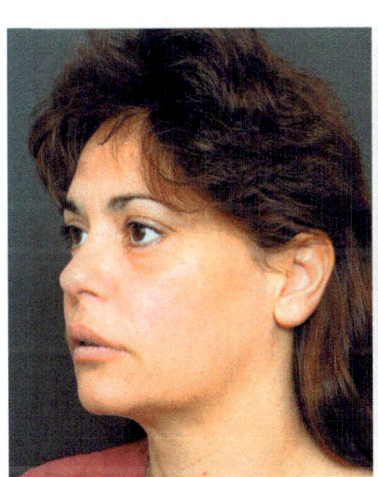
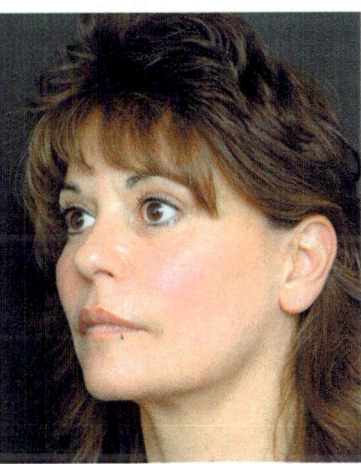

Fig. 29.4 Fat injection of prejowl sulcus. (Reprinted with permission from Lam SM, Glasgold MJ, Glasgold RA: *Complementary Fat Grafting*. Philadelphia: Lippincott Williams & Wilkins; 2007)

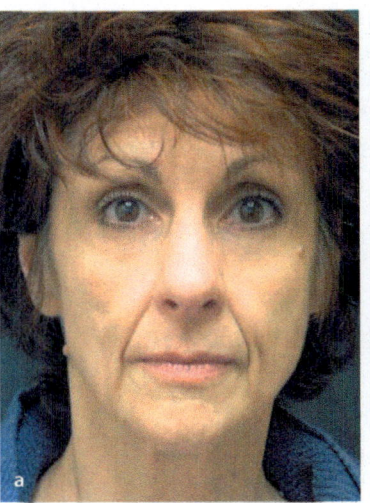
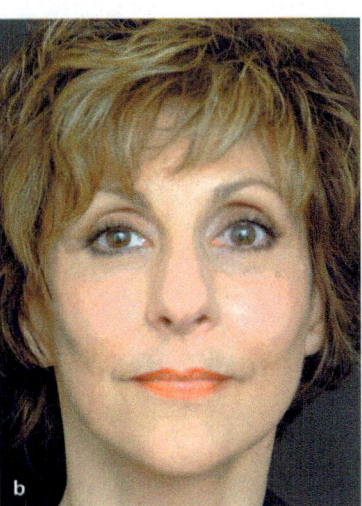

Fig. 29.5 a Preoperatively. **b** Postoperatively after periorbital and midface fat transfer which provided a frame for the eye. (Reprinted with permission from Lam SM, Glasgold MJ, Glasgold RA: *Complementary Fat Grafting*. Philadelphia: Lippincott Williams & Wilkins; 2007)

29.7
Conclusions

This chapter is intended, first and foremost, to challenge the surgeon to rethink his or her aesthetic perspective about the aging face. The operative technique outlined is suggested to provide a simplified and systematic approach to autologous fat transfer and thereby facilitate ease of the operation and minimize morbidity. Volume enhancement should continue to become an increasingly important method for facial rejuvenation and to restore facial harmony.

CHAPTER 30

Facial Volume Enhancement: Decision-Making Between Fat Grafting and Solid Implants

30

Mark J. Glasgold, Robert A. Glasgold, Samuel M. Lam

30.1
Introduction

Recently, facial volume enhancement has been recognized as an important component in overall facial rejuvenation. Gravitational descent is only one mechanism that contributes to the aging process. Many different techniques exist to augment facial volume. Besides temporary injectable fillers that are non-surgical in nature, safe, permanent options can be principally divided into facial fat enhancement and solid-implant insertion. This chapter will focus on an algorithm to help guide a surgeon in deciding when to use autologous fat transfer, solid implants, or a combination of both methods, to achieve ideal facial volume and harmony.

The emphasis will be placed squarely on the preoperative judgment as to the benefits and limitations of each technique rather than a detailed review of methods.

30.2
Discussion

Both autologous fat transfer and solid implants provide effective and beneficial methods of facial volume augmentation; however, the techniques are not interchangeable and carry with them individual benefits and limitations that can be exploited to optimal advantage in a given clinical scenario. At times, combining both techniques judiciously can serve as the preferred method if the patient acknowledges the rationale, cost, and restrictions for doing so. Although aesthetic judgment and success with any method are a personal matter, this chapter will offer some guidelines in the decision-making process based on extensive clinical experience with both techniques.

Autologous fat transfer offers the distinct advantage of easily enhancing complex zones of facial deficiency. For example, periorbital rejuvenation with fat transfer often entails enhancing lateral brow depression and restoring deficiency along the inferior orbital rim, nasojugal groove, lateral canthus, temporal region, anterior malar depression, and lateral cheek. A solid implant typically can only provide a prefabricated augmenta-

tion for a specific deficiency like the lateral and anterior cheek depression. Additional implants would then be necessary to address other concavities like the nasojugal groove, which can be more difficult to efface than with autologous fat transfer. If a solitary cheek implant is used for rejuvenation of the aging face, the result can be less than optimal. As the implant must reside inferior to the exit point of the infraorbital nerve, the implant can actually serve to exacerbate the infraorbital hollow and thereby somewhat worsen the appearance of facial aging. Besides a sensuous volumetric convexity of youth, a seamless confluence of the eyelid and the cheek contour is another essential hallmark. Fat grafting facilitates rejoining the separated appearance of the cheek from the lower eyelid in addition to restoring the full convexity of the cheek contour (Fig. 30.1). A solid implant serves to enhance the volumetric deficiency of the cheek but at the expense of infraorbital hollowing. Therefore, for facial aging in general, autologous fat transfer provides a more comprehensive rejuvenation of the volumetrically depleted aging face.

At times, autologous fat transfer may not be recommended as the sole option for certain clinical circumstances. In particular, an individual who is extremely gaunt may not have sufficient donor fat supply to provide optimal volumetric expansion of the face. In this case, fat grafting can be combined with a cheek implant to provide both seamless contour and volume (Fig. 30.2). A cheek implant used alone in a very thin person may not be advisable, as the attenuated soft-tissue envelope cannot effectively camouflage the visibility of the implant's border. Clinical judgment whether an implant would be warranted in this circumstance should be made cautiously and with proper patient counseling. Unlike cheek implants, a chin implant that is shaped as an extended anatomic style can serve to augment the mentum and in most cases does not reveal any of its borders even in a relatively thin individual.

For patients who are desirous of augmentation of a deficient chin, a chin implant serves as the most assured method of augmentation. Choosing an implant size that matches the patient's particular degree of microgenia permits an almost 1:1 correction of the soft-tissue/bony deficit. Fat grafting can also achieve enhance-

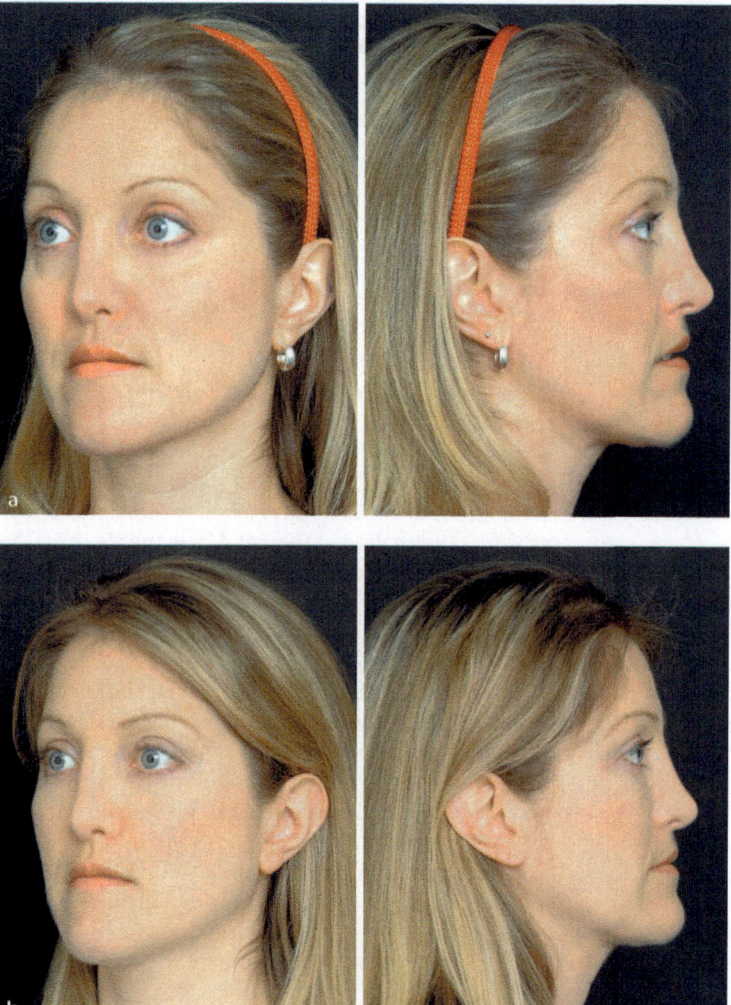

Fig. 30.1 a Preoperative patient who had cheek implants placed approximately 8 years previously. There is a visible volume deficiency just above the implant at the superior orbital rim. **b** Postoperative patient following autologous fat transfer to the inferior orbital rim and cheek. This allowed for creation of a single convexity, eliminating the depression that breaks the lower lid and cheek complex. (Reprinted with permission from Lam SM, Glasgold MJ, Glasgold RA: *Complementary fat grafting*. Philadelphia: Lippincott Williams & Wilkins; 2007)

ment of the mentum but owing to variable resorption over months to years may not be as reliable a method as solid implantation. Fat augmentation of the midface is easier to achieve and more predictable than in the more muscular perioral region (Fig. 30.3). Nevertheless, individuals with only mild chin deficiency or who do not want an alloplast and who may be undergoing simultaneous fat grafting are excellent candidates for fat grafting alone to the chin. Performing additional fat grafting to the chin when concurrent fat grafting is undertaken adds little time and no additional cost. However, the authors do not advocate using a solid chin implant simply to augment a prejowl deficiency that arises almost universally during the aging process. A chin implant in an individual who does not require one can artificially render a change in appearance that can be unacceptable to the patient. The reader is reminded that the ultimate goal of facial rejuvenation is precisely that, to rejuve-

nate the face, not to alter a patient's look unless that is warranted (e.g., in an individual with a deficient chin who desires that change). Even when the anterior face of an extended anatomic chin implant is shaved very thin to remove any unwanted projection, there can still remain some degree of anterior projection of the chin that is undesirable. The prejowl sulcus can be more effectively contoured with autologous fat transfer, as the prejowl sulcus is a three-dimensional entity that should be augmented not only along the anterior border of the mandible but in the immediate inferior edge as well (which a chin implant cannot as effectively accomplish). Prejowl augmentation can be tailored more effectively with variable degrees of fat than with standard-sized chin implants (Fig. 30.4).

Obviously, the ideas espoused in the previous paragraphs are only intended as a framework to guide fruitful dialogue between the surgeon and the patient. Some

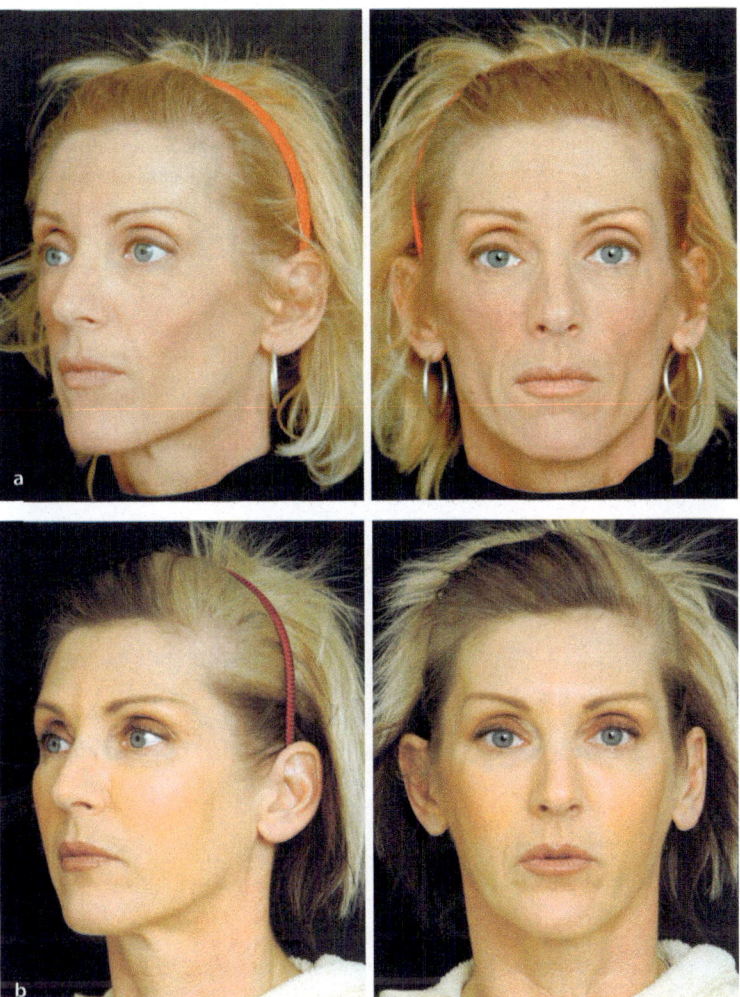

Fig. 30.2 a Preoperative female patient who is an exercise instructor with limited donor fat available and who needed a large amount of fat to address her global facial volume loss. **b** Following placement of a medium Conform Binder Submalar implant and fat transfer to the periorbital region, buccal and submalar regions, including additional cheek augmentation with fat. (Reprinted with permission from Lam SM, Glasgold MJ, Glasgold RA: *Complementary Fat Grafting.* Philadelphia: Lippincott Williams & Wilkins; 2007)

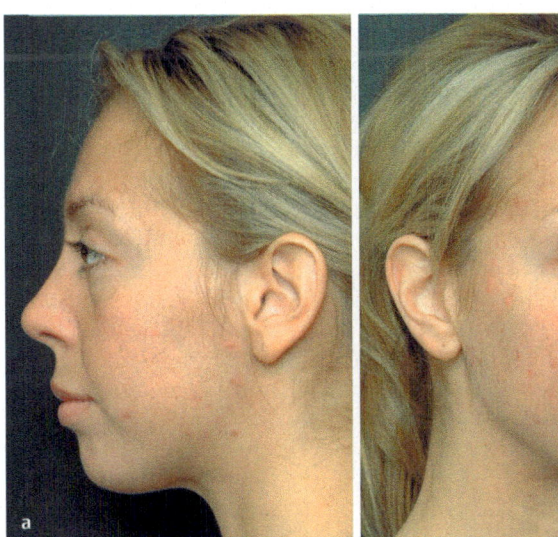

Fig. 30.3 a Preoperative young patient who had a negative vector eye with significant malar volume deficiency and microgenia. *b see next page*

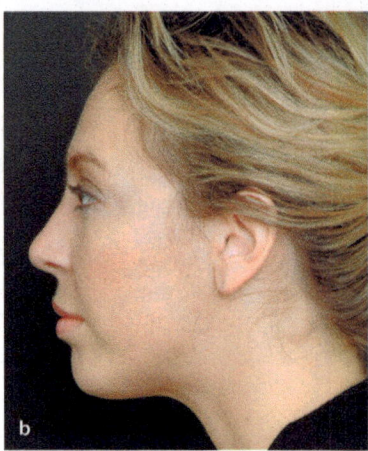
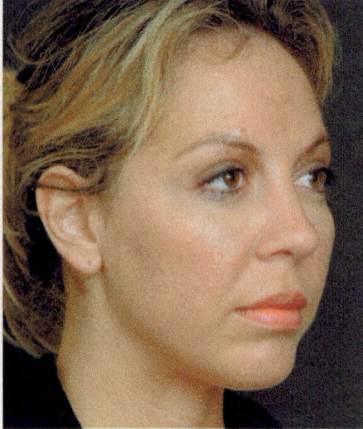

Fig. 30.3 (Continued) **b** Three years following mentoplasty with a medium extended anatomical implant and fat transfer to the cheeks and inferior and superior orbital rim. (Reprinted with permission from Lam SM, Glasgold MJ, Glasgold RA: *Complementary Fat Grafting*. Philadelphia: Lippincott Williams & Wilkins; 2007)

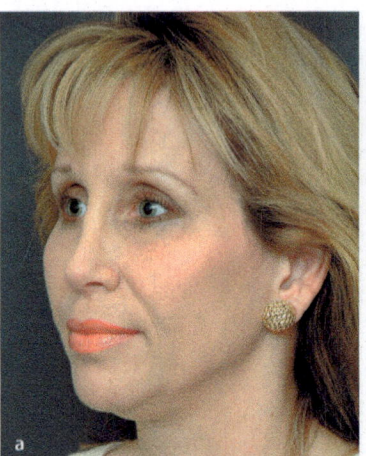
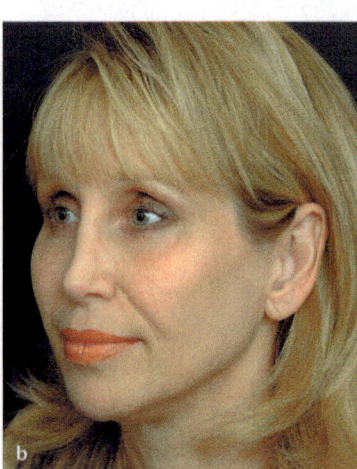

Fig. 30.4 **a** Preoperative patient with isolated volume augmentation of the prejowl sulcus. **b** Postoperative patient following autologous fat transfer. (Reprinted with permission from Lam SM, Glasgold MJ, Glasgold RA: *Complementary Fat Grafting*. Philadelphia: Lippincott Williams & Wilkins; 2007)

patients are adamantly opposed to undergo any kind of alloplast for whatever real or perceived risks that accompany alloplastic augmentation. The recovery time associated with fat grafting is often more substantial and must be communicated during the decision-making process and not after the fact. Patients also may express recalcitrance to undergo fat transfer owing to the potential for ongoing volumetric loss from the variable absorption of transplanted fat and the natural propensity for soft-tissue involution that occurs with aging. The most important point for the surgeon to remember is to articulate all of the salient risks, benefits, and limitations of any procedure so as to ensure patient satisfaction thereafter.

30.3
Conclusions

Hopefully, the proposed construct outlined in this chapter will provide a useful tool for any surgeon approaching a patient desirous of volume enhancement (Table 30.1). Clearly, the authors do not intend any of this information to be absolute but instead it is conclusions based on personal observation and opinion. What works in one surgeon's hands may not in another's owing to idiosyncrasies that lie beyond any systematic explanation. Therefore, the authors refuse any wholesale condemnation or endorsement of a specific technique but offer a rudimentary or sophisticated algorithm depending on the reader's perspective and level of experience.

Table 30.1 Fat grafting versus solid implants

	Fat grafting	Solid implants
Benefits	Permits complex facial sculpting	Potentially more limited recovery time
	Autologous material (limited risk of infection)	More assured 1:1 correction of skeletal/soft-tissue deficiency
	Typically abundant donor supply, no expense for purchase	No resorption over time
	No risk of displacement	
	Easy to add additional fat when undercorrrected	
Drawbacks	Can be absorbed to variable extent over time (therefore, may not provide as definitive a 1:1 correction for specific skeletal deficiencies as a solid implant would)	Risks of infection, displacement, extrusion
	Can have longer recovery times	Initial cost outlays for the implant
		Can exacerbate infraorbital hollow when isolated cheek implants are used
		Can change a person's appearance unfavorably when used simply to create prejowl enhancement when a person does not require anterior chin projection as well
Clinical indications	Facial aging	More definitive correction of microgenia
	Reconstruction of specific defects	Useful for gaunt individuals combined with fat grafting when donor supply of fat is limited
	Can be used in combination with solid implants for very gaunt individuals with a relative deficiency of donor fat	Useful for younger patients who have congenitally deficient skeletal areas

CHAPTER 31

Facial Implants

Benjamin A. Bassichis

31.1
Introduction

Over the past few decades, there has been a paradigm shift in the approach to the treatment of facial aging. This philosophical shift has consisted of a departure from older "subtractive" facial surgery techniques to newer "restorative" techniques and procedures to evoke more beautiful natural-looking results.

Older methods of facial rejuvenation consisted primarily of removing (subtracting) skin and fat and pulling tissues tight. In many instances, this led to a skeletonized and more aged, operated-upon appearance. We now recognize that it is not only the skin that needs to be addressed to correct the signs of facial aging, but also facial soft tissues, including subcutaneous tissue, fat, and facial bones that lose volume and projection over time.

The major architectural promontories of the facial skeleton, including the malar–midface region, nose, and chin, provide the structural foundation for aesthetic facial beauty. The overall harmony of the face is largely determined by the balance, size, shape, and position of these structural fundamentals. A cosmetic surgeon may be able to add facial implants to the facial skeleton to accentuate the areas of the cheekbone or chin. These skeletal augmentations redrape and tighten the skin of the face as well as reorchestrate the elements of facial balance and proportion for an improved cosmetic result. Depending on an individual's specific aesthetic requirements, implant procedures can be performed solo or in combination with other facial plastic procedures to provide a more healthy and youthful appearance. Implant placement surgeries are performed with hidden or invisible incisions so there are no visible scars and the results are immediately evident [1].

Proper selection of implants requires a working knowledge of general size, thickness, and material composition of available implant types. Alloplastic facial implants offer the surgeon many advantages over autogenous tissue, including easy availability of material and simplicity of the operative procedure. Care must be taken to select the proper implant characteristics for the desired aesthetic result, as each synthetic material has unique properties. With all implant types and materials, careful surgical technique is essential to minimize the risks of complications [1].

In the past, a variety of substances have been used for soft-tissue and bony augmentation, including autogenous elements such as iliac and rib bone grafts and nasal cartilage. Varied alloplastic materials including ivory, acrylic, and precious metals remain solely of historical interest. Advancements in biomaterial science have promoted the use of novel, alloplastic implant materials for facial skeletal augmentation [2]. There are several general features that contribute to the biocompatibility of an implant. An ideal implant is composed of materials that do not elicit a chronic inflammatory response or foreign-body reaction, are non-immunogenic, inert in body fluids, and non-carcinogenic. Implant materials must also be non-degradable, yet malleable, such that the shape and position are sustained over time.

Many materials are used for alloplastic implants, including silicone elastomers, expanded poly(tetrafluoro ethylene) (ePTFE), high-density porous polyethylenes, methylmethacrylate, nylon mesh material, bioglass and alumina ceramics, and hydroxyapatite–calcium phosphate material [2]. Currently, the most commonly used materials are solid silicone and ePTFE. Both materials have performed well in terms of the incidence of infection and lack of bony resorption tendencies (when positioned in the correct plane of dissection).

Improved understanding of tissue–implant interface biology has encouraged the development of bioactive implants which allow for biologic bonding of tissue to the implant, which permits natural tissue regeneration as opposed to chronic foreign-body or inflammatory reaction. Evolving material technologies have permitted the creation of better implants; however, the ideal alloplastic material has yet to be formulated [3]. Facial plastic surgeons have been challenged with the development of safe and effective materials for facial contouring and restoration. However, the most significant burden still remains in accurate facial analysis, assessment, and planning to achieve a good surgical outcome.

31.2
Technique

Surgical technique affects both the short-term and more long lasting outcomes in facial skeletal augmentation. General surgical principles relating to implantation technique such as avoidance of contaminated fields, use of perioperative antibiotics, and meticulous intraoperative handling of the implant materials are vital to the success and safety of the operation. Careful preoperative assessment of the recipient site should determine whether adequate vascularity and soft-tissue coverage are present.

31.2.1
Midface Implants

Prominent malar eminences are a canon of beauty in many cultures, conveying the youthful appearance of facial fullness. A hypoplastic flat malar area can make the face appear tired and contributes to a prematurely aged countenance. This tired, sunken look can be secondary to midface hypoplasia and/or atrophy and ptosis of the soft tissues. It can also be accentuated by an overresected facelift procedure. The goal of midface augmentation is to restore the appearance of youth and beauty by enhancing structure and facial contour.

The majority of patients are unaware of the contribution the midface provides in terms of overall facial harmony; instead, many patients focus on the nose, eyes, or lax facial skin. The facial plastic surgeon can educate patients by illustrating how malar augmentation can restore a youthful and balanced facial contour. In patients lacking bony substructure, rhytidectomy alone does not provide sufficient rejuvenation. Volume restoration by means of midface augmentation in conjunction with facelift can provide the scaffolding for a more optimal redraping of facial tissues to achieve a more successful rejuvenation. Malar implantation enhances rhytidectomy or rhinoplasty results by further improving facial balance and harmony.

The majority of malar augmentations are performed on an elective basis. General indications for malar augmentation include posttraumatic and posttumor resection deformities, congenital deformities, aged face with atrophy and ptosis of soft tissues, unbalanced aesthetic facial triangle, a very round full face or a very long narrow face, and midface hypoplasia. Patients may present with changes associated with aging, such as hollowing of the cheeks and ptosis of the midfacial soft tissue. Malar implants can augment cheek hollows and grooves associated with inferior displacement of the malar fat pad and soft tissues secondary to volume depletion of aging. Patients with midface hypoplasia gain aesthetic benefit from enhanced facial volume. Patients with mild hemifacial microsomia may also show improvement. Other patients may request facial augmentation to produce a dramatic high and sharp cheek contour. Flat, thin, and round faces all benefit from malar augmentation, as it balances the face to create a more aesthetically appealing appearance.

Facial analysis, incorporating photographic documentation, is a critical component of patient selection for malar augmentation. Several techniques of facial measurement analysis of the malar region exist; however, the exact location for augmenting the malar eminence is not universally agreed upon, as the type of malar deficiency varies from patient to patient.

After the determination of the appropriate implant size to be used, the patient can undergo the procedure. The most common technique used is via an intraoral route. No external incisions are made on the face. The initial step is to adequately mark the patient, determining the planned placement of the implants. The precise anesthetic solution used is not as important, as long as it contains epinephrine. After infiltration on both sides, a 1.5-cm sublabial incision is made in the vertical direction through all layers down to the bone. Horizontal incisions for the approach are discouraged. Once this incision has been made, a periosteal elevator is used to dissect the periosteum off the bone. Many authors favor the use of fixation to help secure the implant. The author prefers to use precise subperiosteal pockets for implant placement. Therefore, wide undermining is not required, but careful, deliberate creation of pockets allows for precise localization. The infraorbital nerve is not compromised during the dissection. Depending on the implant, the lateral dissection may be extended to the zygomatic arch. Submalar implants or combined implants will necessitate a more inferior dissection from the arch over the masseter muscle. The correct plane of dissection is over the glistening white fibers of the muscle.

Prior to implant placement, an antibiotic solution is used to irrigate the cavity. A 4-0 chromic suture is passed through the lateral edge of the implant. Using an Aufricht retractor, the surgeon identifies the lateral extent of the pocket and the same suture is passed though to the skin surface. With a gentle amount of tension, the implant is inserted into the pocket. The assistant gently pulls on the suture, while the surgeon is guiding from medial to lateral direction. The suture is then gently tied over a bolster, which will be removed after 5 days.

The pocket will "shrink-wrap" around the implant over the next 24–48 h. The incisions are closed in two layers. Attention to detail during the closure cannot be overemphasized as any saliva that penetrates into the wound can lead to infection.

Besides the intraoral route, there are other approaches that may be preferred by other surgeons. The subciliary approach, through a lower blepharoplasty incision, may be used to place smaller implants, especially implants used to augment the nasojugal fold. During facelift surgery, penetration can be made through the subcutaneous musculoaponeurotic system and then carried down to the bone. A subperiosteal pocket can be formed from lateral to medial. This technique limits the access for implant positioning.

31.2.2
Mandibular Implants

The chin has a prominent role in anchoring facial symmetry and aesthetics. Along with the nose, it is a primary determinant of facial balance, especially in consideration of the facial profile. The features of the chin can determine characteristics of the face and even perceptions of personality; a long chin implies strength and power, and a short, small chin portrays weakness.

Abnormalities of the chin are commonly present in patients pursuing cosmetic facial surgery. In fact, chin deformities are the most common abnormality of the facial bones, with microgenia being the most common abnormality; however, with the lack of an associated functional deficit, microgenia often remains untreated. Most commonly, patients present requesting rhinoplasty and are unaware of their associated chin deficit.

When a patient is considered for chin augmentation with an alloplastic implant, it is important to carefully select the proper implant size and shape. It should be noted that some alloplastic chin implants, particularly silicone, will heal with the formation of a fibrous capsule, resulting in thickening of the overlying skin and soft tissues. This should be taken into account when calculating the size of the augmentation. Women are most judiciously treated with undercorrection, to avoid the necessity of removal of an implant that is perceived as too large. This is rarely the case in male patients, where a strong chin is viewed as a positive facial feature [4].

Severe microgenia is a contraindication to augmentation mentoplasty. Other contraindications include labial incompetence, lip protrusion, shortened mandibular height, severe malocclusion, and periodontal disease.

As with all procedures in facial plastic surgery, thoughtful preoperative analysis is crucial to a successful outcome. This analysis involves careful three-dimensional evaluation of the face as a whole, with specific attention directed towards the chin, lips, and nose [5]. The patient is examined from all angles, accompanied by precise photographic documentation in the standard views. Face shape and length and the relationship of the chin and nose to the face are examined. The chin is analyzed for its soft-tissue components and its bony structure. Chin projection and width are noted as are the position and the depth of the labiomental fold. Labial

competence and lip position are evaluated. The lower lip should be located posterior as related to the upper lip. The lower lip should also be in alignment with the anteriormost projection of the chin.

The technique of implant placement for anterior mandible augmentation can be performed through an intraoral or an external route. Similar to the midface augmentation, a precise subperiosteal pocket will allow for minimal migration of the implant. The external approach is preferred by the author, through either a previous scar in the submental region or a novel 1.5-cm incision in the submental crease. The implant is placed along the inferior edge of the mandible. Preoperative marking delineates the midline, inferior edge of the mandible, and lateral extent of the dissection. The lateral dissection is usually carried out 5 cm on each side, but is dependent on the specific implant used. Once the area has been infiltrated with local anesthetic, the submental crease incision is performed. The dissection is carried down through skin and subcutaneous tissue to the periosteum. The midline, inferior edge of the mandible is found and the dissection proceeds superiorly in a supraperiosteal plane for approximately 1.5 cm. During this portion of the dissection, the attachment of the mentalis muscle is carefully dissected. At this point, a no. 15 blade is used to vertically incise the periosteum. With use of a Freer elevator, the dissection is extended 5 cm laterally on both sides. The mental nerve is not routinely identified, but caution is warranted if dissection exceeds superiorly from the inferior edge of the mandible. The central cuff of periosteum will be used for fixation of the implant to provide a small amount of protection against anterior bone remodeling. After the pocket has been created, an antibiotic solution is used to irrigate the cavity. The implant is carefully placed into the pocket on its side and then the opposite side is folded over onto itself to allow for placement.

Once the implant has been positioned, a 5-0 polydiaxanone (PDS) suture is used to fixate the implant to the periosteum in two places. The next layer of wound closure involves reattaching the cut edges of the mentalis muscle back to the periosteum, also performed using 5-0 PDS suture. The following two layers of closure involve the subcutaneous tissue and skin. With meticulous wound closure technique, the incision is very well tolerated by the patient.

31.3
Complications

The complications of using implants for facial augmentation include infection, extrusion, malposition, bleeding, persistent edema, abnormal prominence, seroma, displacement, and nerve damage. Most of the complications listed are due technical error, not due to the implant material used. Extrusion of the implants should not occur if the implants were not forced into the pockets. There should be no folding or spring in the implant after placement. Impaired nerve function, usually temporary, is caused by trauma to the tissues overlying the dissection. Bone erosion beneath the implant can occur, and is more commonly seen in mandibular implants. However, as long as the implant is in the correct position, there have been no reports of clinical significance.

Disfigurement is a risk following a failed implant. This can occur with the formation of a capsule, contracture and scarring, or an abnormally draped mentalis muscle. In the event of a failed implant, treatment is removal. This requires removal of the capsule or de-bridement of the wound in case of infection. Implant replacement is not recommended. Rather, the patient can be reevaluated and recommended for osteoplastic genioplasty.

31.4 Discussion

The role of skeletal changes in facial aging has brought to light the importance of volume restoration in facial rejuvenation. Many patients seek surgery to improve the appearance and balance of facial features to restore a youthful visage. Complete and detailed facial analy-

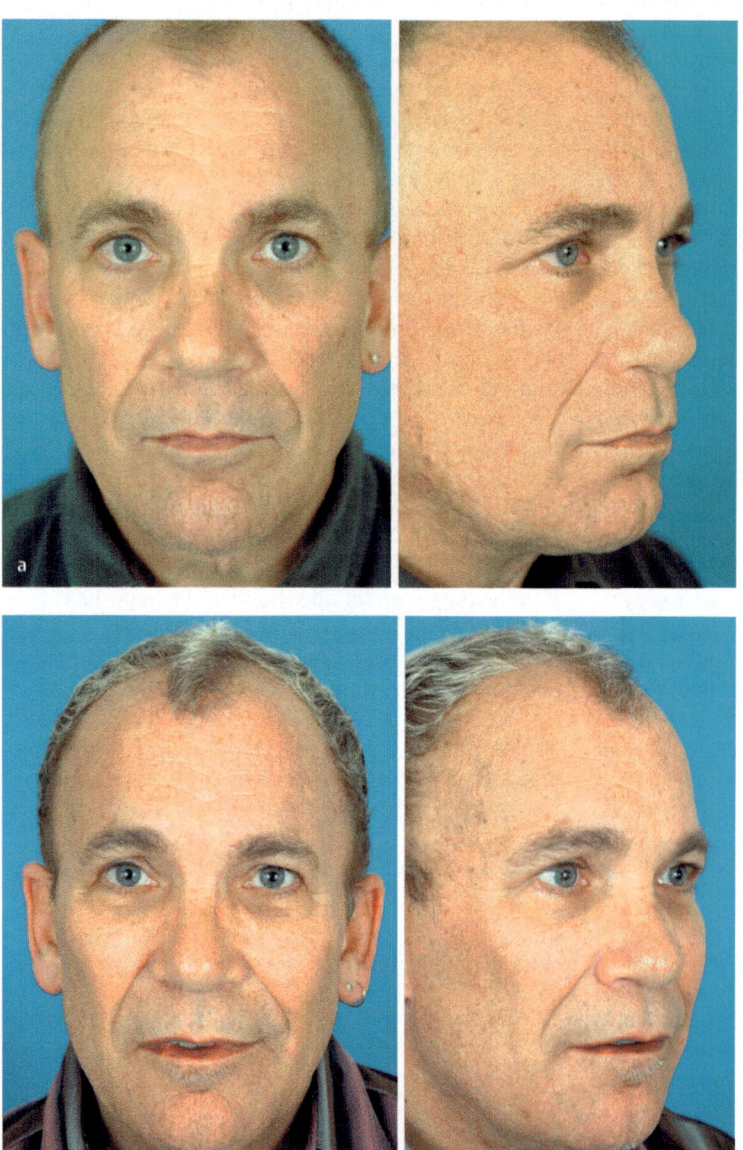

Fig. 31.1 a Preoperatively. **b** After chin implant

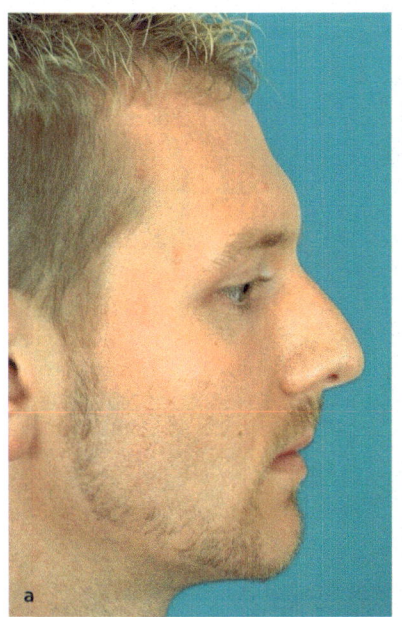 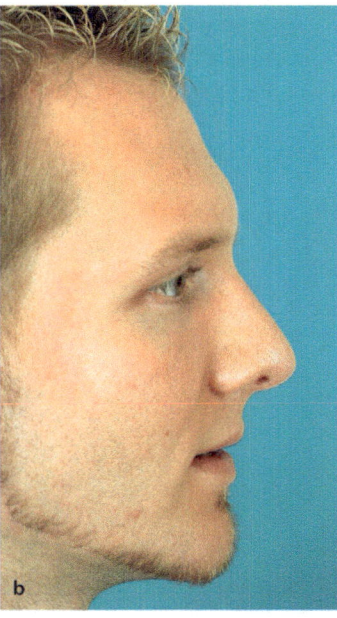

Fig. 31.2 A 26-year-old male patient. **a** Preoperatively. **b** After chin implant and rhinoplasty

sis with appropriate patient expectations is vital in all patients undergoing cosmetic surgery. Alloplastic facial implants offer the facial plastic and reconstructive surgeon many advantages over autogenous tissue, including availability of allograft materials and simplification of the surgical procedure. With all implant types and materials, careful surgical technique is crucial in minimizing the risks of extrusion and infection. Both cheek and chin implants can serve to replace lost volume with relative simplicity and low morbidity (Figs. 31.1, 31.2).

31.5
Conclusions

In properly selected patients, alloplastic facial implantation and can yield highly satisfying results and may complement other facial plastic surgery procedures.

References

1. Eppley BL: Alloplastic implantation. Plast Reconstr Surg 1999;104(6):1761–1783
2. Friedman CD, Costantino PD: Alloplastic materials for facial skeletal augmentation. Facial Plast Surg Clin North Am 2002;10(3):325–333
3. Friedman CD: Future directions in alloplastic materials for facial skeletal augmentation. Facial Plast Surg Clin North Am 2002;10(2):175–180
4. Frodel JL: Evaluation and treatment of deformities of the chin. Facial Plast Surg Clin North Am 2005;13(1):73–84
5. Terino EO: Facial contouring with alloplastic implants: aesthetic surgery that creates three dimensions. Facial Plast Surg Clin North Am 1999;7:55–83

CHAPTER 32

Solid Implants: Mentoplasty and Malar Augmentation

32

Robert A. Glasgold, Samuel M. Lam, Mark J. Glasgold, Alvin I. Glasgold

Alvin I. Glasgold receives royalty payment from Implantech for the Glasgold Wafer™.

32.1
Introduction

Alloplastic solid implants can be used for a wide range of facial enhancement procedures, including augmentation of the cheek and chin as well as of the forehead, temple, nose, lateral mandible, and other folds and depressions of the face. This chapter will focus primarily on the operative considerations for the two principal indications for solid implantation, the cheeks and the chin. These anatomic zones represent the most common reasons for augmentation with solid alloplasts and, for the sake of clarity, will be the only two areas discussed.

Solid implants can be used to correct congenitally deficient bony/soft-tissue facial areas or to improve the lost volume that arises during the aging process. The latter indication was explored in depth in Chaps. 29 and 30. Accordingly, this chapter will discuss more precisely the indications for facial enhancement of the malar and mental regions based on congenital deficiency but can certainly apply to individuals with volume loss from aging, with the caveats enumerated in Chaps. 29 and 30 in mind.

Alloplastic solid implants come in a variety of shapes, sizes, and materials for facial augmentation. Although many types of implants can be used for facial volume augmentation, the senior author (A.I.G.) has had great success for more than 30 years principally with silastic implants in the cheeks and chin. Hence, this chapter will discuss the specific details for facial augmentation with silastic implants in these two areas with the recognition that expanded poly(tetraflouroethylene) (ePTFE) is a suitable alternative among other materials. In fact, the authors generally prefer the use of ePTFE for the nose, where the lighter weight of the implant and the thinner skin of the nose make it a more ideal choice.

The remaining chapter will be divided separately into a discussion of mentoplasty followed by a discussion of malarplasty. Each procedure has its own unique preoperative considerations, implant selection, operative technique, and complications.

32.2
Mentoplasty

32.2.1
Patient Evaluation

The primary goal of mentoplasty is to restore or to establish facial harmony. A deficient chin can have profound aesthetic impact on adjacent facial structures. For example, we have found that approximately 20% of reduction rhinoplasty cases can benefit from some degree of chin enhancement to make the nose appear smaller and to provide improved facial harmony overall (Fig. 32.1). Microgenia can also make the lower lip appear to be overly protuberant, as the lip resides in a solitary anterior position relative to the posteriorly positioned chin.

Evaluating a patient's overall facial shape from a lateral and oblique view can be a valuable part of the initial analysis. Patients are divided into normocephalic, dolocephalic, and brachiocephalic. A dolocephalic ("long head") individual exhibits a greater anterior–posterior cephalic dimension compared with the cephalic width—a feature more commonly found in European races. Brachiocephaly ("short head"), typically found in East Asian races, is defined by a greater cephalic width compared with the anterior–posterior dimension. For instance, a broad brachiocephalic cranium with a narrow chin shape would benefit from a tapered lateral shaped implant to soften the transition from the narrow chin to the wider lateral face.

Aesthetic differences between the male and female gender are very important in preoperative judgment for the surgeon and discussion with the patient. Women look better with a chin that is positioned at or slightly behind a vertical line dropped from the lower lip; whereas men can tolerate some degree of overprojection of the chin anterior to this imaginary line. Use of digital imaging can be very helpful for the patient to evaluate what degree of chin modification is acceptable to him or her, especially when combined with other procedures like rhinoplasty. As most patients do not view their profile very often, they may be completely ignorant of these relationships, and the surgeon can help illuminate these deficiencies for the patient. In fact, many mentoplasty procedures are performed on the basis of advice from

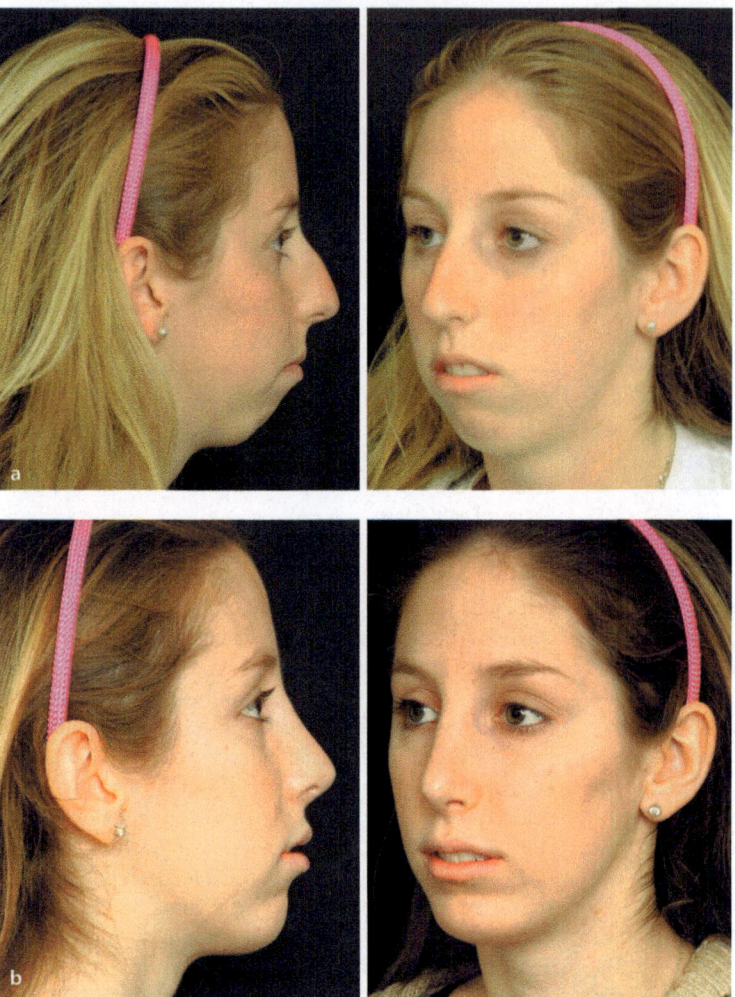

Fig. 32.1 a Preoperative views of a patient whose primary concern was the appearance of her nose, but who would not have gotten as good a result without mentoplasty. **b** Postoperatively following rhinoplasty and mentoplasty. An extra-large extended anatomical implant was used for augmentation

the aesthetic surgeon rather than from initial patient request.

Dental evaluation should be part of every preoperative examination. If a patient exhibits marked orthodontic and/or orthognathic problems, proper referral should be made to an appropriate dental specialist. It is always advisable in these circumstances to seek dental consultation prior to any surgery rather than after the fact. Orthodontic work could be sufficient to correct a problem or alter the degree of chin projection required by an implant. Although orthognathic options may be more invasive and costly, the patient may prefer to have that kind of intervention when warranted, especially if related functional problems coexist, like temporomandibular joint dysfunction.

Other related anatomic attributes that should be evaluated include lip position, depth of the labiomental sulcus, nerve function, and dynamic changes with smiling. As mentioned, the lower lip can appear overly protuberant owing to a deficient chin, which can be pointed out to the patient. A very deep mental sulcus may limit the potential for a greater extent of chin augmentation without concurrent or subsequent soft-

tissue augmentation of the sulcus. The patient should also be examined in smiling and repose, as the former can add additional chin projection in some individuals with microgenia. Accordingly, more conservative chin augmentation should be carried out in these cases so that the chin does not appear overly protuberant during animation. Also, as part of a standard evaluation, the patient's nerve function should be assessed to record preexisting reduction of sensation in the mental nerves and/or compromise in mobility due to facial-nerve impairment. Any preoperative jawline asymmetry and/or cutaneous irregularity should be underscored to the patient so that under critical postoperative scrutiny the patient does not mistakenly believe these conditions arose from the operative procedure.

32.2.2
Implant Selection

Chin implants can be either abbreviated and cover only the central mentum or extended and taper laterally over the prejowl sulcus (Fig. 32.2). The authors prefer the latter type of anatomically extended implant for the following reasons. The extended implant permits partial or complete effacement of the prejowl depression that arises with aging. Use of a more limited sized implant without lateral extension can actually exacerbate the prejowl or in some cases create a visible prejowl sulcus in a patient who did not have it preoperatively. A longer-style tapered implant also permits a more fixed and stable position, reducing the chance of rotation and/or cephalic migration of the implant. We like to conceive of the wider extended implant more as a mandibular-contouring than a chin-contouring implant, as it permits more global rejuvenation of the lower third of the face and more seamless integration with the mandibular body (Fig. 32.3).

Chin implants can be inserted either via an intraoral route or via a submental incision. We prefer to use the submental incision route for three reasons. The longer-style implant is much more difficult to insert via an intraoral route owing to the presence of the intervening position of the mental nerves. Secondly, the implant can be fixated at its inferior aspect to the mandibular periosteum prior to skin closure in order to limit the risk of cephalic displacement. Finally the risk of contamination and subsequently infection is higher with intraoral insertion.

Assessment of appropriate chin projection preoperatively can be difficult, especially for the inexperienced surgeon. Using calipers, sizers, digital imaging, and other ancillary measures can help improve the accuracy of sizing an implant. Nevertheless, the surgeon may find that he or she requires additional projection intraoperatively that would require a larger-sized implant. The senior author has developed a wafer that can be positioned under the central aspect of the chin implant to gain an additional 2 mm of anterior projection if needed without removing the implant or requiring reinsertion of a larger implant. When a surgeon is uncertain as to the precise sizing of the implant, he or she can opt for

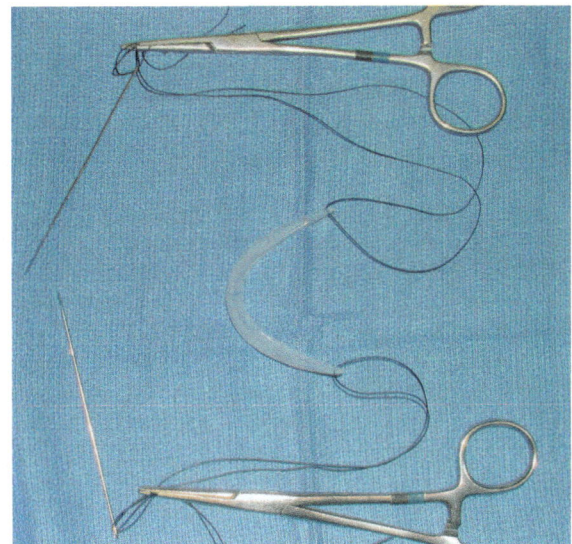

Fig. 32.2 The extended anatomical implant provides anterior projection of the mentum and its lateral extensions fill the prejowl sulcus giving a more natural mandibular contour. This photograph shows the extended anatomical implant after being prepared for insertion by placing a guide (2.0 silk) suture through each tail and threaded through a Keith needle

the slightly smaller size and use a wafer as needed for added projection. Further, if the surgeon finds that the chin is underprojected postoperatively, the surgeon can insert a wafer under the existing implant to enhance projection in an office setting under local anesthesia.

32.2.3
Technique

The patient is marked preoperatively with a circumlinear incision that falls near the submental crease and

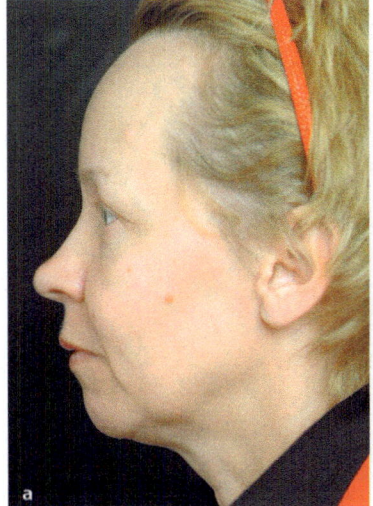
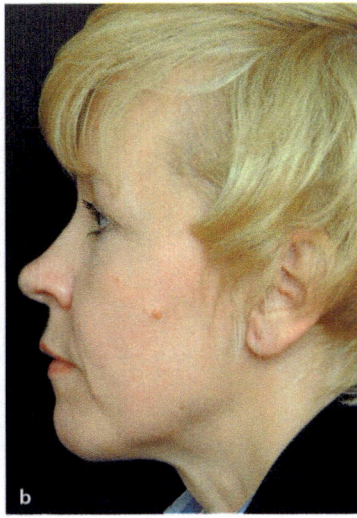

Fig. 32.3 a Preoperative female patient with microgenia and a prejowl deficiency. **b** Postoperatively following mentoplasty with a medium extended anatomical implant which provided anterior projection and recontoured the mandible giving a more defined jawline

curves gently posteriorly following the mandibular contour. The incision typically spans about 2 cm in length for adequate access and should be placed proportionately further posteriorly depending on the implant size, as the implant tends to push the incision farther anteriorly after insertion.

If the implant is not marked along the midline, it is important to either score or mark the implant at the midline to ensure symmetry and proper alignment at the end of the operation. The extended anatomical silastic implant is prepared by threading a 2-0 silk suture affixed to a Keith needle through both ends of the implant at approximately 3 mm proximal to each lateral end of the implant. These sutures are used to guide the implant into the pocket and to limit the chance that the tapered end of the implant will inadvertently fold back onto itself during insertion (Fig. 32.2). The implant is then soaked in either clinadmycin or cefazolin solution in preparation for implantation. It is also advisable to administer cefazolin or clindamycin intravenously prior to the start of surgery.

The cutaneous incision is made with a no. 15 Bard-Parker blade, and dissection is taken down to the periosteum using electrocautery. Use of a wide, double-hooked retractor can be useful to assist in exposure during this phase of the operation. The periosteum is entered along the inferior border of the anterior face of the mandible, leaving a small cuff of periosteum down to which the implant can be sutured toward the end of the procedure. The periosteum along the central mentum is elevated with electrocautery. The lateral subperiosteal pockets are then made. The lateral dissection should not extend more than 1–1.5 cm from the inferior edge of the mandible, as the mental nerves exit the bony foramen at this height. A Joseph elevator is

used to dissect the lateral subperiosteal pockets using the non-dominant hand to guide the progress of the elevator (Fig. 32.4). The elevator should be handled in a slow, deliberate, and controlled fashion to ensure uniform and complete elevation of the periosteum without inadvertent shearing of the overlying soft tissue. Upon completion of the lateral pocket, an Aufricht retractor (0.8 cm × 4.5 cm) is placed within the pocket (Fig. 32.5). If the pocket does not accommodate the complete retractor, then it needs to be enlarged so that it is adequate for implant placement. The same technique is then performed on the contralateral side.

The Keith needle, attached to the implant by the guide suture, is inserted under the Aufricht retractor, aiming toward the angle of the mandible and passed out through the skin laterally along the inferior border of the mandible (Fig. 32.6). The assistant applies gentle traction to the suture and helps to guide the implant into the pocket while the surgeon grasps the implant with a straight clamp and slides the implant into position at the same time. The assistant maintains traction on the implant by holding tension on the silk suture, while the Aufricht retractor is placed in the contralateral pocket and the same maneuver is undertaken to insert the contralateral side of the implant (Fig. 32.7). The implant is confirmed to be in the midline by aligning the central mark with the corresponding skin marking or with the upper central incisors. The implant is then confirmed to be in the proper position both by manual and by visual inspection. At this point, the 2-0 silk guide sutures can be safely removed.

The anterior projection of the implant is confirmed to be adequate before continuing. The surgeon should factor in the added projection caused by the local anesthesia and edema that arises from surgical manipu-

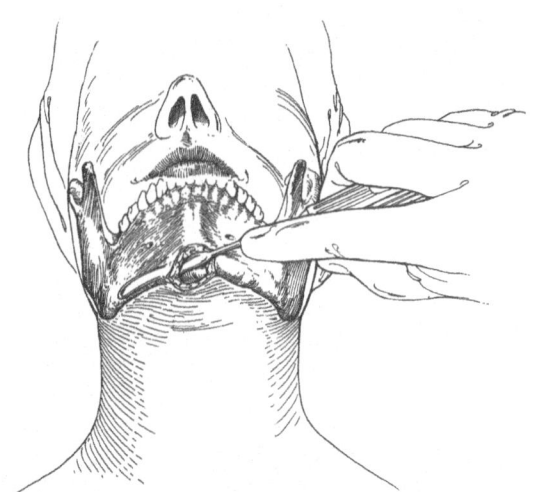

Fig. 32.4 A Joseph elevator is used to elevate the lateral subperiosteal pockets

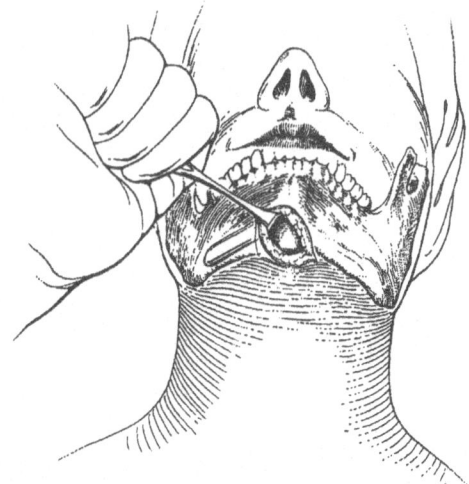

Fig. 32.5 After creation of the lateral pocket an Aufricht retractor is inserted, which ensures the pocket is of adequate size and allows for placement of the implant under the retractor

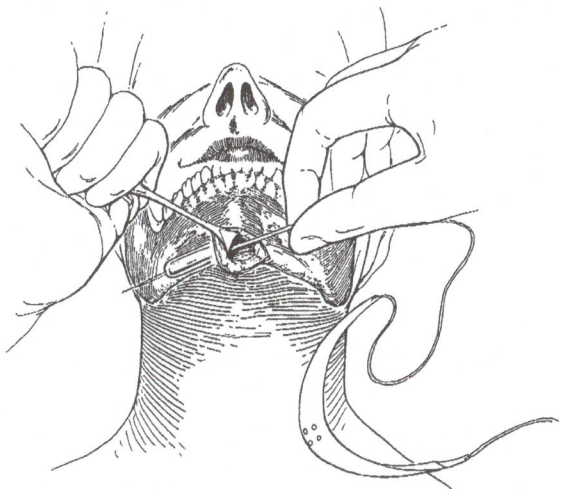

Fig. 32.6 The implant is inserted by passing the Keith needle attached to the implant out through the lateral aspect of the pocket aiming toward the angle of the mandible. The suture is gently pulled to guide placement as the implant is inserted into the pocket

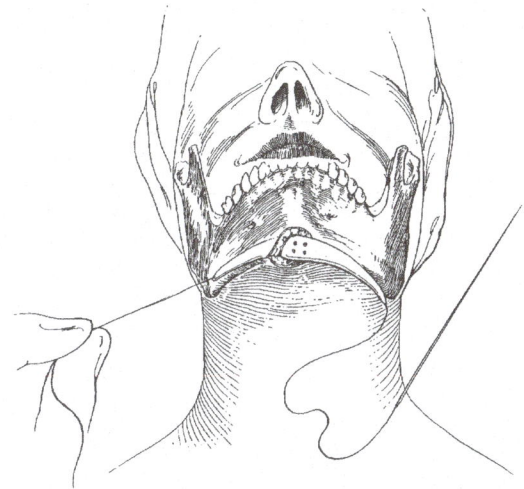

Fig. 32.7 Traction is maintained on the implant to hold it in the pocket while the contralateral side of the implant is placed

lation. The patient's supine position retrodisplaces the jaw and offsets these factors, making the chin appear underprojected. To more accurately judge the degree of augmentation the surgeon should hold the chin forward so that the teeth are in good occlusion during the intraoperative assessment. If the projection imparted by the implant appears to be less than adequate, a silastic wafer (Glasgold Wafer™) that occupies the central mentum can be inserted under the implant to deliver another 2 mm of added projection (Fig. 32.8). The wafer can then be sutured to the overlying implant with two 4-0 polydiaxanone sutures each situated approximately 1 cm from the midline.

Once proper position of the implant has been ensured and adequate projection achieved, the implant is sutured to the inferiorly based cuff of periosteum with a 4-0 polydiaxanone suture 1 cm lateral to the midline on each side. If an extension wafer is used, the implant and the wafer are sutured to the periosteum with the 4-0 polydiaxanone suture. The muscle is closed over the implant with a buried 4-0 polydiaxanone suture. The subcutaneous tissue is then approximated with a few 4-0 polydiaxanone sutures before skin closure with a running 6-0 polypropylene suture.

If a mentoplasty alone is performed, no supportive bandages are required. The patient is discharged after appropriate monitoring and is followed up for removal of skin sutures on the seventh postoperative day. The patient is also placed on prophylactic oral antibiotics, cefadroxyl, or clindamycin for 10 days. Larger implant sizes tend to be associated with a greater degree of postoperative discomfort, which may require narcotic analgesic medications.

32.2.4
Complications

Complications consist of infection, displacement, asymmetry, overcorrection or undercorrection, anesthesia due to mental-nerve injury, motor nerve damage to the marginal mandibular branch of the facial nerve, and mandibular erosion by the implant. Infection remains a relatively rare complication and can occur in the immediate postoperative period or even many months to years after implantation. An infection is typically accompanied by increasing pain, tenderness, and swelling

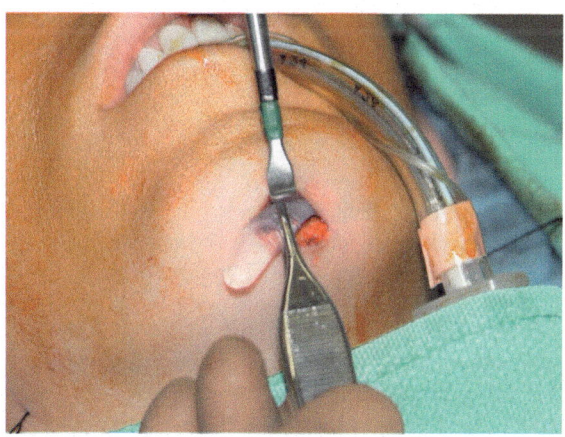

Fig. 32.8 The implant is already in place but additional projection was required in this patient. The retractor is placed under and holds up the extended anatomical implant allowing the extension wafer to be placed under its central aspect

that should be managed with aggressive and early intervention with a broad-spectrum oral antibiotic regimen. If the condition fails this kind of therapy, the implant should be electively removed and reinsertion delayed for 6–12 months in order to allow resolution of edema and the extent of fibrosis and scar to dictate implant resizing.

If the mentum appears to be overcorrected, it is better to wait a minimum of 3 months to observe dissipation of most of the edema before deciding on reoperation. If the size of the mentum appears undercorrected, an extension wafer can be easily inserted under the principal implant as an office procedure to achieve adequate projection.

Asymmetry is most often due to preoperative presence of this condition, a fact that should be carefully evaluated and pointed out to the patient prior to surgery. Use of the submental approach permits wider exposure and periosteal fixation of the implant that should limit the likelihood of this outcome.

Anesthesia and/or paresthesia result most often from excessive traction of the mental nerves and will most likely resolve over a period of several weeks to months. Permanent anesthesia would indicate a more definitive lysis of neural continuity. Similarly, neuropraxia of the marginal mandibular nerve can arise from overzealous traction of the nerve that is most often self-limiting.

Finally, mandibular resorption has been reported with chin implants but oftentimes remains a subclinical radiographic entity. Placement of the implant along the more durable cortical bone that prevails along the inferior aspect of the anterior mandibular face can limit this complication. No conclusive data have revealed any difference in the extent of bony resorption with either subperiosteal or supraperiosteal implant insertion.

32.3
Malar Augmentation

32.3.1
Patient Evaluation

Malar augmentation can play a substantial role in facial enhancement and rejuvenation. Although a chin implant is a relatively safe and reliable procedure in all age groups, cheek implants may be less desirable in the aging face for the reasons enumerated in Chap. 30. Even a younger individual with a relatively thin soft-tissue envelope may predispose toward visibility of the implant either shortly after surgery or in a delayed fashion thereafter. The decision whether to combine fat grafting with solid implantation versus either modality alone was thoroughly discussed in Chap. 30, and the reader is referred there for a more in-depth discussion.

An easy method of analysis for the central third of the face is division of the midface into three principal subcomponents: the superolateral cheek consisting of

the lateral infraorbital region and zygomatic arch, the submalar region inferior to the zygomatic arch, and the anterior cheek where a depression along the malar septum often becomes apparent with midfacial volume loss. A patient who presents with a deficient zygomatic arch or desires "high cheekbones" would benefit from a more superiorly positioned implant (Fig. 32.9). The patient who has some deficit in the submalar/buccal region may be effectively improved by placement of the implant more inferiorly along this depression. For individuals with have a malar depression in the anterior cheek, an implant can be situated for optimal soft-tissue gain. Finally, any combination of these deficiencies may be present that would mandate larger implants that span any or all of these midfacial territories.

32.3.2
Implant Selection

Many configurations of malar implants exist and can serve as reliable alloplasts for midfacial augmentation. The authors have had extensive clinical experience and success with the Binder submalar implant both for the specified submalar region as well as for placement more superiorly across the zygomatic arch. If the implant is intended to span a wider distance across the upper and lower margins of the midface, then the Binder submalar II implant has proven to be an ideal choice given its more expansive superoinferior dimension. Alternatively, the Terino Shell can serve as a suitable implant in these circumstances. Although preoperative asymmetry should be noted and brought to the attention of the patient, it is only rarely that a different-sized implant for each side of the face is required to correct this problem.

32.3.3
Technique

Preoperatively with the patient sitting upright skin markings are made to delineate the desired area of augmentation from the implant.. The position of the implant should be planned so that the superior extent sits just below the infraorbital nerve, the lateral tail extends over the zygomatic arch, and the body or central bulk of the implant fills the anterior cheek malar depression.

The infraorbital nerve is blocked with local anesthesia followed by direct infiltration of local anesthesia into the gingivobuccal sulcus bilaterally. The oral cavity can be gently washed with additional povidone–iodine solution for a reduction in contaminative oral flora along with prophylactic intravenous cefazolin followed by a 10-day course of an oral equivalent antibiotic. The medial aspect of each gingivobuccal incision is scored with an abbreviated cautery mark, and symmetry of the marks is confirmed. The implants should also be bathed in an antibiotic solution before insertion, and the dis-

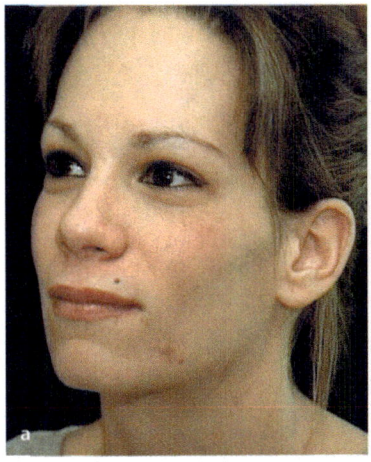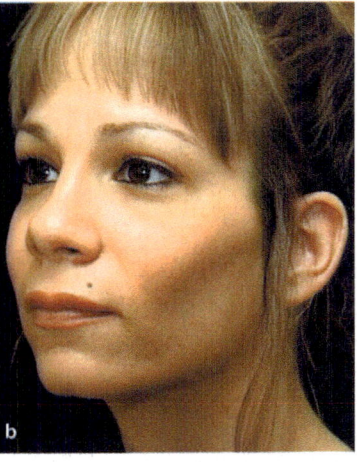

Fig. 32.9 a Preoperatively. **b** Postoperatively following malar augmentation with a Conform Binder Submalar implant (Implantech). The implant created not only a more full anterior cheek but also a more defined zygomatic arch

sected soft-tissue pocket can be irrigated with the same antibiotic solution after implant insertion.

The electrocautery is used to enter the gingivobuccal incision approximately 1.5 cm above the sulcus, leaving an additional cuff of soft tissue before entry into the subperiosteal plane. The remaining dissection is carried out with a Joseph elevator or other periosteal elevator to lift the remaining periosteum toward the zygomatic arch. Using a Binder submalar implant requires a narrow lateral pocket over (or just below) the zygomatic arch in which the implant can be more firmly positioned. For submalar or low placement, dissection is undertaken immediately more vertically before turning laterally toward the zygomatic arch (or just below it). If vertical dissection is initiated, care must be taken to avoid disruption of the superomedially situated infraorbital-nerve bundle. The aforementioned narrow lateral pocket provides a more snug fit for the implant into which the implant is inserted under direct visualization with an Aufricht or Converse retractor and a straight clamp as a guide. The contralateral side is completed in the same manner, and symmetry is verified both visually and manually before closure of the gingivobuccal incision with a 4-0 chromic suture.

32.3.4
Complications

Complications after malarplasty are almost identical to the kinds enumerated for mentoplasty. Infection can arise and mandate implant removal if the patient fails an antibiotic course. Owing to edema, implant symmetry may be the hardest aspect to ensure accurately. In most cases, minor asymmetries go undetected, and preoperative asymmetries should be called to the patient's attention before surgery. The incidence of infection, although low, is higher than that seen with chin implants. This is in part attributable to the intraoral incision. As with chin implants, postoperative infection can occur shortly after the procedure or may manifest months to years later. Management of infection is identical to that described for postmentoplasty infection. Despite these limited complications, malarplasty remains a safe and viable method for midfacial augmentation in the proper patient candidate.

32.5
Conclusion

Alloplasts provide a stable and definitive degree of facial enhancement that does not dissipate with time. Their main drawbacks include the risks associated with synthetic materials like infection, displacement, extrusion, and asymmetry, not to mention cost of the material. Autologous fat transfer can be undertaken to provide facial contouring and does not suffer from the limitations of alloplastic materials. However, fat absorption over time is variable owing to fat-cell survival and dissipation with aging. Careful preoperative judgment and patient counsel should inform every case and help determine the best course of intervention in a given situation.

Part V
Suture Lifts

The History of Barbed Suture Suspension: Applications, and Visions for the Future

33

Donald W. Kress

33.1
Introduction

The ancient Egyptians probably were the first to use embedded sutures to enhance facial appearance. There are references to gold threads placed beneath the facial skin. Some even believe that gold threads were responsible for the beauty of Cleopatra [1]. The mechanism and action of these threads is unknown. In the Orient gold needles and threads were placed beneath the skin either in conjunction with acupuncture or to enhance the "aura." They were sometimes referred to as "charm." In Russia gold threads were placed beneath the surface of the skin to create scarring and tightening of the facial tissues. This has had a renewed popularity in Russia, Japan, Spain, Yugoslavia, and France. Gold threads are most often placed in parallel lines or in a grid pattern. As a mild inflammatory reaction occurs, collagen is deposited around the threads, and when it matures it will contract slightly, giving the desired facial enhancement.

A contemporary modification of this system incorporates an absorbable polyglycol suture with the gold thread [2]. These are also placed in a grid pattern. The polyglycol component stimulates a more powerful inflammatory reaction that in turn increases the lifting or contraction of the overlying facial tissues. Adamyan [3, 4] (Moscow) obtained a US patent in July of 2000 for a "Method of skin rejuvenation" that describes a subdermal placement of gold threads in conjunction with absorbable polyglycol threads for rejuvenation of cheeks, chin, periorbital area, arms, and/or thighs.

The use of smooth sutures to shift facial tissues is extensive. These sutures are primarily used to shift the position of the malar fat pad, the jowls, or for elevation of the brow. In most cases the effects are powerful but short-lived because of the "cheese-wiring" which occurs as the loop of the suture cuts through the supporting tissues. As the suture cuts through the tissues, the effects are gradually lost. A wide variety of deployment methods exist but generally they are used to lift or "loop" either muscular units or fat pads [5–9].

Support of the repositioned tissues with easily implantable materials if the "cheese-wiring" could be eliminated would offer significant advantages. The barbed sutures, which support tissues along their entire length

instead of just the crotch of the loop, hold great promise.

Some of the most significant contributors to this field of barbed suture suspension are reviewed with their inspirations, progression of thinking, techniques at the time of publication, and projections for the future where possible.

33.2
J.H. Alcamo

Alcamo (Camden and Newark, NJ, USA) was a general surgeon and inventor who first filed a patent for barbed sutures in August of 1956 [10]. He received approval in 1964 for what is probably the first US patent which actually describes a "thread" with a roughened or barbed surface [7]. In his patent application, he described the use of his threads, "so formed that it prevents slippage in sutured incisions or wounds…." He further indicated that for holding power the "suture may also be sinuous." His sutures were barbed and unidirectional (Fig. 33.1). There is no evidence that they were ever manufactured or utilized. He had previously developed and patented a sewing machine device for mechanically inserting threads [11].

33.3
H.J. Buncke

Buncke (Hillsborough, CA, USA) (Fig. 33.2), internationally known as the father of modern microsurgery, probably has the next patent "Surgical methods using one-way suture" [12] (Fig. 33.3), which he filed in May of 1997 and for which he received approval in August 1999. In his patent application, he describes various designs of unidirectional and bidirectional sutures, their manufacture, and their deployment. He indicated they would have advantage in general wound closure, tendon repair, and other internal tissue repairs. He may have been the first to recognize the potential for "face-lifts and other cosmetic operations, where the sutures would provide lines of tissue support beneath the skin." His very elegant patent describes different suture de-

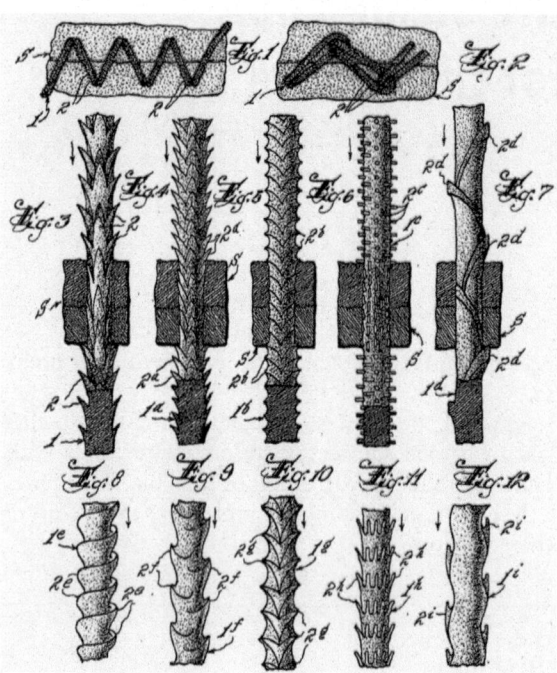

Fig. 33.1 Example of sutures from Alcamo [10]

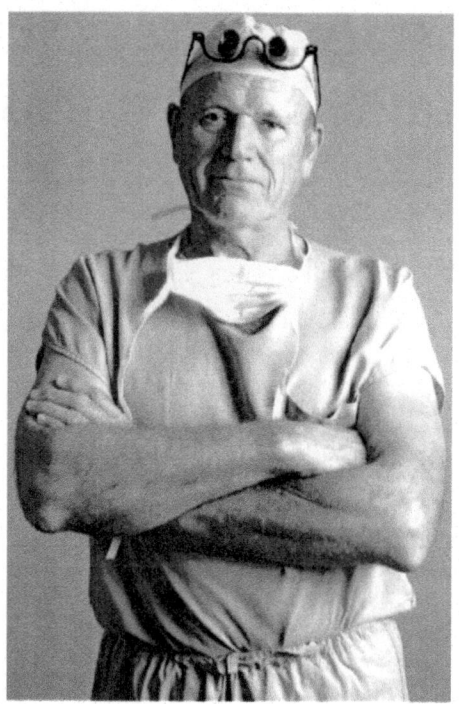

Fig. 33.2 H.J. Buncke (Hillsborough, CA, USA)

signs, methods of deployment, and even proposes manufacturing techniques.

His first interest in the holding power of barbs probably dates to 1945 in the submarine service when he became curious about the structure of sea urchin spines, and again with "stick-tights" which attached to his clothes after hiking in the Sierra mountains. After doing some experimentation with homemade barbed suture material, he considered it a triumph when he was able to swing around a chicken leg held only with a single pass of his barbed sutures passed through the meat of the leg. His patents were acquired by the Quill™ Corporation in 2002 and he is now a member of their Medical Advisory Board.

33.4
N.G. Isse

Isse (Burbank, CA, USA) (Fig. 33.4) [13–16] was searching for a way to improve and simplify his extensive pioneering work with endoscopic procedures. In 2003, while participating in a plastic surgery meeting in Australia, he saw Wu present his work with barbed threads. Wu explained that he developed his thread design by modifying the designs of Sulamanidze (Russia) and his APTOS sutures. After extensive discussions with Wu, and detailed research into the APTOS threads, Isse believed that he could improve on both of these designs by lengthening the sutures and using unidirectional barbs.

His first sutures were called the "Isse Endo Progressive Facelift Sutures". The sutures were 25 cm long with a 10-cm distal portion containing approximately 50 barbs and a 15-cm proximal portion that is smooth and easily fixated to the deep temporal fascia.

Isse, working with Kolster Methods Incorporated, tried several times to file patent applications but each time he had problems with the FDA defining the category of the patent. By defining the suture as a device, the FDA would have required extensive and prohibitively expensive clinical data for approval. His clinical trials started in September 2003. He began with four facial sutures and quickly advanced to six, eight, or ten sutures in men. His concern about the possibility of "cheese-wiring" in the temporal fascia caused him to add initially a reinforcement patch of Gore-Tex® and later Silastic beneath the knot in the temporal area.

Isse's original threads were placed through a hollow needle (20 gauge, 16 cm) in pairs from a small incision in the temple. The threads were positioned to reside in the malar fat pad, while the proximal ends were anchored in pairs over a small Silastic sheet in the temple. The threads were firmly anchored within the malar fat pad so that when traction was applied to the temporal ends, the soft tissue of the midface was lifted. This permits very precise control of the lift and when the desired lift is achieved, the sutures are tied over a Silastic patch in the temporal fascia. Tape is placed over the sutures for one full week to protect them and to discourage facial animation.

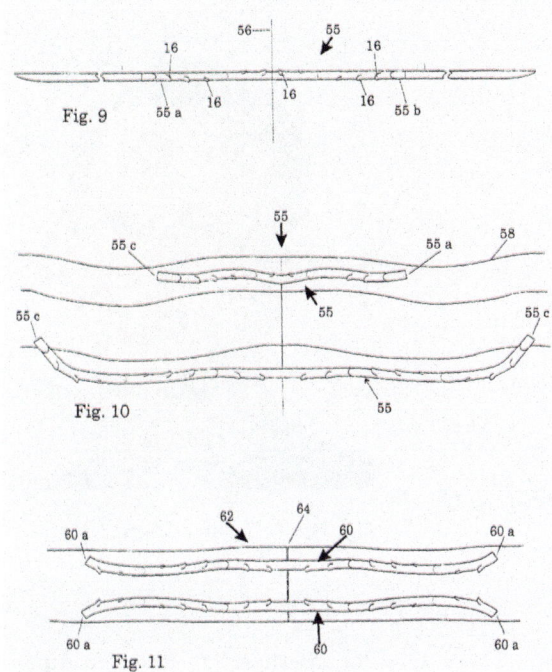

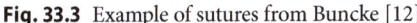

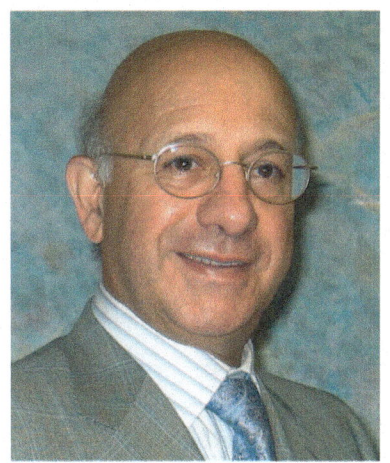

Fig. 33.3 Example of sutures from Buncke [12]

Fig. 33.4 N.G. Isse (Burbank, CA, USA)

The initial results were excellent and the patients were quite satisfied. In spite of this early success, relapse and patient disappointment came much earlier than anticipated. Isse was also dissatisfied that the results did not have the duration he desired. Many of his patients relapsed in as quickly as 6 months. Additionally, his early attempts (February 2005) at elevating the brow were not very successful. There was an unacceptably high incidence of thread breakage secondary to the powerful musculature of the forehead area.

As a former pathologist, Isse began analyzing the problems and addressing the fundamental issues. First, he looked at the tissue reaction to the suture material within the facial issues. Polypropylene, well known as one of the least reactive suture materials, does not elicit a strong inflammatory reaction. Without a strong inflammatory reaction, significant new collagen formation is minimal surrounding a polypropylene suture, and durability is compromised. Second, there still remains the possibility of "cheese-wiring" both at the anchoring knot in the fascia and at the interface of the barbs with the fatty tissues. Third, the materials themselves can be problematic. Polypropylene under the electron microscope appears as a collection of linear bundles. This potentially, over time and the stress of facial animation, predisposes the material to linear shredding of the suture at the cleavage plane where the barbs are cut into the suture. Fourth, the amount of relaxation of the threads for reduction of lift effect is surprisingly very small. By studying the movements of the face, Isse determined that the amount of elevation necessary to create a youthful malar area is only 5–7 mm. If the suture relaxes only 2.5 mm this would result in a 50% loss of the effect.

Taking all of these concerns into account, Isse redesigned his suture, which is pending FDA approved, to create a stronger suture with regularly spaced knots and small floating cones that he refers to as trumpets. This new suture is called the Silhouette Suture® (Figs. 33.5, 33.6). The tiny trumpets serve two very important functions. First, they offer a powerful increase in the holding power of the suture at the time of deployment and, second, they are made of a material that will absorb after 8 months. This absorption of the trumpets will produce

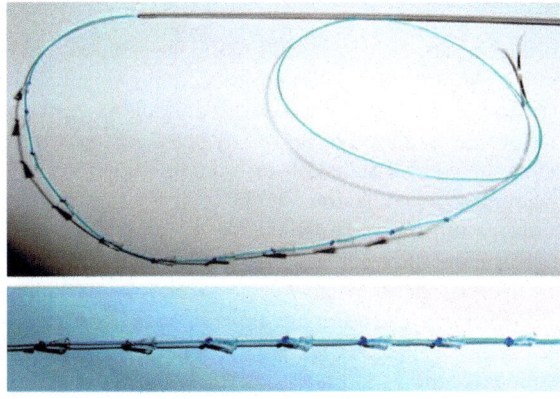

Fig. 33.5 Silhouette Suture by Isse showing knots and "trumpets"

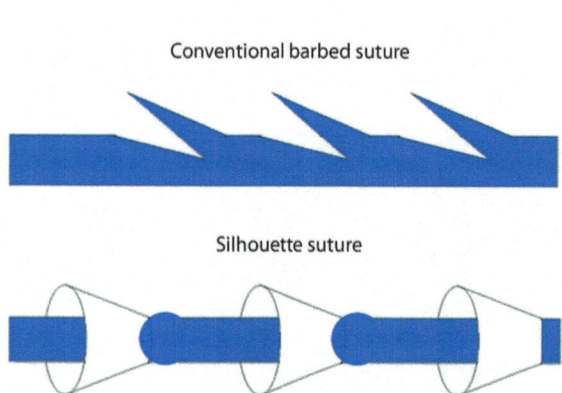

Fig. 33.6 Comparison of Silhouette Suture and barbed poly-propylene suture

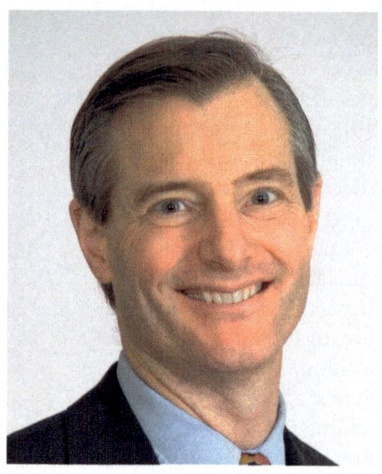

Fig. 33.7 G.L. Ruff (Durham, NC, USA)

an enhanced inflammatory response, an increase in the new collagen surrounding the knots and the threads, and improved longevity of the thread effects. Clinical trials with the new suture are under way, including trials with a heavier version of the Silhouette Suture®, for use on the body.

Isse believes that the ideal thread should last about twice as long as the current fillers and would consider a thread effect of 2 years a success. Even at 2 years, there is a possibility that they could be retightened for an extension of the lift effect. Future work needs to continue to address alternative suture materials, the tissue interface, and deployment methods that are more efficacious.

As his clinical trials continue, Isse will be planning instructional courses which would include lectures, cadaver laboratories, and demonstrations of his technique.

33.5
G.L. Ruff

Ruff (Durham, NC, USA) (Fig. 33.7) was able to draw on his old boy scout days and his undergraduate zoology degree when he was faced with difficult reconstructive problems as a Duke University plastic surgeon. He remembered his fascination with the holding power of the porcupine quills and sought to apply these same concepts to surgical situations. As a lecturer at Duke he was constantly pointing out the hazards of the tissue necrosis that inevitably occurs with knotted loops and tensioned sutures. In an effort to avoid this necrosis, he began to investigate the possibility of cutting barbs into sutures to lift tissues. This would distribute the holding power along the length of the suture and eliminate necrosis at the knot. His first attempts were done in his garage using weed whacker cord into which he manually cut notches or barbs. He also developed

a thin brass tube for inserting this cord and experimented with the holding power of the thread when it was placed in steak. Satisfied with his early trials, he moved on to surgical sutures, which he also had to cut by hand in his garage.

The first clinical test of his new suture using polydioxanone was on a female patient with severe traumatic ectropion. She had been repeatedly repaired with grafting but the ectropion recurred every time. Ruff placed several loop sutures with barbs near the lateral canthus with success.

Ruff eventually went to the Duke University administration and asked to be able to continue this research into sutures on his own. Ultimately, Duke relinquished all rights to the barbed sutures and Ruff resigned his faculty appointment to go into private practice and spend more time developing this new technology.

In June of 2001, he received the first of many patents describing barbed sutures, an inserting device, and several design variations (Fig. 33.8) [17, 18]. He also formed Quill Medical®, a company which would organize ongoing research and control the patents.

Using his first version of the threads, all handmade, Ruff operated on his first 40 patients. This first design

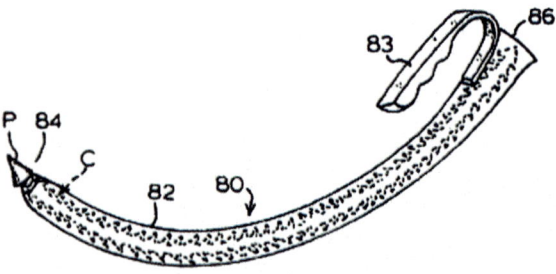

Fig. 33.8 Barbed suture with inserting device from Ruff [18]

was made of polydioxanone, with two straight needles, and bidirectional barbs. One needle deployed a barbed segment of the thread into the scalp to serve as the anchor, while the second needle deployed a longer section of the thread into the facial soft tissues for the lift effect. The preliminary results were good but the gains dissipated rapidly, usually after only 3 months. This led to several revisions of the sutures, including the change to a permanent suture with shallower barbs and different placement techniques. Encouraged by his improved success, Ruff embarked on a systematic and extensive investigation of barb geometry, design, density, and position. He also investigated different placement techniques and suture materials. The strength of the lift, holding power, duration of result, and predictability all improved. One unexpected finding was that placement of the threads in a serpentine manner quadrupled their holding power (first recommended by Alcamo).

In 2003, Quill Medical® signed contracts with Surgical Specialties Corporation to produce and market the sutures under the name Contour Threads™. They made an application to the FDA for approval and because of the similarity to the Endotine™ anchoring system they were given their US FDA clearance in September 2004.

The initial design of Contour Threads™ (Fig. 33.9) is 25-cm 2-0 polypropylene with the barbs in the middle 10 cm. On one end there is a short half-circle anchoring needle and on the other a taperpoint 7-in. straight deployment needle. The sutures are utilized by making a small incision in the scalp, temple or mastoid areas, and the insertion needle is then passed distally in a serpentine manner to below the brow, short of the nasolabial folds, or to just short of the neck midline (Fig. 33.10). These sutures are advanced until the last barbs disappear into the proximal incision. The sutures are then anchored in pairs in a U shape to the deeper fascia of the area. The skin is finally repositioned symmetrically by holding the distal ends and lifting the skin over the sutures, causing the barbs to deploy.

Postoperative instructions include restricted facial animation with or without taping and elevation of the head at night for the first 2 weeks. Complications can include nerve injury, breakage or migration of the suture, infection, bruising, or surface irregularities such as dimpling or grooving. Sometimes, these surface irregularities have been caused by too superficial placement of the sutures. With accurate placement in the subcutaneous fat, small grooves and depressions will resolve within 3 days and the bunching of the skin seen in the posterior neck and temple areas will resolve within 3 weeks.

A more recent version of the Contour Threads™ called "Articulus™" (Fig. 33.11) combines the benefits of two sutures into one. It has two very thin 7-in. straight needles at opposite ends of a 55-cm loop with opposing barbs. This has the advantage of eliminating the need for tying an anchor knot, reduces the number of entry sites to one, and shortens the time of the procedure. The two needles are passed serpentine in the same manner

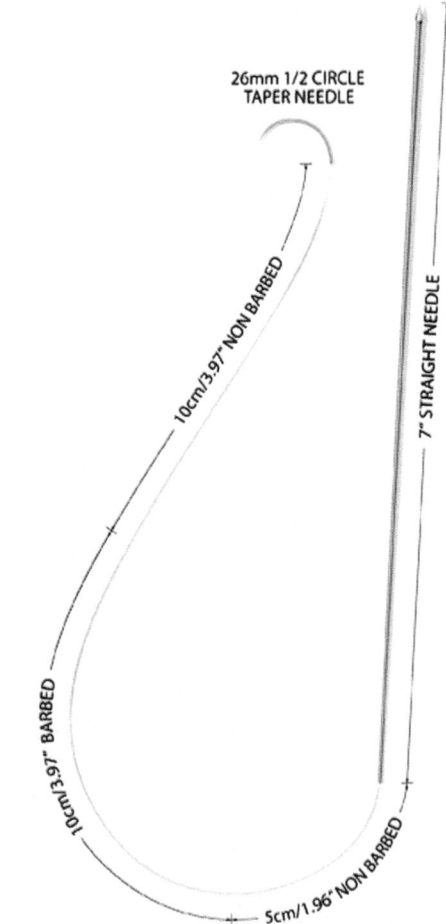

Fig. 33.9 First US FDA-approved Contour Suture. Twenty-five centimeter 2-0 polypropylene with barbs cut in the middle 10 cm

as the original Contour Threads™ but through the same entry site. The clear (non-barbed) central section is reinforced with a Gore-Tex® pledget and takes the place of the breakage- and exposure-prone knot. Combination of this with gentle undermining of the tissues adjacent to the sutures extends the duration of effect along with an anticipated reduction of complications.

Ruff still feels that more work can be done on optimizing the design and geometry of the barbs, on developing new and improved suture materials, and in alternative deployment methods with maximum effectiveness and minimal trauma. He believes a realistic goal for barbed sutures would be a consistent 2-year period of benefit, ideally with an absorbable suture material.

Future applications are already under way with ongoing research into wound closure, breast and body contouring, and tendon repairs. Preliminary work on tendon repair yielded an impressive gain in strength of 8 times a conventional repair using only four threads within the tendon.

Physicians interested in utilizing Contour Threads™ are now required by the FDA to attend a company-su-

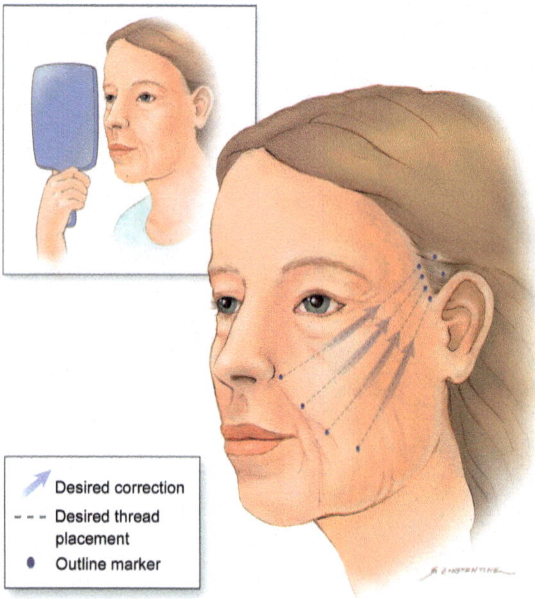

Fig. 33.10 Example of the deployment of the Contour Suture

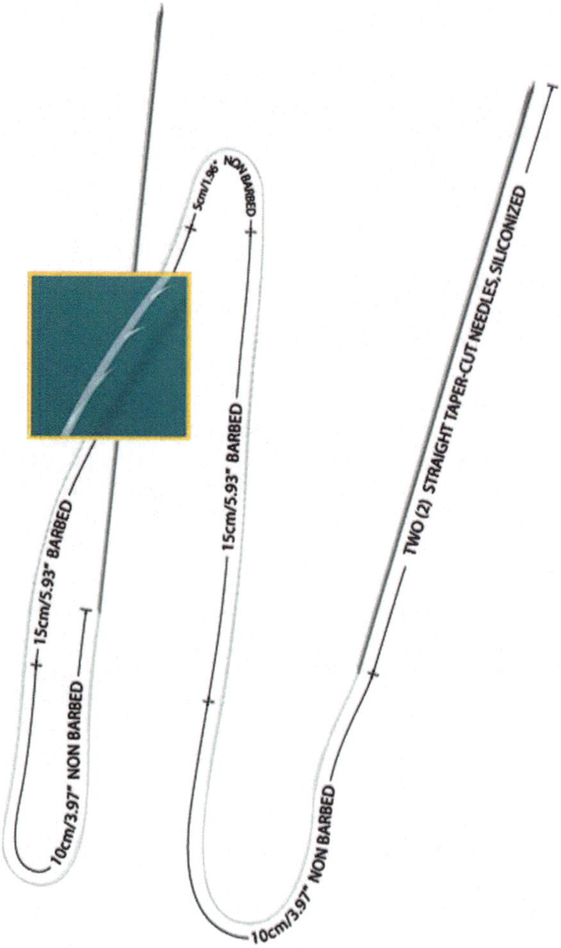

Fig. 33.11 Articulus suture from Contour with two thin 7-in. straight needles, 55-cm loop with opposing barbs, and 5-cm smooth gap

pervised, full-day seminar with didactic sessions, and live surgery demonstrations. Some of the courses also include a cadaver laboratory for hands-on experience.

33.6
M.A. Sulamanidze

Sulamanidze (Moscow, Russia) (Fig. 33.12) [19, 20] recounts that in about 1975 he began searching for new ways of lifting and elevating facial skin which were less invasive and less traumatic than the conventional subcutaneous muscular aponeurotic system procedures. In 1997, he read articles in a newspaper that the French were using small gold threads to reposition facial tissues. While investigating these threads, he developed the idea that they could be made more effective if there were small "cogs" or barbs cut into the sides to increase their holding power. Like all of the other pioneers, he

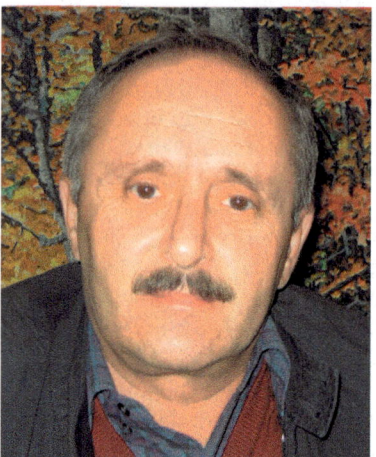

Fig. 33.12 M.A. Sulamanidze (Moscow, Russia)

began cutting the threads himself until he found a pattern which he was happy with. His first patents were through Geneva in 1999 [21–24] and in mid-2000 he began publishing articles about his thread lifts. His papers immediately attracted a lot of attention from European surgeons who visited him in Moscow to learn his technique. His first suture design incorporated monodirectional Prolene and was anchored in the temporal fascia. He quickly became dissatisfied with this design and the poor duration of the effect. He believed that the suture design was not able to hold enough barbs to counteract the powerful muscles of facial animation, particularly when one of the ends was anchored.

His second design combined two unidirectional sutures that were tied together in the midcheek area. This provided some improvement without the fixed anchor but he abandoned this design because of dissatisfaction with the visible incision in the midcheek. Finally, he designed a short bidirectional suture made of 2-0 polypropylene and named it APTOS (Fig. 33.13).

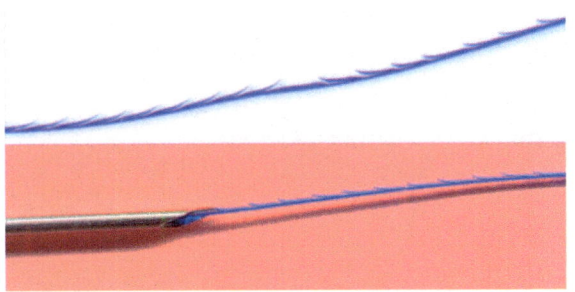

Fig. 33.13 APTOS suture with spinal insertion needle

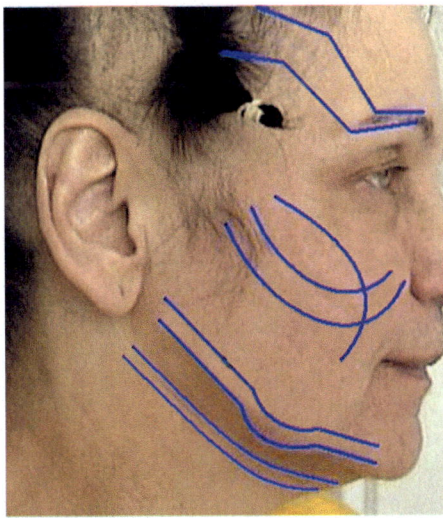

Fig. 33.14 Recommended pattern for APTOS markings

Marking for the APTOS threads is especially important for the line of the introducer (Fig. 33.14). The threads are deployed in curves similar to the lines of aging in the face. The tissues need to be put under aggressive tension for the threads to engage and create the lift effect perpendicular to the line of the introducer. An 18-gauge spinal needle is used in the fatty tissues following the deployment marks and a bidirectional cogged thread (8.5 cm) is carefully introduced into the needle. The tissues to be elevated are compressed manually, the thread centered, and the introducer removed. When the tissue compression is released, the barbs engage and support the elevated tissues. Finally, the exposed ends are trimmed. It is important that the APTOS suture is centered, since an imbalance in the number of cogs on either side of the midpoint can result in late thread migration.

The APTOS suture is most effective in the cheek area with its reduced animation and weak muscle action. It is widely used throughout the world and pirated versions are now being made in Argentina, Korea, China, Romania, and France.

Dissatisfaction with the regular effects of the APTOS threads along the jawline, and the intention to better improve the jowls, led Sulamanidze to develop a completely new product which is called the APTOS Spring® (Fig. 33.15). This product is made of smooth coiled polypropylene which retains its memory and will give lift to the jowls and improve the jawline. Instead of resisting the powerful muscle action in the jaw area, this suture moves with the muscle and continues to provide lift and support to the overlying tissues.

Another of Sulamanidze's innovations is a very long APTOS suture with a unique needle called the APTOS Needle® (Fig. 33.16). Because of this double-ended needle design, the suture can be advanced and directed without having to remove and reinsert the needle. This has the obvious advantage of avoiding the dimples which frequently occur when trying to replace a needle in the exactly the same hole it was removed from. With this new technology Sulamanidze can lift the cheeks

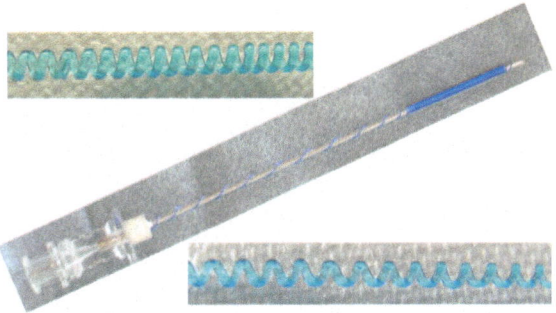

Fig. 33.15 APTOS Spring, usually deployed in very mobile tissues such as the mandibular line

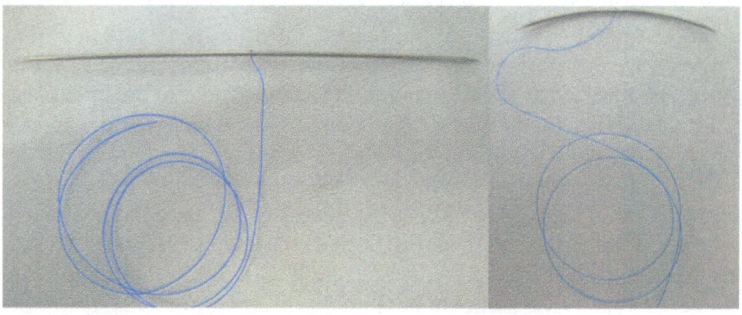

Fig. 33.16 APTOS Needle, used to advance suture without completely removing from the skin

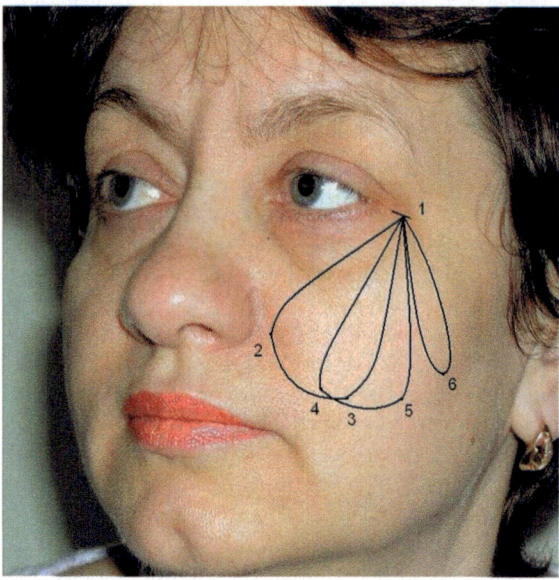

Fig. 33.17 APTOS Needle deployment used for lifting the cheek and midface

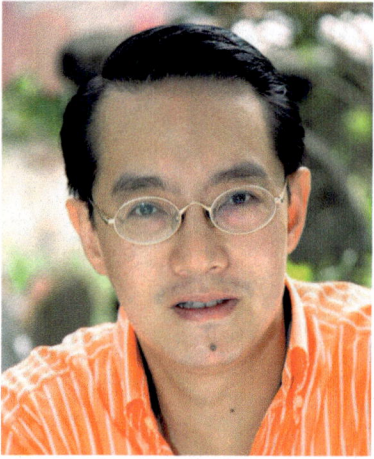

Fig. 33.18 W.T.L. Wu (Singapore)

with two or three loops from a small lateral canthal incision (Fig. 33.17), elevate the neck with multiple passes back and forth across the neck, change the shape of the nose or chin, and elevate moderate breast ptosis. The results of his latest innovation are still new but are quite effective.

Sulamanidze believes that improved material, newer designs, and innovative deployment methods are all important for the future. Training is limited to preceptor courses in Prague and Moscow, although Sulamanidze lectures extensively all over the world.

33.7
W.T.L. Wu

Wu (Singapore) (Fig. 33.18) [25] is a craniofacial surgeon practicing in Singapore. He relates that one of his first experiences with facial rejuvenation came from watching one of the household servants when he was a youth. She wore her hair in a very tight bun and by carefully adjusting her hair, she was able to create an ef-

fective facelift. Later, as a plastic surgeon, he maintained his fascination with simple, minimally invasive methods of facial rejuvenation.

In 2001, after seeing some of the early work by Sulamanidze, he purchased some early APTOS sutures and began to utilize them in his practice. He believed that they were too fine and too easily broken for his purposes. By combining the ideas of Des Fernandes (Capetown, South Africa) and the APTOS suture, he developed his first design. It consisted of a 60-cm length of 2-0 Prolene with two long barbed sections each 20 cm and a 4-cm clear section for the bend. Initial clinical experience with this suture was very successful and he began giving lectures internationally. He called the suture "Woptos Lift" out of respect for APTOS and Sulamanidze. Later Sulamanidze asked him not to use that name and it became simply the Woffles Lift. When presenting in Sydney in 2003, Wu was approached by Isse, who questioned him extensively about his results. Isse also reviewed ideas he had for his own design of barbed sutures. By 2004, Isse had already begun trials on his own version of barbed suture.

The marking procedure and the choice of vectors are critical to all of the versions of the Woffles Lift. Integral to all versions is the suspension of sagging facial tissues to the dense taut tissues of the temporal scalp. In version 1.0 both ends of the long suture are inserted from distal to proximal by using a long 18-gauge needle. The proximal end must be well into the temporal scalp for maximum effect. The loop must be in the clear section and no knots are required when the two free ends are tensioned to lift the tissues. In version 2.0 the "V" is inverted with the free ends in the face. Wu has identified six key facial suspension points for a smooth lift of the face and jawline.

Wu has gone through several iterations searching for continuous improvement. His principal concern is in the duration of the thread lift effect. The weakest point of the suture is the clear section in the bend. This area can still "cheese-wire" through the tissues and weaken the effect. One of his most recent innovations is called the "Version 3.0 X, the Woffles X-lift" (Fig. 33.19). This version takes the problem of the cheese wiring and turns it into an asset. It combines version 1.0 and version 2.0 by interlinking the loops. The sutures are unable to cut through each other and it eliminates completely the risk of "cheese-wiring" by the sutures supporting each other.

Wu believes future improvements will come with stiffer suture materials and better barb designs. He feels we have just begun to explore all the possible applications of threads that would include body lifts, abdominoplasty, breast-lifting, and many open uses. He feels the key to the success of barbed suture lifts is the reduced invasiveness of these procedures. Increased convenience with reduced complications will translate into improved patient satisfaction.

Presently, other than infrequent seminars for small groups, the only way to learn his techniques is to visit his clinic in Singapore.

33.8 Postscript

The old adage that "those who fail to understand history are condemned to repeat it" is still true. It is helpful to all of us to review the thinking, the successes, and the failures of the pioneers of any new procedure. The best and most effective ideas may not have been developed yet. Clearly, our patients are demanding less invasive procedures with effective results. The field of barbed suture suspension can go a long way toward meeting their expectations. The work has barely begun and already we have encouraging results on many fronts.

33.9 Glossary

Adamyan, A.A. Russian plastic surgeon now known as the father of the modern gold thread lifts.

Alcamo, J.H. New Jerseyan general surgeon with the first patent for barbed sutures.

APTOS Needle® An innovative invention of Sulamanidze which permits lifting of large areas such as the cheeks, breast, and abdomen by permitting much easier advancement of a very long APTOS suture.

APTOS Spring® Another innovation by Sulamanidze which consists of a smooth coiled polypropylene suture which is inserted parallel to the jawline for support and lifting of the jowls. By having coils, it is able to adjust to the increased movement and continue to exert its lifting effect.

APTOS threads Sulamanidze's original thread, bidirectional barbs, short thread, needs to be deployed in loops through a hollow needle. After placement in the insertion needle, the tissues are compressed and the needle removed, engaging the barbs of the APTOS suture.

Articulus 400™ Version of Contour Threads™ with two thin straight deployment needles and a large loop with bidirectional barbs and a small central clear area for the bend.

Baramendi, Jose Antonio Encinas Brazilian plastic surgeon and inventor.

Baramendi Sutures Cast version of the APTOS suture which is deployed the same way as the APTOS suture but because the barbs are cast and cannot fold down, the insertion needle requires a much larger diameter.

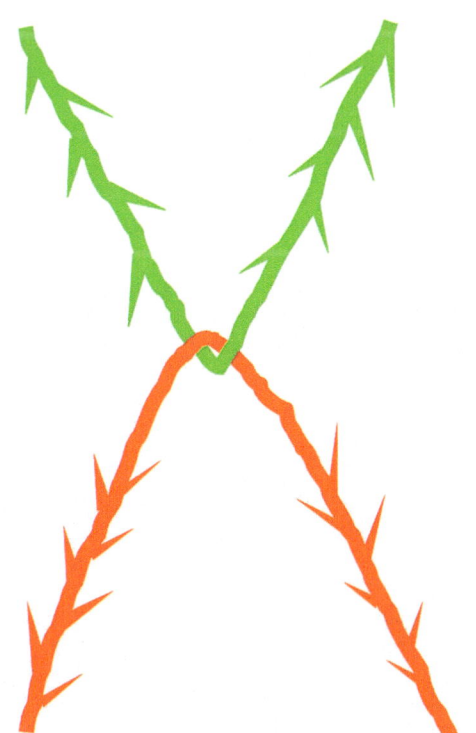

Fig. 33.19 Version 3 Woffles X-lift

Buncke, H.J. Thread inventor and early patent holder; his patents are now owned by Quill Medical®.

Charm Gold needles used in the orient for enhancement of the aura or for acupuncture.

Contour Threads™ Barbed polypropylene suture with a short curved needle on one end for anchorage and a long straight needle on the other end for deployment.

Featherlift™ Market name for the use of the APTOS Russian thread.

Featherlift Extended APTOS thread Isse's early thread design utilizing a longer version of the APTOS suture with unidirectional barbs. It is deployed by passing it into the tissues and then anchoring it to the temporal fascia over a graft.

Isse Endo Progressive Facelift Sutures Early type of unidirectional suture with strong temporal anchorage.

Isse, N. Thread inventor and innovator, Pasadena, CA, USA.

Kolster Methods Incorporated A manufacturer of suture materials (Corona, CA, USA).

Mulholland, R.S. Torontonian plastic surgeon, innovator, and instructor in thread usage.

Quill Medical® The parent company of Ruff that holds the patents for Contour Threads™.

Ruff, G.L. North Carolinan plastic surgeon, inventor, formerly Duke professor.

Silhouette Suture® More modern version of Isse's threads. This suture is a smooth suture with knots and small absorbable "trumpets" to enhance inflammatory response.

Sulamanidze, M. Russian plastic surgeon and inventor.

Surgical Specialties A Pennsylvanian corporation specializing in precision surgical products that has contracts to market and manufacture the Contour Threads™.

Thread Lift™ A company formed by Mulholland to teach various thread-lifting techniques.

Woffles Lift The name used for the non-surgical facelift effect using barbed suture slings. It currently exists in three versions: version 1.0, version 2.0, and version 3.0X.

Woffles Thread A very long bidirectional suture placed through a long hollow needle and then passed again to make a sling.

Woptos sutures An early name for Wu's extended APTOS sutures.

Wu, W.T.L. Singaporean craniofacial surgeon and inventor.

References

1. Connell R. A Golden Stitch In Time Saves Nine Years of Aging. Mainichi Newspapers. http://mdn.mainichi-msn.co.jp/waiwai/archive/news/2005/07/20050706p2g00m0dm019000c.html, 2005
2. Anonymous. Another Demystification Gold-Face. Aesthet News. http://www.gesaps.de/en/Gold-Face.htm, 2005
3. Andamyan AA. Clinical aspects of facial skin reinforcement with special (gold) surgical filaments. Ann Plast Reconstr Aesthet Surg 1998;3:18–22
4. Andamyan AA. Method for skin rejuvenation. US Patent 6,086,578, 2000
5. DeCordier BC, Vasconez LO. Rejuvenation of the midface by elevating the malar fat pad: review of technique cases and complications. Plast Reconstr Surg 2002;110:1526–1536
6. Graziosi AC, Beer SMC. Browlifting with thread: The technique without undermining using minimum incisions. Aesthet Plast Surg 1998;22:120–125
7. Yousif NJ, Matloub H, Summers AN. The midface sling: A new technique to rejuvenate the midface. Plast Reconstr Surg 2002;110:1541–1553
8. Little JW. Three-dimensional rejuvenation of the midface: Volumetric resculpture by malar imbrication. Plast Reconstr Surg. 2000;105(1):267–285
9. Sasaki GH, Cohen AT. Meloplication of the malar fat pads by percutaneous cable-suture technique for midface rejuvenation: outcome study. Plast Reconstr Surg. 2002;110:635–654
10. Alcamo JH. Surgical suture. US Patent 3,123,077, 1964
11. Alcamo JH. Surgeon's suturing device. US Patent 2,988,028, 1961
12. Buncke HJ. Surgical methods using one-way suture. US Patent 5,931,855, 1999
13. Isse NG. Endoscopic facial rejuvenation: endoforehead, the functional lift. Aesthet Plast Surg 1994;18(1):21–29
14. Isse NG. Endoscopic forehead lift, evolution and update. Clin Plast Surg 1995;22(4):661–673
15. Isse NG. Endoscopic facial rejuvenation. Clin Plast Surg. 1997;24(2):213–231
16. Isse NG. Barbed polypropylene sutures for midface elevation. Arch Facial Plast Surg 2005;7:55–61
17. Ruff GL. Insertion device for a barbed tissue connector. US Patent 5,342,376, 1994
18. Ruff GL. Barbed bodily tissue connector. US Patent 6,241,747B1, 2001
19. Sulamanidze MA, Sulamanidze GM. Facial lifting with "APTOS" Threads: Featherlift. Otolaryngol Clin N Am 2005;8(5):1109–1117
20. Sulamanidze MA, Fournier PF, Paikidze TG, Sulamanidze GM. Removal of facial soft tissue ptosis with special threads. Dermatol Surg. 2002;28:367–371
21. Sulamanidze MA. Surgical thread for cosmetic operations. Federal Institute of Industrial Property, Russia. Patent 2139734, 1999
22. Sulamanidze MA. Surgical thread for plastic surgical operations. WIPO Patent WO 2000/051658, 2000
23. Sulamanidze MA. Surgical thread "Aptos" for cosmetic surgery. WIPO Patent WO 2003/103733, 2003
24. Sulamanidze MA. Surgical thread "aptos" for cosmetic surgery. US Patent Appl 20050203576, 2005
25. Wu WTL. Barbed sutures in facial rejuvenation. Aesthet Surg J 2004;24:582–587

CHAPTER 34

Bidirectional, Non-anchored Suture Lifts

34

Samuel M. Lam

34.1
Introduction

Suture lifts have been recently introduced in the USA as an alternative to more invasive techniques for facial rejuvenation. As most trends have moved toward minimally invasive techniques, suture lifts have an undisputed charm. However, as with every new technology, long-term benefit and even short-term efficacy must be carefully evaluated to ascertain the validity and ultimately adoption of the technique into the established armamentarium of methods for facial rejuvenation.

Although there are many competing brands of suture lifts out there, they can be principally classified into three types: non-barbed sutures; bidirectionally barbed, non-anchored sutures; and unidirectionally barbed, anchored sutures. An example of a non-barbed suture is the percutaneous cheeklift that uses a 2-0 polypropylene suture to suspend the cheek, which is sutured superiorly to the temporalis fascia and looped through the malar fat pad inferiorly. The suture is placed through a single inferior skin entry point using Keith needles on either end of the suture, and the loop is buried in the malar fat pad using a temporary pull-out suture that draws the permanent polypropylene through the initial dermal attachments like a Gigli saw. A small expanded poly(tetrafluoroethylene) patch is attached at the base to prevent the suture from eventually cheese-wiring through the tissue.

This chapter will focus only on barbed or cogged sutures and specifically on the bidirectional barbed sutures that remain unanchored, as another chapter in this book is dedicated to unidirectional suture lifting. These bidirectional sutures were originally developed in Russia by Marlin Sulamanidze in 1996 with the appellation APTOS, standing for "antiptosis." The sutures have also been marketed as "Russian threads" and "Feather Lift" as opposed to "endo-APTOS" and "Contour Threadlift" or simply "Threadlift," which refer to the unidirectional variety that are anchored to a superior point of fixation. Like the percutaneous cheeklift, a 2-0 polypropylene suture is used. However, the suture itself is modified with a helical array of tiny cogs that are distributed along the length of each suture. The tiny cogs are fashioned oftentimes with precise laser technology

or old-fashioned hand dissection under magnification, with the latter technique possibly leading to inconsistent tensile strength and a predisposition toward undesirable breakage. The cogs act like little anchor points where the surrounding soft tissue is held in place in an elevated position.

In the unidirectional suture variety, the cogs are only distributed over one end of the suture, with the remaining portion barren of cogs. The cogged side is introduced into the tissue that requires elevation using either a spinal needle or an attached Keith needle. The barren side is tied down to tissue superiorly usually to a paired suture introduced in a similar fashion using an attached curved needle or a French-eye needle. The bidirectional sutures have almost the entire length of the suture covered with tiny cogs that face one direction along half the distance and the opposite direction along the other half. The facial zone that requires elevation is held up manually to the desired position, and a spinal needle is pierced through the skin to keep the tissue suspended in that position. The bidirectional suture is passed through the spinal needle, and the spinal needle is then entirely withdrawn. The engaged cogs support the tissue in the elevated position like a hammock. Accordingly, bidirectional cogged sutures are principally oriented in a horizontal position; whereas unidirectional cogged sutures have some superior or superolateral orientation as the tissue is suspended to a fixed superior-based anchor point. This is not always the case, as unidirectional cogged sutures can be situated primarily in a horizontal direction and bidirectional ones in a more angled course.

34.2
Technique

The technique is straightforward to undertake with a very short learning curve. The procedure can be performed under straight local anesthesia, with oral sedation and oral narcotic medications, or light intravenous sedation. I prefer the latter method with a mixture of Midazolam and fentanyl to achieve optimal patient comfort and some relative amnesia. However, I recognize that this type of anesthesia may not be available in an

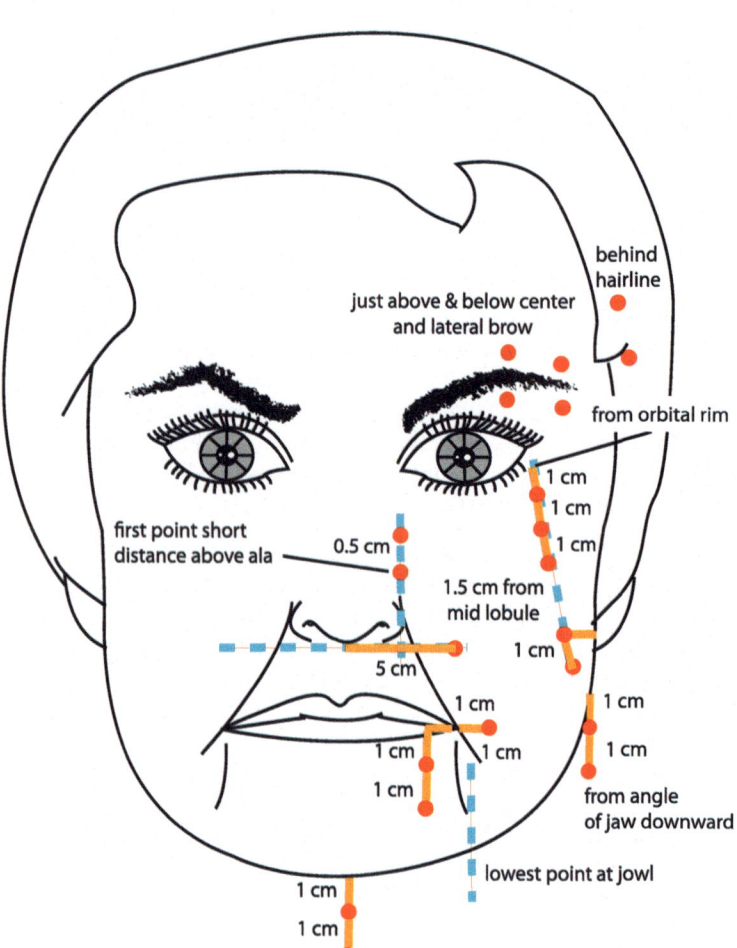

Fig. 34.1 Initial markings on the face that will be used as guide marks for suture placement [Original art created by Samuel M. Lam]

office-based setting owing to state regulations and safety considerations. I own and operate an ambulatory surgery center, which affords me the flexibility to conduct these simple procedures under level II conscious sedation; and I would recommend this approach when feasible. The patient is started on cephalexin, or the equivalent, administered orally the night prior to the operation and this is continued for 5 days to minimize infectious risk.

The first order of business is to establish with the patient the desired areas for facial rejuvenation, which can be basically divided into the brow, midface, jawline, and neck. For the sake of clarity in the following text, we will be referring to how to complete the entire face and neck with these bidirectional threads in a systematic and stepwise fashion.

A permanent marker is used to mark out the entry and exit points where the spinal needle will pass through. Gentian violet is not recommended as a tissue marker owing to its persistent tenacious quality that will irritate most patients. An eyebrow crayon that would otherwise be suitable for marks used in botu-

linum toxin therapy is too temporary to be beneficial and can be easily erased and smudged with the pass of a gauze. All marking is carried out with the patient in an erect, sitting position.

The first marks for brow elevation are situated above and below the hairy eyebrow along the midlength of the brow (v. 34.1). The second marks fall at the lateral terminus of the hairy eyebrow, again above and below the brow. The skin over the lateral brow is then arched upward to the desired position of elevation, and the final two marks are placed in a relatively straight line to the first two marks in this elevated position behind the hairline. In general, two sutures will be used to elevate each brow.

Three sutures will be used for each cheek. The marks for cheek elevation are as follows. Two marks are positioned directly above the nasal ala approximately 0.5 cm above the superior aspect of the ala and then another 0.5 cm above the first mark. A mark is then situated at the horizontal plane of the nasal base at 5 cm lateral to the midline. A ruler is placed on the cheek that extends

Perform both sides like this first.   **Then perform both sides like this.**

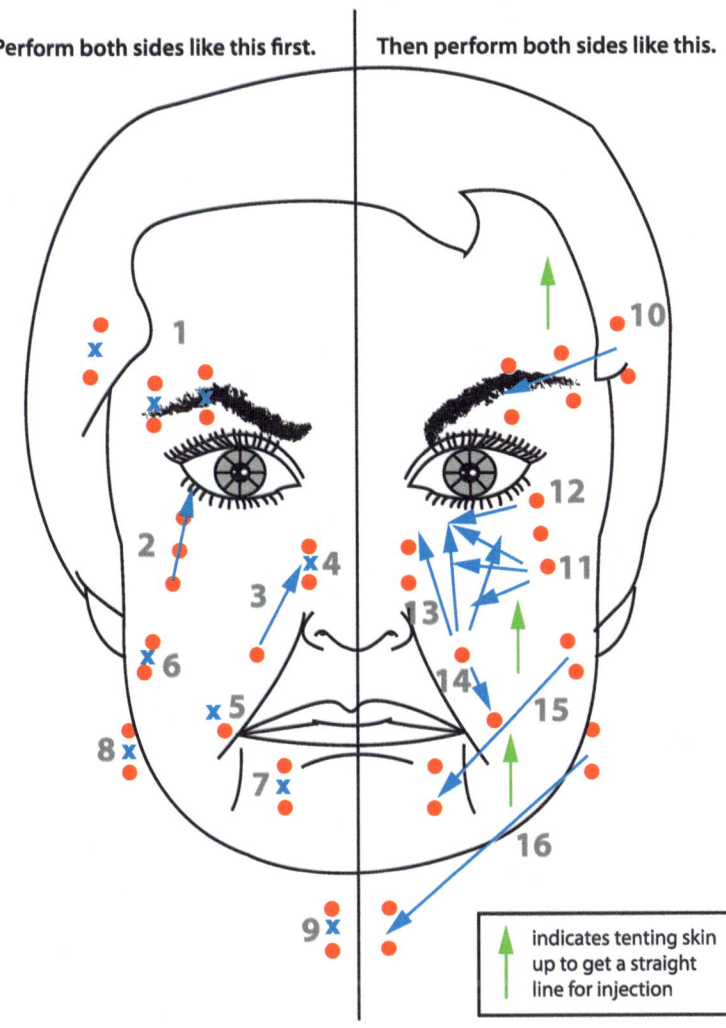

Fig. 34.2 Systematic infiltration of the face with local anesthesia to prepare the face for suture lifting [Original art created by Samuel M. Lam]

indicates tenting skin up to get a straight line for injection

at the 0 mark from the lateral aspect of the inferior orbital rim downward to 1.5 cm anterior to the midlobule of the ear. Marks are placed at 1, 2, and 3 cm, i.e., extending from 1 cm inferior to the inferior orbital rim along the length of the ruler. The final mark for cheek suspension is situated 1 cm lateral to the oral commissure in the same horizontal plane.

The jawline is marked with the lateral dots at the aforementioned 1.5-cm point anterior to the midlobule of the ear and the second mark is approximately 1 cm inferior to the first mark. The medial exit points are positioned 1 cm medial and 1 cm inferior to the oral commissure with the second point 1 cm below the first mark.

The marks for neck elevation are situated 1 cm directly below the lobule, with the second mark 1 cm below the first one. The medial marks fall just medial to any exposed platysmal bands but just lateral to the midline approximately 1 cm below the chin, with the second mark 1 cm below the first one. At times, these marks may be a bit too superior and can be repositioned more inferiorly as needed.

The same marks are made on the contralateral side, and symmetry is confirmed before proceeding. The entire procedure is best carried out with the patient in a semirecumbent position anywhere between 30 and 45° from the horizontal plane.

Typically, I prepare the face for the procedure with the sponge side of a standard chlorhexidine scrub brush. I do not like povidone–iodine solution for bidirectional suture lifting since one is limited in the capacity to clean the face after the procedure owing to the risk of breaking some of the suture cogs. Sterile blue towels are then draped in a turban style around the head and as a V-shape around the neck to maintain a sterile field. I usually only don sterile gloves without a full gown for these types of procedures.

When the patient is adequately sedated, I begin infiltration of the local anesthetic. Five milliliters is used of a mixture that contains 1 ml of sodium bicarbonate and 4 ml of 1% lidocaine with 1:100,000 epinephrine per side of the face and outfitted with a 27-gauge 1.25-in. needle. Both sides of the face are injected on the

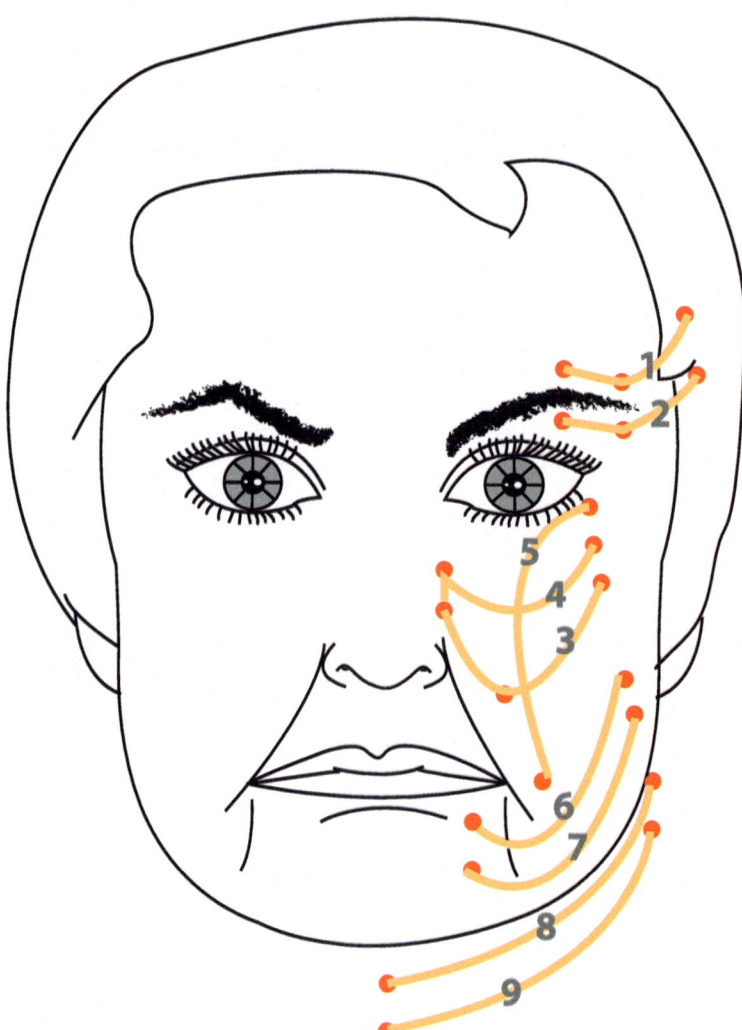

Fig. 34.3 a The order in which suture placement is recommended is from a superior to inferior direction [Original art created by Samuel M. Lam]

left side (Fig. 34.2). The x's in Fig. 34.2 indicate a direct percutaneous injection of anesthetic, and the arrows indicate a subcutaneous threading of injection. Injecting the actual skin markings is carefully avoided to eliminate the possibility for unfavorable tattooing of the skin. After the principal entry and exit points have been anesthetized, the pathways through which the spinal needle will pass are injected (Fig. 34.2). For the brow, jawline, and neck, the tissue is elevated to the desired position using the non-dominant hand. When it comes time to pass the spinal needle, a blanched pathway is visible in the area where the epinephrine has been deposited. When elevating the jawline to the desired position, the focus is lifting the jawline so that the jowl is entirely effaced before injecting the anesthetic solution.

During the 10 min needed for adequate anesthesia and hemostasis from the local anesthetic, the surgeon can prepare the Mayo stand for usage. A sterile paper drape is laid out onto the Mayo stand. It is imperative that a standard blue towel not be used instead since the barbs from the suture will invariably catch on the sur-

gical towel's fabric. The assistant then carefully opens each package of sutures usually only half way so that the sutures do not inadvertently fly out of the package and onto the floor. Toothless forceps are used to withdraw each suture one at a time to be placed on the sterile field. The surgeon should be very careful in placing the sutures in a neat and orderly fashion without them touching one another to minimize the risk of pulling all of them off the field when barbs from one suture catch onto an adjacent one. A sterile package of 4 × 4 gauze must be carefully handled and positioned far away from the sutures, and the assistant should be instructed not to wipe any blood away until the exposed suture ends have been entirely trimmed after introduction. The fibers of the gauze can easily catch the barbs and pull them out of the skin or off onto the floor. The only other instruments needed for the procedure are a single 18-gauge spinal needle and suture scissors.

The brow is addressed first, and subsequent areas are completed from a superior to inferior direction, i.e., brow, then cheek, then jawline, followed by the neck

Fig. 34.3 b For clarity, each zone (brow, cheek, jawline, and neck) has been color-coded [Original art created by Samuel M. Lam]

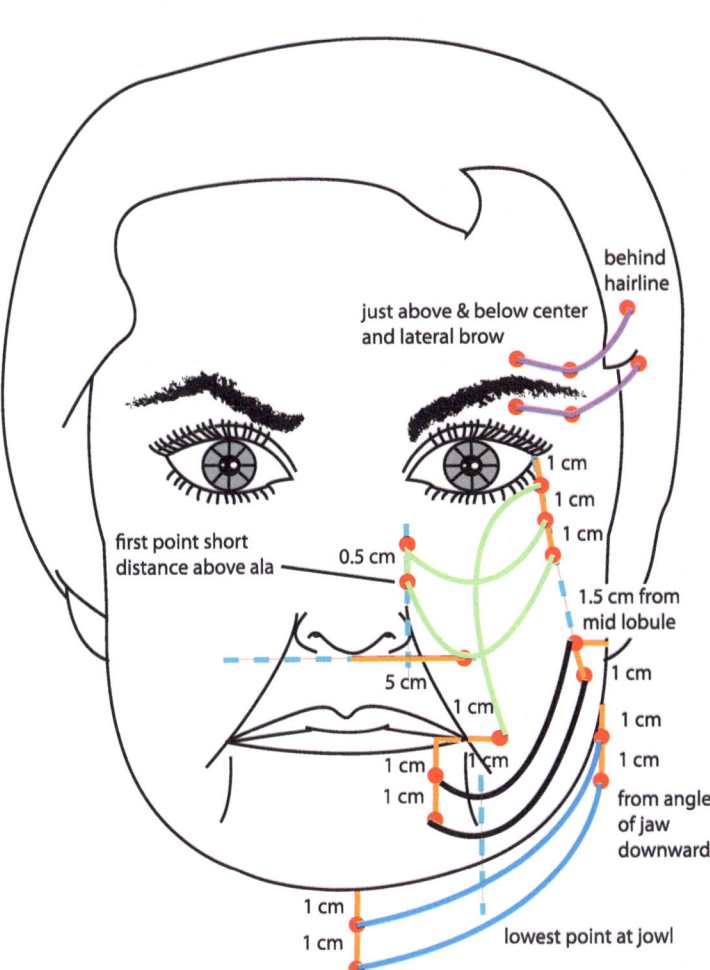

behind hairline

just above & below center and lateral brow

1 cm
1 cm
1 cm

first point short distance above ala — 0.5 cm

1.5 cm from mid lobule

5 cm   1 cm

1 cm

1 cm
1 cm

1 cm   1 cm

1 cm
1 cm

from angle of jaw downward

1 cm
1 cm

lowest point at jowl

(Fig. 34.3). The author tends to do both brows, then both cheeks, etc. in a symmetrical fashion. Alternatively, one hemiface can be completed first before proceeding to the other side. The non-dominant hand is used to elevate the brow skin upward to the desired position, and the spinal needle is inserted into the subcutaneous tissue from the lateral entry point (behind the hairline) through to exit the most medial marked points that are situated at the midlength of the brow. The surgeon can follow the blanched pathway created by the epinephrine as a guide, as mentioned previously. Also, as stated, the needle should not pass through the marked points on the skin to avoid the risk of a permanent tattoo. It is easy to pass the needle just on the inside of each of the marked points, i.e., immediately inferior to the upper marked points and immediately superior to the lower marked points.

After the spinal needle has been introduced, the non-dominant hand can release the suspended tissue since the spinal gauge needle should hold the tissue in an elevated position. The stylet of the spinal needle is removed so that the suture can be introduced. It is far easier to insert the suture through the open hub side of the spinal needle than through the sharp end. The suture should be gently inserted, rotating the suture during insertion to minimize the barbs catching on the needle and pulling back the suture a short distance as necessary when it does catch. When the suture becomes visible from the other side of the spinal needle, the assistant prevents the suture from slipping either with toothless forceps or fingers. The needle is then withdrawn so that the sharp end of the needle almost disappears under the skin but not entirely, while the assistant continues to hold the exposed suture end firmly. At this point, the surgeon adjusts the exposed suture length to ensure that an equal distance of the suture extends from the entry and exit points so that the midpoint of the bidirectional cogs is almost precisely at the center of the subcutaneous tract. With the assistant firmly holding the end of the exposed suture, the surgeon tents up the tissue with the middle finger and and the index finger of the non-dominant hand straddling the needle somewhere along its subcutaneous path and the thumb of the non-dominant hand pinching the skin toward the middle and index fingers. The dominant hand then quickly withdraws the spinal needle with three quick twists in alternating clockwise and counterclockwise directions during removal. Once the needle has been withdrawn, the non-dominant hand can release the tissue, which activates and engages the cogs to hold the tissue in position.

Hopefully, at this point there is an equal distance of suture exposed on both sides. If the suture lengths are slightly asymmetric, the tensile strength should be relatively uncompromised. Significant difference in suture length may need to be reinforced with an additional suture while removing the previous suture or just leaving it in place.

The surgeon should then verify that the suture is properly engaged by gently tugging each exposed side. If there is no movement, then the suture is fully engaged, which can also be evident by the visible lifting action of the tissue. If the suture slides easily when pulled, it needs to be removed because the cogs are damaged or not engaged and a new suture needs to be used to replace it. The exposed suture tails are then trimmed flush with the skin surface. More accurately, the tines of the scissors should be depressed downward onto the skin surface while the non-dominant hand gently pulls upward on the exposed suture tail to ensure that the end of the suture is adequately buried. It may be easier to put both brow sutures on one side in place before trimming all of the exposed suture tails off, but individual surgeon preference will dictate the exact protocol.

Any gross tissue dimpling can be corrected by gently pressing the skin downward until a little pop is felt that reflects breakage of a few cogs that may be implicated in the dimpling. This often occurs where the scissors push down on the skin to trim the suture ends and can be easily corrected with a gentle push on the dimple. If there is only mild dimpling, it is better to leave the dimpling alone for up to 3 weeks postoperatively in order to

preserve as many cogs as possible since at 3 weeks dimpling may have resolved and can still be easily corrected. The cheek is an area that can tolerate more notable dimpling, whereas toleration of the jawline is less so.

The first suture that is passed through the cheek follows the lower arc that exits through the inferior exit point immediately above the nasal ala and captures the point that falls 5 cm from the midline in the horizontal plane of the subnasale (Fig. 34.3). The spinal needle is passed through the subcutaneous tissue in almost a straight line through the prescribed points since the index finger of the non-dominant hand lifts the three points upward into an almost linear arrangement (Fig. 34.4–34.8). In actuality, for maximal lift, the spinal needle can be passed under the skin in a slightly curved arc to recruit more inferior tissue upward. With the spinal needle pierced through the cheek, the cheek is then suspended in the proper elevation. It is hard to overlift the cheek (or brow or any zone for that matter), and some skin dimpling that may be evident either after insertion of the spinal needle or after placement of the suture is well tolerated for the most part in the cheek region. The suture is inserted in the same manner described above for the brow, and the method will be the same for all of the remaining areas of the face. The second cheek suture is inserted in a parallel fashion immediately above the first suture. During insertion of the spinal needle, the surgeon is careful to lift the cheek with the non-dominant hand without pressure on the cheek suture placed immediately prior so as not to disrupt the cogs from the former suture. The final cheek suspension suture is placed in a slightly different vector (Fig. 34.3) and the finger that lifts the cheek does so in a somewhat tangential fashion pushing slightly medially.

The jawline is then addressed next. Just like for the brow, the fingers of the non-dominant hand are used to pull the skin upward until the desired point of elevation (Fig. 34.9). The focus should be at the jowl so that the jowl is effaced during elevation of the tissue. The

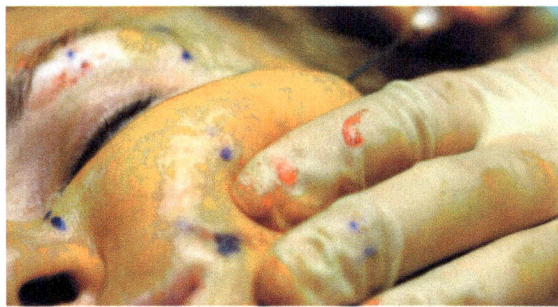

Fig. 34.4 The first maneuver in cheek suspension with the non-dominant hand holding the cheek up to the desired position while the dominant hand inserts the spinal needle through the cheek and malar fat pad

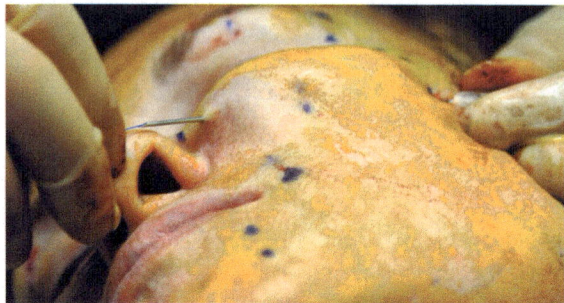

Fig. 34.5 The cheek is suspended in the desired position by the spinal needle with the stylet already withdrawn and the suture being threaded through the barrel

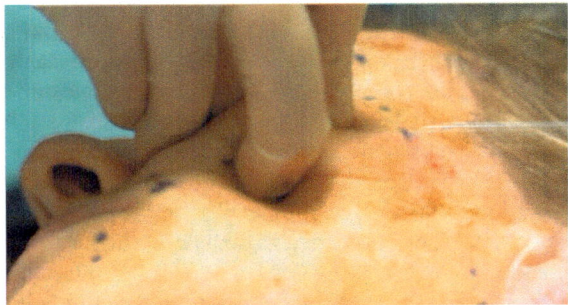

Fig. 34.6 The non-dominant hand straddling the spinal needle in its subcutaneous path with the fifth finger preventing the exposed suture tail from moving (which can be done by an assistant) while the dominant hand removes the spinal needle in a twisting motion, as described in the text. After the spinal needle has been withdrawn, the non-dominant hand can be released, which engages the tiny cogs into the tissue

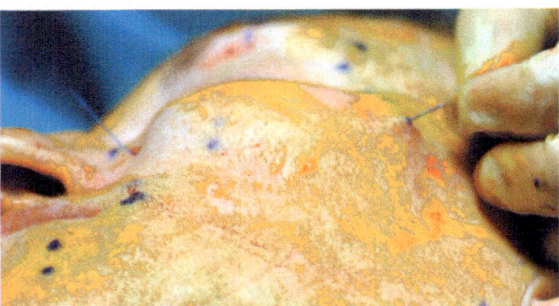

Fig. 34.7 Both ends of the exposed suture are gently tugged to ensure that the cogs are engaged. If they are not and the suture easily slips, the cogs are broken and the suture should be removed and replaced

spinal needle is then passed through the blanched tract resulting from the epinephrine, and the two sutures are inserted in the same manner prescribed above. As mentioned, dimpling along the jawline is less tolerated. If the spinal needle appears to dimple the skin, it should be withdrawn and reinserted until the dimpling disappears. Usually dimpling occurs owing to a too superficial trajectory of the spinal needle.

Finally, the neckline completes the full-facial suture lift. Unlike for all of the preceding areas, the tissue is not elevated with the non-dominant hand prior to insertion of the spinal needle (Fig. 34.10). The skin is simply pierced with the needle, and the remainder of the procedure is carried out as described above.

At the end of the procedure, the surgeon should carefully dab the face with hydrogen peroxide to remove the blood and with alcohol to remove the skin markings. No vigorous wiping should be carried out so that

the integrity of the cogs can be preserved. If any blood or mark is difficult to remove, I leave it alone so as not to disturb the cogs and inform the patient that the skin will be free of these stains after one or two showers (to start the following day).

As part of routine postoperative care instructions, I inform the patient that no excessive smiling, facial animation, or talking should be done on the operative day. Trying to sleep on one's back for the first one to two nights can also minimize disruption of the cogs from pressure and movement of the face on the bed. Liberal use of ice packs for the first 48–72 h and sleeping in a recliner for the first two nights can be helpful.

A very important admonition is to avoid any facial massage for 3 months and to clean or dry the face only with light dabbing rather than wiping motions for the first 3 weeks. I also explain to the patient that he or she may experience popping of a few cogs and that

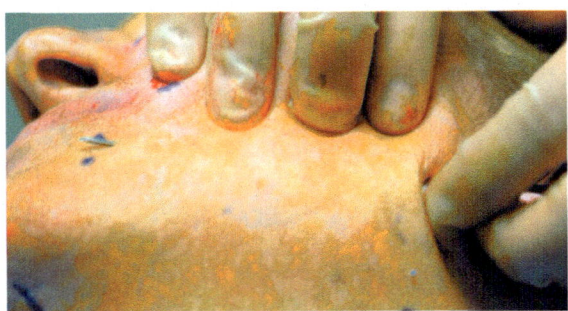

Fig. 34.8 Both suture ends are trimmed by depressing the tines of the scissors downward onto the skin so that the suture ends actually become buried under the skin

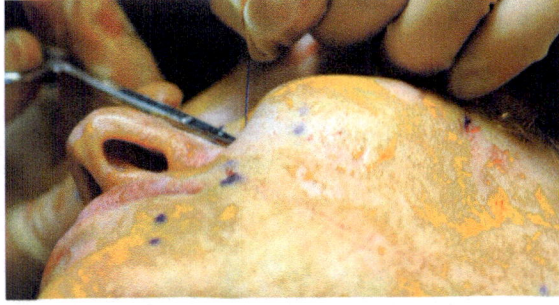

Fig. 34.9 The jawline is elevated for maximal jowl effacement by lifting the tissue upward with the non-dominant hand while the spinal needle is inserted. This technique is the same as advocated for brow elevation but differs from the technique for cheek elevation, as shown in Fig. 33.4

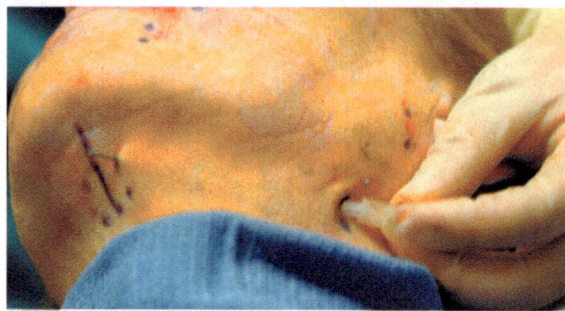

Fig. 34.10 The passage of the spinal needle through the neckline. The technique for passage of the spinal needle in the neck does not require any elevation of tissue by the non-dominant hand, unlike all other facial zones

this should not raise any alarm. Finally, as the scar tissue builds around the cogs over a 3-month period, the patient may notice some ongoing improvement during that time.

34.3
Complications

Patients who are expecting a limited recovery time may experience an extended period of convalescence if ecchymoses develop. If they are severe, they can be socially and/or professionally debilitating. Patients should be cognizant of this outcome so that they can plan or rearrange their calendar accordingly.

Unlike some types of unidirectionally barbed sutures that are anchored, bunching of tissue is rarely encountered except for the occasional dimple or uneven contour that settles out in the same time period of 2–3 weeks. As mentioned, dimpling can occur owing to technical error and can be easily corrected if necessary. Using both index fingers, the surgeon can gently apply skin distraction along the direction of the suture in the area of the dimple to correct the problem. If too many cogs are compromised, an additional suture can be easily inserted but preferably only at a later date after all the edema has dissipated and the final outcome is evident several months later. If dimpling is discovered late, the affected area can be subcised with an 18-gauge Nokor needle or, alternatively, an injectable filler can be used to elevate the depression.

The principal complaint against non-anchored sutures discussed in this chapter relates to the potential for suture migration even many months to years afterwards. If the suture migrates without extrusion, the consequences should be minimal to none. However, the suture can extrude through the skin, which is easily corrected by gently tugging the suture free and removing it. If the suture is visible through attenuated skin, then it should be removed, which may be a slightly more difficult prospect. The best maneuver in this case involves a tiny stab incision with a no. 11 blade or 18-gauge Nokor needle near the non-extruded visible suture, insertion of a crochet hook under the skin to loop the suture, and then pulling the suture out with the hook through the stab incision.

If asymmetry is noted or if the patient is dissatisfied with the degree of lifting, this outcome can be easily corrected by placement of additional sutures in the strategically necessary locations. Obviously, if the patient was expecting the result to be equivalent to that of a standard cervicofacial rhytidectomy, then the result will never be attained with suture lifting. These considerations are discussed more in detail in Sect. 34.4.

The most devastating outcome would be potential nerve damage due to laceration of a motor nerve that lies in the pathway of the spinal needle. Although I have yet to encounter this problem, I have observed some neural fasciculations when the spinal needle exits near the mouth. With this in view, I simply retracted the needle and passed it more laterally without a prob-

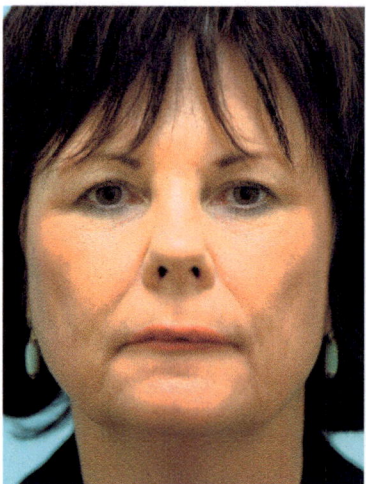
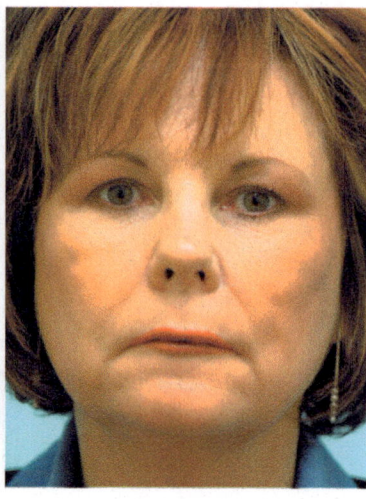

Fig. 34.11 Full-facial suture lifting using 18 bidirectional cogged, non-anchored sutures which shows mild to moderate benefit in each zone

lem. At times, patients can complain of discomfort and tenderness for several days to weeks, and I explain to them that they may experience this sensation as I emphasize to them during preoperative counseling. Theoretically, a small branch of a sensory nerve could also be disturbed. In any case, any discomfort should resolve within several weeks.

34.4
Discussion

Perhaps the most important aspect of suture lifting is appropriate preoperative counseling. Realistic expectations should always be established, especially in this case when the aesthetic gain is significantly more limited than with traditional lifting procedures (Fig. 34.11). Whenever I lecture on suture lifting (whatever kind), I always have a slide that announces, "This is not a facelift. This is not a facelift. This is not a facelift." Patients must fully appreciate the limited benefit they will gain from any kind of suture lift. In addition, the "weekend facelift" sales pitch must be tempered with the very real potential for several weeks of bruising, persistent dimpling, or mild discomfort that may make patients more reticent to undergo the procedure. Longevity of results is hard to estimate given the fact that the aesthetic benefit is less readily apparent than with other lifting methods; however, an estimate is approximately 2– 3 years with some diminution of the result over that period of time. It is best to undersell any results and to defer any claims of longevity.

The author has had moderate success in the midface/cheek region with bidirectional threads but very little success elsewhere, like the brow, jawline, and neck. The author now uses principally unidirectional threads for most of the face when necessary but still relies on bidirectional threads occasionally in the midface. There is some moderate benefit in the brow region when additional sutures are provided in a superoinferior direction across the forehead as support but not remarkable changes. If only bidirectional threads are to be used only in a patient who does not want any work in the midface/cheek region, the author will not do the procedure because the benefit is too small to be appreciated. At times the bidirectional sutures can be beneficial in the midface even more so than the unidirectional sutures, which are harder to position in wider midface structures. The sutures can be used to touch up or correct minor imperfections in my facelifts, browlifts, etc.

The author subscribes to the rule "1+1=3", i.e., when suture lifts are combined with other procedures the overall effect can be more substantial. For example, a formal browlift and lower-face/neck lift can be effectively combined with bidirectional threads in the midface (Fig. 34.12). I have performed numerous procedures in this fashion; however, I prefer to use fat grafting to restore the midface as opposed to a suture lift when possible. Combining a suture lift with other small "no-downtime" options like botulinum toxin therapy or hyaluronic acid injections or, alternatively, smaller operative procedures like blepharoplasty is always a good idea so that the cumulative effect of all these procedures may be more readily appreciated as a discernible aesthetic gain by the patient.

34.5
Conclusions

The reader is cautioned that any procedure that is stated in this text may not necessarily meet with FDA approval. The future of suture lifts is yet to be determined and is contingent upon patient satisfaction, longevity, and the rise of substitute techniques that could be better than what we have today. In that spirit, we are constantly encountering newer and better barbed sutures and combining different types of sutures for optimal aesthetic gain.

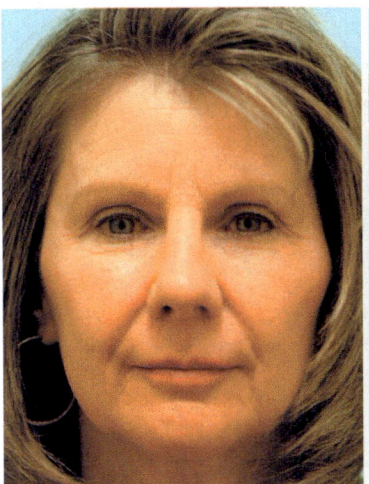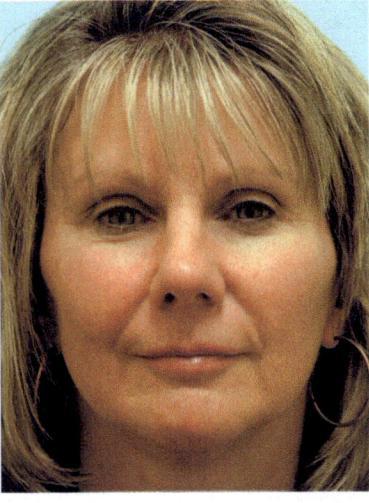

Fig. 34.12 Patient following a formal endoscopic browlift, face and neck lift, combined with six bidirectional threads placed in the cheek

CHAPTER 35

Soft Face Lift Using Threads

Pier Antonio Bacci, Sergio Mancini

35.1
Introduction

Society is changing and consequentially so are tastes, concepts of beauty, and style of life. Patients who were asking surgeons to be transformed or pulled to the maximum to give a youthful appearance now desire less. Today patients ask for mini-invasive and less traumatic surgery, possibly with local anesthesia, and are looking for the best result with the least scar and the least trauma. The scalpel cannot remove "lived" years but it can try to remove a few of the "shown" years and, at the same time, it can help to improve the quality of the life.

A minimal surgery can often bring a smile to a face that has become sad, tired, serious, and severe.

When there is too much excess tissue, it is necessary to use traditional lifting with removal of the tissues and long scars. Prevention of skin alterations and slowing the drooping of skin and tissues can be the true goal of cosmetic medicine and surgery.

Among the new proposals, surgical strategies that use threads for support of the facial tissues are of extreme interest and of great curiosity. The threads produce a soft rejuvenation of the face for the reduction and the improvement of folds and skin drooping that show the course of the years and the history of a patient's life. The threads are proposed for the deceleration of aging and in preventive medicine, but also for the mini-invasive correction of other areas, like the breast, buttocks, abdomen, or thighs.

The term "mini-invasive aesthetic surgery" means a surgery that tries to be minimally invasive and a less bloody solution for aesthetic problems that, very often, constitute real illnesses for the patient, but whose solutions do not always justify extensive interventions with greater risks, greater complications, larger scars, or long convalescences. Superior blepharoplasty, localized liposculpture, or mini lifting can be minimally invasive surgery.

Soft aesthetic surgery means only "the attempt to give good results with noninvasive solutions", because incisions, electrocoagulation, separation of the tissues, or sutures of the different layers are not required. This soft cosmetic surgery offers the surgeon and patient good results with the correct indications and by precise methods.

35.2
Adipose Tissue and Extracellular Matrix

In aesthetic surgery, autologous adipose tissue is used for filling the losses and signs of old age.

Fat tissue involves a true filler that succeeds in filling and constitutes at the same time a bomb of hormones and nourishing substances. Fat is represented in the subcutaneous layer with an adipose pad (Bichat's fat pad) with a typical disposition in the subcutaneous tissue of the cheek area. The reduction of Bichat's fat pad and reduction of the adipose and connective tissue of the check area result in the typical alterations of aging of the face, making it appear sad, serious, and severe.

All tissues have regular metabolic activity that occurs in the extracellular matrix where the fundamental principal vital exchanges occurs. All the microcirculatory and metabolic activities are increased by the anatomic and morphologic regularity of these microstructures. In the processes of aging and in the evolution of the skin excess (ptosis occurs because the skin slips downward as a result of gravity), morphologic and functional alterations of these structures occur and increase principal metabolic alterations of the extracellular matrix. This increases the processes of fibrosis. Prolapse of the adipose tissue of the cheek area and the metabolic alterations of the skin cause the process of aging with:

1. Metabolic alterations causing degeneration of the cutaneous structure
2. Wrinkles
3. Folds
4. Cutaneous excess of the face
5. Depression of the eyebrows and the angles of the mouth
6. Cutaneous excess of the neck
7. Formation of excess cutaneous tissue of the superior eyelid
8. Formation of an adipose bag in the inferior eyelid

Bringing the tissues into their ideal position reduces lymphatic stasis, favors regular morphology of the microstructures, favors oxygenation and nutrition, administers energy, and stimulates the musculature. This constitutes the functional bases to recover normal metabolism of tissues and to slow down the process of aging. Aesthetic surgery of the face uses barbed or nonbarbed surgical threads that are inserted to achieve this goal.

35.3
History

The history of medicine is rich with documents that recount all the clever attempts to discover the best therapies for rejuvenation of the face. Besides the various attempts for lifting the tissues using various types of surgical threads and sutures, including "barbed" threads, it was also careful observation of the typical mantle covering a small exotic animal called *Erethicon dorsatum*, characterized by a dense net of thorns which allows the animal to attach itself well onto plant leaves, that helped the idea of barbed threads to be conceived.

35.3.1
The Beginnings

In 1956, a work by Buttkewitz [1, 2] was published concerning the correction of nasolabial wrinkles using strips of nylon. Galland and Clavier, in 1966, started using a new method where catgut threads and Reverdin needles were used in order to lift up the tissues and secure them onto tendons or fibrous tissues using local anesthesia. This method was developed and improved further by Guillemain [3], who named this the "curl lift." It was an interesting technique but with inconsistent and nonlasting results over time. Guillemain did not believe, at that time, that his method was the mother of all other methods using threads.

35.3.2
The Double-Tip Needle

In the 1980s, Capurro patented a type of needle with two tips, thus allowing a double entry. This particular device allows the introduction of surgical threads deep into the tissues without having to make other cutaneous incisions in order for the thread to come out. This type of needle, together with a thread that is more or less elastic, was perfected by Capurro [4, 5], while other researchers have developed interesting personal modifications.

In 1986, Yanai et al. [6] and Boo-Chai [7] described their instrument and methods but Mendez Flores and Fournier later developed this typical method of facial rejuvenation, particularly in order to rejuvenate the forehead and cheeks [8–10].

35.3.3
Serdev's Threads

Serdev started using spineless smooth threads characterized by short elasticity. These are inserted into the tissues and affixed by knots, thus creating a "tobacco-like bag" shape. Such suturing results in augmentation of volume and further projection of the tissues. The suture described by Serdev utilizes a new idea in order to lift up and to fix the tissue in the face and other areas of the body [11–13].

The surgical thread used is made of a semielastic, antimicrobial, and slowly reabsorbable polycaproamide substance (with a resistance of 60 N), made in Bulgaria by Polycon® and widely used in Eastern countries in stomach and abdomen surgeries. With use of particular needles, it has been possible to attach the thread to fibrous and stable structures of the body that would limit the destruction of the suture itself. The threads are used for the subcutaneous musculoaponeurotic system (SMAS) in the face, the trabecular system for the gluteus, the fascia and muscular tendons for the breasts, and other fibrous structures such as fascia, tendons, or ligaments in other areas. This technique has proven itself to be very useful for the correction of the cheeks, chin, and buttocks.

35.3.4
APTOS Threads

Sulamanidze, in the 1990s, started perfecting a nonabsorbable surgical thread which has a double line of thorns that are arranged one against the other like two ears of wheat facing each other. Such characteristics give the thread a self-supporting capacity once it has been inserted in the tissues.

In 1999, Sulamanidze patented a new type of thread that allows for a simple surgical method to be applied in order to improve facial tissues [14–16]. This thread is made by making use of new polymers or biological materials, which allow tissues to be set in new and more harmonious positions. Such threads, called "APTOS" (antiptosis) threads, have been shown to be of use in some methods of facial rejuvenation.

35.3.5
Unidirectional Barbed Threads

In 2002, the author began to use absorbable and nonabsorbable barbed threads characterized by a single line of unidirectional thorns. This allows for fibrosis to occur within the tissues. As a result, the thread is used to provide traction, which limits sectioning or detachment of skin tissue.

This unidirectional barbed thread introduces new advantages. The barbed side of the thread anchors to

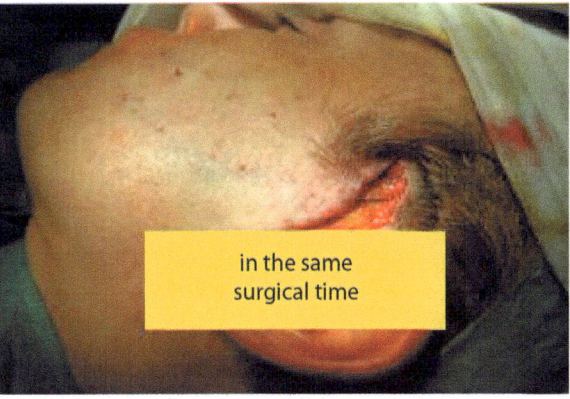
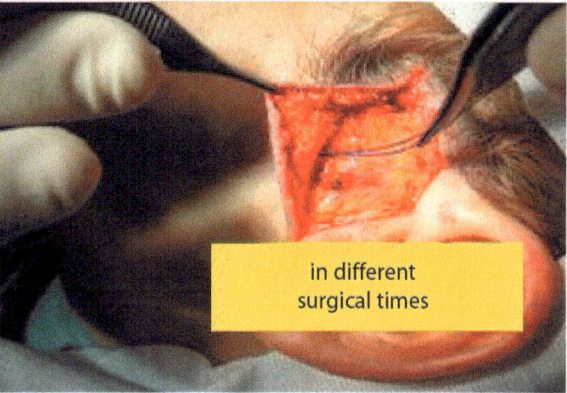

Fig. 35.1 Threads can be used to pull the tissue and subcutaneous musculoaponeurotic system without separation

the tissues and allows traction of the tissues. Thread from the nonbarbed side can easily be removed. With use of nonabsorbable threads the tissue can be lifted and ptosis corrected. Absorbable threads allow temporary fibrosis to be created with an increase in the physiological cellular activities.

New horizons open up with the use of the method of lifting in two phases. First, the thread is positioned and, then, after some weeks with only a small incision, one can retie the thread and increase the traction of the tissues without causing any detachments of the fibrosis (Fig. 35.1).

The author's complete surgical kit may be used for the introduction of the different surgical threads (barbed and nonbarbed, absorbable and nonabsorbable, and normal surgical threads) into the tissues and is particularly useful in soft and mini-invasive cosmetic surgery of the face and neck (Fig. 35.2).

This surgical kit contains:

1. An interchangeable handle for different uses and that is easy to use for precise introduction
2. A short (15-cm) and a long (20-cm) needle characterized by a nontraumatic point and with two tunnels for threads (thread no. 0/0 can be used)
3. A short (15-cm) and a long (20-cm) needle characterized by a mini-invasive point and with two tunnels for threads (thread no. 0/0 can be used)

The interchangeable handle allows for the use of different needles at the same time as the use of the different methods and various threads. These different needles (with mini-invasive or nontraumatic points) allow for the introduction of the threads in different layers, such as skin, subcutaneous tissue, fascia, muscle, or tendon.

With the use of different threads, even with unidirectional threads and different methods, good results can be obtained for various cosmetic problems and the threads can also be used in conjunction with fillers or lipofilling to improve the results for the treatment of folds and wrinkles.

Absorbable threads allow stretching to take place with tissue repositioning in such a way as to slow the dropping of the tissues [17, 18]. The author calls this method "T3–biolifting," to indicate the typical application of absorbable linked hyaluronic acid in three layers in conjunction with, when necessary, barbed absorbable threads or lipofilling [19, 20].

The new position of the face tissues can recover the activity of the microcirculation and of the extracellular matrix with new good function of metabolism. With new production of physiologic collagen and connective tissue, the time until old age can be extended.

35.3.6
A New Era

For over 10 years, Ruff has been testing materials and methods and this has resulted in recognition by the Food and Drug Administration (FDA) of a peculiar barbed surgical thread for the rejuvenation of the face

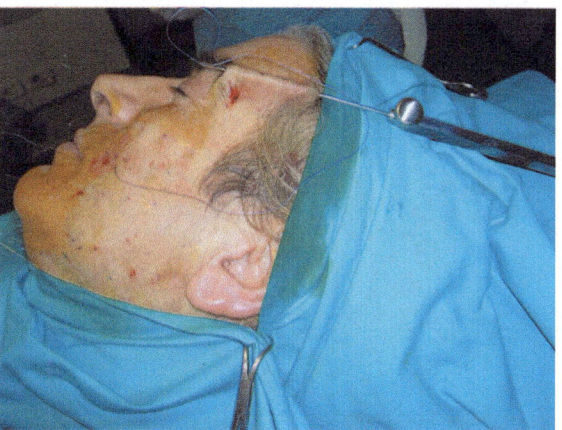

Fig. 35.2 Instrument used to introduce different threads

and the neck areas [21–32]. The FDA has also approved the typical application method, which has definitely opened the doors to the development of a new soft and mini-invasive aesthetic surgery strategy. Using this new method, called Contour ThreadLift™, it is possible to lift up all facial tissues directly using threads or by sliding the skin over the threads, because there is a real point of anchorage for the knot (Fig. 35.3).

The FDA has requested that physicians who intend to use this new approved method participate in suitable practical training sessions in order to apply the new method at its best.

For such purpose, the company has appointed some international opinion leaders. The Documentation Center of Aesthetic Pathologies and Cosmetic Surgery in Arezzo was the first center of excellence in Italy for the use and training of the Contour ThreadLift™ method.

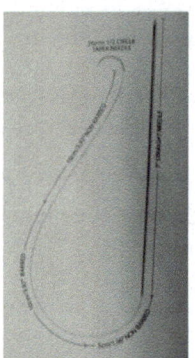

• Using this method we can a point of anchorage for the threads.

• We have not only the traction of the threads but we use the lines of the threads to lift up all parts of the skin.

Fig. 35.3 The new American Contour ThreadLift

35.4
Goals

The goals of aesthetic surgery of the face are:
1. Spatial recovery of the adipose zygomatic tissue
2. Recovery of the SMAS and the platysma
3. Reduction of the cutaneous excess
4. Harmonization of the eyebrows and the angles of the mouth

For these goals, traditional plastic and aesthetic surgery offers a vast range of solutions, more or less invasive. Of these solutions, there are well-known advantages regarding side effects and complications. In particular cases and in selected patients, different mini-invasive solutions can be offered with the use of unidirectional barbed threads. It is possible "to bring the tissues (skin—subcutaneous layer, adipose tissues, and muscle) into their best position, increasing the physiological restructuring of the tissues and avoiding cutaneous excisions and subcutaneous surgical separation" (Figs. 35.4, 35.5). To achieve this goal particular threads can be used that are anchored to the deep tissues and that allow, in one or more sessions, the tissues to recover and to improve normal metabolic and structural arrangement. Any alteration in the morphological structure can cause bending or reduction of the capillary bed that can reduce the speed of flow of arteriolar blood. But it is especially on the venous-lymphatic side that there are the alterations that cause metabolic damage. These alterations activate the process of oxidative stress with evolution toward typical fibrosis.

Functionally every attempt for recovering the anatomical structure in a better position will slow down the

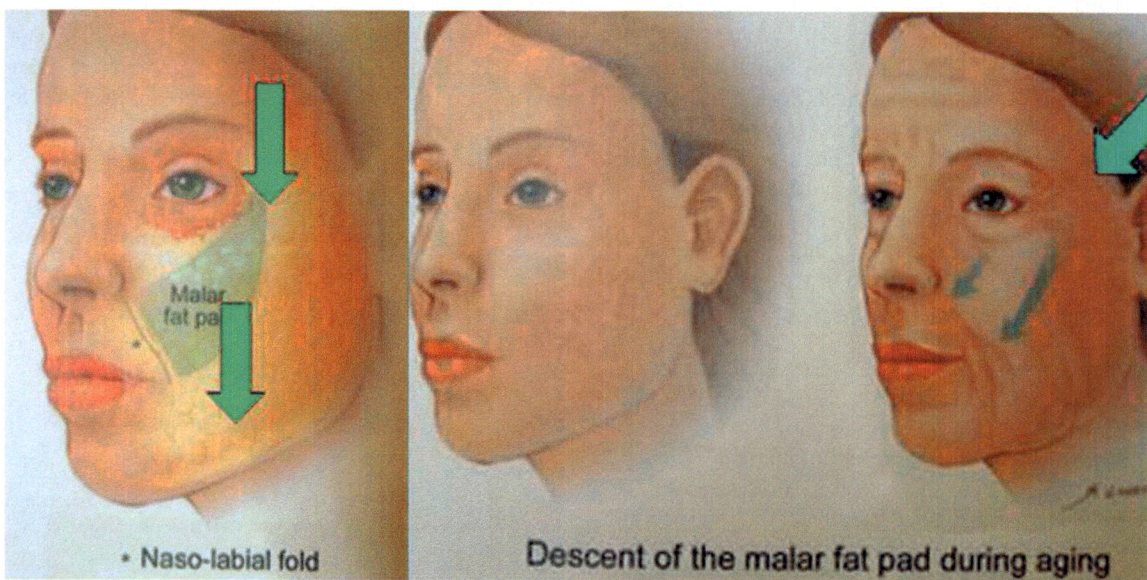

Malar fat pad

• Naso-labial fold

Descent of the malar fat pad during aging

Fig. 35.4 When tissues fall down there are wrinkles and folds and the face shows aging lines

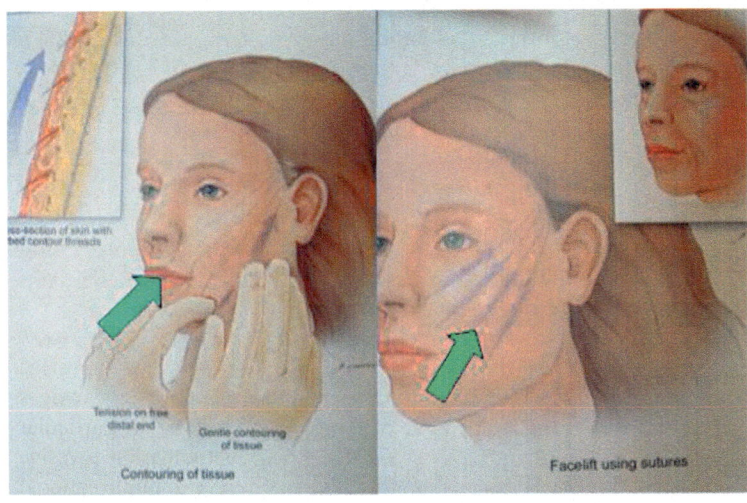

Fig. 35.5 Replacing the tissue position and contouring of the face using Contour Threads

process of oxidative stress and will cause an improvement in microcirculation and metabolism, therefore reducing the processes of aging and tissue degeneration. Using the Contour ThreadLift™ method can give the best results.

35.5
Strategy

There are various surgical solutions using different surgical threads.

1. Guillemain technique: This is called the "curl lift" technique and is the simplest and most intelligent method to lift the ptotic tissues since it allows anchorage and lifting of the tissues with simple surgical threads that are in daily use, absorbable or nonabsorbable. Various technical variations or particular tools can be used, such as Capurro's needle, the Mendez Florez method, or Bacci's tools.

2. Sulamanidze technique: This method uses some gentle surgical threads that introduce thorns, like ears of wheat, that are self-sustaining in the tissues.

3. Serdev method: Taking the idea of Galland and Clavier, Serdev uses threads that are semielastic and absorbable over time as well as particular needles to anchor the tissues to solid and fixed structures.

4. Ruff method: This represents the new era in cosmetic surgery, being the first method officially approved by the FDA for the rejuvenation of the face and the neck. It uses barbed and unidirectional threads, similar to those used in our experience, but in partnership with particular needles that create a true point of anchorage for the threads, similar to rails of the track, on which one can contour and slide the skin.

All these methods offer advantages and indications, but they can become synergistic when an integrated treatment is used, not only with the use of different threads and methods but also in association with more traditional surgical techniques.

35.6
T3–Soft Face Lifting

In 2002, the author worked with two integration methods, threads of support and surgical lifting by departing from the use of absorbable or nonabsorbable unidirectional barbed threads. It is possible to form temporary fibrosis along the path of the threads in 3–6 weeks with the mini-invasive method used in two sessions, named "T3–soft face lifting." "T3" means "traction threads treatment," which is treatment that uses the traction on surgical threads to lift the tissues.

This method consists of two mini-invasive surgical sessions with local anesthesia:

1. First session: This involves the application of threads of support, barbed or nonbarbed, absorbable or noabsorbable, according to the indications, using the author's particular needles or mini cannulas with two holes. This session is often associated with lipofilling that allows the activation of tissue metabolism because of the hormonal push given by the autologous fat tissue and from the new position of the tissues partially obtained with the support of the threads.

2. Second session: When necessary, this is performed after 3–6 weeks with the purpose of giving time for the connective tissues to become organized and, therefore, to allow good traction on the threads. Depending on the extent of the skin excess, an incision is performed (the smallest possible) along the classical lines before and behind the ear, then with the least dissection to find the tails of the threads giving the traction. The tissues are brought into their ideal position and the subcutaneous tissue and SMAS are

sutured with Monocryl or Monoswift 3/0 or Prolene 4/0. Such a method allows traction of the tissues, avoiding extensive dissection. This method has given good results in cases of minimal or medium ptosis without skin excess. Good results have also been obtained using the Contour ThreadLift™ method.

35.6.1
Method

To apply the threads few surgical tools are necessary:
1. Local anesthesia, usually with small drops along the marked lines
2. Some particular needles or cannulas of various sizes
3. A selection of threads of different structure and caliber
   (a) Semielastic smooth and long-duration absorbable threads of polycaproamide (no. 2–2/0) (Serdev)
   (b) Absorbable thread, barbed or not barbed, nos. 2/0, 3/0 (Vicryl, Monocryl, or PDS)
   (c) Nonabsorbable barbed unidirectional thread (2/0–3/0) (Contour ThreadLift™)
   (d) Nonabsorbable bidirectional barbed thread (2/0–3/0) (Sulamanidze)

The use of different threads depends on the indication and on the experience of the surgeon. The use of absorbable threads is useful for preventive purposes such as with corrections and surgery in two sessions. Nonabsorbable threads are initially used for the principal indications. Experience has allowed the identification of a precise protocol of treatment according to the method used.

35.6.1.1
Guillemain Method

After local anesthesia, a thread is passed on the peripheral sides to lift them up. Using the double-point needle of Capurro, subcutaneous and muscular passages can be performed (described by the Mendez Florez method). The same needles or mini cannulas with two holes allow the passing of the threads and anchoring them to solid points or the tying of knots where necessary. The author prefers to use threads of Vicryl or Monocryl that are anchored to the fascia, ligaments, or the periosteum. A shorter session after 3–6 months will make the result stable for a long period of time. Such a strategy is interesting before possible lifting to appraise the results for medium ptosis and, above all, for the recovery of the tissues.

Interesting results have been obtained using the T3–biolifting, where this is performed in association with fillers positioned in the zygomatic area or with lipofilling. In these cases the absorbable threads allow improvement of the aesthetic result, lengthening the life of the positioned tissues.

35.6.1.2
Sulamanidze Method

This involves use of bidirectional barbed threads utilizing local anesthesia and the use of particular needles where the thread is inserted.

As a rule the thread is inserted in a "Z" in such a way as to fix the thread making traction around two tails. The bidirectional thorns will fix the positioned thread (usually a couple of threads to strengthen the support) and after 2–3 weeks the thread will be stable and give more lasting support. The method is suitable above all for the "brow lift" and for the forehead.

The author no longer uses APTOS threads.

35.6.1.3
Serdev Method

This method is founded on three characteristic principles:
1. The semielastic and delayed reabsorption structure of the threads that allows the tissues to sustain their position without cutting them
2. The formation of so many "tobacco-like purses" that have the ability to project the tissues
3. The fixation of the thread to fixed and solid structures

With use of particular small needles the thread is anchored to a solid and fixed structure and the thread is passed building a "tobacco-like purse."

The tissues become anchored and projected so that the final result is support of the lifted tissues and projection with the effect of "increase of volume." Such a method is most typically indicated for the correction of the zygomatic region and for mini-invasive surgery of the buttocks and the breast.

35.6.1.4
Ruff Method

This method, called Contour ThreadLift™, represents the conclusion of a long period of study and search. The value of the method depends on certain principal characteristics:
1. A complete surgical thread with a linear and circular needle of high quality and with unidirectional small thorns that allow a strong and immediate anchorage of the tissues.
2. The possibility of lifting all ptotic skin at the same time, creating a true point of anchorage.

3. A precise method of application expressly approved by the FDA for the rejuvenation of the face and the neck.
4. The ability to remove the thread with extreme ease at any time.

After local anesthesia with small drops along the path, the thread is inserted with the smooth part fist that is connected to a linear needle that has the same dimension as the barbed thread. Such technique avoids the formation of hematoma and tunnels that can reduce the anchorage of the thorns to the tissues (Fig. 35.6). Using the circular needle, which is connected to the other tail of the thread instead, a point of anchorage is created using a knot. Making traction on the peripheral tail

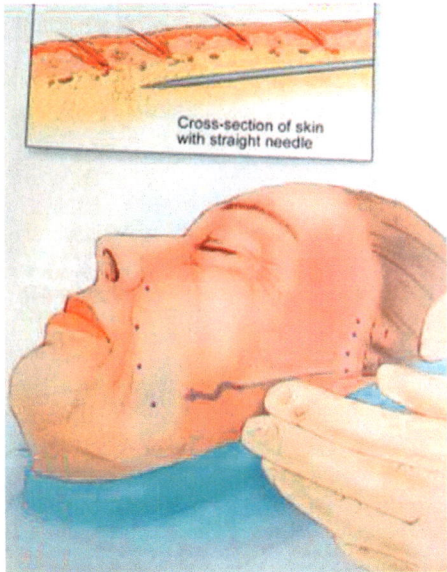

Fig. 35.6 Introduction of straight needle and thread

of the thread, which on the other side is anchored to a fixed structure, the surgeon slips the skin on the thorns, to lift the skin to the best position. Such positioning is performed with the patient sitting and provided with a mirror, so that the patient appraise and determine the result (Fig. 35.7).

Using Bacci's tools and different threads, we can improve the result or make corrections. After 3 weeks the small cutaneous indentations, expression of the excess of the skin, will be reabsorbed as a spontaneous result of the improved metabolism and of the improved microvascular net created by recovering all the positions of the tissues (skin—subcutaneous, adipose tissue, and muscular fascia).

Steri-Strips and ice are applied postoperatively for some time. The patient is told to avoid smiling and to perform a lot of facial mimicry for a few days to favor the stabilization of the tissues.

35.6.2
Indications and Contraindications

The advantages of the "soft face lift with threads" can be described as:
1. Mini-invasive surgery with local anesthesia
2. Outpatient intervention
3. Possibility of improvement in multiple sessions
4. Possibility for easy removal of the thread
5. Long duration of the result
6. Absence of true complications
7. Absence of scars or risk of keloids
8. Recovery of the anatomical structures

The typical indications are:
1. Patient with important public activity
2. Patient who expressly asks for it
3. Patient who refuses traditional surgery

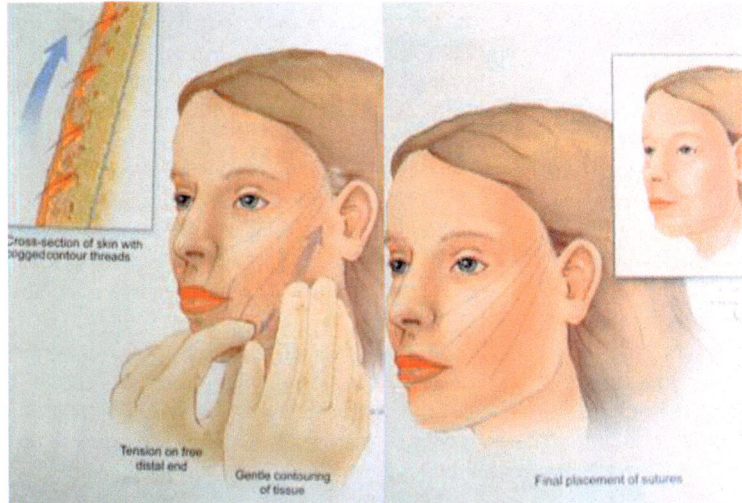

Fig. 35.7 Sliding skin by the Contour Threads to lift the skin

4. Patient who does not want scars
5. Patient with increased risk of keloids or allergies
6. Patient with psychological alterations or who is not very motivated
7. Patient with initial or not very advanced ptosis
8. Patient who requires appraisal of the possible results before lifting

The typical contraindications can be:
1. Patient who requires to be changed and to be pulled to the maximum
2. Patient who requires traditional lifting
3. Patient with very advanced ptosis
4. Patient who requires immediate results

35.6.3
Results

There have been no complications apart from small hematomas, slight asymmetries, and ptosis for retouches or additions of threads. These retouches or new sessions, together with the attainment of the best result over time, constitute the true essence of the mini-invasive strategy that uses threads of support.

The author has had interesting results in the aesthetic corrections of paralytic or posttraumatic asymmetries:
1. From 2002 to 2005 there were 31 procedures of T3–soft face lift with absence of true complications and total satisfaction of the patient.
2. From 2004 to 2005, 62 cases were treated (46 with Contour ThreadLift™ and 16 with the mixed method), with satisfactory results in most of the cases. No complications have occurred. Changes, corrections, or improvements are easily performed. Two patients asked for the thread to be removed to have traditional lifting.

35.7
Conclusions

Aesthetic surgery of the face offers an ample range of surgical solutions. It is possible to get rejuvenation of the face and the neck with mini-invasive or soft methods without scars. New solutions using different surgical threads appear to be a valid solution. This is a noninvasive and ambulatory surgery, with a high level of safety, good and lasting results, and a minimum of social and physical uneasiness with few complications.

Every phase is important for a good result with this intervention. The most important factor is the choice by the patient and the respect for the indications. This surgical strategy may not be able to offer the same results as that of traditional surgery, but it does not introduce the same risks and complications.

The soft face lift using threads will allow, in suitable cases, the patient to achieve good and lasting results. Above all, it will slow aging, making the patient appear hostile and more smiling.

References

1. Buttkewitz H.: Die Nade Tecnik der subcutanen Gewebsrafung einer schnittlosen Korrekturmethode bei kosmetischen Brust und Gesichtoperationen. Zentralbl Chir 1956;81(29):1185–1192
2. Ulloa M.G.: The Ageing Face. Turin, Piccin 1983
3. Guillemain R.: Le" Curl Lift", le profession medical. Chir Plast Estét Mar 1970
4. Capurro S. Jr.: Un ago a due punte. Paper presented at the 32nd national congress, Palermo, 13–17 September 1983
5. Capurro S. Jr.: The double tipped needle. Plast Reconstr Surg 1987;79(6):1006
6. Yanai A., Fukuda O., Hirabayashi S.: Double tipped center-threading suture needle for subcuticular suturing. Plast Reconstr Surg 1986;78(3):411–413
7. Boo-Chai K.: Plastic construction of the superior palpebral fold. Plast Reconstr Surg 1973;31:74–78
8. Fournier P., Flores M.: Le lifting invisible. Rev Chir Esthet Langue Fr 2003;27(113):9–20
9. Fournier P.: Historie de l'aguille a deux pointes. Rev Chir Esthet Langue Fr 2004;28(115):19–27
10. Hernandez Perez E., Abbar K.: A percutaneous approach to eyebrowlift: the Salvadorian option. Dermatol Surg 2003;29(8):852–855
11. Serdev N.: Own method scarless breast lift by suture and needles perforations only. Int J Cosmet Surg 2001;1(1):1–41
12. Serdev N.: Serdev suture for scarless buttock and ultrasonic liposculpture of the buttocks. Int J Cosmet Med Surg 2003;5(1):27–34
13. Serdev N.: Scarless Serdev suture methods in brow and face lifts. Int J Cosmet Med Surg 2001;3(1):9–15
14. Sulamanidze M.A., Fournier P., Sulamanidze G.: Removal of facial soft tissue ptosis with special threads. Dermatol Surg 2002;28(5):367–371
15. Sulamanidze M.A., Shiffman M.A., Sulamanidze G.: Facial lifting with APTOS threads. Int J Cosmet Surg Aesthet Dermatol 2001;4:275–281
16. Sulamanidze M.A., Fournier P., Paikidze T.G., Sulamanidze G.M.: Removal of facial soft tissue ptosis with special threads. Dermatol Surg 2002,28:367–371
17. Bacci P.A.: T3 soft face lifting and bioresurfacing. Paper presented at the cosmetic surgery congress, Varna, June 2003
18. Bacci P.A.: T3-soft face lifting. Paper presented at the aesthetic medicine congress AGORA, Milan, October 2004
19. Bacci P.A.: T3-soft face lifting. Paper presented at the 29th world congress of cosmetic and dermatology surgery, Manila, February 2004

20. Bacci P.A., Mancini S.: Chirurgia estetica mini invasiva: i fili di sostegno (Not invasive aesthetic surgery using threads). Minelli, Arezzo 2006;45–180

21. Ruff G.L.: insertion device for a barbed tissue connector. US Patent 5, 342, 376, 1994

22. Leung J.C., Ruff G.L., Megaro M.A.: Barbed bidirectional medical sutures: biomechanical properties and wound closure efficacy study. Soc Biomater Trans 2002;25:724

23. DuBois J.J.: A technique for subcutaneous knot inversion following running subcuticular closures. Mil Med 1992;157(5):255

24. Scott D.W., Miller W.H., Griffin C.E.: Small Animal Dermatology, 5th Ed. Philadelphia, Saunders 1995:55–174

25. Nilsson T.: Effect of increased and reduced tension on the mechanical properties of healing wound in the abdominal wall. Scand J Plast Surg 1982;16:101–105

26. Alcamo J.H.: Surgical sutures. US Patent 3,123,077, 1964

27. Tang J.B., Gu Y.T., Rice K.: Evaluation of four method of flexor tendon repair for postoperative active mobilisation. Plast Reconstr Surg 2001;107(3):742–749

28. McKenzie A.R.: An experimental multiple barbed suture for the long flexor tendons of the palm and fingers. Preliminary report. J Bone Joint Surg 1967;49(3):440–447

29. Barry L., Bazan C., Poletti E., Treen B.: The emerging technique of the antiptosis subdermal suspension threads. Dermatol Surg J 2004;30:41–44

30. Kazinnikova O.G., Adamian A.A.: Age specific changes in facial and cervical tissue: a review. Ann Plast Reconstr Surg 2000;1:52–61

31. Ingle N.P., King M.W., Leung J.C., Batchelor S.: Barbed suture anchoring applicability to dissimilar polymeric materials. Soc Biomater Trans 2003;26:100

32. Bacci P.A.: Restyling tessutale. Tema Med 2005;10(2):29–33

Chapter 36

Anti Gravity/Elevation Lift: Facelifting Without Incisions

36

Longin Zurek

36.1
Introduction

In recent years, different facelift techniques using threads have become increasingly popular [1–5]. Patients are seeking the simplest and least invasive cosmetic procedures, not only for the purpose of rejuvenation, but also in order to maintain their youthful appearance and prevent the development of signs of aging.

The first phenomenon in the aging process of the face is ptosis related to diminished support against gravity. Although ptosis has traditionally been treated by facelift, attempts to improve the signs of aging without incisions were made over five decades ago.

In 1956, Buttkewitz [6] reported his method of elevating tissues by means of subcutaneously applied nylon thread (Fig. 36.1).

In 1999, Sulamanidze, described a novel technique of lifting soft tissue of the face with barbed threads called APTOS (antiptosis) sutures [7, 8]. The original APTOS sutures were made from 2/0 polypropylene monofilament with convergent dents, which allowed one-way movement of the threads in the soft tissue of the face. These sutures were implanted along special lines, which produced uniform gathering of soft tissue and resulted in some repositioning and support against gravity.

Barbed sutures were first developed in the 1960s [9]. In 1967, McKenzie [10] reported the use of experimental multiple barbed sutures for tendon repair in the hands. Also the idea of reinforcing facial skin with special gold filaments had been described earlier [11].

As the original APTOS sutures were not available in Australia, the author devised a handcrafted version customized to the design of the barbs and the length of each thread. The modification was named the Anti Gravity/Elevation Filament (AGE Filament; Fig. 36.2) and was registered as a trademark in March 2003.

36.2
Technique of Manufacturing AGE Filaments

36.2.1
Materials

1. Polypropylene suture, 2/0 Prolene blue monofilament from Ethicon
2. Personna Plus no. 15 blade
3. Wooden tongue depressor
4. Sterilization pouches

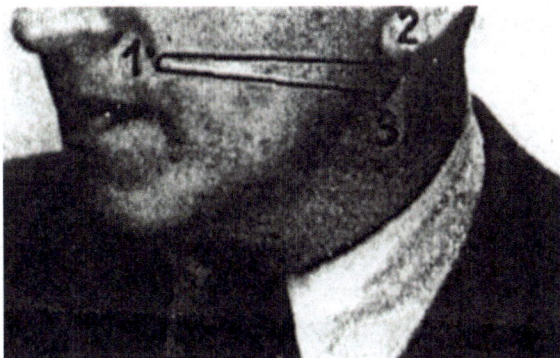

Fig. 36.1 Buttkewitz method of elevating tissues by means of subcutaneously applied nylon thread shown in the correction for the drooping buccolabial fold. (Courtesy of Pierre F. Fournier)

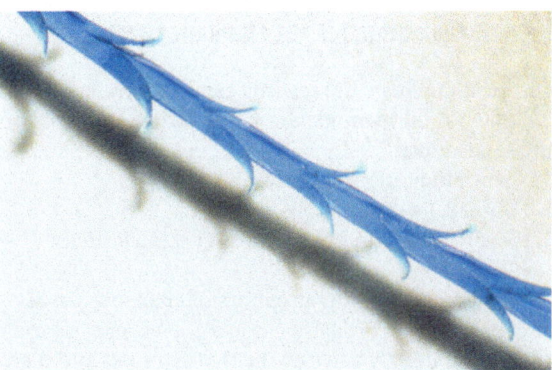

Fig. 36.2 Anti Gravity/Elevation Filament™ (AGE Filament™). Under magnification

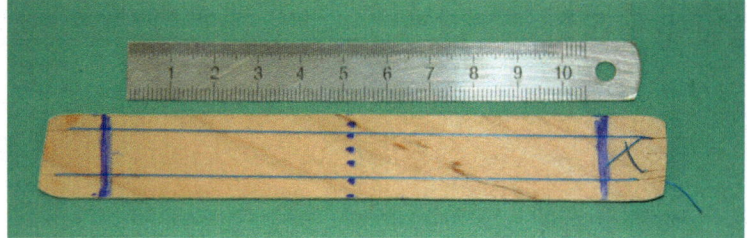

Fig. 36.3 The Prolene suture is stretched on previously sterilized tongue depressors a few days prior to cutting, allowing the thread to remain straight, which facilitates implantation

36.2.2
Method

Full aseptic technique is observed. Surgical cap, mask, gown and sterile gloves are worn. Good lighting and magnifying loops are necessary. It is important that the technician is able to sit in an ergonomic position using an appropriate table and chair.

The Prolene suture is stretched on previously sterilized tongue depressors a few days prior to cutting, allowing the thread to remain straight, which facilitates implantation (Fig. 36.3). The tongue depressor is marked with the length of the threads to be notched. The mid point of the length is also marked where the notches would converge or diverge. Notches are made on the thread approximately 1 mm apart at an appropriate angle around 45° (Fig. 36.4). By rotating the thread, the thumb of the non-dominant hand allows the barbs to be escarped in a spiral fashion. The same process is repeated on the opposite aspect of the thread, resulting in a double-helix configuration. The ends of the thread are cut and removed from the tongue depressor. The tensile strength of every thread is tested by manually stretching it.

The threads are then washed in sterile distilled water, placed into sterilization pouches and autoclaved in a standard manner. The sterilization process does not affect the integrity of the device.

36.3
Patient Evaluation for AGE Filament Lift

The ideal candidate has realistic expectations, good skin elasticity, mild to moderate facial laxity, and mild to moderate ptosis.

Contraindications include:
1. Unrealistic expectations
2. Severe photodamage with loss of skin elasticity
3. Severe laxity and ptosis
4. Very thin faces with atrophic subcutaneous tissue

There is a category between the two extremes and there is always an exception from the general rule. The purpose of the AGE Filament lift is to provide or restore some support, as well as to elevate and reposition the soft tissue of the face to some degree.

36.4
Instruments

1. Spinal needle 18 gauge, 3.50 in. (1.2 mm × 90 mm)
2. 27-gauge, 0.5-in. needle (0.40 mm × 13 mm)
3. 25-gauge 1.5-in. needle (0.50 mm × 38 mm)
4. Luer-Lok 3-ml syringe
5. Curved iris scissors
6. Curved hemostat
7. Sterile towels and swabs

Local anesthesia is done with 1% lidocaine containing 1:200,000 epinephrine freshly mixed.

36.5
Surgical Technique

The concerns of the patient are identified and the face is then examined in front of a three-way mirror. Skin quality, degree of facial laxity, ptosis and thickness of subcutaneous tissue are assessed.

For the purpose of AGE Filament lift, the face is divided into four zones:

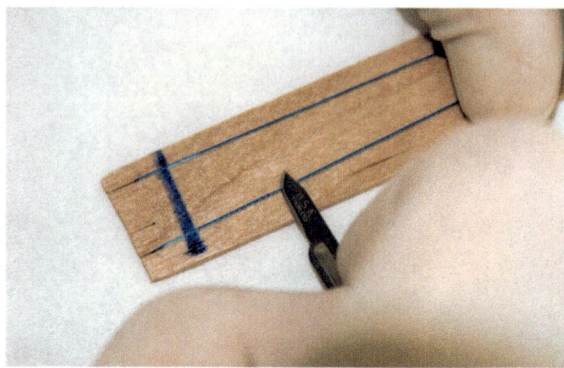

Fig. 36.4 Notches are made on the thread approximately 1 mm apart at an appropriate angle at around 45°

1. Eyebrow
2. Mid face
3. Lower face
4. Neck

Consent forms are discussed and signed and standardized photographs are taken. Skin markings are drawn (Fig. 36.5).

36.5.1
Medications

Cephalexin (500 mg) is given and then continued with 1 capsule twice daily for 4 days. Diazepam (5–10 mg) is given as a sedative and paraecetamol (500 mg) plus codeine phosphate (30 mg) is given for analgesia.

36.5.2
Preoperative Instructions

Patients are advised not to take any aspirin or other medications that could compromise coagulation 2 weeks prior to the procedure. Patients are not to wear any makeup.

36.5.3
Postoperative Instructions

Patients are advised to avoid excessive movements and any manipulation of the face for up to 2 weeks after the procedure. Antibiotics are to be taken twice daily for 3 days. Ice packs can be applied to relieve swelling and

discomfort, protecting the skin with a hand towel. An appointment to return within 1 week is scheduled.

36.5.4
Surgical Skin Markings

36.5.4.1
Eyebrows

Two parallel lines are drawn in the shape of a lazy "S" at various angles in relation to the midline. This is done in order to attain appropriate elevation of the mid and lateral portion of the eyebrow.

36.5.4.2
Mid Face

The shape of the cheeks is marked by two parallel lines commencing at the superior and inferior margins of the zygoma, continuing horizontally for not more than 1 cm (bearing in mind the location of temporal branches of the facial nerve in the mid zygomatic region) and continuing along the gentle curvature of the cheek. It is helpful to ask the patient to smile in order to visualize the natural shape of the cheek.

36.5.4.3
Lower Face

Depending on the degree of elevation desired, the two parallel markings start in the preauricular region corresponding to the superior and inferior borders of the

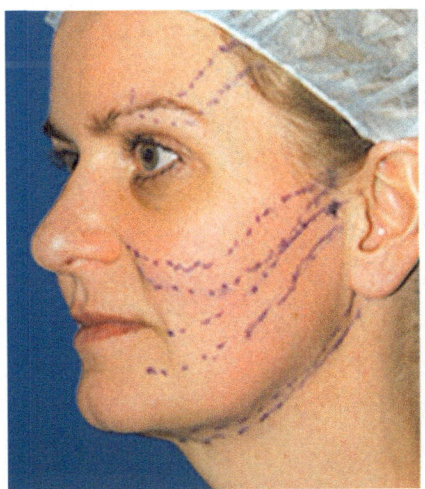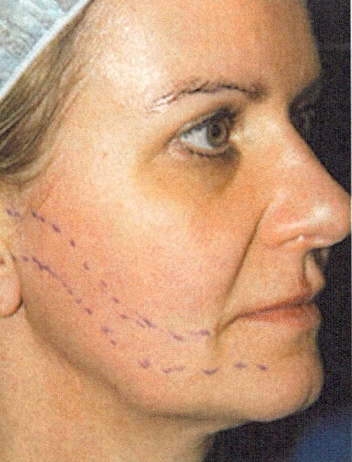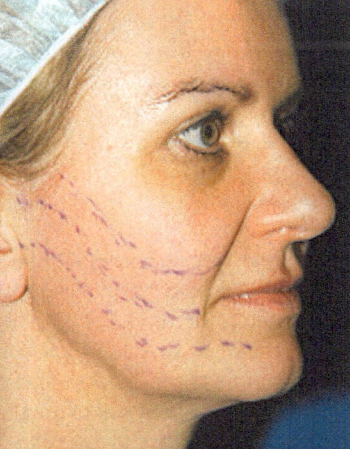

Fig. 36.5 Skin markings are drawn

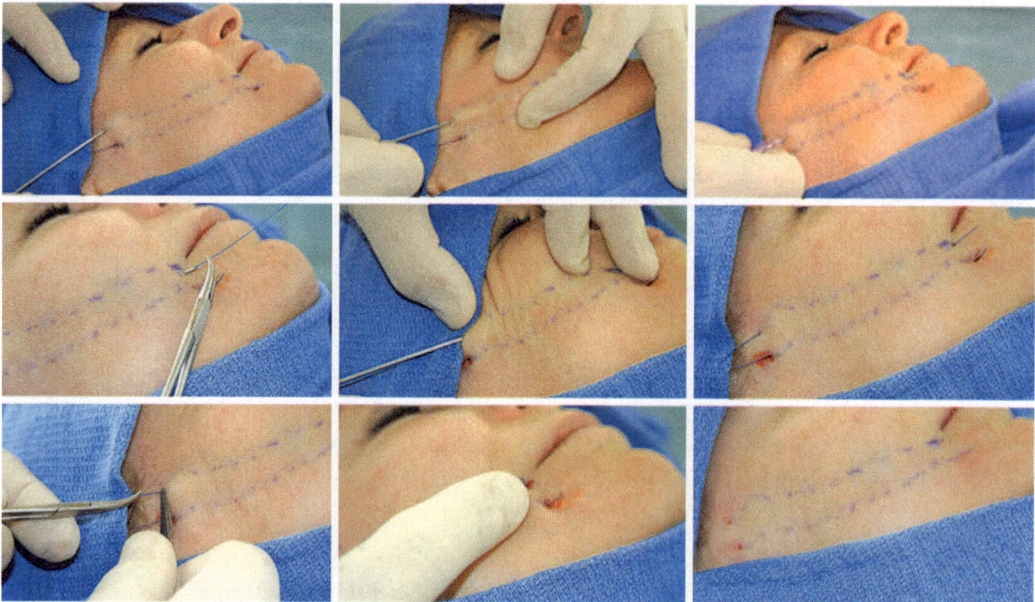

Fig. 36.6 Implantation of AGE Filaments

tragus. They can also be placed in a higher position at the superior and inferior borders of the zygoma (these lines must not extend more than 1 cm horizontally). The lower line follows the line of the mandible, finishing in the chin. The upper line is usually placed parallel to the lower line, however it can be directed towards the angle of the mouth. Occasionally an additional thread can be planned superiorly and follows the curvature of the cheek.

36.5.4.4
Neck

The midline of the neck is marked and two diverting lines are drawn from the mastoid process along the cervical mental angle and submental region.

36.5.5
Technique of Implantation

The skin is prepared using 10% povidone–iodine solution or 0.1% chlorohexidine aqueous solution. Ice may be applied to the injection sites to reduce discomfort of infiltration and produce vasoconstriction. A small amount of local anesthetic is injected intradermally at the point of entry and exit of the spinal needle using the 27-gauge needle. The planned tracks are infiltrated using the 25-gauge long needle. About 10 min is allowed for vasoconstriction to establish.

The implantation of AGE Filaments is described next (Fig. 36.6).

36.5.5.1
Brow

Penetration of the skin begins at the temporal hairline starting with the inferior line. The spinal needle is advanced in an immediate subdermal plane, along the skin markings, proceeding deeper to include the mass of the outer brow to the point of exit just above the brow.

It is important to feel some resistance during this maneuver in order to ensure effective anchoring of the device and prevent migration of the thread. After removal of the introducer from the spinal needle, the thread is inserted using a curved hemostat. Tissue above the needle is infolded by pinching with the thumb and index finger of the non-dominant hand, while the fifth finger is used to secure the end of the thread. The spinal needle is then withdrawn following the curve of the skin

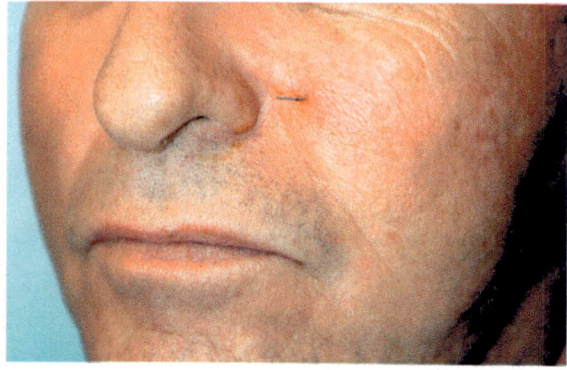

Fig. 36.7 Extrusion

marking. The effective anchoring is checked by pulling both ends of the thread with the hemostat. The same process is repeated to implant the superior thread.

The gathered tissue is then adjusted manually by applying gentle, even, pressure with the index and middle finger of the dominant hand along their course. Care is taken to prevent accidental inclusion of hair in the temporal region.

The ends of the threads are then grasped with a curved hemostat and are cut with curved iris scissors flush to the skin. Care must be taken not to "buttonhole" the skin.

36.5.5.2
Cheek

After the skin has been penetrated vertically, the needle is advanced horizontally for not more than 1 cm and continues along a deeper plane above the superficial musculoaponeurotic system. While the needle is advancing, the malar area is pinched between the index finger and thumb of the non-dominant hand, gently "feeding" it. Extreme care is taken to prevent an uneven course of the needle, which would produce dimpling, by constantly checking and adjusting the uniformity of the tissue above it.

36.5.5.3
Lower Face

The same technique is employed except the depth of implantation is more superficial but still ensuring adequate and uniform coverage of the device.

36.5.5.4
Neck

The entry of the spinal needle is perpendicular to the mastoid process and includes periosteum, while advancing along the lines in the immediate subcutaneous plane. The correct depth is confirmed by some resistance on advancement and good, even coverage on elevation of the needle.

36.6
Complications

Extrusion (Fig. 36.7) incidence is approximately 5%, migration (and extrusion) (Fig. 36.8) incidence is 0.005%, chronic inflammation and superficial skin loss (Fig. 36.9) occurs in 0.010% of cases, hematoma (Fig. 36.10) in 0.002% of cases, scarring (Fig. 36.11) in 0.003% of cases, and infection (Fig. 36.12) in 0.003% of cases.

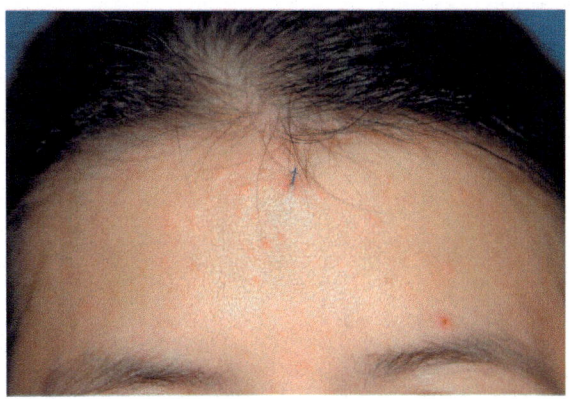

Fig. 36.8 Migration (and extrusion)

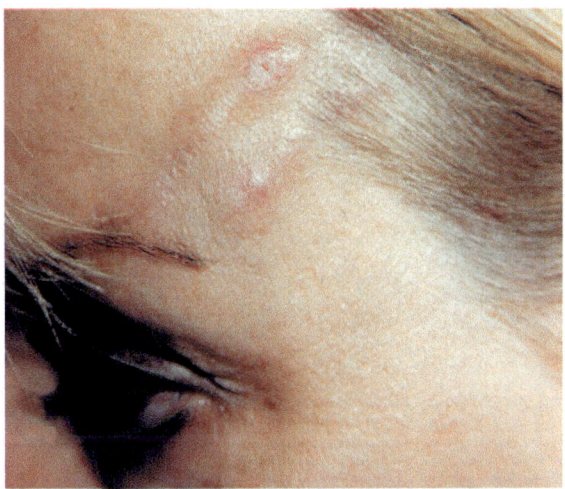

Fig. 36.9 Chronic inflammation and superficial skin loss

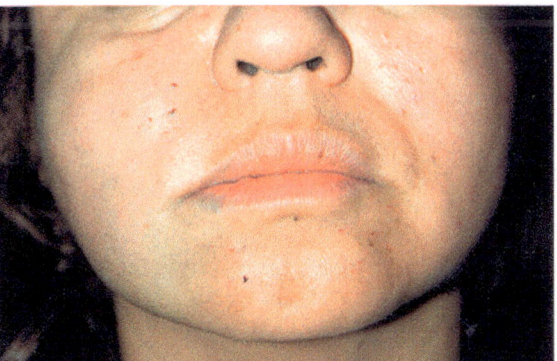

Fig. 36.10 Hematoma

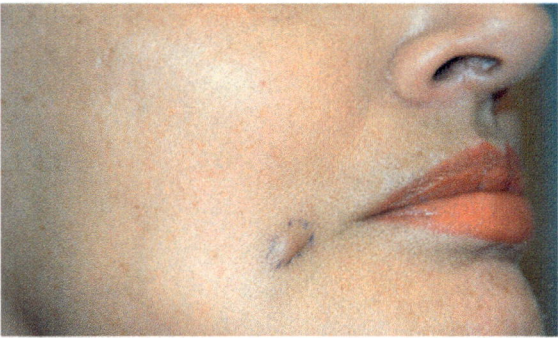

Fig. 36.11 Scarring

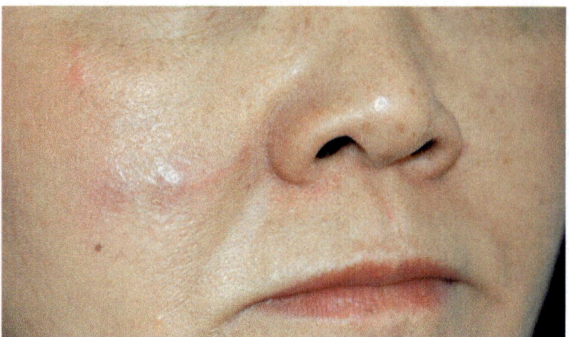

Fig. 36.12 Infection

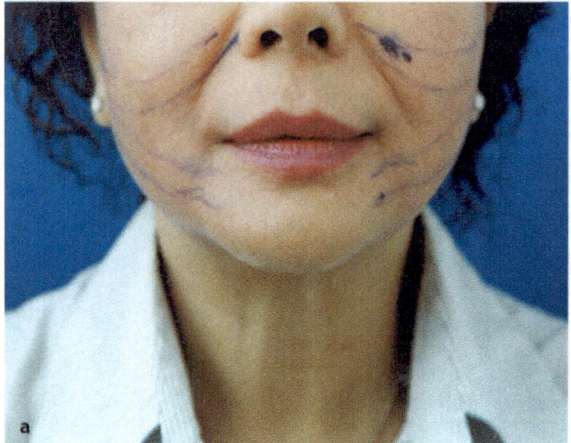

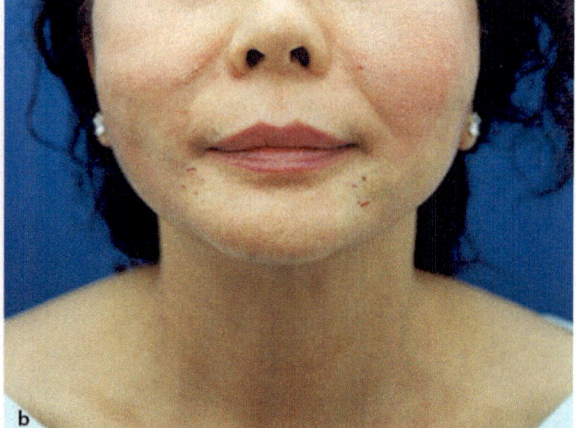

Fig. 36.13 a Before and **b** Immediately after AGE Filament lifting of the mid and lower face

36.7
Discussion

The author has performed over 1,000 facelifting procedures using barbed sutures and finds they are effective in providing a degree of support against gravity as well as some elevation and repositioning of facial tissue (Fig. 36.13) [12–17]. The AGE Filaments have a higher density of barbs that result in a more secure self-anchoring and a higher degree of fibrosis.

Histopathological examination of the AGE Filaments 6 months after implantation showed fibrosis.

Surveys showed a high degree of patient satisfaction exceeding 90%. Currently surveys are being conducted to examine long-term results. Many patients continue to present usually after 12 months requesting additional AGE Filaments in order to maintain the results.

There is large potential in applying this device in Asians since these patients are very suitable owing to their facial configuration and lesser degrees of ptosis and skin laxity. Asian patients are also reluctant to undergo surgery owing to cultural factors and the tendency for unfavorable scars.

36.8
Conclusions

Barbed suture facelifting is an evolving technique. Although the experience is relatively short and limited, the technique is promising with growing interest around the world.

The barbed suture lifts are safe, effective and relatively easy to perform. The ability to manually prepare a barbed device gives the surgeon an opportunity to further improve as well as customize the device.

References

1. Badin AZ, Forte MRC, Silva OL. Scarless mid- and lower face lift. Aesthet Surg J 2005;25(4):340–347
2. Haiavy J, Leventhal MS. Facial rejuvenation with barbed sutures: A retrospective analyses of technique and results. Am J Cosmet Surg 2005;22(4):39–247
3. Isse NG, Fodor PB. Elevating the midface with barbed polypropylene sutures. Aesthet Surg J 2005;25(3):301–303

4. Belo VG, Buse EB, Cayetano RJ, Flores MA. Seamless face-lift with aptos thread: The Belo medical group experience. Am J Cosmet Surg 2005;22(3):182–186

5. Fournier PF. A Rediscovered Technique: The Curl Lift. Curl Lift training course at the 21st International Congress of French Society of Aesthetic Surgery, Paris, France, 16 May 2004

6. Buttkewitz H. Needle technic of subcutaneous drawing-together of tissues; cosmetic surgery of the breast and face without incision. Zentrabl Chir 1956;81(29):1185–1192

7. Sulamanidze MA, Fournier PF, Paikidze TG, Sulamandize GM. Removal of facial soft tissue ptosis with special threads. Dermatol Surg 2002;28:367–342

8. Sulamanidze MA, Fournier PF, Paikidze TG, Sulamanidze GM. Facial lifting with APTOS threads. Int J Cosmet Surg Aesthet Dermatol 2001;3:257–280

9. Alcamo JH. Surgical suture. US Patent 3,123,077, 1964

10. McKenzie AR. An experimental multiple barbed suture for the long reflexor tendons of the palm and fingers. J Bone Joint Surg 1967;49(3):440–447

11. Adamyan AA. Clinical aspects of skin reinforcement with special (gold) surgical filaments. Ann Plast Reconstr Aesthet Surg 1998;3:18–22

12. Zurek LH. Facelifting with Self Anchoring Polypropylene Sutures. Australasian College of Cosmetic Surgery and Cosmetic Physicians Society of Australia Annual Conference, Australia 2003 & 2004

13. Zurek LH. Age filament lift instructional courses with live surgery presentations. Seoul, Korea, Dec 2003

14. Zurek LH. Age filament lectures. Korean Society of Aesthetic Surgery Conference. Seoul, Korea, Dec 2003

15. Zurek LH. Age filament lift surgical demonstration. The Philippine Society for Cosmetic Surgery workshop on Minimally Invasive Suture Techniques. Quezon City, Philippines, Feb 2005

16. Zurek LH. Facelift techniques live surgery workshops. 5050 Aesthetic Surgery Clinic, Seoul, South Korea 2003, 2004, 2005, 2006

17. Zurek LH. Surgical demonstration of age filament lift technique. Cosmetic Surgery Clinic. Taipei, Taiwan, Dec 2005

CHAPTER 37

The Curl Lift: a Rediscovered Technique

37

Pierre F. Fournier

37.1
Introduction

The idea of lifting selected parts of the face with subcutaneous sutures is not new. The aim is to tighten the subcutaneous tissues as well as the overlying skin. This procedure has the advantage of lifting the desired parts of the face or the upper neck without scar, under local anesthesia, with little downtime and minimal discomfort and complications as it is a minimally invasive procedure.

The results are not as dramatic as a surgical procedure but are good results in selected cases with young or mature patients who do not want and do not need major surgery. They only want maintenance of youth or beauty and not radical rejuvenation or embellishment.

A special needle is inserted under the skin with a polypropylene thread of suture material. One loop of this thread will lift the chosen part of the face and a second loop of the same thread will moor it to the more resistant tissues of the scalp. The advantage of this technique is to have two anchoring points. The result obtained is instant and leaves only a little scar in the scalp near the hairline. Should it be necessary to modify the result obtained, the procedure is reversible with tightening or relaxing by adding or removing sutures under local anesthesia.

Folds of skin may be seen above the places treated and usually flatten over a period of 2–3 weeks. Dimples on the lifted area on the face are avoided with experience.

37.2
History of the Curl Lift

Ulloa [1], in 1983, mentioned a technique of elevating the tissues on the face by means of subcutaneously applied nylon threads stitches. Buttkewitz [2] described this technique in 1956 and there is a picture that demonstrates the correction by suture of a "drooping buccolabial fold."

In 1970, Guillemain [3] described a similar technique named the curl lift. He used a spinal needle or a long Reverdin needle to elevate with a rein tendon, a kangaroo tendon, or a nylon thread the tail of the eyebrow, the cheekbone area, the lower part of the face, or the upper neck. With the patients under local anesthesia, a suture was placed in the subcutaneous tissue and firmly anchored above and below. The patients were mostly men who did not want a major operation. His partner Galland and their pupil Clavier have used this technique since 1966.

This technique was not widely used in the 1970s, not because of the results, which were usually good, but because at this time most of the patients were mature or more advanced in age and needed major techniques of rejuvenation or embellishment. It was performed only occasionally but was known by many cosmetic surgeons in France.

In 2002, Sassaki and Cohen [4] described a similar technique with two needles. They used it either during a surgical lifting to improve its duration or as the closed procedure.

In 2003, Mendez Florez [5] described and improved the technique using a double-bevel needle of his own conception and also a special maneuver also of his own conception to simplify the operation. He gives many surgical details that many cosmetic surgeons use today and he has taught his procedure to many surgeons during the past 3 years.

This double-bevel needle is similar to the needle used for a very long time by upholsterers. And needles with two tips, curved or straight, small or large, with one central eye were often used in the past by general or plastic surgeons [6–10].

In 1986, Yahai et al. [11] described the use of a curved needle with two tips and one central eye. In 1983 and 1987, Capurro [12, 13] described the use of a double-tipped needle. Such needles with two tips and a central eye allow the surgeon easily to place sutures subcutaneously or to place long portions of threads subcutaneously without an incision (Fig. 37.1).

Double-tipped needles have also been used by orthopedic surgeons (meniscus surgery) and plastic surgeons (cleft-palate surgery). Also subcutaneous sutures with a normal curved or straight needle with a nylon thread have been used to ligate small varicose veins or in cosmetic surgery, and in Oriental upper blepharoplasties by Boo-Chai [14, 15], who started in 1952. Mathay (J.

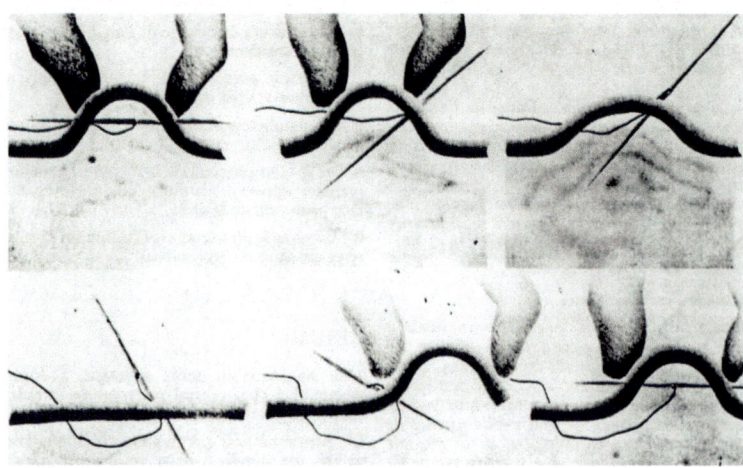

Fig. 37.1 Capurro method demonstrating the use of the double-pointed needle with a central eye

Mathay, Makati Medical Center, Manilla, 1974, personal observation) used subcutaneous sutures to narrow large tips of the nose in Orientals. Serdev [16–18] described this technique with an elastic suture [19–21].

Since the rediscovery of this technique and the publication of the reports by Sassaki and Cohen [4] and Mendez Florez [5], many cosmetic surgeons have used it and many different names have been proposed, such as the thread lift, the nonsurgical facelift, the stitch lift, the suture lift, the suspension lift, the invisible facelift, and the filting [22].

The author keeps the name the "curl lift" chosen by Guillemain [3], who popularised the technique.

37.3
Indications

1. The best indication is a young patient with one or several "weak points" on his/her face or upper neck due to the aging process:
   (a) Eyebrow ptosis
   (b) Significant nasolabial sulcus
   (c) Significant labiomental sulcus
   (d) Mild ptosis of the lower face with pseudojowls
   (e) Mild skin excess on the upper neck
2. Young patients wanting to modify their appearances especially by brow lifting or lifting of the cheek bone area responsible for a too deep nasolabial sulcus or labiomental sulcus (marionettes). More mature patients who do not want a major procedure.
3. Patients complaining of an unsatisfactory result shortly after a surgical cervicofacial lifting.
4. The curl lift is not indicated in a patient with a lot of skin excess even if slight improvement is possible. Only moderate skin excess can be corrected satisfactorily.
5. Most patients want improve only one part of face (upper, middle, lower) or upper neck but several parts can be treated at the same time .

37.4
Technique

1. Marking the patient seated or standing
2. Local anesthesia
3. Hydrotomy
4. A 5-mm incision in the scalp , near the hairline
5. Insertion of the needle either below the lower anchoring point or in the upper one in the scalp
6. Placement of the thread in the eye of the needle
7. Partial removal of the needle
8. Rotation of the needle by 180° degrees on its axis (Mendez Florez's maneuver)
9. Needle pushed back parallel to the first track through the incision in the scalp
10. Removal of the threads from the eye of the needle
11. Lift of the weak point and estimation of the desired correction (with or without a mirror given to the patient)
12. Surgeon's knot after additional or no additional anchoring
13. Suturing the scalp incision
14. Moderately compressive dressing for 24 h

37.5
Facial Analysis and Marking the Patient

As with other procedures that are performed on the face or neck, a thorough facial analysis has to be done at least at two different consultations 2 weeks apart. All information will be given to the patient, oral and written (reflection period for the patient and for the surgeon).

Patients having outward aging (tissue proliferation, tension and pressure wrinkles) are not a good case even if improvements can be made. Patients having inward aging (tissue involution, sag and shrinkage wrinkles) are good cases. In this latter case, facial ptosis may be due to sagging without loss of volume or to sagging with a loss of volume mostly of the fatty framework of the face

and volume surgery, and therefore lipofilling should be done as well at the same time or in two sessions. Books with chapters on facial analysis are very useful [23–26].

When marking the patient for the treatment of the nasolabial sulcus, the patient should be standing or seated and not horizontal. With a mirror in his or her hand, the patient will explain what he or she wants, with the right index finger on the place to be lifted on the cheekbone area, and then the degree and direction of the lifting that wanted.

The surgeon will then study if a "curl lift" is possible. The surgeon marks the place giving the desired lift on the cheekbone area (point L for lifting). Two centimeters below this point L another point will be marked (O for "out"). A third one will be marked on the scalp, close to the hairline (I for "in") (Fig. 37.2). All such points should be on the same straight line as the future track of the needle and the thread. This line when treating the nasolabial sulcus should be more or less perpendicular to the sulcus. The same marking has to be done in the different places needed to be lifted:

1. Tail of the eyebrow
2. Lower part of the face
3. Upper part of the neck

37.6
Anesthesia and Hydrotomy

The author always uses local anesthesia with infiltration (4 ml of Xylocaine 1% with 1:200,000 epinephrine mixed with 6 ml of normal saline, in a 10-ml syringe). Solutions are kept in the refrigerator before use (4°C). The complete track of the needle is infiltrated gently using a 30-gauge needle and giving small taps on the skin with the fingers of the left hand to decrease the slight discomfort of the infiltration. Emla® cream can also be used beforehand to reduce pain. Ten milliliters of the mixed solution is enough on each side to be treated.

After waiting 10 min, with a clock in the hand, the surgeon performs hydrotomy is to elevate the skin from

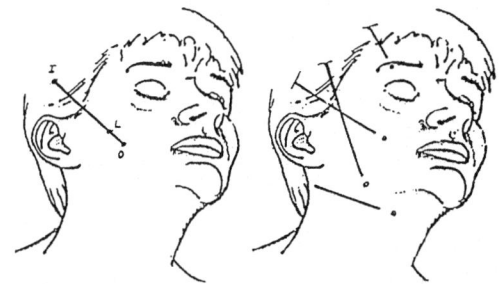

Fig. 37.2 Marking the patient when using Mendez Florez technique. *Left*: Marking to lift the cheekbone area. *Right*: Marking of others places of the face and upper neck

the deeper structures. Ten milliliters of chilled normal saline is infiltrated along the future track of the needle before making the small incision in the scalp. No sedation is necessary but it could be used with some patients. The best preparation is the psychological one (vocal sedation).

37.7
Surgical Technique

In the following the personal technique of Mendez Florez [5] is outlined.

37.7.1
Anesthesia

The solution used is 2% lidocaine in a 20-ml vial with 1:80,000 epinephrine in 20 ml of normal saline.

Half a tablet of midazolam (15 mg) is given before local anesthesia. A nerve block of the facial zone to be treated is performed. No more than 20 ml of the solution is necessary for good anesthesia of the desired zone.

37.7.2
Operation

Florez Mendez uses a special double-beveled needle of his own conception. Three lengths are 8, 10 or 12 cm. A 0.5-cm incision is made in the scalp near the hairline. The needle is inserted through this incision into the subcutaneous tissue and incompletely removed at a point 0.2 cm below the place to be lifted (point L). The threads on the upper bevel remain subcutaneously at the place to be lifted (Fig. 37.2). A special maneuver has to be done at that time that requires a rotation of 180° of the needle on its axis on the right or on the left side, and after this the needle is pushed up parallel to the first track until the upper incision and removed. A lower curl is the obtained by grasping firmly the part to be lifted. The thread is then detached from the needle and after traction a surgeon's knot is made with or without additional anchoring . The thread may or may be not anchored through the galea or to the periosteum. The incision is closed. The sutures used are polypropylene 4/0 or 5/0.

The procedure has two anchoring points, with one below and the other above. The result obtained is instantaneous. This double-beveled needle and the 180° rotation should be credited to Mendez Florez [5].

This technique is used on the forehead to lift the tail of the eyebrow, in the cheekbone area, and in the lower face or upper neck. The action in this technique is in the tension applied and securing it. There is a pull.

With APTOS threads [27–29], another excellent technique with the same indications, the action is to support the lifted structures once they have been repositioned. Such APTOS threads could be compared to crutches. They have no anchoring and no mooring of the repositioned tissues.

An excellent result depends on:

1. The type of the thread used (absorbable or nonabsorbable, smooth or braided)
2. The degree of tension
3. The precise placement
4. The pull in the good direction

37.7.3
Variations of the Technique

Since the popularization of this technique, others variations have been used.

37.7.3.1
Use of a Long Straight Needle

All the aforementioned facial or cervical areas may be lifted with a long straight needle with one distal eye (regular needle) for the thread. The needle is passed through a small incision in the scalp and removed completely at the point to be lifted. When the needle is out, it has to be reinserted through the same punctured point in the skin to be moved completely 2 cm further. Again through this last puncture point through the skin, the

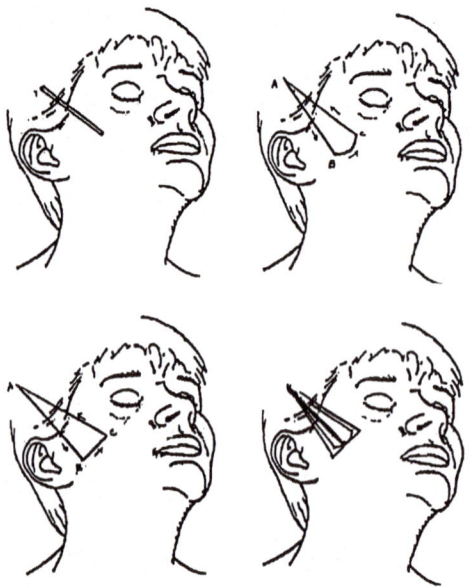

Fig. 37.3 The lower curl has a different grip according the tool used. **a** Needle of Mendez Florez. **b** Curved needle. **c** Straight needle. **d** Comparison of the different curls

needle is inserted to reach the upper incision. Needle and thread are removed and after the desired traction a knot is tied with or without additional anchoring (Fig. 37.3).

37.7.3.2
Guillemain Technique

Guillemain [3] used a similar technique either with a long straight Reverdin needle or with a spinal needle.

37.7.3.3
Variation of the Hook Technique

Currently, the author uses a variation of the hook technique (Fig. 37.4). At the chosen point to be lifted (point L), a thread is mounted on a curved needle through the skin. After the loop has been made, the subcutaneous thread is grasped on each side with a blunt hook inserted through the incision in the scalp. The best hook is easily made with a modified upholsterer needle. One end of the loop is then removed through the incision in the scalp. The other side of the loop is removed in the same manner through the same scalp incision or through another small one near the first one if desired.

One end of the threads is finally mounted on a curved needle and anchored deeply to the periosteum before the surgeon's knot is tied after putting the desired tension on the thread.

The thread used is polypropylene 2/0 but it is possible also to use a braided nylon (Mersuture®Ethicon) thread that may give longer-lasting results, as scar tissue will pass through it. A larger lower loop can be made with a straight threaded needle if desired. Folding the skin where the skin has been punctured will avoid unpleasant dimples.

With this technique, a larger lower loop and a larger surface of subcutaneous tissue between the two loops will give more resistance, a stronger grip at the lower level and less tension in the subcutaneous tissue where the traction is applied.

In all cases a dressing has to be used that is occlusive and with moderate pressure for 24 h.

37.7.3.4
The Barbed Thread Technique

The barbed thread technique combines the advantages of the curl lift and the APTOS threads with use of a modified thread.

After the future tracks of the thread have been carefully studied, small incisions are made on the thread with a no. 11 blade, on one or both sides of the thread. Such modifications are only on the descending and ascending parts of the thread (Fig. 37.5).

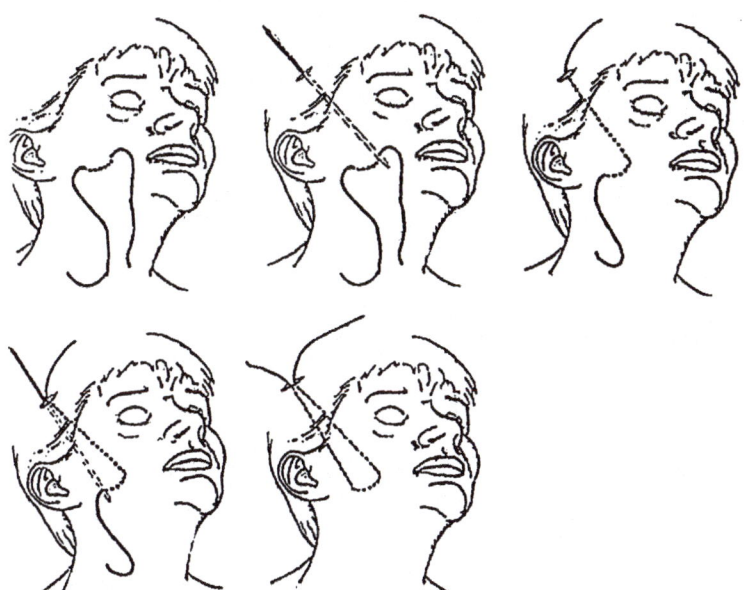

Fig. 37.4 The hook technique. Different steps

To pass this thread, an epidural needle is used. The operation has three steps:

1. The epidural needle is passed from B to A. The thread is then passed from B to A and this section of the thread has hooks on most of its length. After the nonhooked portion of this thread has been grasped in the scalp incision, the epidural needle is removed.
2. A similar maneuver is performed from C to B. The remaining hooked and nonhooked section of the thread is passed through the needle from B to C. The needle is removed.
3. The epidural needle is inserted finally from A to C and the last portion of the hooked and nonhooked section of the thread is passed from C to A. A surgeon's knot is tied after applying the desired tension to the part to be lifted (Fig. 37.5). Anchoring or not anchoring is left to the judgment of the surgeon.

This type of makeshift thread has the advantages of the pull of the curl lift and the support of the APTOS threads.

According to the results of the facial analysis, a syringe for lipofilling may be used at the same time if volume surgery is also needed. APTOS threads [27–29] can be

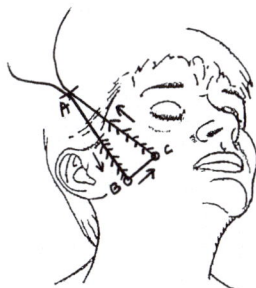

Fig. 37.5 The barbed thread technique

used to reinforce the result obtained in case of hyperlaxity of the cutaneous layer.

37.7.4
Complications

This procedure, being minimally invasive, has minimal complications:

1. The results are of short duration.
2. Too tight sutures damage the subcutaneous tissue, dividing the fibrous ligament and the retinaculum cuti connecting the subcutaneous muscular aponeurotic system to the skin.
   (a) A good and lasting result in patients having a moderate ptosis can be obtained with moderate tension of the treated place of the face or on the upper neck.
   (b) Using the hook technique will decrease the complication as the surface of soft tissue between the thread is much wider in the lower anchoring point. A new thread has to be placed again to treat this complication.
3. Dimples above the lower curl may be observed. They may disappear after a few days or more. They may be treated by subcision with a sharp needle, local hydrotomy or a small fat graft. When using the "hook technique," folding the skin between before using the curved needle or the straight needle in the subcutaneous tissue of the lower anchoring point will avoid this inconvenience.
4. Folds of the skin above the lower curl are frequently more or less important depending on the tension or with patients having a major facial ptosis. They flatten over a period of 2–3 weeks. They are less important if the distance between the two anchoring

points is large; consequently, when this complication is feared, the distance between the two anchoring points should be increased and the upper anchor point should be placed higher in the scalp, instead of placing it too close to the hairline. Should some excess skin remain, a new shorter suture may be placed above the first one.

5. An asymmetrical result is always possible. This is avoided with experience. A small excision in the scalp has also been proposed to correct the asymmetry or residual folds. Should one side be asymmetrical, it is always possible to improve one side by placing another thread to increase the result obtained or to remove a too tight suture and replace it with an adequate one. The patient should be informed of such possibilities and that the operation is reversible.

6. A suture that is too tight may cause pain and should be removed. A less tight one will be placed immediately after this removal.

7. Edema is moderate, usually for a few days.

8. Ecchymoses may be seen but are infrequent.

9. Discomfort or a slight pain is possible for a few days and weak painkillers are given for 3 days.

10. Potential complications include damage of the facial muscles, vessels, nerves or salivary glands. A careful hydrotomy can avoid this as well as thorough knowledge of the facial anatomy and of the danger zones. Infection is possible, but has not been reported, as well as hematoma.

11. No sequelae have been described.

37.7.5
Postoperative Care

1. The mild compressive dressing is removed after 24 h.
2. Vibramycine (100 mg) twice a day for 5 days.
3. Anti-inflammatories for 1 week.
4. Light painkillers for 2 or 3 days.
5. Makeup may be used after 2 days but care must be taken.

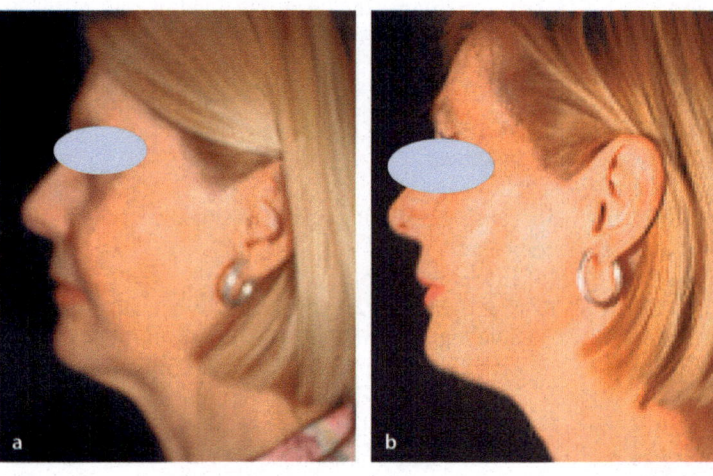

Fig. 37.6 a Preoperatively. **b** Following neck curl lift

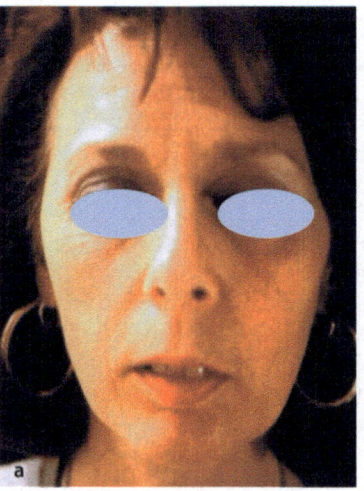
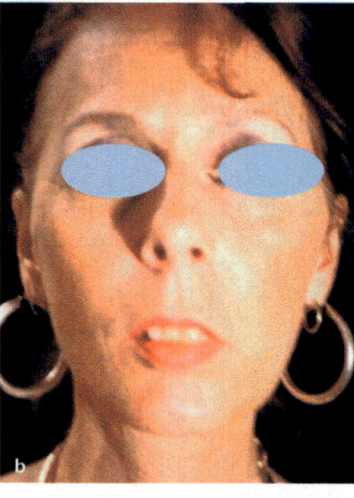

Fig. 3w7.7 a Preoperative. **b** Following cheek area curl lift

6. Yawning and laughing too much should be avoided.
7. Facial massage should be avoided for 2 months and has to be always very prudent after that time, should the patient consider it useful.

37.8
Conclusions

A rediscovered technique comes back for a new life. If mature or older patients need and request a conventional surgical facelift they need a major operation. Today a large group of young patients or middle-aged patients want to improve their appearance with a minor noninvasive, ambulatory procedure under local anesthesia with little downtime (Figs. 37.6, 37.7). They want to treat the first signs of the aging process, given by "father time," the first "weak point" and not the whole face or neck as with older patients. Many of them want also to improve what "Mother Nature" has not given them, such as a horizontal eyebrow or a too significant nasolabial sulcus.

The needle today is challenging the scalpel in offering patients what they desire. Avoiding the scalpel for youth and beauty maintenance is the present policy in cosmetic surgery.

References

1. Ulloa, M.G.: The Ageing Face. Piccin, Turin 1983
2. Buttkewitz, H.: Die Nadel Technik der subcutanen Gewebsrafung einer schnittlosen Korrekturmethode bei kosmetischen Brust und Gesichtoperationen. Zentralbl Chir 1956;81:1185
3. Guillemain, R.: La profession médicale. Le "Curl lifting." Chir Plast Esthét Mar 1970
4. Sassaki, G.H, Cohen, A.T.: Meloplication of the malar fat pad by cable-suture technique for midface rejuvenation. Outcome study (392 cases—6 years experience). Plast Reconstr Surg 2002;110(2):635–654
5. Mendez Florez, M., Rossani, G.A., Ivan Hernandez, P.: Face up: minilifting subcutaneo no quirùrgico con suturas de polipropileno. Tecnica personal
6. Fournier, P.F.: Le lifting invisible. Rev Chir Esthét Langue Fr 2003;27(113):9–20
7. Fournier, P.F.: Histoire de l'aiguille à deux pointes. Rev Chir Esthét Langue Fr 2004;28(115):19–27
8. Levy, I.: Histoire anecdotique des Instruments médicaux. Josette, Lyons
9. Orsini, P.: Principes et Techniques de la Chirurgie. Masson et Cie, Paris 1957
10. Anonymous: Catalogue d'instruments médicaux chirurgicaux, 5th edn. Haran, Paris
11. Yanai, A., Fukuda, O., Hirabayashi, S.: Double-tipped center-threading suture needle for subcuticular suturing. Plast Reconstr Surg 1986;78(3):411–413
12. Capurro, S. Jr.: Revista Italiana di chirurgia plastica: un ago a due punte. Paper presented at the 32nd National Congress of the Italian Society of Plastic Surgery, Palermo, 13–17 September 1983
13. Capurro, S. Jr.: The double tipped needle. Plast Reconstr Surg 1987;79(6):1006
14. Boo-Chai, K.: Buried mattress sutures placed transconjonctivally. Oriental cosmetic blepharoplasty. Further experience with cosmetic surgery of the upper eyelid. In: Transactions of the 3rd International Congress Plastic Surgery, Washington, DC, 13–18 October 1963. International Congress Series no 66. Excerta Medical Foundation, Amsterdam, pp 518–524
15. Boo-Chai, K.: Plastic construction of the superior palpabral fold. Plast Reconstr Surg 1963;31:74–78
16. Serdev, N.: Serdev suture for scarless buttock lift and ultrasonic liposculpture of the buttocks. Int J Cosmet Med Surg 2003;1:1–8
17. Serdev, N.: Scarless Serdev suture methods in brow and facelifts. Int J Cosmet Med Surg 2003:9–15
18. Serdev, N.: Cirugia ambulatoria de levantamiento de gluteos mediante una sutura sin cicatrices de incision. Int J Cosmet Med Surg 2003;5(1):27–34
19. Lewis, J.R., Jr.: Direct brow lift. In: The Art of Aesthetic Plastic Surgery, Lewis J.R. Jr. (Ed), Little Brown, New York 1989:705–707
20. Hernandez-Perez, E., Hassan, A.K.: A percutaneous approach to eyebrowlift : the Salvadorean option. Dermatol Surg 2003;29(8):852–855
21. Erol, O.O., Sozer, S.O., Velidedeoglu, H.V.: Brow suspension a minimally invasive technique in facial rejuvenation. Plast Reconstr Surg 2002;109:2521–2532
22. Zarem H.A.: Brow suspension , a minimally invasive technique in facial rejuvenation. Plast Reconstr Surg 2002; 109:2533 (discussion)
23. Little, J.W.: Three dimensional rejuvenation of the midface: volumetric resculpture by malar imbrication. Plast Reconstr Surg 2000;105(1):267–285
24. Bassereau, G.: Le filting (lifting non invasif par fils en boucle de suspension): principe technique et résultats preliminaries. J.J.P. S.O.F.C.P.R.E., Paris Mar 2004
25. Fournier, P.F.: Body Sculpturing U.S.A. Rolf 1987
26. Fournier, P.F.: Liposculpture: The Syringe Technique. Arnette, Paris 1991
27. Fournier, P.F.: Liposculpture: Ma Technique. Arnette, Paris 1989
28. Fournier, P.F.: Liposculpture: Ma Technique, 2nd edition. Arnette Blackwell, Paris 1996
29. Sulamanidze, M.A., Fournier, P.F., Paikidze, T.G., Sulamanidze, G.M.: Removal of facial soft tissue ptosis with special threads. Dermatol Surg 2002;28:367–371

CHAPTER 38

Barbed Thread Facelift: a Personal Journey

38

Oscar M. Ramírez, Vincent C. Giampapa, Eugenio Pacelli Chapa

This article is dedicated to the memory of Feliciano Blanco M.D., a young rising star in plastic surgery whose life was cut short in July 2005 in Monterrey, Mexico.

38.1
Introduction

Surgeons and patients alike are constantly searching for methods of facial rejuvenation that can be done with minimal invasion of tissues, with the least amount of anesthesia and with "no" downtime. This is the holy grail of aesthetic surgery. One of the latest players in this field is the barbed thread lift; however, the use of suture suspension during lifting has been successfully done for around two decades [1–4]. However, this type of suture suspension for the midface and neck required an open or a semiopen procedure. The mechanical reason why in these cases the suture suspension worked was because of the wide undermining and repositioning of the soft tissues in the elevated position, which was held long-term by these sutures until the scar formation allowed tissue reattachment in the new position. When this suture suspension was applied in a percutaneous fashion, the general complaint was that this suture tended to act like a cheese wire cutting through the tissues and diminishing the effect over a period of time. The reason for this was that these sutures were smooth without barbs. The advent of the barbed suture was a new concept in facial lifting because of the ability of the barbed suture to hold and support tissues along its entire length rather than just the loop made by the smooth sutures. This mechanical advantage of the suture has made it possible to use it without tissue undermining.

The mechanical principle of the barbed suture is to make it easy to insert it in one direction and difficult to move it in the opposite direction. Once the suture has been introduced in the soft tissues, these can be lifted to a position in one direction and the barbs of the sutures will theoretically prevent the tissues from dropping to the original position. Although, in principle, this made a lot of sense, in practice the early configuration of the barbed sutures was not reliable enough and other ingenious surgeons modified and improved the configuration with the barbed sutures as well as the surgical prin-

ciples. The senior author (Ramirez) initially tried the technique and did a few procedures without significant improvement in the quality of rejuvenation. Later on, after becoming involved in a couple research projects with poor results and almost abandoning the technique and technology, one of the coauthors (Giampapa), after modifying several key points of the technique, was able to obtain better results which convinced the senior author to become an advocate of the operation, albeit with some limitations.

38.2
History of Non-barbed Sutures

Since the early 1980s as the senior author developed the subperiosteal techniques of facial rejuvenation, a concept was introduced of suture suspension in the deep layers to allow a reliable lifting and remodeling of the soft tissues [1, 2]. The smooth suture suspension was also applied to the author's endoscopic procedures [3]. Subsequently, following the work of Giampapa, a suture suspension technique was added to my cervicoplasties [4, 5] (see Chap. 80); however, these operations needed open or semiopen techniques. Subsequently, other surgeons introduced the suture suspension to their techniques, such as Keller et al. [6], Sasaki and Cohen [7], and DeCordier and Vasconez [8]. They showed good results, but the surgery still required some type of tissue dissection. Other smooth suture elevations performed by Graziosi and Beer [9] and Erol et al. [10] provided simple solutions for the forehead and midface elevation with little morbidity. However, the long-term results were unpredictable. The cut-through or cheese-wire effect was very common.

38.3
History of Barbed Sutures

The earliest available reference to the invention of the barbed sutures is the one attempted by Alcamo [11], who in 1964 patented a roughened suture that offered resistance to only one direction. However, there is no reference of its actual clinical use. The next important reference is that by Fukuda [12], who in 1984 patented the surgical barbed suture. There is also no reference to the clinical use of these barbed sutures.

The next important landmark is the work done by Sulamanidze et al. [13–15], who, during the period from 1986 to 1998, studied a series of subdermal thread insertions using threads from 5- to 18-cm long. Sulamanidze's report is also the first clinical report of the concept and technique of the use of barbed sutures. He described the application of the barbed sutures in the subcutaneous plane without undermining [13]. He called the threads APTOS (antiptosis). These sutures were introduced in the USA with the name of Feather-Lift sutures; however the FeatherLift did not gain Food and Drug Administration (FDA) approval until June of 2004.

In the USA in the late 1990s, Ruff [16] invented what is now called Contour Thread. The difference between the FeatherLift and Contour Thread sutures is that the former is a bidirectional, free-floating device that does not require specific anchoring, while the latter is a unidirectional barbed suture with needles attached to either end. The FeatherLift requires a hollow cannula for insertion and is not anchored to a fixed structure. It is a self-anchoring device with one barbed segment used to lift the lower tissues while the upper barbed segment and its cogs engage the tissues, providing support in a usually higher position. The first generation Contour

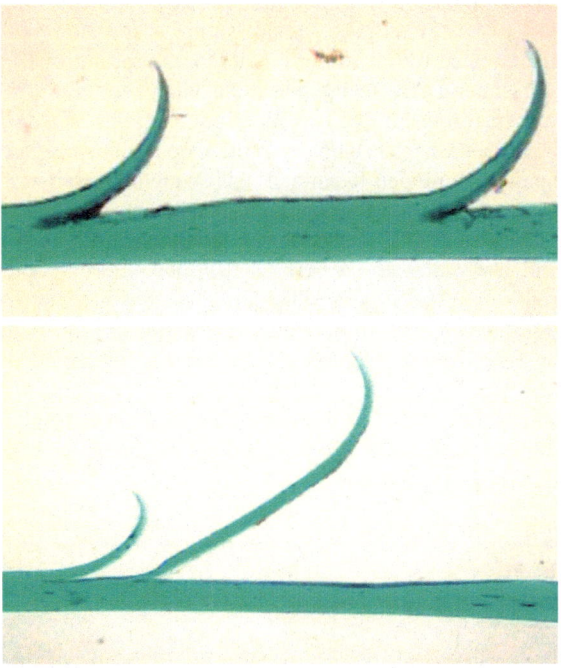

Fig. 38.1 The APTOS thread seen at ×10 magnification (original picture). *Top*: The unused suture. Observe the suture stem-to-barb ratio. *Bottom*: The used suture. Delamination of the barbs is common

Thread, on the other hand, has a unidirectional barb configuration and two needles, one attached to each opposite end. One long straight needle is used for threading the suture into the tissues that you want to lift (e.g., cheek) and the other end is used to anchor the thread in a fixed structure (e.g., temporal fascia proper). Subsequently, Leung and Ruff patented other variations and configurations of sutures, such as bidirectional barbed sutures with different varieties of needles and length of sutures [17].

Other surgeons, such as Wu and Lee, have designed a particular type of configuration on their threads [18, 19]. Wu has also designed different modes of suture application that he calls Woffles I and Woffles II type of lifting. Sulamanidze, Ruff, and Wu do not use any undermining, however Lee uses his barbed sutures during the endoscopic submuscular lift, in which he performs undermining.

There are also other sutures in the international arena. Beramendi in Brazil has designed semirigid sutures with a variety of configurations [20]. There are also absorbable barbed sutures made in Italy.

38.4
Biomechanics of the Barbed Suture

Not all barbed sutures are the same. That is certainly true for the APTOS suture versus a Contour Thread. The APTOS barbed sutures come in 3-0 blue polypropylene with the cogs relatively longer and thinner than the Contour Thread cogs. On the other hand, the Contour Thread suture comes in 2-0 clear polypropylene. The ratio of the stem-to-barb of the suture seems to be higher for the Contour Thread. Reversing the factors of the equation, the barb-to-stem ratio is lower for the Contour Thread. This particular configuration of the APTOS thread may make it more susceptible to delamination (Fig. 38.1).

The APTOS thread is introduced with a hollow cannula of diameter larger than the suture diameter, while the Contour Threads have attached needles of diameters very slightly larger than the suture diameter. This allows the introduction of the APTOS suture in a wider channel, which at least theoretically might make the cog engagement a bit looser. The Contour Thread, on the other hand, having an appropriate needle diameter, widens the channel where the suture is placed. The flexible needle configuration of the Contour Thread also allows the introduction of the suture in a zigzagging direction, which will anchor better the tissues into the barbs of the suture. Biomechanical studies have also shown that the shorter the length of the barbs, the stronger the grip of the tissues. It is like comparing the ends of a long branch of a tree, which will hold less weight than the short stem of the branch of the tree. The APTOS suture has long branches. The Contour Thread has shorter branches. The double-needle attachment at the end as well as the bidirectional barb configuration offer additional versatility for changing directions at the end of the path (more anchor), to apply suture knots if needed or to anchor in a loop of the central non-barbed segment. The newest sutures with a helicoidal distribution of the cogs offer the additional advantage of better grip. Newer designs that are in the pipeline are absorbable sutures that can be used in the semiopen or open methods of tissue lifting.

38.5
Personal Experience

In March 2004 while the senior author was lecturing at the International Facial Rejuvenation Meeting in Monterrey, Nuevo Leon, Mexico, Blanco and Pacelli Chapa presented five patients who were recently operated upon by two experienced surgeons during a workshop with a live surgery demonstration. They used the original APTOS threads. At that point, the patients were at about the 1 month postoperative stage. Since there

was no significant difference between before and after the procedure, I urged them to follow up the patients for at least 1 year to see if the claimed phenomenon of later improvement due to scar/capsular formation and contracture would occur. These patients were followed up for a period of 12 months. No visible improvements were seen during this time. Blanco reported this study at the Annual Meeting of the Society of Aesthetic Plastic Surgery at New Orleans in March 2005 (Fig. 38.2).

In the study of Blanco et al., the technique used was as originally described by Sulamanidze. A typical patient received one to two threads to the tail of the brow, three or four threads to the midface and jowl, and two threads to the neck. An average of 12 sutures were used per patient. The APTOS threads were introduced using a hollow 20-gauge cannula. The sutures were of 3-0 polypropylene. The ends were cut flush to the level of the skin with a slight pulling to allow the 2–3-mm retraction into the depths of the soft tissues. Paper tape and bandages to the face were used for support. The patient was instructed to sleep on her back, avoiding pressure on the side of her face, and also to avoid excessive

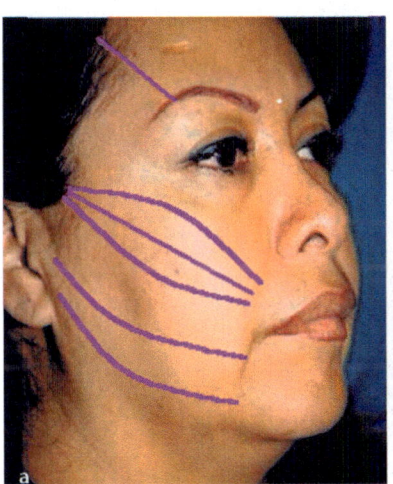
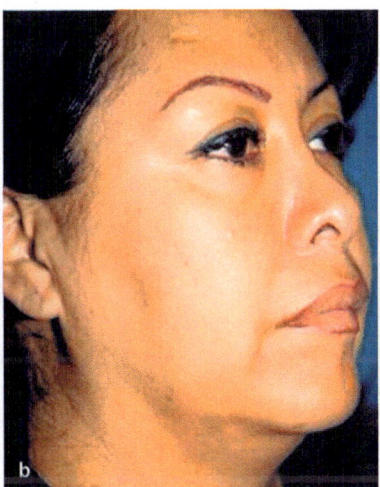
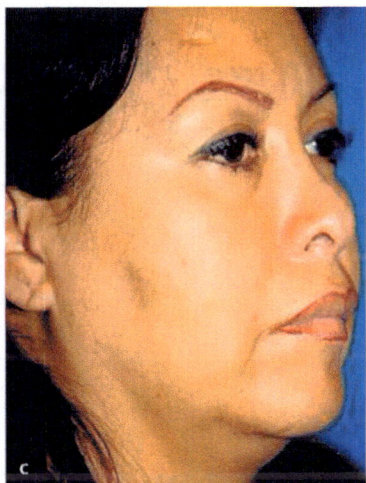
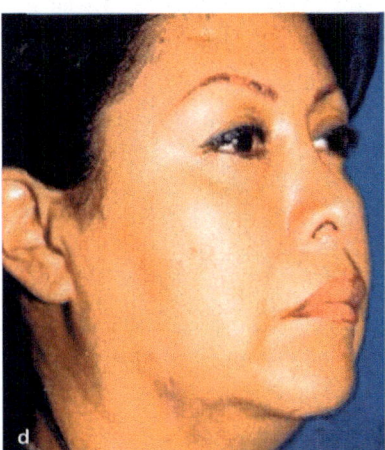
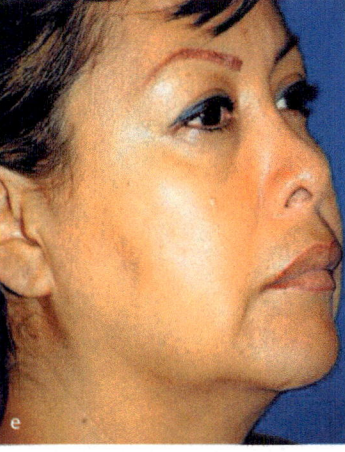

Fig. 38.2 a Observe the location and the number of APTOS thread sutures in a typical patient from Blanco's study. This patient received one suture on the forehead, three sutures on the midface, and two sutures on the lower face and jawline. **b** A 47-year old patient from Blanco's study. Observe the brow ptosis and sagging of the cheek, nasolabial folds, and jowls. **c** Six weeks postoperatively. No significant improvement is noted. **d** Six months postoperatively. No improvement is seen. At this stage according of the theory of "delayed improvement by scar/fibrosis formation" the patient should show significant facial lifting. **e** One year postoperatively. No improvement is seen

mastication and facial animation, which were forbidden for a period of 1 month.

Other presentations at national meetings were not convincing enough for us to embrace the procedure as it was described. Those experiences were the input to do another study in which we decided to use the Contour Thread in undermined flaps and to apply the threads in a deeper plane.

38.6
Subperiosteal Non-endoscopic Technique

Ramirez and Pacelli Chapa conducted this study. The procedure was a non-endoscopic subperiosteal undermining of the forehead and midface with deep fat/subperiosteal suspension using the Contour Thread barbed sutures. Thirteen consecutive patients were operated on at the Plastika Surgery Center in Monterrey, Mexico. The first eight patients were operated on by Ramirez and the remaining five patients were operated on by Pacelli Chapa using the same technique and protocol. There were 12 female patients and one male patient. The age range was 40–59 with an average of 45.5 years. Three days prior to surgery, the patient had an injection of Botox to the corrugators and crow's-feet areas to prevent early pull down of the brows by muscle hyperactivity. Each patient had a non-endoscopic subperiosteal undermining for the frontal area via two paramedian incisions. The area surrounding the supraorbital and supratrochlear nerves were not undermined, with the lower limit of dissection 2 cm above these nerves (Fig. 38.3). However, the glabella and the tail of the brows were aggressively dissected and periosteal spreading was done with tip up (no. 7 Ramirez elevator made by

Snowden Pencer–Tucker, GA, USA). The midface was approached via a 2-cm temporal incision and a 2.5-cm intraoral Caldwell–Luc type of incision. Once the temporal fascia proper had been identified, the dissection of the temple was done over this fascia until the superior border of the zygomatic arch at its anterior third was reached. Dissection of the zygomatic arch on the anterior third was done in a blind fashion. This limited dissection of the zygomatic arch was to prevent injury of the frontal branch of the facial nerve that crosses the arch on its medial third. The midface was approached via an intraoral incision and was dissected under direct visualization using a fiberoptic-lit retractor. The masseter fascia elevation was included for 1 or 2 cm; however the zygomatic arch was dissected only on the anterior third. Frontal fixation was done with a bidirectional Contour Thread introduced in each paramedian incision at the subperiosteal–galeal plane interface and with the needle pulled through the tail of the brow. The opposite end of the suture with the barbed segment in the opposite orientation was threaded and fixed to the non-undermined scalp posterior to the paramedian incision and the corresponding needle was pulled through the intact scalp. Another suture was threaded from the temporal incision into the suborbicularis oculi fat (SOOF) and malar periosteum. Bichat's fat pad and the modiolus were anchored to this barbed thread. The other end of the thread was anchored to the temporal

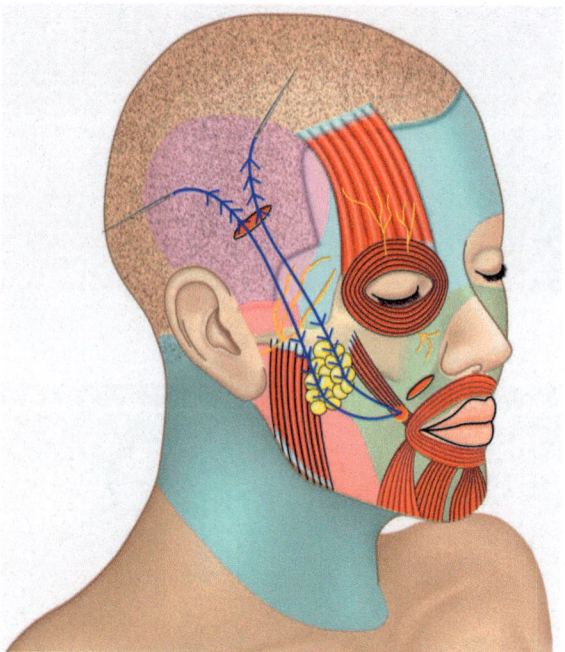

Fig. 38.4 The dissection across the zygomatic arch is only on its anterior third. The proximal anchoring for support is in the temporal fascia proper and in the non-undermined scalp. The lifting segment of the suture is placed in the deep fat–periosteal layer

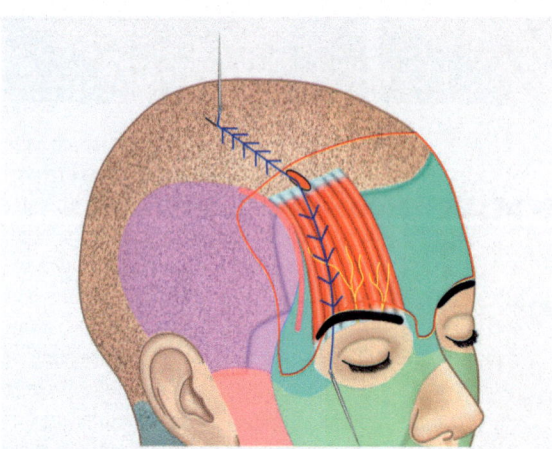

Fig. 38.3 Observe the extent of the dissection for the non-endoscopic superiosteal forehead rejuvenation. There is no dissection around the supraorbital/supratrochlear nerves. Observe the placement of the barbed sutures and the orientation of the cogs

fascia proper and the superior temporal scalp (Fig. 38.4). No endoscope was used and no upper or lower blepharoplasty or fat grafting was performed. One patient suffered from unilateral frontal neuropraxia, which lasted 1 month. One patient had extrusion of the barbed suture on the forehead. These patients were followed up for a period of 1 year. Although the early results were very encouraging, after a period of about 5–6 months we started to see significant relapse that was not seen in comparable endoscopic cases (Fig. 38.5). Although there was still some improvement at the 12-month mark, the improvements were not comparable with those of the lifting and remodeling that were are able to achieve using endoscopic techniques.

To explain this unseemingly paradoxical result two factors were hypothesized as possible explanations:

1. The undermining was not as complete as with the dissection done for the endoscopic techniques. The area around the supraorbital nerves and supratrochlear nerves were not dissected. No corrugator resection was done. Only the anterior third of the zygomatic arch was dissected for tunneling between the temporal and midface pockets.

2. The mechanism of tissue lifting with the sutures is by telescoping rather than imbrication and in-mass mobilization common to the endoscopic techniques. The imbrication will probably allow healing and reattachment in a better mechanical position and these will therefore be less prone to relapse. The telescoping, on the other hand, does not allow an effective in-mass mobilization.

Giampapa, on the other hand, was working on different variations of the "non-undermining" version and applying the sutures in different ways. The newer configurations of the barbed sutures also contributed to the improved results of the procedure. He actually convinced me that the technique actually works, giving about 50% of improvement when compared with the open methods.

38.7
Newer Approaches to Facial Rejuvenation Using the Contour Thread

The original FDA clearance for the FeatherLift sutures as specified in the 510 (K) Summary of Safety &. Effectiveness says: "they are indicated to use in midface suspension to fixate the cheek subdermis in an elevated position." Consequently, surgeons have been using these devices in the subcutaneous plane. The only initial variation of the Contour Thread from this was the anchoring of one end of the suture to the temporal fascia proper where a small incision was made. In early reports at national meetings, no significant difference could be seen between the patients before and after the

procedure who were presented during these lectures. For that reason, we started looking for better options to take maximal advantage of the technology. From a regulatory point of view, at this point in time these applications can be considered "off-label" use of the sutures.

38.7.1
Subcutaneous Muscular Aponeurotic System Insertion of the Contour Thread

This technique is excellent for the treatment of the midface using the same vectors as in the traditional subcutaneous muscular aponeurotic system (SMAS) operation. The Contour Threads are introduced through a small incision in the upper medial ear area, more precisely at the level of the root of the helix. Three to four unidirectional barbed sutures are introduced with the straight needle piercing the parotid fascia; more anteriorly this follows the SMAS layer in which the needle is weaved. At the level of the malar fat the needle is introduced into this fat and exits just lateral to the nasolabial fold or marionette line, respectively. Three sutures are directed in a vertical distribution to the nasolabial fold and two to the marionette line. The proximal ends of the sutures are tied (two and two) deep to the parotid fascia to bury the knots deep. The cartilage is used as an anchoring element for better support (Fig. 38.5).

38.7.2
Biplanar Needle Positioning Using the Contour Thread for Midface Rejuvenation

In this technique, the preoperative topographical marking is very important to guide the surgeon for the correct placement of these sutures. Typically two sutures are used for the upper cheek and tear-trough area, one suture for the corner of the mouth, and another suture for the marionette line.

Each needle is introduced through a small 1–2-cm incision made in the hair-bearing area of the temporal scalp. The path of the unidirectional suture is in two planes. Above the zygomatic arch this is at the subcutaneous plane and below this arch it is at the SMAS–muscle plane. The proximal end of each suture is anchored to the temporal fascia proper. Two adjacent sutures at the non-barbed segment are tied deep under the scalp. The knot can also be buried under the temporal fascia proper. Appropriate digital advancement of the soft tissues over the sutures is made until the engagement into the cogs achieves the desired elevation and shape of the tissues. The excess material at the distal end is trimmed flush to the skin and an additional push on the skin in an upward direction is made to disengage the last few barbs from the subdermal plane to prevent excessive indentation. Sutures are kept lateral to the na-

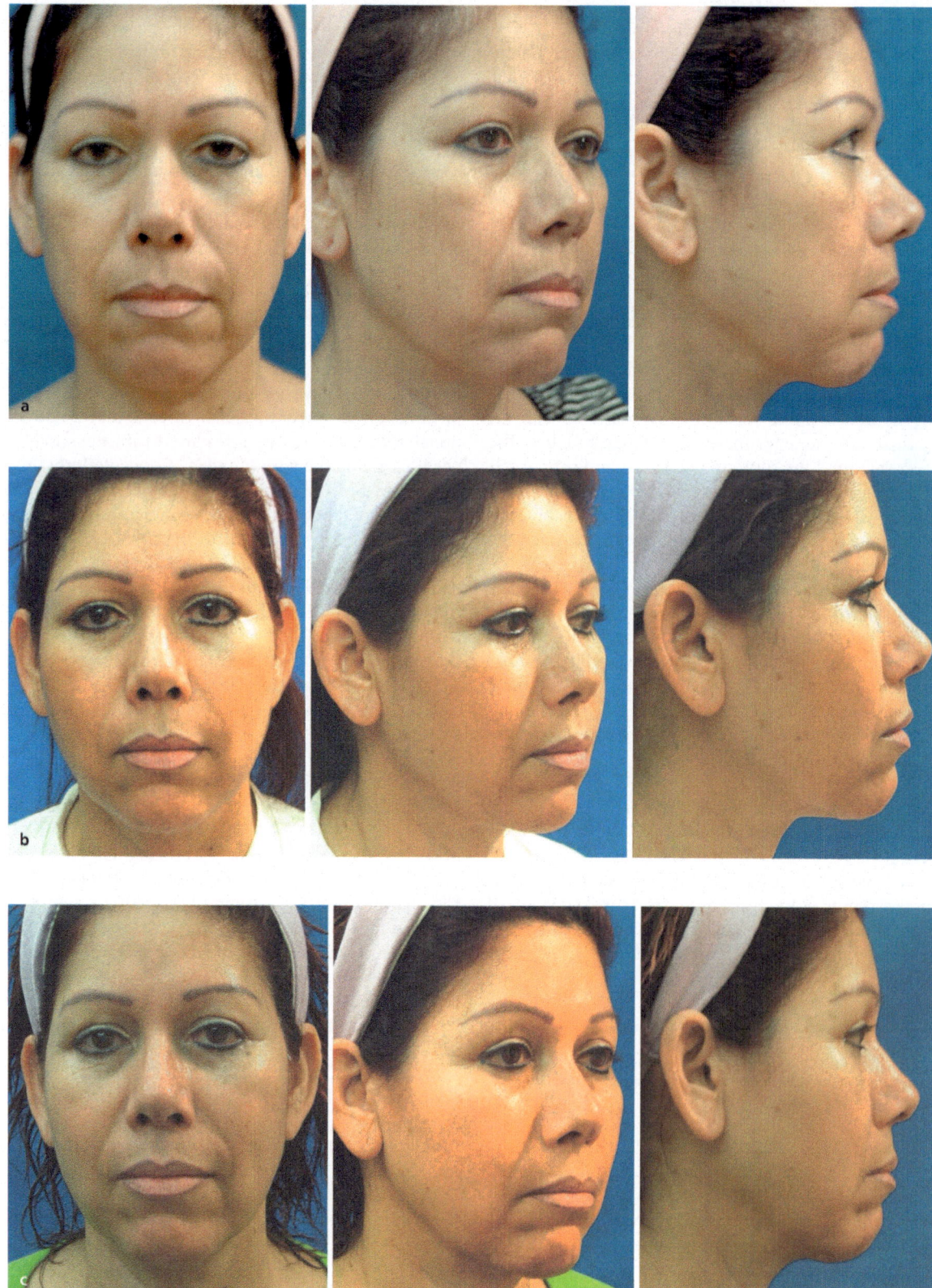

Fig. 38.5 a Preoperative 49-year-old female patient. Observe the degree of facial aging. **b** Three months postoperatively. There is a significant improvement at every level. At this point the degree of facial rejuvenation achieved was encouraging. The brow position, tear-trough-deformity correction, and cheek volume are excellent. **c** Ten month post operatively. There is significant relapse and the initial improvement obtained is almost completely gone

solabial fold. A well-contoured flesh-colored micropore tape is applied to the face. Facial motion is restricted for 1 month. The results seen after 1 year are good to moderately good (Fig. 38.6).

38.7.3
Biplanar Neck Lift

The neck can be lifted without undermining. For this, a small 1–1.5-cm incision immediately over the mastoid grove is made on both sides. Through this incision the straight needle of the first Contour Thread is placed completely subcutaneously along the lower border of the mandible and exits at the medial border of the platysma near the midline. The second, third, and fourth Contour Threads are placed parallel to each other initially at the subcutaneous plane and after passing the level of the mandibular angle the needle is traversed into the deep muscular plane. The needle exits at the medial border of the platysma near the cervical midline. The curved needle on the opposite end of the suture is passed through the mastoid fascia and two adjacent sutures are tied together. These sutures are pulled prior to tying until the cogs can be felt engaging the neck envelope. Additional digital contouring is done as needed while gentle tension is applied on the free distal end of the suture. The sutures are then trimmed flush to the skin. The indentations are manipulated as previously described. Contouring tape is also applied to the neck. The results seen after 1 year are considered to be from good to excellent.

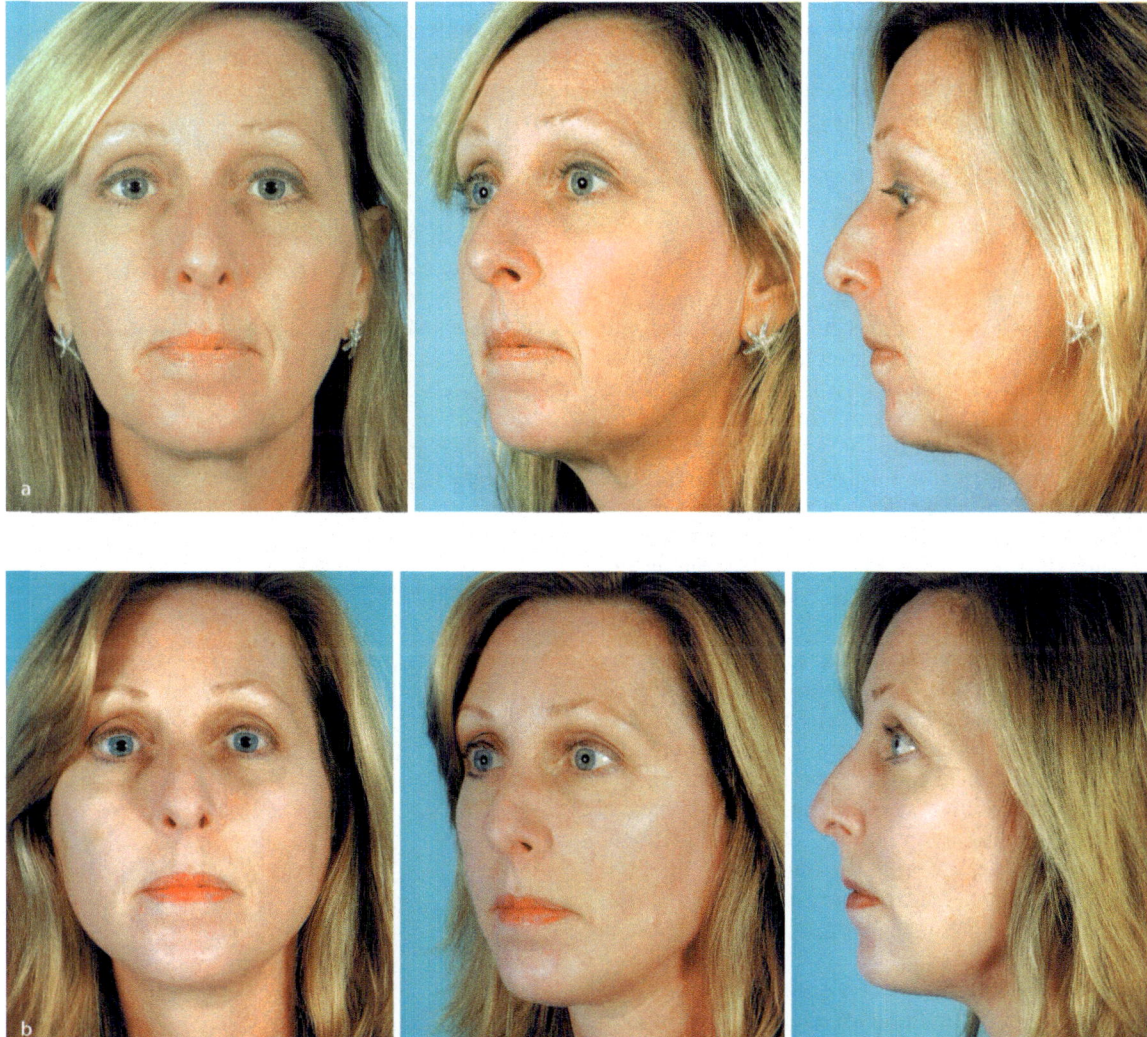

Fig. 38.6 a Preoperative patient with aging at the level of the periorbital area, nasolabial fold, marionette areas, and the jowls. **b** Postoperatively. Observe the improvement obtained in the areas mentioned. The periorbital area is the area with less improvement

When the face and neck are done either separately or together a well-contoured neck and face soft bandage is applied for 48 h.

38.7.4
Use of Contour Thread Sutures for Facial Suspension During Open or Minimally Invasive Semiopen Midface Lift

The Contour Thread can be incorporated into the standard-open or the small-incision-open facelift. This allows the extent of the dissection on the central oval of the face and the length of the facelift incision to be decreased. The suture suspension with the barbed threads can also be incorporated into the endoscopic procedure to make easier the SOOF lift. The leading needle is engaged into the malar fat pad and SMAS during standard techniques and into the SOOF-periosteum during the endoscopic approach. The proximal needle is anchored to the temporal fascia proper. The rest of the maneuvers are similar to those of the closed technique. Usually two sutures are required for each cheek.

38.8
Discussion

Like any new procedure the surgical techniques and technology of barbed sutures have evolved and will continue to evolve. The final chapter on the barbed suture has not been written yet. It will find its proper place in the surgical armamentarium. The applications of the current procedures and current suture technology have to be seen in the correct perspective. This is important for the surgeon and for the patient, so the expectations of what the procedure may achieve can be set on a realistic level. This will prevent unhappiness, frustration, and potential litigious situations. The "closed" procedure at best can provide "at half of the cost, half of the lift of a facelift, and half of the duration." The lifting relaxes by about 50% in the first 6–12 weeks. It is not a replacement for more enduring and proven techniques. It is not a lunchtime procedure either. It is not a procedure like Botox injection or a Restylane type of filler. It is still a surgical procedure that require local anesthesia and in some cases oral or intravenous sedation. The degree of facial edema, ecchymosis, discomfort, and tightness can be significant. Furthermore, some patients have significant dimpling at the exit points of the sutures, uneven contour of the facial curvatures with grooving along the cheeks, and waviness and skin folding along the hairline and around the ears (Fig. 38.7). Patients are not ready to return to work or engage in social activities until at least the seventh to tenth postoperative day. During the early postoperative period significant care is important but this is also restrictive. The face has to be protected to avoid disengagement of the cogs from the tissues that have been lifted. Patients are instructed to sleep on their backs. Excessive facial mimicking, talking, and chewing are to be avoided. This may restrict a patient's function at work or socially. Facial and scalp cleansing and washing have to be done in a cranial direction. The patient may need another person to help with this. All of these may be necessary for about 3 weeks, at which time the connective tissue around the cogs may be strong enough for the patient to engage in more liberal activities.

If we understand the limitations in the degree of facial rejuvenation and the need to allow time for postoperative recovery, then the procedure is placed in the right position among all the procedures in the wide spectrum of options for surgical rejuvenation. I usually tell my patients that this is only a way to postpone a more traditional surgical procedure for different lengths of time. The longevity of the rejuvenation obtained depends of the age of the patient and the quality of the facial anatomy that you work with. The best result is obtained in a younger individual who shows the first signs of facial aging and the face is not too thin or too fat. Patients with strong skeletal support also show better results and have results with more longevity. The worst patient is the older individual with excessive sagging, a lot of redundant skin, and poor skeletal support. Heavy-face or thin-face patients regardless of their age are also poor candidates for this surgery.

38.9
Conclusions

A historical personal evolution with the use of the Contour Thread has been presented. An unbiased appraisal

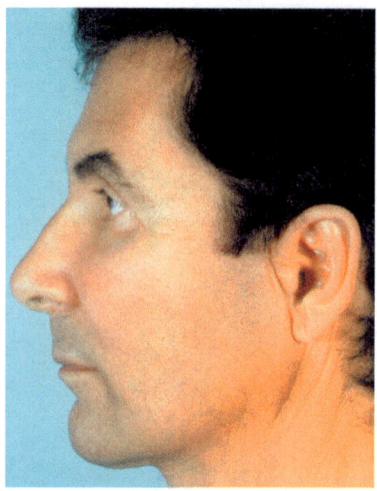

Fig. 38.7 Note the amount of redundancy of skin in the preauricular area following a Contour Thread surgery. Most patients redrape this excess skin in about 6–12 weeks. Occasionally some patients may require a secondary skin excision

of the surgical results has been made. The use of barbed sutures in general is still in its early stages and like many other techniques improvements and refinements are expected. In the final analysis, the barbed suture technology will find its proper place among all the options available in the surgical rejuvenation of the face.

References

1. Ramirez OM, Maillard GF, Mussolas A. The extended subperiosteal facelift: a definitive soft tissue remodeling for facial rejuvenation. Plast Reconstr Surg 1991;88:227–236

2. Ramirez OM. The subperiosteal rhytidectomy: The third generation face lift. Ann Plast Surg 1992;28:218–232

3. Ramirez OM. Endoscopic full face lift. Aesthetic Plast Surg 1994;18:363–371

4. Giampapa VC, DiBernardo BE. Neck recontouring with suture suspension and liposuction: an alternative for the early rhytidectomy candidate. Aesthet Plast Surg 1995;19(3) 217–223

5. Ramirez OM. Cervicoplasty: Non-excisional anterior approach. Plast Reconstr Surg 1997;99:1576–1585

6. Keller GS, et al. Elevation of the malar fat pad with a percutaneous technique. Arch Facial Plast Surg 2002;4:20–25

7. Sasaki GH, Cohen AT. Meloplication of the malar fat pads by percutaneous cable-suture technique for midface rejuvenation: outcome study (392 cases, 6 years experience) Plast Reconstr Surg 2002;110: 635–654

8. De Cordier BC, Vasconez LO. Rejuvenation of the midface by elevating the malar fat pad: review of technique cases and complications. Plast Reconstr Surg 2002;110:1526–1536

9. Graziosi AC, Beer SMC. Browlifting with thread: The technique without undermining using minimal incisions. Aesthet Plast Surg 1988;22:120–125

10. Erol OO, Sozer SO, Velidedeoglu HV. Brow suspension, a minimally invasive technique in facial rejuvenation. Plast Reconstr Surg 2002;109:2521–2532

11. Alcamo JH. Surgical suture. US Patent 3,123,077. 1964

12. Fukuda M. Surgical barbed suture. US Patent 4,467,805. 1984

13. Sulamanidze MA, Fournier PF, Paikidze TG, Sulamanidze GM. Removal of facial soft tissue ptosis with special threads. Dermatol Surg. 200;28:367–371

14. Sulamanidze MA, Shiffman MA, Paikidze TG, Sulamanidze GM, Gavasheli LG. Facial lifting with APTOS threads. Int J Cosmet Surg Aesthet Dermatol 2001;4:275–281

15. Lycka B, Bazan C, Poletti E, Treen B. The emerging technique of the antiptosis subdermal suspension thread. Dermatol Surg 2004;30:41–44

16. Ruff GL. Barbed bodily tissue connector. US Patent 6,241,747B1. 2001

17. Leung JC, Pritt S. Barbed, bidirectional surgical sutures: in vivo strength and histopathology evaluations. Soci Biomater Trans 2003;26:100

18. Wu WTL. Barbed sutures in facial rejuvenation. Aesthet Surg J 2004;24:582–587

19. Lee S, Isse N. Barbed polypropylene sutures for midface elevation. Arch Facial Plast Surg 2005;7:55–61

20. Badin AZ, Campelli-Forte MR, Loyola e Silva O. Scarless mid- and lower face lift. Aesthet Surg J 2005;25:340–347

CHAPTER 39

Transcutaneous Facelift

Enrique Hernández-Pérez, Hassan Abbas Khawaja

39.1
Introduction

Facelifting has undergone considerable changes in technique recently with a trend towards the simpler ones over the radical ones. The idea is to have a simpler, safer and certainly a procedure whose results might be nicer. Some examples are S-lift, delta-lift, lower superficial musculoaponeurotic system (SMAS)-platysma facelift and facial lifting with APTOS threads [1–6]. Transcutaneous facelift (TCFL) is one of the simplest of all known facelift techniques. It is suitable for individuals requiring a moderate to mild facelift. The idea of this procedure came to us when we saw the satisfactory results obtained with the percutaneous approach to eyebrow lift, recently published [7].[7]

39.2
Technique

Patients with ASA I or II must be preferred. As we are going to use epinephrine, it is imperative to avoid aspirin or beta blockers. TCFL is carried out on highly motivated healthy adults.

Step 1: 1% lidocaine with 1:400.000 epinephrine is used as anesthesia for the line AB in the temporal region and for points C, D, E and F (Fig. 39.1). We use the Khawaja–Hernandez (KH needle, somewhat similar to the Keith needle, but relatively longer, thinner and with a pointed end but not sides). The length of the KH needle is 9 cm, the width is 1 mm at the broadest part and 2 mm at the eye of the needle. It tapers towards the end. However, a Keith needle or a Thui needle with similar dimensions can also be used for the procedure.

Step 2: Incision is made on the line AB.

Step 3: The KH needle with Prolene 2/0 attached to the eye of the needle is passed from line AB towards point C. The needle track is very superficial and straight in the suprazygomatic portion where the temporal branch/branches of facial nerve crosses/cross the zygomatic arch. In the infrazygomatic portion, the needle takes bites of SMAS but relatively superficially in a side-to-side zigzag manner. This is done by gently swaying the needle sideways. Below the lobe of the ear, the bites are relatively deep in an upside-down fashion (troughs

and valleys). The skin can be pulled up somewhat with the other hand to facilitate the maneuver. The idea is to take bites of SMAS, rather than pursuing a straight course. The needle exits at point C.

Step 4: From point C to D, the needle takes a similar zigzag course.

Step 5: From point D back to the same point on line AB, the needle follows exactly the same pattern as while coming down from line AB to point C, i.e., relatively deeper course below the lobule, a relatively superficial course until the zygomatic arch and very superficial at the zygomatic arch.

Step 6: The SMAS is pulled up vertically and a knot is tied. It is important to make four to five passes in the knot to make it more secure.

In a similar manner, the second suture starts from the line AB towards points E and F and back to the same point on line AB, and is tied at an angle of 45° after pulling it up superolaterally. It is important to tie the knots in the deeper periosteum of temporal bone to provide a stable lift. Closure of the line AB is performed with

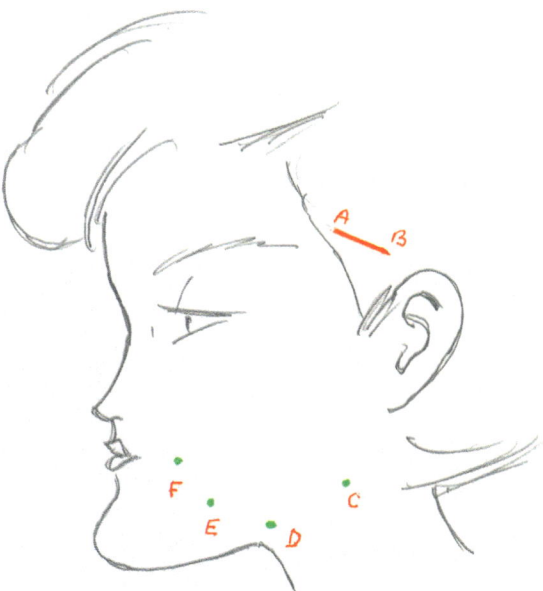

Fig. 39.1 Anesthesia is injected in these points

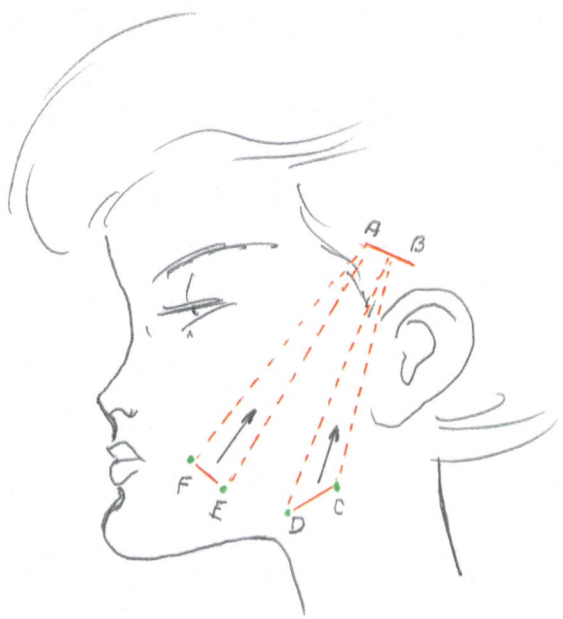

Fig. 39.2 The suture is attached in the deeper periosteum of temporal bone. The needle passes very superficially above the zygoma and deeper below it

Prolene 4/0 interrupted stitches (Fig. 39.2). Lifting on the other side is carried out in a similar manner.

The distance between the points C and D and E and F varies from 1.5 cm to a few millimeters, depending on the nature of the lift. If more pull is required, it is mandatory that the distance between the points is reduced, otherwise humps will form between the points. The entry and exit points can coincide, i.e., points C and D can merge, and similarly points D and F can merge if more lift is required. On the other hand, if tissues are pulled excessively, unaesthetic transverse wrinkles appear on the face. Though these are temporary and disappear with the passage of time, these create worry for the cosmetic patients,who do not want to wait long for the results. It is best to keep the pull mild to moder-

ate to avoid this problem. Different surgical facelifting techniques (S-lift, delta-lift, etc.) should be considered when excessive lift is required.

39.3
Results

All the patients have been satisfied with the results (Figs. 39.3). Postoperative follow-up ranged from 18 to 24 months . The degree of satisfaction and postoperative results were same after passage of that time.

39.4
Complications

Mild and transitory edema was the only problem observed in some 10% of patients. It was settled in no longer than 1 week. Minor and very limited bruising was noted in less than 2% of patients.

39.5
Discussion

TCFL is a very simple, quick method of facelifting without surgical undermining, but with plication of the SMAS using the KH needle. We have not seen any major complication with this facelift; however, it is good to mark beforehand pathways of the marginal mandibular and frontal branches of the facial nerve [8]. It is necessary to avoid the pathway of the marginal mandibular nerve and to take a relatively superficial course along the frontal nerve pathway, staying very superficial on the zygomatic arch. For best results, it is necessary to combine it with other noninvasive or mini-invasive modalities of facial rejuvenation, i.e., correction of nasolabial folds using fillers, liposuction of chin area/platysmal bands plication, transcutaneous brow lifting (the Salvadorian option), orally administered isotretinoin [9], fat injections, topically applied tretinoin, chemical peels

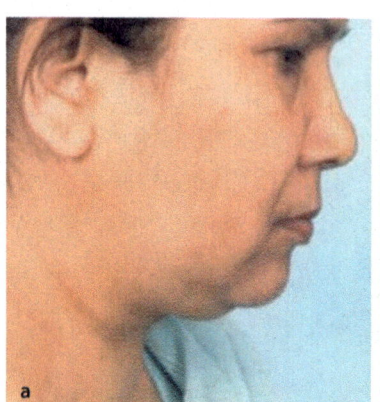
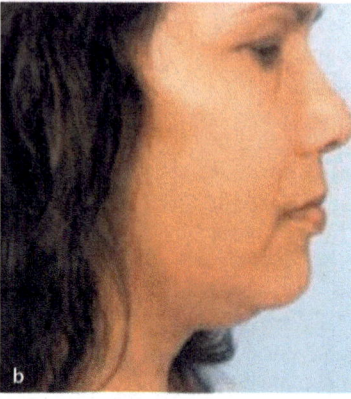

Fig. 39.3 a Before transcutaneous facelift. **b** After transcutaneous facelift. Note the improvement in the mandibular angle

[10], sunscreens and Botox for crow's-feet, glabellar frown lines and transverse forehead lines. By the way, frequently we have combined successfully TCFL with percutaneous eyebrow lift.

An argument concerning this technique of facelift can be that it is not possible to make a successful lift without undermining; however, our experience in this regard points to the contrary. Plicating the SMAS with the KH needle, and then lifting it, and attaching it to the periosteum of temporal bone makes a reasonable lift possible. As with aging, laxity of skin and SMAS continues and perhaps, after several years, it could be necessary to repeat the procedure, which takes only 20 min. Skin and SMAS are most lax in the lower third of face, moderately lax in the mid face and least lax in the upper face. Owing to this peculiar anatomy of skin and SMAS, it is possible to grip and feel the thickened SMAS at and below the zygomatic arch. However, as we proceed from the mid to the lower face, the grip of the SMAS becomes progressively narrower. For this reason, the results of transcutaneous lift, which aims at providing a maximum lift to the lower third of the face, a moderate lift to the mid third and the least lift to the upper third of the face, correspond to the peculiar anatomy of skin and SMAS, which act together as one unit as a result of the deep dermal connections between skin and SMAS [11]. Therefore, lifting the SMAS without skin lift also lifts the skin. In contrast, if skin lift is performed with undermining which destroys the dermal connections between skin and SMAS without SMAS plication or lifting, the results are not so good. Skin tightening takes place, but SMAS and subcutaneous tissues sag as a result of laxity and gravity. More so, it is not possible to lift the skin without undermining. If subcutaneous dissection is carried deep to the SMAS, damage to the branches of facial nerve can take place [9].

The frontal (temporal) branch of the facial nerve is liable to be damaged at the mid zygomatic arch [8, 11]. It can be caught in suture, if suture is taken close to the bone. No bites should be taken at the zygomatic arch, and the needle should pass superficially. On the other hand, a compression paresis can take place, if the suture compresses the frontal branch; however, this is usually temporary. Damage to zygomatic and buccal branches of the facial nerve can take place, but clinically paresis does not take place owing to a number of cross-connections between the zygomatic and buccal branches [11]. Damage to the marginal mandibular nerve is rare as needles stay away from the marginal mandibular nerve pathway.

Sometimes, while the needle is being passed, the patient complains of pain. The whole needle track pathway is marked beforehand. If the patient complains of pain, a little more lidocaine with epinephrine can be administered in the needle track.

Wrinkles and puckering of tissues can take place with excessive lift. This is usually temporary. Only drops of patience are all that are necessary, or in order to shorten this, subcision may be used.

If excessive lift is required, it is wise to reduce the distance between the facial points considerably. This will eliminate the wrinkling of tissues between the facial points [8]. The distance can be reduced even to a few millimeters or the needle may be reintroduced through the same orifice (this way, points C and D should become the same). An additional suture can be passed instead of two in these cases, using six points on the face. On the other hand, in cases of moderate lift, it is not necessary to reduce the distance between the points; however, sutures should not be pulled up too tightly.

In order to avoid asymmetry, it is necessary for less-experienced surgeons to mark the facial points and needle track pathways exactly on both sides of the face, taking measurements from the angle of the mandible and from the mid lower jawline (point halfway from the angle of the mandible and center of the chin). Asymmetry can also take place if tissues are pulled up excessively on one side compared with the other. For achieving the best results, it is necessary to keep the pull mild to moderate. However, it is also necessary to take into consideration prior asymmetry of the face to adjust the pull accordingly.

In the case of APTOS threads, support is provided by the thread with bilateral (converging) direction of the cogs [4]. In fact, the threads provide a sort of volume augmentation and slight lift to the sagging tissues; whereas in case of TCFL, mild to moderate lift of the SMAS is provided by attaching Prolene thread to the thick temporal fascia or periosteum of temporal bone, thereby providing a reasonable and stable lift. Therefore, in patients who require a volume augmentation and slight lift, APTOS threads are suitable, and in cases of somewhat more sagging, TCFL can be done to provide a moderate stable lift (Fig. 39.3).

39.6
Conclusions

TCFL is a quick, safe, mini-invasive surgical method of facelifting [12]. It can be carried out on persons of all age groups. For achieving best results, it is necessary to keep the lift moderate along with Botox, fillers, liposuction of the chin, fat transfer, topically applied tretinoin, sunscreens, orally administered isotretinoin, and microdermabrasion [10].

References

1. Saylan Z. The S-lift for facial rejuvenation. Int J Cosmet Surg 1999;7:18–24

2. Khawaja HA, Hernandez-Perez E. The delta lift: A modification of S-lift for facial rejuvenation. Int J Cosmet Surg Aesthet Dermatol 2002;4(4):309–315

3. Serdev NP. Total ambulatory SMAS lift by hidden minimal incisions part 2: Lower SMAS-platysma face lift. Int J Cosmet Surg Aesthet Dermatol 2002;4(4):285–292

4. Sulamanidze MA, Shiffman MA, Paikidze TG, Sulamanidze GM, Gavasheli LG. Facial lifting with Aptos threads. Int J Cosmet Surg Aesthet Dermatol 2001;3(4):275–281

5. Graziosi AC, Canelas Beer SM. Browlifting with thread: the technique without undermining using minimum incisions. Aesthet Plast Surg 1998;22:120–125

6. Erol OO, Sozer SO. Brow suspension, a minimally invasive technique in facial rejuvenation. Plast Reconstr Surg 2002;109:2521–2532

7. Hernández-Pérez E, Khawaja HA. A percutaneous approach to eyebrow lift: the Salvadorean option. Dermatol Surg 2002;29:852–855

8. Salasche SJ, Bernstein G. Surgical Anatomy of the Skin, 1st edition. Stamford, Appleton and Lange 1988:89–139

9. Hernandez-Perez E, Khawaja HA. Oral isotretinoin as part of the treatment of cutaneous aging. Dermatol Surg 2000;26:7:649–652

10. Hernandez-Perez E. Resorcinol peel as a part of a facial rejuvenation program. Am J Cosmet Surg 1997;4:35–40

11. Chaurasia BD. Human Anatomy Regional and Applied, 2nd edition. Delhi, Jain Bhawan 1992:39–49

12. Hernández-Pérez E, Khawaja HA. Percutaneous eyebrow lift: Simplifying the technique. Cosmet Dermatol 2005;18:716–720

CHAPTER 40

Biolifting and Bioresurfacing

Pier Antonio Bacci

40.1
Introduction

All during history men and women have always had the desire to improve their own appearance, beginning with improving the state of the skin, so we could say that "Aesthetic surgery of the skin is as old as humankind" [1]. In primitive societies, shells and details stones were used for engraving and to smooth the skin. Egyptians used a cream of sulfur and resorcine to smooth the skin and thanks to animal oils and alabaster, regeneration of skin was improved. In the papyrus of Edwin Smith (1700 bc) and in the papyrus of Ebers (1600 bc) magic prescriptions are found for the hair or for the cutaneous lesions. In Mesopotamia the Babylonians became experienced in surgery as noted in the code of Hammurabi (2000 bc), in China medicine and Chinese surgery blossomed as noted in the *Canon of the Medicine* (2600 bc). In the *Rig Veda* (1500 bc), Indian surgeons pointed out their particular interest in the reconstruction of the nose cut off thieves. In ancient Greece physicians developed care of the skin and the hair, with ancient physicians being specialized in the art of cutaneous exfoliation. The Renaissance Europeans studied exfoliation of the skin through translating ancient Greek manuscripts, giving greater development of aesthetics in dermatology, medicine, and surgery.

Today there is a tendency to confuse aesthetic surgery with plastic surgery that evolved after the First World War from dentistry and adopting techniques from ancient dermatology and general surgery. Plastic surgery is surgery for the recovery of form and function, while aesthetic surgery is more like dermatologic surgery and is surgery of the physical aspect and the desires to be better-looking. Aesthetic surgery overlaps many disciplines and is not within any specific specialization.

40.2
Patient Desires

One of the principal objective of aesthetic medicine and surgery is the rejuvenation of the face, where the years and various diseases have left the signs of tissue and metabolic alteration as wrinkles, loss of elasticity and skin tone, alterations of the hair, and the aesthetic anomalies tied to alterations of the quantity and quality of the fat tissue.

Alterations of the basal activities of cells and vital systems constitute signals sent by those structures that dysfunction for the regulation of metabolic exchanges and constitute the beginning of chronic and degenerative diseases as well as the processes of aging. Maintaining the state of health with regard to aesthetic anomalies belongs to "medicine for the health and the comfort of the patient" through maintenance of the functional harmony of the whole body and of the patient's own image.

40.3
Aging of the Face

The observation of an aged face asks for a careful reflection both of the trials that have provoked the various modifications and of the nature of the same alterations. In aging, the face suffers changes in the principal structures: the bony skeleton, the adipose tissue, and the musculocutaneous system.

According to the rules of universal proportions [2], the face can be separated into three equal segments: the first one from the joining of the hair to the eyebrow, the second from the glabella to the subnasal furrow, and the third one from this line to the chin.

Aging provokes a slow but continuous resorption of the bony structure with reduction of mass, so an unbalance is provoked between bony mass and cutaneous tissue and there is too much skin and subcutaneous tissue. Such disproportion is most evident in the inferior part of the face from the retraction of the jaw and reduction of the dental structure.

Dzubow and Coleman [3] noted that aging provokes alterations and degeneration (Fig. 40.1).

The continuous hormonal and circulatory modifications induced from the style of life, particularly by improper feeding, sedentariness, and smoking, provoke alterations in the metabolism of all the tissues, ending in the reduction of the quantity of water and subcutaneous adipose tissue (typical of the young face) as well as the muscular and cutaneous vascularization that their structural and metabolic reduction provokes. All these

Growing old

The proportions change with the alterations of the structures

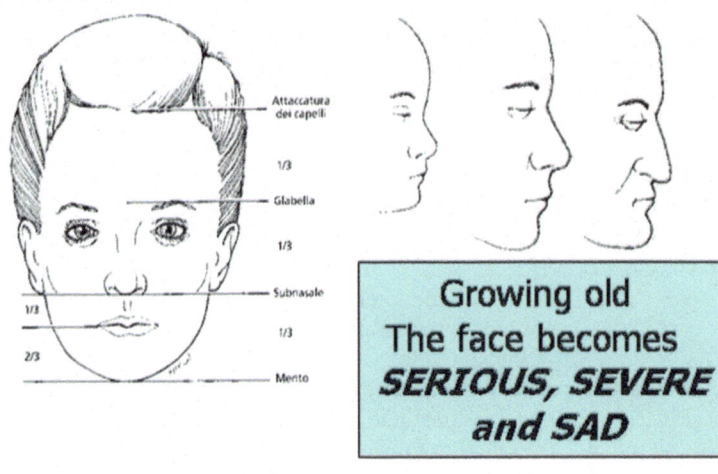

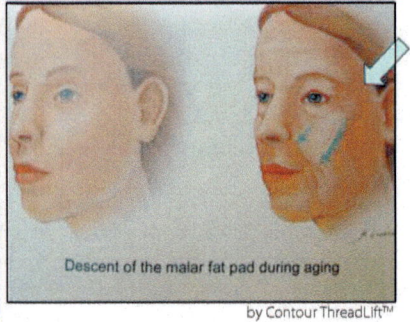

Fig. 40.1 The process of aging of the face

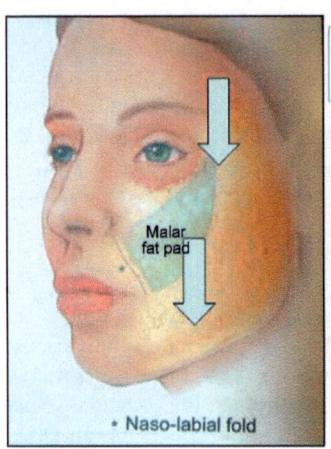

Fig. 40.2 Prolapse of the adipose and connective tissues.

modifications provoke a change in the muscular structure that manifests itself in the reduction of the fibers with reduction of the tone and of tropism with consequent prolapse of the tissues caused by gravity.

At the same time and in the same way there is a decrease of the metabolic and vascular activities of the skin and subcutaneous tissue that provokes reduction of the structure and the cutaneous tone, where we have less soluble and more rigid collagen, a fragmented elastic net, and regression of the microcirculation with reduction of the "cells to veil," i.e., of the lymphoadipose and microvascular system that surrounds and nourishes the same microcirculatory system. All of this provokes reduction and atrophy of the skin and the systems of support with consequent low glide in gravity. It is this low glide of the tissues, caused by gravity and altered metabolism that increases the initial vascular, metabolic, and aesthetic alterations of the face (Fig. 40.2).

The process of aging of the face is from a series of mechanical, physical, and physiological chemical alterations induced by the stress of life that reduces the

metabolic activities and vascular function that activate those alterations of chronic degenerations characterized by cutaneous excess, reduction of fat and the glide of the fat tissue, and atrophy of the skin.

Changes, usually induced by feeding, smoking, hormones, and intestinal dysfunctions, alter the equilibrium of the interstitial matrix, with increase of free radicals, alteration of metalloproteases, alteration of the production of collagen, reduction of the microarterial circulation, increase of the microlymphatic stasis, and finally activation of the processes that will result in degeneration of aging characterized by fibrosis [3–5]. Various degenerative changes due to gravity and loss of glide of the tissues evolve into the typical alterations as a result of aging (Fig. 40.3).

The process of evolution of the suborbicularis adipose bulge is typical. While cutaneous excess of the superior eyelid with relative adipose bulge depends in the most part on prolapse of the frontal structures and from reduction of the eyebrow fat, in the lower eyelid the prolapse of the malar structure with reduction of

Evolutions of folds and wrinkles

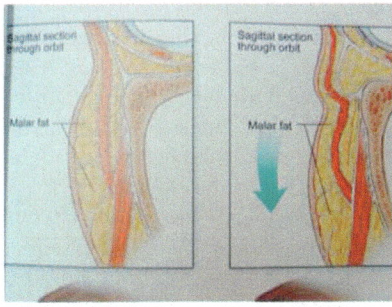

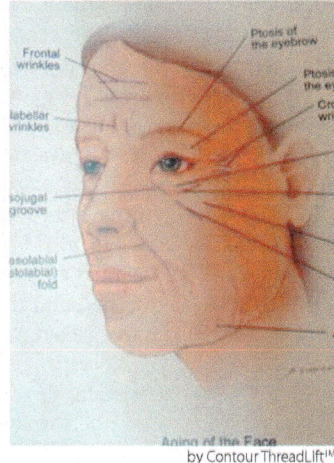

Fig. 40.3 Mechanism of formation of the lower-eyelid bulge

New position of the tissue using Contour ThreadLift™

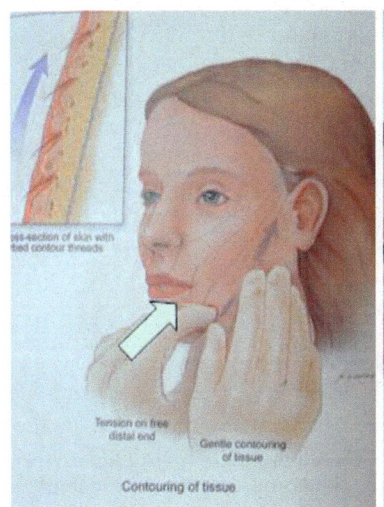

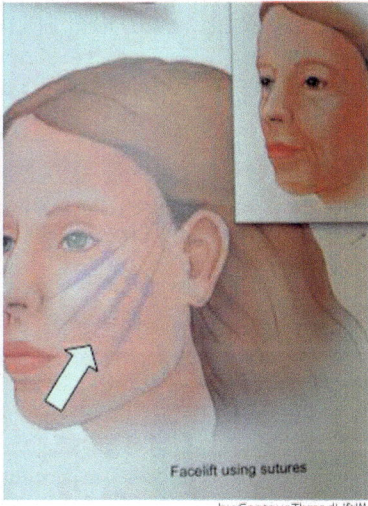

Fig. 40.4 Contouring of the tissues by the mini-invasive method using Contour ThreadLift™

the adipose tissue and its prolapse stretches the ligament and suborbicular septum, provoking formation of the bulge and the cutaneous excess.

While the tissues droop, there are some morphological alterations (in the temporal and spatial position) of the microvascular systems of nutrition and purification of the tissues of the neurological and metabolic systems, which give rise to signals and the production of the structural substances, among which are collagen and elastin. It is this association of metabolic alterations with the mechanical alterations induced by the droop of the tissues that is key to the interpretation of these changes [6].

Bringing the tissues to a more juvenile, more pleasant, and less severe appearance to the face reduces the annoying wrinkles and cutaneous excess folds (Fig. 40.4). Bringing the tissues to their best position means slow-ing down the processes of aging and improving oxygenation, decreasing the lymphatic stasis and the tissue toxicity, reducing free radicals and the oxidative alterations, reducing the alterations of the metalloproteases as well as the process of fibrosis. It means returning normal function to the extracellular matrix.

Depending on the type and of the degree of aging of the face different treatments can be used, such as surgical or dermatologic cosmetic treatments. A fundamental rule is to make a basic classification to plan the correct therapeutic procedure.

1. Excess of skin: When the face has cutaneous excess, surgical treatment must be used to allow tissue recovery and elimination of the cutaneous excess. Traditional lifting, in its various modifications, provides a new position of the deep tissues with duplication and fixation of the superficial muscular

aponeurotic system to guarantee a more lasting result, but not an eternal one. Aesthetic surgery results in about 5 years (between 3 and 8 years depending on the type of skin, of the age, and of the lifestyle) of improvement. In selected patients the mini-invasive solution using surgical barbed or nonbarbed threads can give good results but they should give a new good position of the skin, reducing all processes of aging. These soft methods are indicated as the most diffuse and suitable treatments particularly for the nonadvanced phases and for preventive indications with their mini-invasiveness in multiple sessions and with almost no complications or scars.

2. Reduction of volume
   (a) When there is no true skin excess but the aesthetic anomaly is characterized by reduction of the skin structure with reduction or regression of the adipose and the connective tissues, surgery is not suitable and can only be of help in particular cases.
   (b) The elective treatment is the use of substances to fill and thereby increase the volume and to redraw the contours of the face. The principal fillers are found in the family of hyaluronic acid, which has the principal characteristic of being absorbable and practically without complications. Except for particular cases, it is best to avoid nonabsorbable fillers because of their complications. When it is necessary to use nonabsorbable fillers it is better to use a solid prosthesis, such as solid silicone or Gore-Tex.

3. Skin aging: In the case of patients without skin excess or reduction of the volume, but with underlying irregularity and degeneration of the cutaneous structure (the true cutaneous aging), it is necessary to adopt a noninvasive dermatologic cosmetic treatment protocol that reduces the skin irregularities and improve the external aspect that favors a resumption of the microcirculation, of the oxygenation, and of the production of physiological connective tissues [7–10].

When there is prolapse of the tissues, the angles of the mouth go down and, often, there may be formation of white saliva at the angles that interferes with the patient's relationships. Aesthetic treatment allows the patient to achieve the desire to maintain his/her own dignity and role in society.

40.4
T3–Bioresurfacing

Old age causes modifications, both physical and functional, of the organisms that, in the past, were considered as a sad and disheartening decadence of the bodily harmony and human activities. From such a feeling was born the instinctive impulse for man to fight against the senile phenomenon.

In the case of patients with neither cutaneous excess nor reduction of volume, but who have underlying cutaneous aging with irregularity and degeneration of the dermoepidermal structure, dermatologic cosmetic and noninvasive treatment protocols are used to reduce these irregularities and improve the external aspect favoring improvement of the metabolism. Such a protocol has been named by the author "T3–bioresurfacing," meaning an attempt to rejuvenate the skin by stimulating the natural physiological regeneration with a triad of integrated treatments.

„Bioresurfacing" uses an integrated protocol of different methods to regulate the activity of the skin:

1. Endermologie® LPG: Physical therapy finalized to vascularize and to drain the lymph
2. Transderm® method: To regulate and to stimulate the superficial tissues
   (a) Crystal microdermabrasion: To regulate and to eliminate the horny layer
   (b) Dermoelectroporation: To introduce substances and to stimulate activity
3. Intense pulsed light (IPL): To provide energy and to activate the cellular functions

The integration of these methods has produced interesting results with limited complications and interruption of working activity.

40.4.1
Endermologie® LPG System

The LPG system represents a true revolution in the field of physical therapy and aesthetics, both in the idea and in the practical application. It deals with patented equipment that uses air in the phases of aspiration and compression and a head with two rolls that allows traction on the tissues to perform some maneuvers and has physiotherapeutic applications. Such treatments allow the morphological and functional reconstitution of the connective and the adipose tissue [11–14].

The LPG system acts on the skin and on the subcutaneous tissue to improve the connective tissue, the fat tissue, and the arteriolar, venous, and lymphatic microcirculation, and the blood flow containing the hormones. With LPG the therapist can increase the therapeutic results by use of a "palper-rouler" characterized by movements of compression and tissue rotation, allowing the return of elasticity of the tissues (Fig. 40.5). This allows better function by producing stimulation of metabolism and vascularization and, secondarily, lymphatic drainage and purification of the tissues [15, 16]. The application of the different possibilities of treatment achieves the best results.

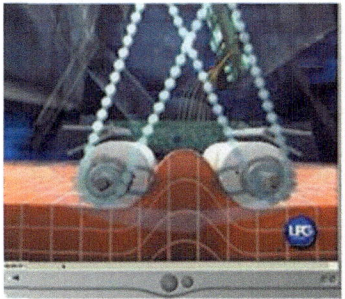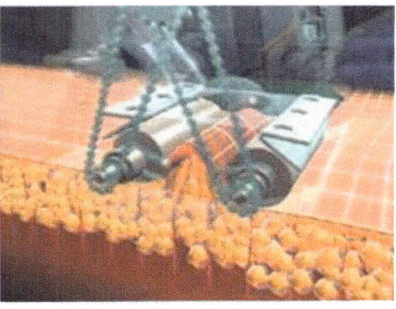

Fig. 40.5 The LPG system allows better function by producing stimulation of metabolism and vascularization and, secondarily, lymphatic drainage and purification of the tissues. *Left*: Typical LPG method. *Right*: Stimulation and compression of tissues

40.4.2
Transderm® Method

The Transderm® method is the union of noninvasive treatment to regulate the cutaneous irregularities, as results of acne or cutaneous atrophy, and the introduction of nutritional substances avoiding the use of needles. For this purpose it uses an association of superficial microdermabrasion with crystals of corundum and dermoelectroporation.

40.4.2.1
Superficial Microdermabrasion

Dermabrasion is one of the most important weapons in the hands of the dermatologic surgeon [17–19]. It is generally used to remove the epidermis and some layers of the dermis, depending on the irregularities needed to be treated. The author uses it only for the treatment of the horny layer.

For aesthetic anomalies characterized by skin irregularities and dystrophies, such as acne, wrinkles, stretch marks, sagging of the skin, treatment with dermoelectroporation is preceded by surface microdermabrasion treatment performed by a system using corundum powder crystals (aluminum oxide in a sterile, disposable package) that produces removal of the corneous layer with simultaneous vascularization of the tissue by mechanical stimulation (light suction–light pressure–dermabrasion).

When dermabrasion treatment needs to be deeper and might cause pain, a session of dermoelectroporation treatment is used first to introduce an anesthetic (2% lidocaine percutaneously without epinephrine). Removal of the corneous layer smoothes the skin and facilitates dermoelectroporation treatment that is performed immediately after microdermabrasion by applying substances containing elastin, collagen, and amino acids. The same protocol is used for the treatment of cellulite. The treatment is integrated into the protocol.

40.4.2.2
Dermoelectroporation

The skin has an exchange function with the outside environment, which is also used as a means of introduction of drugs [20–24]. Endermic diffusion is a passive phenomenon: in fact the skin behaves like a passive membrane. Penetration of the substances takes place in two stages characterized by:

1. Dormancy stage, in which the dermal layer is charged, usually electrically
2. Flow stage, in which the flow becomes constant

Dermoelectroporation treatment is a method that enables absorption using equipment that generates electric pulses allowing the opening of special "electric gates" promoting the passage of substances of adequate size. The apparatus used for medical and aesthetic purposes is Transderm Ionto® from Mattioli Engineering. Dermoelectroporation treatment is applied by a discharge given by an electric inductor charged with a controlled current and then discharged with a typical kind of reversible exponential voltage wave [25–30].

The reason why the method works well only after dermabrasion of the horny layer is because the high voltage in the classic electroporation produces partly poration of the horny layer and partly poration of the dermis (with the residual energy after having perforated the horny layer).

Dermoelectroporation eliminates the need for a high voltage because the horny layer is eliminated with dermabrasion and so the voltage needed to porate the dermis is lower. It works like high-voltage electroporation; however, it replaces the dangerous and hard-to-control effect of the high voltage on the horny layer with the safer dermabrasion. The lower energy is used only in order to open watery channels in the dermis Basic nutritional substances of the tissues, such as amino acids or sodium hyaluronate, introduced by microneedles in the dermal layer, provide the stimulation of the physiological new connective tissue, such as elastin and collagen.

All of this has opened a new frontier in the antiaging protocols of regeneration and rejuvenation, reducing the use of needles and bloodier methods. Immediately after microdermabrasion, active substances such as collagen, hyaluronic acid, amino acids, and elastin or their precursors are introduced by means of dermoelectroporation treatment.

40.4.3
Intense Pulsed Light

IPL technology is an evolution of laser technology since it does not send forth continuous-wave light, which strikes water or other elements with direct surgical action, but it uses a photon as a flash, which strikes particular photodermoreceptors that are stimulated or altered.

Suitable mainly for affecting hemoglobin and dark colors, it has shown an ability to transfer energy to the tissues that directly stimulate the principal vital reactions of the extracellular matrix and the new production of physiological collagen [31–35].

IPL is used at the end of the Transderm session (crystal microdermabrasion and dermoelectroporation) where it guarantees the transfer of a quantity of such energy to favor the use of the introduced substances and the activation of the tissue reactions of the matrix. Energy is produced in the form of heat that allows important microarteriolar vascularization that favors the oxygenation of skin that it is found in state of microcirculatory deficiency, particularly in people who smoke or use the estrogen–progestin pill or drugs.

The author prefers to use a wavelength around 640–690 nm in association with a lower wavelength (530–580 nm) in most cases. Normally, in patients with Fitzpatrick skin types 5 or 6 IPL is not used. The scheme for the use of IPL in bioresurfacing is:
1. Endermologie® treatment
2. Superficial microdermoabrasion and dermoelectroporation
3. IPL: 640 nm, 23–27 J/cm²; 560 nm, 24–28 J/cm²; sessions at 15, 21, and 30 days

The patient is treated with a cold cream (BIAFIN) and, in particular cases, a mask of vitamin C is used.

T3–bioresurfacing allows the patient to use makeup around 20 min after the procedure. Particularly in winter, the patient uses a nighttime cream based on phytic acid and vitamin C, and alternates, sometimes, with a mix of base ointments of retinoic acid (0.0025%) and cortisone cream in low dose.

40.4.4
T3–Bioresurfacing: Treatment Protocol

The treatment is used for the improvement of irregularities of the skin and for the signs of aging by stimulating the production of new collagen and stimulating the extracellular matrix.

Different sessions at 15, 21, and 30 days take place:
1. Lymphatic drainage, skin vascularization, and connective tissue stimulation with the use of the Endermologie® LPG system
2. Transderm® method using superficial microdermabrasion with crystals of corundum to smooth the skin and to open the horny layer, followed by the introduction of precursor substances of collagen, elastin, and hyaluronic acid using dermoelectroporation connected to the Ultrapeel Transderm® instrument (Mattioli Engineering, Italy) that allows opening of the pores that are the watery channels
3. Energy administration by IPL provided by a Quantum IPL instrument with an energy of 532–695 nm that allows stimulation of the cellular function and the extracellular matrix

At the end, an antiherpetic cream or lenitive substances can be applied for therapy or cosmetic action. Such a protocol will not produce immediate visual effects from the surgery or from the use of fillers but it will favor a slow but continuous improvement of the aspect and the tropism of the skin with progressive rejuvenation of the face.

40.4.5
T3–Biolifting

In patients without true cutaneous excess and tissue prolapse and where the aesthetic anolmalies are characterized by a reduction of the "structure" and of the "tropism" of the skin with reduction or regression of the adipose and the connective tissue, surgery is not always suitable and is not the first treatment indicated, even if it can sometimes be of help. These cases, as a rule, represent the large majority of the patients from 25 to 40 years old. These patients do not have an indication for traditional surgery with traction and excision of the tissues. They are patients with "nasogenal wrinkles " that begin to become "nasogenal folds" and, especially in hyperactive subjects, where the crows'-feet and the peribuccal irregularities are in association with the true and deep wrinkles. As a rule, these patients are found in the central phase of their social evolution and working activity. They normally request lesser treatments and above all wish improvements without changing. The treatment of choice is dermosurgical, mini-invasive treatments, and the use of filler substances to increase the volume and to redraw the contours of the face.

The substances that the author prefers are the traditional "fillers" that have the characteristic of being natural and of being reabsorbed in different periods of time, but they are always absorbable substances. These substances belong to two major groups: the family of collagen and that of hyaluronic acid. Collagen was initially derived from tendons of ox and horse and required testing for the dangers of allergies and complications. Today such risks are reduced and synthetic collagen is now available.

In every case, the author prefers hyaluronic acid that has the principal characteristic of being natural (not derived from animals), absorbable, and without complications. Nonlinked hyaluronic acid constitutes a substance of great use in ophthalmology and orthopedics. The nonlinked form has a duration of a few days when inserted in the dermal layer and does not behave as a filler, but as a substance of stimulation for the production of physiological collagen, particularly if associated with precursors of collagen, elastin, or hyaluronic acid.

In the linked form, named "cross-linked," it is hooked to benzyl alcohol and has a more complex form, so it is reabsorbed more slowly. Depending on the concentration and of the type of application it can last from 2 to 8 months.

As a rule, these products do not give true complications in comparison with the nonabsorbable substances. The author believes that we must avoid the complications of nonabsorbable substances. It is better to use a solid prosthesis such as solid silicone or Gore-Tex.

"Biolifting" is a treatment that has the tendency to restructure the skin and to increase the lost volume in the process of aging.

40.4.5.1
Method

In synergy with treatments by bioresurfacing, treatment can be performed that allows the stimulation of the tissues and increases the volume with new harmony of the contours of the face. In this sense of "tissue fullness " and of "good hydration" it will give a juvenile aspect to the face. Using only absorbable substances such as hyaluronic acid in different concentrations increases the length of time it will be effective.

The author uses Teosyal 27 or 30, from the Swiss company Teoxane, which contains 25 mg of reticulated hyaluronic acid in a phosphate buffer at pH 7.3. This is normal hyaluronic acid that introduces different concentrations of a linked substance. This product contains a low quantity of proteins that limits the production of free radicals, reduces inflammation, and therefore increases of the length of time for which the product is effective.

This substance with different concentrations and three layers of insertion gives different characteristics. That is why this protocol is called T3–biolifting since there are three layers: superficial, middle, and deep. Using this method improves the quality of the skin, reduces wrinkles, improves the expression of the eyes, and harmonizes the external aspect (Fig. 40.6) [36].

Superficial Layer

Nonlinked hyaluronic acid is introduced by mesotherapy (drop by drop), by lines in the dermoepidermal layer, or in superficial intradermal layer. Good results can be obtained in the treatment of the neck, acne, and in superficial irregularities of the skin.

Middle Layer

Linked hyaluronic acid is used in low concentration introduced drop by drop in the middle dermal layer. Good results are obtained for the treatment of the middle wrinkles and for cutaneous restructuring.

Deep Layer

Linked hyaluronic acid used in high concentration is introduced into the deep dermal layer or into a submuscular layer in the treatment of the zygomatic area (where it improves the contours) or in the eyebrow area, where it increases the brightness of the look.

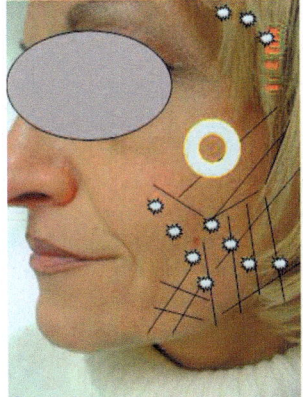

T3-Biolifting
Different layers

Using different layers we can have the best results

1. Improvement of skin structure
2. Reduction of the skin folds
3. Reduction of the wrinkles
4. Improvement of the brightness of the eyes
5. Improvement of the youth of the face
6. Harmonization of external aspect

Fig. 40.6 Different layers for different concentrations of the filler

Threads of Support

Prolapse of the tissues (tissue ptosis) causes contortion of the morphological anatomy and of the functional anatomy of the microstructures with alteration of the metabolic functions of the extracellular matrix with consequent formation of local lipolymphedema. Morphological alterations of the microvessels cause deceleration and lymphatic stasis that alters the metabolic functions of the tissue and increases the free radicals, with metabolic damage to the extracellular matrix that activates the process of oxidative stress with microedema, formation of lipoperoxidation, mitochondrial and metalloprotease damage, alteration of the collagen, inflammatory and chronic evolution toward pathological fibrosis. Repositioning of the tissue provides new metabolism and new life for the same tissues.

When it is necessary, that is when an initial prolapse of the skin results in irregularities and cutaneous depressions (not yet requiring lifting or mini lifting), surgical threads can be used. Surgical unidirectional barbed threads, absorbable or nonabsorbable, can be used. The author uses the Contour ThreadLift™. This method gives rapid improvement without complications, giving a more juvenile aspect of the face and lengthens the lifetime of the substances, reducing the free radicals and the vascular and metabolic alterations thanks to the new spatial position of the tissues [37].

40.4.5.2
Indications

The typical indications for biolifting are the treatment of wrinkles and harmonization of the face.

Together with bioresurfacing, it offers good results without complications for patients. It is necessary to have correct indications and to interview the patient prior to treatment in order to have the best results and satisfaction of the patient.

References

1. Coleman P.W., Hanke C.W.: Storia della chirurgia estetica dermatologica. In Coleman P.W., Hanke C.W., Alt,T.H., Asken S. (eds): Chirurgia Estetica Dermatologica, Rome, Verduci 1999:1–6
2. Dzubow L.: L'invecchiamento del volto. In Coleman P.W., Hanke C.W., Alt T.H., Asken S. (eds): Chirurgia Estetica Dermatologica, Rome, Verduci 1999:7–17
3. Bacci P.A.: Le Celluliti. Arezzo, Alberti 2000:17–73
4. Albergati F.G., Bacci P.A., Mancini S.: La Matrice Extracellulare, Arezzo, Minelli 2005:71–301
5. Goldman M., Bacci P.A., Hexsel D., Liebaschoff, G.: Cellulite: Pathophysiology and Treatment, New York, Taylor & Francis 2006:7–75
6. Ball P., Knuppen R., Haupt M., Breuer H.: Interactions between estrogens and catecholamines. 3. Studies on the methylation of catechol estrogens, catecholamines and other catechols by the catechol-O-methyltransferases of human liver. J Clin Endocrinol Metab1972:34(4):736–746
7. Bacci P.A.: Il tessuto adiposo. In Bacci P.A. (ed): La Celluliti, Arezzo, Alberti 2000:45–50
8. Albergati F.G., Bacci P.A., Mancini S.: Il trasporto di membrane. In Bacci P.A. (ed): La Matrice Extracellulare, Arezzo, Minelli 2005:45–53
9. Bacci P.A.: Il lipoinfedema. Flebogia Oggi 1998;2:31-40
10. Adcock D., Paulsen S., Shack R.B.: Analysis of the cutaneous and systemic effects of Endermologie in the porcine model. Aesthet Surg J 1998:18(6):414–422
11. Fodor P.B., Watson J., Shaw W.: Physiological effects of Endermologie: a preliminary report. Aesthet Surg J 1999;19(1);1–7
12. Bacci P.A.: La fascia superficial. In Baci P.A., Liebaschoff G. (eds): Las Celulitis, Buenos Aires, Medical Books 2000:77–79
13. Bacci P.A.: La fascia superficiale. In Bacci P.A. (ed): Le Celluliti, Arezzo, Alberti, 2000;4:79–82
14. Numberger F., Muller G.: So-cal;led cellulite: an invented disease. J Dermatol Surg Oncol 1978;4(3):221–229
15. Binazzi M., Papini M.: Aspetti clinico istomorfologici. In Ribuffo C., Bartoletti C.A. (eds): La Cellulite, Rome, Salus 1983:7–15
16. Brizzio E.O.: La riabilitazione in flebolinfologia. In Mancini S. (ed): Trattato de Flebologia e Linfologia, Turin, UTET 2001:399–403
17. Alt T., Coleman W., Hanke C., Yarborough J.: Dermabrasion. In Coleman P.W., Hanke C.W., Alt T., Asken S. (eds): Cosmetic Surgery of the Skin, St Louis, Mosby Year Book 1997:147–196
18. Dzubow L.M.: Dermabrasion. J Dermatol Surg Oncol 1994;20(5):302
19. Benedetto A.V., Griffin T.D., Benedetto E.A.: Dermabrasion: therapy and prophylaxis of the photoaged face, J Am Acad Dermatol 1992;27(3):439–447
20. Asbill C.S., El-Kattan A.F., Michniak B.: Enhancement of transdermal drug delivery: chemical and physical approaches. Crit Rev Ther Drug Carrier Syst 2000;17(6):621–658
21. Suhonen T.M., Bouwstra J.A., Urtti A.: Chemical enhancement of percutaneous absorption in relation to stratum corneum structural alteration. J Controlled Release 1999;59:149–161
22. Pausnitz M.R., Bose V.G., Langer R., Weaver J.C.: Electroporation of mammalian skin: a mechanism to enhance transdermal drug delivery. Proc Natl Acad Sci USA 1993;90(22):10504–10508
23. Pacini S., Peruzzi B., Gulisano M.: Qualitative and quantitative analysis of transdermic delivery of different biological molecules by iontophoresis. Ital J Anat Embryol 2003;18(Suppl 2):127–129
24. Lombry C., Dujardin N., Préat V.: Transdermal delivery of macromolecules using skin electroporation. Pharm Res 2000;17(1):32–37

25. Tezel A., Sens A., Mitragotri S.: Incorporation of lipophilic pathways into the porous pathway model for describing skin permeabilization during low-frequency sonophoresis. J Controlled Release 2002;83(1):183–188

26. Kontturi K., Murtomaki L.: Mechanistic model for transdermal transport including iontophoresis. J Controlled Release 1996;41:177–185

27. Bacci P.A.: The role of dermoelectroporation. In Goldman M., Bacci P.A., Hexsel D., Liebashoff G. (eds): Cellulite: Pathophysiology and Treatment, New York, Taylor & Francis 2006:291–301

28. Costello C.T., Jeske A.H.: Iontophoresis. Phys Ther 1995;75:554–563

29. Pacini S., Peruzzi B., Gulisano M., Bernabei et al: Analisi microscopica, qualitativa e quantitativa del trasporto transdermico di farmaci e macromolecole biologiche mediante un nuovo tipo di dermoelettroporazione. In La Flebologia in Pratica, Arezzo, Alberti, 2004:132–136

30. Bacci P.A., Liebaschoff G.: Pathophysiology of cellulite. In Goldman M., Bacci P.A., Hexsel D., Liebashoff G. (eds): Cellulite: Pathophysiology and Treatment, New York, Taylor & Francis 2006:41–75

31. Maimon T.: Stimulated optical radiation in ruby. Nature 1960;187:483

32. Anderson R.R., Parrisch J.A.: Selective photothermolysis: precise microsurgery by selective absorption of pulsed radiation. Science 1983;22:524–527

33. Walsh J, Flotte T, Anderson R.: Pulsed CO_2 laser tissue ablation: effect of tissue type and pulse duration on thermal damage. Laser Surg Med 1988;8(2):108–118

34. Fitzpatrick R., Ruiz-Esparza J., Goldman M.: The depth of thermal necrosis using the CO_2 laser: a comparison of the superpulsed mode and conventional mode. J Dermatol Surg Oncol 1991;17(4):340–344

35. Garden J.M., Tan O.T., Polla L.L.: The pulsed dye laser: its use at 577 nm wavelength, J Dermatol Surg Oncol 1987;13(2):134–138

36. Bacci P.A.: Biolifting. In Bacci P.A., Mancini S. (eds): Chirurgia Estetica Mini-Invasiva con Fili di Sostegno, Arezzo, Minelli 2006:147–184

37. Bacci P.A.: I fili di sostegno. In Bacci P.A., Mancini S. (eds): Chirurgia Estetica Mini-Invasiva con Fili di sostegno, Arezzo, Minelli 2006:214–282

CHAPTER 41

Percutaneous Eyebrow Lift

41

Enrique Hernández-Pérez, Hassan Abbas Khawaja

41.1
Introduction

Brow ptosis is one of the commonest stigmata of facial aging. Frequently it evokes the impression of a tired, sad or bored face. Besides age, heredity is a factor of great importance in provoking brow ptosis.

A myriad of techniques have been proposed to improve such a condition [1, 2]; however, practically all of them leave scars or visible deformities. Direct eyebrow lift leaves a permanent scar immediately above the hairy area that is difficult to hide. This scar is fine in the beginning, but later on it becomes wide and the patient becomes unsatisfied [3]. Conventional coronal lift with a pretrichial incision can lead to elevation of frontal hairline, and a wide unaesthetic forehead [4]. In addition, traumatic alopecia, partial paralysis of the forehead, areas of necrosis, deepening or widening of scars, hematoma, extensive necrosis and lagophtalmus can take place [3, 4]. In 2002, Erol et al. [5], reported a technique for eyebrow lift which was simple and effective. With the intention to simplifying it further, we utilized a Keith needle instead of a catheter [6]. This method has undergone some modifications, in order to make it easier still.

41.2
Methods

The authors propose two different and very simple methods in order to improve this condition:
1. With the patient comfortably seated and after careful asepsis with povidone–iodine, the actual position of the eyebrow is assessed. The actual form of the eyebrow tail is marked on the skin. A similar line is marked in the temporal region immediately behind the hairline. Anesthesia is performed with 1% lidocaine and 1:400,000 epinephrine using 1-ml syringes and 30-gauge needles. Two small papules are made in the proposed entry and exit sites of the needle. Then anesthesia is done along the whole subcutaneous path of the procedure. Anesthesia is repeated similarly on the other side (Fig. 41.1).

Prolene, 3-0, or a similar nonabsorbable material directly attached to a straight needle is utilized. Traction is made in an upward and lateral direction. The end point of such movement depends on the form of the eyebrow and the general proportion of face of the patient. However, it is important from an aesthetic point of view to proceed with caution, and not to overcorrect since " in cosmetic surgery better less than more." After waiting for about 15 min for the effect of epinephrine, the surgeon inserts the needle from upward to downward subcutaneously (from the marked temporal point to the eyebrow point). The posterior end of Adson forceps is used to help exit at the marked point of the eyebrow, and an assistant pushes the skin firmly but not excessively in a contralateral direction. Such countertraction is always helpful in these procedures. Entry is from point A and exit is at point B (Fig. 41.2). Reentry

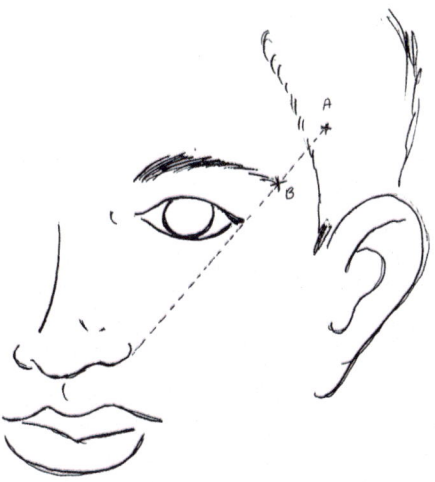

Fig. 41.1 A line is placed between the alae nasi, the outer canthus of the eye and the lateral eyebrow. This method makes it very easy to mark points *A* and *B*

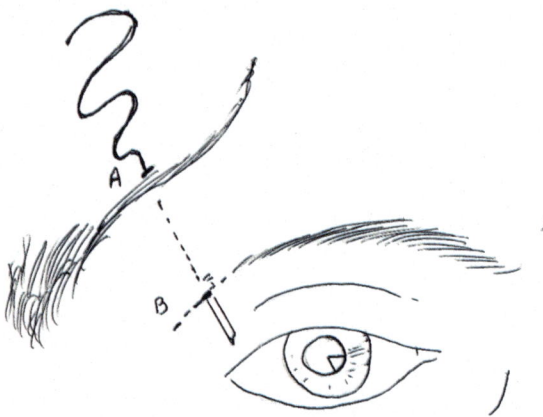

Fig. 41.2 The needle enters at point *A* and exits at point *B*

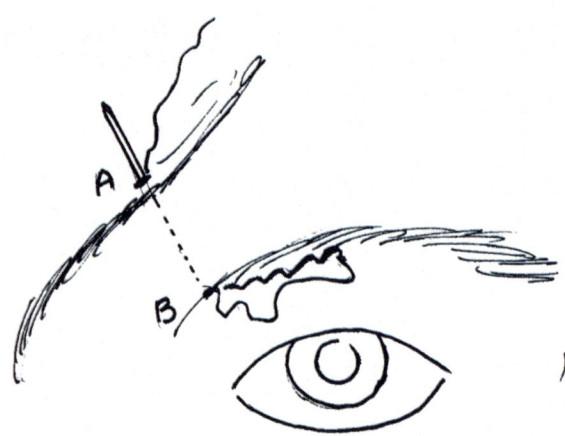

Fig. 41.3 The needle enters at the point *B* and exits back at the initial point *A*. A knot is tied here, avoiding excessive traction

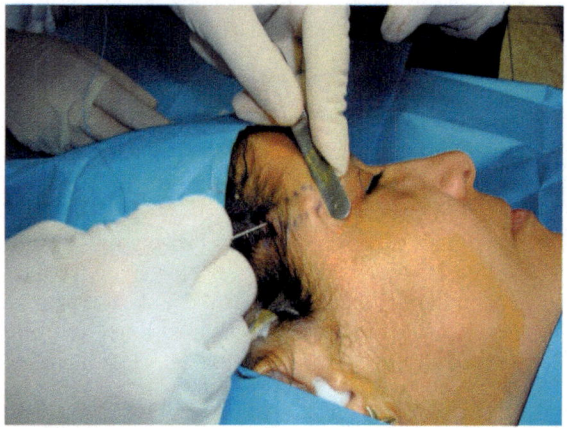

Fig. 41.4 The needle is going from point A to point B

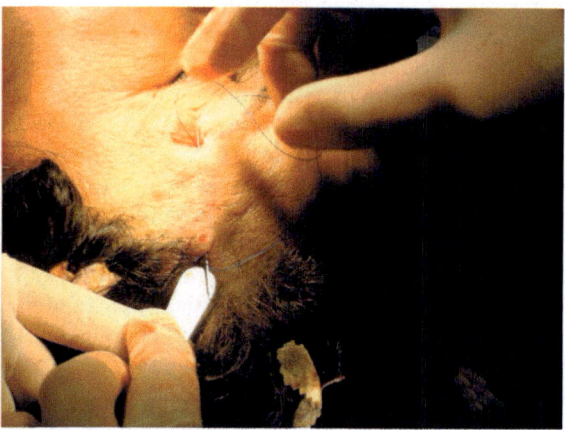

Fig. 41.5 Needle going back from point B to point A

is through the same point B, and exit is back at the initial point A (Fig. 41.3). A knot is tied with as much traction as necessary but without excessive overcorrection (Figs. 41.4, 41.5). The assistant cuts the ends of the thread short and the knot is buried subcutaneously using the tail of the same straight needle. If necessary, the procedure is repeated at two more points, C and D, 2–3 mm medially, not only in the eyebrow but also in the temporal hairline. The same procedure is repeated on the opposite side. The surgical procedure is completely ambulatory and does not need any special preoperative or postoperative care. The only complications have been transitory edema and minor bruising that fades spontaneously in 3 or 4 days. There has not been motor or sensory nerve problems. Excluding anesthesia time, the procedure takes no longer than 5 min for each eyebrow.

2. The second modification is similar to the previous one. Asepsis and anesthesia are utilized in the same

manner. However, instead of drawing only one line, that is to say, A to B and vice versa, two lines are drawn, both parallel and separated by 5 mm. Point A is marked medial and superiorly, becoming point B in the middle of the hairs of the eyebrow. Points C and D must be parallel below and above, respectively (Fig. 41.6). Prolene, 3-0, attached to a straight needle is used. The needle enters at point A, and running through a subcutaneous course, exits at point B; then it reenters at the same point B and exits at point C; reentering at point C, and making a rectangle, it goes to point D, and finally, after being inserted at point D, the needle emerges at point E, which is the former point A. Very small incisions are made with a no. 11 blade scalpel to make the exiting of the needle easier. The other end of the suture is pulled and a knot is tied at this point, raising the eyebrow. The knot is buried in the skin, and 5-0 blue monofilament nylon is sutured at the entry point. Care is also taken that the suture is buried at other points and is

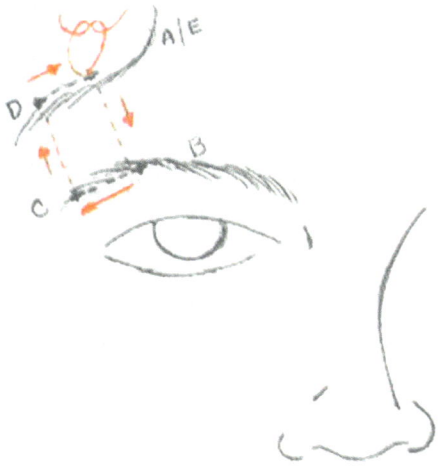

Fig. 41.6 The needle is inserted in the direction of the *arrows*, from point *A* to point *E*. At the end, the knot is made at point *E*, which coincides with point *A*

not exposed. How high the position of the eyebrow is depends on the tension placed on the knot at the initial entry point. The same procedure is repeated on the opposite side. The 5-0 monofilament nylon at the temporal hairline is removed on the seventh day. This simple method of eyebrow lift can be repeated along the entire length of the eyebrow.

41.3
Results

This surgical procedure has been simple, safe and effective in more than 40 patients operated upon so far (Fig. 41.7). In spite of the fact that this technique was

oriented primarily for improving the eyebrow tail, it also is used for raising central and medial parts of the eyebrows using more suture points. Complications are all minor and transitory and there have not been any foreign-body reactions, extrusion, fibrosis, palpable cordlike tracts or tattoos as a result of thread staining. Patient satisfaction was classified as very good in 80% and good in 20% of the cases. The follow-up at 6 months and 1 year showed sustainable results in all patients. The longest follow-up has been for 3 years.

41.4
Discussion

With use of these very simple techniques, upper-lid blepharoplasty could become unnecessary or be minimized. A possible argument against the use of the techniques is that sutures could cut through the tissues. However, if the surgeon remains in the subdermal plane and uses correct traction and a careful technique, such events do not take place. Experience of other surgeons getting good and persistent results without deep fixation and costly undermining confirms that these sutures can sustain prolonged lifting of tissues [5, 7]. Sometimes a very tiny dimple could be seen on the entry points of the needle, like a small skin bite; it usually will disappear in a couple of weeks or a simple subcision can be performed if the patient wishes to shorten the time. The procedure can be easily repeated or revised in every case.

Satisfaction of the patients has been very high and the postoperative observational period has been longer than 3 years. This confirms that deep fixation is not always necessary to lift the tissues for prolonged periods.

Facial aging is a complex process and an isolated procedure cannot resolve it; therefore, it is necessary to

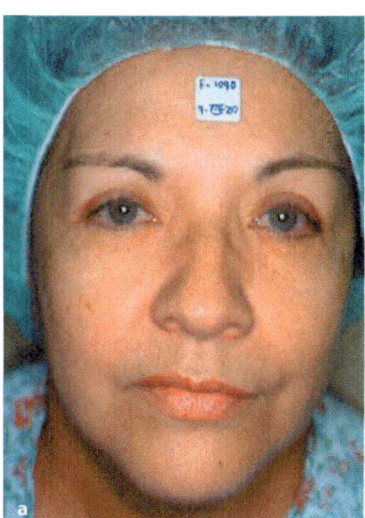
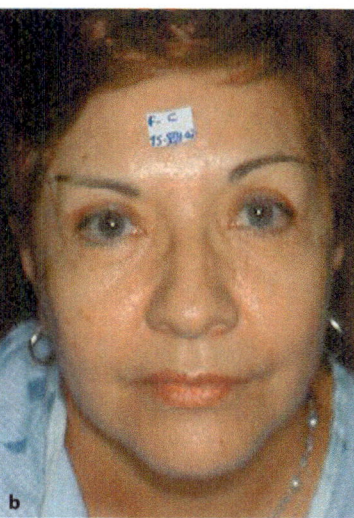

Fig. 41.7 a Preoperatively. **b** Postoperatively

combine different techniques or specific programs to get better results [8].

41.5
Conclusions

This technique seems to be simple, safe and effective. It is worth recommending it combined with other procedures in a program of facial rejuvenation.

References

1. Barton EE Jr, Kenkel JM. Direct fixation of the malar pad. Aesthet Plast Surg 1997;21:239–242
2. Graziosi AC, Canelas Beer SM. Browlifting with thread: the technique without undermining using minimum incisions. Aesthet Plast Surg 1998;22:120–125
3. Kinize DM. Limited incision foreheadplasty. Plast Reconstr Surg 1999;103:271–274
4. Rees TD, Aston SJ, Thorne CHM. Blepharoplasty and facialplasty, including forehead-brow lift. In: MacCarthy JG. Plastic Surgery. Philadelphia: Saunders 1990:2320–2414
5. Erol OO, Sozer SO, Velidedeoglu HV. Brow suspension, a minimally invasive technique in facial rejuvenation. Plast Reconstr Surg 2002;109:2521–2532
6. Hernández-Pérez E, Khawaja HA. A percutaneous eyebrow lift: The Salvadorian option. Dermatol Surg 2003;29:852–855
7. Zarem HA. Brow suspension, a minimally invasive technique in facial rejuvenation. Plast Reconstr Surg 2002;109:2533–2536
8. Hernández-Pérez E, Khawaja HA. Oral isotretinoin as part of the treatment of cutaneous aging. Dermatol Surg 2000;26:649–652

Chapter 42

Suture Lift of the Nasal Tip

42

Chelso G. Cueteaux, Melvin A. Shiffman

42.1
Introduction

Cosmetic surgery of the nose frequently produces unsatisactory results that require modifications. The surgeon should carefully evaluate the nose and its relationships and determine the patient's desires before deciding on a surgical procedure. One utilizes the concepts of harmony, balance, symmetry, and proportions. Surgery uses procedures to refine proportions, contours, silhouette, and volume.

There are diverse techniques in surgery to modify and alter the disproportions of the nose. The surgeon should consider any breathing problems as well as aesthetic defects. The nose determines an individual's appearance and may affect interpersonal relationships.

Patients are presently more interested in short procedures, under local anesthesia and in an ambulatory setting, with low cost, low risk, and a fast recovery time.

42.2
Problems Requiring Surgical Treatment

Surgical problems encountered that require surgical therapy include reduction of the large hooked nose, augmentation of the nasolabial angle, elevation of the nasal tip, shortening of the nose, and reducing the wide nose.

42.3
Patient Examination

The nose should be examined and evaluated as to:
1. Nasofronal angle
2. Bony triangle
3. Alar cartilages
4. Nasal tip
   (a) Projection
   (b) Rotation
   (c) Symmetry
   (d) Position and definition
5. Nasal ala (wing of nose–the flaring cartilaginous expansion forming the outer side of each naris)
   (a) Width
   (b) Retraction
   (c) Relation with alar cartilages
6. Nasolabial angle and columella
7. Nasal examination
   (a) Internal valves
   (b) Septum
   (c) Nasal vestibule

42.4
Objectives in Nasal Surgery

The obectives in nasal surgery are:
1. Return the nose to normal proportions and harmony
2. Have accord with the physical aspects of the face
3. Reduce the size of the nose
4. Change the form of the tip of the nose
5. Change the entry angle of the nose and the upper lip
6. Reduce the dorsal hump
7. Modify the form of the nasal fossae
8. Modify the nasomental angle
9. Diminish the size of the nasal fossae
10. Have realistic expectations
11. Minimal risk

42.5
Technique

The technique conists of the following:
1. Antibiotic (Microcyn)
2. Complete sterility
3. Mark those areas of the nose to be treated
4. Local anesthetic: 2% lidocaine with epinephrine, maximum 5 ml
5. Number 11 blade
6. An 18-gauge spinal needle
7. 3-0 Proline suture
8. Wullstein dissector
9. Micropore tape 1 cm, skin color
10. Camera, preferably digital

42.6
Surgery

If the patient is an acceptable candidate for nasal lift surgery, preoperative photographs are taken. Local anesthesia is used, 1 ml in the base of the nose for cutting the depresor, 1 ml each side in the area between cartilage and bone of the anterior nose, 1 ml in the nasofrontal area, and 2 ml in the upper side of nose (Fig. 42.1). An incision is made in the inferior nasal vestibule, across the clumella, and exposing the nasla depressor muscle. This muscle is transected with the Fournier technique. There is an immediate elevation of the nasal tip. Further correction is necesary to maintain the elevation.

An incision is made on the nasal tip anterior and superior to the nasal vestibule and an incision (or two 16-gauge needle holes on each side) is made in the area of the frontonasal angle at the level of the nasal bone. The Wullstein dissector is used to detach the superficial tissues from the nasal cartilages through the nasal tip incision. An 18-gauge double-pointed needle is intro- duced into the nasal tip and passed superiorly on the left side of the nose superficial to the cartilages exiting at the nasofrontal angle on the left. A hook needle is passed from the right side of the nasofrontal angle to the left side catching the periosteum and the Prolene suture is inserted into the opening in the hook needle and pulled across the space. A double-pointed needle is inserted through the tip of the nose incision and passed along the right side superficial to the cartilage to the nasofrontal angle and the suture is attached to the needle and then pulled back through the tissues exiting at the nasal tip. The suture is tied with sufficient tension to lift the nasal tip to the proper position and tied. The knot is pushed under the skin.

42.7
Postoperative Care

The patient can begin activities immediatley after surgery. Anti-inflammatory medication is started with an

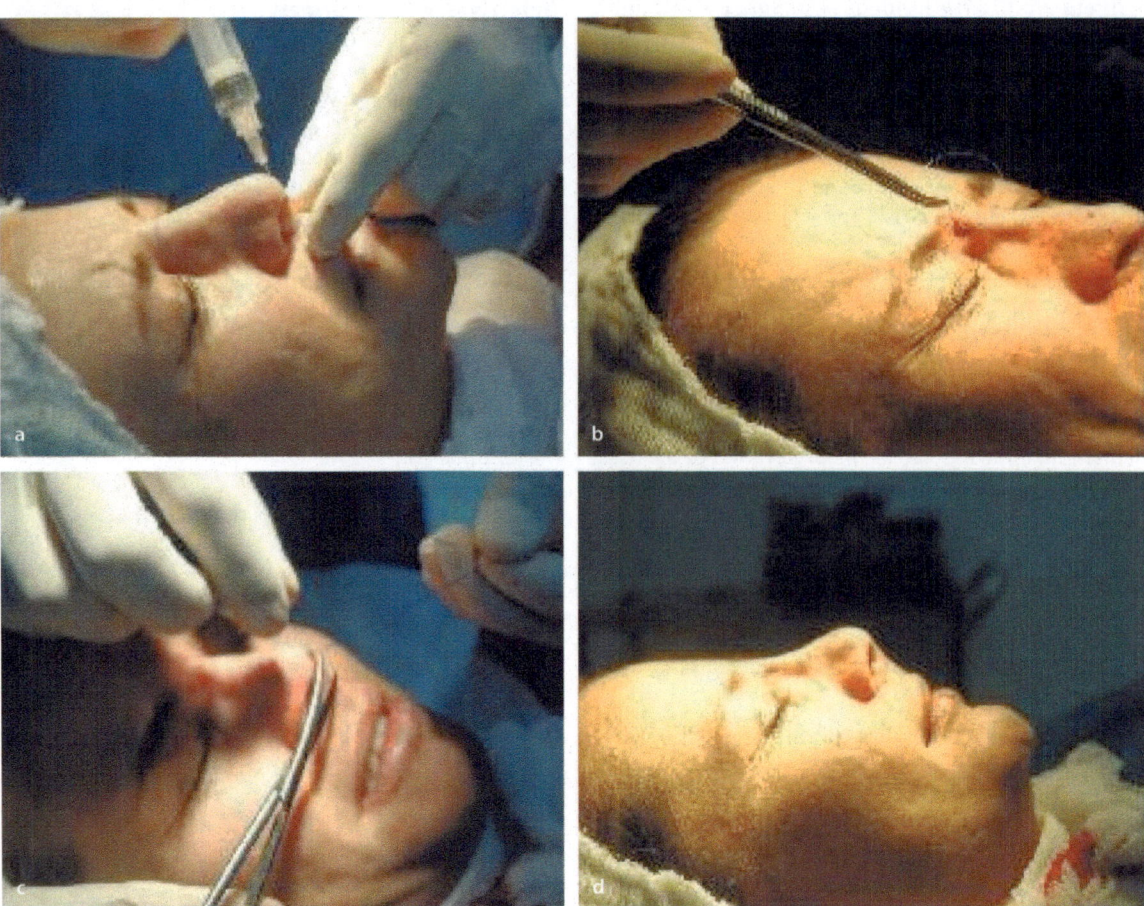

Fig. 42.1 a Injection of local anesthesia. **b** Suture passed on the right side to the nasofrontal fold. **c** Suture being tied at the nasal tip. **d** Final result

antibiotic (ciprofloxacin) and taken for 5 days. For pain a patient may need one tablet of ketoralac every 8 h. The edema and discomfort may last up to about 8 days.

42.8 Complications

There were 72 patients that had suture nasal tip lift, with 62 women and 13 men. The ages ranged from 18 to 58 years. There were three cases of slight edema that lasted 3–7 days. Eight cases had hematomas. Most patients were very satisfied with the results (Figs. 42.2, 42.3)

42.9 Conclusions

The suture nasal lift is an alternative, simple procedure with a drooping tip. The surgery is exclusively aesthetic and should not be used for nasal ventilation problems. The technique is easy to learn and can be done under local anesthesia in an ambulatory setting with low cost to the patient.

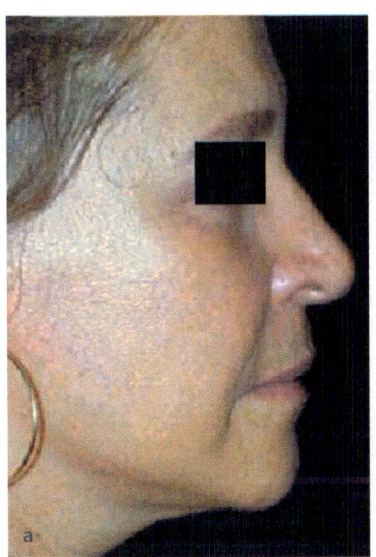
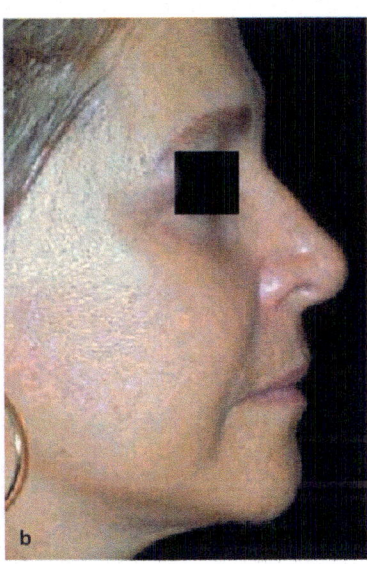

Fig. 42.2 a Preoperatively. **b** Postoperatively

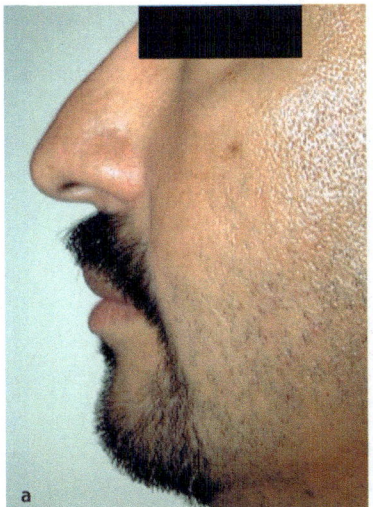
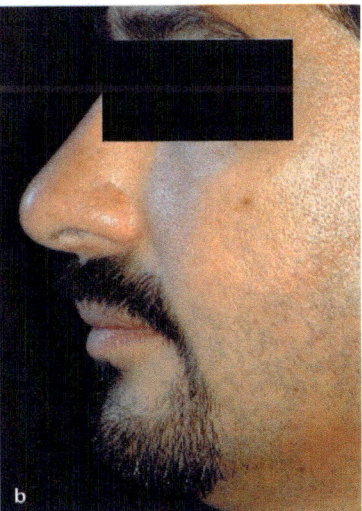

Fig. 42.3 a Preoperatively. **b** Postoperatively

Selected Reading

1. Achauer, B.M., Eriksson, E., Guyuron, B., Coleman, J.J. III, Russell. R.C., Vander Kolk, C.A.: Plastic Surgery: Indications, Operations, and Outcomes. Primary and Secondary Rhinoplasty, Volume 5. St. Louis, Mosby 2000:2631–2683

2. Anderson, J.: On the selection of patients for rhinoplasty. Otolaryngol Clin North Am 1975;8(3);685–688

3. Beekhuis, G.J.: Surgical correction of saddle nose deformity. Trans Sect Am Acad Ophthalmol Otolaryngol 1975;80(6):569–607

4. Bonne, O.B., Wexler, M.R., De-Nour, A.K.: Rhinoplasty patients' critical self evaluations of their noses. Plast Reconstr Surgery 1996;98(3):440–441

5. Conley, J.: Intranasal composite grafts for dorsal support. Arch Otolaryngol 1985;111(4):241–243

6. Constantian, B.F.: Grafting the projecting nasal tip. Ann Plast Surg 1985;14(5):391–402

7. Goin, J.M., Goin, M.K.: Changing the Body Psychological Effects of Plastic Surgery. Baltimore, Williams & Wilkins 1981

8. Jonson, C., Jr, Alsarraf, R.: The Aging Face: A Systematic Approach. Philadelphia, Saunders 2002:112

9. Nique, T.A., Kai Tu, H.: Anesthesia for Facial Surgery. Thieme, New York 1993

Part VI
Surgical Variations: Face

CHAPTER 43

Short Access Facial Elevation: a Modified S-Lift   43

Longin Zurek

The author has no financial interest or support from any manufacturers of the products mentioned in this article.

43.1
Introduction

There is a growing interest today in less invasive facial rejuvenation. The majority of people considering a facelift are not prepared to accept the high risk of complications and prolonged convalescence associated with aggressive procedures.

The following is a brief overview of the history and evolution of facelifting procedures, which began as "minilifts" and progressed gradually to very aggressive procedures with extensive dissection, deep plane and subperiosteal. However, in recent years there has been a reversal in this trend, leading to minimal intervention.

Although it is uncertain who performed the first facelift, the procedure was being done almost 100 years ago by a number of surgeons, including Holländer (1912), Lexer (1931) and Joseph (1921) in Germany, and Passot (1919) (Fig. 43.1), Noel (1926), Bourguet (1921) and others in France. The majority of the early efforts involved excision of strips of skin in front of and behind the ears, with or without minimal undermining (minilifts).

In 1907, an article by Miller was published dealing with the removal of facial wrinkles by subcutaneous sectioning of facial muscles. In the 1950s, owing to an increased demand for facelifts, many surgeons in the USA, South America and Europe concentrated on procedures to remove facial wrinkles. At that time some surgeons thought that longevity of results was directly proportional to the extent of undermining [1].

Skoog [2] was the first to include deeper planes of the face during facelift surgery. The concept of the superficial musculoaponeurotic system (SMAS) was established by Tessier of Paris and defined by his students Mitz and Peyronie [3]. The SMAS was described as a continuous fibromuscular layer surrounding and interlinking the muscles of facial expression and contains fibrous septae that extend through the subcutaneous fat and attach to the overlying skin (Fig. 43.2) [4]. Underneath the SMAS there is a loose areolar plane [5, 6].

Subsequently a number of facelift techniques involving deeper plane and extensive dissections were

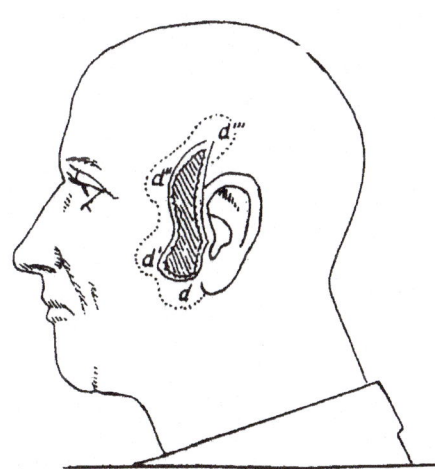

Fig. 43.1 Passot (1919): Preauricular skin excision with little or no skin undermining (minilift) abandoned by most surgeons as the results were short-lived

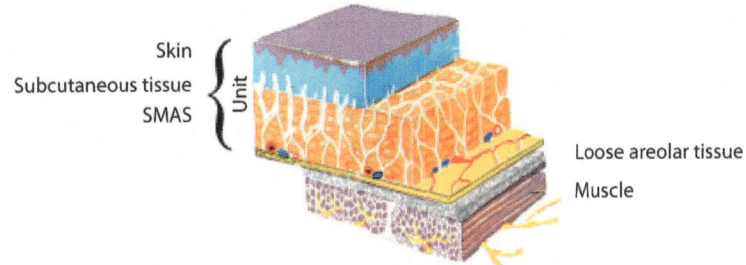

Skin
Subcutaneous tissue
SMAS
Unit
Loose areolar tissue
Muscle

Fig. 43.2 The skin, subcutaneous tissue and superficial musculoaponeurotic system (*SMAS*) can be considered as a unit

developed; however, a high incidence of complications including facial nerve injury were reported. In the early 1990s some surgeons began to question the justification of this approach [7]. A prospective comparative study of facelift techniques conducted in 1996, involving 21 patients, explored this issue. A conventional facelift was performed on one side of the face and on the other side the patients underwent an extended/deep-plane procedure. No discernable differences were noted after 6 and 12 months. This study further reinforced the doubt regarding the justification of aggressive facelifts [8]

Ansari combined the S-shaped incision described by Passot and Lexer with manipulation of the SMAS, and developed a technique of facelift which he called the "S-lift" (Fig. 43.3) [9, 10]. The author incorporated the S-lift into his practice in 1998 after an instruction course [11].

By early 2000 after over 300 S-lift procedures the author modified the S-lift. This showed overall satisfaction of 91%; however, 4% of cases had temporary dysfunction of the frontal branch of the facial nerve [12]. This was one of the reasons behind further modifying the technique. The point of anchoring of the SMAS plication sutures was changed from the zygoma to the deep temporal fascia, 2 cm above the zygoma and not more than 1 cm in front of the helix. To obtain access to this point the upper "S" incision was extended to the temporal region initially in a shallow arc and finally in almost a semicircular shape. This incision also allows excision of excess skin following advancement and rotation of the flap and hiding the scar away from the temporal hairline.

The modification of the S-lift, was named the S-access facial elevation (SAFE) and was reported at a number of meetings in Australia and overseas (Fig. 43.4) [13–20].

Salyan [21, 22] (Saylan, Berlin, October 2004, personal communication) modified and widely popularized the S-lift (Fig. 43.5). Tonnard et al. [23–25] (Fig. 43.6) modified the S-lift and called it the minimal-access cranial suspension lift (MACS).

43.2
Patient Evaluation

Prior to consultation patients are asked to complete a consultation form (Table 43.1) and medical history data form (Table 43.2).

During the initial consultation the author precisely identifies the patient's concerns and expectations, as well as motivations for seeking cosmetic surgery. The Hippocratic principal is "not to make things worse" and there is a surgical duty to protect patients from unnecessary surgery. The author feels that successful cosmetic surgery often improves patients' quality of life. Today the majority of cosmetic surgery clients are seeking the least invasive procedures which carry minimal risks and downtime. People are also looking for a natural result

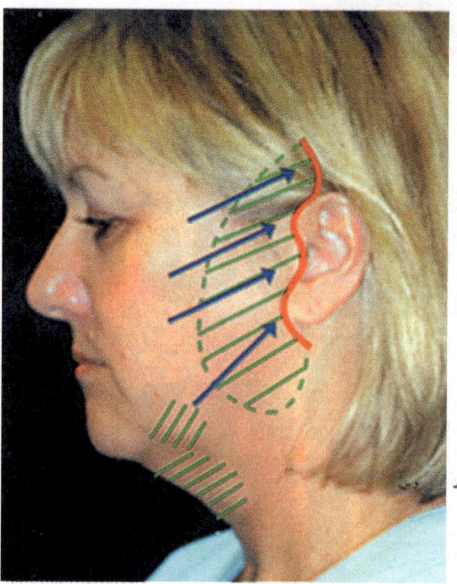

Fig. 43.3 Ansari: S-shaped incision, limited skin and SMAS undermining. Extensive blunt subplatysmal dissection and lipoplasty of the jowls and neck

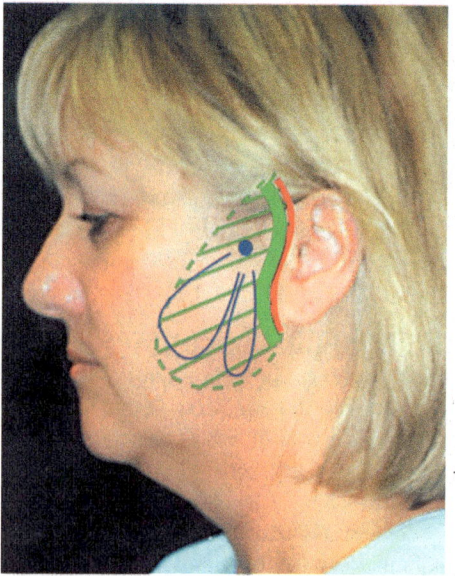

Fig. 43.4 Zurek: S-access facial elevation (SAFE). An S shaped incision starting in the posterior hairline above the level of the eyebrow and following the helical rim in front or behind the tragus (preserving the incisura of the tragus in posttragal incision) and follow the earlobe approximately 2 mm distal to its junction with the cheek skin, extending behind the lobe and the concha groove depending on the degree of skin laxity in the neck. Immediate subcutaneous undermining 4 cm anteriorly and to the angle of the mandible inferiorly. Three plication sutures anchored to the deep temporal fascia. Skin redraped as an advancement rotation flap and excess skin excised. Wound repaired without any tension with a single layer of vertical mattress sutures

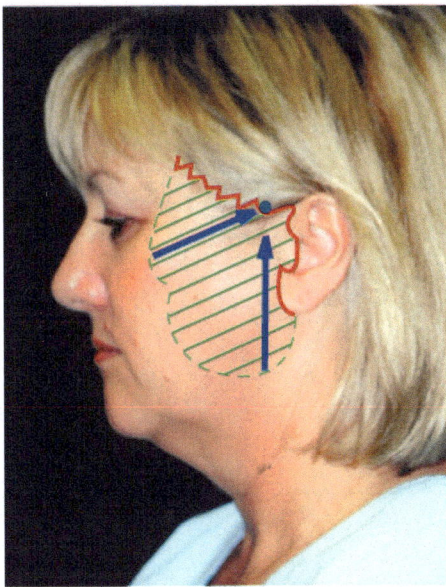

Fig. 43.5 Salyan: Excision of a predetermined strip of skin in front of the ear recently abandoned by him. Undermining medially 5–7cm. SMAS plication by two U- and O-shaped sutures (recently just by one butterfly-shaped suture) and anchored to the periosteum of the zygoma. Wound closure under some tension

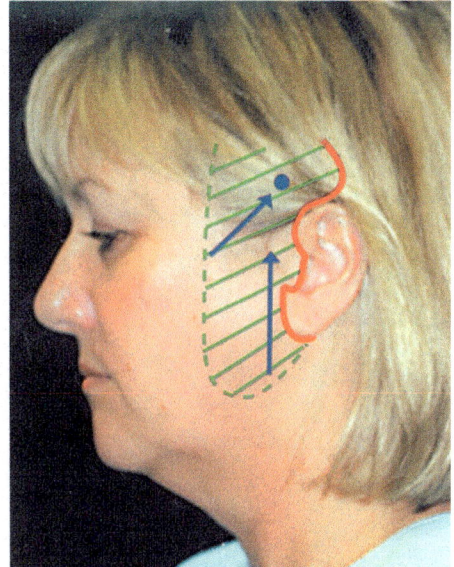

Fig. 43.6 Tonnard et al.: Minimal-access cranial suspension lift (MACS lift and extended MACS lift). Preauricular incision extended to the temporal hairline, subcutaneous undermining 5 cm anteriorly and inferiorly to the mandibular angle. Two purse-string sutures, narrow U- and open O-shaped anchored to deep temporal fascia. Extended MACS lift, extended incision along the temporal hairline with supplementary area of undermining over the malar fat pad. Third purse-string suture suspending the malar fat pad

with a "refreshed" appearance and no obvious stigma of intervention. Many surgeons realize that often more can be achieved by doing less, which benefits both the patient and the surgeon.

43.3
Examination

Following the interview, the patient sits in front of a three-way mirror with standardized lighting. The patient is asked to precisely identify his/her concerns, e.g., loose skin in the neck, jowls, droopy eyelids.

Physical examination involves assessment of skin quality and skin excess. The cheeks are pinched and pulled horizontally in order to classify the amount of facial laxity as mild, moderate and severe (Fig. 43.7).

To address moderate to severe skin laxity a form of facelifting procedure would have to be considered, allowing the removal of some excess skin. A mild degree of laxity with ptosis may be suitable for support, e.g., barbed sutures and/or volume replacement, e.g., fat transfer. In the neck, submental fat deposit is assessed by a pinch test, preplatysmal or subplatysmal location is identified and platysmal bands are evaluated. A range of options are given to address the patient's concerns (including no intervention at this stage), and the antici-

pated effects on the face is demonstrated in front of the mirror.

43.4
Patient Education

A well-informed patient is a better patient. When the patient requests the SAFE procedure (with or without submental liposculpture) and he or she is considered to be a suitable candidate, thorough patient education is provided. The principles of the procedure are explained and possible complications are discussed. The patient is given preoperative and postoperative instructions as well as an informed consent form to take home for perusal (Table 43.3). The patient is invited for a second consultation and given an opportunity to meet with former patients who underwent similar procedures.

43.5
Technique

On the day of the procedure the patient is given the opportunity to ask any further questions and the informed consent form is signed. Preoperative instructions (Table 43.4) are checked and postoperative information (Table 43.5)

Table 43.1 Consultation

DR. LONGIN ZUREK   COSMETIC SURGICENTRE OF SYDNEY
Certified Cosmetic Surgeon   St George Private Hospital
Australasian College of Cosmetic Surgery   1 South Street, Kogarah. 2217
International Board of Cosmetic Surgery

Confidential

Consultation & Medical History Data

Date: _____

Mr/Miss/Ms/Mrs/Dr _____

First Name _____ Surname _____

Date of Birth: _____

Home Address: _____

_____

Telephone: (Home) _____ (Work) _____

(Mobile) _____ (E-mail) _____

Marital Status: _____ Spouses Name: _____

Your Occupation: _____

How were you referred, or how did you hear about our centre? _____

In which surgical procedures are you interested ? Please indicate

- ADVANCED S-LIFT (SAFE) _____
- FACE LIFT WITHOUT INCISIONS (AGE FILAMENTS) _____
- EYEBROWS _____
- EYELID UPPER/LOWER _____
- NOSE RESHAPING _____
- LIPS _____
- CHIN _____
- NECK _____
- EAR & EARLOBES _____
- CHEMICAL PEEL / DERMABRASION _____
- LIPOSCULPTURE Area _____
- BREAST Enlargement _____

Reduction _____

What specifically do you wish to have improved? _____

When did you begin to consider surgical improvement? _____

Have you consulted any other doctor about this, and when? _____

Have you had any previous cosmetic / plastic surgery? Yes / No _____

When, and what was done and who performed the surgery? _____

Were you satisfied with the results? Yes / No. _____

If not, why? _____

Have you had any other prior surgery? Yes / No. If yes, what was done and when was it performed?

_____

Were there any complications in the surgeries performed? Yes / No _____

If yes, explain _____

_____

Table 43.2 Medical history data

MEDICAL HISTORY (Please circle appropriate response)

No Yes   Are you taking any medication?
List them if you can _____
_____

No Yes   Are you allergic to any medication, cream, tape, etc.?
List them if you can _____
_____

When was your last physical examination? _____

No Yes   Have you had a blood test recently?

Who is your family doctor? _____

No Yes   Would you object to our contacting him/her for information pertaining to your health?

No Yes   Have you recently received local anesthesia by a dentist or doctor?

No Yes   Did you have a "reaction" to any anesthetic ?
If yes, explain _____

No Yes   Do you have any history of excessive bleeding / bruising ?
If yes, explain _____

No Yes   Do you a tendency to delayed / poor healing ?
If yes, explain _____

No Yes   Do you have a history of excessive scarring ?
If yes, explain _____

No Yes   Do you suffer from asthma?

No Yes   Do you have frequent pains in the chest?

No Yes   Do you smoke? If so, how many cigarettes per day?

No Yes   Do you usually take 2 or more alcoholic drinks per day?

No Yes   Are you easily upset or irritated?

No Yes   Do you often feel unhappy or depressed?

No Yes   Have you ever received medical treatment for a "nervous breakdown"?

No Yes   Have you ever been under the care of a psychiatrist or psychologist?

No Yes   Do you have any medical problems which have not been covered?
If so, please explain _____

Signed: _____
Date: _____

Thank you, the information you have provided is essential in the comprehensive evaluation of your care.

Table 43.3 Informed consent for S-lift *(Continued next page)*

DR LONGIN H. ZUREK
MD, DPD, FACCS
DIP. INTERNATIONAL BOARD OF COSMETIC SURGERY
COSMETIC SURGEON

Cosmetic Surgicentre of Sydney   Tel (02) 9553 6237
St George Private Hospital   Fax (02) 9553 9639
Level 5, Suite 7c   After hours No: (02) 9331 6018
1 South Street, Kogarah 2217   Email: zurek@ozemail.com.au

INFORMED CONSENT FOR S-Lift

Patient Name: ....
Date: ....

I hereby request Dr Longin Zurek to perform an S-Lift procedure on me. I fully understand this procedure and its limitations. I am aware that the practice of medicine is not exact science, and that no guarantees have been made to me as to the result of the procedure.

Dr Longin Zurek has discussed in details with me the information that is briefly summarised below:

a _____ Nature and purpose of S-Lift.
S-Lift is a surgical procedure by which ptotic (drooping) tissue of the lower face and neck is elevated and excess skin is removed. Following this the skin is redraped and sutured in place.

b ____ Risks
I understand that among the known although minimal risks are, bruising, lumpiness, dimpling, sagging of the skin, some raising of the natural sideburns, scarring, numbness, minor depressions and swelling. A second procedure may be needed in the future. I am aware that in addition to the risks specifically described above, there are other risks such as loss of blood and infection that may accompany any surgical procedure, as well as injury to nerves that may lead to weakness of facial muscles.

c_____ I understand that the two sides of the human body are not the same and can never be made the same.

d _____ Anaesthesia
I understand that this procedure will be performed under local anaesthesia and oral sedation if required. I consent to the administration of local anastehesia and I am aware oft the risks involved such as allergie or toxic reactions to the anaesthetic, and cardiac arrest.
e ____ Alternatives to Face-lift/S-Lift
Alternative methods of removing excessive skin do not exist, although chemical/laser peeling and/or dermabrasion may improve the wrinkles and tighten the skin, they do not remove the excess loose skin.

f ____ Informed Consent
I have had sufficient opportunity to discuss my condition and proposed surgery and all of my questions have been answered to my satisfaction. I believe that I have adequate knowledge on which to base an informed consent to the proposed treatment.

g ____ Photographs
I consent to be photographed before, during and after the treatment; these photographs shall be the property of Dr Zurek and may be published in scientific journals or books, and shown for educational, informative or promotional purposes, and to be shown to prospective surgery patients.

Table 43.3 *(Continued)* Informed consent for S-lift

h _____ Co-operation
I agree to keep Dr Zurek and his staff informed of any change in my permanent address, and I agree to co-operate with them before, during and after the surgery. I understand that I should not smoke or drink alcoholic beverages for at least 2 weeks before surgery, both of which can jeopardise the surgical procedure and the healing afterwards.

i _____ This Paragraph Pertains to Smokers
Smokers are recognised to have a significantly higher risk of post-operative wound healing problems as well as operative and post-operative bleeding, it can also lead to skin necrosis. Although it helps to stop smoking for several weeks before and after surgery, this does not eliminate the increased risk resulting from long-term smoking.

Please initial each paragraph and sign below.

Patients' Signature: .... Witness: .... Date: ....

Table 43.4 S-lift preoperative instructions form *(Continued next page)*

DR LONGIN H. ZUREK
MD, DPD, FACCS
DIP. INTERNATIONAL BOARD OF COSMETIC SURGERY
COSMETIC SURGEON

Cosmetic Surgicentre of Sydney
St George Private Hospital
Level 5, Suite 7c
1 South Street, Kogarah 2217

Tel (02) 9553 6237
Fax (02) 9553 9639
After hours No: (02) 9331 6018
Email: zurek@ozemail.com.au

S-LIFT

Pre Operative Instructions

1. _____ No aspirin-containing medications, vitamin E, nonsteroidal anti-inflammatory medications or excessive alcohol 2 weeks prior to the procedure as these promote bleeding.

2. _____ If you are a smoker, stop smoking at least 2 weeks prior to and, after the procedure.

3. _____ Arrange transportation home on the day of the procedure.

4. _____ Shampoo hair 1 day before the procedure and do not use hairspray before or after the procedure. You may wish to have your hair tinted prior to surgery as it may be 4 weeks before you can colour the hair again.

5. _____ Light breakfast/lunch, no coffee as this is a stimulant.

Table 43.4 *(Continued)* S-lift preoperative instructions form

6. _____ Arrange a few days supply of food that requires little chewing eg. yoghurt, soup, bananas, mashed potato, ice cream, jelly etc.

7. _____ Wear a garment with an open front or a large opening in order for it to be removed easily after the procedure when you get home. Wear flat comfortable shoes.

8. _____ Remove all jewellry (earrings and neck ornaments) prior to arrival and leave at home.

9. _____ All trace of face/neck makeup and cream should be thoroughly washed off.

10. _____ Bring a large solid coloured scarf or hooded jacket to cover the support garment.

11. _____ Arnica tablets (homeopathic remedy that will help minimize bruising and swelling) is recommended. Two tablets three times a day sucked or chewed (not swallowed) for seven days prior to surgery and seven days after surgery. Please purchase 84 tablets (6 x 14 days) from your chemist. However this is optional.

Table 43.5 S-lift postoperative instructions form *(Continued next page)*

DR LONGIN H. ZUREK
MD, DPD, FACCS
DIP. INTERNATIONAL BOARD OF COSMETIC SURGERY
COSMETIC SURGEON

Cosmetic Surgicentre of Sydney   Tel (02) 9553 6237
St George Private Hospital   Fax (02) 9553 9639
Level 5, Suite 7c   After hours No: (02) 9331 6018
1 South Street, Kogarah 2217   Email: zurek@ozemail.com.au

S-LIFT

Post Operative Instructions

1. _____ No aspirin or alcohol for 3 days after the procedure.

2. _____ Take antibiotics (cephalexin), 1 capsule every 12 hours, for 3 days.

3. _____ Mild to moderate pain is expected after surgery. To relieve pain, you may take Panadine Forte or Capadex (one tablet every 6 hours as required) you may also take a sedative or medication against nausea if necessary these will be supplied to you.

4. _____ Avoid excessive chewing, talking and movement of the jaw.

Table 43.5 *(Continued)* S-lift postoperative instructions form

5. _____ After surgery, the wound area will be numb for several weeks and you may burn yourself unknowingly by applying hot packs etc, using curling irons or even blow-drying your hair on or near your operated skin. Avoid baths and take a warm rather than hot shower.

6. _____ For the first few nights it is advisable to sleep on your back with your head elevated to prevent swelling and bruising around your eyes.

7. _____ Please return the day after the procedure for change of dressings.

8. _____ Male clients, please refrain from shaving until day 3.

9. _____ You may shampoo your hair after 3 days avoiding hot water any harsh rubbing or combing to the incision. No other dressings will be required It is advisable to continue wearing the head support with the special sponges as much as possible until the sutures are removed and occasionally beyond that time if you find it helpful.

10. _____ All skin sutures will be removed usually 7 days after surgery.

11. _____ If you wear makeup, please refrain from doing so for at least the first week after surgery. Makeup may cause skin irritation or adversely affect wound healing. The same applies to perfume and cologne.

12. _____ Do not have any permanent waves or hair colouring for four weeks post-operatively.

13. _____ We would like to see patients 6 to 12 months after surgery. As we conduct regular surveys following surgery, you may be contacted by the office and your cooperation will be greatly appreciated.

14. _____ In case of emergency, please contact Dr Zurek on his after hours number (9331 6018).

Strenuous physical activities should be avoided for approximately 2 weeks after procedure. *Remember, a good basic rule is:* _____ "IF IT HURTS, DON'T DO IT".

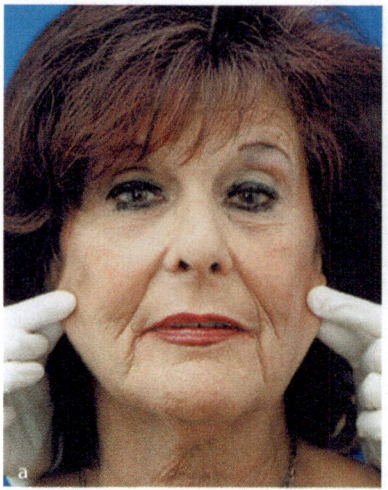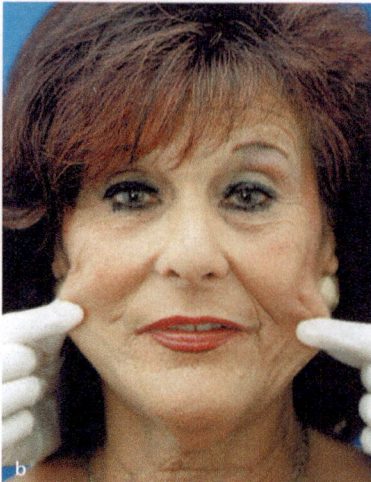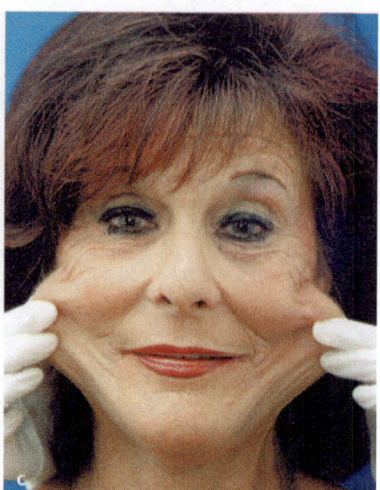

Fig. 43.7 a Mild, **b** moderate and **c** severe facial laxity

is reinforced. Standardized photographs are taken and skin markings are drawn.

The oral medications are as follows:

1. Antibiotic: Cephalexin (500 mg) immediately followed by one capsule twice daily for 4 days
2. Sedatives, hypnotics: Zopiclone (7.5mg) and diazepam (5–10mg)
3. Analgesic: Codeine phosphate (30 mg) and paracetamol (500 mg)
4. Antiemetic: Prochlorperazine (5–10mg)

The skin is prepared with a 10% solution of povidone–iodine or a 0.1% aqueous solution of chlorhexidine.

The local anesthetic used is 0.5% lignocaine with 1:200,000 epinephrine (100–150ml freshly prepared). A typical formula is 25ml 2% lignocaine, 0.5ml 1 mg/ml epinephrine and 74.5 ml sodium lactate (Hartmann's solution).

43.5.1
Instruments and Suture Material

Until late 2003, 2-0 polypropylene (Prolene reference no. 8833) was used; however, in several cases patients complained of nodules caused by multiple knots at the anchorage point in the temple. The sutures were removed after approximately 6–12 months and were always noted to be loose, and the removal did not compromise the "lifting" effect. This led to the use absorbable sutures, polydioxanone (PDS II from Ethicon reference no. Z333), that are expected to be completely absorbed within 6 months.

Three pairs of toothed hemostatic forceps are used to secure a square of gauze to the edges of the hair-bearing skin flap. The author prefers the Snowden–Pencer Diamond Jaw Baumgartner (reference no. 32-0110) needle

holder for plication. For skin repair three pairs of 12-cm Olsen–Hegar needle holders with various jaws for 4/0, 5/0 and 6/0 nylon sutures are used.

43.5.2
Technique of the SAFE

The principal of the SAFE is based on maintaining the skin, subcutaneous tissue and SMAS unit, joined by the retaining ligaments by limited undermining (sectioning the retaining ligaments) to a maximum of 4 cm. The lifting of the SMAS then results in elevation and repositioning of soft tissue and skin [26].

It is critical to visualize in your minds eye the course of the temporal branch of the facial nerve in the middle section of the zygoma. The danger area is located approximately 2 cm behind the lateral orbital rim and 1.8 cm from the helix as the rami lying in the SMAS crosses the zygomatic arch (Fig. 43.8). The skin marking for facial undermining is limited to maximum of 4 cm.

The operative field is infiltrated using 0.5% lignocaine with 1:200,000 epinephrine, approximately 40–50 ml per side. The author prefers a 3-ml Luer-Lok tip syringe and a 27-gauge 0.5-in. (0.40-mm×13-mm) needle. Start with intradermal ring block along the incision line and the boundaries of undermining and then continue injecting the remaining area by infiltration into the immediate subdermal plane, producing hydrodissection of skin from the underlying SMAS. Allow 10 min for vasoconstriction to take effect (Fig. 43.9).

The preauricular S-shaped incision on the right is the mirror image of the S on the left. The upper S is extended to the temple and the retroauricular lower S is extended, using a no. 15 Personna Plus blade. Subcutaneous undermining is performed with Metzenbaum scissors. The edges of the wound are held with toothed hemostat forceps and the middle finger of the nondominant hand is used to guide the depth and the limit of undermining ("smart" finger, like a smart hand in liposculture). Undermining of the temporal flap is done under direct vision to prevent injury to the hair follicles (Fig. 43.10).

Meticulous hemostasis is with bipolar electrocautery. Any potential bleeder is secured by suture ligature using a 4/0 braided polyglycolic acid suture. The hair-bearing temporal flap is turned out using a gauze square and three pairs of toothed hemostatic forceps in order to keep the hair out of the wound. A paraffin gauze plug is placed in the external auditory meatus (Fig. 43.11).

The point of anchoring of the plication sutures is infiltrated with a small amount of anesthetic solution (Fig. 43.12).

The first vertical plication suture starts at the point approximately 2 cm above the zygoma and 1 cm anteriorly to the helix by taking a deep bite of temporalis muscle (touching the temporal fossa, taking care not to break the tip of the needle) and directed superiorly (Figs. 43.13, 43.14). The "bite" includes the strong superficial layer of the deep temporal fascia and is strong enough to allow the whole head to be lifted. It is unnecessary to have additional trauma from dissection in order to visualize the deep temporal fascia when absorbable sutures are used (Fig. 43.15). The needle is then reversed and continues inferiorly (Fig. 43.16). Strong bites of the SMAS are taken. At the angle of the mandible several horizontal bites include the platysma muscle. The needle is then redirected superiorly to the starting point (Fig. 43.17).

The first square double-throw knot is carried down, allowing several seconds to infold (pile up) the narrow tear-shaped purse-string-like suture (Figs. 43.18, 43.19). Infolding (piling up) acts as a mini-imbrication (advancement and overlapping) where subsequent fibrosis will produce shortening and reinforcement of the SMAS producing elevation and repositioning of soft tissue of the face. The knot is tied to maximum tension with the assistant's hand supporting the vertical movement of the face; this produces elevation of the neck and face of on average about 3–4 cm (Fig. 43.20). This knot is secured by several additional throws. The second plication suture is directed toward the angle of the mouth (Fig. 43.21). The third wider encircling plication suture further supports the already-infolded SMAS (Fig. 43.22). The knots in the temple are secured in a flat position by a single PDS suture. The redundant skin is redraped over the ear and temple, and is secured with a temporary key stitch above the ear (Fig. 43.23). Only the redundant skin is excised, starting from preauricular area then the postauricular area, utilizing a "Burow's triangle" if necessary (Fig. 43.24).

Finally the temple flap is addressed. The skin is redraped as an advancement rotation flap starting inferiorly in a vertical direction and changing the vector to horizontal at the level of the temple (Figs. 43.25, 43.26).

The wound is repaired with a single layer of vertical mattress sutures with no tension on the wound edges, which are handled in an "atraumatic manner," minimizing the use of toothed forceps (Fig. 43.27), starting from the preauricular segment using 5/0 and 6/0 nylon and continuing in the postauricular area and finally in the temple region using 4/0 nylon.

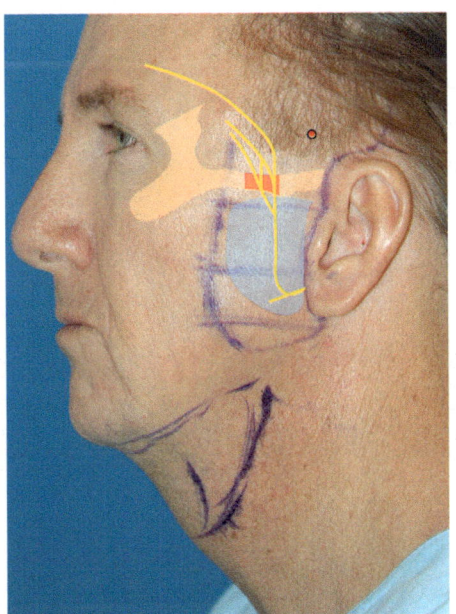

Fig. 43.8 It is critical to visualize in your minds eye the course of the temporal branch of the facial nerve in the middle section of the zygoma. The danger area is located approximately 2 cm behind the lateral orbital rim and 1.8 cm from the helix as the rami lying in the SMAS crosses the zygomatic arch. Note skin marking. Facial undermining is limited to a maximum of 4 cm

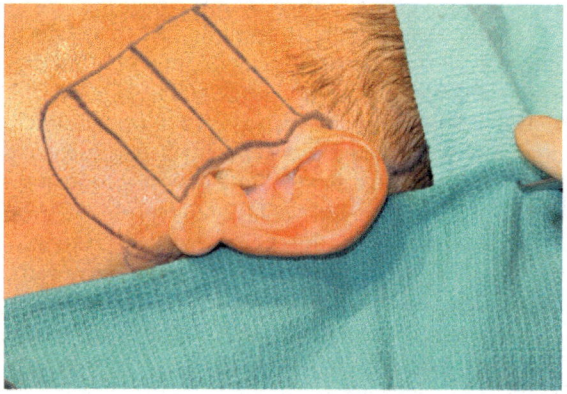

Fig. 43.9 Operative field infiltrated using 0.5% lignocaine with 1:200,000 epinephrine, approximately 40–50 ml per side. I prefer a 3-ml Luer-Lok tip syringe and a 27-gauge 0.5-in. (0.40-mm×13-mm) needle. Start with intradermal ring block along the incision line and the boundaries of undermining and then continue injecting the remaining area by infiltration into the immediate subdermal plane, producing hydrodissection of skin from the underlying SMAS. Allow 10 min for vasoconstriction to take effect. Preauricular S-shaped incision on the right (mirror image of S on the left). Upper S extended to the temple and retroauricular extension of the lower S, using a no. 15 Personna Plus blade

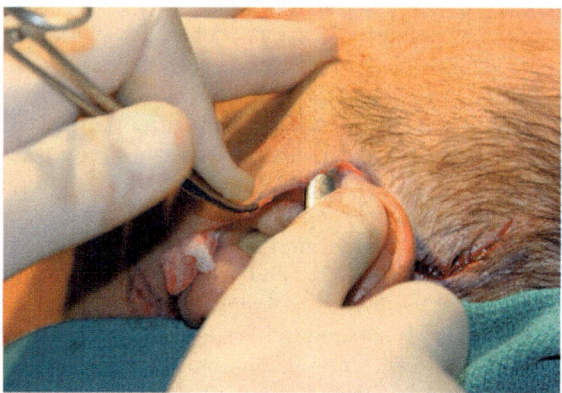

Fig. 43.10 Immediate subcutaneous undermining with Metzenbaum scissors. Note the holding of the edges of the wound with toothed hemostat forceps also using the middle finger of the nondominant hand to guide the depth and the limit of undermining ("smart" finger, like a smart hand in liposculture). Undermining of the temporal flap under direct vision to prevent injury to the hair follicles

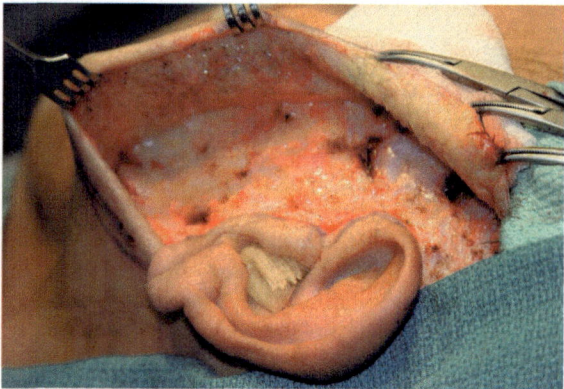

Fig. 43.11 Meticulous hemostasis by bipolar electrocautery. Any potential bleeder secured by suture ligature using 4/0 braided polyglycolic acid suture. Note the hair-bearing temporal flap turned out using a gauze square and three pairs of toothed haemostatic forceps in order to keep the hair out of the wound. Paraffin gauze plug in external auditory meatus

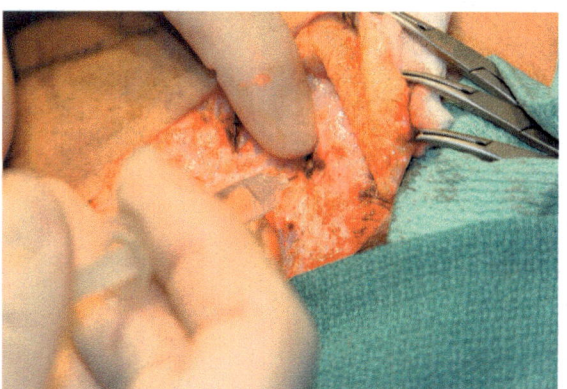

Fig. 43.12 The point of anchoring of the plication sutures is infiltrated with a small amount of anesthetic solution

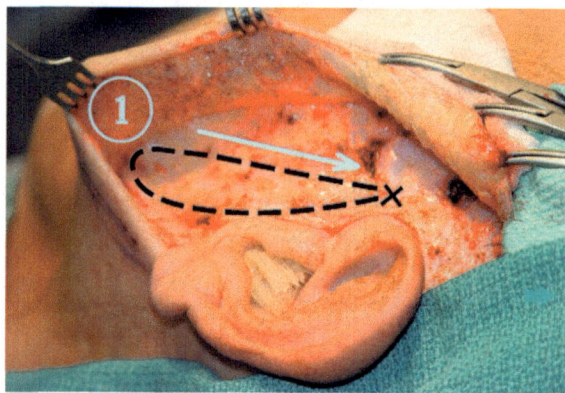

Fig. 43.13 The first vertical plication suture

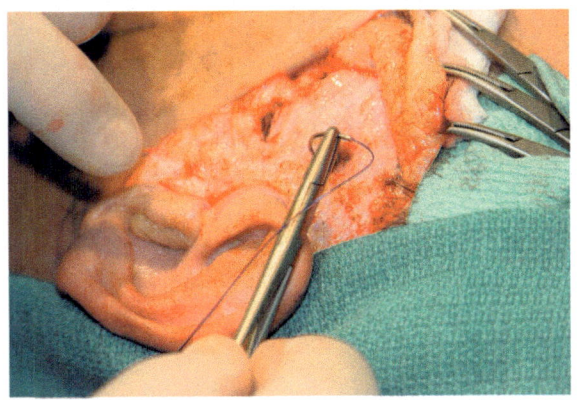

Fig. 43.14 The first vertical plication suture starts at the point approx. 2cm above the zygoma and 1cm anteriorly to the helix by taking a deep bite of temporalis muscle(touching the temporal fossa, taking care not to break the tip of the needle) and directed superiorly

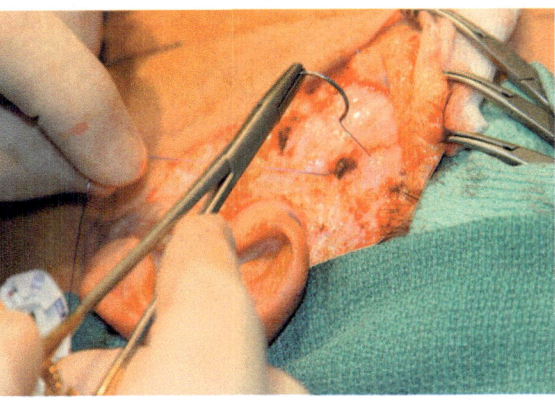

Fig. 43.15 This "bite" includes the strong superficial layer of the deep temporal fascia and is strong enough to allow the whole head to be lifted. I find it unnecessary to dissect additional trauma in order to visualize the deep temporal fascia when I use absorbable sutures

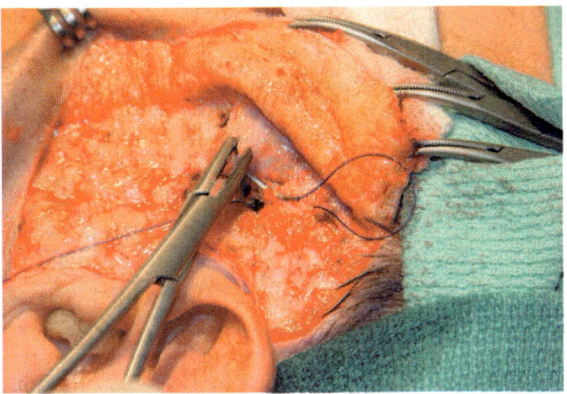

Fig. 43.16 The needle is then reversed and continues inferiorly

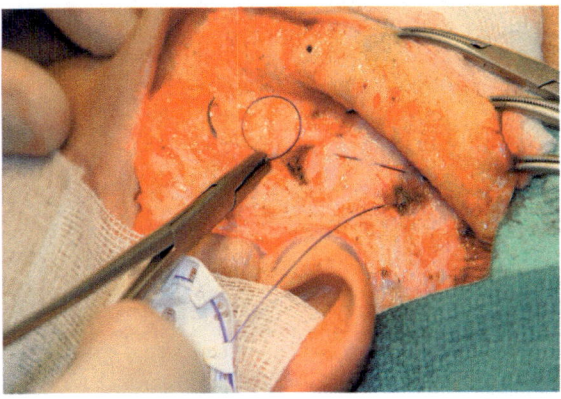

Fig. 43.17 Strong bites of the SMAS are taken. At the angle of the mandible several horizontal bites include the platysma muscle. The needle is then redirected superiorly to the starting point

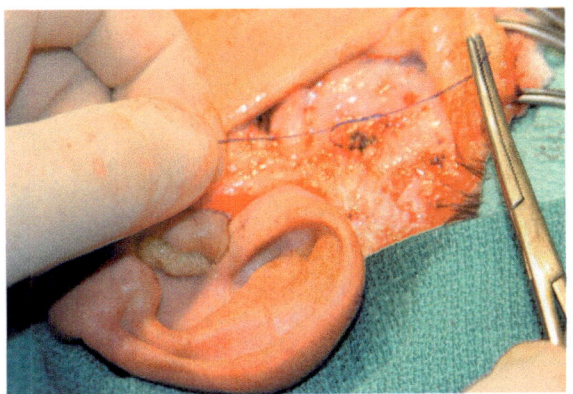

Fig. 43.18 The first square double-throw knot is carried down allowing several seconds to infold (pile up) the narrow tear-shaped purse-string-like suture. Infolding (piling up) acts as a mini-imbrication (advancement and overlapping) where subsequent fibrosis will produce shortening and reinforcement of the SMAS, producing elevation and repositioning of soft tissue of the face

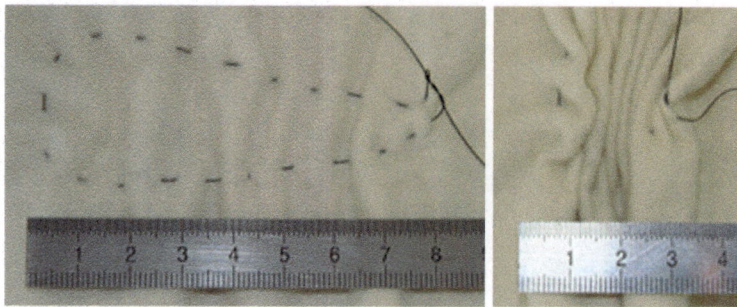

Fig. 43.19 Model of "purse-string" plication suture

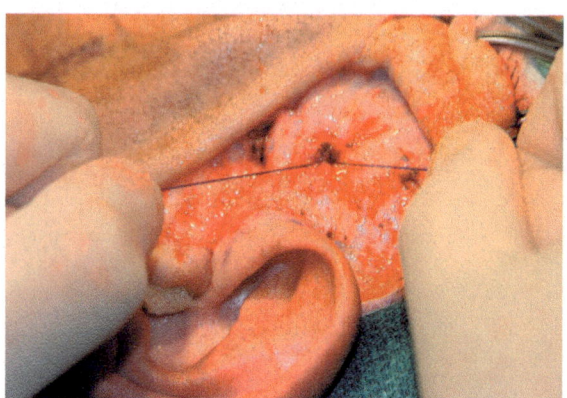

Fig. 43.20 The knot is tied to maximum tension with the assistant's hand supporting the vertical movement of the face. This produces elevation of the neck and face of on average about 3–4 cm. This knot is secured by several additional throws

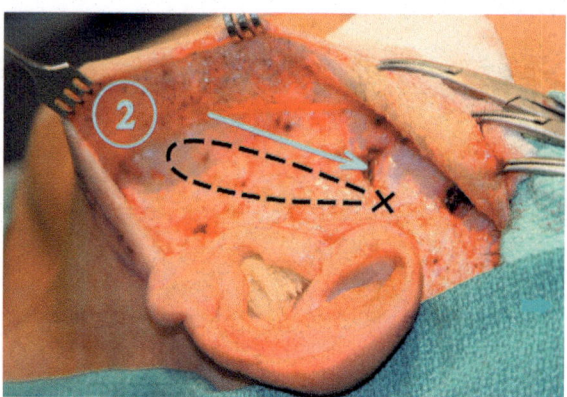

Fig. 43.21 The second plication suture is directed toward the angle of the mouth

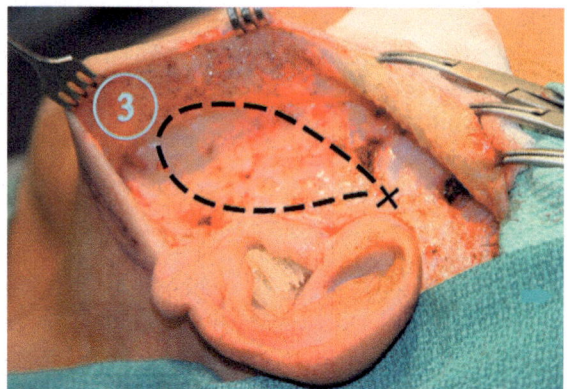

Fig. 43.22 The third wider encircling plication suture further supports already-infolded SMAS. The knots in the temple are secured in a flat position by a single PDS suture

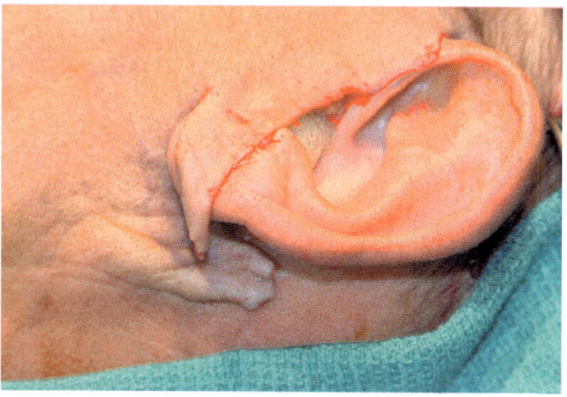

Fig. 43.23 The redundant skin is redraped over the ear and temple, and is secured with a temporary key stitch above the ear

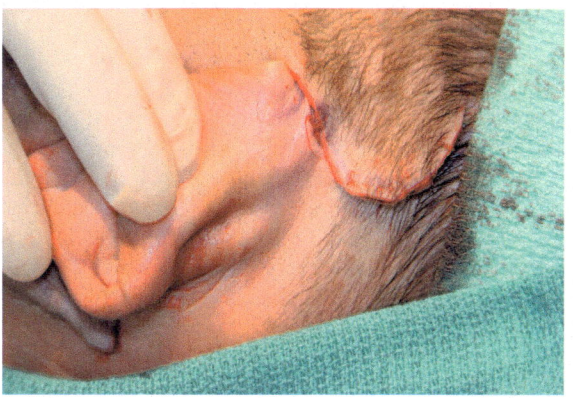

Fig. 43.24 Only the redundant skin is excised, starting from preauricular area, then the postauricular area, utilizing a "Burow's triangle" if necessary

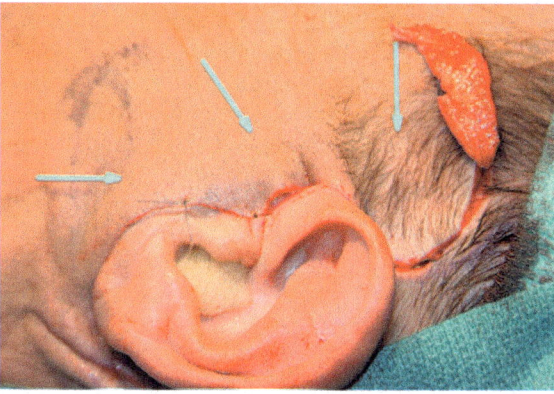

Fig. 43.25 Finally the temple flap is addressed. The skin is redraped as an advancement rotation flap starting inferiorly in a vertical direction and changing the vector to horizontal at the level of the temple

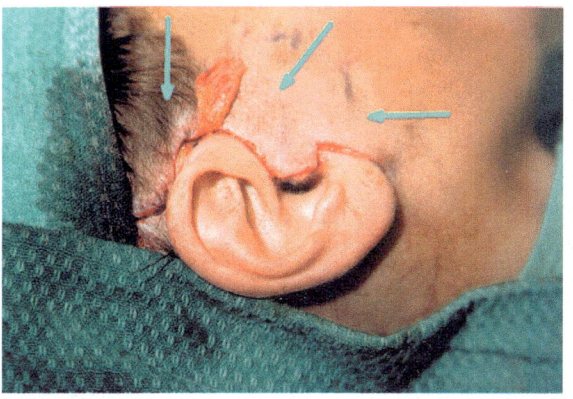

Fig. 43.26 Posttragal example. Note the minimal elevation of the sideburns and maintenance of the hair-bearing line above the ear

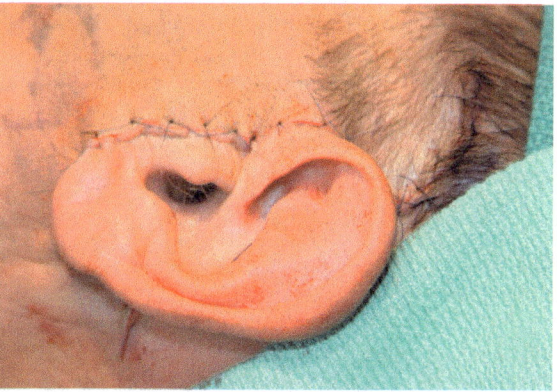

Fig. 43.27 The wound is repaired with a single layer of vertical mattress sutures with no tension on the wound edges, which are handled in an "atraumatic manner," minimizing the use of toothed forceps, starting from the preauricular segment using 5/0 and 6/0 nylon and continuing in the postauricular area and finally in the temple region using 4/0 nylon

43.5.3
Dressings

Antibiotic ointment is applied to the wound, followed by a strip of sterile paraffin gauze and then a nonadherent pad. A silicone-backed adhesive foam pad is placed on the side of the face, followed by 7.5-cm×7.5-cm gauze squares. The dressings are secured by a head-support garment fastened with two adjustable Velcro straps.

The patient remains in the facility for observation for 2 hours postoperatively and is then discharged home.

The patient returns to the office the next day and the dressing is removed. The wound is cleaned with hydrogen peroxide and antibiotic ointment is applied to the suture line. Any blood/anesthetic fluid collection under the flap is aspirated using a blunt microcannula or a large-bore needle inserted via a gap in the suture line. Seven days postoperatively, the patient returns for removal of sutures.

43.5.4
Complications

43.5.4.1
Hematoma

Hematoma is the most common complication. In a series of 1,000 procedures performed between 1998 and 2005 there was only one case of expanding hematoma in a male patient. This developed about 1 h postoperatively as a result of a bleeding branch of the superficial temporal artery; it was controlled by suture ligation (incidence 0.1%). To prevent hematoma, it is critical to control the patient's blood pressure and pain and to prevent nausea and vomiting.

43.5.4.2
Postoperative Edema

To prevent excessive swelling 8 mg dexamethasone intramuscularly is given preoperatively. Patients are instructed to elevate the head of the bed postoperatively. Occasionally a short course of dexamethasone administered orally is given.

Silicone-backed adhesive foam pads, e.g., EPIfoam from Biodermis, applied to the sides of the face and supported by the head straps may be helpful in reducing swelling by intermittent compression action of the sponge. Arnica tablets may also assist in minimizing swelling and their inclusion in the preoperative instructions is recommended. Two weeks postoperatively manual lymphatic drainage may assist in resolving residual swelling. No incidence of infection was noted.

43.5.4.3
Nerve Injury

In the initial series (approximately 300 cases) when the SMAS plication suture was anchored to the zygoma there was a 4% incidence of neuropraxia of the frontal branch of the facial nerve. Since the anchoring has been changed to the temporal fascia (approximately 700 cases) there has been no incidence of any nerve injury.

43.5.4.4
Flap Necrosis

There was one case of skin slough when the patient presented 4 weeks postoperatively with a "scab" on the side of her face (Fig. 43.28). After surgery, she had been using an infrared lamp in order to "accelerate" healing as she had a previous good result with that modality following gynecological surgery. The wound was cleaned daily and allowed to granulate and reepithealize spontaneously. Patients are warned not to apply any heat, including use of hairdryers, etc., for several weeks after surgery.

43.5.4.5
Scarring

Owing to meticulous atraumatic technique and wound repair without any tension by a single layer of vertical mattress sutures, the scars are imperceptible. The SAFE as a secondary procedure has proven to be effective in removing unfavorable scars due to wound closure under tension.

43.6
Discussion

SAFE can be classified as a minimally invasive facelift. Patient safety is paramount in cosmetic surgery and, as there have not been any significant complications in over 1,000 procedures preformed by me, I am comfortable using the SAFE abbreviation. Every surgical intervention carries inherited risks; however, in less invasive procedures these risks are reduced.

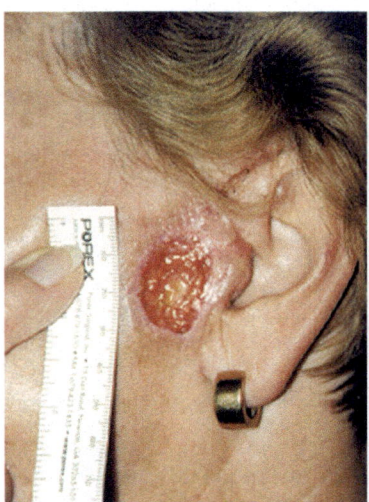
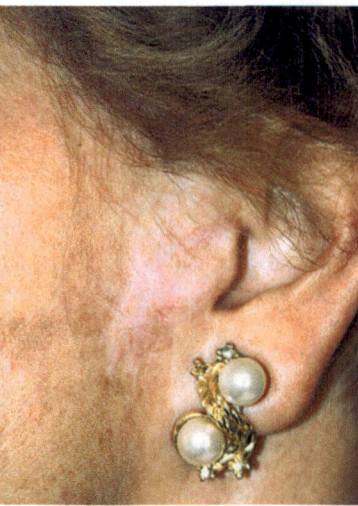

Fig. 43.28 Full-thickness skin loss due to burn from an infrared lamp and appearance after 12 months

The procedure is performed under local anesthetic and oral sedation in an office setting with the assistance of one nurse. Patients return home after surgery and then return the next day for a follow-up visit. The downtime on average is 7–10 days, and in that time most people's appearance is socially acceptable.

After 3 weeks, most scars are imperceptible. The first vertical SMAS plication suture elevates the neck and lower face and the second oblique suture results in some elevation of the midface.

This elevation and repositioning of soft tissue results in a natural refreshed appearance without stigma of facelift, e.g., wind-tunnel look, pixie ears, visible scars, obvious elevation of sideburns.

The procedure has been used in rejuvenation for all degrees of the aging face using Baker's classification type I to type IV (Figs. 43.29–43.31) [27].

Cervical liposculpture/undermining is advised in almost all cases in order to produce skin contraction and redraping. About 10 min after infiltrating the neck with tumescent anesthetic solution, liposculpture of the neck is performed using a Tulip SL 3.0 spatula cannula attached to a 10-ml Luer-Lok syringe, through a single submental access. An adjustable Velcro support with a silicone-backed adhesive foam pad is applied after surgery and is kept on for 2 weeks.

As facial aging is a continuing process, the author prefers to classify facial aging as early, moderate and severe

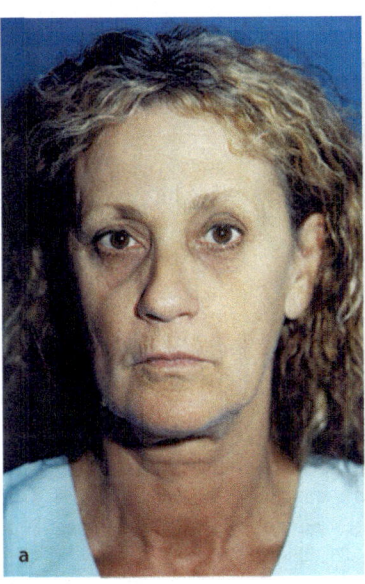
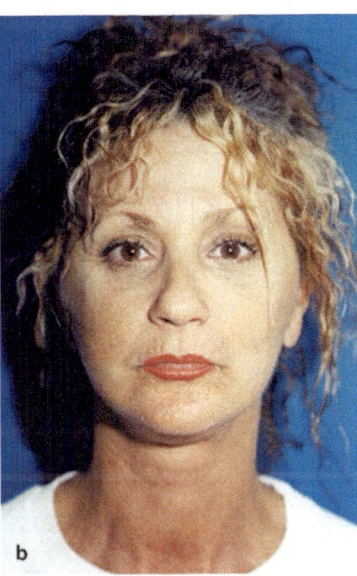

Fig. 43.29 Type I: the ideal candidate. **a** Before surgery. **b** One week after SAFE

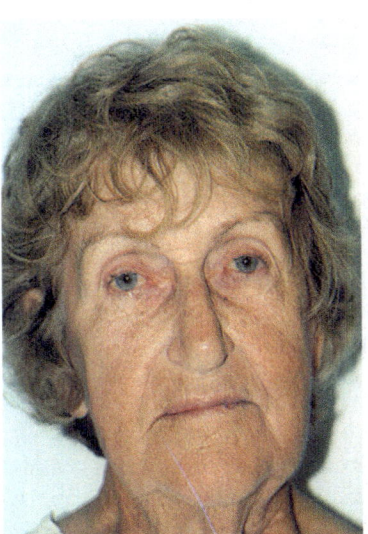
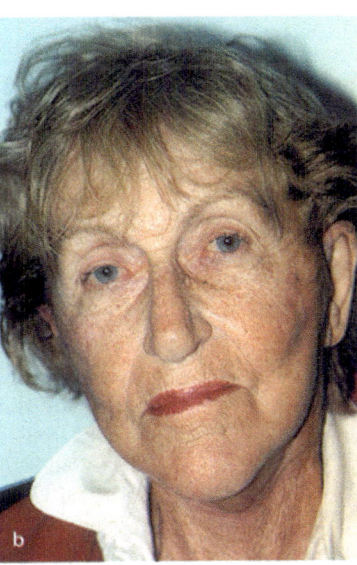

Fig. 43.30 Type II: the good candidate. **a** Before surgery. **b** Three years after SAFE

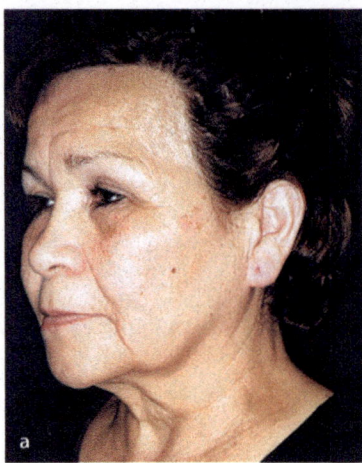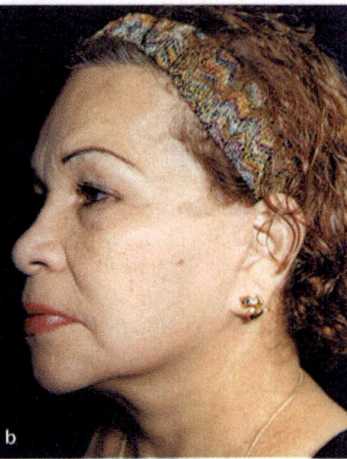

Fig. 43.31 Type III: the fair candidate.
a Before surgery. **b** Seven days after SAFE

(the end point "aged face") [29]. Longevity of the results appear to be comparable with that from conventional facelifts, especially in cases with early facial aging.

43.7
Conclusions

The ultimate goal of successful cosmetic surgery is a happy patient and surgeon. In that complex process, appropriate patient selection is critical. Patients have to be appropriately motivated, understand the benefits as well as the limitations of cosmetic procedures, and be prepared to maintain the results by ancillary procedures.

The SAFE modification of the S-lift is effective, low risk and economical with short downtime. The procedure is relatively easy to perform and already a number of surgeons have adapted the technique and are pleased with the results.

References

1. Mayer DM, Swanker WA. Rhytidoplasty. Plast Reconstr Surg 1950;6(4):255–263
2. Skoog T. Plastic Surgery: New Methods and Refinements. Philadelphia: Saunders 1974
3. Mitz V, Peyronie M. The superficial musculo-aponeurotic system (SMAS) in the parotid and cheek area. Plast Reconstr Surg 1976;58(1):80–88
4. Larrabee WF, Makielski KH. Surgical Anatomy of the Face. New York: Raven 1993:45–48
5. Owsley JQ. Facelift. Masters Series I. Plastic Surgery 2005, Chicago, September 2005
6. Webster RC, Smith RC, Papsidero MJ, Karolow WW, Smith KF. Comparison of SMAS placation with SMAS imbrication in face lifting. Laryngoscope 1982;92(8 Pt 1):901–912
7. Duffy MJ, Friedland JA. The superficial plane rhytidectomy revisited. Plast Reconstr Surg 1994;93(7):1392–1403
8. Ivy EJ, Lorenc ZP, Aston SJ. Is there a difference? A prospective study comparing lateral and standard SMAS face lifts with extended SMAS and composite rhytidectomies. Plast Reconstr Surg 1998;101(2):549–551
9. Ansari P. Neue Methode der Gesichts- und Halsstraffung. Kosmet J 1983;8:14–15
10. Ansari P. Elimination of the retroauricular incision in face lifts. Aesthet Surg 2003;23(1):14–19
11. Ansari P. Instructional course: short scar facelift. The European Academy of Cosmetic Surgery, London, May 1998
12. Zurek L. S-lift patient survey. Int J Cosmet Surg Aesthet Dermatol 2000;2(4):235–241
13. Zurek L. Modified S-Lift Zurek's Technique. Australasian College of Cosmetic Surgery Annual Conference, 2000, 2001, 2002, 2003, 2004, 2005
14. Zurek L. Survey of Randomly Following the S-Lift Procedure. EACS 5th Annual Meeting on Cosmetic Surgery Berlin, May 2001
15. Zurek L. Live Surgery Workshops: Face Lift Zurek's Technique. 5050 Aesthetic Surgery Clinic, Seoul, South Korea September 2003, 2004, 2005, 2006
16. Zurek L. Instructional Course: SAFE 2nd World Congress of Cosmetic Surgery Mumbai, December 2003
17. Zurek L. Live Surgery Workshop: SAFE, 4th World Congress on Cosmetic and Dermatology Surgery. Manila, February 2004
18. Zurek L. SAFE International Congress of Advanced Cosmetic Surgery Ho Chi Minh City, August 2004
19. Zurek L. Instructional Course: SAFE, 49th Meeting and World Congress of the International Academy of Cosmetic Surgery. Lisbon, September 2004
20. Zurek L. SAFE Instructional Course and Live Surgery Presentation. The 1st World Congress of the Taiwan Academy of Facial Plastic and Reconstructive Surgery, Taipei, December 2005

21. Saylan Z. Workshop: Facelift and the New S-Lift, Dusseldorf, January 1999

22. Saylan Z. The S-lift: less is more. Aesthet Surgery J 1999;19:406

23. Tonnard P, Verpaele A, Monstrey S, Van Landuyt K, Blondeel P, Hamdi M, Matton G. Minimal access cranial suspension lift: A modified S-Lift. Plast Reconstr Surg 2002;109(6):2074–2086

24. Tonnard P. Instructional Course: MACS, Congress IPRAS, Sydney 2003

25. Tonnard P, Verpaele A. The MACS-Lift Short-Scar Rhytidectomy. QMP 2004

26. Massiha H. Short-scar face lift with extended SMAS platysma dissection and lifting and limited skin undermining. Plast Reconstr Surg 2003;112(2):663–669

27. Baker DC. Minimal incision rhytidectomy (short scar facelift) with lateral SMASectomy: Evolution and application. Aesthet Surg 2001;21:14

28. Austin H, Weston G. Rejuvenating the aging mouth. Perspect Plast Surg 1994;8:1

CHAPTER 44

The Delta Lift: a Modification of S-lift for Facial Rejuvenation

44

Hassan Abbas Khawaja, Enrique Hernández-Pérez

44.1
Introduction

The results of conventional facelift are unnatural, and a masklike appearance is common. Elongation of the ear lobe with a triangular deformity, separation of the ear lobe on one side, adherence of the inner border to the skin on the other side, or sometimes large keloid scars behind the ear can all occur. Hair loss as a result of scarring and traction alopecia is also common. Nasolabial fold correction is limited, with most facelifts, thereby creating a limiting factor to the facelift. Attempts at removal of the crease can result in a number of complications, such as damage to the branches of the facial nerve [1]. In addition, a number of slips of the muscles of facial expression become attached to the nasolabial fold. Failure to divide some of these slips during facelift can result in asymmetry of the smile [2]. Only the most radical subperiosteal facelift as described by Hamra [3] can have a longer-lasting effect on the nasolabial fold. Perhaps the first description of the minilift was provided by Passot. Preauricular skin excision accompanied by little or no skin undermining was abandoned by most surgeons because the results were short-lived [4]. S-lift has recently regained popularity in Europe and in the Americas as a result of its simplicity and short operating time, but is has one important drawback: facial nerve palsy can develop in some patients when operated on by inexperienced surgeons [5]. The delta lift is a modified version of the facelift of Passot and the S-lift. It is very safe and has none of the drawbacks of its predecessors. In addition, the results are superior to those of all conventional and radical facelifts.

44.2
Superficial Musculoaponeurotic System and Related Facelift Anatomy

Attention to the superficial musculoaponeurotic system (SMAS) concept is essential for a successful facelift. The SMAS represents an extension of the superficial cervical fascia into the face. It forms a continuous sheath throughout the face and neck. Is thickness varies from patient to patient and from region to region. It is dense and thick over the parotid. As the facial layer is traced superiorly to the zygomatic arch, it is termed temporoparietal fascia within the temporal region and galea within the scalp, both of which are substantial in terms of thickness. As it is traced medially into the cheek overlying the masseter and buccal fat pad, it tends to become thinner and less distinct. Within the malar areas, it is quite thin and comprises the fascia of the elevators of the upper lip. The SMAS invests the superficial mimetic muscles (platysma, zygomaticus major, zygomaticus minor, and risorius) and fibrous septa connect the SMAS to the overlying dermis of the skin. The mimetic muscles, SMAS, and skin function therefore as a single anatomical unit in producing movement of the facial skin.

The deeper layer of cervical fascia continues into the face as the parotid-masseteric fascia. Somewhat confusingly, it is also termed a part of the SMAS by some authors. The significance of this anatomical layer lies in the fact that the facial nerve branches and the parotid duct always lie deep to the deep fascial layer. As long as the integrity of this layer is maintained, facial nerve injury will not result from dissection [6]. The superficial and deep cervical fascia are intimately adherent to one another by dense fibrous attachments along the zygomatic arch, thereby dividing the SMAS into a suprazygomatic and an infrazygomatic portion.

The frontal branch of the facial nerve, unlike other nerve branches that lie deep to the deep fascial fascia, is an anomaly. Once the frontal branch crosses the zygomatic arch, it traverses the temporal region along the undersurface of the temporoparietal fascia and then peripherally penetrates this layer to innervate the frontalis muscle along its deep surface. Therefore, if the temporoparietal fascia is violated during dissection, injury to this nerve can take place. The area at greatest risk for damage to the temporal branch can be more easily demonstrated by drawing a line from the ear lobe to the lateral edge of the eyebrow and from the tragus to a point just above and behind the highest forehead crease. The temporal branches are at equal risk in the area defined by these lines, especially where they cross the zygomatic arch. At this point over the zygomatic arch, the frontal nerve/branches are particularly vulnerable because they lie in the SMAS just beneath the subcutaneous fat and over the bony prominence [7].

The approximate path of the ramus to the frontalis muscle can be traced by drawing a line from 0.5 cm below the tragus to a point 1.5 cm above the lateral eyebrow. It is most vulnerable as it crosses the mid zygomatic arch [6, 7]. Damage to the temporal branch results in loss of function of the frontalis muscle, which derives its sole innervation from one solitary ramus that 85% of the time has no cross branches with the zygomatic nerve. The forehead appears flat, the eyebrow falls to a lowered ptotic position, and there is inability to raise the eyebrow. There is no interference, however, with closure of the eyelid. Innervation of the upper part of orbicularis oculi and corrugator supercillii shows little functional or cosmetic deficit. Single branching patterns exist; however, in some cases as many as six nerve branches can be traced crossing the zygomatic arch. Despite the variety of branching patterns, these nerve fibers are always medial and inferior to the frontal branch of the superficial temporal artery. The frontal branch of the superficial temporal nerve is easily palpated and therefore is a useful landmark in identifying the frontal nerve.

The marginal mandibular nerve exits the parotid approximately 4 cm beneath the base of the ear lobe near the angle of mandible. In 81% of patients, the nerve lies above the mandibular border. In 19% of cases, it lies inferior, although only in the region posterior to the facial vessels. The marginal mandibular nerve then crosses the facial artery and vein, and from this point anteriorly its runs superior to the mandibular border. Where the facial artery and vein cross the mandibular border is a very useful landmark. The facial artery can be palpated just anterior to the angle of mandible, along the anterior masseter border, and serves as a quick method for localizing the marginal mandibular nerve. In this location, the nerve is superficial as it crosses over the facial vessels and it is at this point that marginal mandibular nerve injury can take place [8]. The subcutaneous dissection remains superficial to the SMAS and platysma, so motor nerve injury will be prevented.

The spinal accessory nerve is the most important structure in the posterior triangle of the neck. Its exits the skull through the jugular foramen, most posteriorly, crosses the internal jugular vein, and passes downwards and posteriorly, to the upper part to the sternocleidomastoid approximately 4 cm below the mastoid process and then passes beneath or through the muscle. The nerve leaves the muscle at its mid portion and crosses the posterior triangle situated between the superficial and prevertebral layers of deep cervical fascia to pass under the anterior border of the trapezius supplying both muscles. Its overall course is diagonal, but is nearly vertical in the posterior triangle. The exit point of the spinal accessory nerve coincides with that of several cervical plexus nerves at a site known as Erb's point [8].

44.3
Technique

Keeping the basic anatomical realities in mind, we conceive of this facelift as a three-step procedure.

44.3.1
Step 1: Correction of Prominent Nasolabial Folds

Six to eight Gore-Tex CV 0 sutures are used for each nasolabial fold/furrow using a needle similar to the Keith needle with a pointed end, not sides, to decrease the chance of fistula formation. The number of Gore-Tex threads used depends on the depth of the furrow/fold [9]. Preoperative assessment of the fold is important. Careful inspection is done after insertion of the Gore-Tex threads if the fold is still prominent. Careful subcutaneous insertion and feathering of the ends of the Gore-Tex threads are important as well as following a very careful antiseptic technique. The upper part of the nasolabial fold constitutes a portion of the danger area of face. Infection from this area can lead to cavernous sinus thrombosis [10].

Fillers, like siloxane with the microdroplet technique and poly(methyl methacrylate), are used plus subcision of the folds to get rid of the crease.

44.3.2
Step 2: Liposuction of the Chin Area/Correction of Platysma Bands

Anesthesia, 1% with epinephrine, is used chilled for the incision sites in the central submental crease. Chilled Klein's solution (150–250 ml; 1,000 ml with 25 ml 2% lidocaine and 1 ml 1% epinephrine) is used for infiltration using a Lamis syringe [10]. A 15.3-mm flat spatula cannula is utilized for liposuction in this area using a suction machine. Marking the marginal mandibular nerve and facial vessels is done beforehand. Platysma band correction is performed via a small (2–3-cm) submental crease incision only if there is significant platysma laxity. Edge-to-edge anastomosis or overlapping of the two bellies is performed in cases of excessive laxity using 3/0 interrupted Prolene sutures.

44.3.3
Step 3: The Delta Lift

The superficial temporal artery is palpated and the path of the frontal branch of the facial nerve is marked beforehand in addition to the marginal mandibular nerve and facial vessels. The spinal accessory nerve in the posterior triangle and the greater auricular nerve are also marked. Marking of the skin excision is done in the form of a delta (Fig. 44.1) and up to a 6±1-cm dotted line indicating that the extent of undermining is marked. No sedation is used. Chilled lidocaine (1%) without epinephrine is used for incision sites and chilled Klein's solution for the area to be operated on using a Lamis syringe (Fig. 44.2). Klein's solution is prepared fresh; using chilled solution is very important to provide good anesthesia and analgesia [11].

After the skin has been excised and the flap has been raised, the SMAS is identified. A vertical 2/0 Prolene suture is started at the level of the lower end of the parotid gland, taking multiple small bites in the SMAS up to the lower end of the platysma and then backis tied (Fig. 44.3). This pulls the platysma muscle upwards and restores the cervicomental angle. The bites should be superficial to the parotid-masseteric fascia and the deep cervical fascia. Plication should be in a superolateral direction. A second horizontal suture of 2/0 Prolene starting 2 cm in front of the tragus towards the marionette line and the lower part of the nasolabial fold and back is tied at an angle of 45°, pulling the SMAS superolaterally. Another similar suture towards the mid and upper nasolabial fold is tied superolaterally well away from the path of the frontal nerve. This suture lifts the malar fat pad upwards, thereby creating an appearance of youth (Fig. 44.4).

After careful checking of hemostasis, three 3/0 Prolene sutures are tied to approximate the skin. It is important that the skin suture closure follows the SMAS closure (Fig. 44.5). The lowest suture is tied vertically and superolaterally and is tied at an angle of 45° follow-ing the SMAS closure and is under moderate tension. The upper suture is tied superolaterally in the direction of SMAS closure and is under the least tension. Closure is performed using a 6/0 continuous Prolene suture in women and 5/0 in men (Fig. 44.6) Closure is performed from below upwards so that the dogear, if it forms, is hidden in the hairline and not behind the ear. A similar procedure is followed on the other side.

The skin and subcutaneous vectors should be at an angle of 45° (superolateral). The conventional facelift has separate vectors of tension on the skin and the SMAS. The SMAS flap is pulled in a different direction and the skin is draped differently. It is important that the skin and SMAS be considered as one unit and closure of the SMAS should follow skin closure. Only in this way can a natural result be achieved and the mask and wind-tunnel look of the conventional facelift be avoided (Fig. 44.7).

The other important point to understand is that dissection should stay away from the frontal branch of the facial nerve and therefore should be well below the zygomatic arch. There is reason to believe that suspending the SMAS to the periosteum of the zygomatic bone, as in an S-lift, can result in increased incidence of frontal nerve damage and painful neuromas by breaking the temporoparietal fascia and incorporating the frontal nerve or its branches in the suture. For maximum safety, the SMAS should be plicated well below the zygomatic arch, away from the frontal nerve pathway. Another point to consider is that while inserting the vertical and horizontal sutures, the path of marginal mandibular nerve should be kept in mind. The bite of the sutures

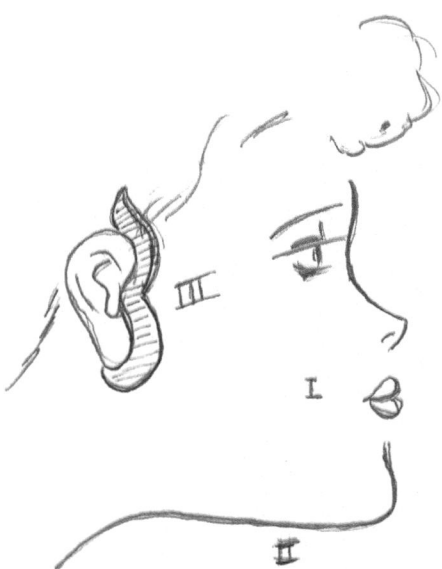

Fig. 44.1 Three steps of the delta lift procedure

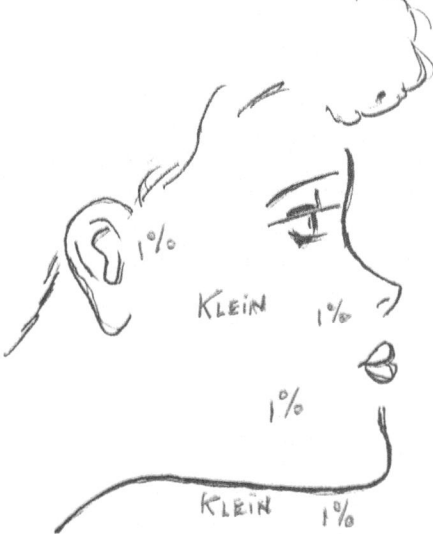

Fig. 44.2 Administration of anesthesia

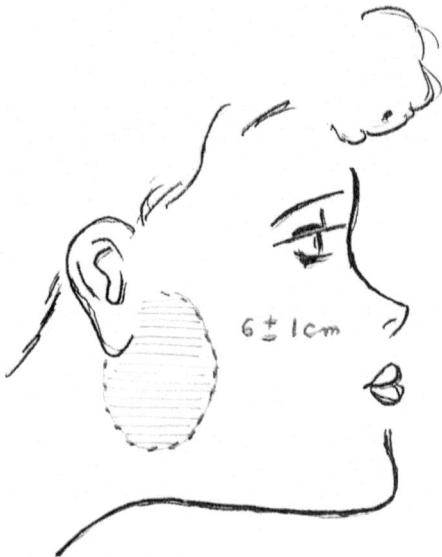

Fig. 44.3 Extent of undermining

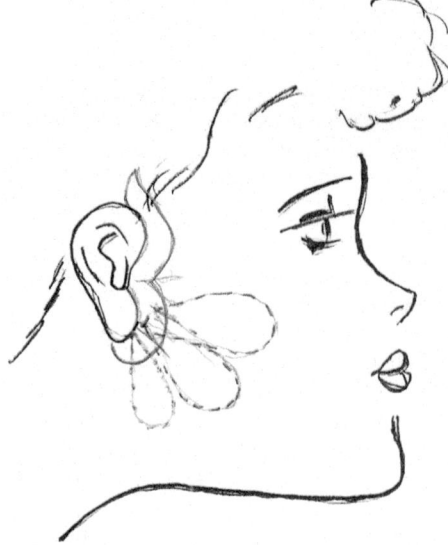

Fig. 44.4 The superficial musculoaponeurotic system plication

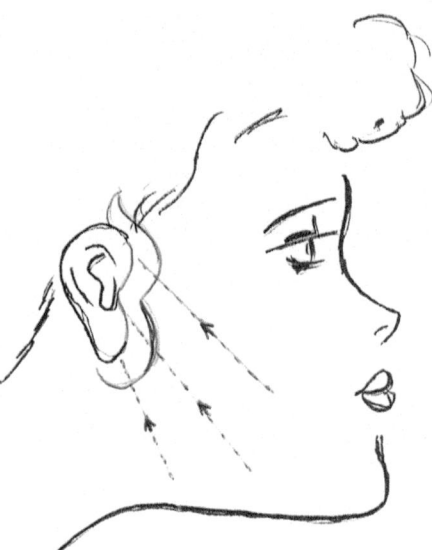

Fig. 44.5 The angles of skin pull

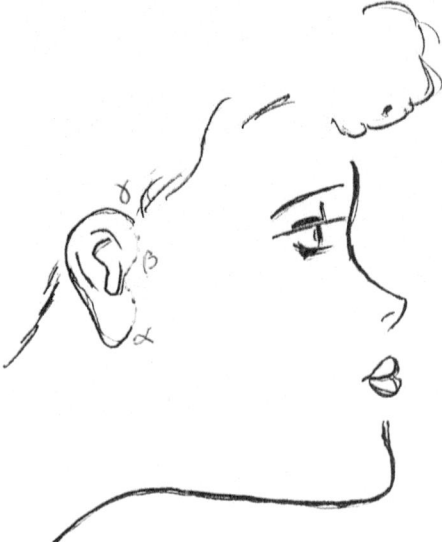

Fig. 44.6 Final closure for the delta lift procedure

near the marginal mandibular nerve should not go deep to the SMAS and platysma. It is better to omit one or two bites in the vicinity of the marginal mandibular nerve. No bites should be taken where the marginal mandibular nerve is superficial near the facial vessels. Because dissection is well away from the posterior triangle and posterior neck flaps are not created, the spi-

nal accessory nerve in the posterior triangle as well as the greater auricular and lesser occipital nerves are not in danger as in a usual facelift procedure.

The upper part of the delta lift can be extended backwards for a posterior neck pull. The extension can be made in the hairline above the mastoid. However, in most cases it is unnecessary.

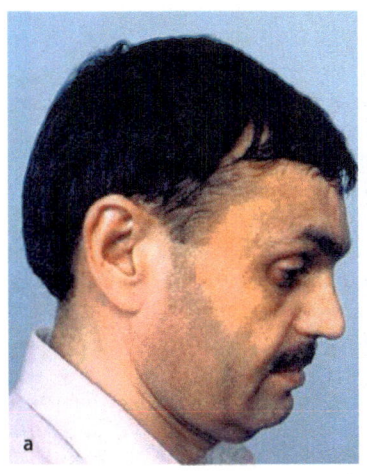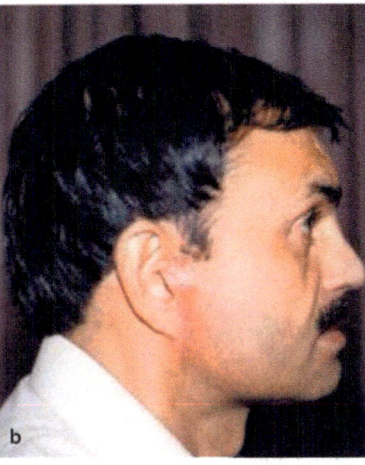

Fig. 44.7 **a** Appearance before steps I, II, and III (delta lift). **b** Appearance after steps I, II, and III (delta lift)

44.3.3.1
Retroauricular Extension

Retroauricular extension of a delta lift is required only in some cases of:
1. Lobular deformity with a long lobule
2. Excessive mid-face lift with an inferior scar below the lobule, pulling it downwards
3. Excessive inferolobular neck skin laxity

44.3.3.2
Temporal Extension

In cases of posterior neck skin laxity, an upper extension of the delta lift can be made in the hairline above the mastoid. In this way, a retroauricular scar will be avoided. However, it cannot fully correct a lobular deformity, which is better corrected using a retroauricular incision.

44.3.4
Complications

No serious complications were encountered using the delta lift such as facial nerve palsy, hematoma, skin necrosis, and infection. The only problems encountered with this procedure may be prominent scars in front of the ear and dogear in the hairline (Table 44.1). The dogear disappears spontaneously in a few months in most cases. A dogear plasty can be performed in other

Table 44.1 Complications from conventional lift, S-lift, and delta lift

Conventional lift	S-lift	Delta lift
Facial nerve/branches damage	Facial nerve palsy	Prominent scar
Greater auricular and spinal accessory nerve damage	Hematoma	Dogear in the hairline
Pulmonary embolism	Tension and pain in the pretragal region	
Skin necrosis	Soft-tissue dimpling inferior to ear lobe	
Hematoma		
Edema		
Infection		
Scarring		
Hair loss		
Ear-lobe deformity		

cases. Prominent scars can be improved by resurfacing or scar-revision techniques. There is sometimes extrusion of one or two Gore-Tex threads. These can be reinserted if some difference is noted in the nasolabial folds later on.

44.4
Conclusions

The delta lift is a safe ambulatory procedure with aesthetic results superior to those of all conventional and radical facelift procedures. It has minimal or no complications. It is suitable for younger, middle-aged, and elderly patients alike. It can be combined with treatment using blepharoplasty, peels, sunscreens, topically applied tretinoin, orally administered isotretinoin, fat and collagen injections, and Gore-Tex and Botox as part of a facial rejuvenation program [12–18].

References

1. Peck G.C.: Complications and Problems in Aesthetic Plastic Surgery, 1st edition. New York, Gower Medical Publishing 1992:3.2–3.15
2. Barton F.E. Jr, Gyimesi I.M.: Anatomy of the nasolabial fold. Plast Reconstr Surg 1997;100(5):1276–1280
3. Hamra S.T.: Subperiosteal face-lift. Plast Reconstr Surg 1995;96(2):493
4. Rees T.D., Wood-Smith D.: Cosmetic Facial Surgery, 1st edition. Philadelphia, Saunders 1973:151
5. Saylan Z.: The S-lift for facial rejuvenation. Int J Cosmet Surg 1999;7:18–24
6. Salasche S.J., Berstein G.: Surgical Anatomy of the Skin, 1st edition. Stamford, Appleton and Lange 1988:89–97
7. Robinson J.K., Arndt K.A.: Atlas of Cutaneous Surgery, 1st edition. Philadelphia, Saunders 1996:5–14
8. Baker T.L., Gordon H.L.: Surgical Rejuvenation of the Face, 2nd edition. St. Louis, Mosby-Year Book 1996:153–179
9. Lassus C.: A surgical solution to the deep nasolabial fold. Plast Reconstr Surg 1996;97(7):1473–1478
10. Beeson W.H., McCollough E.G.: Aesthetic Surgery of the Aging Face. St. Louis, Mosby, 1986:76–77
11. Klein J.A.: Tumescent technique for local anesthesia improves safety in large volume liposuction. Plast Reconstr Surg 1993;92(6):1085–1098
12. Kaye B.L.: Facial Rejuvenative Surgery, 1st edition. Philadelphia, Lipincott 1987:45–46
13. Hernández-Pérez E.: Resorcinol peel as a part of a facial rejuvenation program. Am J Cosmet Surg 1997;14:35–40
14. Hernández-Pérez E.: Implantes de grasa autóloga. In: Camacho F., Dulanto F. (eds). Cirugía Dermatológica. Madrid, Biblioteca Aula Médica 1995:563–569
15. Hernández-Pérez E., Henríquez A., Marroquín Burgos R.: Isotretinoin en el acné vulgar. Experiencia en 4,000 casos. Dermatol Rev Mex 1994;38:263–266
16. Kligman A.G., Grove G.L., Hirose R., Leyden J.: Topical tretinoin for photoaged skin. J Am Acad Dermatol 1986;15(4 Pt 2):836–859
17. Schoenrock L.D., Repucci A. D.: Goretex in facial plastic surgery. Int J Aesthet Restor Surg 1993;1:63–68
18. Carruthers J.,Carruthers A.: Treatment of glabellar frown lines with C. botulinum-A exotoxin. J Dermatol Surg Oncol 1992;18(1):17–21

CHAPTER 45

Easy Lift

45

Sid J. Mirrafati

45.1
Introduction

Many types of facelifts are available to patients, from the traditional facelift to deep plane facelift and to modified facelifts and thread lifts. Each has its indications according to the patient's physical appearance of aging and the patient's desires regarding cost, postoperative recovery time, pain and discomfort, and length of time the results last.

Depending on the age category and the need of the patient, the surgeon should suggest the procedure that would give the best results with the fewest complications. The "easy" lift procedure is a combination of a cheek lift with a modified S-lift, and mesh platysmaplasty. It is certainly not the treatment of choice for every patient, but 85% of the author's patients prefer this procedure. Patients can return to work in less than 1 weak with virtually no complications and no incision in the back of the head along the hair line.

45.2
Patient Consultation

Different types of facelift procedures are offered to the patient depending on the patient's needs and desires along with their expectations of the procedure. There are three factors that must be considered: (1) the invasiveness of the procedure and the patient's health conditions that would allow such surgery; (2) the time off work or their expected recovery time; (3) the budget allowed for the procedure.

Rejuvenating a face to a more youthful, rested, and younger look does not always require a facelift procedure. It does depend on the degree of the result the patient is expecting, such as fat transfer or volume filling to the face. The author offers patients three levels of facelift: suture lift, "easy" lift, and the three-dimensional facelift.

The suture lift or the feather lift is mainly for minimal lifting. It should generally be used for patient in the 30–40 age group. The recovery is 3–5 days with minimal complications.

The "easy" lift procedure is a midface lift with a moderate result. This is basically a noninvasive lift with a moderately fast recovery (5–7 days) and little chance of complications. The procedure can be done under local anesthesia or tumescent anesthesia. This is especially helpful for the patient who is either afraid or hesitant of having general anesthesia or whose health conditions do not allow for outpatient general anesthesia especially for an elective case.

45.3
Initial Consultation

The patient should be told about the risks and the benefits of the different treatment options. The patient's facial aging and the patient's expectation should be evaluated and a treatment plan should be proposed that both the patient and the surgeon agree upon.

45.4
Procedure

Preoperative photographs are taken. The operative procedure can be done under local anesthesia or general anesthesia. If the patient is having the procedure under general anesthesia there should be appropriate monitoring with an anesthesiologist or certified registered nurse anesthetist.

Preoperative marking is done for the S-lift, the upper and the lower part of the tragus, and the angle of the jowl line. A line is drawn vertically down at the posterior edge of the zygoma. This will limit the undermining of the flap to the line or in some cases about 1 cm beyond the line in men with large facial features. Another line is drawn at an angle, 0.5 cm lateral to the nasolabial fold up to the temporal region passing at the level of the inferior edge of the zygoma. This will be the tract for the cheek lift procedure. The markings are made for the mesh platysmaplasty procedure.

The patient is placed in a supine position and the head and the neck are prepped and draped in a sterile fashion. Sterility must be carefully maintained. The incision is made following the preoperative marking along the side of the ear and extending about 1 in. into the temporal region. In men the incision is in front of the tragus and in women it is inside the tragus. The incision

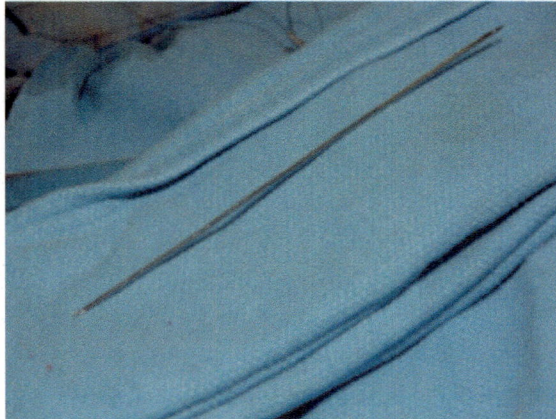

Fig. 45.1 Double-pointed needle

is extended around the ear lobe in the natural crease and behind the ear up to the level of the tragus in most cases. Another incision is made in the submental crease. Tumescent fluid, consisting 1 l of lactated Ringer's solution, 500 mg of lidocaine, 1:500,000 epinephrine, and 1 g of Ancef, is injected into the neck and the face in the area where the undermining will be done. On aver-

age about 200 ml of tumescent fluid is injected into the neck and the face area.

A 2.5-mm Mercedes cannula on a 20-ml syringe and vented 5 ml is used to liposuction the neck, jowl, and face. The liposuctioning should remain below the level of the cheek lift marking.

The face flap is raised making sure that there is a fatty layer on the subdermis. If the skin and fat layer are too thin, some patients may be able to feel the sutures underneath. A 2-0 Prolene suture is used starting at the inferior edge of the zygomatic arch forming a purse string of the subcutaneous musculoaponeurotic system (SMAS) in an O shape. The purse string pulls the SMAS vertically at several points. The facial skin is pulled in a superoposterior direction, the excess excised, and the skin sutured close.

The double-pointed needle (Fig. 45.1) with 2-0 nylon threaded through the proximal end is passed through in the subcutaneous layer along the cheek lift marking. The needle is brought out medially, 0.5 cm lateral to the nasolabial fold. The needle is pulled until 1 cm of the distal end is felt under the skin, then the needle is angled vertically down to the zygomatic bone and the needle is looped through, grabbing the malar fat pad, finally bringing the needle out from the incision and anchoring to the deep temporal fascia. The tissue

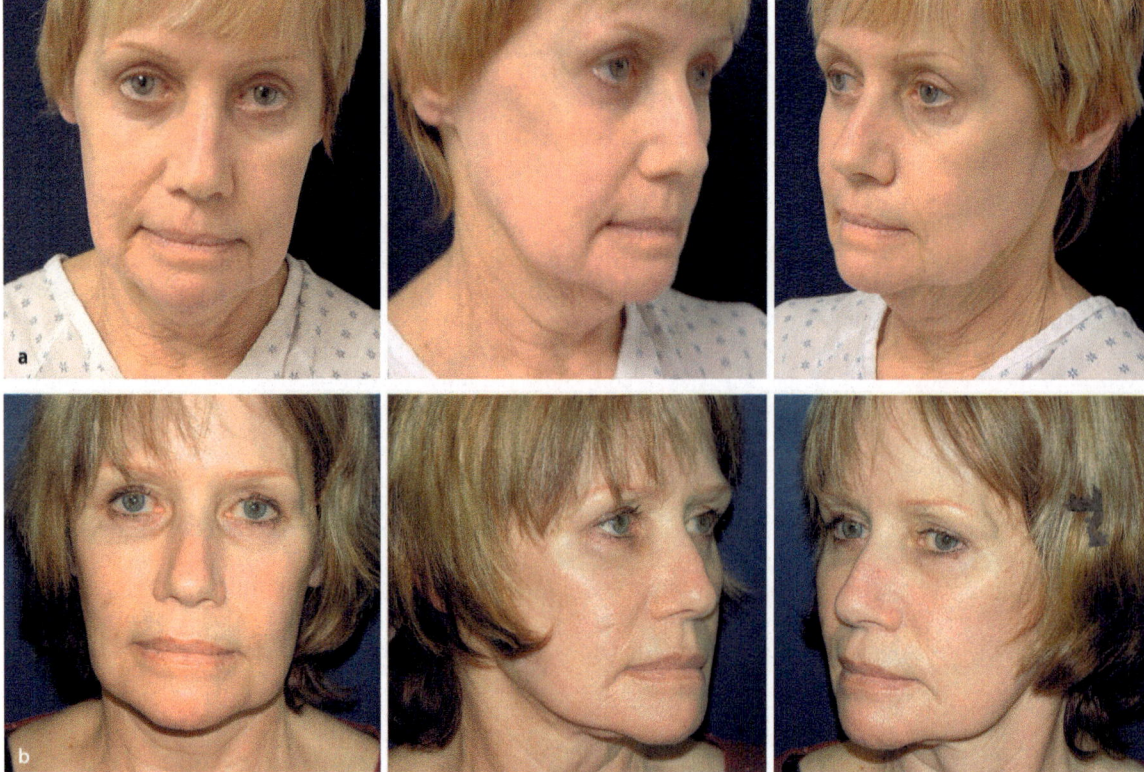

Fig. 45.2 a Preoperatively. **b** Postoperatively after "easy" lift

should be lifted beyond the desired level because as the nylon warms to body temperature it expands and the lift relaxes slightly. The cheek lift elevates the malar fat pad, providing volume to the cheek, and gives an overall pleasing appearance. The mesh platysmaplasty procedure is then performed. Foam and a compression dressing are applied to the neck and the jowl area.

45.5
Postoperative Care

The patient is told to lie at 45° and apply ice to the face area. Use of antibiotic (Keflex) as well as vitamin C (usually 2,000–3,000 mg/day) is continued. The patient is given a Medrol dose pack and the patient starts this on the day of the surgery and continues for 5 days. Generally the patient wears the neck band dressing for 3 days. The patient can also take a shower on the third postoperative day.

The sutures in front of the ear are removed in 5–6 days and those behind the ear in 7–8 days. Sometimes,

owing to the cheek lift procedure, the patient may have a slight indentation at the point of the pull. This will resolve in a few days but in some instances it can persist for a few weeks.

45.6
Complications

There has been no motor or sensory nerve deficit, infection, seroma, or skin necrosis in over 40 patients. All the patients were very happy with the results (Figs. 45.2, 45.3). One of the patients decided to have a neck lift 1 year later.

45.7
Conclusions

The "easy" lift procedure is well accepted by patients and complications have virtually been nonexistent. The recovery time is moderately short (6 days on average).

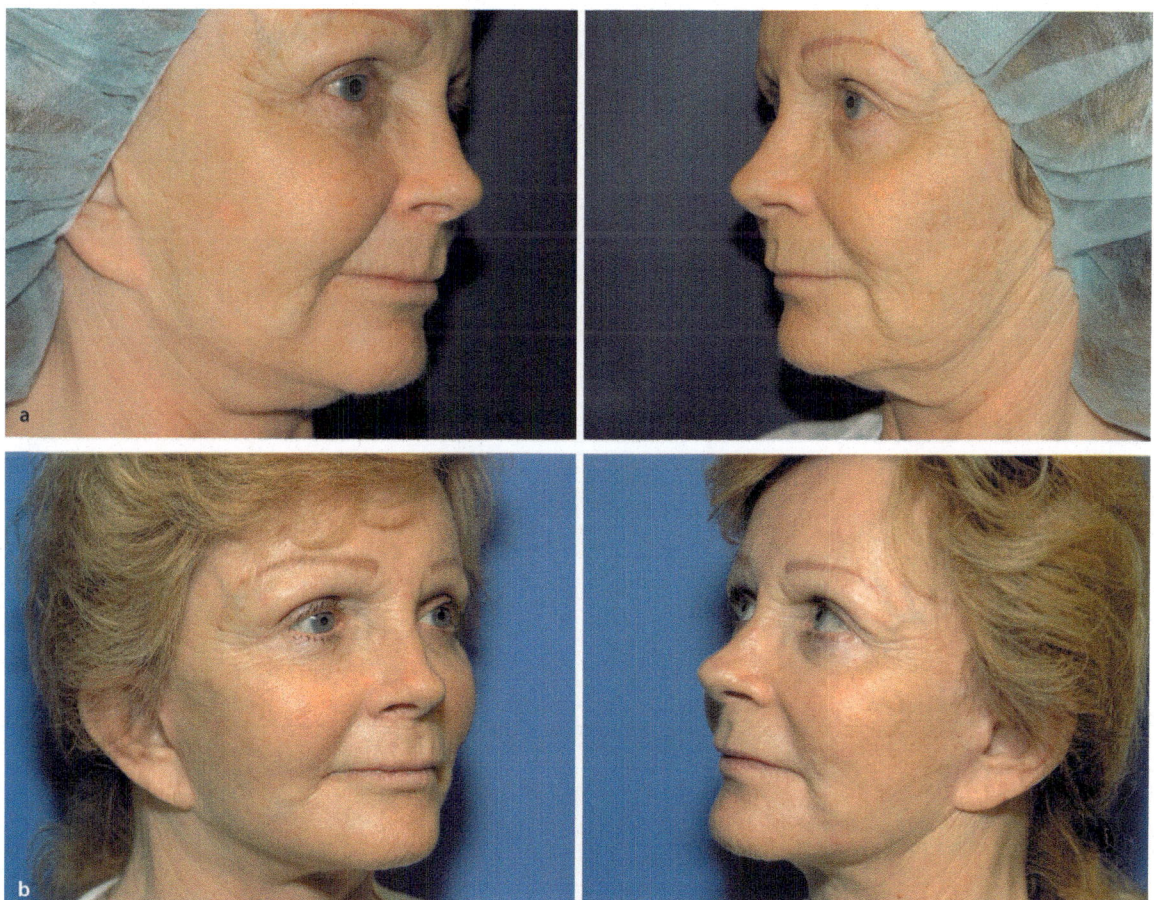

Fig. 45.3 a Preoperatively. **b** Postoperatively after "easy" lift

Chapter 46

Simplified S-Lift

Enrique Hernández-Pérez, Hassan Abbas Khawaja

46.1 Introduction

Simplified facelifts are the trend of the new century [1, 2]. Conventional facelifts resulting in "mask face" or "wind-tunnel face" are outdated. Patients prefer ambulatory surgery and minimal convalescent period [3]. The subperiosteal facelift, composite rhytidectomies, triple facelifts, and deep-plane facelifts can result in a prolonged recovery period with hospitalization, and a number of complications [4, 5].

S-lift requires preauricular skin excision, and a modified superficial musculoaponeurotic system (SMAS) plication (Fig. 46.1) [6, 7]. Correction of nasolabial folds can be achieved either before or after the procedure by means of a tissue filler. In general we perform first some subcision and then we use injections of filler substances.

46.2 Technique

All of our patients, irrespective of age, are sent to a cardiologist for a cardiac and vascular checkup, mentioning especially that we are going to use epinephrine. Blood tests are performed, consisting of complete blood count, bleeding and coagulation tests, hepatitis B surface antigen and HIV tests in addition to other relevant tests. Administration of cefadroxil monohydrate is started orally 1 day prior to surgery. Patients begin using povidone–iodine shampoo for the scalp and a Betadine face wash 3 days before surgery (clorhexidine if allergic to iodides). One hour prior to surgery we use 0.1 mg clonidine orally when the blood pressure is not less than 100/60 and the pulse rate is above 60 per minute. Because the patient is fasting and he/she will have undergone intravenous sedation, we also use oral administration of 15 ml ranitidine and 50 mg dimenhydrate. Comfort of the patient is crucial. The operating room must be fully equipped, and there should be complete monitoring under the supervision of a certified anesthesiologist.

46.2.1 Submental Liposuction and Platysmal Band Plication

Anesthesia (1%) with 1:400.000 epinephrine is used for a point in the centralsubmental crease and in the preau-

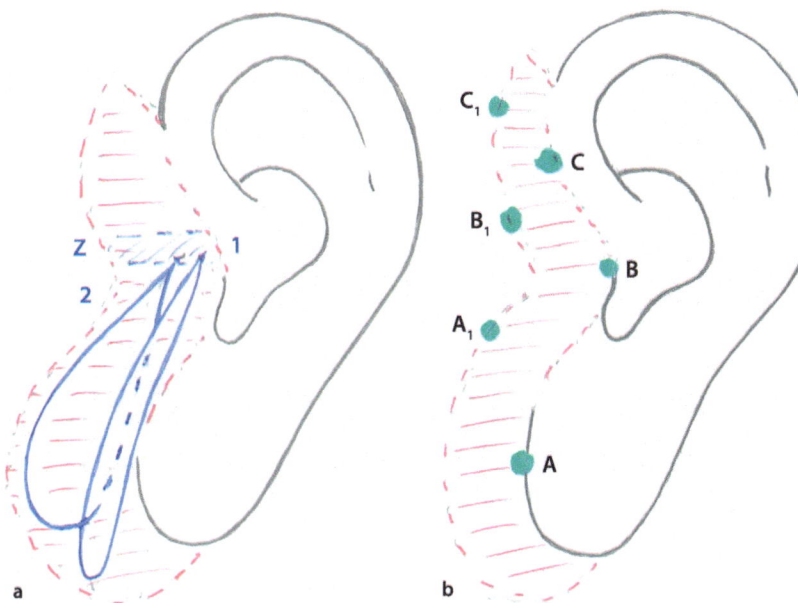

Fig. 46.1 a After a lazy "S" has been removed in front of the ear and undermining is complete, two sutures are performed, one "U" (*1*) and one "O" (*2*) and are attached to the zygoma (*Z*).
b The points in *green* are sutured using Vicryl 3/0

ricular area. A Lamis infiltration syringe is used to provide tumescent anesthesia. A 150-ml aliquot of chilled Klein solution is infiltrated subcutaneously in the neck, as well as the same amount in each side of the face, to get tumescence [8]. During this part of the procedure, the patient must have a kind of pillow below his/her shoulders, in an hyperextended position with the intention to make the maneuvers easier. Liposuction of the chin is performed using a machine and a 3- or 4-mm flat spatula cannula (Fig. 46.2).

Care is taken regarding the marginal mandibular nerve, which is marked beforehand. An assistant places his/her hand in the junction between the mandibular angle and the masseter with that aim. After that we make several passes with a dissector in a "V". The idea is to undermine completely the skin and a some of the fatty tissue from its muscular plane. At this moment the free plane will be reached and you will feel it when you put your cannula and the dissector inside in different directions. Liposuction is avoided close to the facial vessels and nerve.

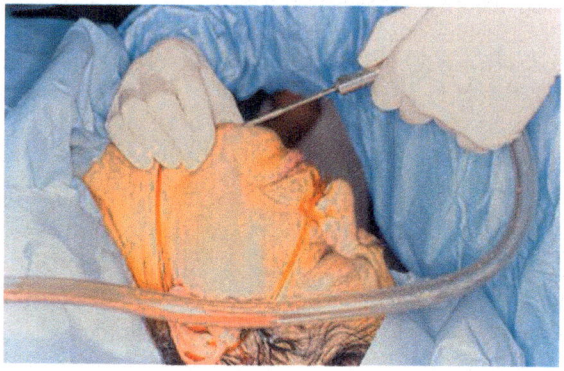

Fig. 46.2 Submental liposuction is performed with a flat spatula cannula. The right hand of the surgeon protects the marginal mandibular nervev

Platysmal band correction is performed via a small 2-cm submental crease incision, only if there is excessive platysmal laxity. Edge-to-edge anastomosis, or overlapping of the bellies, is performed in these cases using three or four Prolene 2/0 interrupted stitches [9].

46.2.2
The S-Lift

The skin is marked in the form of a lazy S in the preauricular region [6] in the preanesthetized area, and the skin and subcutaneous tissue are removed using tenotomy scissors and a no. 15 scalpel blade (Fig. 46.3). The incision follows the lobule and auricular creases, and the tragal margin. A retrotragal incision may be used. The complete marked skin S is excised. Undermining (5±1 cm away from the auricle) is performed using a 4-mm flat spatula cannula (Fig. 46.3). Dissection is made on skin and subcutaneous tissue below the zygomatic arch (the tragus is taken as a marker point). Above the zygoma the dissection is made only in the skin to protect the temporal branch of the facial nerve. Once the plane of the dissection has been reached, the rest of the fibrous trabeculas are severed using very gently Metzenbaum scissors whose tip is directed to the skin above (like a shot in the air) (Fig. 46.4). It is good to remember that when working below the zygoma care must be taken with the parotid gland and to protect the branches of the facial nerve that lie deep in the gland.

Open liposuction is performed using a vacuum cleaner technique, with the help of a 6-mm flat spatula cannula [6]. Prolene 2/0 is used for SMAS plication. The first suture starts at the periostium of the zygomatic arch. It takes small bites of the SMAS in the direction of the upper and the mid nasolabial fold. It goes back to the periostium in the form of an O, where, after plication, knots are tied [6, 9]. The other vertical suture

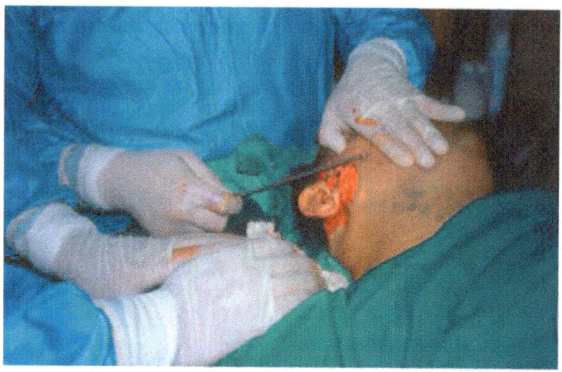

Fig. 46.3 The skin has been removed. Undermining is performed with the cannula. The surgeon's left hand shows the extension of the undermining

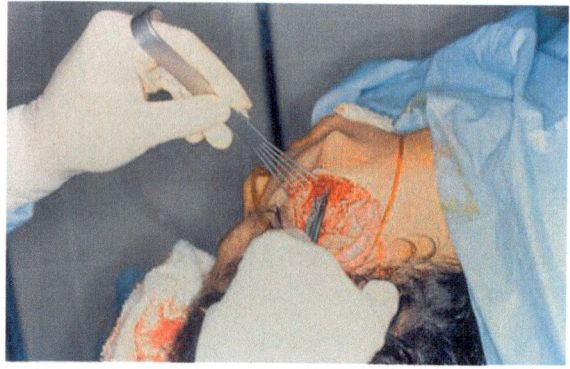

Fig. 46.4 Remaining fibrous trabeculas are gently severed with Metzenbaum scissors

starts close to the first one at the zygomatic arch. It goes down vertically taking small bites of the SMAS, in the direction of the mandibular angle. It ascends again in the form of a U, and goes back to the same point at the periostium of the zygomatic arch, where after plication, knots are tied (Fig. 46.5). Subcutaneously, Vicryl 3/0 sutures are used for points a to a1, b to b1, and c to c1. Most traction is placed on point a1, moderate traction on b1, and the least traction on c1 [9]. Four or five mattress nylon 4/0 sutures are used to close the incision and then a 5/0 continuous suture. The authors usually start inferiorly, behind the lobule of the ear, and go up in the temple, so that if a dogear forms, it is hidden in the scalp. If that occur, a simple plasty is performed to correct it.

The other side is operated on similarly. Triple antibiotic ointment and sterile dressings are applied over the sutures. Tight compression bandages are used for 24 h. At that time they are removed and a neck and face girdle is placed, with daily changes, for 5 days. After that, the girdle is used only 12 h/day, in the morning or at night, according to the convenience of the patient. Cold compression is started immediately, and the patient is advised to continue it for the next 4 days after surgery. This decreases considerably the postoperative inflammation and edema. Cefadroxil monohydrate for 1 week and prednisone per os postoperatively are used by the patient (20 mg/day for 4 days). Stitches are removed postoperatively in about 5–7 days.

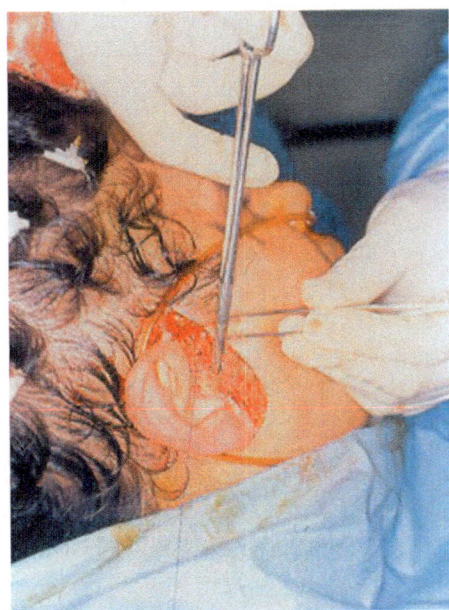

Fig. 46.5 Plication of the superficial musculoaponeurotic system is performed through two sutures ("U" and "O") which are fixed to the zygoma

46.2.3
Chin Implant

To make the chin more prominent, at the end of the procedure, and to make the cervicomental angle sharper and more defined, the authors use 8–10 ml of fat transferred to the chin, using a fat-transfer cannula through one or two very small needle incisions in both sides of the chin (Figs. 46.6, 46.7).

46.3
Complications

46.3.1
Facial Nerve Palsy

Facial nerve palsy is a possibility, and has been reported with a secondary S-lift; however, it usually disappears with time [6]. The authors have never seen this complication. This might be due to the fact that the zygomatic branch of the facial nerve is often in the form of several filaments, and there are cross-connections between these filaments [10]. Even if one or two filaments are caught in the sutures, as a result of cross-connections

and increasing number of branches, nerve palsy does not take place.

46.3.2
Hematoma

Hematomas can take place if you use syringes for infiltration instead of a Lamis syringe. Klein tumescent fluid preoperatively and cold compression postoperatively are not used. Patients having a family history, taking Aspirin or beta-blockers, and smokers can end up with hematomas [11]. Therefore, it is important to perform coagulation studies preoperatively.

46.3.3
Seroma/Sinus Formation

If large-volume fat transfer is performed in the face in conjunction with facelift, this can result in the formation of seromas. The chance of seroma formation is increased if a non-tumescent technique and general anesthesia are used. Serum exudation can continue from the suture line, or a skin sinus can form as a result of fat necrosis [12]. These seromas should be managed conservatively. However, they may take several weeks or months to resolve; therefore, it is imperative that the amount of fat transferred to the face should not exceed the recommended amounts.

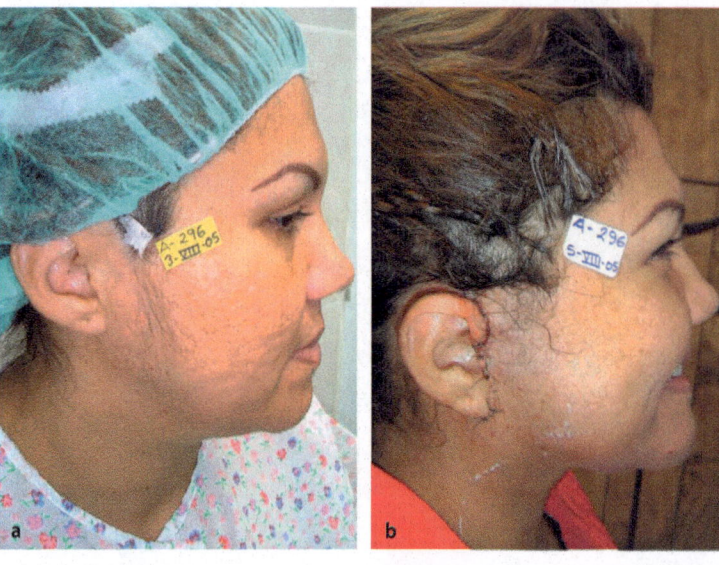

Fig. 46.6 a Preoperatively. b Postoperatively

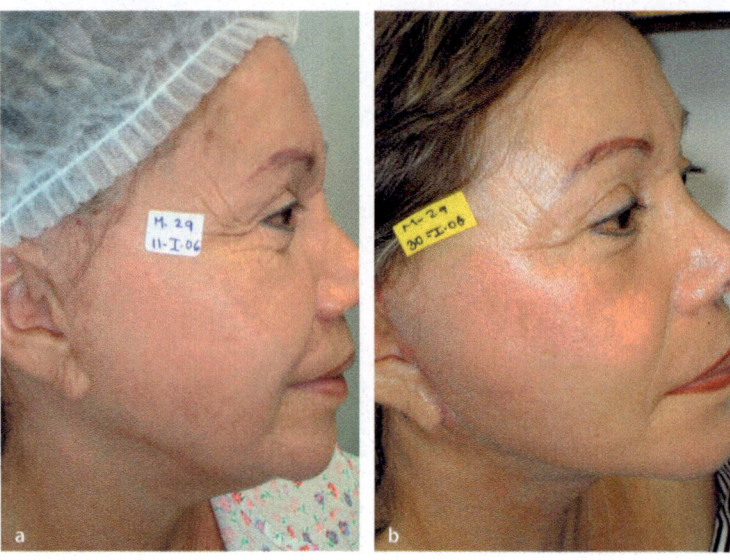

Fig. 46.7 a Preoperatively. b Postoperatively

46.3.4
Pain and Pretragal Tension

Pain and pretragal tension can take place; however, these are transitory and disappear in a few weeks.

46.3.5
Dogear

A dogear can form behind the lobule or in the temple. It improves considerably in the coming weeks. To prevent it, a lower to upper suture technique should be used. Continuous sutures should be started from behind the lobule, and should end at the temple. As skin in the temple is thick, dogear formation is less. However, in resistant cases, a dogear plasty can be done later.

46.3.6
Skin Necrosis

The authors have never had skin necrosis in any of their cases. As skin is excised first, and undermining is performed later using the tumescent technique, skin necrosis does not take place.

46.4
Discussion

The simplified S-lift is much safer and has superior results than conventional and radical facelifts (Figs. 46.2, 46.3). It is a simple, safe, and quick method of facelifting, suitable not only for younger patients (as originally proposed by Saylan), but for all age groups. In older patients, where the skin is more lax and wrinkled, the size of the marked S has to be increased considerably, depending on the skin laxity. As most skin laxity is in the mid to lower face and jowl areas, retroauricular and temporal extensions of facelift are rather unnecessary. With the tumescent technique, there is much less bruising and inflammation. There is quick and rapid recovery with a more natural look. The total procedure takes less than 3 h, including neck surgery, chin implant, and sedation/anesthesia.

Though facial nerve damage can take place as a result of placement of sutures in the zygomatic arch periosteum, in practice we have never seen this happen, because of the reasons mentioned earlier [10]. There is very little chance of skin necrosis as the skin is excised prior to undermining. Secondary and tertiary S-lifts can be conveniently performed.

The authors usually combine the S-lift with other modalities of facial rejuvenation, like blepharoplasty, chemical peels, sunscreens, topically applied tretinoin, orally administered isotretinoin, fat injections, fillers and Botox [13].

46.5
Conclusions

The simplified S-lift is a rapid and safe method of face-lifting. The recovery is quick, and complications are minimal. It is suitable for patients of all age groups requiring a facelift. The complex facelifts, like subperiosteal facelift , composite rhytidectomies, and deep-plane facelifts, are risky and extreme procedures. The S-lift can be combined with other forms of facial rejuvenation. However, we insist that the S-lift must always be performed with lifting of the neck and chin implants. That is the way to get better results.

References

1. Khawaja HA, Hernandez-Perez E. Transcutaneous face-lift. Dermatol Surg 2005;31:453–458
2. Serdev NP. Total ambulatory SMAS lift by hidden minimal incisions part 2: lower SMAS-platysma lift. Int J Cosmet Surg Aesthet Dermatol 2002;4:285–292
3. Sulamanidze MA, Shiffman MA, Paikidze TG, Sulamanidze GM, Gavasheli LG. Facial lifting with Aptos threads. Int J Cosmet Surg Aesthet Dermatol 2001;3(4):275–281
4. Hamra ST. Subperiosteal face-lift. Plast Reconstr Surg 1995;96:493–506
5. Rees TD, Wood-Smith D. Cosmetic Facial Surgery, 1st edition. Philadelphia, Saunders 1973:151
6. Saylan Z. The S-lift for facial rejuvenation. Int J Cosmet Surg 1999;7:18–24
7. Schoenrock LD, Repucci AD. Goretex in facial plastic surgery. Int J Aesthet Restor Surg 1993;1:63–68
8. Klein JA. Tumescent technique for local anesthesia improves safety in large-volume liposuction. Plast Reconstr Surg 1993;92:1085–1098
9. Khawaja HA, Hernandez-Perez E. The delta lift : A modification of S-lift for facial rejuvenation. Int J Cosmet Surg Aesthet Dermatol 2002;4:309–315
10. Salasche SJ, Bernstein G. Surgical Anatomy of the Skin, 1st edition. Stamford, Appleton and Lange 1988:89–97
11. Peck GC. Complications and Problems in Aesthetic Plastic Surgery, 1st edition. New York, Gower Medical Publishing 1992:3.2–3.15
12. Khawaja HA, Hernandez-Perez E. Fat transfer review: Controversies, complications, their prevention and treatment. Int J Cosmet Surg Aesthet Dermatol 2002;4:131–138
13. Hernandez-Perez E, Khawaja HA. Oral isotretinoin as part of the treatment of cutaneous aging. Dermatol Surg 2000;26(7):649–652

CHAPTER 47

The Round-Lifting Technique

Ivo Pitanguy, Henrique Nascimento Radwanski, Natale Ferreira Gontijo de Amorim

47.1
Introduction

During the aging process, the aspect of the skin changes gradually, from tight and wrinkle-free in youth to an irregularly colored and drier surface in older age. Senescence also involves skeletal and muscular atrophy, laxity of the subcutaneous tissue and consequent flaccidity of the skin with the accentuation of furrows and rhytids. Different factors are responsible for these changes, such as excessive sun exposure, stress and personal habits such as alcohol consumption, smoking and poor nutrition.

The surgeon should understand that the purpose of any procedure for the aging face is to help the individual cross with enhanced self-confidence the sometimes difficult path to a mature age, and not to return the patient to an earlier stage of life. In our beauty-centered culture, where life is face-paced and people are rapidly judged as regards their appearance, the face is frequently the main focus of anxiety, especially in individuals who have attained a certain stage in their lives. In these cases, job competition, interpersonal relationships and physical well-being are reasons that many times motivate the patient to come to the plastic surgeon, seeking for a more youthful look. Experience is necessary to investigate and appreciate these subjective motivations. This evalu-

ation requires both empathy and openness towards the patient.

In the last few decades, facial aesthetic surgery has undergone enormous progress. A greater understanding of anatomy, mainly of deep structures such as the malar fat pad and the superficial musculoaponeurotic system (SMAS), allows the surgeon to enhance his/her results. Knowledge of the details of different surgical approaches and variations thereof are fundamental in the planning of each individual case.

47.2
Surgical Technique

A satisfactory outcome of an aesthetic facial procedure is obtained when signs of an operation are undetectable and anatomy has been preserved. Visible scars and dislocation of the hairline are among the most common complaints and everything should be done to avoid these stigmas.

The senior author's personal approach to surgical treatment of the aging face is presented, giving emphasis to the correct traction applied to the facial flaps (the "round-lifting" technique) and the forehead (the "block" lifting or the juxta-pilose subperiosteal lifting),

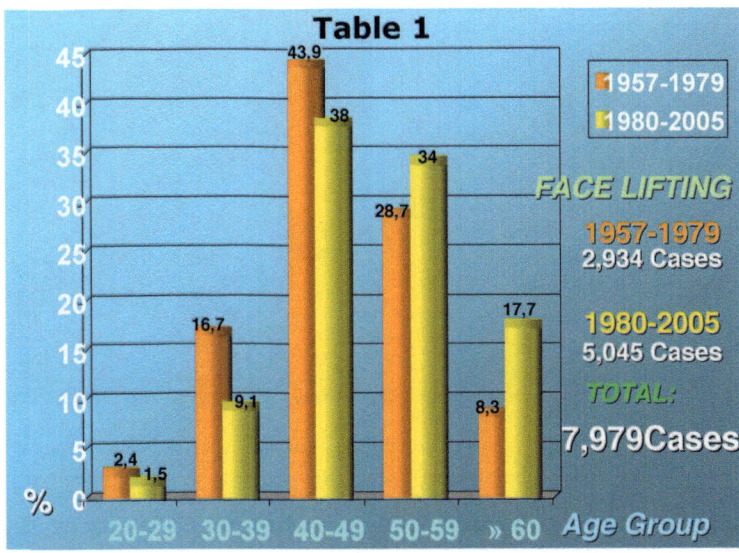

Table 47.1 Different age groups are shown, in two distinct periods in the senior author's experience

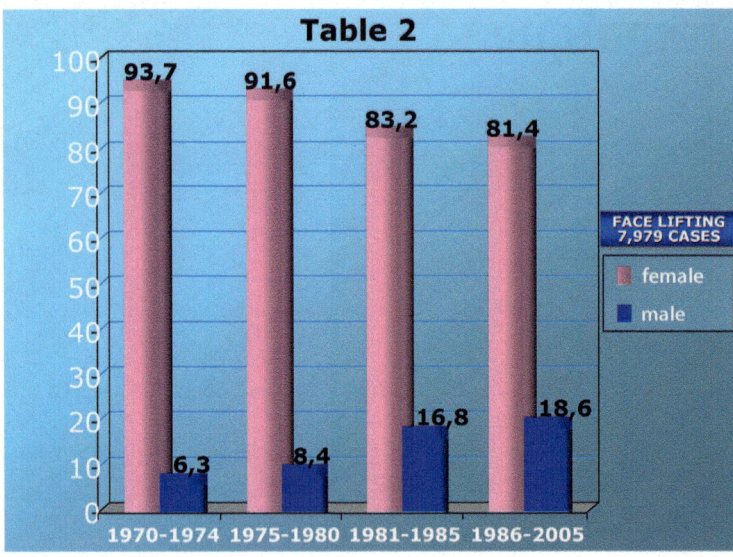

Table 47.2 Distribution of patients according to gender

ensuring that all anatomical landmarks are precisely preserved. These principles, which have evolved in over 40 years of experience, have offered consistent and satisfactory results.

47.2.1
Round-Lifting Technique

Rhytidoplasty is one of the most frequently performed surgeries in the senior author's private practice. A total of 7,979 personal consecutive cases have been analyzed to date (Table 47.1), with a noticeable increase in male patients noted. In the 1970s, men represented 6% of face-lifting procedures; in the 1980s, approximately 15%; currently, 20% of patients who seek aesthetic facial surgery are men (Table 47.2).

Local infiltration is performed and the standard incision is demarcated, beginning in the temporal scalp, and proceeds in the preauricular area in such a way as to respect the anatomical curvature of this region. The incision then follows around the earlobe, and, in a curving fashion, finishes in the cervical scalp (Fig. 47.1). This S-shaped incision creates an advancement flap that prevents a step-off in the hairline, allowing the patient to wear the hair up without revealing the scar.

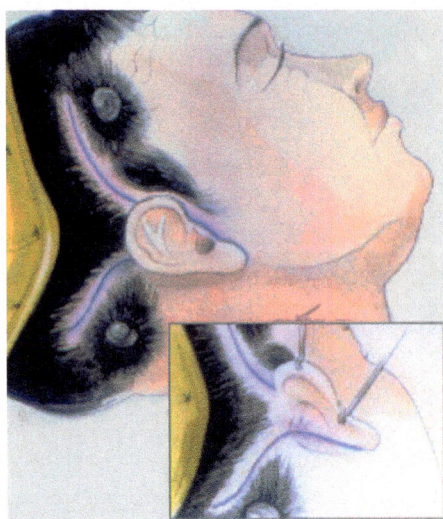

Fig. 47.1 The classic incision, as described for the round-lifting, curves around the anatomical landmarks, and finishes in a sinuous italic "S" in the cervical scalp

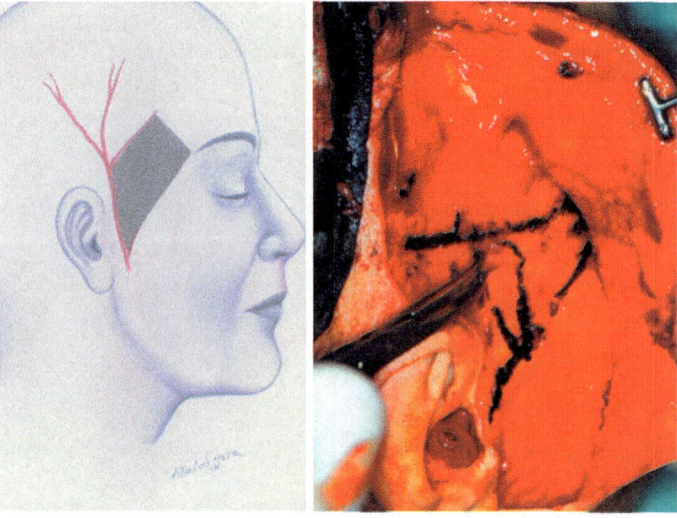

Fig. 47.2 The variation in the anatomical distribution of the frontal branch of the facial nerve determines an area called "no man's land," where this nerve is particularly vulnerable to lesion by eletrocoagulation

Variations of this incision are chosen depending on each case. The choice of which incision is most appropriate should have the following goals in mind: the treatment of specific regions for optimal distribution of skin flaps; the resection of previous scars in secondary rhytidoplasty; and the maintenance of anatomical landmarks. Secondary face-lifts commonly present elements that require different incisions according to each case.

Undermining of the facial and cervical flaps is performed in a subcutaneous plane, the extension of which is variable and individualized for each case. A danger area lies beneath the non-hair-bearing skin over the temples, which we have called "no man's land," where most of the temporofrontal branches of the facial nerve are more superficial. Dissection and hemostasis over "no man's land" should be carefully performed. Larger vessels should be tied (Fig. 47.2).

The treatment of the very heavy, fatty neck requires that the dissection proceed all the way to the other side under the mandible. With the advent of suction-assisted lipectomy, submental lipodystrophy is mostly addressed by liposuction, in a crisscross fashion (Fig. 47.3). Sometimes this is still done with direct lipectomy using specially designed scissors, defatting the submental region, as has been described historically. Following this, treatment of medial platysmal bands is carried out under direct vision. Approximation of diastasis is done with interrupted sutures, plicating down to the level of the hyoid bone.

Undermining of the facial flaps is extended over the zygomatic prominence to free the retaining ligaments of the cheek. Dissection of the deeper elements of the face has evolved over the past 20 years. Almost no treat-

ment was advocated before the publications that first described the SMAS. Approach to this structure has been a topic of much discussion. Currently, we determine whether to plicate the SMAS only after subcutaneous dissection has been completed. Pulling of the SMAS is done, noting the effects on the skin. The same maneuver is done with the malar fat pad, and has given satisfactory and natural results (Fig. 47.4). The durability of this maneuver is relative to the individual aging process. Tension on the musculoaponeurotic system allows support of the subcutaneous layers, corrects the sagging cheek and reduces tension on the skin flap.

Techniques that treat the pronounced nasolabial fold include traction of skin flaps and traction on the SMAS, or the fascial fatty layer, and have variable results. Filling with different substances may also be done at the end of surgery, either with fat grafting or with other material. Direct excision of the nasolabial fold is reserved for the older male patient. In very select cases this technique

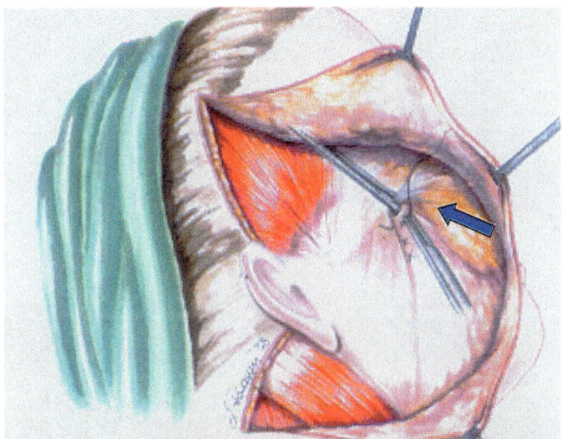

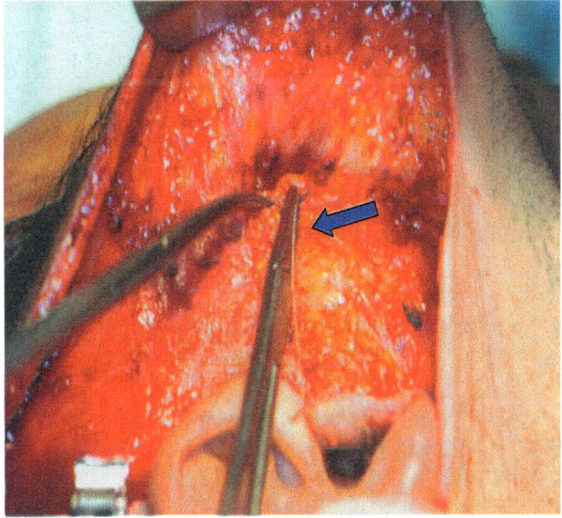

Fig. 47.4 Repositioning of the malar pad is done after subcutaneous dissection has been completed

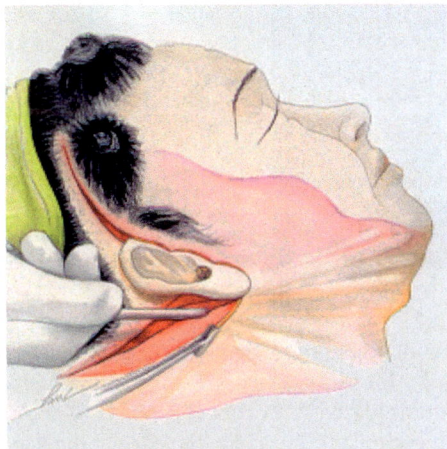

Fig. 47.3 Liposuction has been useful to complement a face-lift, and permits the removal of fatty tissue from the cervical region. This maneuver should be done in a crisscross fashion to ensure an even plane of subcutaneous tissue

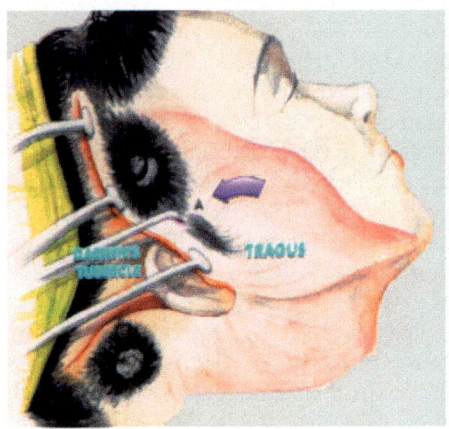
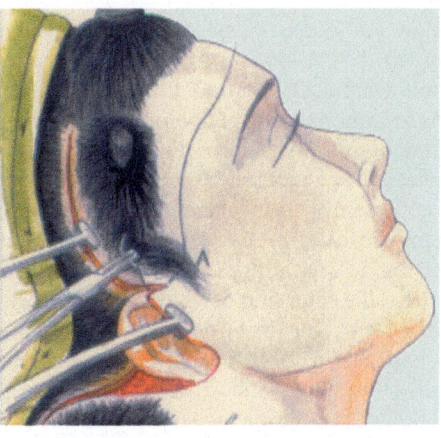

Fig. 47.5 The direction of traction of the anterior or facial flap follows a vector that connects the tragus to Darwin's tubercle. Excess tissue is marked with a Pitanguy flap demarcator. A key suture is placed over point *A*

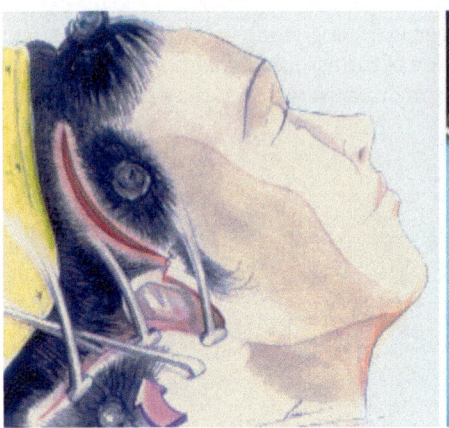
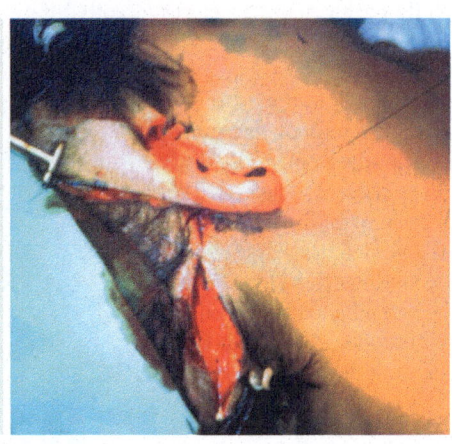

Fig. 47.6 The posterior flap has been rotated and fixed at point B

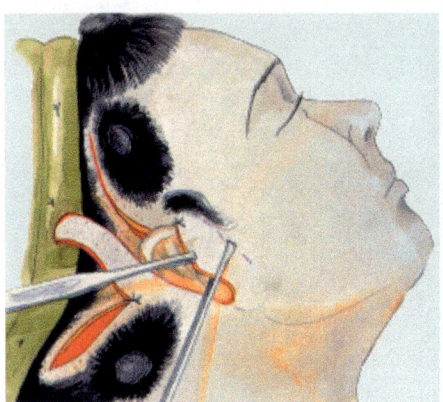
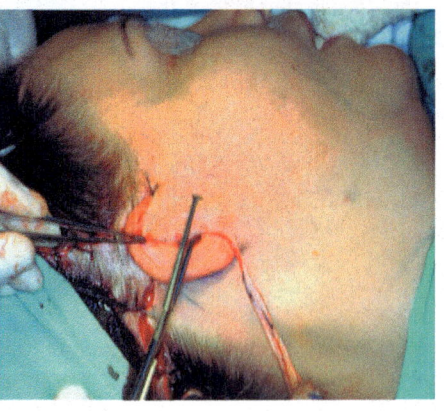

Fig. 47.7 Excess facial skin is demarcated with no tension on the flap

gives a definite solution to the nasolabial fold, with a barely noticeable scar that mimics the nasolabial fold itself.

The direction of traction of the skin flaps is a fundamental aspect of the "round-lifting" technique. In this manner, the undermined flaps are rotated rather than simply pulled, thus acting in a direction opposite to that of aging, and ensuring a repositioning of tissues with preservation of anatomical landmarks. A second advantage in establishing a precise vector of rotation is that the opposite side is repositioned in the exact manner.

This vector of traction connects the tragus to Darwin's tubercle for the facial (or anterior) flap. A Pitanguy flap demarcator is placed at the root of the helix to mark point A on the skin flap (Fig. 47.5). The edge of the flap is then incised along a curved line crossing the supraauricular hairline so that bald skin, not pilose, is resected. A key suture is located here. Likewise, the cervical flap should also be pulled in an equally precise manner, in a superior and slightly anterior vector of traction, to avoid a step-off of the hairline. Key stitches are placed to anchor the flap along the pilose scalp at point B so

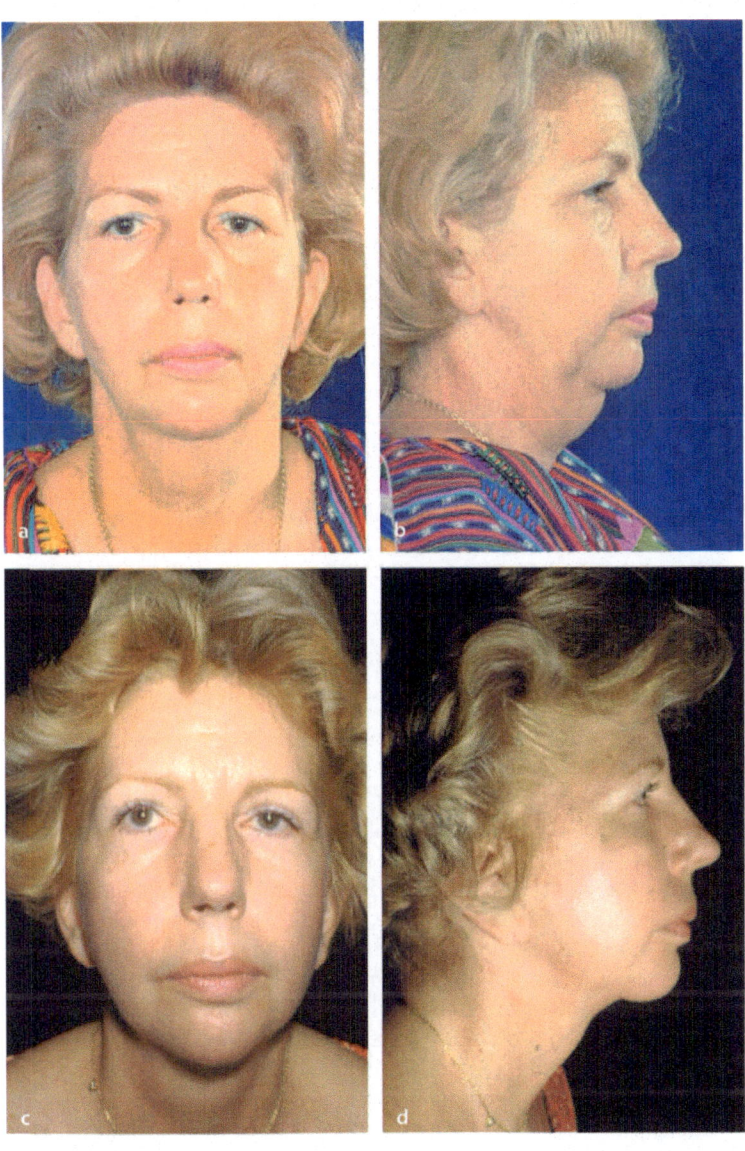

Fig. 47.8 Submental lipectomy was a primary concern in this 58-year-old patient. This was done by ample liposuction and open lipectomy, together with a round-lifting technique to reposition facial and cervical tissues. **a, b** The patient preoperatively. **c, d** The patient at 2 years follow-up

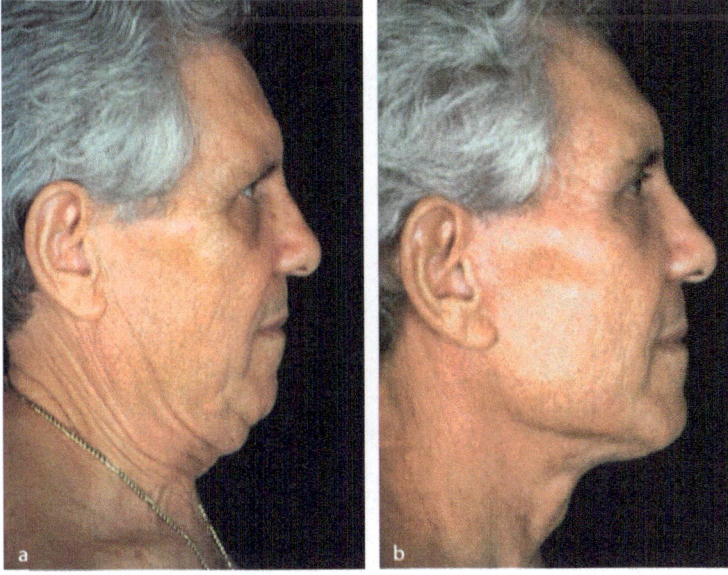

Fig. 47.9 Male patients have become more frequent in the office of the plastic surgeon, and many seek rejuvenation procedures. This 63-year-old man had a face-lift with blepharoplasty, with special attention given to correction of platysmal bands. **a** The patient preoperatively. **b** The patient at 2 years follow-up

that there is no tension on the thin skin at the peak of the retroauricular incision (Fig. 47.6).

Only when the temporary sutures have been placed will excess facial skin be resected. Skin is accommodated and demarcated along the natural curves of the ear, with no tension whatsoever (Fig. 47.7). Final scars are thus not displaced or widened. The tragus is preserved in its anatomical position, and the skin of the flap is trimmed so as to perfectly match the fine skin of this region.

When performing a brow lift using the block technique, placing these key sutures at points A and B is mandatory before any traction is applied to the forehead flap, essentially "blocking" the facial flaps (Figs. 47.8, 47.9).

47.2.2
Forehead Lifting

Aging in the upper face becomes evident with a descent in the level of the eyebrow and the appearance of wrinkles and furrows, sometimes from an early age. These are a direct consequence of muscle dynamics, responsible for the multitude of expressions so characteristic of man, and are also due to loss of skin tone. Elements of the upper face that must be considered preoperatively for any procedure are the length of the forehead and the elasticity of the skin; muscle force and wrinkles; the position of the anterior hairline and the quality and quantity of hair.

An important decision to be made regarding a brow lift is the placement of incisions. There are basically two classic approaches: the bicoronal incision and the limited juxta-pilose incision. The first allows for treatment of all elements that determine the aging forehead while hiding the final scar within the hairline. Certain situations, however, rule out this incision. Patients with

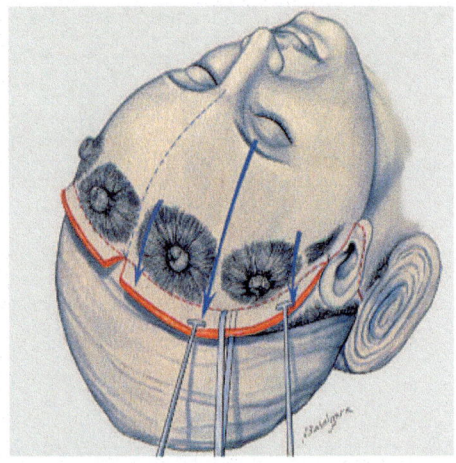

Fig. 47.10 Positioning of the forehead flap is only done after the facial flaps have been rotated and "blocked." This avoids excessive elevation of the facial tissues and alteration of the hairline

a very long forehead or those who have already been subjected to previous surgery should not be considered for this incision, because they will have an excessively recessed hairline if the forehead is further pulled back. The final aspect will be displeasing, giving the patient a permanent look of surprise.

Having "blocked" the facial flaps at points A and B, as described above, the forehead may be pulled in any direction, either straight backwards or more laterally (Fig. 47.10). The amount of scalp flap to be resected is determined by the length of the forehead and the effect that traction causes on the level of the eyebrow. The midline is positioned, demarcated, incised and blocked with a temporary suture. Sometimes no traction is necessary and no scalp is removed in the midline. Two

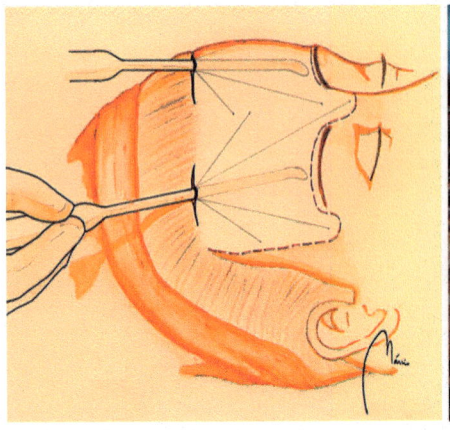
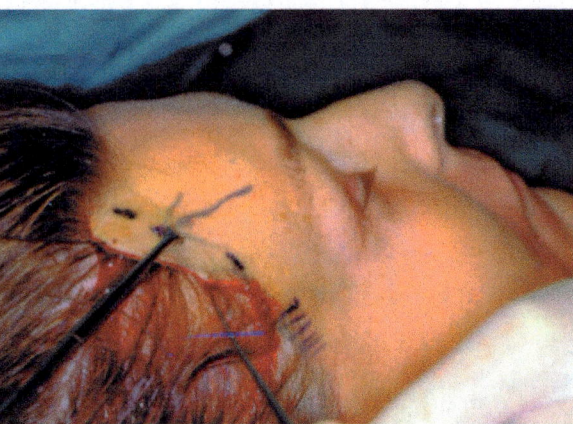

Fig. 47.11 The midline of the forehead flap is fixed, and each lateral flap is pulled according to the amount of correction required

symmetrical flaps are created, and lateral resection can now be performed allowing the eyebrow to be raised as necessary (Fig. 47.11).

The second approach is the juxta-pilose incision, performed when the patient presents with ptosis of the lateral eyebrow and scant lines of expression of the forehead. The short distance required to reach the eyebrow region is easily achieved by subperiosteal blunt dissection (Fig. 47.12). Endoscopic instrumentation has permitted treatment of the brow through minimal access, and has proved useful in select cases.

47.3
Complications

Complications in rhytidoplasty are infrequent, yet can bring great distress to the patient and to the surgeon. It is essential to eliminate patients who continue to smoke, as the risk for skin slough is greatly increased. Smoking must be stopped completely at least 2 weeks in advance. In the immediate postoperative period, blood pressure must be constantly monitored by the nursing staff to prevent hypertension and consequent hematoma formation. If an expanding hematoma is diagnosed, the surgeon may initially attempt to drain the collection at the bedside. Early identification and treatment of large hematomas is essential to prevent sequelae. Nerve injuries, dehiscence and other complications are infrequent and should be treated conservatively.

References

1. Pitanguy, I., Ramos, A.: The frontal branch of the facial nerve: The importance of its variation in the face-lifting. Plast Reconstr Surg 1966;38:352–356

2. Pitanguy, I.: Ancillary procedures in face-lifting. Clin Plast Surg 1978;5:51–69

3. Pitanguy, I.: Frontalis-procerus-corrugator aponeurosis in the correction of frontal and glabellar wrinkles. Ann Plast Surg 1979;2:422–427

4. Pitanguy, I.: The aging face. In: Carlsen, L., Slatt, B. (eds). The Naked Face. Ontario, General Publishing 1979:27

5. Pitanguy, I., Ceravolo, M.P., Dègand, M.: Nerve injuries during rhytidectomy: Considerations after 3.203 cases. Aesthet Plast Surg 1980;4:257–265

6. Pitanguy, I., Ceravolo, M.: Hematoma post-rhytidectomy: How we treat it. Plast Reconstr Surg 1981;67:526–528

7. Pitanguy, I.: Indication for and treatment of frontal and glabellar wrinkles in an analysis of 3,404 consecutive cases of rhytidectomy. Plast Reconstr Surg 1981;67:157–166

8. Pitanguy, I.: Les Chemins de la Beauté. Un Maitre de la Chirurgie Plastique Témoigne. Paris, Lattes 1983

9. Pitanguy, I.: The face. In: Aesthetic Surgery of Head and Body. Berlin, Springer 1984:165–200

10. Pitanguy, I.: Forehead lifting. In: Aesthetic Surgery of Head and Body. Berlin, Springer 1984:202–214

11. Pitanguy, I., Salgado, F., Radwanski, H.N.: Submental liposuction as an ancillary procedure in face-lifting. FACE 1995;4(1):1–13

12. Pitanguy, I., Brentano, J.M.S., Salgado, F.; Radwanski, H.N., Carpeggiani, R.: Incisions in primary and secondary rhytidoplasties. Rev Bras Cir 1995;85:165–176

13. Pitanguy, I., Pamplona, D.C., Giuntini, M.E., Salgado, F., Radwanski, H.N.: Computational simulation of rhytidectomy by the "round-lifting" technique. Rev Bras Cir 1995;85:213–218

14. Pitanguy, I., Amorim, N.F.G.: Treatment of the nasolabial fold. Rev Bras Cir 1997;87:231–242

15. Pitanguy, I., Pamplona, D.C., Weber, H.I., Leta, F., Salgado, F., Radwanski, H.N.: Numerical modeling of the aging face. Plast Reconstr Surg 1998;102:200–204

16. Pitanguy, I., Radwanski, H.N.: Rejuvenation of the brow. Dermatol Clin 1998;15:623–635

17. Pitanguy, I., Radwanski, H.N., Amorim, N.F.G.: Treatment of the aging face using the "round lifting" technique. Aesthet Surg J 1999;19:216–222

18. Pitanguy, I., Soares, G., Machado, B.H., de Amorim, N.F.G.: CO2 laser associated with the "round-lifting" technique. J Cutan Laser Ther 1999;1:145–152

19. Pitanguy, I.: The round-lifting technique. Facial Plast Surg 2000;16(3):255–267

20. Pitanguy, I.: Facial cosmetic surgery: A 30-year perspective. Plast Reconstr Surg 2000;105:1517–1529

21. Pitanguy, I., Amorim, N.F.G.: Forehead lifting: The juxtapilose subperiosteal approach. Aesthet Plast Surg 2003;27:58–62

CHAPTER 48

The QuickLift™ and Lateral Subcutaneous Browlifting

48

Dominic A. Brandy

48.1
Introduction

In June of 2004, the author introduced a modification of the S-lift of Saylan [1] called the QuickLift™ [2]. The original procedure differed from the S-lift in that the incision was radically different and customized, the undermining was more aggressive in the neck and temporal regions, the advancement vector was much steeper, and one large O-shaped purse-string was utilized for subcutaneous muscular aponeurotic system (SMAS) and platysmal tightening instead of a U-shaped and O-shaped purse-string (Fig. 48.1). These changes created better cosmetic results in the neck, jowl, and mid-face regions, which allowed the purse-string plication concept to move into the realm of treating individuals with more significant aesthetic problems (i.e., older patients).

Recently, the author revised the QuickLift™ with an encircling double purse-string plication technique (Fig. 48.2) that has been found to create better improvement of the mid-face and periorbital region; eliminate bulging of subcutaneous and SMAS tissue; provide stronger SMAS and platysmal support; and create a backup support in case one of the purse-strings pulls through [3]. This article also recommended liposuction of the neck and/or jowl with a 3-mm Coleman cannula combined with a submental tuck (Fig. 48.3). At the time of this writing the 1-year results have been extremely gratifying (Figs. 48.4, 48.5) with patient satisfaction being very high. In short, the QuickLift™ offers the advantage of being able to be performed in 1–2 h with local anesthesia, while creating significant long-term improvements in the neck, jowl, mid-face and periorbital regions, with minimal morbidity and complication.

Although the QuickLift™ does give significant facial and neck improvement, it does not address the degeneration of the brow, bone, fat and muscle that occurs with age. Ptosis of the lateral brow is especially one characteristic that creates an unattractive look as one ages. In the young patient it has been stated that the distance between the eyebrow and the mid pupil should be approximately 2.5 cm [4]. But as we all age this distance diminishes and starts to create the illusion that there is an excessive amount of skin on the upper eyelids. In fact, patients with sagging lateral brows usually mention excessive eyelid skin as their primary complaint, when in essence it is a ptotic lateral brow that is causing the problem.

This lateral forehead region is unique because it is the only area on the forehead that is void of musculature (Fig. 48.6) unlike the medial aspect, which is covered extensively by the frontalis muscle. This muscle is important in the context of facial aging because its contractile state helps keep the medial brow elevated in a more youthful position as one ages. Conversely, the lateral brow region has minimal musculature to help keep it in an elevated state. It is therefore more subject to skin photodamage and intrinsic skin aging. Because of these facts, the lateral brow is the first area to show the affects of aging and as this degenerative process continues, the lateral region usually sags more intensely than the medial aspect.

Because aging in the lateral forehead region is primarily a cutaneous problem, the author thinks that addressing skin only is the best and safest way to manipulate this area. This chapter describes a modification of previously reported subcutaneous browlifts [5–7] that can easily be added to the QuickLift™ procedure, without significantly increasing operative time or postoperative morbidity and complication.

48.2
Technique

At the consultation the consent forms are reviewed and the patient takes them home for further study. The night before the procedure the patient washes his/her hair and face with povidine shampoo and takes 1 mg of lorazepam before bedtime. In the morning the patient again washes the scalp and face with povidine shampoo and reports to the surgical facility. At the clinic the consent forms are again reviewed, questions answered, and the forms are signed. Diazepam (10 mg) is then administered orally, and a combination of 2.5 mg of midazolam and 50 mg of meperidine hydrochloride is given intramuscularly.

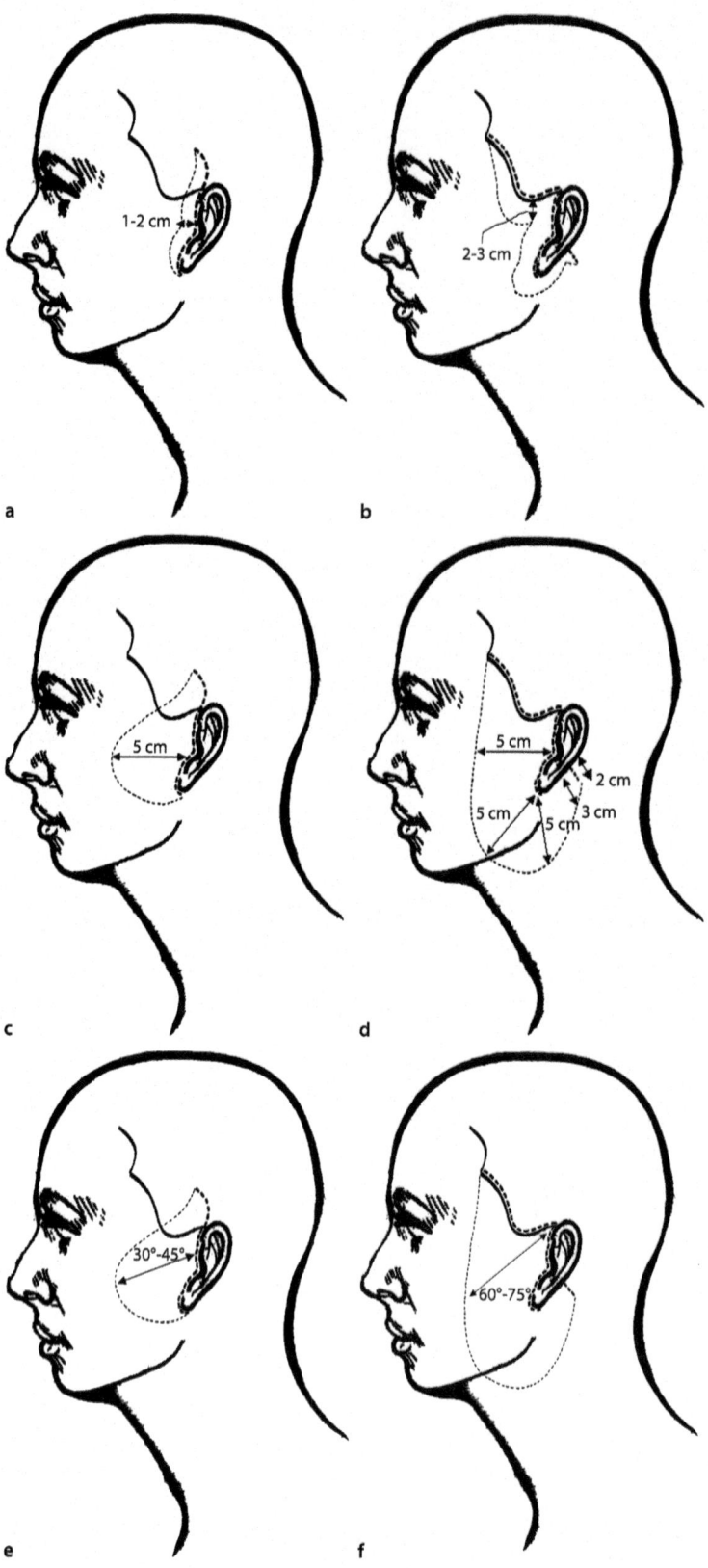

a

b

c

d

e

f

Fig. 48.1 a The S-lift incision is shaped like a lazy S and is extended into the temporal hair. Usually 1–2 cm of skin is removed at a 3045° angle. **b** The QuickLift™ incision extends 3 mm behind the temporal hairline to the most anterior aspect of the temporal peak. It also extends 4 cm along the posterior crease of the earlobe and has a hockey stick that follows Langer's lines. This incision is customized to the individual and allows for a 60–75° angle of advancement with 2–3 cm of skin removal throughout. **c** The S-lift undermining is 5 cm anterior to the incision with little to no undermining inferior to the earlobe. **d** The QuickLift™ undermining is 5 cm anterior to the tragus in the horizontal axis, 5 cm anterior to the earlobe (along the angle of the mandible) 5 cm inferior to the bottom of the earlobe and 1.5–2.5 cm below the hockey stick in the postauricular region. In the temporal region the undermining is usually 2.5 cm from the inferior aspect of the temporal hairline. **e** Because of the shape of the S-lift incision, the surgeon is primarily limited to a 30–45° angle of flap advancement. This fact limits the effect that can be accomplished at the cervical region. **f** The QuickLift™ incision allows for a 60–75° angle of flap advancement, which creates significant improvement in the neck region without aggressive undermining. This more superior advancement also prevents a pulled-back appearance and counters the normal gravitational downward pull of aging

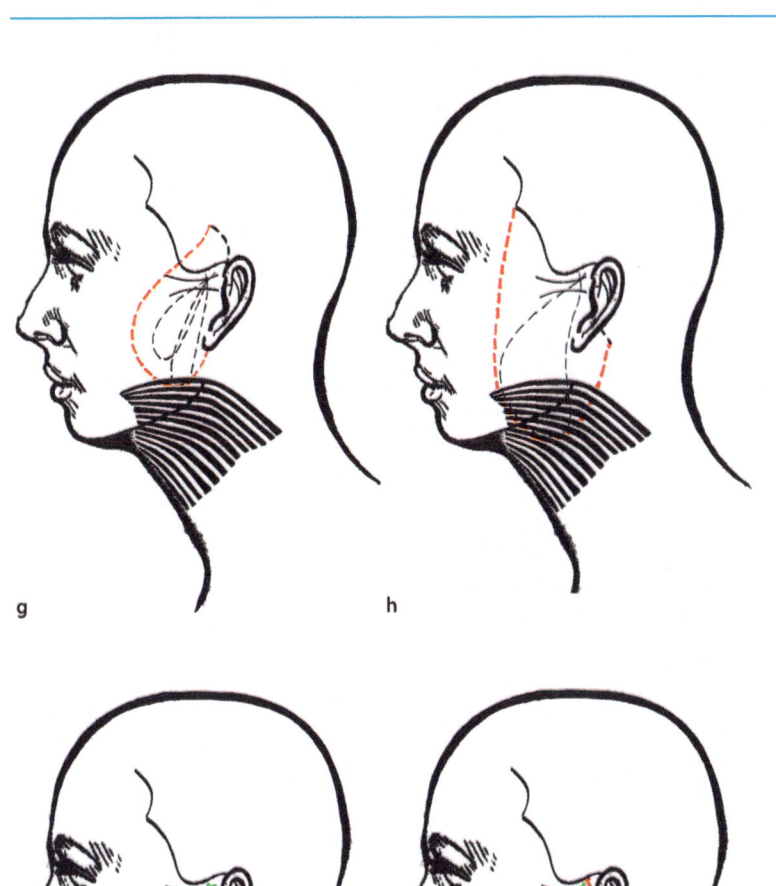

Fig. 48.1 *(continued)* **g** The S-lift purse-string plication consists of a deep 2-0 braided nylon anchor suture at the zygoma with a U-shaped and O-shaped purse-string applied to the subcutaneous muscular aponeurotic system (SMAS) and superior aspects of the platysma to create tightening of the subanatomy. **h** The original QuickLift™ purse-string consisted of one anchored large O-shaped purse-string that followed the area of undermining. There is a much greater degree of platysmal tightening and neck improvement with this approach

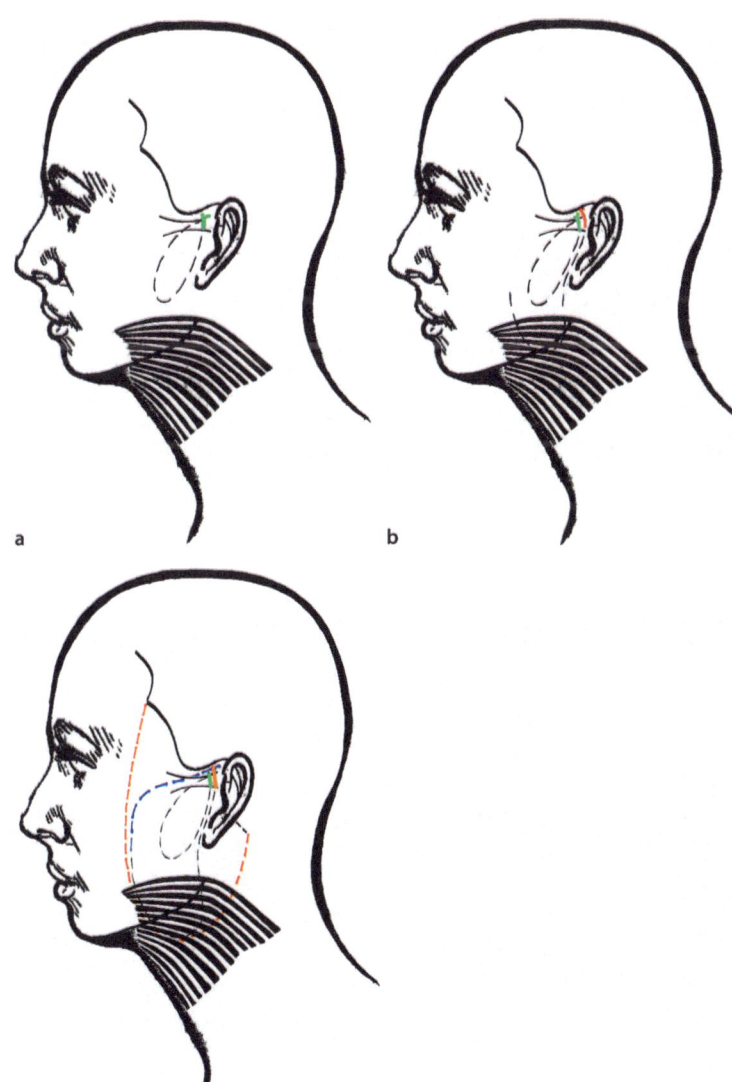

Fig. 48.2 **a** The newer encircling double purse-string plication technique involves first performing a 2-0 braided nylon anchor suture 1.5 cm away from the skin edge (indicated in *green*). This anchor suture is directly over the zygomatic arch, passes all the way to the bone and is 1.5 cm in length. Three to four more 1.5-cm superficial grasps of the SMAS are taken toward the bottom of the jowl, one 1.5-cm grasp is made perpendicular and medial to the latter, then five 1.5-cm grasps of the SMAS are made toward the anchor suture. Five throws of the suture are made and a 2-mm suture end is left. **b** The second 1.5-cm anchor suture (indicated by *red*) starts 3 mm superior and 3 mm lateral to the first anchor suture's knot. Four to five 1.5-cm-long grasps of the SMAS are made in a directly inferior direction. The next four 1.5-cm-long grasps will be of the platysma and should follow directly behind the edge of skin undermining. **c** The second purse-string differs from the original Quick-Lift™ purse-string in that the 1.5-cm SMAS grasps are continued more superiorly to affect the mid face (indicated by *blue*). Once the surgeon has reached the same height as the superior aspect of the second anchor suture, superficial grasps are made directly toward the second anchor suture. The last grasp of tissue before hitting the second anchor suture will be the third anchor suture and should be 3-mm deep (indicated by *orange*). The second and third anchor sutures will thus create a V-shaped anchoring point for the platysma, jowl and mid face

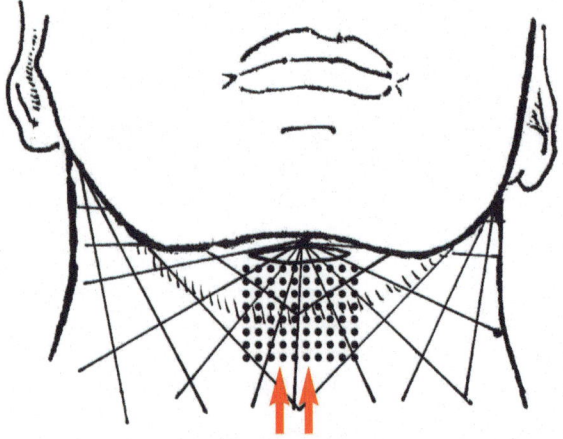

Fig. 48.3 The revised QuickLift™ involves liposuction of the neck and/or jowl with a 3-mm Coleman cannula combined with a submental tuck

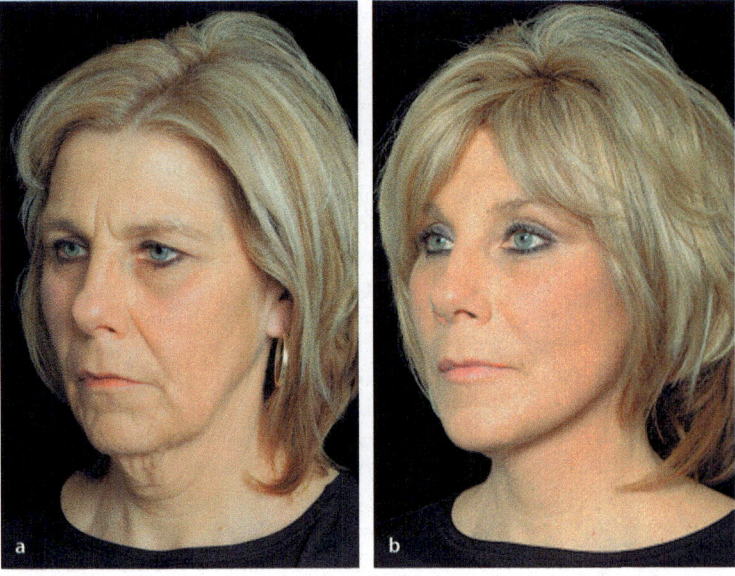

Fig. 48.4 a A patient before the QuickLift™ with the encircling double purse-string plication technique. **b** Twelve months after the procedure

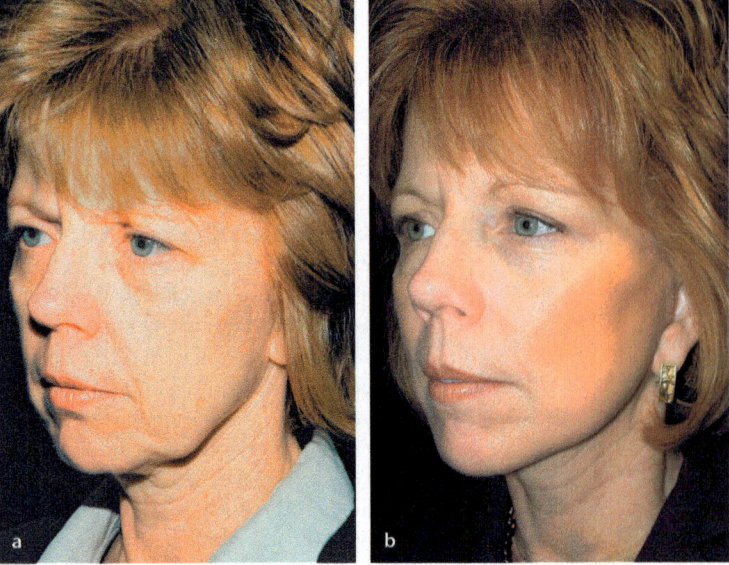

Fig. 48.5 a A patient before the QuickLift™ with the encircling double purse-string plication technique. **b** Fifteen months after the procedure

48.2.1
Marking

The scribing for the proposed incision line is then begun with a Pilot Marker®. This marker is utilized because it has been found to contain ink that gets the surgeon through the surgery without major portions of the markings being removed. The author utilizes a surgical technique that places the incision on the tragus (not posterior or anterior); therefore, the scribing is begun on the tragus. From that point, the anatomy of the ear is followed so that a straight line is not drawn in the preauricular region (Fig. 48.7). If one looks at Fig. 48.6, the marking moves in and out of the ear anatomy to create a meandering incision line. This wavering line makes the visibility of the postoperative scar very difficult to perceive.

In the area behind the ear, the marking is brought 2 mm above the earlobe crease for a distance of 4 cm and a hockey stick is drawn to project from that crease line in one of Langer's lines (Fig. 48.7). This hockey stick is usually 2.0 cm in length, but can be shorter or longer depending upon the amount of excess posterior neck skin available for Burrow's triangle excision during the procedure.

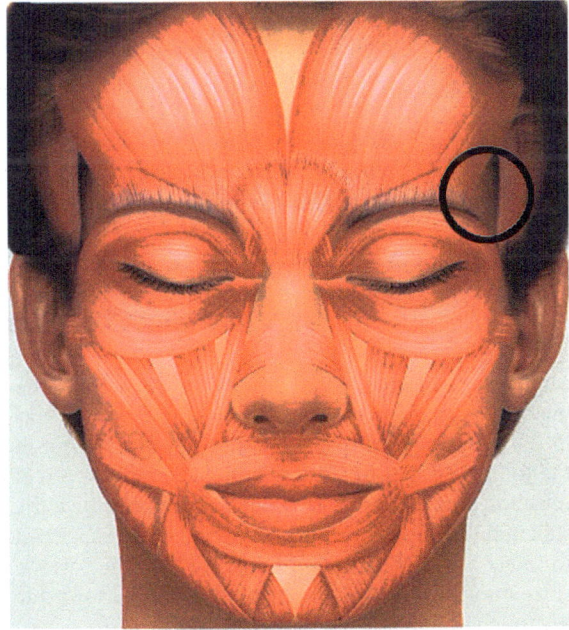

Fig. 48.6 The lateral forehead region has minimal musculature (indicated by the *circle*), which makes the lateral brow more prone to ptosis because there is no musculature to keep it in an elevated state. The lateral brow is thus very prone to sag secondary to skin photodamage and intrinsic dermal aging. Conversely, the medial forehead has the frontalis muscle, which keeps the brows fairly elevated throughout life because of its contractile state

From the top of the preauricular line (superior attachment of the ear), the line proceeds 3 mm behind the anterior edge of the temporal hairline all the way to the end of the temporal peak. It is critical that magnifying loupes be used at this point so that the temporal line is marked exactly 3 mm behind the anterior edge of any existing hair follicles. This distance has been chosen because it will normally contain enough hair follicles to make a 45° bevel technique effective at camouflaging the scar at a later time (Fig. 48.8). If a 45° bevel is begun 3 mm behind the anterior edge of the temporal hairline and a similar bevel is performed on opposite side, a significant number of hairs will be trapped beneath and anterior to the incision line upon closure (Fig. 48.8). Normally, these trapped hairs will go into anagen effluvium for 3 months owing to surgical trauma, but after this period of time, the follicles will start growing through and anterior to the scar (Fig. 48.8).

Once the temporal hairline aspect of incision has been marked, the lateral forehead incision is scribed. At this point the author has the patient raise his/her forehead, at which time the lateral forehead wrinkles are discerned. A line that follows Langer's lines (Fig. 48.7) is then drawn in red ink along one of the lateral forehead wrinkles (Fig. 48.9). This line can be easily extended from the temporal hairline incision. This red line is extended as far medially as needed to create the amount of elevation that is desired, but is always lateral to the supraorbital nerve and vessels. If one brow is slightly lower than the opposite brow, it is not uncommon to extend the incision above the lower brow slightly more medial. If both brows need to be raised equally, a point is drawn at the midline of the forehead, and it is made certain that the distance from the midline to the end of each forehead incision marking is equal.

After the red lines have been completed, the Pilot Marker® is used to draw a line above the red line in accordance with the amount of skin the surgeon judges should be removed above the given eyebrow. For example, if the surgeon predicts that 2 cm of skin will be removed at the lateral forehead, the Pilot Marker® blue line will be drawn in a fusiform shape 1 cm above the red line (Fig. 48.9). Conversely, if only 1 cm was predicted to be removed, the blue line is drawn 5 mm above the red line. This is done so that after the fusiform excision of excess lateral forehead skin, the incision line is exactly in the position of the former wrinkle.

The area of undermining is now scribed with a Bonnie Blue ink. A vertical line is drawn from the end of the red line to a point that is 1 cm below the inferior aspect of the brow (Fig. 48.9). The QuickLift™ undermining points are then drawn 5 cm anterior to the tragus incision line, 5 cm anterior to the earlobe along the angle of the mandible, and 5 cm inferior to the earlobe. These anterior points are connected with the Bonnie Blue ink and are then extended to meet the vertical line underneath the brow (Fig. 48.9). The point 5 cm below the

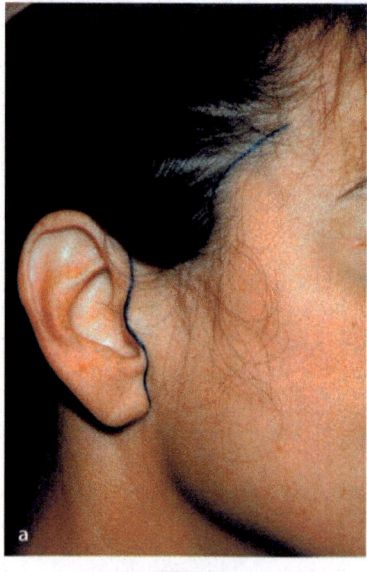
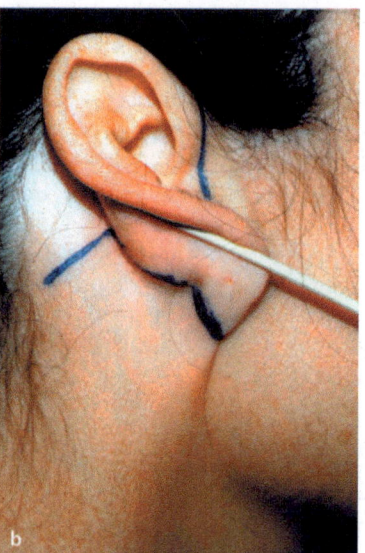
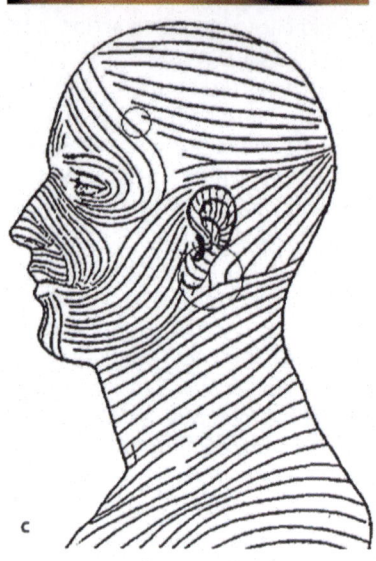

Fig. 48.7 a The markings are begun on the tragus and extend along the front the ear and 3 mm behind the temporal hairline. Notice how the line meanders along the anatomy of the ear. This creates a much less detectable scar. **b** The line is extended 2 mm above the posterior earlobe crease and is 4 cm in length. The hockey stick is usually 1.5–2.5 cm in length but will vary in size depending upon the amount of excessive posterior neck skin available for Burrow's triangle excision during the procedure. This line should be made in Langer's lines so that healing is optimal. **c** The hockey-stick and forehead incision usually heal extremely well because they follow Langer's lines

earlobe is then connected to the end of the hockey stick behind the ear.

If the patient is concerned about a scar in a forehead rhytid, one can extend the incision into the anterior hairline using the bevel technique (Fig. 48.9). Also, if the patient is concerned about a scar in a forehead rhytid and has a minimal brow ptosis problem, one can extend normal undermining to the lateral brow from the normal QuickLift™ incision (Fig. 48.9), so that a mild superior lateral elevation is achieved.

48.2.2
Surgery

The patient is brought into the operating room, at which time the face is prepped with povidone solution. The area to be undermined is infiltrated with 0.2% lido-

caine hydrochloride with 1:200,000 epinephrine utilizing a 21-gauge spinal needle and making certain to stay in the subcutaneous space. It is also important to push the solution slowly because it is often the rapid speed of injection that causes most of the discomfort. Once the subcutaneous space has been injected, it is important to inject along the incision lines and into the earlobe since hooks will be used to manipulate the earlobe during much of the procedure.

The incision is begun at the most medial aspect of the right forehead marking. At the onset, the no. 15 blade is held with an inward 45° bevel so that maximal eversion will be accomplished at the forehead wrinkle at the time of closure. However, when the temporal hairline is reached, it is critical to change the bevel to a 45° angle in the opposite direction, so that the hair follicles anterior to the incision will be preserved (Fig. 48.8). This latter bevel continues up to the superior aspect of the attach-

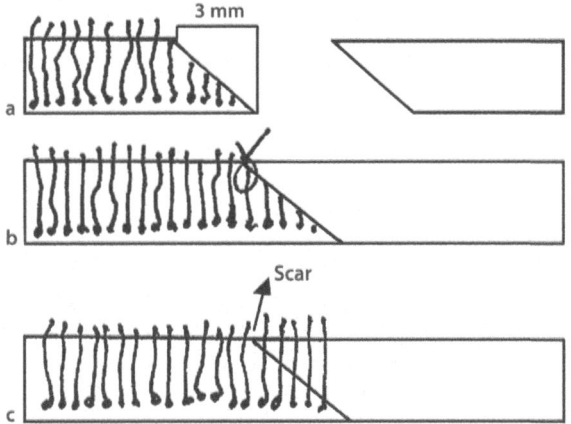

Fig. 48.8 a A 45° beveled incision is made 3 mm behind the anterior edge of the temporal hairline. This bevel will trap many hair follicles beneath the scar and the area anterior to it. The opposite side should also be beveled in the same direction when the excess skin is removed during the procedure. **b** When the skin edges are approximated, notice how the hair matrices are trapped below and anterior to the sutured incision. It is imperative that these incisions be closed with ×2.5–3.5 magnification under minimal tension for this technique to work well. **c** In 3 months (after anagen effluvium is completed) hair will start growing through and anterior to the scar line

ment of the pinna. At this point, the bevel is changed to the opposite direction throughout the remainder of the incision (anterior to the ear, inferior and posterior to the earlobe). Once again, this is done to create maximal eversion upon closure, which will improve the cosmetics of the scar.

Undermining is begun with a no. 15 blade in the V-shaped area at the superior aspect of the ear and is continued for 1 cm down to the anterior aspect of the earlobe. Once this has been accomplished, the superior V-shaped aspect of this newly created flap is grasped with a Lahey clamp and pulled away from the temporal forehead region and toward the surgeon. As this vector of tension is created with the Lahey clamp, undermining is performed with a facelift scissor in the area immediately above the zygoma and continues toward the most medial aspect of the forehead incision. The assistant spreads with his/her fingers on the lateral forehead skin and pulls the lower brow away from the surgeon with the thumbs. This tension helps keep the skin turgid so that accurate undermning can be performed in the forehead region. The forehead undermining is performed with the tips of the facelift scissors pointing upward to avoid the temporal branch of the facial nerve. Tunnels are made 1 cm apart and the 1-cm bridges are then cut with facelift scissors with the points facing upward. It is important to undermine 1 cm below the inferior aspect

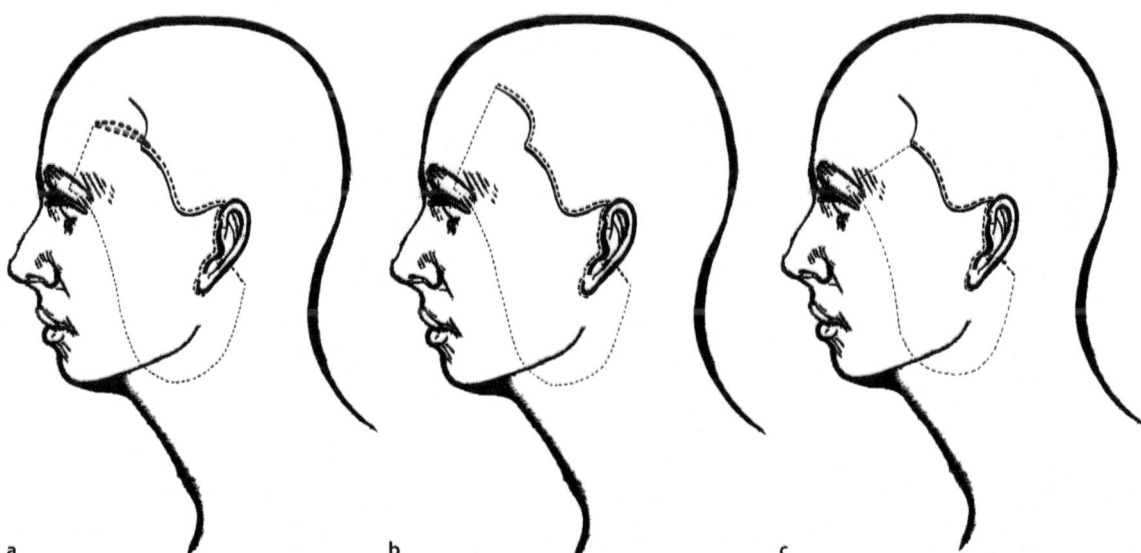

Fig. 48.9 a The patient is asked to raise his/her forehead and a lateral forehead rhytid is chosen for the lateral forehead extension of the QuickLift™. This wrinkle is drawn in red. After the amount of forehead skin excision has been predicted, a blue line is drawn above the red line so that the final incision, after fusiform excision, will end up exactly at this red wrinkle line. The undermining should be 1 cm below the inferior border of the brow, 5 cm anterior to the tragus parallel to the floor, 5 cm anterior to the earlobe along the mandible, 5 cm directly inferior to the earlobe and 1.5–2.5 cm away from the earlobe crease. **b** If the patient is concerned about a scar in the forehead crease, the incision can be brought up along the anterior hairline. **c** If the patient is concerned about a scar in the forehead and has a minimal lateral brow ptosis, one can undermine over from the conventional QuickLift™ incision and slightly raise the lateral brow

of the lateral brow so that the scarring mechanisms will keep the brow in its new position.

Once the forehead undermining is complete, the remainder of the facial undermining is performed similarly with facelift scissors; with the tips of the scissors primarily facing downward. The most critical aspect of the remaining undermining is to make certain that the flap is thick at the predicted site where the V-shaped advanced flap opposes the scalp at the superior attachment of the pinna. It is not unusual for the author to actually draw this area preoperatively. This region is most susceptible to necrosis and should be as thick as possible.

Undermining in the area below and behind the earlobe is performed with the tips of the scissors primarily pointing upward. This position of the tips of the scissors helps undermining go more quickly and prevents injury to the greater auricular nerve. Upon completion of all of the aforementioned undermining, thorough hemostasis is accomplished throughout.

At this point in the procedure, the encircling double purse-string SMAS plication is performed (Fig. 48.2). But before this aspect is completed, the author injects a combination of 1% lidocaine hydrochloride and 0.25% bupivocaine into the site of the anchor sutures. These injections are performed with a 1-in. 30-gauge needle and are extended all the way down to the zygomatic arch 1.5 cm away from the skin edge of the tragus. The initial 2.0 braided nylon anchoring suture is placed 1.5 cm away from the skin edge, directly over the zygomatic arch (indicated by green in Fig. 48.2). The suture needle should go down to bone and should grasp a 1.5-cm length of tissue. Three 1.5-cm long, more superficial grasps of the SMAS are then taken toward the inferior aspect of the jowl. One 1.5-cm grasp is made perpendicular to the latter suture and subsequently five 1.5-cm grasps are taken back to the original anchor point. Five throws are made to create a firm knot and a 2-mm tag is left in place (Fig. 48.2).

The second anchoring 2-0 braided nylon stitch is now performed (noted by red in Fig. 48.2b). The needle enters 3 mm above and 3 mm medial to the knot of the first purse-string. This anchor suture is deep over the zygoma, similar to the first anchor suture. Four to five 1.5-cm-long grasps of the SMAS are taken in a directly inferior direction (Fig. 48.2). The remainder of the 1.5-cm-long grasps follow the outer edge of the undermined zone toward the perioribital region. The first four grasps along the line of undermining will tighten the platysma, with the remaining grasps tightening the SMAS.

When the second purse-string arrives at the same height as its origin anchor suture (noted in blue), 1.5-cm grasps of the SMAS are made toward this higher anchor suture (3 mm above the first anchor suture). The last grasp, before meeting the second anchor suture, should be a third anchor suture creating a V-shaped double

anchoring point for the larger second purse-string suture (noted by orange in Fig. 48.2c). This third anchor suture is not as deep as the first two but should at least be 3-mm deep. Once again, five throws of the suture are made and a 2-mm suture end is left.

Once the encircling double purse-string has been completed, thorough hemostasis is accomplished and the excess skin is excised. The step during the skin removal is to grab the V-shaped area at the superior insertion of the ear with a Lahey clamp and mildly pull in a superior direction. The author looks underneath the skin and marks where the line of excision will be. An inwardly beveled incision is then made at this marking and the skin edges are temporarily stapled together. The author then applies a D'Assumpaceo clamp to the scalp and superior forehead edge and sees how much advancement should be performed at the forehead region. Marks are made with the D'Assumpaceo clamp and the author makes a line connecting the indentations made by the clamp. An incision is then made at the forehead line with a 45° inward bevel for eversion and this bevel is continued throughout the temporal hair (Fig. 48.8). These skin edges are then temporarily stapled together.

The remainder of the facelift is done by advancing small segments, looking underneath to evaluate advancement, drawing the appropriate lines, excising, and stapling. At the region behind the earlobe the skin is advanced as firmly as possible, then a Burrow's triangle is created to removed this excess skin. The length of the hockey stick will depend on the amount of skin that is removed (the more skin removed, the longer the hockey stick).

After all areas have been stapled in their appropriate positions, the staples are removed one by one and are replaced by deep 5-0 PDS sutures. The lateral forehead sutures are the most important in this procedure. The initial three deep sutures (Fig. 48.10) are tacked down to the periosteum. The remaining deep sutures from the temporal hairline to the superior attachment of the ear are tacked down to the temporalis fascia (Fig. 48.10). These tacking sutures are critical for stabilization and anchoring of the superior forehead and scalp. Once these have been completed, the 5-0 PDS sutures are inserted throughout the length of the remaining incision. After all deep sutures have been placed, the skin is sutured with a running 6-0 fast absorbing gut under ×2.5 magnification. A mild pressure dressing is applied and the patient is seen the next day. At 1 week, the patient can apply water-based makeup to all incision sites.

If a patient desires a lateral subcutaneous browlift with no QuickLift™, the incision should begin at the superior aspect of the pinna and should extend into a forehead rhytid, the anterior hairline or the most anterior aspect of the temporal peak (Fig. 48.11).

The technique was retrospectively analyzed by photography and satisfaction levels of 28 patients over an

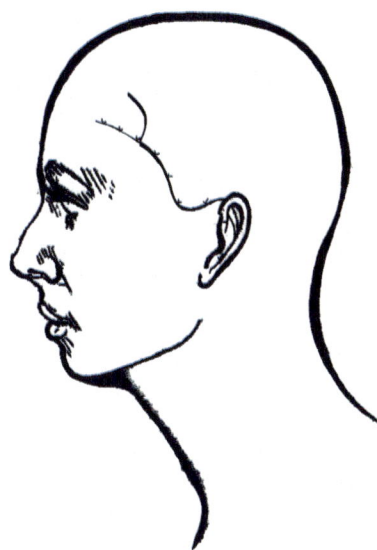

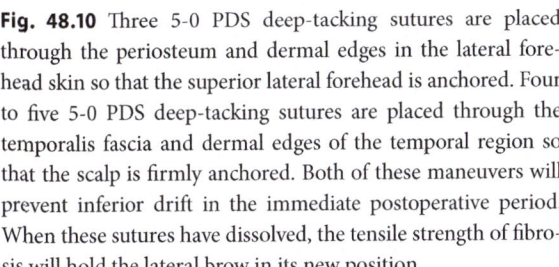

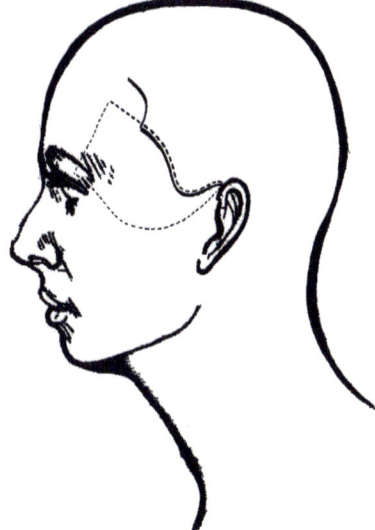

Fig. 48.10 Three 5-0 PDS deep-tacking sutures are placed through the periosteum and dermal edges in the lateral forehead skin so that the superior lateral forehead is anchored. Four to five 5-0 PDS deep-tacking sutures are placed through the temporalis fascia and dermal edges of the temporal region so that the scalp is firmly anchored. Both of these maneuvers will prevent inferior drift in the immediate postoperative period. When these sutures have dissolved, the tensile strength of fibrosis will hold the lateral brow in its new position

Fig. 48.11 If a patient desires a lateral subcutaneous browlift with no QuickLift™, the incision should begin at the superior aspect of the pinna and should extend into a forehead rhytid, the anterior hairline or the most anterior aspect of the temporal peak

18-month period. Overall, the satisfaction rate was extremely high, short and long-term.

48.3
Complications

All patients who had a cutaneous browlift with the QuickLift™ experienced some upper-eyelid ecchymoses in the immediate postoperative period, but these usually resolved within 2 weeks. There was one case of a small necrosis (smaller than 1 cm²) that was near the incision line at the temporal hairline and healed spontaneously without any corrective action being required. When the QuickLift™ was performed without the browlift ($n = 812$), there was a 1.0% incidence of necrosis (larger than 1 cm²) at the preauricular area. When liposuction and submental tuck were added to the procedure, the incidence was 3.5%. There were four cases of cellulitis that resolved quickly with antibiotics and one temporary buccal nerve paresis. All patients had areas of temporary anesthesia that resolved in approximately 3 months. The incidence of hematoma that needed evacuation was 0.5% ($n = 4$).

Because the results have been so good, the author now performs this lateral cutaneous browlift on ap-

proximately 5% of his QuickLift™ patients. The results have been especially gratifying to the patients and to the author.

48.4
Discussion

Browlifts are primarily classified according to the plane of dissection and the way of entering the given plane of dissection. The three primary planes of dissection are:
1. Subperiosteal
2. Subgaleal
3. Subcutaneous

The five primary locations for entering the plane of dissection are:
1. Behind the hairline (bicoronal, temporal or endoscopic)
2. Hairline incision
3. Mid forehead
4. Suprabrow
5. Upper eyelid (browpexy)

Friedland et. al. [8] preferred to categorize browlifts into four generations: the first is limited to direct skin excisions without extensive undermining; the second is a bicoronal approach with subgaleal separation and musculature modification; the third is extensive subperiosteal dissection; and the fourth is the endoscopic approach with various planes of dissection .

In most recent years, the main goal of cosmetic surgeons had been to limit the long scar of the bicoronal and hairline approaches. Thus, the endoscopic approach has had significant emphasis during the past 20 years. This technique requires only three to five different short scars, but also requires expensive endoscopic equipment with intensive training. Many different planes for dissection can be utilized and various ways for anchoring the soft tissue to the scalp and skull have been widely discussed in the literature [9–13]. All of this expense and training toward limiting the scar length, however, can lead to unsatisfied patients owing to early recurrence of brow ptosis secondary to limited exposure, inadequate shrinkage of the scalp, or failure of the anchoring system.

Connell [14] made the anterior hairline incision popular, but his plane of dissection was subgaleal. His claim was that the hairline incision prevented the danger of causing alopecia. Beveling the incision at a 45° angle spares hair follicles and causes hair follicles buried underneath the incision to start growing through the scar 3 months after the procedure (Fig. 48.8).

Ullmann and Levy [5, 7] further emphasized the anterior hairline approach, but they performed their dissection in a subcutaneous plane. They felt that the subcutaneous approach offered better results with the added benefit of the prevention of persistent scalp anesthesia and paresthesia commonly recorded after the subgaleal approach [6]. According to Ullmann and Levy the most important advantage of undermining in the subcutaneous plane is that it prevents the most frightening complication of all—facial temporal nerve injury.

The author's approach incorporates both the beveled hairline approach with the mid-forehead approach by extending the beveled temporal incision in one of the lateral forehead wrinkles. As previously alluded to, intrinsic skin aging and photoaging are the primary causes of lateral forehead aging. It is the author contention that the periosteum and galea are not significant aspects to lateral forehead aging. It therefore makes little sense to put the patient at increase risk and make the procedure more difficult, if the main component of lateral forehead aging is skin, not periosteum or galea.

One question that the author has received from observers of this technique is "Why can't the incision be made to extend along the temporal hairline into the frontal hairline instead of being brought into a lateral forehead wrinkle?" That approach can be utilized and is the approach that has been utilized by other surgeons (Fig. 48.9) [5–7]. In fact, if the patient has concerns about the forehead scar, the hairline approach is utilized. Also, if the ptosis is minimal, the undermining to the lateral brow can be reached from the normal QuickLift™ incision (Fig. 48.9). It is the opinion of the author that the closer one is to the area that he/she is trying to affect, the better the result that will be accomplished. For example, if one were performing a medial thigh lift, the results nearer to the incision line would be much better than the areas closer to the knee. Likewise, during a browlift, the closer the incision is to the brows, the better and more permanent the uplift.

The forehead scar should not be a problem if one uses an effective eversion technique, makes certain that the incision is directly in a wrinkle line and uses at least ×2.5 magnification for closure. The scars should be barely perceptible with the naked eye at a 3-month period from the time of the procedure if the precautions are taken. Therefore the risk-to-benefit ratio is much in favor of the benefit. Also, patients can start applying makeup over the incision at 1 week. At 4 weeks, dermabrasion or laser resurfacing can be performed if it is felt necessary. Additionally, the forehead incision is rarely used on patients under 50 years of age because scar formation is well known to be more intense in patients younger than 50.

Looking at the longevity of the procedure, it appears that this approach gives as good a lasting effect as any browlifting procedure to date. The mechanism for this is that the brow is totally detached 1 cm below its inferior border, and is elevated into a new position with the scarring mechanisms holding the brow in this new position. The tacking sutures in the periosteum and temporalis fascia are also very important because they keep the skin from drifting inferiorly in the immediate postoperative period. After 1–2 months, fibrosis will take over to keep the brow in its newly elevated position.

If the patient desires a lateral subcutaneous browlift without the QuickLift™, the incision begins at the superior aspect of the pinna and extends superiorly into the forehead rhytid, the anterior hairline or the anterior aspect of the temporal peak (Fig. 48.11). When browlifting is not performed, the results have also been extremely good and long-lasting. The author feels strongly that neck liposuction with a submental tuck adds longevity to the procedure through anterioposterior skin removal and increased fibrosis.

48.5
Conclusions

The technique describes a lateral cutaneous browlift that is extended into a lateral forehead wrinkle from the QuickLift™ incision. The browlift can also be performed from the QuickLift™ incision without an extension (mild ptosis) or alone without the QuickLift™. Because there is no musculature with its concomitant contractile activity in the lateral forehead region, aging of the lateral forehead is much more aggressive than that of the medial forehead and this aging is primarily cutaneous in nature. The author therefore believes that lateral brow ptosis should be treated with a lateral subcutaneous lift rather than a more dangerous subgaleal or subperiosteal approach. When a lateral cutaneous browlift is not performed with the QuickLift™ for indicated patients, the results have also been very gratifying to the patient and physician.

In this era of deep-plane forehead undermining with its concomitant morbidity and complication, the concept of subcutaneous forehead lift is introduced that is combined with the QuickLift™. This combined approach has created consistently excellent results while being safe, reproducible and long-lasting. The Quick-Lift™ offers a modification of the S-lift that gives results that are comparable with those of an extensive facelift without the downtime and morbidity.

References

1. Saylan Z: The S-lift for facial rejuvenation, Int J Cosmet Surg 1999;7(1):18–23

2. Brandy DA: The QuickLift: A modification of the S-lift. Cosmet Dermatol 2004;17:251–360

3. Brandy DA: The Quicklift™: Featuring an encircling double purse-string plication technique with blunt neck/jowl undermining for tightening of the sagging SMAS, platysma and skin. Am J Cosmet Surg 2005;22(4):223–232

4. McKinney P, Mossie RD, Zukowski M: Criteria for the forehead lift. Aesthet Plast Surg 1991;15(2):141–147

5. Ullmann Y, Levy Y: In favor of the subcutaneous forehead lift using the anterior hairline incision. Aesthet Plast Surg 1998;22(5):332–337

6. Vogel JE, Hoopes JE: The subcutaneous forehead lift with anterior hairline incision. Ann Plast Surg 1992;28(3):257–265

7. Ullmann Y, Levy Y: Superextended facelift: our experience with 3,580 patients. Ann Plast Surg 2004;52(1):8–14

8. Friedland JA, Jacobsen WM, TerKonda S: Safety and efficacy of combined upper blepharoplasties and open coronal browlift. A consecutive series of 600 patients. Aesthet Plast Surg 1996;20(6):453–462

9. Vasconez LO, Core GB, Gamboa-Babadilla M, Guzman G, Askern C, Yamamoto Y: Endoscopic techniques in coronal brow lifting. Plast Reconstr Surg 1994;94(6):788–793

10. Toledo LS: Video-endoscopic facelift. Aesthet Plast Surg 1994;18(2):149–152

11. Ramirez OM: The anchor subperiosteal forehead lift. Plast Reconstr Surg 1995;95(6):993–1003

12. Ramirez OM, Pozner JM: Subperiosteal minimally invasive laser endoscopic rhytidectomy: The SMILE facelift. Aesthet Plast Surg 1996;20(6):463–470

13. Toranto IR: The subperiosteal forehead lift. Clin Plast Surg 1992;19(2):477–485

14. Connell B: Brow ptosis. Local resections. 3rd International Symposium on Plastic and Reconstructive Surgery of the Eye and Adnexa. Williams and Wilkins: Baltimore 1982:338

CHAPTER 49

The Curl Lift Combined with Skin Resurfacing

James E. Fulton Jr.

49.1
Introduction

It would be helpful to have a safe and effective method to reverse the early signs of facial laxity. This early sagging of the jowls, eyebrows, and neck does not require a full facelift. The curl lift provides a good alternative for lifting the face and returning to work in 1 week [1]. This procedure can also be combined with chemical peels [2] or laser resurfacing [3], treatment of the anterior neck [4], augmentation with adipose tissue [5], a browlift, or blepharoplasty [6].

49.2
Method

49.2.1
Informed Consent

The risks and benefits of the procedure and the alternatives are reviewed with the patient. Photographs are taken and blood tests, including complete blood count, chemical profile, hepatitis screen, HIV, prothrombin time, partial thromboplastin time, and bleeding time, are done. The patient signs the informed consent form and all questions are answered. The patient is told to avoid aspirin, vitamin E, and nonsteroidal anti-inflammatory drugs for 10 days before and after the procedure. The patient is also instructed to wash the face and scalp the night before and the morning of the procedure with liquid antibacterial soap. The patient is given a prescription for antibiotics (cephalexin, 500 mg, twice a day) and antiviral medications if skin resurfacing is done (famciclovir, 500 mg, three times a day) for the 7 days following the surgery.

49.2.2
Skin Resurfacing (Optional)

If skin resurfacing is planned along with the curl lift, it is done at this time. The combination of Jessner solution and trichloroacetic acid gives a safe and effective peel for rejuvenation [7], or if further rejuvenation is

needed, the Ultrapulse CO_2 laser is used [8]. Some patients with acne or traumatic scars may require laser-assisted chemabrasion [9].

49.2.3
Treatment of the Anterior Neck (Optional)

Rejuvenation of the anterior neck is completed at this time if the submental fat pad or the platysma bands are significant (Fig. 49.1) [4]. After infusion of the modified tumescent solution (Table 49.1) [10], liposuction and/or plication with a running locked braided nylon suture (4-0) of the anterior platysma bands is completed. Bands below the line of placation are excised. Hemostasis is achieved. The incision site is left open until the end of the procedure to permit a second look. Then the site is closed with 5-0 polyethylene interrupted sutures.

49.2.4
The Curl-Lift Procedure

The first step is to draw an accurate diagram of the extent of the curl lift. After pinching and marking, the lines are drawn in the direction of the lift (Fig. 49.2). To facilitate the lifting, three or four key sutures are planned. These landmark sutures are placed deep into the fascia in the hairline and/or at the zygoma. The incision points A and B are injected with local anesthetic, 2% lidocaine with epinephrine (1:200,000). The temple, cheek, and lateral neck lines are then hydrodissected with 50–100 ml of modified tumescent solution (Table 49.1, Fig. 49.3) [10]. After a 15-min waiting period, a

Table 49.1 Modified tumescent solution

Lactated Ringer's solution	500 ml
Lidocaine	25 ml
Epinephrine (1:1,000)[a]	2.5 ml

[a]The result is an epinephrine concentration of 1:250,000. This may be diluted further for a thinner or older patient who may be sensitive to epinephrine

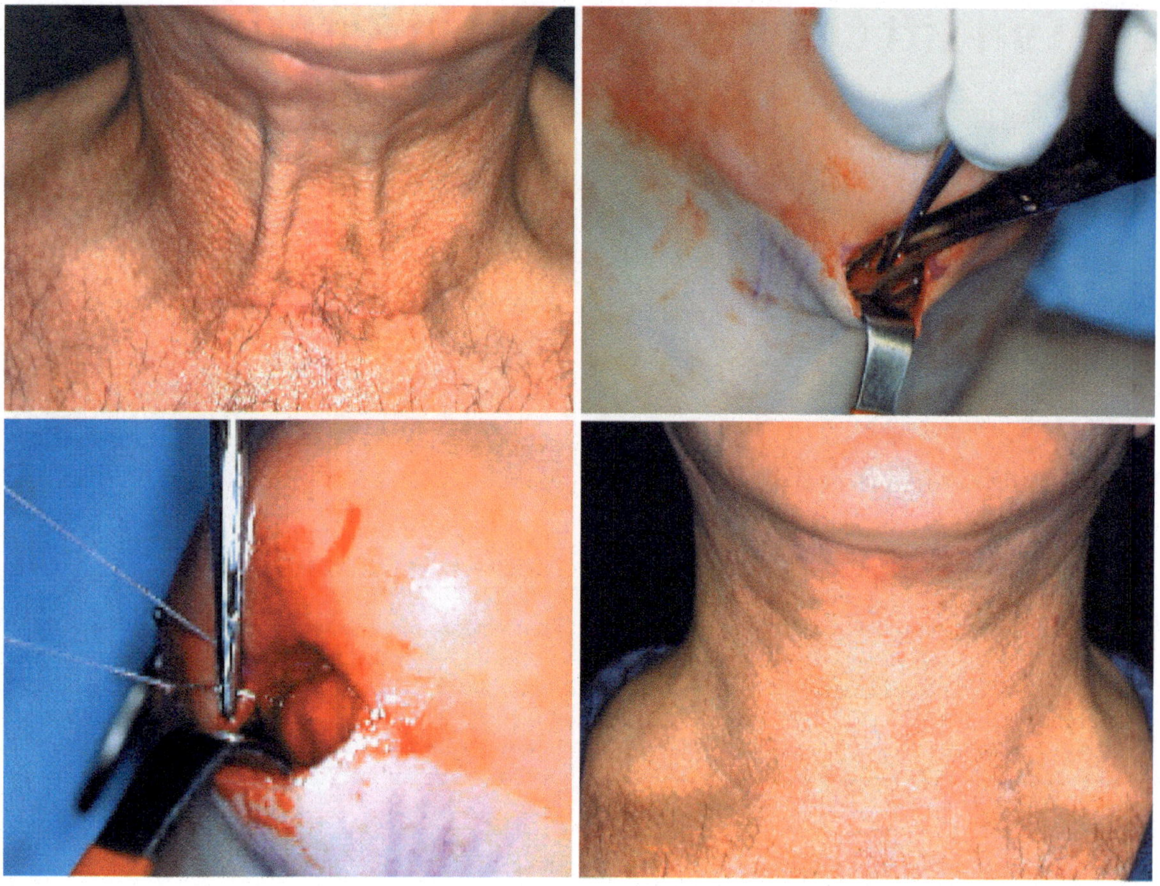

Fig. 49.1 The platysmaplasty provides a support for the curl lift

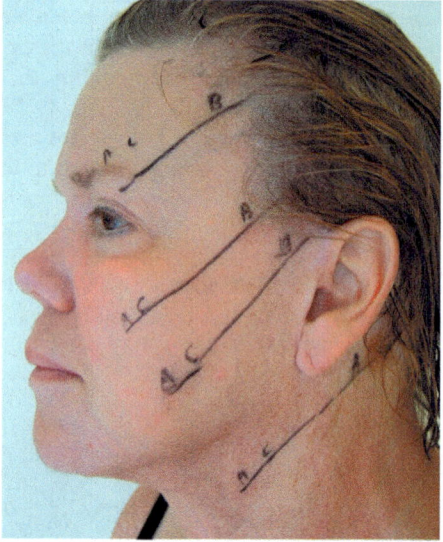

Fig. 49.2 The markings for the curl lift. The skin anterior to the zygoma, anterior to the temporal, and the mastoid fascia are marked *A*, *B*, and *C*

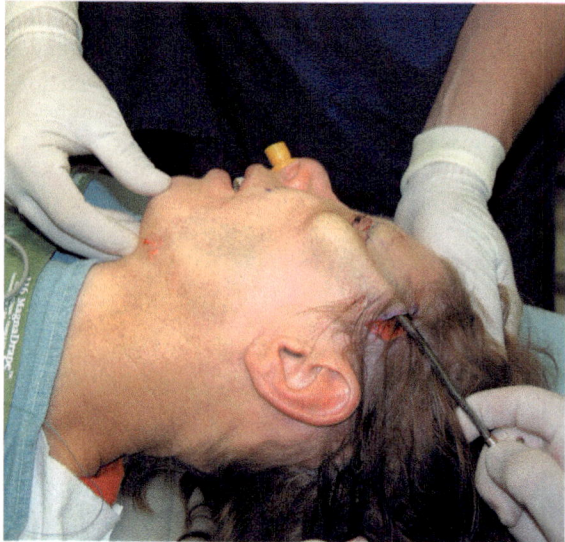

Fig. 49.3 Tumescent infiltration. The lateral cheek is hydrodissected with the modified tumescent solution. To provide extra vasoconstriction the epinephrine concentration is increased to 1:250,000

subcutaneous tract is developed from point A to point B with a 1.5-mm × 15-cm Newport cannula. This blunt dissection elevates the natural trabeculae of the face. Reduced-pressure liposuction is used, if necessary, to reduce large fat pads in the jowl area [11]. At point B the cannula tip is loaded with a 3-0 braided polyglactin 910 suture and a 3-0 polyethylene suture. The Newport cannula is pulled back to point C and, then, rotated (the curl) 180° and returned to point B. The sutures are released from the cannula. The cannula is removed. The resulting lift is tested. The braided polyglactin suture is used as a dissector to loosen up any fascial depressions before suturing both sutures into the deep fascia with a curved needle.

The skin incisions are then approximated with 5-0 polyethylene sutures or staples.

49.2.5
Postoperative Dressings

Following the procedure, a dressing is applied over the suture sites. If the face has been resurfaced with the CO_2 laser or dermabrasion, silicon sheeting is applied to the deepithelialized tissue [12]. Surgical tube gauze no. 6 is applied to yield positive pressure. The patient is moved to the recovery station and reminded as he/she is discharged to avoid any unnecessary coughing or straining. The patient comes in the next day for the dressings to be checked and a new tube gauze to be put on. Tube gauze is changed daily for 3–4 days. After this, the dressing is removed and gentamycin ointment is applied to the suture lines with a cotton-tipped applicator to keep crusts from forming. The superficial sutures are removed in 7 days. The patient continues to apply the ointment to the suture line as needed. After 3 days the patient begins walking exercises and returns to work in 1 week.

49.3
Results

The curl lift provided a lift to the temporal, jawline, and neck area in the 23 cases studied (Fig. 49.4). There was rejuvenation, especially when combined with skin resurfacing such as chemical peel in 12 patients (52%) (Fig. 49.5) or laser resurfacing in eight patients (35%) (Fig. 49.6). Adipose tissue augmentation also filled out the central compartment of the face in 16 patients (70%).

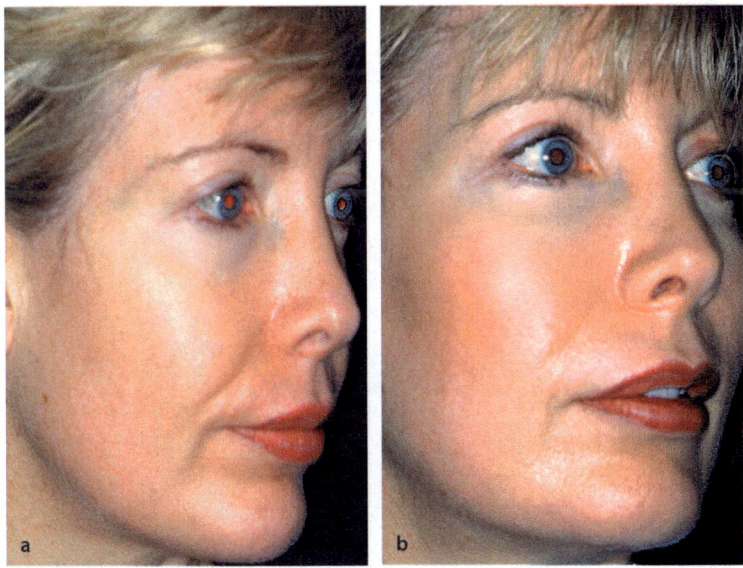

Fig. 49.4 a Before procedure. **b** After procedure. Note the elevated nasolabial fold and accentuated cheekbone area

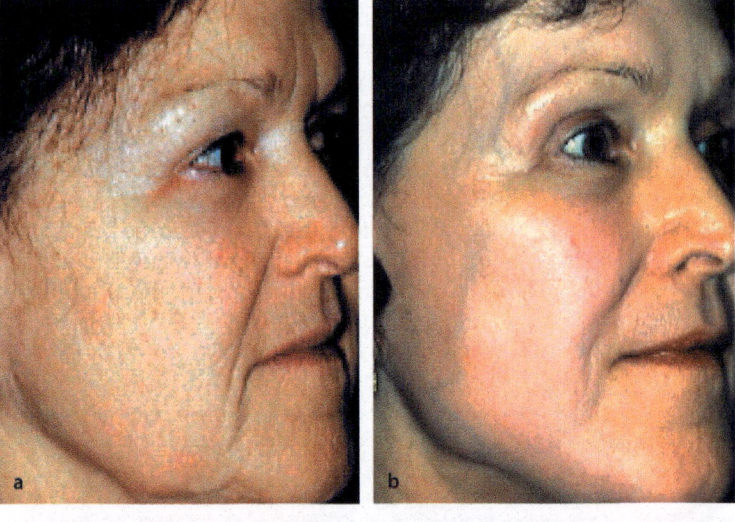

Fig. 49.5 a Before procedure. **b** After procedure. In addition to the curl lift the skin is often freshened with a Jessner solution–trichloroacetic acid peel and/or dermabrasion

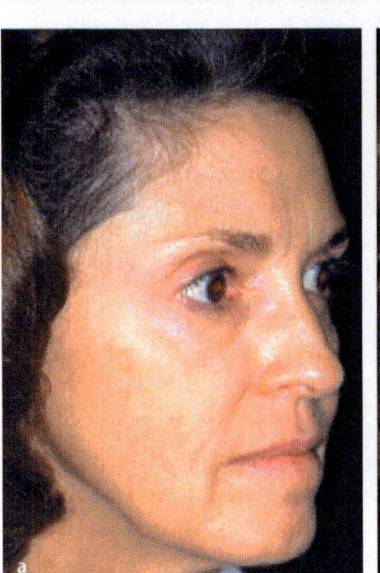
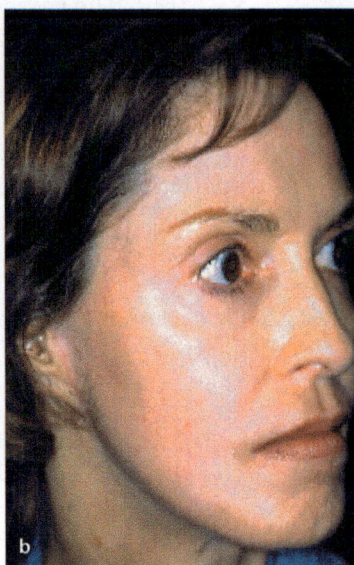

Fig. 49.6 a Before procedure. **b** After procedure. A more dramatic change is noticed when the curl lift is combined with CO_2 laser resurfacing

49.4
Complications

Complications have been minimal (Table 49.2). No seromas or hematomas have developed. Crusting was evident at the sites of the skin sutures until we began to use occlusive dressings. Then this problem diminished. Several patients had dysesthesias in suture areas that resolved over several weeks. One patient developed intermittent, unilateral spasms of the massester muscle that also resolved after 2 weeks. There has been no flap necrosis, loss of skin texture, or dyspigmentations. During the 6-month follow-up period there has been no recurrence of the tissue laxity, indicating that the curl-lift sutures have remained intact.

Table 49.2 Complications of the curl lift (summary of 23 cases)

Type	Percentage
Persistent edema[a]	26
Ecchymoses	22
Dysesthesias	17
Hematomas	8
Massester spasm	4
Suture spitting	4
Skin slough	0

[a]Significant edema lasting more than 2 weeks

49.5
Discussion

The curl lift combines a facial rejuvenation with short recovery periods. This has been especially important with busy patients who must be back at work in 1 week. The face may still look puffy at this point; however, this appearance gradually softens in the following weeks. This fullness has not been a problem for these patients returning to work and often is a conversation piece leading to patient referrals. The procedure is often combined with skin resurfacing (87%). The chemical peel is used for those patients who prefer a fresher look; laser resurfacing and/or dermabrasion is chosen for more dramatic rejuvenation.

The complications have been minimal as this surgery is not extensive. There has been no skin necrosis. No large hematomas, seromas, or infections have developed. This technique appears to the patient as a minor surgery compared with a full facelift. There is avid patient interest in these lesser procedures as opposed to full facelift where the patients are nervous and concerned about extensive recovery, skin texture changes, and loss of work.

The key to the success of the procedure is the internal suturing. The sutures elevate the neck, jowls, and temporal areas. There are no tragal pulldowns or earlobe deformities. These sutures are safe, as they are placed laterally where there are no superficial motor nerves. Other adjuncts are the hydrodissection with tumescent solution and liposuction at reduced pressure, if necessary. The 2.0-mm Newport cannula opens the pocket in the fatty subcutaneous plane and guides the placement of the sutures. We have found that the instrument is also useful whenever blunt dissection is needed.

The author combines the method with monitored anesthesia care anesthesia. Intravenous sedation with Propofol does not depress the central respiratory center and there is no significant nausea and vomiting after the procedure. Reduced-pressure liposuction debulks the submental area without excessive tissue trauma or bleeding. The placation of the anterior platysma bands provides a sling to support the bilateral sutures.

49.6
Conclusions

The curl lift combined with skin resurfacing is less demanding on the surgeon and the patient. The time in the operating room is about 1–2 h instead of the 4–6 h often required for a conventional facelift. Complications are lessened. The patient returns to work in 1 week with an improved profile.

Before attempting this procedure the physician must visit a surgeon doing this technique.

References

1. Sulamanidge MA, Fournier PF, Paikidz TG, Sulamanidze GM. Removal of facial soft tissue ptosis with special threads. Dermatol Surg 2002;28(5):367–371
2. Fulton JE, Porumb S. Chemical peels: their place within the range of resurfacing techniques. Am J Clin Dermatol 2004;5(3):179–187
3. Fulton JE Jr. Simultaneous face lifting and skin resurfacing. Plast Reconstr Surg 1998;102(7):2480–2489
4. Feldman JJ. Corset platysmaplasty. Plast Reconstr Surg 1990;85(3):333–343
5. Fulton JE Jr, Suarez M, Silverton K, and Barnes T. Small volume fat transfer. Dermatol Surg 1998;24(8):857–865
6. Fulton JE Jr. Rejuvenation of the orbital complex. Int J Aesthet Restor Surg 1996;4:43–48
7. Monheit GD. The Jessner's + TCA peel: a medium-depth chemical peel. J Dermatol Surg Oncol 1989;15(9):945–950
8. Fitzpatrick RE. Facial resurfacing with the pulsed CO_2 laser. Facial Plast Surg Clin 1996;4:231–420
9. Fulton JE Jr, Silverton K. Rejuvenation of the acne scarred face. Am J Cosmet Surg 1998;15:281–289
10. Fulton JE Jr, Rahimi D, Helton P. Modified tumescent liposuction. Dermatol Surg 1999;25(10):755–766
11. Elam MV, Parker D, Schwab J. Reduced negative pressure liposuction interaction. J Aesthet Restor Surg 1997;5:101–104
12. Suarez M. Fulton JE Jr. A novel occlusive dressing for skin resurfacing. Dermatol Surg 1998;24(5):567–570
13. Friedberg B. Propofol-ketamine technique. Aesthet Plast Surg 1993;71:297–300

CHAPTER 50

Three-Dimensional Facelift

50

Sid J. Mirrafati, Melvin A. Shiffman

50.1
Introduction

Most cosmetic surgeons refer to the words "facial rejuvenation" to mean either facelift or facial laser resurfacing. The word "lifting" only implies pulling up what has fallen or tighten up what has loosened. If facelifting means only these methods, the result will be an unnatural tightened (pulled) appearance. A pulled, tight look is not aesthetically pleasing and does not give the appearance of youth.

In the past 20 years the techniques utilized mainly involve pulling the superficial musculoaponeurotic system (SMAS) to Hamra's [1] deep-plane composite facelifting to the most recent Saylan's [2] S-lift (a modified facelift). The face is three-dimensional and lifting in the vertical and horizontal directions is two-dimensional and will result in a flat, pulled, and aesthetically unnatural look.

50.2
The Aging Face

When a face ages, there are different causes that must be addressed:
1. Volumetric deflation of the facial fat pad (fat atrophy) and repositioning of the facial fat pad. This also involves bone resorption including the cranial and alveolar bones. The problem is particularly noticeable in the buccal area, which results in repositioning of the upper lips.
2. The gravitational and looseness of the facial ligaments, which results in hanging jowl and deepened nasolabial folds.
3. The actinic damage of the facial skin itself.

The combination facial rejuvenation addresses all these concerns except the bone resorption, which is not easily rectified. The combination results in a natural and youthful look. Most importantly, it is safe and postoperative recovery is fast.

50.3
Methods

In this study there were 25 patients. Five were male and 29 were female. The average age was 49 years. The longest follow-up was 4.5 years for a female patient and 3.5 years for a male patient. There was no significant past medical history for any of the patients. Three were smokers who did not stop smoking during their recovery period and the rest were non-smokers or patients did not smoke 1 month before surgery and 1 month after the surgery.

The preoperative laboratory work included tests for complete blood count, Chem-20, prothrombin time, partial thromboplastin time, HIV, and pregnancy in women, and EKG for patients older than 55 years of age. All patients were started on 1,000 mg of vitamin C preoperatively and were told to stop all aspirin, vitamin E, garlic, and any herbal medications 10 days before surgery. Keflex, 500 mg twice daily, was started the day before surgery and was continued for 9 days. Patients who were to have chemical peeling or laser resurfacing were started on 500 mg Valtrex daily starting 3 days before surgery and this was continued for 9 days.

Each patient had facelift, liposuction of the neck and jowls, and fat transfer to the cheeks, nasal jugular groove, nasolabial fold, and the marionette line. The patients were given a choice whether or not to have laser resurfacing of the face and chemical peel of the neck. A discussion was held with each patient explaining each procedure for facial rejuvenation and the possible risks and complications.

The patients were told not to take any food after midnight before surgery. On the day of surgery, preoperative photographs were taken and skin marking was done. All patients were given general anesthesia. The surgery was performed in an outpatient surgical facility. Five of the patients were admitted to an outpatient facility for 24-h observation purely on the decision of each patient.

50.4
Procedure

Following administration of general anesthesia, the patient's neck was prepped with acetone using three passes. Then three passes of Jessner solution were used followed by three passes of 20% trichloroacetic acid. Generalized frosting of the neck up to the jowl line was the end point. The patient's neck and face was tumesced using the tumescent solution (1 l of lactated Ringer's solution, 50 ml of 1% lidocaine, and 2 ml of 1:1,000 epinephrine).

Laser resurfacing of the face was performed using a Coherent CO_2 Ultrapulse laser (Palo Alto, CA, USA). The forehead and the face up to lateral zygomatic line were treated with three passes of the laser. Beyond that area, which would later be lifted as a flap, two passes were made. The laser setting was 300 mJ, 60 W of power, and at a density of 5. The eyes were lasered at 250 mJ, 50 W of power, and a density of 4.

The neck and jowls were liposuctioned using a 3-mm Giorgio Fisher cannula under 15 mmHg of vacuum.

If platysmal bands are present, a small incision is made in the submental crease, and the flap is raised above the platysma down to the hyoid bone. The band is plicated using 5-0 nylon and the band below the hyoid bone is transected in a horizontal fashion. The skin is closed using a running 5-0 nylon suture.

About 50 ml of fat is harvested from either the lower abdomen or the lateral thigh. An incision is made along the preoperative marking in the posttragal area in female patients and in the pretragal area in male patients. The flap is raised above the SMAS to the lateral zygomatic line. The SMAS is lifted according to Saylan's S-lift techniques using the U and O purse-string 2-0 Ethibond suture with the exception of starting the U from the mastoid fascia. In some patients with a full buccal area, the buccal fat pad is removed. Care is used to only remove the fat that is extruded and not to pull the fat out or else an indentation of the area will result. The skin is lifted, 2 cm is resected, and then the skin is closed using 2-0 chromic in the subcutaneous tissues and 5-0 nylon on the skin.

Fat is then transferred to the face, after washing with saline and decanting, using a 16-gauge blunt needle through a skin opening made by a non-coring 16-gauge needle. On average, 5–6 ml of fat is transferred into each cheek and each nasolabial groove, 1–2 ml of fat is transferred to the medial side of the nasolabial fold, and

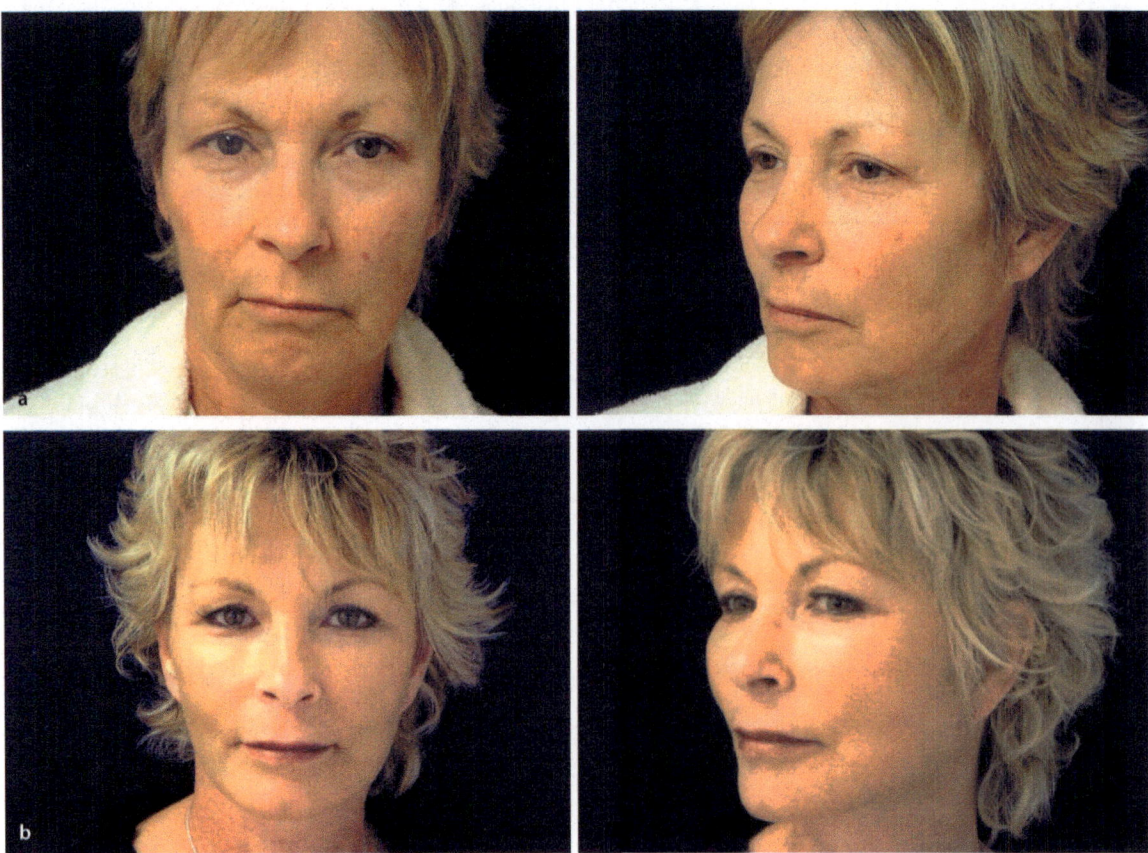

Fig. 50.1 a Before. **b** After

1–2 ml is injected into the marionette line. The fat is transferred in a retrograde fashion into different planes, above the bone, into the muscle, and into the subcutaneous tissues.

Silon TSR dressing is applied to the face, foam compression is applied to the neck, tube netting is applied to hold everything in place, and the neck is wrapped with an ACE bandage to apply pressure.

Following recovery from the anesthetic, the patient is sent home or to aftercare for 24 h of observation if requested by the patient. The patient is seen the first postoperative day to adjust the Silon dressing, the ace wrap is removed, and a neckband is applied for 3 days. The Silon dressing remains in place for another 3 days. After the third postoperative day, the patient applies a petrolatum ointment and washes his/her face with a gentle cleanser, such as Cetaphil cleanser, three times daily until the fifth postoperative day, at which time washing is reduced to twice daily. The sutures are removed on the fifth postoperative day. After the tenth postoperative day, the patient applies sunscreen with moisturizer daily. This is followed, in darker skin types, with a bleaching lotion applied from the 15th to the 20th postoperative day before the skin turns dark.

50.5 Conclusions

The combination three-dimensional facial rejuvenation will result in a more natural and younger more rejuvenated face (Figs. 50.1, 50.2). The younger face is not a pulled face but is a fuller face. The face is a three-dimensional figure that needs to be pulled horizontally (U suture) and vertically (O suture) and raised outward (fat filling), which result in a three-dimensional lifting of the face.

References

1. Hamra, S.T.: The tri-plane face lift dissection. Ann Plast Surg 1984;12(3):268–274
2. Saylan, Z.: The S-lift for facial rejuvenation. Int J Cosmet Surg 199;7(1):18–23

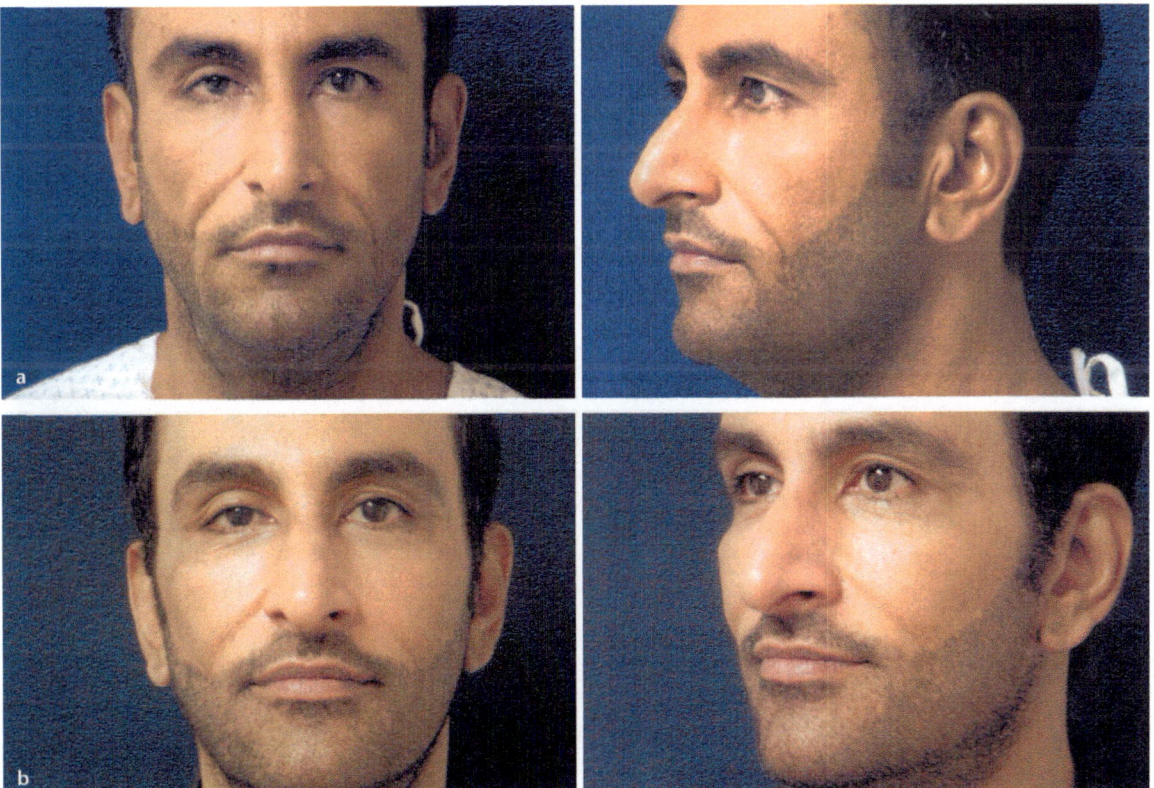

Fig. 50.2 a Before. **b** After

CHAPTER 51

Mini Facelift

Phillip R. Langsdon, Matthew R. Stumpe

51.1
Introduction

Humans, by nature, have always been concerned about their appearance and the effects of aging. In ancient times, various acidic-type washes derived from wine and fruit were used in an attempt to improve damaged skin [1]. The search has continued for these age-defying potions. Over the last century, the quest moved not only into physician's offices but also into the operating room, where various approaches have been developed.

Holländer [2] provided an account of a surgical lift performed in 1901 for removal of excess facial skin or wrinkles. Joseph [3] was the first to emphasize the effect of aging skin on women trying to gain employment and the benefits of cosmetic surgery.

The facelift has continued to evolve for over a century. Techniques include simple skin dissection, superficial musculoaponeurotic system (SMAS) suspension, SMAS undermining, "deep plane", and extensive skin undermining; all with several different variations and ancillary procedure additions.

The mini lift is simply a more minor version of facial suspension and, like the facelift, surgeons have various approaches and modifications.

51.2
Basic Principles and Rationale for Mini Facelift

Knowledge of the SMAS is essential when performing facial rejuvenation surgery. The layer is deep to the subcutaneous fat of the skin and superficial to the parotid fascia and invests the mimetic musculature of the face and neck. It is generally thought to be continuous from the temporoparietal fascia to the platysma [4–6]. The SMAS is also inclusive of the orbicularis oculi and orbicularis oris muscles [4–6]. This connection and investment system allows for plication and/or imbrication of the SMAS to support the sagging system and add longevity and efficacy to a facelift. The SMAS is directly connected to the skin in the central portion of the face, contributing to support in this area when the system is suspended lateral and/or superiorly. The senior author (P.R.L.) feels that skin suspension alone does not provide as good longevity of results.

Many different names are used for promoting the mini facelift procedure, and many surgeons may have their own variation of some portion of the mini lift; however, the procedures are designed to accomplish the same basic mission. The basic goals include a shorter recovery period with less "downtime", possibly a shorter scar (when compared with a full or lower facelift), and possibly less bruising and edema. In general, this abbreviated mini lift appeals to a patient's search for a less invasive, less morbid, and less costly technique to achieve facial rejuvenation.

The mini facelift involves limited skin undermining; this is an advantage in patients who smoke and desire some facial rejuvenation. Hematoma formation is also less likely with a short skin flap.

51.3
Technique

51.3.1
Patient Selection

Patients who are candidates for a mini-lift-type of procedure should demonstrate an understanding of the differences between a mini lift and a "full" or lower-face lift. Mini lifts appeal to the desire for reduced morbidity, downtime, and cost. But, it is very common for the patient candidate to both need and desire more extensive results. Of course, it is not possible to have it both ways. Therefore, the patient candidate must demonstrate a comprehension of the limitations of the mini-lift procedure. The author usually discusses the details of the differences of the various procedure on three occasions prior to surgery. Additionally, the patient must understand that no surgical rejuvenation procedure can remove facial asymmetries, improve the general facial deflation that occurs with aging, halt aging, remove wrinkles or facial expression lines, or restore the deteriorated condition of skin. Other techniques, not included with the mini-lift procedure, might be considered or needed to address facial atrophy, wrinkles, skin deterioration, asymmetries, and/or future aging.

Mini lifting will also not improve any condition or region of the face not included in the procedure. For instance, significant submental tissue and platysmal banding will not be improved as it would with a lower-face lift along with submental muscular plication and extensive skin redraping. Other procedures might be needed and/or recommended and the patient should understand that volume replacement and skin resurfacing will not occur with a mini lift. It should be fully explained what reasonable results are possible with differing techniques.

A mini facelift targets early to moderate jowling. It is reasonable to perform a mini facelift on a patient needing a more extensive surgery if the patient understands and accepts the limitations of this procedure. The physician is always able to recommend what surgical procedure is deemed best for the patient.

51.3.2
Anesthesia

Anesthetic techniques for this procedure vary from surgeon to surgeon, from surgical facility to surgical facility, and from patient to patient.

Sedation should only be undertaken in a state-approved (or legitimate regulatory organization) and yearly-inspected setting that is restricted by safety guidelines. All emergency equipment, proper personnel, and appropriate emergency medications should be present.

In the authors' facility, 1 h prior to surgery the patient is administered 20 mg diazepam orally, 200 mg dramamine orally, and 40 mg prednisone orally. The patient is also administered an oral antibiotic. It may take 1 h or slightly longer for the diazepam to have full effect. Local anesthesia is undertaken with 1% Xylocaine containing 1:100,000 epinephrine buffered with $NaHCO_3$ to include the incision lines and the circumferential periphery of the flap margins. The area to be undermined is injected with 0.5 % Xylocaine containing 1:200,000 epinephrine. Intravenous sedation is optional, but can be very helpful during the injection of local anesthesia. Intravenous sedation may be offered and must be monitored in an appropriate setting. It is usually delayed until the orally administered diazepam has been fully absorbed. Intravenous sedation is accomplished with diazepam in 2.5-mg doses and/or hydromorphone in 0.5- or 1.0-mg doses administered in 5-min intervals until the patient is relaxed. The 5-min interval allows for complete circulation and time for the physician to adequately observe the impact of the dose, before additional sedation is administered.

51.3.3
Marking (Male vs. Female Incision)

The temporal sideburn is preserved at the level of the superior portion of the ear; herefore, a horizontal mark

is usually placed in this location to prevent the migration of hair to a point superior to the cephalic portion of the ear. The resulting incision may then be reused in future facial rejuvenation procedures without elevation of the sideburn area and loss of temporal hair.

The marking is continued in the preauricular groove found just in front of the curvature of the auricle. In female patients, a posttragal mark is incorporated to hide the scar, 1–2 mm behind the tragus. In male patients, the incisional mark is usually carried in front of the tragus in a preauricular crease. An area of non-hair-bearing skin can be left between the tragus and sideburn in male patients. The mark then curves around the earlobe (Fig. 51.1).

Postauricularly, the incisional mark is carried into the postauricular sulcus. Some surgeons stop the incision mark low in the postauricular sulcus; however, this may result in bunching of the skin that is unsatisfactory to the patient in the early postoperative period. Therefore, the incisional mark is extended up the postauricular sulcus and on to the posterior hairline, forming a short gentle curve along the hairline. This extension of the postauricular incision allows for removal of excess skin and the prevention of bunching.

The extent of skin undermining is marked approximately 4 cm from the incision site.

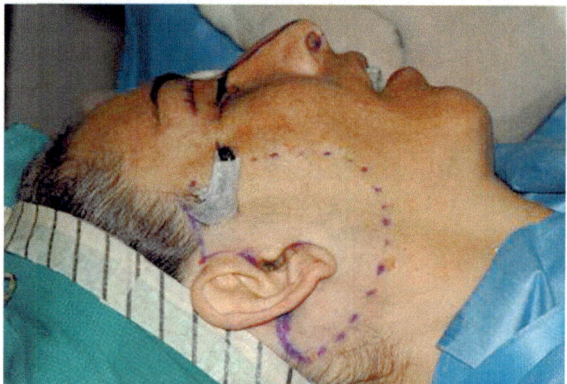

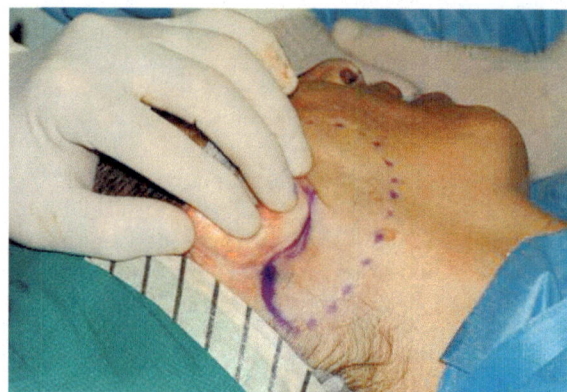

Fig. 51.1 Preoperative marking

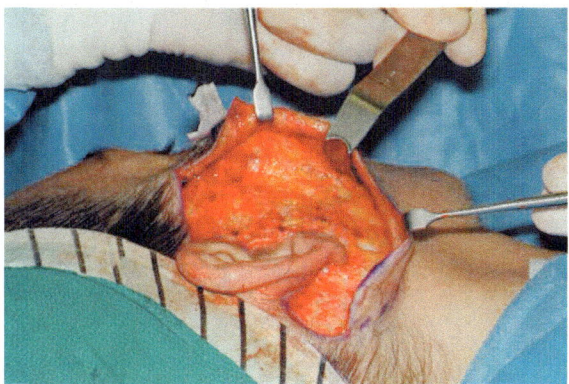

Fig. 51.2 Flap raised

51.3.4
Basic Principles

A no. 15 blade is used to make the incisions in the preoperative periauricular markings. The incision is carried through the dermis and is beveled across the direction of the hair follicles in hair-bearing temporal and posterior hairline skin. This maneuver allows the hair to grow through the incision line. The skin is then undermined beginning at the tragus; leaving as much subdermal tissue as possible attached to the deep tissue. A thin tragal flap minimizes tragal contracture during the postoperative healing phase. The remainder of the facial skin is then fully undermined in a supra-SMAS (subdermal) layer to a point averaging 4 cm from the incision, following the preoperative marking plan (Fig. 51.2). Hemostasis is achieved with bipolar cautery under direct visualization.

51.3.5
Materials

With the skin flap adequately elevated, the SMAS is plicated in a posteosuperior vector using a 2-0 Ethibond® suture (Fig. 51.3). The suture is secured at the zygomatic periosteum and placed through the SMAS, creating a "purse-string" loop. The suture is first continued inferiorly, then directed anteriorly, and then posterosuperiorly to return back to the zygomatic periosteum; creating a teardrop loop. This SMAS suture often leaves a trough deformity that is closed with interrupted plication sutures across the depression (Fig. 51.4). Free fat grafts are placed as necessary to fill suture depressions.

The skin is draped in a posterosuperior vector and secured at the highest postauricular point with an interrupted 2-0 nylon suture. This is followed by a second securing suture at the junction of the horizontal tem-

poral incision and the superior extent of the preauricular incision. The redundant skin is then resected in a manner creating minimal skin tension. The neotragal skin is left redundant to avoid forward displacement of the tragus by skin contracture. The earlobe is placed in a position that is about 0.5–0.75 cm superior to the position where it naturally lies, in the unrepaired state. This overcorrection prevents the lobe from being pulled too far inferiorly during the natural healing process, thus preventing the pixie earlobe deformity. Skin edges are approximated with a 5-0 plain gut suture, using a 4-0 Vicryl suture for additional support as necessary. The senior author finds that the 4-0 Vicryl suture is rarely needed and reserves its use for situations where it is determined there might be a slight excess of tension at a wound-closure site. The postauricular closure, above the posterior portion of the earlobe and below the level of the hairline, is performed in a manner that leaves 1-cm gaps between sutures (Fig. 51.5). This helps prevent the accumulation of blood beneath the flaps.

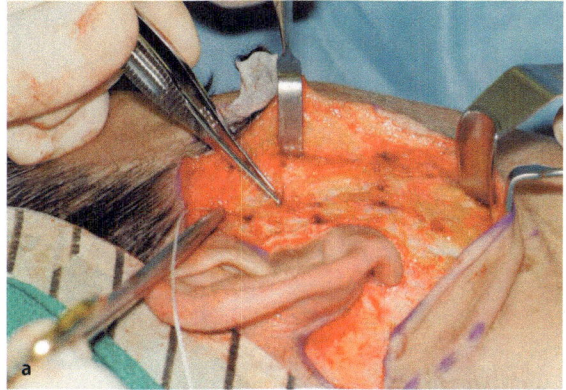

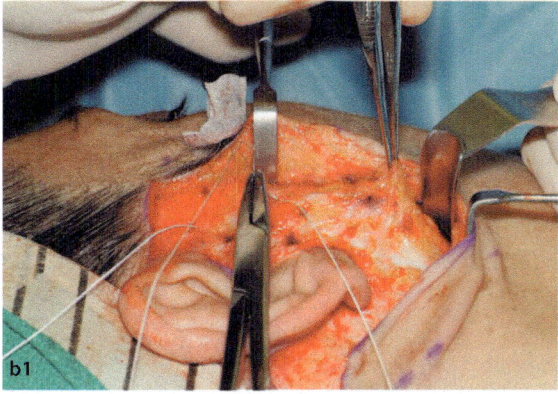

Fig. 51.3 a Beginning suture in the zygomatic arch. **b** Suture going inferiorly. *c, d, e see next page*

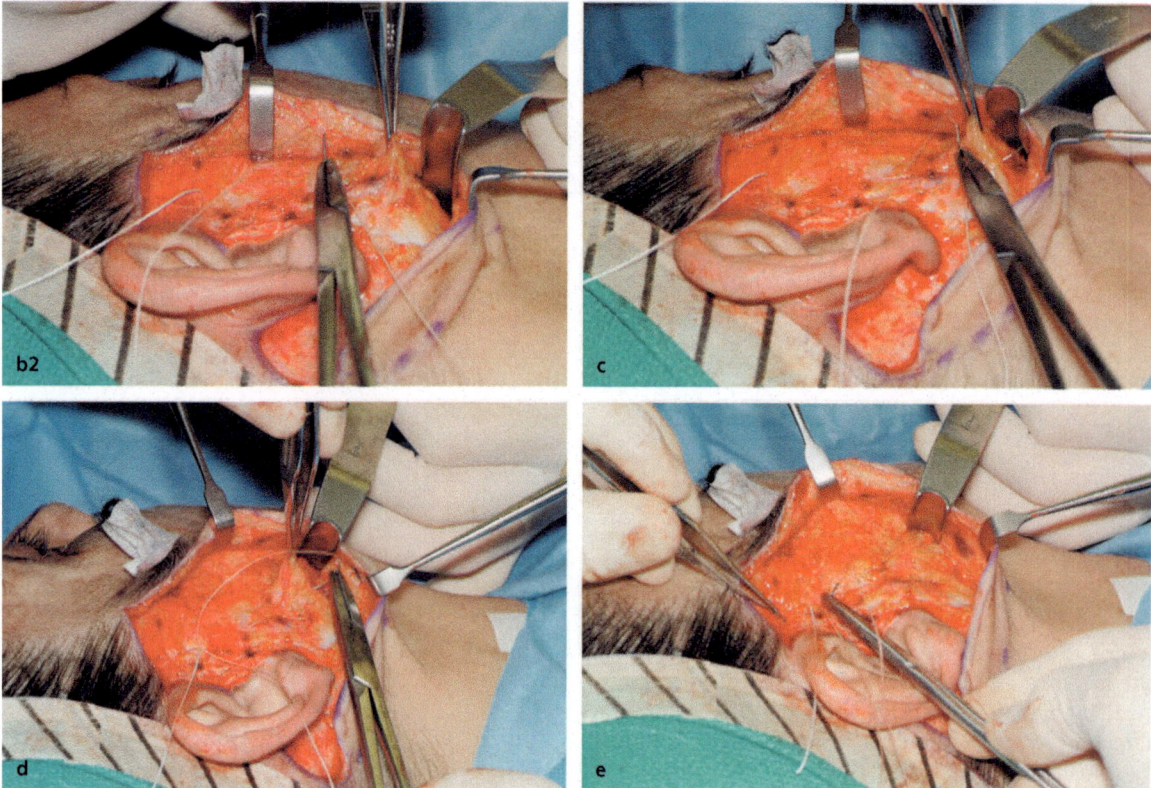

Fig. 51.3 *Continued* **b** Suture going inferiorly. **c** Suture beginning to go anteriorly. **d** Suture going back superiorly. **e** Suture going back in the zygomatic arch

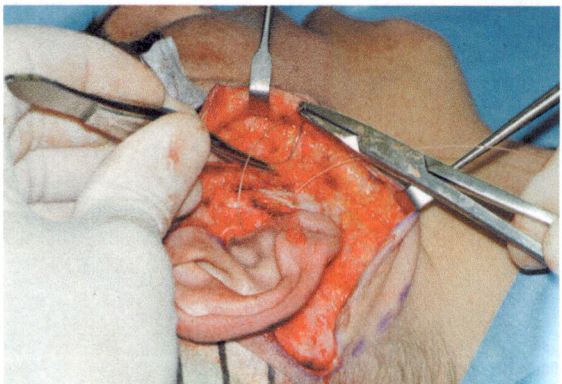

Fig. 51.4 Suture plicating the depression created by the lifting suture

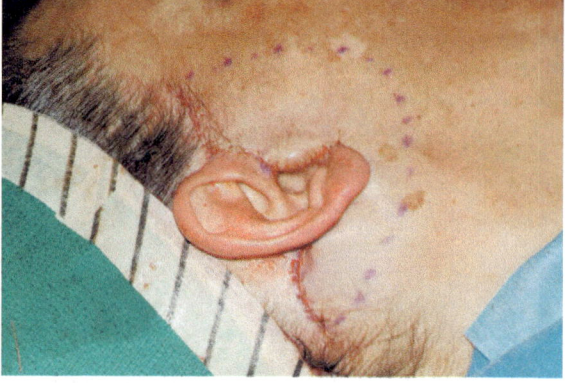

Fig. 51.5 Skin repaired and patient ready for dressing. The nylon suture was not used in this patient

51.3.6
Dressing

Any collected blood is expressed from under the flaps via the postauricular closure gaps. A light dressing is applied with 4 × 4 gauze pads and a cotton wrap, applying only very gentle pressure. A light elastic wrap is placed over the dressing. The elastic wrap is removed 4 h after placement. The patient is evaluated the following day. The remaining dressing is removed and the incisions are cleaned with hydrogen peroxide and dressed with Vaseline®.

51.4
Limitations

The mini facelift is appropriate for any patient requiring minimal to moderate rejuvenation. The mini facelift is also appropriate for a patient who is a candidate for a more aggressive procedure, but elects for a mini lift and understands the limitations of the procedure. The mini facelift does not address platysmal banding or neck sagging.

51.5
Ancillary Procedures

Ancillary procedures such as neck liposuction with or without platysma plication, chin augmentation, forehead procedures, and upper and lower blepharoplasty may, of course, be preformed along with the mini lift.

51.6
Complications

Complications occur in any surgical procedure and the mini facelift is no exception. However, mini facelift surgery has less opportunity for complications than full facelift surgery. Hematoma formation is possible but can be minimized with meticulous surgical hemostasis, proper patient selection, and the cessation of all medications, herbs, vitamins, and red wine that may cause bleeding. All patients should be counseled to discontinue medications, herbs, vitamins, etc. that may cause bleeding, 2 weeks prior to surgery. Large hematomas should be treated to avoid skin flap necrosis, but the senior author has not seen large hematomas associated with this limited flap procedure. If a small accumulation of blood is seen the following morning it is usually easily expressed through the postauricular skin closure gaps.

Flap necrosis might occur at the distal ends of flaps where blood supply is most tenuous. This is a very infrequent occurrence with limited flap elevation and would most commonly be an issue in heavy smokers; who are not consciously accepted as patients. Caution should be exercised in smokers or patients with diabetes, collagen vascular disease, or Raynaud's disease. However, the senior author does not consider these situations or conditions necessarily contraindications to mini lifting. Smokers should be counseled to reduce or discontinue smoking at least 2 weeks prior to surgery.

Nerve injury may be sensory or motor. Sensory reduction is common and not considered a complication; rather a normal consequence of surgery. The senior author has never experienced a major motor or sensory nerve injury. Masterful knowledge of facial nerve and greater auricular nerve anatomy will prevent most major nerve injuries. Compression nerve injuries usually resolve with time.

Deep infection is rare, as is cellulites. Antibiotic prophylaxis is used routinely.

51.7
Conclusions

The mini facelift is not a replacement for a classic facelift, but provides an option for patients who do not present with advanced facial aging or those unwilling to undergo a more extensive procedure. It provides the advantage of less risk, less morbidity, less surgical time, and less downtime for the patient. Patients also enjoy the reduced postoperative restrictions. The mini lift has proven to provide a high degree of patient satisfaction for those who understand the limitations, are realistic, and are emotionally stable (Fig. 51.6).

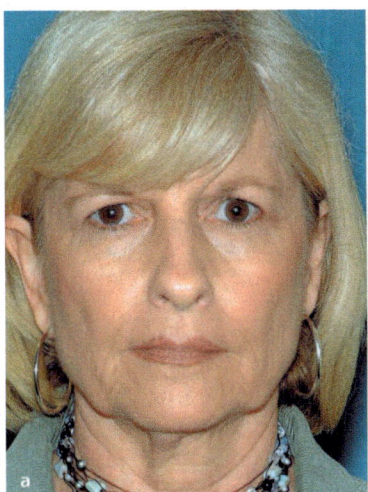 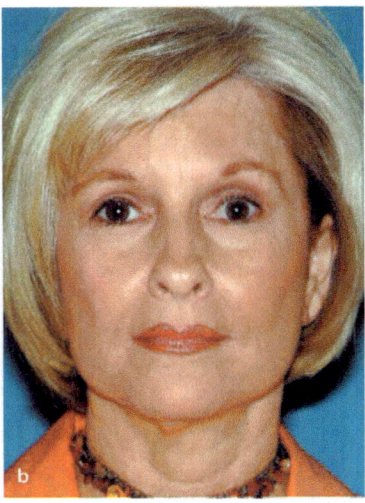

Fig. 51.6 a Preoperatively. **b** Postoperative mini-lift patient with forehead lift

References

1. Yarborough JM, Beeson WH. Aesthetic Surgery of the Aging Face. St. Louis, Mosby 1986:142
2. Holländer E. Plastische (kosmetische) Operation: Kritische Darstellung ihres gegenwärtigen Standes. In Klemperer G, Klemperer F (Eds), Neue Deutsche Klinik. Berlin, Urban and Schwartzenberg 1932
3. Joseph J. Verbesserung meiner Hängewangenplastik (Melomioplastik). Dtsch Med Wochenschr 1928;54:567
4. Gossain AK, Yousif NJ, Madiedo G, Larson DL, Matloub HS, Sanger JR. Surgical anatomy of the SMAS: a reinvestigation. Plast Reconstr Surg 1993;92(7):1254–1263
5. Ghassemi A, Prescher A, Riediger D, Axer H. Anatomy of the SMAS revisited. Aesthet Plast Surg 2003;27(4):248–264
6. Accioli de Vasconcellos JJ, Britto JA, Henin D, Vacher C. The fascial planes of the temple and face: an en-bloc anatomical study and a plea for consistency. Br J Plast Surg 2003;56(7):623–629
7. Tonnard PL, Verpaele A, Gaia S. Optimising results from minimal access cranial suspension lifting (MACS-lift). Aesthet Plast Surg 2005;29(4):213–220
8. Fulton JE, Saylan Z, Helton P, Rahimi AD, Golshani M. The S-lift facelift featuring the U-suture and O-suture combined with skin resurfacing. Dermatol Surg 2001;27(1):18–22
9. Saylan Z. The S-lift: Less is more. Aesthet Surg J 1999;19:406
10. Duminy F, Hudson DA. The mini rhytidectomy. Aesthet Plast Surg 1997;21(4):280–284
11. Onizuka T, Hosaka Y, Miyata M, Ichinose M. Our minifacelift for Orientals. Aesthet Plast Surg 1995;19(1):49–58
12. Baker TJ, Gordon HL. The temporal face lift ("mini-lift"). Plast Reconstr Surg 1971;47(4):313–315
13. Stephenson KL. The "mini-lift," an old wrinkle in face lifting. Plast Reconstr Surg 1970;46(3):226–235

CHAPTER 52

Complications of Facelift

52

Melvin A. Shiffman

52.1
Introduction

A standard facelift can have many types of complications. The composite or deep-plane facelift is more prone to complications especially with inexperienced cosmetic surgeons. The modified facelift reduces the risks and complications; however, the results may not be as long-lasting.

52.2
Complications

52.2.1
Asymmetry

Asymmetry results from excess excision of skin from one side of the face or from unequal pull on the flaps, not in the same direction, on each side. Distortion of the earlobe is common if the closure is performed under any tension around the bottom of the ear. Revision surgery may have to be performed.

52.2.2
Bleeding

Postoperative bleeding may occur if the vessels are not completely ligated or electrocoagulated.
Other causes of bleeding include:
1. Surgical technique
2. Aspirin or non-steroidal anti-inflammatory drugs
3. Hypertension
4. Anticoagulation drugs (coumadin)
5. Blood dyscrasia
6. History of easy bruising

52.2.3
Dehiscence

Tight wound closure with tension may result in wound dehiscence. This may require resuturing but if the tissues are friable, the wound may have to be allowed to heal with secondary intention.

52.2.4
Dog-Ear

A dog-ear may occur in the temporal region or the posterior neck. Most of them will tend to resolve over a few months. It is easier to repair the dog-ear at the end of the surgical procedure, but revision may be performed at a secondary surgery.

52.2.5
Ear Deformities

Excessive tension is the usual cause of ear deformity. Excision of skin around the ear should be performed after tension sutures have been inserted above the ear and behind the ear. Secondary surgery may be necessary to correct a deformity.

52.2.6
Edema

Edema usually subsides within the first few weeks. Chronic edema should be investigated for causes other than the surgery. Diuretics are not usually recommended.

52.2.7
Hair Loss

Hair loss can occur as the result of a tight closure and tension on the hair-bearing tissues. Most of the time the hair will regrow over time. Repair of the area of chronic hair loss may require excision (after 6 months) of the bare region or hair transplantation can be performed.

52.2.8
Hematoma

An expanding hematoma (pain and swelling of the side of the face) is a surgical emergency and requires early wound exploration with evacuation of the hematoma, ligation of bleeder, and probably needs to be drained at the time of closure [1].

52.2.9
Infection

Infection is rare (11 in 6,166 cases, or 0.18% [2]). Inflammation may be treated with topical steroids and any infection should be treated with appropriate antibiotics. Heat applied locally is helpful.

52.2.10
Irregularities

Irregularities may be the result of coming too close to the skin in developing the facial flap. Indentations of the skin following facelift surgery can be treated with a filler, preferably autologous fat. In one case indentation occurred from a very tight S suture in a modified facelift (S-lift) (Fig. 52.1). This resolved over a couple of months without treatment, except massage of the area.

52.2.11
Necrosis

Necrosis can be the result of the flaps being too thin or the closure being too tight. Smokers are very suscep-

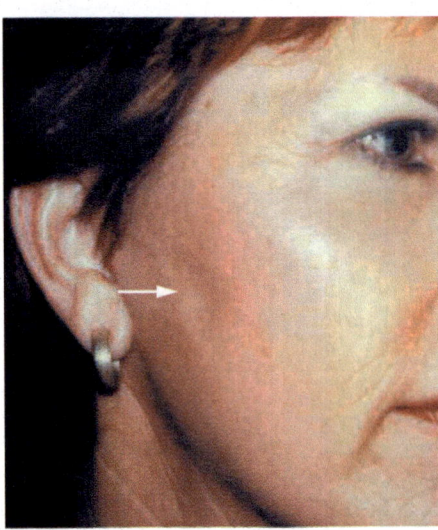

Fig. 52.1 This patient had an S-lift and 1 week after surgery began to notice a swelling of the right cheek. On examination there was a soft swelling that became an indentation when compressed by the finger. Simple observation with mild massage of the area allowed the problem to resolve that originated from too tight a closure of the purse-string S suture in the parotid fascia

tible to flap necrosis if the smoking is not completely stopped prior to and after surgery [3]. Especially dangerous is electrocoagulation of bleeders on the skin flap. The oozing of blood on the skin flap should be treated with compression only.

52.2.12
Neurological

Any of the facial sensory or motor nerves in the area of the facelift may be injured. Especially susceptible are the branches of the facial nerve and the anterior and posterior auricular nerves. Prevention is a necessity. The surgeon should understand facial anatomy and the three dimensional relationship of the nerves.

Temporary paresis can occur with injection of local anesthesia into the area of the nerve or from traction on the nerve. This type of paralysis can be observed until it clears. If there is any question of motor nerve transection then studies should be performed to establish nerve conduction. Early repair of a transected nerve will aid in more complete and earlier return of function.

52.2.13
Pain

Persistent facial pain is rare. If pain is acute following surgery, this may suggest an expanding hematoma. If it is chronic, branches of the sensory cervical nerves may have been injured. The pain will usually subside within 6 months. Nerve blocks may give temporary relief.

52.2.14
Pigmentation Changes

Hyperpigmentation may follow facial ecchymoses even with full resolution of the bruising. Sunlight exposure may increase the possibility of hyperpigmentation.

In patients with telangiectasias more hyperpigmentation may develop after rhytidectomy.

52.2.15
Salivary Fistula

Sutures placed deep in the parotid fascia (part of the superficial musculoaponeurotic system) can result in a salivary fistula (rare) (Fig. 52.2). Treatment would require removal of the offending suture, bland diet, and Donnatol four times daily to reduce the salivary flow. The fistula usually heals very readily with this treatment.

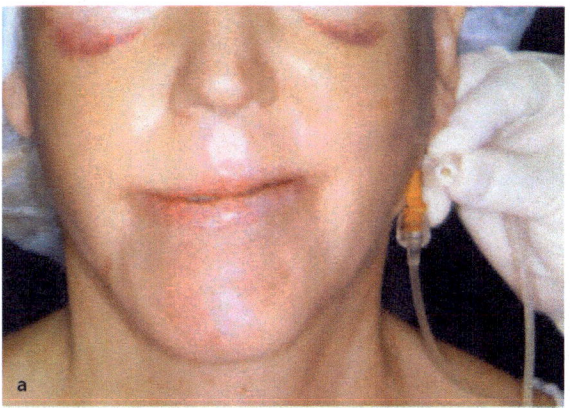

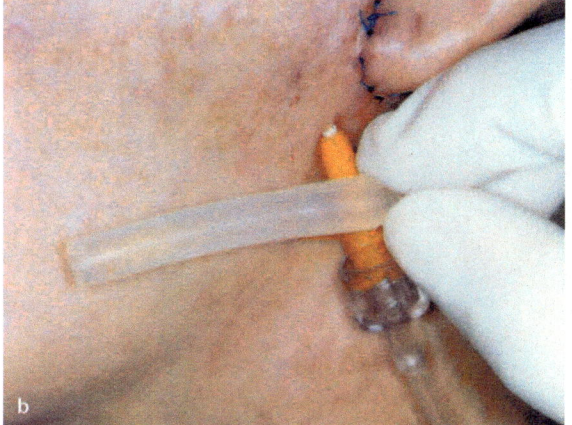

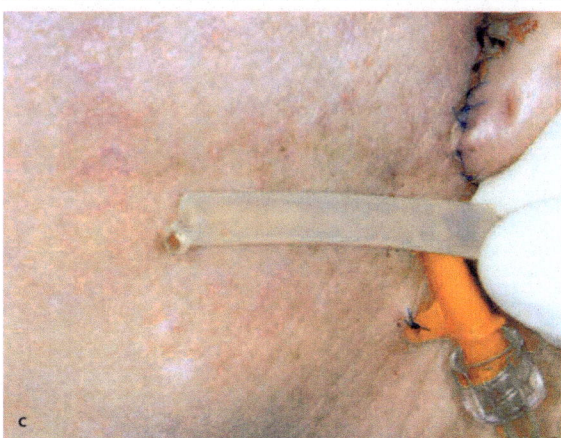

Fig. 52.2 a Patient developed a soft swelling a few days after a modified facelift. This was drained with a suction catheter. The wound drained 120 ml clear fluid daily. **b** Following removal of the vacuum reservoir, there was no drainage after 1 min. **c** Following biting of a wedge of lime, there was drainage at the end of the catheter within 5 s. The diagnosis of salivary fistula was confirmed

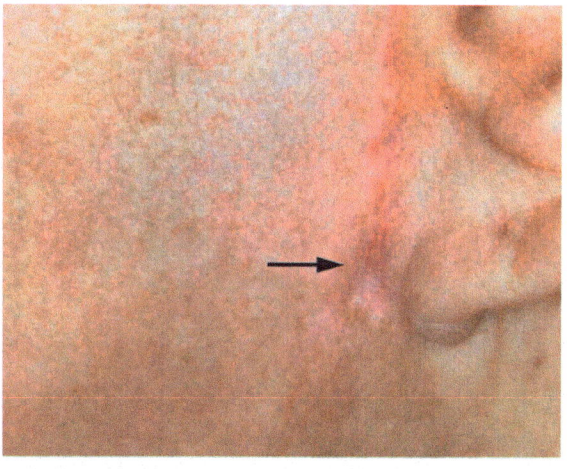

Fig. 52.3 Scar at the anterior inferior portion of the ear following S-lift. Surgical revision was necessary

52.2.16
Scar

Scars are usually a physiologic response to injury and may be hypertrophic or keloid. Keloid scars can be hereditary. Tight closure can contribute to a widened scar (Fig. 52.3).

There are a variety of treatments for keloids and hypertrophic scars, including steroid injection, surgery, 5-fluorouracil injection, silicone gel sheeting, bleomycin injection, or a combination of these.

52.2.17
Seroma

Seroma may occur following an unrecognized hematoma under the skin flap. Use of a syringe with needle drainage followed by compression may resolve the problem. Open drainage with suction catheter can be used for persistent seroma.

References

1. Niamtu, J. III: Expanding hematoma in face-lift surgery: Literature review, case presentations, and caveats. Dermatol Surg 2005;31(9 Part 1):1134–1144
2. LeRoy, J.L., Rees, T.D., Nolan, W.B. 3rd: Infections requiring hospital readmission following face lift surgery: incidence, treatment, and sequelae. Plast Reconstr Surg 1994;93(3):533–536
3. Rees, T.D., Liverett, M.D., Guy, C.L.: The effect of cigarette smoking on skin-flap survival in face lift patient. Plast Reconstr Surg 1984;73(6):911–915

Part VII
Surgical Variations:
Hair, Brow, Eye,
Ear, Nose, Lips, Chin, Neck

CHAPTER 53

Aesthetic Principles for Hair Restoration

53

Samuel M. Lam, Emina Karamanovski

53.1
Introduction

Oftentimes, when contemplating the dynamics of facial rejuvenation, hair restoration is overlooked. However, a comprehensive approach to facial rejuvenation should consider the important role that hair restoration can play. Part of the problem lies in the relatively few qualified surgeons who perform the procedure. This fact has more to do with the paucity of training programs that are currently available and with the necessity of having an experienced and dedicated hair-transplant team to make the venture a success than with the difficulty of the procedure itself. Unlike other methods of facial rejuvenation that almost solely rely on the expertise and skill of the surgeon, successful hair restoration is equally contingent on the surgeon's skills as those of the supportive team. Proper graft preparation and placement are critical to attain uniformly excellent results.

Besides the technical facets of operative technique, preoperative evaluation and aesthetic design are integral to success. There are intricacies of designing patterns that mimic nature so that operative results remain seamlessly undetectable. Oftentimes, judgment as to proper hairline, lateral hump, temporal points, and crown design can be more difficult than simply the technical operative creation of the recipient sites themselves. Understanding how hair naturally grows and is lost will guide the surgeon in a correct determination of how to reconstruct every component of hair loss. Judgment cannot be taught in a simple chapter but is accrued over years of experience. This chapter is only intended to serve as a framework for a prospective surgeon contemplating undertaking hair-restoration surgery or desirous of refining his or her already-established fund of knowledge and it should benefit both the neophyte and the advanced hair-restoration surgeon.

53.2
Technique

53.2.1
Hairline Design

The most important area for hair restoration is unequivocally the anterior hairline for many reasons. First, it is the area that is most conspicuous for both the patient and the casual onlooker. Second, the hairline serves as an aesthetically important frame for the face. A strong, full hairline draws the attention of a viewer back toward the patient's face, whereas a weak, thin, or non-existent hairline attracts unwanted attention and pulls the viewer's eyes up toward and beyond it. Third, a properly designed and executed hairline rejuvenates the face by reestablishing ideal, youthful facial proportions, as Leonardo da Vinci conceived, in which the face is divided into equal vertical thirds. For patients with extensive alopecia from the hairline all the way through to the crown, the surgeon may only possess a sufficient number of grafts from the occipital donor site to construct the hairline and frontal central tuft of hair. This area remains the primary goal for any hair-restoration surgeon. Hair loss is a progressive process with two caveats that should be issued: the possibility of exposing the transplanted hair in an unnatural or unfinished manner and the possibility of eventually depleting the donor area and thereby limiting future hair-restoration efforts. Unlike the vertex/crown, a properly designed hairline can accommodate for the progression of further hair loss and still maintain a natural result, as will be discussed further.

What constitutes the hairline? The rim of hair that frames the face consists of two areas: the anterior or frontal hairline and the lateral or temporal hairline. It is important to mention that the word "line" is only an expedient term, as the hairline represents in reality a 2–3-cm-wide zone of hair that appears as a cragged, irregular, and undulating region and that provides a transition from the bare forehead scalp to the hair-bearing midscalp.

Frontal hairline design, i.e., the general shape and location of the anterior hairline, has to be considered. The position of the anterior hairline is a necessary starting point. In general, the cardinal sin is creating a hairline that will look unnatural with further aging and will fail to accommodate the ongoing progression of hair loss, e.g., creating a hairline that is too low or too wide. A hairline may be too low if it breaks the rule of vertical thirds or is situated on the vertical plane of the forehead. A hairline that is too wide arises when it is drawn to extend laterally past an imaginary line that runs vertically through each lateral canthus. From the profile view with the patient in the Frankfurt horizontal plane, a hairline should appear parallel to the ground or slightly tilted upward, i.e., the posterior, lateral portion is situated more superiorly than the anterior, central portion of the hairline. Placing a hairline at an aggressively low starting point may seem all right for the present time, but as the patient ages, this low hairline may not match the patient's age or with the extent of future hair loss may appear unnatural. The ethical responsibility that the surgeon has toward any patient is not only to perform a beautiful and seamless restoration but also to look forward into the future for expectant hair loss. This responsibility is twofold: first, in planning proper hair restoration to ensure an adequate donor supply to cover the needs of possible subsequent hair restoration session(s) and, second, combining surgical restoration with appropriate medical management (finasteride and/or minoxidil) to retard the progression of a patient's hair loss. One should always recall that a hairline can be easily lowered but not so easily elevated after hair-restoration surgery.

Proper position is determined with the placement of the central, anterior point. Many different formulas have been advocated for the placement of the anterior point of the hairline. Using a combination of different formulas can help guide the beginning and even the advanced hair-restoration surgeon in establishing the proper initial height. The rule of thirds establishes that by classical dogma the anterior face should be elegantly divided into equal vertical thirds: from the menton to the subnasale, from the subnasale to the glabella, and from the glabella to the anterior hairline. Although this rule serves as a good starting guide below which the hairline should not extend, this point may at times be too low given the patient's age and extent of hair loss. A more conservative measurement placed more superiorly may be preferable in most cases. The hairline can be created more posteriorly at first and then adjusted anteriorly in the midline by jutting out a small widow's peak to reach this line if such a shape matches the patient's head shape (see later for more details). Another rule that is very useful involves drawing a line 45° from the point of intersection of the horizontal and vertical planes of the scalp, as inspected from a lateral profile view (Fig. 53.1). Again, these rules serve only as guiding principles. Facial proportions and progression of hair loss will determine the lowest point that is acceptable for the anterior hairline.

After the anterior point of the hairline has been established, the lateral extent of the hairline should be outlined next. The lateral extent of the hairline terminates at an imaginary line drawn through the lateral canthus of each eye. The best way to measure this point is to stand immediately in front of the patient and close one eye while holding a pen at arm's length. After one side has been measured in this fashion, the surgeon then stands behind the patient and inspects the head from behind with the head tilted back. A point is made in the mid-

line, and a tape measure is used to mark the distance from this lateral point to the midline and the same distance is measured to the contralateral point (Fig. 53.2). The same relative anteroposterior position of each lateral point should be maintained for symmetry. The lateral terminus of the hairline is a very important concept, as the eye perceives any hair lateral to this point as temporal-region-bearing hair. The lateral terminus is the point where the frontal hairline curves back allowing a natural-looking connection with the temporal hairline. If the surgeon extends the hairline laterally beyond the prescribed lateral terminus point, the parted hair would resemble an unnatural "comb over." The hairline at the frontotemporal angle should appear to be unzipping so that the angle on the hairline side matches the angle on the temporal side. After the three critical points (anterior midline and two lateral ends of the hairline) have been satisfactorily undertaken to define the position of the hairline, the shape of the hairline can be designed by connecting these three points. In general, there are two basic hairline shapes: a suppressed, bell shape and a rounded contour (Fig. 53.3). The curve of the bell shape transitions approximately at the midpupil from a medial convexity to a relative lateral concavity. The rounded

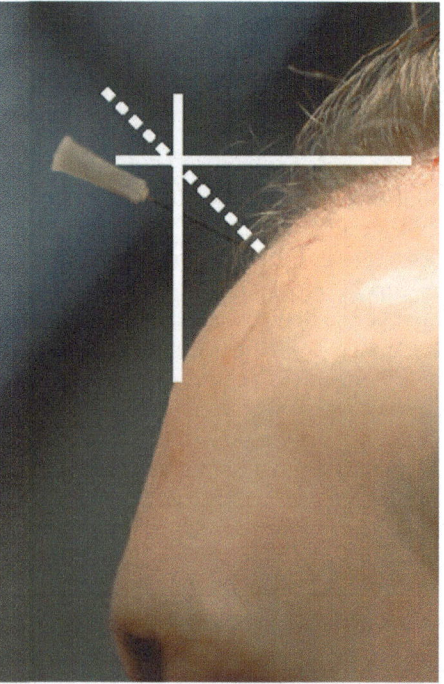

Fig. 53.1 The 27-gauge needle is inserted at the anterior, central midline of the hairline to demonstrate the proper starting point of the hairline. As indicated by the *dotted line*, the central, anterior midpoint should fall at a 45° intersection of the horizontal and vertical planes of the forehead, i.e., where the vertical plane transitions into the horizontal plane

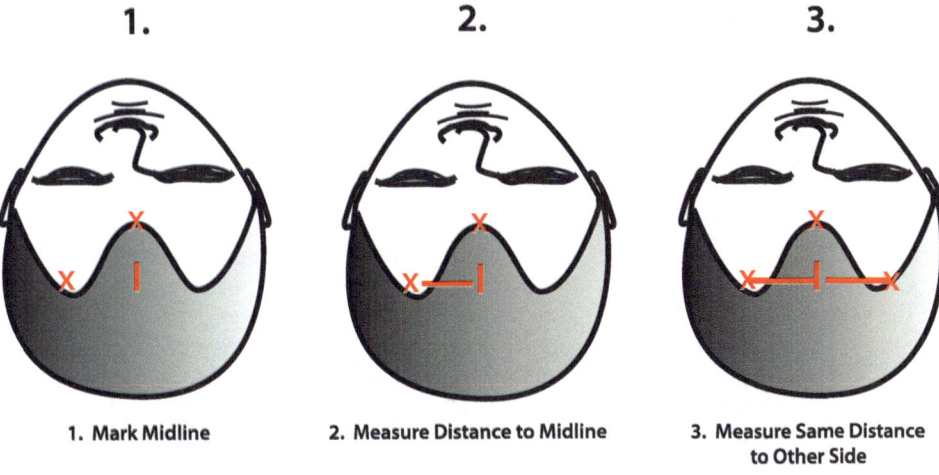

1. **2.** **3.**

1. Mark Midline   **2. Measure Distance to Midline**   **3. Measure Same Distance to Other Side**

Fig. 53.2 After the anterior, central midpoint has been established (Fig. 53.1), the lateral point of the hairline that corresponds with a line that runs vertically through the lateral canthus is drawn. The midline is marked, and the distance is measured from the lateral point to the midline. The same distance is measured to the contralateral lateral point. These three points will establish the overall hairline shape (Fig. 53.4). (Original art created by Samuel M. Lam)

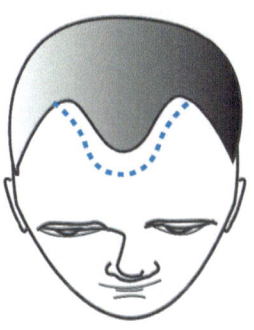 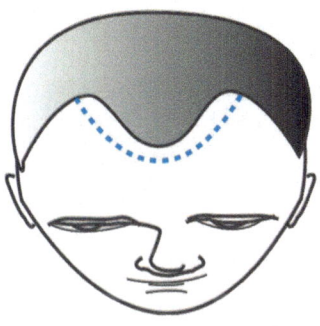

Bell Curve Design
1. Narrower Head
2. Graft Conservation
3. Temporal Recession

Round Design
1. Wider Head
2. Mature, Stable Temporal Hair

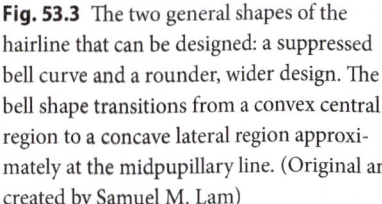

Fig. 53.3 The two general shapes of the hairline that can be designed: a suppressed bell curve and a rounder, wider design. The bell shape transitions from a convex central region to a concave lateral region approximately at the midpupillary line. (Original art created by Samuel M. Lam)

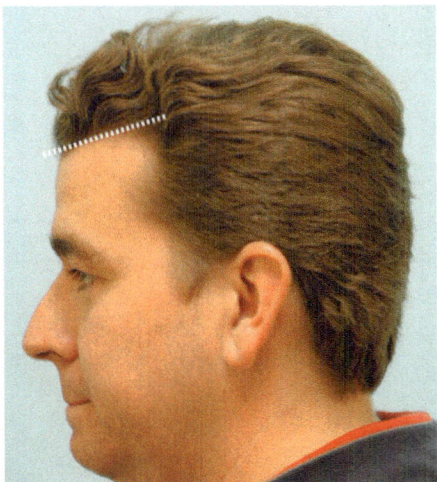

Fig. 53.4 The hairline when viewed in profile should be relatively flat or upsloping but never downsloping in order to ensure a natural result

shape is designed by connecting the midpoint and the two lateral points in a simple convex shape without the transition at the midpupil. The more rounded shape should not appear like a saucer or bowl but should still have some lateral concavity or should be fading posteriorly to match the temporal recession. With either design, from the side view, the hairline should be parallel to the ground or slightly tilted backward (Fig. 53.4). Deciding which hairline shape is appropriate for the patient is contingent upon aesthetic judgment and preoperative discussion with the patient. As a general rule, a patient with a relatively narrow head may look better with the former bell shape, whereas a wider head may be more suited to the wider rounded shape. After the hairline shape has been created, the surgeon should review the shape for symmetry from three angles: (1) in front of the patient, (2) from both sides of the patient; and (3) from behind the patient while holding a mirror in front of the patient. Looking at a mirror in this fashion can give the surgeon the perspective that the patient will have when examining his/her own hairline and at the same time corroborate with the patient the acceptability of the design.

53.2.2
Hairline Execution

So far what has been discussed is the macroshape of the hairline; however, the equally important constituent elements of a hairline concern the placement of the sites and the grafts themselves. The grafts should not fill in this hairline rigidly, otherwise the shape of the hairline will be too well defined and appear as an artificial wall of hair. The purpose of a good hairline is to constitute a naturally proportional frame to the face without the appearance of any linearity and to provide a soft transition from the bare forehead scalp to the denser central hair. The hairline is actually not a line of hair but rather a zone of hair with two objectives in mind: first, to provide a progressive increase in hair density achieved over the first 2–3 cm and, second, to create a soft transition from the bare forehead skin (Fig. 53.5). The creation of the hairline should be started at the most posterior point of the transition zone, i.e., approximately 2–3 cm behind the intended anterior line (Fig. 53.6). From this point, there is advancement forward toward the line creating little irregularities like a coastline in which tiny

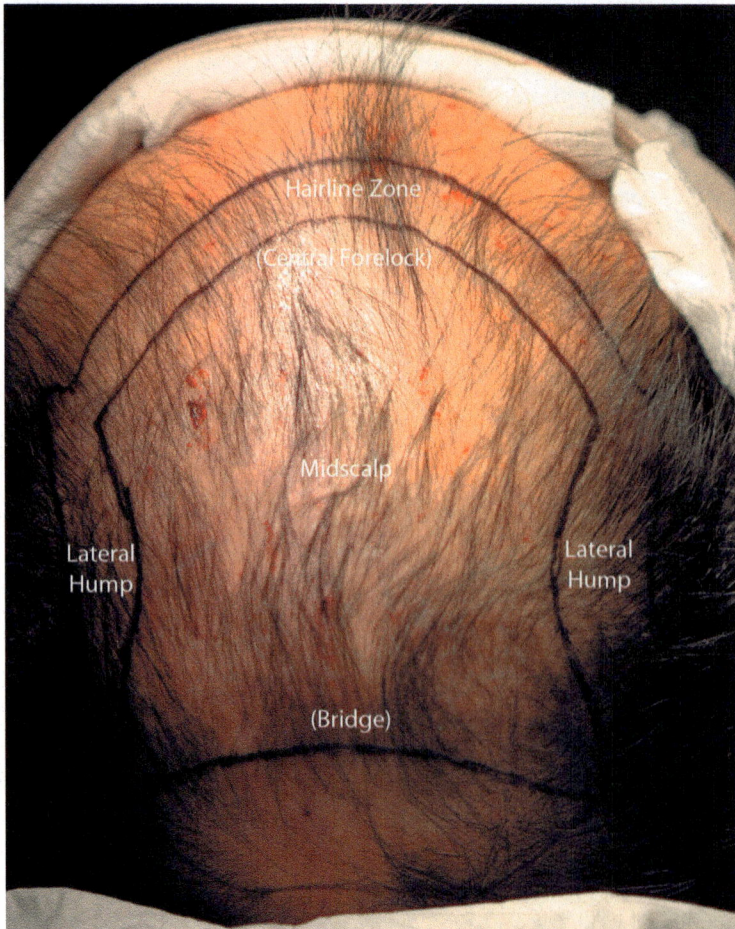

Fig. 53.5 The markings show the anterior hairline with a line drawn several centimeters behind the hairline that constitutes the posterior limit of the hairline zone. The central zone represents the midscalp where multiple follicular-unit grafts are planned. The lateral borders are marked out for lateral-hump reconstruction

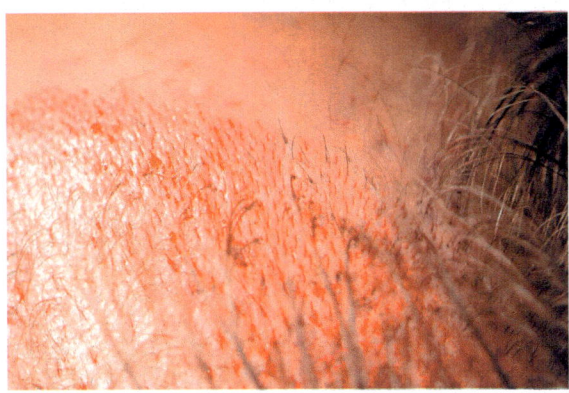

Fig. 53.6 The recipient sites across the hairline zone and midscalp should be oriented principally forward in an anterior direction except at the frontotemporal apex, where they should begin to diverge laterally to transition to the temporal hairline

placed at a very low anterior angle along the hairline and, for that matter, for most of the transition zone into the midscalp. The angle refers to the placement of the blade (or needle) as it relates to the scalp. A low angle permits the transplanted hair to "shingle", i.e., for the hairs to lie on top of each other, establishing a stronger shadow over the scalp and thereby creating less of a "see-through" effect. Transplanted hair that exits the scalp at a very low anterior angle provides the illusion of more density.

The second attribute that should be recalled when creating recipient sites is direction. Whereas angle refers to the relative elevation of the created site from the scalp, the direction is defined by the way that the graft points when exiting the scalp, e.g., anteriorly or toward the left or right. Generally speaking, the grafts should aim directly anteriorly for almost the entire hairline with the exception near the transition laterally toward the temporal area (Fig. 53.6). At the frontotemporal apex, the hairs begin to splay out and point slightly laterally in a progressive fashion to match the direction of the hair on the temporal hair-bearing side. Except for this small region of transition, the majority of the hairline should exhibit hairs that are placed facing straight forward in order to minimize the see-through effect that would be engendered by splaying the hairs to any extent laterally from the midpoint.

archipelagoes and jetties are present while all the time maintaining the overall desired shape of the hairline and always making sure the sites interlock (Fig. 53.7). The first few rows of sites are to accommodate three-hair follicular-unit grafts (FUGs), then the next few rows anteriorly will accommodate two-hair FUGs and finally the most anterior sites are designed for one-hair grafts. At the conclusion of site creation, the design is completed by placing scattered "sentinel" one-hair grafts sporadically in front of the densely packed sites to ensure a softer natural appearance of the hairline.

Besides hairline shape and location, the angle, direction, and distribution of the recipient sites are equally important in maximizing density, minimizing graftiness, and mimicking nature. All recipient sites are

Distribution constitutes the final attribute in recipient-site creation and refers to the placement of the sites relative to one another. All sites should be distributed in a tight, interlocking fashion for several reasons. First, the see-through effect is diminished as the grafts are staggered one row behind the other rather than in the same picket-row alignment. Second, a greater number of sites, and thereby grafts, can be placed per square centimeter when they are interlocked. Similarly, it is

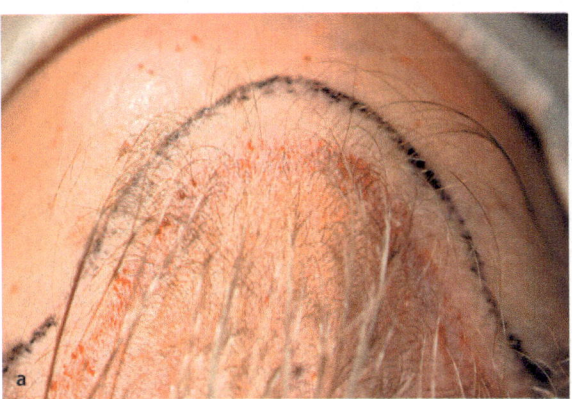
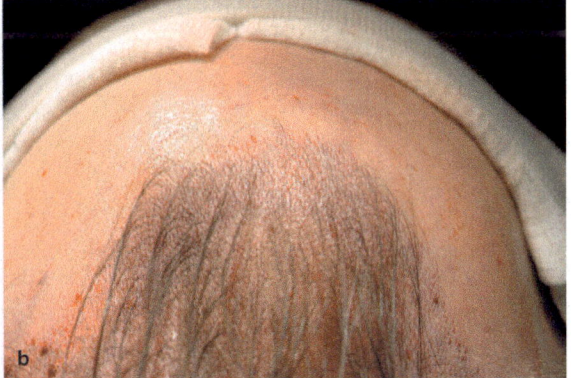

Fig. 53.7 a Rather than begin creating the recipient sites for the hairline immediately, the authors prefer to start several centimeters behind the anterior hairline at the posterior limit of the hairline zone and march forward toward the anterior hairline. This method permits the creation of a less linearly arranged hairline but one that exhibits an undulating and irregular pattern while maintaining an overall symmetric shape and a tight, interlocked grid. **b** Completion of the recipient sites for the anterior hairline

easier to place grafts in this fashion since they compete less for the surrounding space/tissue. Third, the transplanted hair grows more naturally as the individual grafts are evenly distributed and the hair to bare-skin ratio is more uniformly consistent.

53.2.3
Hairline Design in Women

There are three principal patterns of hair loss in women. The first type of hair-loss pattern is a diffuse thinning of the midscalp. The second type is a Christmas-tree pattern of hair loss across the midscalp with the apex of the tree situated posteriorly. The third type of hair loss in women is a recession of the hairline with a conspicuous absence of the frontotemporal hair. Any combination of the aforementioned female hair-loss patterns can also be observed. Restoration of lost hair in women mandates an understanding not only of how hair is lost in women but also how hair grows in women, especially concerning frontotemporal hair loss. Unlike in most men who have hair that is more uniformly directed anteriorly along the hairline, the pattern of hair growth is more complex in women. Women tend to exhibit a "cowlick" in which there is a small, central widow's peak with hair directed in a radial fashion throughout most of the anterior hairline (Fig. 53.8). A careful analysis of a woman's existing hairline can help guide a surgeon to mimic this swirling pattern more accurately so as to blend it in with the patient's natural pattern (Fig. 53.9). Whereas the frontotemporal hair may or may not need reconstruction in men, it is almost always necessary for women with the anterior hair-loss pattern (Fig. 53.9). To reconstruct this type of lost hair in women, we primarily select finer donor hair and transplant it via single FUGs. In the case of the other two types of female hair loss, if the hairline is thin combination grafting is used

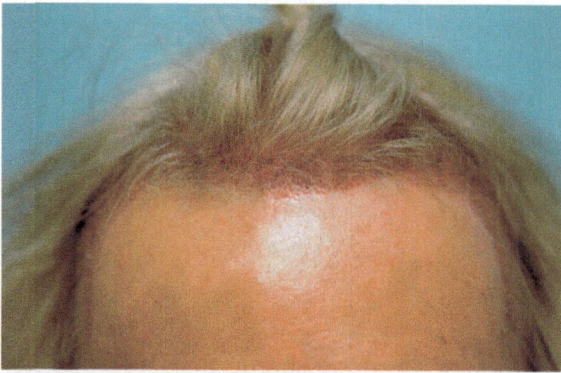

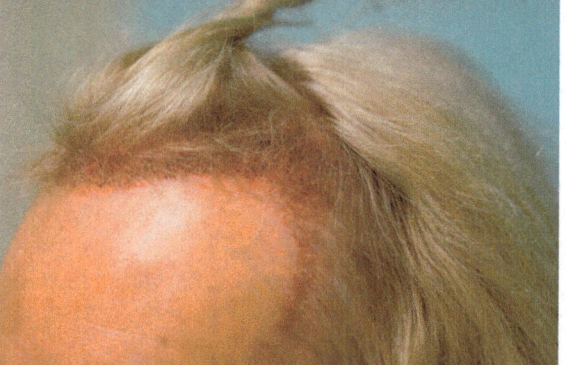

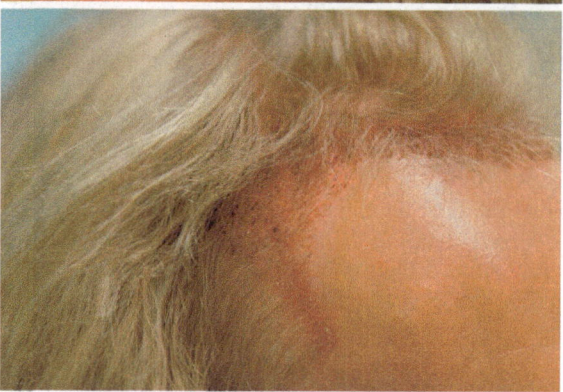

Fig. 53.9 Reconstruction of the central cowlick of the female hairline and the temporal recession that is characteristic of one type of female hair loss

and if the hairline is intact the reconstruction may require exclusively the use of larger multiple FUGs, which are grafts containing more than a single follicular unit. These subtleties mandate a different strategy and technique for women.

53.2.4
Temporal Point Design

Hairline design is intimately associated with the design of temporal points, as they complete the discussed frame for the face. Having a hairline that extends ag-

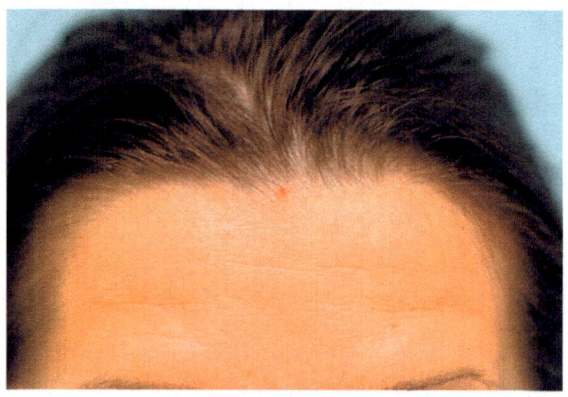

Fig. 53.8 Women tend to exhibit a "cowlick" in which there is a small, central widow's peak with hair directed in a radial fashion throughout most of the anterior hairline

gressively in an anterior position with a weak and posteriorly oriented temporal fringe appears unnatural. In fact, oftentimes toupees (also known as hairpieces or hair systems) appear unnatural because the hairline is positioned far too anteriorly to match the receded temporal hairline. The hairline and anterior temporal region should always be designed together so that there is harmony and balance. The reconstruction of the temporal points is extremely complex owing to the sharp and changing hair angle found in that area. Considering that temporal points are exposed and difficult to conceal if done incorrectly, a beginner surgeon is encouraged not to attempt this type of reconstruction early in his/her career.

The direction of the hair in the temporal area differs from person to person. Nevertheless, the hair should be oriented almost flat against the scalp in an even more acute angle than the anterior hairline in almost every case. Studying the flow of temporal hair in individuals with strong (or even weak) temporal hair can provide a better understanding of the matter. The inexperienced surgeon is encouraged to evaluate the pattern of as many people as possible before embarking on temporal reconstruction to begin to grasp how best to recreate the temporal area in a natural manner. Even in a particular patient desirous of temporal reconstruction, the surgeon can still use the remaining temporal hair as a very useful guide in determining how to design the pattern to match the existing hair. Additionally, the reader is cautioned, as the scalp is extremely thin in the temporal region, making site creation and graft placement more difficult. The major temporal blood vessels that course through this area also elevate the technical challenge.

53.2.5
Lateral Hump Design

The lateral hump refers specifically to the temporal hair-bearing region that falls behind the anterior temporal border and extends upward toward the midscalp and reaches the midscalp at a specific apex. Like the anterior temple, all hair that encompasses the temple and lateral hump falls on a line lateral to the lateral canthus. In patients with a thick, full head of hair, this apex is obscured but becomes increasingly more exposed with ongoing hair loss. Over time, with more extensive hair loss, the lateral hump falls away from the midscalp, mandating simultaneous reconstruction to rejoin the lateral hump with the midscalp (Fig. 53.10).

The direction of the hair in the lateral hump should again be very acutely angled near the scalp and follow the continuity of the anterior temporal border. The unzipping described earlier in which the hairline and the anterior temporal border exhibit progressive divergence should be continued further posteriorly along the bor-

der that separates the midscalp from the lateral hump. These hairs then continue to fall progressively downward until they are nearly or completely oriented in a sagittal manner posteroinferiorly (Fig. 53.11).

53.2.6
Midscalp Design

The midscalp is an ill-defined entity in that it can be defined in many ways. In this case, we have defined it as the area that extends behind the hairline all the way posteriorly to the beginning of the crown and terminating laterally at the junction with the lateral hump (Fig. 53.7). Although the midline zone that falls immediately behind the hairline is more accurately recognized as a distinct region known as the central forelock, we have included it within the domain of the midscalp. The main goal in hair reconstruction of the midscalp

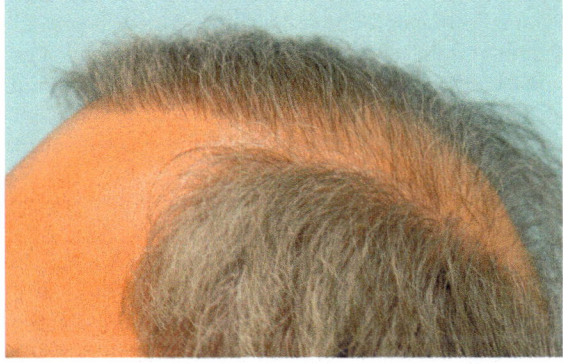

Fig. 53.10 This patient had undergone multiple hair transplantations in the past and now presents with an unnatural looking result, as the lateral hump has fallen away from the denser central midscalp, a condition that does not appear in nature

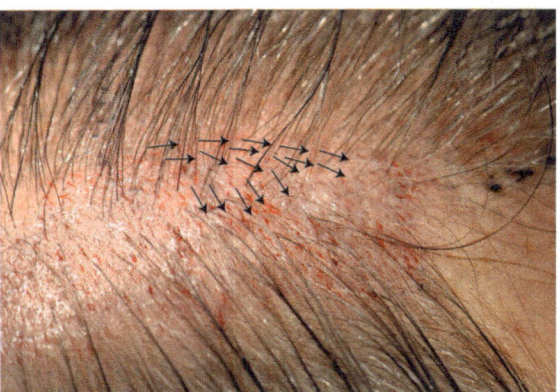

Fig. 53.11 Right-sided lateral-hump reconstruction showing the unzipping pattern of the recipient sites that mimics what is found naturally in non-balding individuals

is to provide coverage, thereby visual density, and to reinforce the hairline. The most posterior limit of the midscalp ends at the point where the scalp begins to assume a vertical orientation and where the swirl of the crown hairs becomes evident. This posterior limit of the midscalp is another important anatomic zone, which we will refer to hereafter as the bridge. The central forelock (the anterior midline border of the midscalp) and the bridge are very important areas to reconstruct with appropriate hair density because of their significant impact on creating visual density.

The central forelock can be seen when a bystander is looking at the patient head-on as well as from the left and right sides; therefore, it offers maximal camouflage of the scalp from all anteriorly viewed angles and should be a central concern when constructing the midscalp. Similarly, the bridge (or posterior limit of the midscalp) is also very important, as it constitutes the wall through which individuals standing behind the patient can peer into an exposed midscalp. Consequently, both areas create a shadow that prevents light from reflecting onto the scalp, which thereby decreases the see-through effect, enhancing visual density. When possible, the surgeon should try to provide a tight and focused reconstruction of both areas, though considering the central forelock of higher importance than the bridge.

Another important consideration in the midscalp concerns how the patient typically parts the hair. With a left-sided to right-sided parting, the surgeon should focus added density along the left border of the midscalp, i.e., along the parting of the hair, and decreased density (if needed to economize grafts) along the way in a progressive fashion to the right side of the midscalp. The reason for doing this is twofold. First, greater density along the parting of the hair provides more visual camouflage of naked scalp where the hair is parted. Second, the hairs situated near the left side of the scalp travel a greater distance as they are combed to the right side of the head than are the hairs that are situated on the far-right side of the head. This phenomenon is known as the "cascade effect" and should be exploited to optimal advantage when the patient's hair parting style is known and donor hair is limited.

For the most part, hair in the midscalp is oriented at a low angle and in an anterior direction as described for the anterior hairline. The midscalp hair can assume a slightly more elevated angle progressively as the surgeon approaches the posterior bridge of the midscalp. Nevertheless, keeping a relatively low angle (below 45°) is optimal to achieve improved shingle and to minimize the exposure of the grafts themselves as discrete surgical entities. Although almost all of the recipient sites should be created with a rigidly anterior direction, the few rows near the lateral limit should splay slightly laterally to blend progressively with the temporal hair and lateral hump (Fig. 53.12).

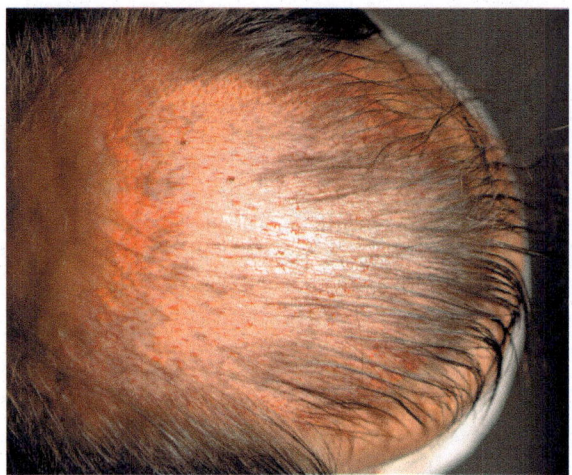

Fig. 53.12 Recipient-site creation principally in the midscalp using an SP91 blade to accommodate multiple follicular-unit grafts with a tight wall of interlocking follicular-unit grafts along the posterior limit, which we have termed the "bridge". The transition over to the lateral humps is also demonstrated, which are reconstructed with follicular-unit grafts

53.2.7
Crown Design

The crown is perhaps the most complex area to reconstruct. Hairs must remain at very low angles to the scalp like in the temporal area, but the hairs must be oriented in a progressive spiral from a central swirling point (Fig. 53.13). If the patient has some existing miniaturized hair in the crown, the surgeon can carefully follow the pattern of the existing hair when designing the swirl. If the patient is fully bald in this area, the surgeon must create a spiral of hair from scratch (Fig. 53.14). If the patient parts the hair from the left to the right side, it may be wise to situate the center of the swirl somewhat toward the left side and to orient the swirl to radiate in a clockwise fashion. Doing so permits the hair to arch forward and over to the right to camouflage the parting more effectively. Like the "cascade effect" described before for the midscalp, the greater density of hair should be situated along the upper arch of the swirl where hair can fall across and over to provide maximal camouflage of the crown. There should not be any abrupt transitions in direction from one hair-bearing area to another; therefore, the swirl should arch up and forward and blend seamlessly with the anterior orientation of the bridge of the midscalp.

The patient's crown should not be attempted in most cases as a patient's first-time outing for several reasons. First, the patient and others see the loss of hair across the anterior hairline much more frequently. Also, the anterior hairline provides a necessary frame for the face. Second, the crown can be a relatively unstable area where ongoing recession is the norm. It is important to observe this region of the scalp for some time before contemplating reconstruction, particularly if the patient is not on medical management, is younger, or has poor donor density to provide necessary future restoration. Third, to achieve a naturally looking vertex, a significant number of hairs need to be transplanted to construct an adequately dense hair-swirl pattern. Different from the frontal or midscalp hair that shingles easily, the hair in the vertex has a tendency to open or splay by exposing the scalp and look unnatural if sparse. For the same reason, it is also not wise to reconstruct the entire scalp during one session owing to the risk of creating artificially thin coverage. If the patient runs out of donor hair and the crown was reconstructed earlier on but now the patient does not have enough hair for either the increasingly exposed crown or the midscalp to be completed, the result can be devastatingly unnatural. Planning ahead for future hair loss is essential when contemplating crown reconstruction. If the hair is grossly miniaturized with an abundance of vellus hair, it is also wise to have a patient start a program of finasteride and possibly minoxidil, if the patient is compliant, for 6–12 months before embarking on the crown, which is particularly susceptible to temporary shedding of native hair after hair transplantation.

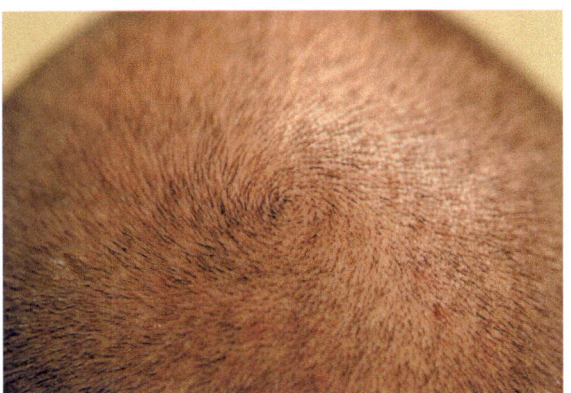

Fig. 53.13 A natural (unoperated on) crown showing the characteristic swirling pattern from a central radial point that must be recreated during crown reconstruction

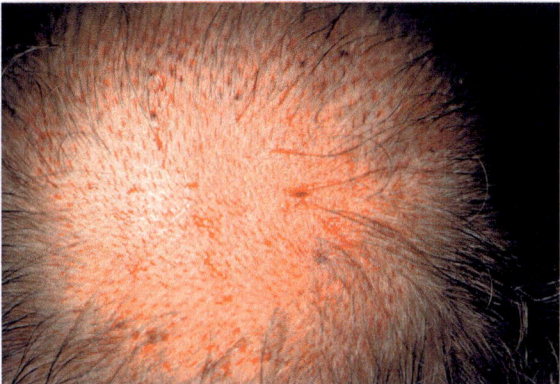

Fig. 53.14 Crown reconstruction undertaken by following the very scant residual natural crown pattern and with blending and smooth transitions into the lateral hump and midscalp

Chapter 54

Follicular-Unit and Multiple-Follicular-Unit Hair Restoration

54

Samuel M. Lam, Emina Karamanovski

54.1
Introduction

The history of hair restoration can be traced back to the early nineteenth century when Dieffenbach [1] recorded his efforts at transplanting hair and feathers in animal subjects. However, the modern era of hair transplantation began with Okuda [2] in 1939 and Tamura [3] in 1943 by covering shameful hair loss in the pubic region with scalp hair. Orentreich [4] should be accorded the rightful epithet "the father of hair restoration," as our current methods stem back to his work in 1959 that involved transplantation of hair from the back of the head, an area that would never undergo hair loss, to the front of the head and the transplanted hair would retain the native characteristics of the donor scalp, i.e., the hair would not undergo loss when transplanted to the new site. However, the subsequent three decades in which Orentreich's punch-grafting method was popularized have been associated with unsightly "plugs" and created much damage in the public's mind about the unnatural appearance of the transplanted hair.

The 1980s ushered in a new era when hair restoration was undertaken with much smaller grafts known as minigrafts and micrografts. Headington's [5] seminal thesis in 1984 provided the foundation for a change in technique. He studied scalp hair and noticed that hair grew in discrete clusters of one to four hairs, which he termed "follicular units." These follicular units are observed in close scrutiny of the scalp and during graft dissection, hair grafts created in respect to those groupings. Follicular-unit transfer has become the mainstay for modern hair restoration and has ended the era of pluggy grafting.

Although single follicular-unit grafts (FUGs) are uncompromisingly used to create a naturally looking hairline, it is my experience that they do not provide adequate hair density to cover the midscalp. The authors use FUGs principally along the hairline and other exposed perimeter zones and prefer, at times, multiple FUGs (MUGs), formerly "minigrafts", to yield unsurpassed visual density in the region of the central midscalp. A MUG is a single graft composed of two to four follicular units. How is this different from a plug then? The size, shape, and placement of these grafts are very distinct from those of the old plugs of yesteryear. While plugs were round clumps of hair loosely distributed and comprised 16–20 hairs per graft, MUGs are much smaller sized grafts that contain five to ten hairs per graft and are distributed in a linear, tightly interlocked fashion. They are also positioned at a very low angle to the scalp so that the graft cannot be easily detected. Finally, they are never placed in an exposed area like the frontal hairline but are rather blended and camouflaged behind smaller FUGs. Again, they may not look as undetectable as FUGs upon very close inspection, but the reason why MUGs have become an important component of our hair-restoration practice is that when used strategically they provide unparalleled hair density in a single session that would otherwise be difficult to achieve with a standard session of single FUGs.

MUGs are used selectively and judiciously in our practice. On rare occasion, such as female hair loss that requires increase in midscalp density only, MUGs may be used in isolation without supporting/camouflaging FUGs. At times, hair restoration calls for use of FUGs alone. For example, if a patient only requires reconstruction of the frontal hairline or the patient's existing hairs are too closely spaced to permit use of larger instruments needed for MUG creation, then FUGs would be preferable. Because of their smaller size, FUGs are more forgiving than MUGs and are highly recommended for the beginning hair-restoration surgeon.

Owing to the complexity of judgment/planning, site creation, graft dissection, and placement, the beginning hair-restoration surgeon should be encouraged to undertake only single follicular-unit transfer until such time that he or she feels comfortable advancing to use MUGs in conjunction with FUGs. As mentioned in Chap. 53, the success of hair-restoration surgery is contingent upon the skill of the surgeon but also on the dedicated hair-transplant team, which is knowledgeable about how to dissect grafts and place them as well. Graft dissection and placement of MUGs requires extra skill and attention that a junior team would most likely not be able to undertake well and may compromise an already tedious operation. Also, the surgeon is liable for a mistake with MUGs, as MUGs that are poorly distributed and angled can appear "pluggy." If one attempts to use MUGs, we suggest starting with white or fine-caliber donor hair, which is much more forgiving. It should be recalled that using larger grafts could amplify both good and poor results. Although this chapter will explore the differences between FUGs and MUGs, the entire procedure outlined in Sect. 54.2 can be undertaken with FUGs alone.

54.2
Technique

54.2.1
Consultation

The surgeon should establish with every prospective patient what areas of the scalp the patient desires to have the transplant and also what prior experience with medications, surgery, and hairpieces the patient has had in the past. The patient's age and rate of hair loss are very important aspects to consider when contemplating hair transplantation. For instance, a younger patient in his 20s with rapid loss of hair may not be a suitable candidate for hair transplantation for fear of depleting the donor hair without being able to maintain a natural hair pattern all the while chasing the progression of his hair loss. In these younger patients, it is best to carefully observe them over many years on medical management, such as finasteride and minoxidil, before committing to operate on them. We always counsel a patient about future hair loss, the possible need for more transplantation sessions, the extent of donor hair available today and in the future, and the need for FDA-approved medical management to retard ongoing hair loss.

With shaving one's entire head in vogue, a patient may become interested in eventually shaving his head. This option may not be suitable after transplantation, and this limitation should be communicated. The linear donor scar that may be imperceptible when camouflaged with hair could become notably exposed when the overlying hair is shaved clean. Further, shaving the hair in the region of transplanted grafts may reveal a small amount of skin dimpling at each graft location that would become visible with a shorn head. Transplanted grafts are also more resistant to eradication with laser hair-removal technology. It is particularly important to communicate these considerations especially to younger patients who may try to explore these options in the future.

During the process of hair loss, susceptible hairs that are prone to fall out not only simply leave the scalp but also undergo a process of miniaturization in which thicker, terminal hairs convert to tiny, vellus hairs. If the patient exhibits a significant proportion of these vellus hairs in the zone for transplantation, he is more likely to sustain temporary traumatic shedding of his existing hair postoperatively, known as telogen effluvium, and would benefit from maintenance with finasteride and minoxidil for 6 months or more to stabilize these

hairs before transplantation. This is particularly true of the crown area, which should be undertaken only cautiously for the reasons outlined in Chap. 53.

Besides careful evaluation of the recipient area, the surgeon should study the donor hair for hair density, color, texture, scalp elasticity, and the presence of any previous scars. The importance of hair density has already been discussed. Color and texture play an important role in making results appear even more natural, as finer, curly, lighter-colored hair blends more seamlessly than thicker, darker, and straighter hair. Nevertheless, proper technique can make even difficult hair appear completely natural if done right. Good scalp elasticity predisposes toward better wound closure and may facilitate a shorter interval between hair-transplant sessions if the patient desires a second session early. Unfavorable scars from previous sessions may need to be removed in conjunction with the current proposed session, which may compromise either hair yield or wound closure. In such a case, the surgeon should discuss the situation with the patient preoperatively to determine his or her priority and decide accordingly.

54.2.2
Planning

After the surgeon and patient have agreed upon the area of the scalp for transplantation, the surgeon should plan the number of grafts needed to cover the desired area and how much donor area needs to be harvested to achieve that objective. Many variables are considered to accurately assess the number of grafts needed for transplantation in any given area, e.g., hairline, midscalp, or vertex. On average, 25–30 FUGs and ten to 15 MUGs per square centimeter are considered densely packed. Typically, a transition zone of a hairline will require approximately 350–450 follicular units to achieve progressive coverage and 400–600 MUGs, (depending on the recipient and grafts size) or 800–1,200 FUGs across the central midscalp behind the hairline zone.

Solid-core needles of 16, 17, 18, and 19 gauge are used to create various-sized recipient sites that accommodate FUGs versus an SM no. 62 or an SP no. 91 blade for MUG recipient sites.

The authors prefer a multiblade handle to remove donor hair in order to facilitate ease of graft dissection; however, using a multiblade instrument without proper scalp preparation with tumescent solution risks a higher transection rate and must be undertaken with greater caution than use of a standard freehand ellipse. The technique for using a multiblade handle correctly is discussed in the following section.

Table 54.1 gives the projected number of grafts available for a 5-cm-long, 5.0-mm-wide strip of donor hair based on different donor-hair density. Although the table gives values for both FUGs and MUGs, the reader can simply ignore the second column and base his or

Table 54.1 Calculation of donor hair for harvesting for a 5-cm × 5.0-mm strip

	Follicular-unit grafts	Multiple follicular-unit grafts
Low density	120	40–45
Medium density	120–150	50–60
High density	150–200	70–75

her calculation on FUGs. The numbers in each column relate to the number of follicular units available for harvest in the specified donor strip based on perceived donor density.

54.2.3
Operation

54.2.3.1
Setup

Although the procedure can be easily accomplished with only an oral sedative and narcotic, it is significantly more comfortable for the patient to be under level II conscious sedation using a mixture of intravenous midazolam and fentanyl titrated as needed. The only part of the procedure that is truly uncomfortable for the patient is administration of the anesthetic ring block and donor harvesting. The patient does not require any further titration of intravenous sedation for the remainder of the procedure. Midazolam also provides the benefit of amnesia, so any discomfort the patient should express will most likely not be recalled afterward. As hair-restoration procedures can be quite lengthy, the intravenous sedation can lessen patient restlessness by reducing the time that the patient is actually required to be awake and absolutely still. The reader is advised to adhere to all state regulations that pertain to the administration of level II anesthesia.

Patient positioning is crucial to the ease of the procedure. A dental chair that can position the patient in an erect, semierect, and supine position is indispensable for various aspects of the procedure. Also, the headrest of the dental chair should be relatively compact and permit access circumferentially around its perimeter. This feature becomes particularly important for the individuals placing the grafts. For donor harvesting, the headrest should be able to be removed entirely or moved out of the way to permit access to the occiput.

A positive patient experience can be enhanced by having a selection of DVD films available during the afternoon so as to reduce the perceived length of the procedure and to distract the patient. Obviously, this would be unnecessary for shorter procedures like only hairline reconstruction.

54.2.3.2
Donor Harvesting

After the calculated distance of the donor strip(s) has been outlined, the assistant can shave a bandwidth of hair (approximately 1.5–2-cm wide) along the occiput to facilitate donor harvesting and ensure clean closure. In order to harvest the maximal number of grafts possible without compromising donor closure in the patient who requires a large number of grafts, we often harvest from temple to temple. The temple provides finer hairs that can be used for the hairline and can also be an excellent donor site for patients who have had only their occiput depleted of usable grafts from prior transplantation sessions done elsewhere. The preferred area for occipital harvesting resides just above the nuchal ridge but can be adjusted based on previous scarring and scalp elasticity. In order to expose the donor area, the hair that resides above the area for harvesting should be taped up with 1-in. clear plastic tape, which can be removed at the end of donor harvesting. A circumferential ACE bandage should be secured that resides immediately below the proposed hairline anteriorly and below the shaved occiput. Folded 4 × 4 gauze is placed between the scalp and the ACE wrap and is used to catch any bloody soilage during the procedure. At this point, the hairline and other areas of the scalp for hair transplantation should have already been designed according to the principles outlined in Chap. 53. The patient should check using a mirror that the design matches his or her aesthetic objectives before proceeding. Although no formal sterile preparatory solution is required, the patient is asked to wash the hair the night before and the morning of the procedure with Hibiclens.

When the patient has been properly sedated, the surgeon can at this point administer the local anesthetic ring block that contains buffered 1% lidocaine with 1:100,000 epinephrine. Typically, 20 ml is required to cover the entire circumference of the head. If only the hairline is to be reconstructed, the anesthetic can be delivered just immediately below the donor area and immediately anterior to the hairline without the need to traverse the entire head circumference. Before donor harvesting commences, the forehead immediately above where the local anesthetic was injected is infiltrated with 10 ml of a mixture containing 0.01% lidocaine with 1:200,000 epinephrine and 0.4 mg/ml triamcinolone and an additional 10–20 ml of the same mixture is infiltrated subcutaneously into the entire area planned for transplantation, i.e., the recipient scalp. This solution facilitates hemostasis by virtue of the epinephrine and reduction in postoperative edema owing to the steroid component.

The donor site is then generously infiltrated with tumescent solution for two reasons. First, the tumescent solution will help straighten the follicles out to minimize transection, which is particularly important when using the less forgiving multiblade instrument. Second, the tumescent solution raises the follicles away from the deeper vital structures of nerves and blood vessels so as to minimize their injury. The tumescent solution contains 0.01% lidocaine with 1:200,000 epinephrine. Typically, we infiltrate approximately 150–200 ml of tumescent solution to acquire the necessary turgor before harvesting begins, all depending on the size of the area harvested. The plane of infiltration is very important and should be in the immediate subcutaneous plane and not subgaleal. A blanching effect of the scalp is often an indication of the proper infiltration. The tumescent infiltration should continue until the scalp is tense and indurated and uniformly flat throughout. Additional tumescent solution can be infiltrated directly into the dermal plane to further straighten the hair follicles and to achieve added turgor. The surgeon should not be concerned with follicular transection with the injection needle during dermal infiltration, as this complication simply does not arise. Very little time should transpire between completing tumescent infiltration and donor harvest, as tumescent solution can be rapidly absorbed.

A multiblade instrument is used for harvesting in order to facilitate graft dissection. A Tori handle of the multiblade instrument can accommodate various number of no. 10 blades with spacers between the blades to adjust the size of each donor strip. We have found that Personna blades are far superior to the standard Bard–Parker blades for donor harvesting and graft dissection. For a right-handed surgeon, it is easier to begin harvesting from the right side of the head and progress toward the left side. With proper tumescence, the hair shafts should be almost perpendicular to the scalp but may be slightly still angled downward. The surgeon should try to visualize the angle of the hair shafts and match the blade to parallel these shafts (Fig. 54.1). After passage of the blade through a short distance of the scalp, the surgeon should lift the superior flap of tissue with the non-dominant hand to evaluate whether any follicular transection is observed on the harvesting strip. If the follicular bulbs (the base of the hair shaft) appear to be principally transected, the blade handle is too high and should be adjusted downward. By moving the handle downward, the blade tips move in the opposite upward direction. If the upper portion of the hair shaft appears primarily transected, the handle should be moved upward so that the angle of the blade is adjusted in the opposite direction to minimize transection. Slow, deliberate progression through the scalp with frequent inspection for transection can limit follicular transection (Fig. 54.2). A high transection rate reduces the number of usable grafts and can compromise the projected number of grafts to be transplanted. Besides visual inspection, the surgeon can actually feel transection as the blade slices through the tissue, i.e., the resistance that the blade encounters when dragged through hair shafts is higher than through the butterlike tissue free of any ensnared follicles. During harvest, the surgeon

should also ensure that the length of the blade is at an appropriate depth: not so deep that the blood vessels and nerves are injured or too superficial that the blade does not extend past the hair follicles. At times, the depth of the exposed blades must be adjusted on the handle if they are too recessed to permit adequate tissue penetration. Care must be particularly exercised when harvesting from the thinner temporal region, where inadvertent injury to the temporal artery may compromise blood supply and lead to decreased graft survival, excessive telogen effluvium, or frank tissue necrosis.

After the multiblade has traversed the entire arc of donor scalp, both ends must be tapered to a single point with a no. 10 blade taking care to avoid transection of the follicles with the blade. The donor strip can then be removed with Metzenbaum scissors, being careful to ensure that the tines of the scissors pass immediately below the hair bulbs without being excessively deep (with too much subcutaneous fat removed) or too superficial (with either exposed bulbs at the bottom of the strip or, worse, transected bulbs). Generally 1–2 mm of fat should be left below the bulbs. The assistant should hold the patient's head steady during harvesting and also elevate the superior flap to expose the follicles to facilitate donor strip removal. The assistant can also dab any excessive blood that would obscure the surgeon from seeing the base of the follicles during donor strip removal.

At this point, the open donor wound should be inspected for any signs of excessive bleeding. If a disrupted vessel is encountered, the surgeon can judiciously cauterize the vessel with bipolar forceps, being careful not to apply excessive thermal injury to the surrounding tissue. Many blood vessels are intimately paired with a nerve that could be damaged with exuberant cauterization. If the bleeding emanates proximal to a follicle, the bleeding should not be cauterized in order to avoid injury to the follicle. When hemostasis is achieved, the surgeon can close the incision. Before closing, we prefer to perform what is known as a trichophytic closure, which entails removal of approximately 1 mm of skin along the inferior edge of the wound (Fig. 54.3). Microserrated scissors facilitate easy removal of this thin strip. This trichophytic closure permits possibly a better wound closure by allowing the hair follicles to grow through the cut incision and thereby to camouflage the incision line more effectively, similar to the technique used for closure of a trichophytic browlift.

Closure of the incision is carried out with a running, non-locking 3-0 nylon (or polypropylene) suture (Fig. 54.4). Prior to closure, the wound is cleaned of any entrapped hair, and towel clamps are applied intermittently across the entire length of the incision in order to relieve tension on the incision line. The towel clamps also serve to decompress the remaining tumescent solution out of the donor scalp and thereby facilitate ease of wound closure. With a trichophytic closure, a slightly smaller bite of tissue should be taken along the inferior wound edge compared with the upper wound edge in order to promote 1 mm of overlap over the exposed trichophytic edge. If a trichophytic closure is not planned, then the wound is closed with a larger bite of tissue along the inferior wound edge and a relatively smaller bite of tissue along the superior flap so that the wound edges appear well approximated without significant overlap of the edges (since the wound edge is typically slightly beveled superiorly to match the angle of the hair follicles). To reduce the aggravation of the suture knot on the wound edge, the knots at both ends of the running suture can be affixed to the scalp approximately 1 cm distal to both ends of the wound. Prior to continuing, the surgeon or assistant should ensure that none of the

hairs are trapped under the sutures, which can be very irritating to the patient during the postoperative period. Additionally, the wound can be cleaned gently with a spray bottle containing saline, and the saturated pieces of gauze that are held by the circumferential ACE bandage can be exchanged for clean, fresh ones as needed.

At this point, the surgeon should administer longer-acting 0.25% bupivacaine with 1:200,000 epinephrine as a ring block to reinforce the effect of the lidocaine that typically begins to dissipate at that juncture. Like for lidocaine, about 20 ml of bupivacaine is generally required to cover the entire circumference of the head. The dental chair can then be repositioned with the patient in a supine position to facilitate recipient-site creation.

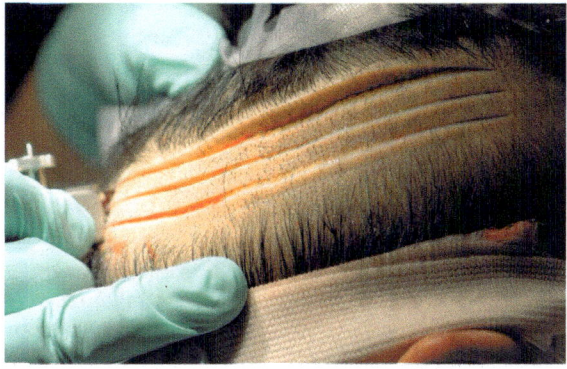

Fig. 54.1 A multiblade handle is used to remove donor strips from the occiput. With proper tumescent solution, very little bleeding should be observed, as the follicles are elevated away from the underlying vasculature. The angle of the blade must be constantly adjusted to ensure limited follicular transection

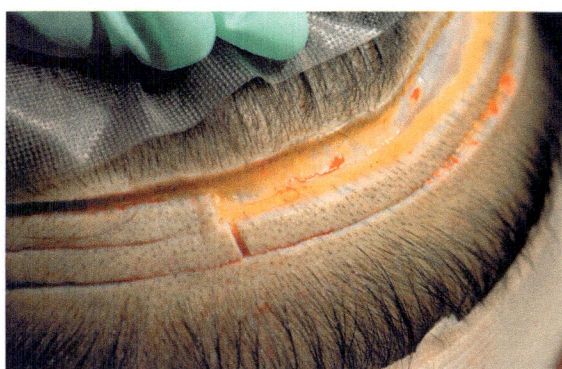

Fig. 54.2 There is limited to no transection of follicles with one strip already removed from the donor site for better view

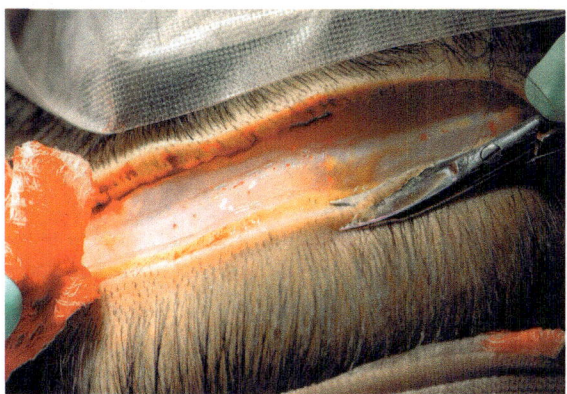

Fig. 54.3 A trichophytic closure facilitates hair growth through the scar and thereby better camouflage of the donor scar. Microserrated scissors are used to trim approximately 1 mm of skin from the inferior wound edge

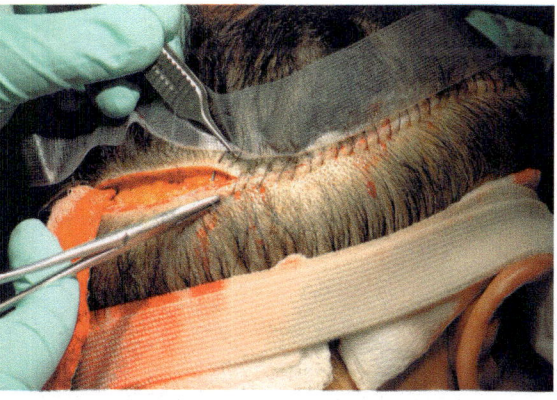

Fig. 54.4 The wound edge is approximated with a running, non-locking 3-0 nylon suture with minimal tension ensuring that no hairs become entrapped under the suture or inside the wound itself. A slightly smaller bite of tissue is taken on the inferior wound edge compared with the upper wound edge to promote 1 mm of overlap to cover the exposed trichophytic edge

54.2.3.3
Recipient-Site Creation

With the patient positioned supine, the surgeon should then administer a generous amount of recipient-site tumescent solution to reinforce and supplement the initial application (0.01% lidocaine, 1:200,000 epinephrine, and 0.4 mg/ml triamcinolone). Again, the infiltration should be in the subcutaneous plane in order to elevate the skin away from the underlying vasculature so that the instruments used to create the sites do not damage the blood supply below. Preservation of the blood supply is particularly important toward the midline of the scalp where vascularity is more tenuous. In any case, it is always wise to have readily available topical nitropaste that can immediately alleviate any incipient violaceous changes before the onset of possible frank necrosis. Typically, we use between 60 and 100 ml of recipient-site tumescent solution, which we apply periodically throughout the time that recipient sites are created, i.e., the entire amount of tumescent solution is not delivered at one time like in the donor area.

Proper recipient-site creation is contingent upon the correct angle, direction, and distribution of the sites (Fig. 54.5). These details were elaborated in Chap. 53. The reader is encouraged to review these principles when designing and creating recipient sites.

54.2.3.4
Graft Dissection and Placement

To ensure graft survival and proper growth, the donor tissue and individual grafts have to be handled properly, i.e., gently manipulated and not left to dry out. Donor

tissue has to remain moist at all time whether by periodically spraying the tissue with saline solution during dissection or by keeping it immersed in a chilled saline bath. After the donor strip has been measured, the tissue is segmented into smaller 2–5-cm sections that are easier to manipulate. The first cut through the tissue is known as slivering, the purpose of which is to expose follicular units and thereby facilitate further dissection. This cut is performed gently by sliding or teasing the blade through the space between the follicular units, making sure that slivers are uniform and that the hair units remain intact. As the dissection progresses, grafts containing the same number of hair are grouped together, i.e., one-hair group, two-hair group, three-plus hair group; and these groups are arranged on 2 × 2 Telfa pads and placed into Petri dishes filled with chilled saline solution. We use a tongue depressor soaked in saline solution as a cutting surface, jeweler no. 3 forceps to hold the tissue, and a Personna Prep blade or a no. 10 blade to dissect the tissue.

Regarding graft placement, jeweler no. 5 forceps are preferred. During placement, individual grafts are held by the cuff of fatty tissue below the follicles (the grip of the forceps should be gentle yet deliberate), inserted into individual sites, and then dabbed with a folded 4 × 4 gauze. Further, one should pay attention not to crush or injure hair follicles by squeezing the graft or forcing it into the site because this inappropriate manipulation may cause poor hair growth or the appearance of kinky hair. Also, grafts have to be placed by matching their size to the appropriate-sized site. If a graft is too small for a site it will slide inside off the site and appear as a "pitted" graft. If a graft is too large for a site, it will appear compressed when it grows in. Although sites are created with the desired hair angle in mind, appro-

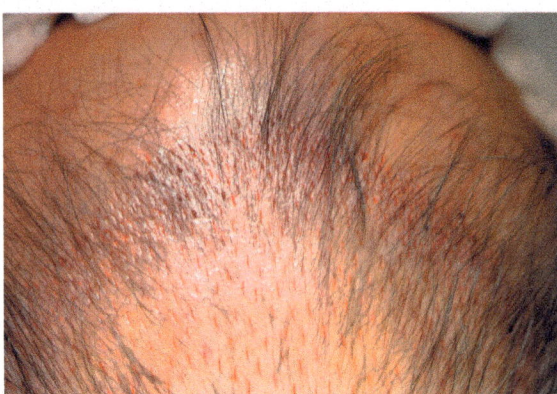

Fig. 54.5 Tightly, interlocked, and forward-angled recipient sites that increase in size progressing posteriorly are shown with a natural undulating hairline. The larger posterior sites are created with an SP91 blade and are designed to accommodate multiple follicular-unit grafts (MUGs)

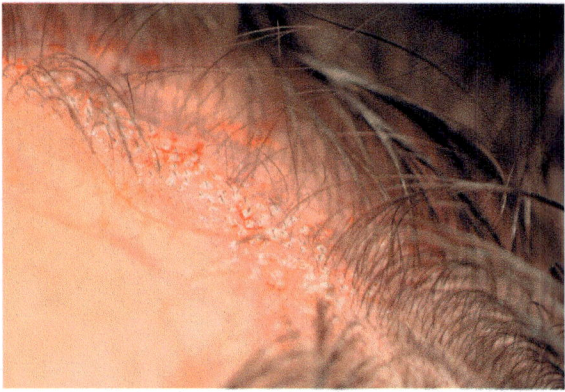

Fig. 54.6 Grafts should be placed into the recipient sites so that the grafts rest just above the surrounding skin surface

priate graft orientation is important and even more so when placing MUGs. One should also be mindful when placing grafts in-between existing hair so that no native hair becomes trapped under the grafts. Finally, to ensure more uniformly seamless healing, grafts should be placed slightly (approximately 1 mm) above the skin level (Fig. 54.6).

54.3
Postoperative Care

Postoperative care is relatively simple. To minimize postoperative edema, the patient is instructed to sleep preferably in a semierect position like in a recliner for the first 2–3 nights and to apply an ice pack on the forehead and the donor area for 20 min on and 20 min off while awake for the first 1–2 days. However, the patient is cautioned not to apply the ice pack directly on the grafted areas. The patient is also supplied with a small package of 4×4 gauze for direct and sustained local pressure for 5 min, in case any bleeding is encountered the first night. Showering should be deferred for 24 h but can be started by allowing use of only a low-pressure faucet and gentle cleansing for the first week. Thereafter, the patient can resume normal showering habits. No specialized shampoo formula need be used. The patient will develop scabbing over each graft, which should not be disturbed during the first week. After that time, the patient is encouraged to vigorously rub these scabs off, as they can impair graft viability after the first 10 days. During the initial postoperative visits, the normal shedding of transplanted hair and the natural 2–3-month waiting period for the new hair growth cycle to begin are once again explained to the patient.

Donor sutures are removed on the tenth postoperative day. Patients then return 3 months after the procedure, as early growth may become apparent at this time. Generally speaking, any growth at this juncture is sporadic and limited. By the fifth to sixth postoperative month, patients typically exhibit considerable growth and may finally begin to express satisfaction with the result. Ongoing benefit is observed through the ninth to tenth postoperative month with a diminution of gain over the following 2 months. Accordingly, patients are seen 3, 6, 9, and 12 months postoperatively and then semiannually to annually thereafter.

54.4
Complications

Hair restoration is easy to perform but hard to perform well. The complications in hair-restoration surgery can be poor or unnatural hair growth, poor donor or recipient scalp healing, prolonged scalp anesthesia, and frank necrosis or extensive postoperative effluvium. Even if the surgeon harvests grafts skillfully, closes the donor incision beautifully, and makes seamlessly perfect recipient sites, the operative team could affect results by cutting or handling grafts poorly, which could compromise graft survival and ultimately graft appearance. Accordingly, the surgeon and his or her operative team must be equally adept to achieve excellent results (Figs. 54.7, 54.8).

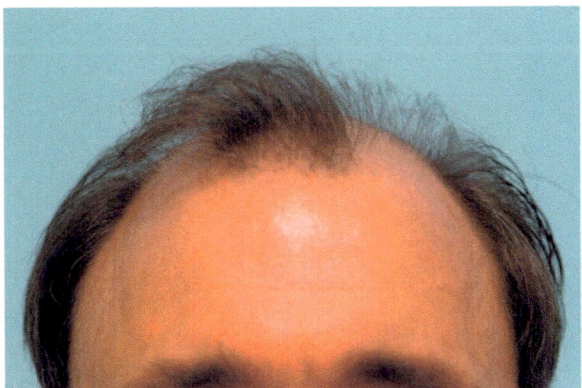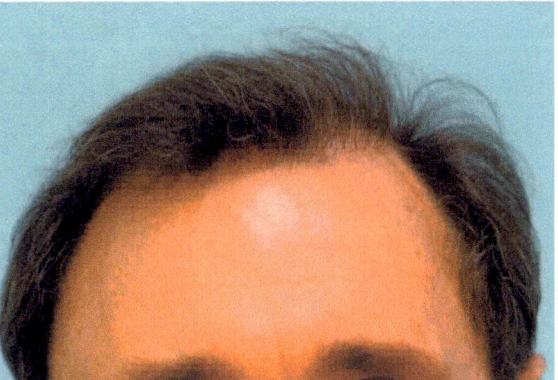

Fig. 54.7 This 42-year-old male patient underwent hair transplantation with 1,001 grafts comprising 596 follicular-unit grafts (FUGs) and 197 MUGs to yield 4,526 hairs and is shown 9 months after that session with notable aesthetic improvement

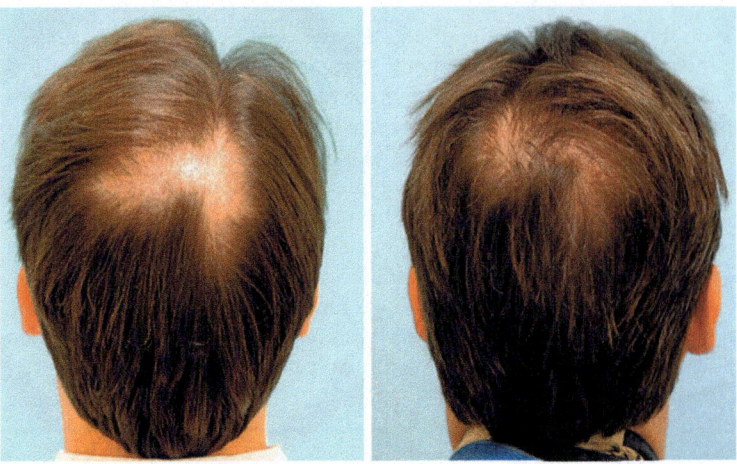

Fig. 54.8 This 56-year-old male patient underwent hair transplantation with 791 grafts all of which were FUGs to yield 2,002 hairs and is shown 8 months after that session with notable aesthetic improvement

References

1. Dieffenbach, J.F.: Nonulla de Regeneratione et Transplantatione. Dissertation 1822
2. Okuda, S.: Clinical and experimental studies of transplantation of living hairs. Jpn J Dermatol Urol 1939;46:135–138
3. Tamura, H.: Pubic hair transplantation. Jpn J Dermatol 1943;53:76
4. Orentreich, N.: Autographs in alopecias and other selected dermatoloical conditions. Ann N Y Acad Sci 1959:83:463–479
5. Headington, J.T.: Transverse microscopic anatomy of the human scalp. A basis for a morphometric approach to disorders of the hair follicle. Arch Dermatol 1984;120(4):449–456

Chapter 55

Mesotherapy for Treatment of Male-Type Alopecia

55

Oh Sook Kwon

55.1 Introduction

Male-type alopecia is called androgenic alopecia or bald hair and this type usually begins to show in the late 20s or 30s. The patients have thin and soft hair from the frontal to the vertex area of the head instead of thick and healthy hair. This happens from the effects of male hormones and only thin, soft and short hair shows because of the short period of the anagen stage (Fig. 55.1). Male-type alopecia usually starts with an M shape that starts from the frontal area of the head or starts from the vertex of the head. But the posterior hair and temporal hair remain because of the effects of male hormones.

The main causes of alopecia include male hormones and age. There are other causes, such as local circulation (Fig. 55.2), mental stress, unbalanced nutrition, and cradle cap. Alopecia is the action of androgen on the hair follicles. Testosterone is transformed to dehydrotestosterone by an enzyme called 5α-R. The activity of 5α-R is much higher in alopecia patients.

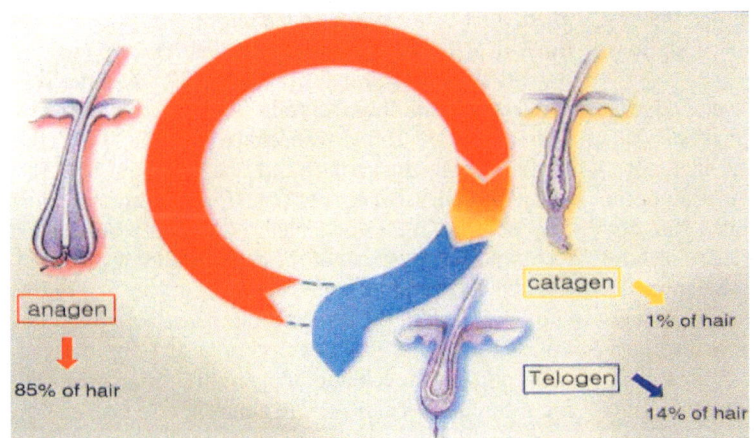

Fig. 55.1 Phases of hair growth. Anagen-stage hair constitutes 85% of the entire hair. Those anagen-stage hairs proceed to the talogen stage through the catagen stage. The alopecia index is defined as the ratio of anagen-stage hair to talogen-stage hair. Normal hair has a value over 5. A value lower than 5 is an indication for treatment

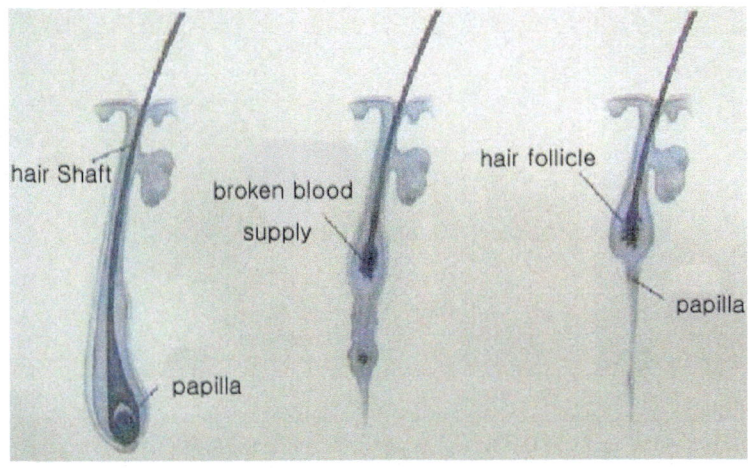

Fig. 55.2 The importance of blood supply. The hair follicle shrinks and the hair is getting thinner. Alopecia can be caused by poor blood circulation

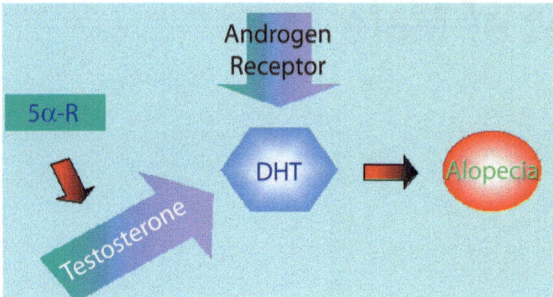

Fig. 55.3 Progress of alopecia. The hormone that causes alopecia is dihydrotestosterone (*DHT*), which is transformed from testosterone by *5α-R*. If too much is secreted, this causes reduction of hair follicles and interrupts regeneration and differentiation of follicles. So, eventually it causes alopecia

Alopecia is often though to be just a sign of aging (Fig. 55.3). Many treatments have been introduced but there have been no permanent and effective alternatives. There are two ways to treat male alopecia. One is a surgical and the other is a nonsurgical method. Nonsurgical methods include finasteride, applying hormone products, mesotherapy or general intravenous therapy, ultraviolet (UV) irradiation, local hair tonic, scalp massage, and diet.

Since hair autotransplantation was developed and proved its merit, it has become popular; however, hair autotransplantation has many problems so it is not a good fundamental alternative for treatment of alopecia. A new method has been introduced called mesotherapy that requires exact indications and knowledge of how to perform it. The basic concept of mesotherapy is to stimulate the local blood circulation to supply enough nutrition to hair follicles in order to promote the regeneration of hair follicles in alopecia areas, delay the degeneration, and lower the activation of androgen.

55.2
Instrument Description

To deliver the drug effectively, needle treatment is used first with a mesogun and second with a mesoroller. The syringe is prepared with a drug cocktail and used with the mesogun and then with the mesoroller (Fig. 55.4). The cylinder contains 192 tiny needles that make multiple injections possible. There are various needle lengths: 0.2, 0.5, 1.0, 1.5, and 2.5 mm. Among of them, 0.5-mm needles are most often used for alopecia treatment by the physician and 0.2-mm needles are for personal care at home.

55.3
Technique

The most important point of mesotherapy is to deliver drugs to the hair follicles by needle stimulation. To maximize the treatment effect, the scalp of the patient is steamed. Through this step it is easier to remove the horny layer and the pores are enlarged. The next step is scaling. This removes the horny layer and dirt in the pores. Immediately after this step, mesotherapy is applied. First is the mesogun technique. The cocktail is a mixture of 2 ml buflomedil (vasodilator), 2 ml vitamin B_5, and vitamin B complex including 2 ml biotine. This is injected 1 mm into the scalp. The direction of the injection is from frontal to occipital (Fig. 55.5) and the angle between the syringe and scalp is about 45°. The injection interval is about 1 cm. The starting direction may be from the right or left. Next is the mesoroller technique. The cocktail of the drugs is 1 ml copper peptide, DNA and RNA (diluted with 2 ml normal saline and 1 ml $NaHCO_3$), and 2 ml amino acid. The length of the needle is 0.5 mm. The injection is at 1-cm intervals starting from the left and applying the drugs with rolling technique. For the severe alopecia area such as the

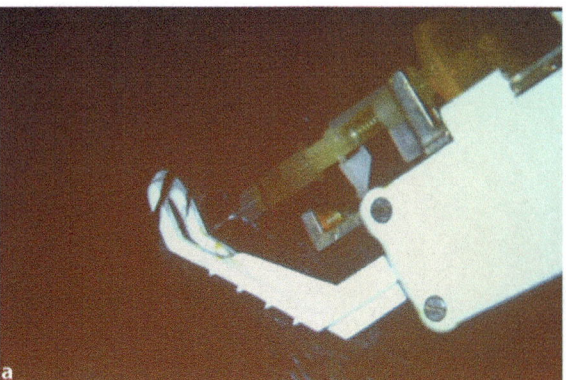
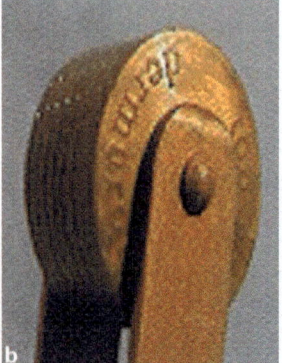
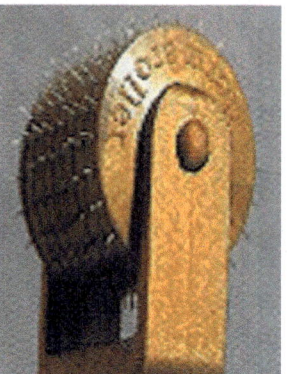

Fig. 55.4 **a** Injection technique. This is the manual technique, injecting by hand with a 30-gauge needle, 4 mm in length. **b** Mesoroller that gives multineedle stimulation. This makes possible multichanneling and enables effective drug delivery

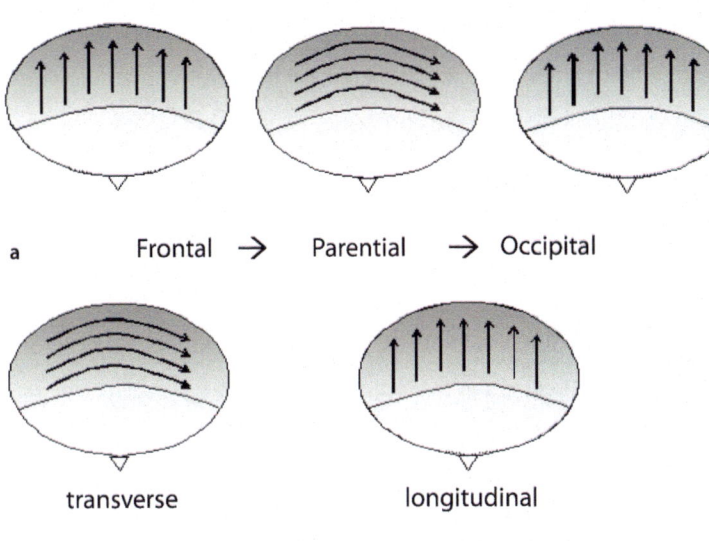

a   Frontal → Parential → Occipital

transverse   longitudinal

b   Frontal → Parential → Occipital

Fig. 55.5 a Method of injection. The direction of injection does not really matter. For convenience, usually start from frontal to occipital. Proper injection interval is 1 cm. Inject in the alopecia area and also around it. **b** Method of injection. Transverse and longitudinal are possible directions for the injection, but from frontal to occipital is recommended

frontal and vertex areas, injection (mesogun and meso-roller) is done more closely. After the drugs have been administered, it is necessary to wait a while to suppress the scalp.

The patient is cautioned not to wash the hair after treatment and not to get a hair perm and coloring for 24 h.

55.4
Complications

There are almost no side effects. There may be a little bit of discomfort with bleeding and pain when injecting and there may be a minor side effect like drug allergy.

55.5
Discussion

Each individual cell has a nucleus in its center. A nucleus has plenty of DNA inside it. DNA participates in the gene phenomena of the existence of living things and is in charge of protein synthesis. RNA exists in the cytoplasm and it synthesizes protein by the order of DNA. In other words, RNA (1) takes an order from DNA as to what kind of protein it should make, (2) gathers amino acid, which is a component of protein, and (3) becomes a protein manufacturing factory itself. DNA has genetic information and RNA synthesizes protein that is essential for the human body in accordance with the genetic information contained in DNA.

Because it is quite complicated for many reasons, the cause of gray hair and alopecia is not known in detail. Even though people have the same problems of gray hair and alopecia, the causes are different. Alopecia is caused by a male hormone, in other words, the hormone dehydrotestosterone interferes with the synthesis of ATP (amino acid ingredient), which provides the energy for hair growth. Stress causes alopecia in many cases by creating a lot of active oxygen that is not helpful for hair growth, so in the end enough nutrition is not supplied to follicles by a poor blood stream because of active oxygen. Too much sebum in the scalp will cause alopecia. Around the follicle there is a lot of RNA and this RNA eventually is reduced because of low liver function by aging and strong UV radiation. If is RNA reduced, protein that is the ingredient of hair cannot be made.

This will lead to alopecia. No matter what the reason for alopecia is, it is strongly related to nucleic acids. There are reasons that are not related to nucleic acids, but it is still worthwhile to try to eat nucleic acids and to apply low molecular weight nucleotides on the scalp.

55.6
Conclusions

Mesotherapy is suitable for male-type androgenic alopecia, stage 6 of the Hamilton classification, the female-type androgenic alopecia, and stage 3 of the Ludwig classification. Mesotherapy is especially effective for postpartum alopecia. In this treatment, it is very important to supply vitamins, minerals, amino acids, and DNA and RNA that improve local microcirculation and this will slow down the degeneration of hair follicles.

More than 90% of patients experience no more loss of hair after four treatments and after 3 months of treatment the hair grows back again (Figs. 55.6, 55.7). Younger patients experience their hair growing faster than older patients.

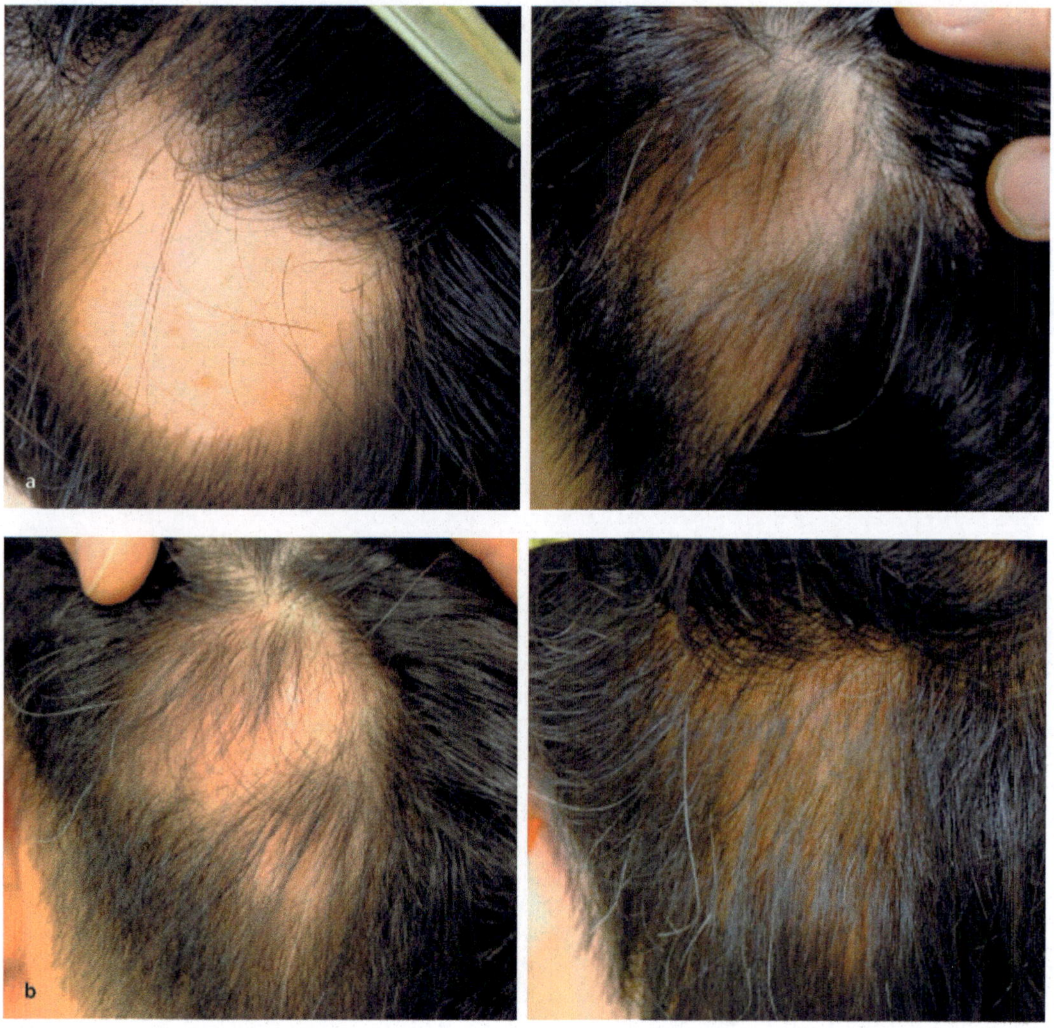

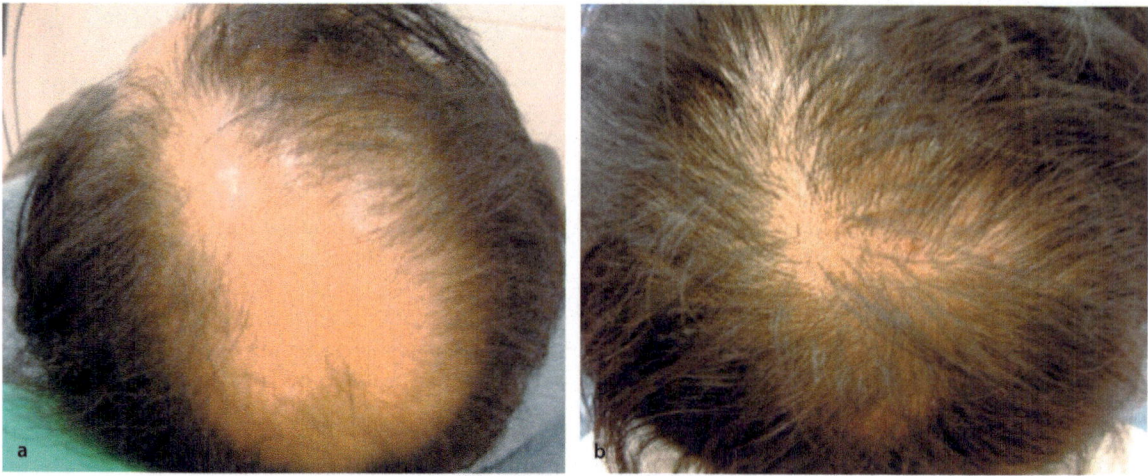

Fig. 55.6 Alopecia. **a** Before. **b** After 20 weeks, roller needle depth 0.5 mm, age 36

Fig. 55.7 Alopecia. **a** Before. **b** After 16 weeks, roller needle depth 0.5 mm, age 55

Mesotherapy is one of the best and most effective methods that can be used with other treatments. It contributes to slowing down of the androgenic phenomenon. Mesotherapy is excellent for postpartum alopecia. The important thing with mesotherapy is continuous treatment like with other aesthetic treatments. Mesotherapy is the most effective treatment to achieve hair growth. In some cases, younger patients can have better results from the treatment but actually the age does not really matter. In the case of the male patient, there would be need for an accompanying treatment such as minoxidil treatment and in the case of the female patient hormone treatment. It is very crucial and necessary for the patient to manage heavy stress.

Suggested Reading

1. Ahn SK, Hwang SM, Jiang SJ, Choi EH, Lee SH: The changes of epidermal calcium gradient and transitional cells after prolonged occlusion following tape stripping in the murine epidermis. J Invest Dermatol 1999;113(2):189–195

2. Ahn SK, Jiang SJ, Hwang SM, Choi EH, Lee JS, Lee SH: Functional and structural changes of the epidermal barrier induced by various types of insults in hairless mice. Arch Dermatol Res 2001;293(6):308–318

3. Choi EH, Kim MJ, Ahn SK, Park WS, Son ED, Nam GW, Chang I, Lee SH: The skin barrier state of aged hairless mice in a dry environment. Br J Dermatol 2002:147(2):244–249

4. Jiang SJ, Koo SW, Lee SH: The morphologic changes in lamellar bodies and intercorneocyte lipids after tape stripping and occlusion with a water vapor-impermeable membrane. Arch Dermatol Res 1998;290:145–151

5. Jiang SJ, Hwang SM, Choi EH, Elias PM, Ahn SK, Lee SH: Structural and functional effects of oleic acid and iontophoresis on hairless mouse stratum corneum. J Invest Dermatol 2000;114(1):64–70

6. Parienti IJ: Mésothérapie, 2nd Ed. Masson, Paris 1995

7. Pistor M: Mésothérapie Pratique. Masson, Paris 1998

8. Le Coz J: Traité de Mésothérapie. Masson, Paris 2004

9. Min BK: Diagnosis and Treatment of Hair and Scalp Disorders. Seoul, Korean Academy of Medical Sciences, Seoul 2005

10. Park YW: Cellulite and Aesthetic Mesotherapy. Seoul, Korean Academy of Medical Sciences, Seoul 2004

CHAPTER 56

Mid Forehead "Buttonhole" Eyebrow Elevation   56

Harry Mittelman, David S. Chrzanowski, Adam D. Schaffner

56.1
Introduction

At one time, surgery for the aging face was limited primarily to rhytidectomy and blepharoplasty [1], ignoring the contribution of the position of the brow in its relation to beauty and youth. The addition of surgery for rejuvenation of the upper third of the face has brought more balance to facial aesthetic surgery. This began with the introduction of coronal forehead lifts. However, the length of the incision and postoperative sequelae, such as alopecia, made this technique less popular with facial aesthetic surgeons and patients. The search for less invasive surgery popularized other techniques, such as endoscopic browlifts. Endoscopic browlifts were more technically difficult, but more acceptable to patients.

The goals of browlift procedures are superior repositioning of the eyebrow, an improvement in the contour of the eyebrow, minimal neurological and vascular morbidity, and a scar acceptable to the patient. In addition, the procedure should be long-lasting and dependable with a firm type of fixation. In the opinion of the senior author, the buttonhole mid forehead browlift best meets the goals of browlift procedures. It is technically easier to perform than endoscopic browlift techniques, appears to have equal or better longevity compared with other techniques, and the resulting incision scar when reapproximated meticulously is very acceptable to patients.

When performing a browlift with a blepharoplasty, consideration may be given to including a trans-upper-lid blepharoplasty brow suspension technique. This separates the palpebral and orbital portions of the orbicularis oculi muscles. Theoretically, this should increase the longevity of any browlift procedure by decreasing some of the downward pull on the orbicularis oculi muscle and the brow, when closing the eyes.

56.2
Anatomy

The ideal shape and position of the eyebrow has been described. The medial brow should be thicker, having a club shape, which gently tapers laterally [1]. It should begin at a position superior to the medial canthus of the eye, in line with the nasal alar groove, slightly above the orbital rim [2, 3]. In women, it should gently arch superiorly between the level of the lateral limbus and the lateral canthus, while in men the arch should not be as prominent. The lateral extent of the eyebrow can be determined by a line extended from the nasal alar groove through the lateral limbus of the eye [2, 3]

The layers of tissue in the forehead consist of skin and subcutaneous connective tissue, the frontalis muscle and galea aponeurosis, loose connective tissue, and periosteum covering the frontal bone [4]. While multiple muscles are responsible for brow depression, only the frontalis muscle elevates the brow. Brow depressors include the corrugator supercillii, procerus, and medial supercillii portion of the orbicularis oculi muscles. The strongest depressor of the mid and lateral brow is the orbital portion of the orbicularis oculi muscle.

The temporal branch of the facial nerve supplies motor innervation to the frontalis muscle. This nerve branches off the superior half of the facial nerve after leaving the stylomastoid foramen. It travels superiorly above the zygoma immediately deep to the temperoparietal fascia to innervate the frontalis muscle from the undersurface of the muscle. The sensory innervation is by the first division of the trigeminal nerve, via the supraorbital and supratrochlear nerves. These travel through notches (or less often in foramina) located on the medial portion of the superior orbital rim [4]. The blood supply to the forehead originates from the supratrochlear artery and travels parallel to the sensory nerves.

56.3
Preoperative Assessment

Elasticity of the forehead develops with aging, and causes the eyebrows to fall inferiorly from their ideal position. Patients often present to the facial aesthetic surgeon with complaints about redundant eyelid skin, making them look tired. The astute surgeon should also determine if eyebrow ptosis is playing a role in causing this perception of fatigue [5, 6].

Often patients with eyebrow ptosis will initially seek consultation for treatment of their deep horizontal forehead lines. Severely ptotic eyebrows, at or below the superior orbital rim, may cause the patient to continually elevate their brows in order to improve their vision. The continued contraction of the frontalis muscle may accentuate horizontal forehead lines. Treatment of horizontal forehead rhytids with a paralytic-like botulinum toxin can actually exacerbate the eyebrow ptosis, especially when it is used in the lower portion of the forehead. Methods of elevating the lateral brow with botulinum toxin can help this problem.

When counseling a patient, the facial aesthetic surgeon must assess the degree of eyebrow ptosis and preoperative asymmetry of eyebrow position [7]. It is important to note preoperative motor and sensory function of the forehead. The position of the hairline, age and gender of the patient, and degree of preoperative horizontal forehead rhytids all play a role in determining the optimal method of brow elevation [7, 8]. It is important to assess the need for browlift alone versus the need for combining browlift with upper-lid blepharoplasty. It is also important to assess the patient's skin type, whether it is thin or thick, as incisions may be more visible in patients with thicker skin. Men with male-pattern baldness and women with a high hairline are better candidates for mid forehead browlift procedures [9].

It is important to counsel the patient on the appropriate procedure and to discuss the risks and benefits as well as the limitations of each method. Patients must understand that browlifts as a rule are not permanent procedures. Even in the hands of the best of surgeons, the lasting effects of this surgery are not very predictable and can be disappointing to the patient and the surgeon. Asymmetry of the resulting eyebrow elevation with endoscopic techniques is not unusual. This is true for other approaches as well.

Photographic documentation is an essential part of the consultation and preoperative planning for any browlift procedure. Standard frontal views with adequate lighting over a blue or black background are taken. In addition, closeup photographs of the eyelids should be considered especially when a blepharoplasty procedure is planned. It is important to eliminate any excess function of the frontalis muscle during digital photography, so that the actual degree of ptosis and preoperative asymmetry can be recognized and documented. This can be achieved by having the patient gently open the eyes after closing them fully.

56.4
Choice of Procedure

The objective of browlift procedures is superior repositioning of the brow. The goal is to create a long-lasting, dependable, and reproducible result with a firm type of fixation. Neural and vascular injury should be minimized. In addition, the morbidity of the procedure should be minimal and the resultant scar should be acceptable to the patient. In the observations of the senior author, such a technique has not been developed, but the mid forehead "buttonhole" eyebrow elevation procedure is less difficult to perform and has minimal morbidity than comparable procedures.

Multiple types of browlift procedures have been developed over the past few years. These include browpexy, direct browplasty, mid forehead browlift, posttrichial coronal forehead lift, pretrichial/trichophytic coronal forehead lifts, bilateral temporal lift, endoscopic forehead lift, minimally invasive brow suspension, and FeatherLift/"hish hook" suture techniques [4–6, 9, 10]. There are many advantages and disadvantages of each procedure.

In the experience of the senior author, the optimal procedure for eyebrow elevation without corrugator or procerus muscle resection, in most patients, regardless of gender, is the mid forehead buttonhole browlift procedure. This may be combined with a trans-upper-lid blepharoplasty eyebrow suspension procedure. Although the mid forehead incision creates a permanent horizontal scar in the forehead, when designed correctly and reapproximated meticulously without tension, the incision is virtually invisible with time, even without camouflaging cosmetics.

The senior author believes that many published techniques for endoscopic forehead lifts may elevate the hairline, may cause small areas of alopecia, may result in some numbness around the incision, and may not be as long-lasting as other procedures. The rationale for the mid forehead lift procedure is based on the principle that the closer the incision to the area addressed, the more effective the procedure. In this procedure, where one suspends the attachments of the eyebrow to a fixed point (the periosteum of the frontal bone), this principle is very important. When this rationale is employed, the effects may be similar to or better at times than those for the endoscopic approach, but with less morbidity, fewer complications, and less difficulty.

In a noteworthy study by Ahn et al. [11], the effect of botulinum toxin type A injected into the depressor muscles of the forehead of patients was compared with the effected produced in patients who had undergone some type of browlift procedure. They found that the amount of brow elevation was approximately equal in both patient subsets 1 year following the surgical procedures. Therefore, botulinum toxin type A injections to the brow depressor muscles may be considered as an alternative to surgery. Even with eyebrow elevation surgical procedures, the authors are very strong proponents of using botulism toxin type A for eyebrow depressor muscle paresis rather than cutting or resecting the depressor muscles.

56.5
Surgical Technique

56.5.1
Mid Forehead Buttonhole Browlift

After reviewing preoperative notes and photographs, the surgeon must determine the optimal amount of skin to be excised if any, and the location of the brow in need of superior repositioning. The incision is usually planned in a natural forehead crease a few centimeters above the area of the brow to be addressed (Fig. 56.1). If both the medial and the lateral brow are to be addressed, separate incisions should be planned. Commonly, an ellipse of forehead skin is excised in addition to the eyebrow suspension. The surgeon then marks the patient, with the patient sitting completely upright. After the patient has been marked for all planned procedures, the patient is sterilely prepped and draped in the usual manner.

When performed in conjunction with an upper-lid blepharoplasty, the browlift is always performed first. The area of dissection on the forehead is injected with a 50:50 mixture of 1% lidocaine and 0.25% Marcaine with 1:200,000 fresh epinephrine. When injecting, great care must be taken to avoid capillary networks, which can cause bruising and may obscure the proper surgical plane during the procedure.

The planned elliptical incision is made and appropriate forehead skin and subcutaneous tissue are excised.

The dissection is carried inferiorly, in a subcutaneous plane, to the superficial surface of the orbicularis oculi muscle. The undermining is performed about 1 cm medial and lateral to the most medial and lateral portions of the incision in a trapezoidal shape. The plane of dissection is immediately subcutaneous, superficial to the frontalis muscle (Fig. 56.2). Dissection continues inferiorly to the level of the superior hairs of the brow. It is imperative that this dissection toward the eyebrow is under the skin but above the orbital orbicularis oculi muscle. The orbicularis oculi muscle is identified and preserved. The dissection inferiorly must not go below the level of the superior hairs of the eyebrow. The procedure will not be effective if undermining is extended past this landmark. Generally no dissection is carried out superior to the incision. Hemostasis is controlled using bipolar electrocautery.

Next, a 5-0 Prolene suture is placed through the periosteum at the superior portion of the incision laterally (Fig. 56.3). The suture is then placed through the lateral portion of the orbicularis oculi muscle that was previously identified (Fig. 56.4). The suture is looped through the muscle in a purse-string fashion to avoid tearing the muscle when tension is placed on the suture (Fig. 56.5). The suture is then tightened for the appropriate degree of brow elevation with slight overcorrection. A similar suture is placed medially between the periosteum and the orbicularis oculi muscle, using the same purse-string suture technique through the orbicularis oculi muscle.

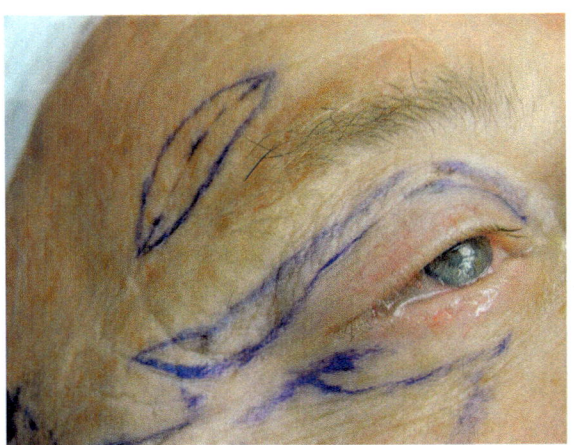

Fig. 56.1 The mid forehead browlift incision is planned a few centimeters superior to the brow in a natural forehead crease

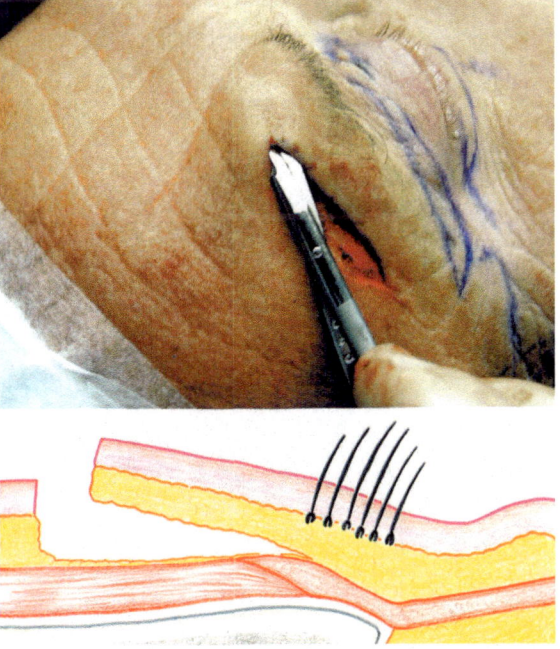

Fig. 56.2 Dissection is continued inferiorly in the subcutaneous plane until the orbicularis oculi muscle is in view medially

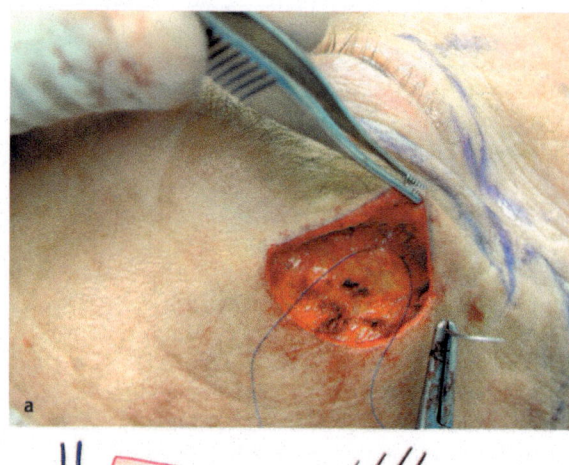

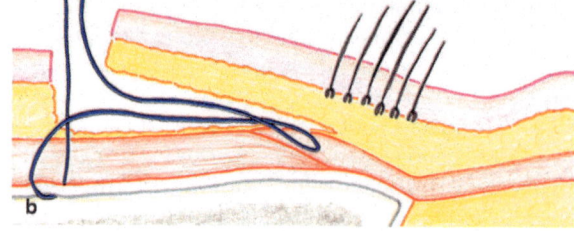

Fig. 56.4 a Suture is passed through orbicularis oculi muscle. **b** Lateral view shows suture placed in the periosteum and the orbicularis oculi muscle

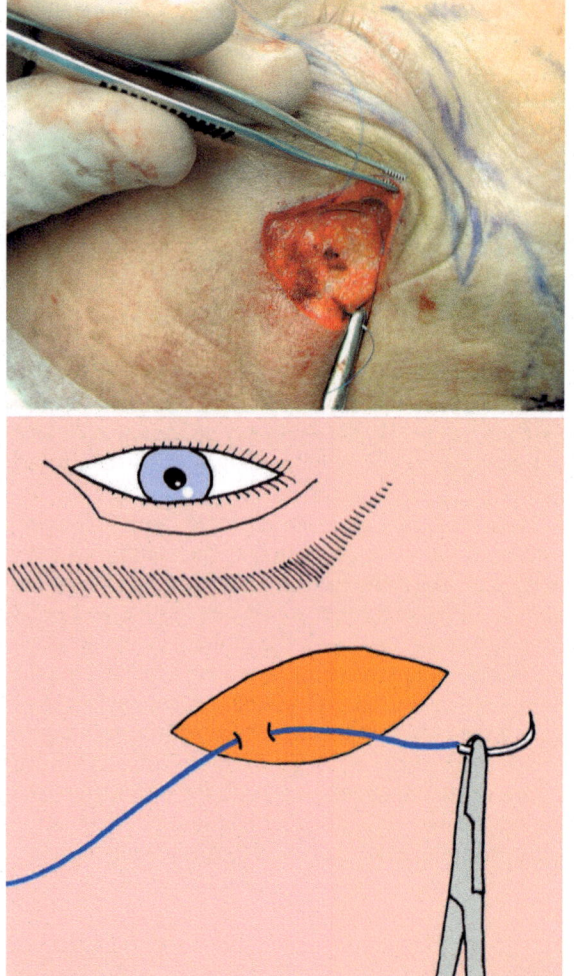

Fig. 56.3 Suture is passed through the periosteum at a superior portion of the incision

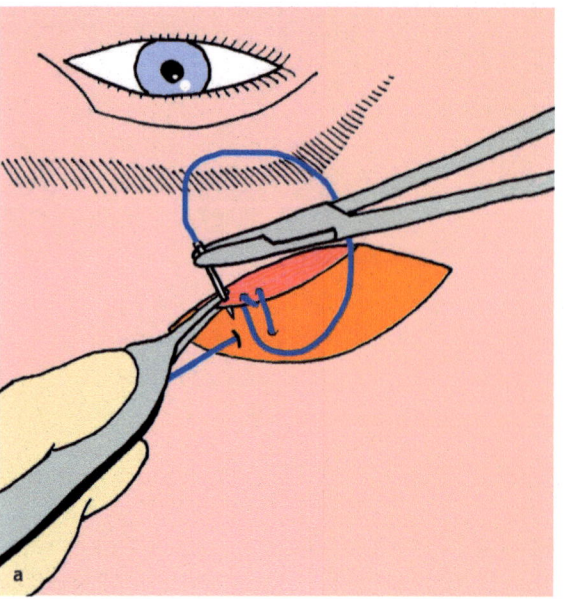

Fig. 56.5 a Orbicularis oculi muscle is sutured using purse-string technique. *b, c see next page*

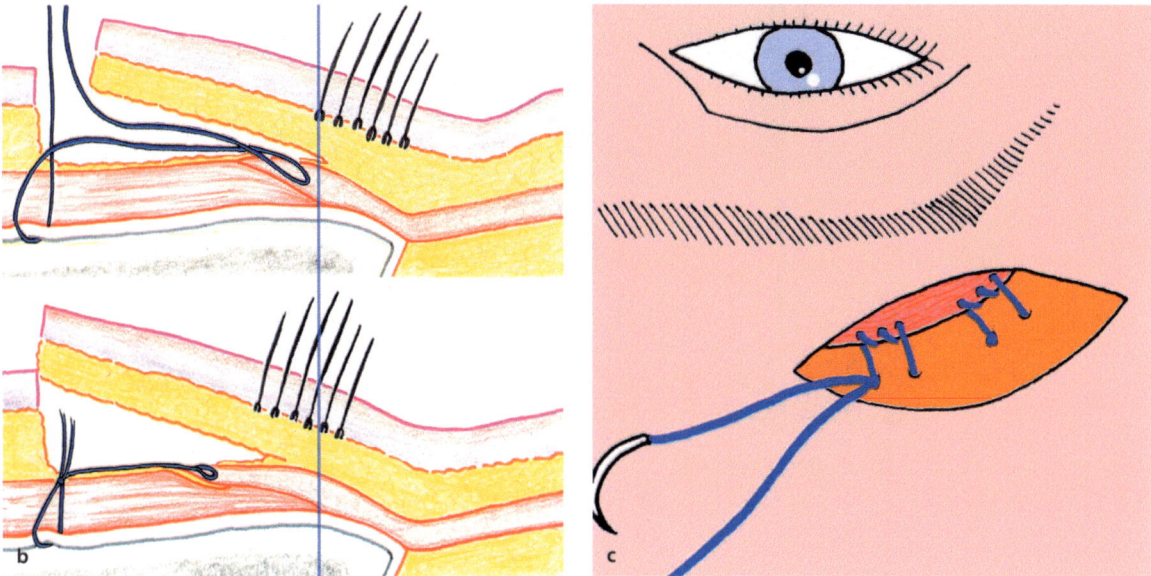

Fig. 56.5 *(Continued)* **b** Tightening of the suture pulls the mobile orbicularis oculi muscle with attached skin and brow superiorly toward the immobile periosteum, thereby elevating the eyebrow. The *blue line* demonstrates the amount of superior elevation of the brow. **c** Both medial and lateral sutures have been placed between the periosteum and the orbicularis oculi muscle

The incision must be meticulously closed with interrupted subcuticular 6-0 Monocryl sutures. Following placement of these sutures, the incision should appear closed (Fig. 56.6). Next, 6-0 Prolene interrupted sutures are used to reapproximate the skin edges, first with a couple of vertical mattress sutures and then with simple interrupted sutures. The most time-consuming part of the procedure is closing the incision in such a way as to keep the skin flap flat and avoid any "ripple" effect at either end of the closure. The procedure is then repeated

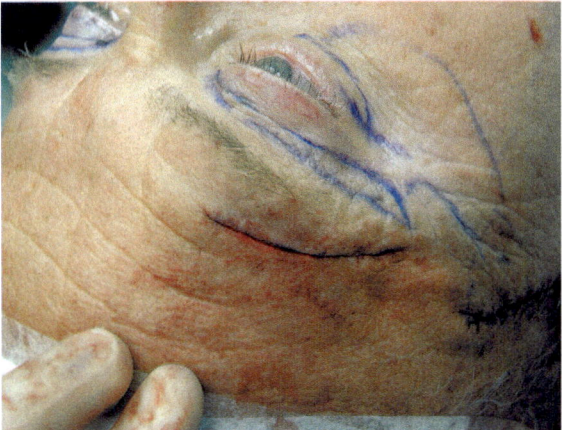

Fig. 56.6 The incision is closed under no tension using buried 6-0 Monocryl sutures

on the opposite side. Sterile strips are placed across the incision and a light-pressure dressing is placed between the incision and the eyebrow, which limits postoperative edema.

56.5.2
Trans-Upper-Lid Blepharoplasty Brow Suspension

Following the mid forehead browlift procedure, a trans-upper-lid blepharoplasty brow suspension may be performed. Prior to the procedure, the preoperative photographs and surgical notes should be reviewed. The planned incision, a standard blepharoplasty incision, is marked in the usual manner, and the area of dissection on the upper lid is injected with a 50:50 mixture of 1% lidocaine and 0.25% Marcaine with 1:200,000 fresh epinephrine. Again, great care must be taken to avoid capillary networks, which can cause bruising. The incision is made in the upper lid and the appropriate amount of skin, muscle, and/or fat is removed according to the surgeon's preoperative determination.

If only skin was excised or an incomplete incision was made in the orbicularis oculi muscle, then it is necessary to make a complete incision in the orbicularis oculi muscle (Fig. 56.7). Hemostasis is precisely controlled using bipolar cautery. Next, the superior portion of the muscle is identified and undermined with blunt dissection (Fig. 56.8) and sutured to the periosteum of the superior orbital rim using 5-0 Prolene. The incision is then closed using interrupted cutaneous 6-0 Prolene

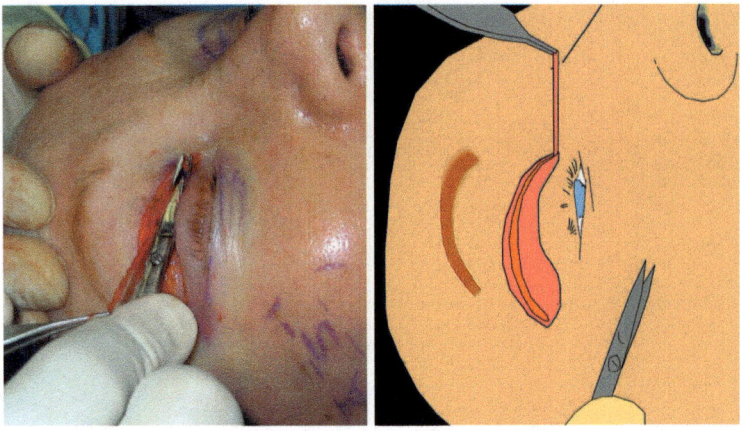

Fig. 56.7 A small strip of orbicularis muscle is removed

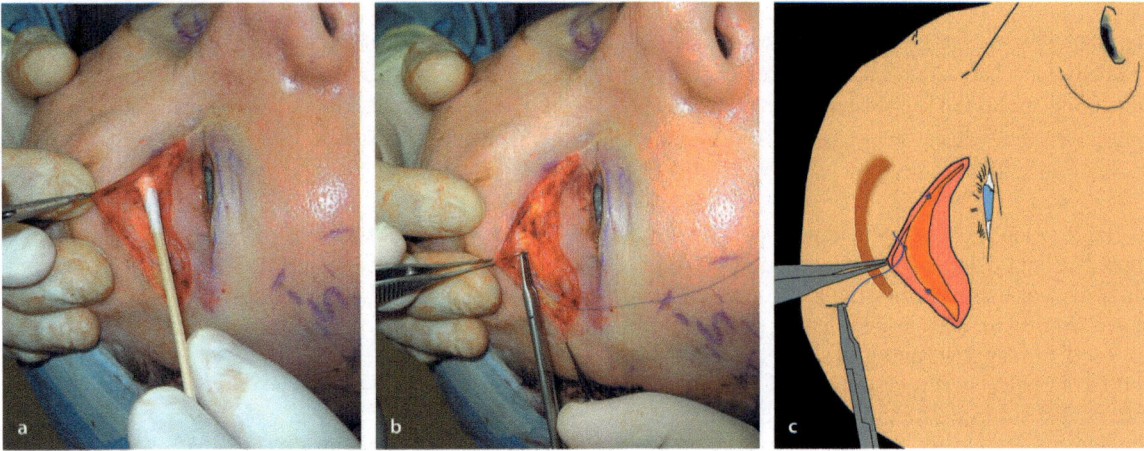

Fig. 56.8 a The superior portion of the orbicularis oculi muscle is undermined with blunt dissection. **b** The superior portion of the orbicularis oculi muscle is sutured to the underlying periosteum of the superior orbital rim. **c** Three sutures are shown with the orbicularis oculi muscle sutured to the periosteum of the superior orbital rim

sutures in the upper lid, followed by a running subcuticular 6-0 Prolene suture from the medial to the lateral incision. A sterile strip is placed across the incision lateral to the lateral canthus to prevent widening of the incision. Finally, flucinolone ointment is placed on the upper-lid incisions.

56.6
Postoperative Care

When the mid forehead buttonhole browlift is performed, the dressing is removed the following day. The patient is instructed to clean the incision twice daily and place ointment over the incision. The patient is allowed to wash his/her face 48 h following the proce-

dure as long as a gentle cleanser is used. The majority of sutures are removed on postoperative day 4, and the remainder of the sutures by postoperative day 7. Sterile strips are replaced when sutures are removed. This prevents any widening of the scar postoperatively. The patient must anticipate normal postoperative sequelae with proper postoperative counseling. It is normal to have several days of edema superior to the brow, but the surgeon should be aware if a small hematoma or seroma develops. When the sutures are removed, the incision is barely visible; however, as collagen is remodeled the incision will become red and raised, and this will subside over the course of the next several months.

When the trans-upper-lid blepharoplasty brow suspension is performed, iced saline gauze compresses are used to decrease postoperative swelling and bruising immediately following surgery and their use is continued for 48–72 h. A mild steroid ointment such as 1% flucinolone is used on the upper-lid incisions, and the patient is instructed to clean the incisions with warm water and replace the ointment twice daily. The portion of the incision lateral to the lateral canthus is taped with sterile strips. The interrupted cutaneous sutures are removed on postoperative day 4, with the exception of several laterally placed sutures. On postoperative day 7, all sutures are removed, including the running subcuticular suture. The patient may start using camouflaging cosmetics on postoperative day 4 and may resume use of contact lenses after 2 weeks.

56.7
Future Considerations

Many methods exist for rejuvenation of the brow. Mid forehead buttonhole eyebrow lift with or without trans-upper-lid blepharoplasty brow suspension gives a dependable result, with a firm type of fixation. Reevaluation of this and other browlift procedures must continue in order to discover the long-term results and sequelae of each procedure.

References

1. Quatela VC, Graham HD, Sabini P. Rejuvenation of the brow and midface. In: Facial Plastic and Reconstructive Surgery, second edition. Papel, I.D. (Ed), New York, Thieme 2002:173
2. Roth JM, Metzinger SE. Quantifying the arch position of the female eyebrow. Arch Facial Plast Surg 2003;5(3):235–239
3. Rafaty FM, Brennan HG. Current concepts of browpexy. Arch Otolaryngol 1983;109(3):152–154
4. Netter FH. Atlas of Human Anatomy. Philadelphia, W.B. Saunders. 1989 Plates 20, 21
5. Miller PJ, Wang TD, Cook TA. Rejuvenation of the aging forehead and brow. Facial Plast Surg 1996;12(2):147–55
6. Morgan JM, Gentile RD, Farrior EF. Rejuvenation of the forehead and eyelid complex. Facial Plast Surg 2005;21(4):271–78
7. McKinney P, Mossie RD, Zukowski ML. Criteria for the forehead lift. Aesthet Plast Surg 1991;15(2):141–147
8. Paul MD. The evolution of the brow lift in aesthetic plastic surgery. Plast Reconstr Surg 2001 108(5):1409–1424
9. Cook TA, Brownrigg PJ, Wang TD, Quatela VC. The versatile midforehead browlift. Arch Otolaryngol 1989;115(2):163–68
10. Johnson CM, Waldman SR. Midforehead lift. Arch Otolaryngol 1983;109(3):155–159
11. Ahn MS, Catten M, Maas CS. Temporal brow lift using botulinum toxin A. Plast Reconstr Surg 2000. 105(3):1129–1135

CHAPTER 57

Endoscopic Forehead Lifting

Omer Refik Ozerdem, Patricio Andrades, Luis O. Vasconez, Jorge de la Torre

57.1
Introduction

The methods for forehead lifting can be classified as endoscopic, open, or combined (biplanar) (Fig. 57.1). The procedure is not standardized and there is a wide variation of the techniques (Fig. 57.1) [1–11]. Endoscopic brow lifting is one of the first clinical applications of the endoscope in plastic surgery. There are many advantages of endoscopic brow lifting, including avoidance of most of the problems associated with the coronal approach such as increased operative time, long scalp scar, scalp dysesthesia, and alopecia. It is a minimally invasive technique and is simple to perform in experienced hands. It offers fast recovery and can easily be combined with other facial procedures and can be used as a safe secondary procedure.

The main goal of rejuvenation of the upper third of the face is to improve the transverse forehead wrinkles and the glabellar frown lines and to raise the eyebrows

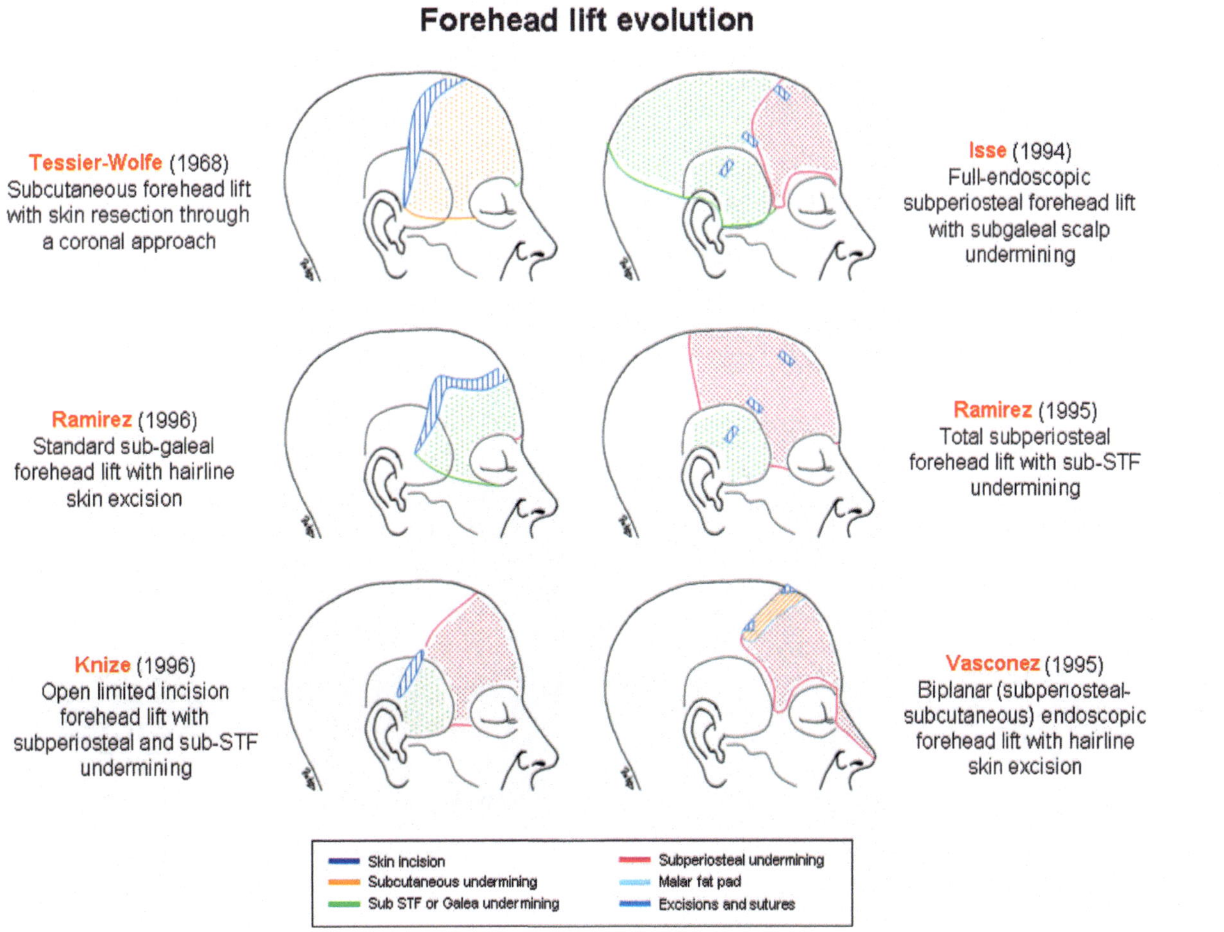

Forehead lift evolution

Tessier-Wolfe (1968) Subcutaneous forehead lift with skin resection through a coronal approach

Isse (1994) Full-endoscopic subperiosteal forehead lift with subgaleal scalp undermining

Ramirez (1996) Standard sub-galeal forehead lift with hairline skin excision

Ramirez (1995) Total subperiosteal forehead lift with sub-STF undermining

Knize (1996) Open limited incision forehead lift with subperiosteal and sub-STF undermining

Vasconez (1995) Biplanar (subperiosteal-subcutaneous) endoscopic forehead lift with hairline skin excision

Skin incision
Subcutaneous undermining
Sub STF or Galea undermining
Subperiosteal undermining
Malar fat pad
Excisions and sutures

Fig. 57.1 Forehead lift evolution

and the eyelids in patients who have eyebrow and eyelid ptosis. In addition to an endoscope, angled elevators and retractors, grasper forceps, an endoscopic carpal tunnel knife, a high-resolution monitor, a VCD recorder, and an adequate cable length are required. Four- and 5-mm scopes are used with a tissue guard and with an angle of 30°, so that when the endoscope enters the frontal cavity parallel to the bone, the angled scope shows the area of interest. The monitor is placed at the patient's feet, and the surgeon and the assistant stay at the patient's head.

There are various incision, dissection, and suspension-fixation methods:

1. The authors prefer to complete the blepharoplasty operations first, considering that the edema that occurs owing to the endoforehead operation would compromise the blepharoplasty operation.
2. The forehead dissection should be limited to the area between the pretrichial line and the supraorbital rims and between the vertical lines at the lateral orbital rims. However, dissection is extended to the nasal tip at the midline, which improves the results by detaching the procerus muscle and by slightly elevating the nasal tip.
3. Incisions are placed in front of the hairline, eliminating the risk of alopecia and providing easy entrance and manipulation of the endoscope.
4. The periosteum must be released completely at the inferior border of the dissected area.
5. After release of the periosteum and ablation of the depressors, the less opposed activation of the elevators will provide the desired pulling force so that sutures or screws are not necessary for suspension; however, staples are used for external suspension for several days.

Then the eyebrow depressors (the corrugator, depressor supercilii, and procerus) are removed with grasper forceps between the supraorbital and the supratrochlear nerves and medial to the supratrochlear nerves (Fig. 57.4). At the end of the procedure, the incisions are closed transversely. The staples are placed on the incisions and 3–5 cm behind them. Then each vertical pair of staples is approximated to each other with 3-0 nylon sutures for suspension (Fig. 57.5). These staples are kept in place for several days.

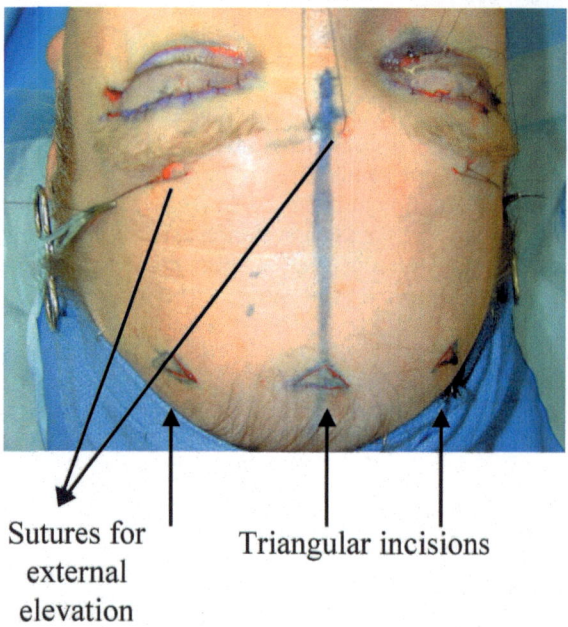

Fig. 57.2 Triangular incisions, sutures for external elevation

57.2
Authors' Preferred Method

Three triangular incisions are marked anterior to the frontal hairline, so that more room is obtained for the entrance of the endoscope and the closure of the wound sites will provide extra elevation of the eyebrows (Fig. 57.2). After local infiltration, the marked skin and subcutaneous tissue are excised above the musculoaponeurotic tissue. The galea and the periosteum are separated with a hemostat with care being taken not to damage the local sensory nerves. After entering the subperiosteal plane, the dissection is carried out with a blunt elevator. The periosteum is elevated off the supraorbital ridge, taking care not to damage the nerves and the vessels. The dissection is performed to the level of the lateral orbital rims on both sides and to the tip of the nose inferiorly. The supraorbital periosteum is divided completely to the level of the lateral orbital rims with an endoscopic carpal tunnel blade (Fig. 57.3).

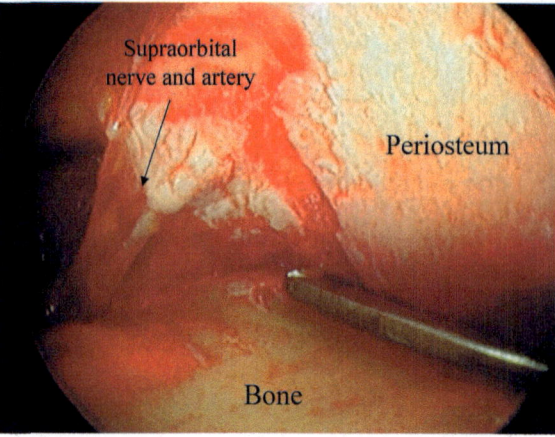

Fig. 57.3 The periosteum is divided by an endoscopic carpal tunnel blade. Supraorbital nerve and artery on the *left*, periosteum on the *right*

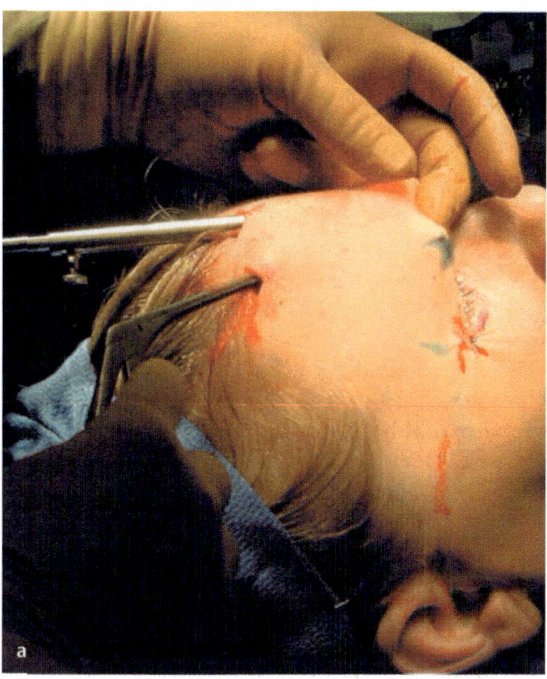
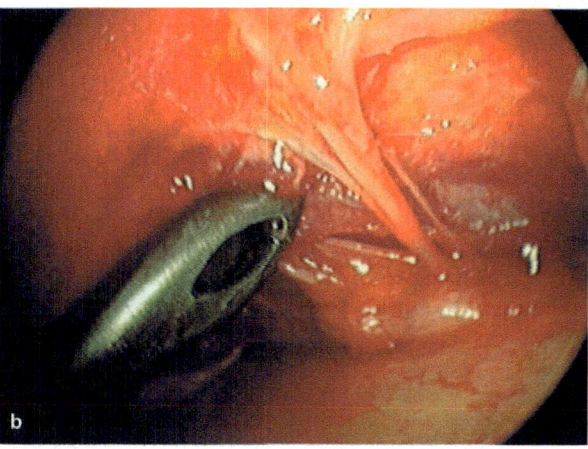

Fig. 57.4 The depressors of the eyebrow are removed with grasper forceps: **a** bimanual manipulation is important; **b** the neurovascular structures should be preserved

The effectiveness of the endoforehead technique may be restricted by the following situations: very ptotic eyebrows, deep transverse wrinkles, high forehead, and asymmetric eyebrows. In these clinical situations the biplanar endoscopic forehead lift (Fig. 57.1) is preferred, particularly if the patient is older than 55 years. In this technique, a frontal pretrichial incision is performed and the skin flap is raised 3–4 cm anterior to the hairline. Then three vertical slit incisions are made on the musculoaponeurotic tissue to gain access to the subperiosteal plane and for the entrance of the endoscope and other instruments (Fig. 57.6). Dissection and muscle ablation steps are done as in the endoscopic method. At the end of the operation, plication of the frontalis muscle is performed and the excess skin is trimmed.

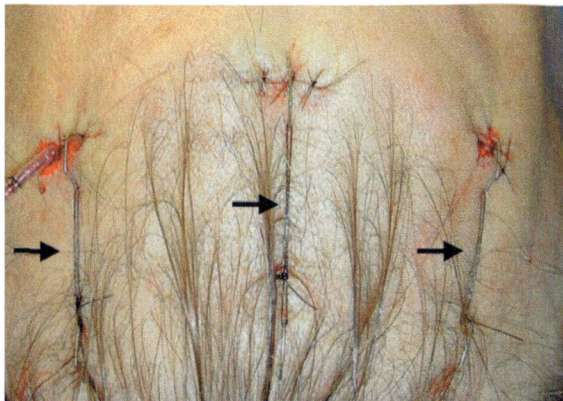

Fig. 57.5 The staples are placed and approximated to each other with 3-0 nylon sutures (*arrows*)

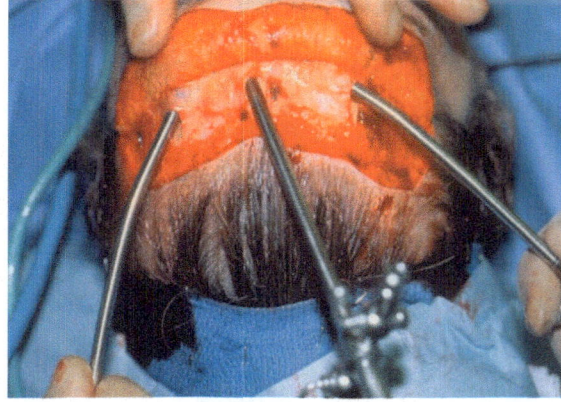

Fig. 57.6 Biplanar technique: the elevators and the endoscope were inserted through the slit incisions

57.3
Results

Between the dates of January 1994 and July 2003, 726 endoscopic forehead lifting procedures were performed in 715 patients (11 patients had the endoscopic forehead lift repeated). Of these, conventional procedures were carried out in 634 cases and the biplanar technique in 92 cases. Sixty three cases had coronal frontal lifting previously. Concomitant procedures were as follows: rhytidectomies 86%, blepharoplasties 50%, tip rhinoplasties 39%.

Attenuated transverse forehead wrinkles, reduced glabellar frown lines, raised eyebrows, and widened appearance of the eyes were commonly seen with endoscopic or biplanar technique (Figs. 57.7, 57.8). Some frowning ability was retained in the patients. Pruritus and numbness, although temporary, were possible problems. Overelevation of the eyebrows with the fixation has not been observed.

Unsatisfactory results included forehead irregularities (2%), persistent horizontal forehead wrinkles (1%), and persistent glabellar frown lines (2%), with a total of 4.5%. In addition, 11 patients (1.5%) needed a redo procedure. Complications included persistent forehead dysesthesia (2.2%), alopecia (0.2%), periorbital problems (10.2%), forehead hematoma (3.5%), and frontal nerve injury (1.8%). Forehead dysesthesia was not observed in none of the biplanar forehead lifting cases. Periorbital problems were seen in 10.2% of the patients, including difficult eye closure (7.0%), eye irritation (8.3%), upper-eyelid asymmetry (7.8%), and eyebrow malposition (2.5%). The complication rate was quite acceptable and did not significantly increase with the addition of other facial procedures. The exception was the concomitant ptosis correction because it resulted in a definitive increase of periorbital complications, which improved spontaneously.

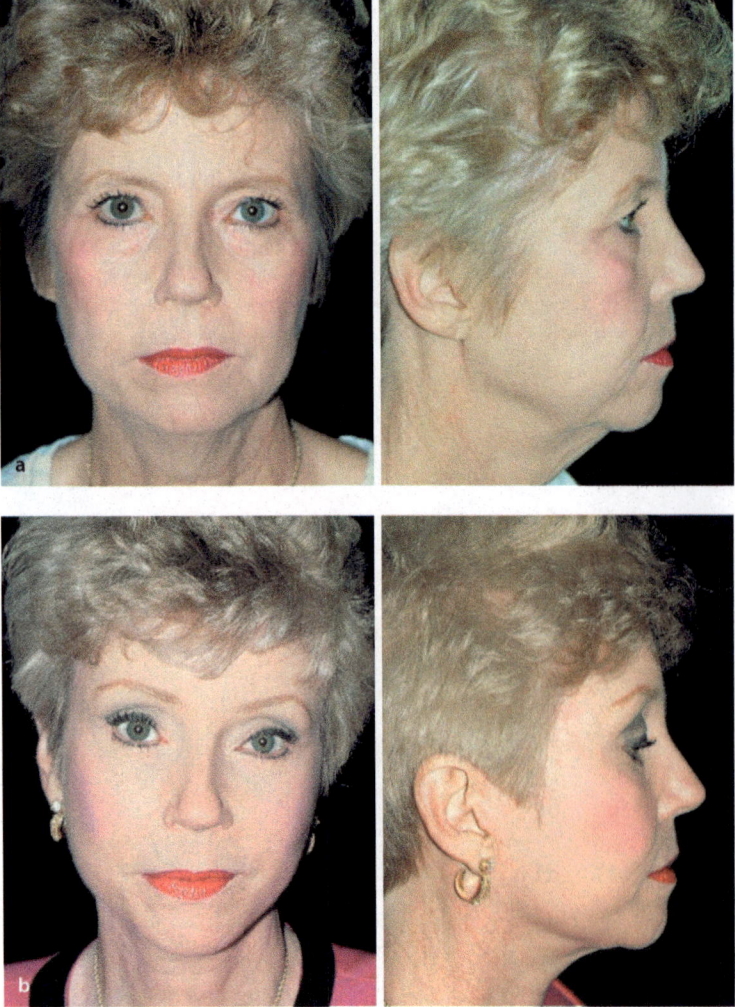

Fig. 57.7 a Preoperatively. **b** Postoperatively following blepharoplasty and cervicofacial and endobrow lifting procedures

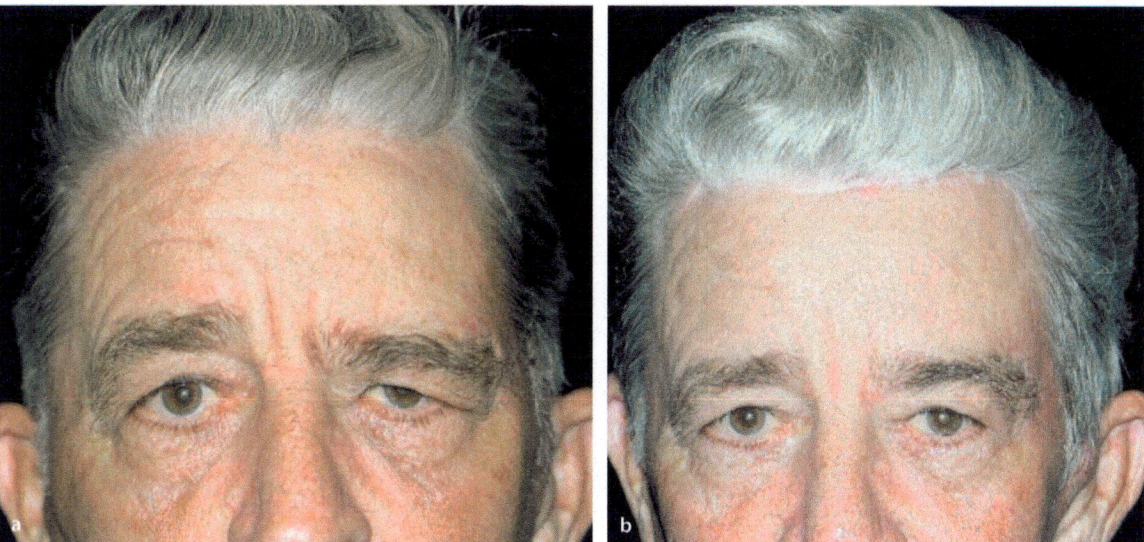

Fig. 57.8 **a** Preoperatively. **b** Postoperative patient folllowing biplanar endoforehead lifting for correction of eyebrow asymmetry due to frontal branch paralysis

References

1. Ozerdem OR, Vasconez LO, de la Torre J. Upper face-lifting. Facial Plast Surg Clin North Am 2006;14(3):159–165
2. Tessier P. Ridectomie frontale: Lifting frontale. Gaz Med Fr 1968;75:5565
3. Wolfe SA. The subcutaneous forehead lift, revisited. Plast Reconstr Surg 2000;105(1):449–450
4. Wolfe SA, Baird W. The subcutaneous forehead lift. Plast Reconstr Surg 1989;83(2):251–256
5. Vasconez LO, Core GB, Oslin B. Endoscopy in plastic surgery. Clin Plast Surg 1995;22(4):585–589
6. Core GB, Vasconez LO, Graham HD III. Endoscopic browlift. Clin Plast Surg 1995;22(4):619–631
7. Ramirez OM. Classification of facial rejuvanation techniques based on the subperiosteal approach and ancillary procedures. Plast Reconstr Surg 1996;97(1):45–55
8. Ramirez OM, Robertson KM. Update in endoscopic rejuvenation. Facial Plast Surg Clin North Am 2002;10(1):37–51
9. Ramirez OM. Endoscopic subperiosteal browlift and facelift. Clin Plast Surg 1995;22(4):639–660
10. Ramirez OM. Endoscopic assisted biplanar forehead lift. Plast Reconstr Surg 1995;96(2):323–333
11. Oslin B, Core GB, Vasconez LO. The biplanar endoscopically assisted forehead flap. Clin Plast Surg 1995;22(4):633–638

CHAPTER 58

Reduction of the Supraorbital Ridges

58

Jean-Paul Lintilhac

Published posthumously

58.1
Introduction

Although it is possible that some plastic surgeons have reduced a prominent supraorbital ridge for either asymmetry or abnormal prominence, there have not been many reports in the medical literature on this subject [1].

The author's original intent was to reduce a thick, protruding superciliary ridge in male transsexuals in order to give the ridge a more feminine appearance. After success with male transsexuals, the operation was extended to women with a thicker, low, or downward-slanting lateral portion of the supraorbital ridge giving them a "hard" or "sad" appearance. The bone reduction may be useful in some men who have a very thick and low supraorbital ridge giving them a "suspicious" appearance.

58.2
Preoperative Examination

The examination should consist of:

1. Inspection
   (a) To determine the general shape, thickness, and protrusion of the supraorbital rim that may be more or less hidden by excess skin or fatty hernias of the eyelid and will be best appreciated by elevating the eyebrow with the finger.
   (b) To determine the level of the supraorbital ridge in relation to the eye whether low or high or slanting more or less downward in its lateral half.
   (c) To determine the level of the eyebrow in relation to the orbital ridge. In young individuals it can be at the same level, above or under it; however, there is no doubt that with age the eyebrow has a tendency to fall.
      • When the eyebrow is low and the supraorbital ridge is also low and prominent, the upper eyelid has generally a normal convex appearance, a marked flexion crease, and is usually sagging. This corresponds to the usual masculine type of supraorbital ridge hypertrophy.
      • When the eyebrow is high and the supraorbital ridge is rather high but prominent and

slanting downward in its lateral part, the upper eyelid is generally concave and quite hollow under the roof of the orbit. In this case there is usually no flexion crease or the upper eyelid. This hollow eye corresponds more to a feminine type of supraorbital ridge hypertrophy.
      • The importance of the supraorbital ridge must be compared with other bony structures of the face (nose, chin, cheek bone). It is not just mere chance if most patients already had previous nose and chin reductions.

2. Palpation: Palpation will allow appreciating the shape and contours of the supraorbital ridge. Many men (and transsexuals) have a bony protuberance immediately above the frontomalar suture.

3. Roentgenograms: While not absolutely necessary, X-rays will help to study the thickness of the bone, the position of the supraorbital foramen, and the extension of the frontal sinus.

4. Photographs: Preoperative frontal and lateral views should be taken.

The examination for existing scars might reveal a tendency to hypertrophy or keloid formation. In this case the palpebral approach should be preferred.

The usual blood tests and preoperative checkup should be utilized.

58.3
Technique

The operation is performed under local anesthesia with 1 or 0.5% Xylocaine with epinephrine after the usual premedication. Neuroleptanalgesia or general anesthesia can also be given to apprehensive patients as the use of the chisel and mallet is noisy and unpleasant, although not painful.

If the eyebrow needs to be raised, the bone is approached through an incision above the eyebrow (superciliary approach). If the eyebrow is already high, the approach is through an incision (or excision) on the upper eyelid (palpebral approach).

58.3.1
Superciliary Approach

58.3.1.1
Skin Excision Above the Eyebrow

The two skin excisions are performed above the eyebrow after marking the areas to be excised (Fig. 58.1). The upper incision starts from the middle of the eyebrow or somewhat medially on the vertical passing through the pupil. It describes a regular curve extending 1–2 cm outside the tail of the eyebrow. At its peak it reaches 3–6 mm (or more) above the eyebrow according to the degree of elevation needed. The lower incision follows the upper border of the eyebrow exactly, turning at its extremity to join the upper incision laterally. The upper and lower incisions should be different in shape although equal in length, the upper being regularly concave and the lower should have a double curve. The incisions are performed with a no. 10 or no. 15 blade cutting all the way through the skin and the whole thickness of skin excised. Some superficial veins and occasional arteries are electrocoagulated.

58.3.1.2
Skin Undermining

The skin is undermined at the lower edge of the excision taking care not to interfere with the hair follicles of the eyebrow. The undermining is initiated with the scalpel and continued with the scissors. It should reach the level of the supraorbital ridge.

58.3.1.3
Incision of the Muscle

Five millimeters above the orbital ridge, as controlled by palpation, the orbicularis oculi muscle is incised following the direction of its fibers from the level of the external canthus to the middle part of the orbit (Fig. 58.2). Both sides of the muscle are retracted using skin hooks or two prong nasal retractors (which should be blunt because of the vicinity of the eye).

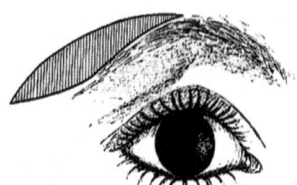

Fig. 58.1 Skin excision above the eyebrow

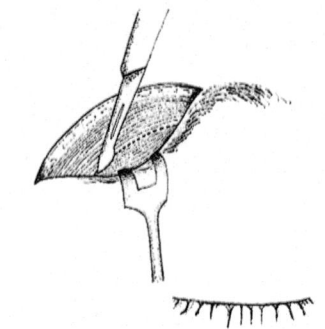

Fig. 58.2 Incision of the orbicularis oculi muscle after skin undermining

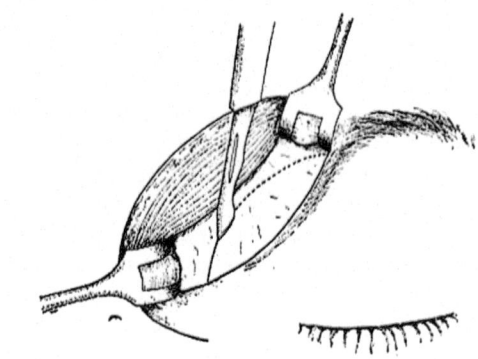

Fig. 58.3 Incision of the periosteum

58.3.1.4
Incision of the Periosteum

After incising through the layer of connective tissue where one generally encounters some blood vessels, the incision is carried through the periosteum down to the bone 5 mm above the lower margin of the supraorbital ridge (Fig. 58.3). This incision should extend from immediately above the external canthal ligament to the midline of the orbit or even a little further depending on the shape of the bony ridge, but it should avoid the supraorbital foramen and the emergence of the supraorbital nerve.

58.3.1.5
Elevation of the Periosteum

The periosteum of the lower lip of the incision is raised with a periosteal elevator. Mosquito forceps grasp the periosteal flap as soon as it appears, facilitating its elevation (Fig. 58.4). The periosteal elevation should extend from a point between the external canthal ligament (which must not be seen) and the frontomalar suture (clearly visible once the periosteum is elevated) to past the midline of the orbit.

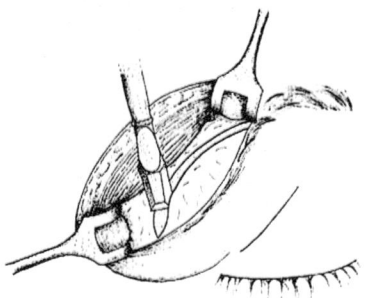

Fig. 58.4 Elevation of the periosteum on the supraorbital ridge

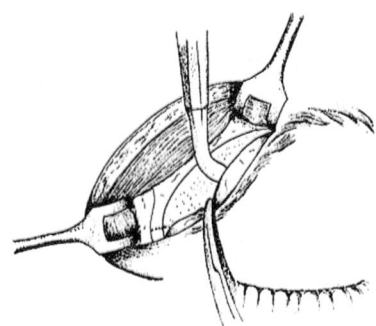

Fig. 58.5 Elevation of the periosteum under the supraorbital ridge toward the roof of the orbit

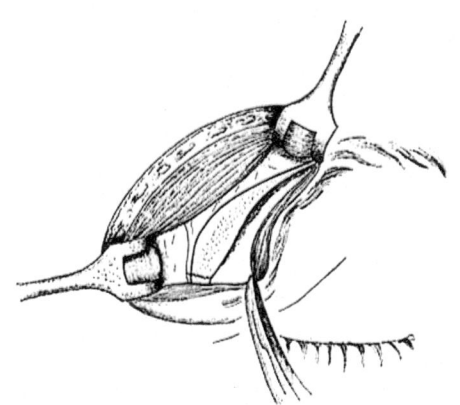

Fig. 58.6 Exposed hypertrophic supraorbital ridge

The lower aspect of the supraorbital ridge (this means toward the roof of the orbit) must also be freed of its periosteum, for which a cleft-palate periosteal elevator is generally used. The upper lip of the periosteal incision is also elevated from the prominent part of the bone (Fig. 58.5).

The supraorbital ridge appears fully exposed in its external half and the surgeon can appreciate it shape, thickness, and the aspect of the tubercle often existing in its outer part (Fig. 58.6).

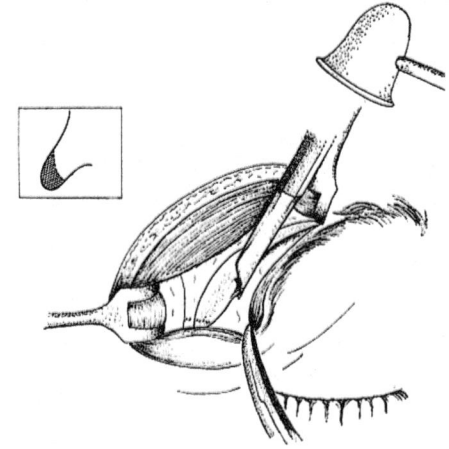

Fig. 58.7 The supraorbital ridge is resected and reshaped with an osteotome and a mallet. The *insert* shows a lateral view of a section of the supraorbital ridge and the way its hanging and protruding part should be resected

58.3.1.6
Bone Resection and Reshaping of the Supraorbital Ridge

The author uses a fine 8-mm chisel or osteotome and mallet to resect the bone but any other sort of mechanical device could be employed. The hanging part of the bone is first removed and the orbital ridge reshaped so that the lateral upper quadrant of the orbit will take a nice regular shape (Fig. 58.7). The bone resection is limited laterally by the external canthal ligament, which must be avoided, and medially by the supraorbital foramen. Some of the bone thickness responsible for the forward protrusion of the orbital ridge is also removed so that the bone takes a beveled shape that will produce a better appearing supraorbital ridge.

58.3.1.7
Incision, Draping, and Suturing of the Periosteum

By pulling the periosteum upward with mosquito forceps the former shape of the periosteum will not come in contact with the newly formed supraorbital ridge (Fig. 58.8). To release and drape the periosteum over the new bone contour, two incisions must be made in the periosteal flap with a no. 15 blade from its free margin up to the bone and perpendicular to it (Fig. 58.9). The incision is only in the periosteum and care must be taken not to open the orbit letting the orbital fat appear in the incision. If the orbital fat appears, the excess fat must be removed without suturing.

By pulling on the medial periosteal flap with mosquito forceps, the periosteum can be seen to drape neatly over the new bone structure. A few millimeters of the medial flap, which is now too long, is cut off (Fig. 58.10) and two 3-0 catgut sutures are used to fix it to the superior lip of the periosteal incision, which has also been slightly elevated (Fig. 58.11). One catgut suture on each lateral flap is sufficient for fixation.

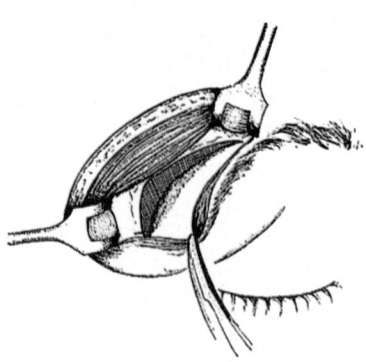

Fig. 58.8 The *checkered area* represents the newly cut bone, the periosteum retains its former shape

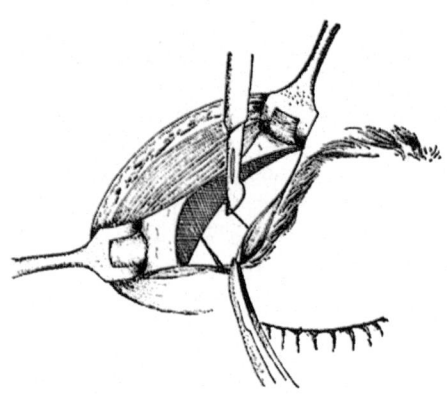

Fig. 58.9 Incision of the periosteum to allow for its draping on the new bone contour

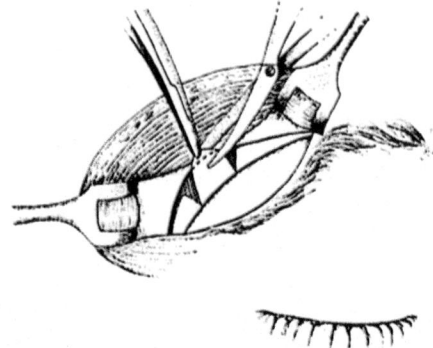

Fig. 58.10 Scissors cutting the excess length of the periosteal medial flap

58.3.1.8
Orbital Muscle Resection and Suturing

A crescent strip of about 3 mm is excised with scissors from the upper margin of the incision in the orbicularis oculi muscle (Fig. 58.12). Three 4-0 catgut sutures will approximate the two margins (Fig. 58.13).

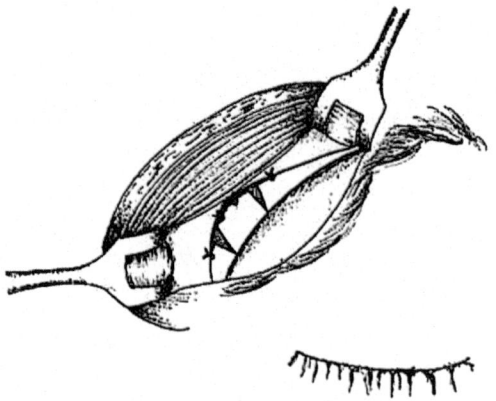

Fig. 58.11 Suturing of the periosteum

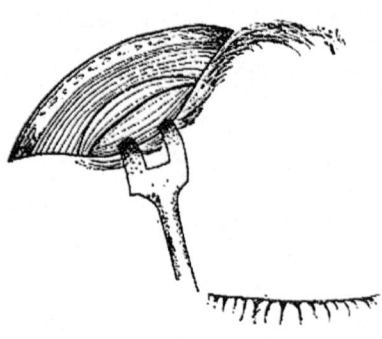

Fig. 58.12 Excision of a crescent-shaped strip of the orbicularis oculi muscle

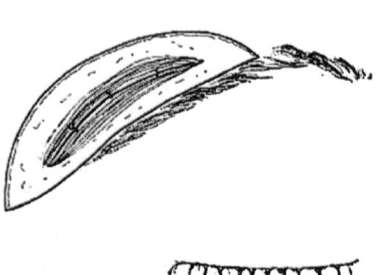

Fig. 58.13 Suturing of the muscle

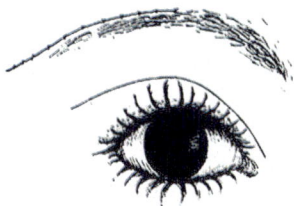

Fig. 58.14 Skin suturing

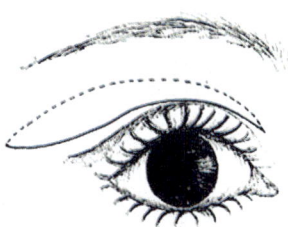

Fig. 58.15 The *solid line* shows simple incision. The *dotted line* shows the extent of excision

58.3.1.9
Skin Suturing

Owing to the extensive undermining and muscle resection and suture, the skin margins are approximated with 8-0 silk without tension (Fig. 58.14).

58.3.2
Palpebral Approach

When the eyebrow is high or in normal position, the approach is through the upper eyelid (Fig. 58.15). If the upper eyelid has no excess skin, the palpebral approach will be through a simple incision. The incision follows the normal flexion crease when it exists but extends laterally and upward for 1–2 cm. If there is no definite crease, the incision lies in the concavity of the upper eyelid and extends outward and upward across the hypertrophied supraorbital ridge.

If the upper eyelid is wrinkled and sagging with excess skin, the palpebral approach will be through a skin excision (Fig. 58.15) comparable to that of the usual upper-eyelid blepharoplasty extending across the supraorbital ridge. This excision will expose the orbicularis oculi muscle and the prominent supraorbital ridge.

Orbularis oculi resection is omitted but incision of the muscle and periosteum and bone resection are similar to the superciliary approach.

58.4
Postoperative Care

A light dressing is applied on the eye for the first night after the surgery. Antibiotics and an anti-inflammatory drug are generally given.

There is usually no pain after surgery. Swelling and ecchymoses of the upper eyelid are usually present for a few days. The skin sutures are removed after 6 days in the superciliary approach and after 4 days in the palpebral approach.

After 10–15 days, edema of the upper eyelid has disappeared but some thickening of the tissues operated on will persist for 1–2 months. It will take about 3 months until the end results are finally obtained.

58.5
Results

The cosmetic result of the surgery has been highly satisfactory to the surgeon and the patients (Figs. 15.16–15.18). The scars are practically invisible. The eyebrow is raised when it is necessary and the supraorbital ridge is also made higher and less prominent suppressing the "hard", "suspicious",or "sad" appearance.

The only limitations to this operation is at the inner part of the supraorbital ridge when it is especially prominent, thus giving a deep-set, sunken eye that cannot be treated with this procedure because of the presence of the supraorbital nerve and the frontal sinus that might present difficult problems.

58.6
Complications

There is the possibility of injury to the supraorbital nerve or hematoma. The author has had no complications in 60 procedures.

58.7
Conclusions

Reduction of the supraorbital ridge is indicated in a prominent or overhanging supraorbital ridge giving a "hard" or "sad" appearance. The approach is through a skin excision above the usually low eyebrow, thus raising it. When the eyebrow is high, the approach is through the upper eyelid. After separation of the orbicularis oculi muscle and elevation of the periosteum, the prominent portion of the prominent lateral part of the supraorbital ridge is resected with a chisel. The periosteum must be properly incised and well draped on the new bone structure.

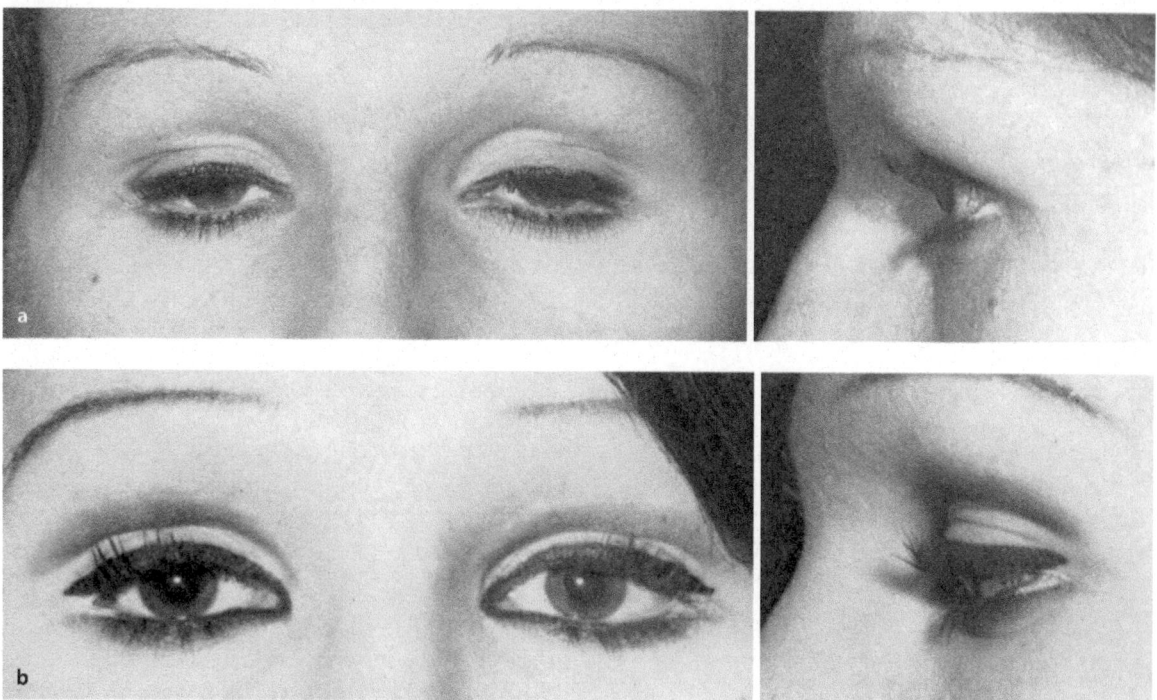

Fig. 58.16 a Preoperative transsexual with a low, thick, prominent supraorbital ridge. **b** Postoperative resection using a superciliary approach

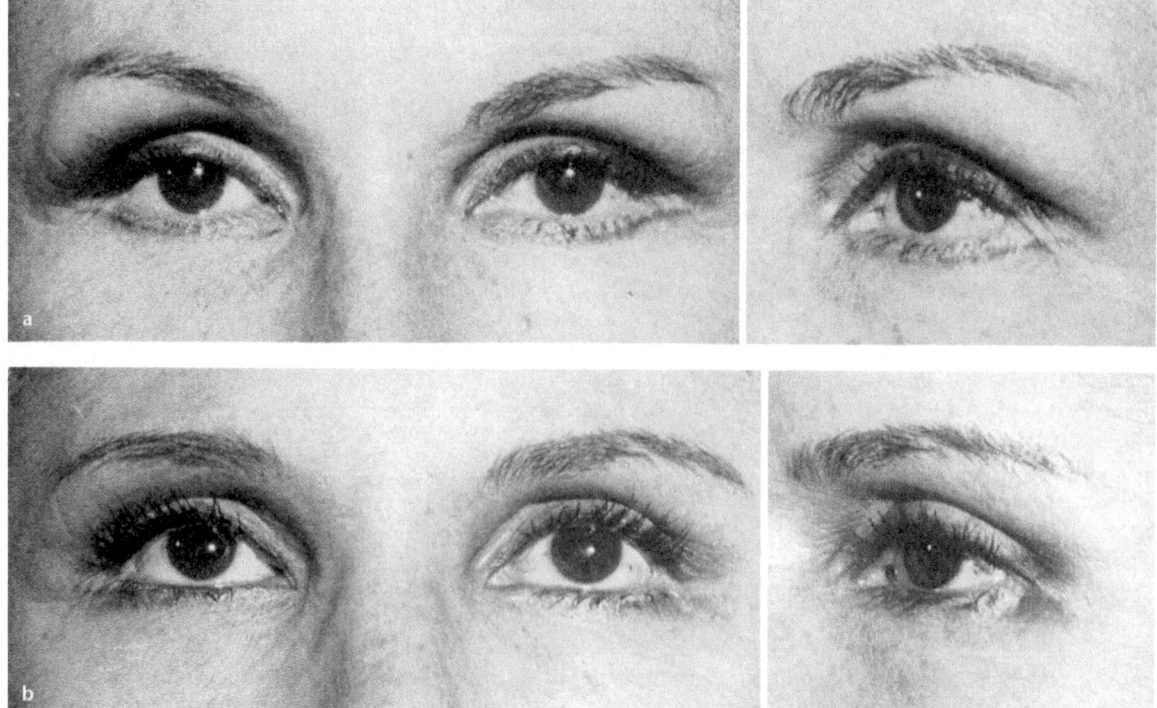

Fig. 58.17 a Preoperative female patient with a low, thick supraorbital ridge giving a hard, suspicious appearance. **b** Postoperative resection using a palpebral approach

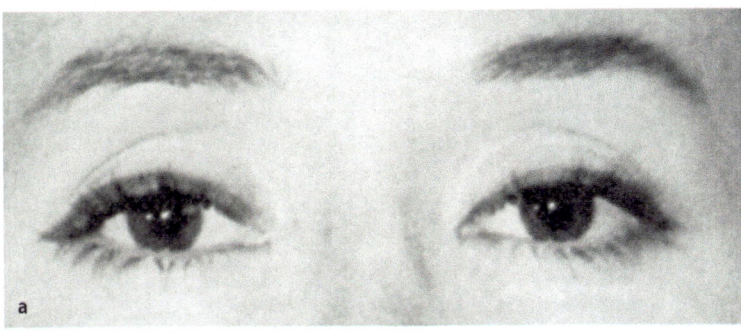

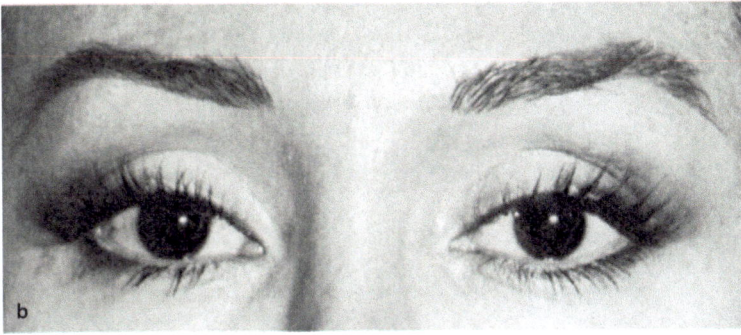

Fig. 58.18 a Preoperative female patient with supraorbital ridge slanting slightly downward, whereas the eye slants upward. **b** Reduction of the supraorbital ridge through a superciliary approach emphasizing the slanting eye and improving the exotic appearance

Reference

1. Whitaker L.A., Morales L. Jr., Farkas L.G.: Aesthetic surgery of the supraorbital ridge and forehead structures. Plast Reconstr Surg 1986;78(1):23–32

CHAPTER 59

Asian Blepharoplasty in the Creation of a Double Eyelid

59

Young Kyoon Kim

59.1
Introduction

In general, two broad categories of double-eyelid surgery exist: incision and non-incision technique. But both are strictly dependent on skin-to-levator aponeurosis fixation for creation of double eyelids. In a conventional full-incision method, the lower skin flap is debulked by removing some of the tissue that lies between eyelid skin and the levator aponeurosis, including the orbicularis oculi muscle, and the skin-to-levator aponeurosis fixation can be made more securely than in the buried-suture method. But it has the disadvantages of a postoperative adhesive scar and prolonged edema. In contrast, in a conventional buried-suture method, the skin-to levator aponeurosis fixation cannot be ensured because the normal tissues (including dermocutaneous tissue, orbicularis oculi muscle, levator aponeurosis, tarsus) are captured in the trap of a suture knot, even though it has the advantages of technical simplicity, immediate ambulation, and short recovery time. Therefore, a partial-incision technique is another alternative. A partial-incision technique is selected for generally younger patients with relatively thin palpebral skin without skin redundancy to include all of the ad-

vantages of both conventional methods as mentioned above, but a full-incision technique is selected for aged patients with thick and/or redundant palpebral skin.

59.2
Waikiki Partial-Incision Technique

The desired crease line and its width are estimated using a curved wire and calipers with the patient sitting in an upright position. A dot is placed on each crease at the level of the pupil. The patient is instructed to remain in a supine position on the operation bed. The distance between the ciliary margin and the dot is measured with calipers. Generally, the height of the crease is approximately 7–8 mm on average. A natural crease is made by placing the curved wire on the marking. A line is drawn on this crease, starting from the level of medial limbus and proceeding laterally for 15 mm (Fig. 59.1). A dot and line are marked on the contralateral crease in the same fashion.

A solution of 2% lidocaine with 1:100,000 epinephrine is used for anesthesia. Just 0.3 ml of anesthetic with a 30-gauge insulin needle per side is infiltrated into the central region of the marking subcutaneously (Fig. 59.2).

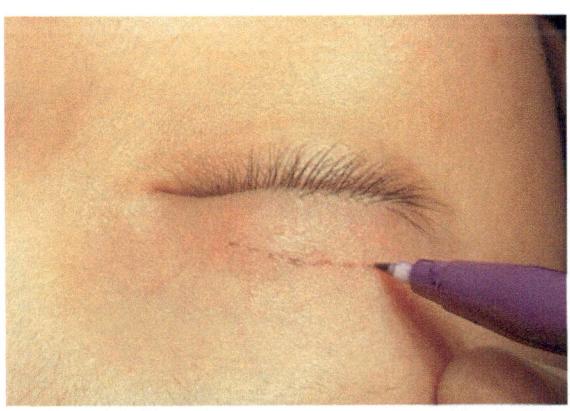

Fig. 59.1 Several dots are marked along the natural crease, starting from the level of the medial limbus and proceeding laterally for 15 mm. An incision line is then drawn on the dots

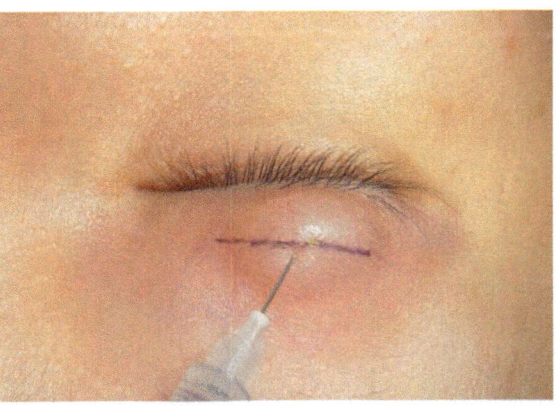

Fig. 59.2 Local anesthesia (0.3 ml 2% lidocaine with 1:100,000 epinephrine) is infiltrated with a 30-gauge needle and a 1-ml insulin syringe by placing the needle superficially in the midline of the incision and raising a wheal

After injection, the skin is carefully pinched with the thumb and index finger, then squeezed and infiltrated bilaterally to prevent vessel injury and consequent hemorrhaging. At least 10 min is needed to pass to achieve maximal hemostasis and anesthesia.

An incision is made through both the skin and the orbicularis oculi muscle with a CO_2 laser, starting from the level of the medial limbus and proceeding laterally for 10–15 mm. A 0.1-mm spot-sized hand piece is prepared and a power setting of 5 W and 10–20 mJ in the ultrapulse mode is used. For hemostasis, the laser mode is changed to continuous wave with a power setting of 5 W. Hemostasis is achieved by defocusing the laser beam. Needle-point Bovie electrocautery can additionally be used to achieve hemostasis (Fig. 59.3).

The orbital septum is incised with a CO_2 laser until the underlying orbital fat is exposed. The utmost lateral aspect of the orbital septum is picked up with fine-toothed forceps, and a small window is created with fine tenotomy scissors (Fig. 59.4). The preaponeurotic adipose tissue of the middle fat compartment is gently teased out through the septal defect until a glistening whitish surface of the levator aponeurosis is partially exposed. Tenotomy scissors are inserted through the septal window and the orbital fat septum is transected with a CO_2 laser along the length of the incision from a lateral to a medial direction. The underlying levator aponeurosis, which has a glistening silky white surface, is then exposed (Fig. 59.5). Once the levator aponeurosis has been fully exposed on one side, the contralateral side is addressed in same fashion before resecting orbital fat.

With bilateral fat pads exposed, the amount of fat to be excised is estimated about 10 mm above its exposed base in a symmetrical fashion (Fig. 59.6).

When a fixation is done, a single skin-to-levator aponeurosis suture is placed in the central aspect of the incision using 7-0 nylon in a buried fashion. The needle captures not only dermis but also the adjacent epidermis 0.5–1.0 mm from the inferior skin edge of

the incision and the skin edge including cornified epidermis, which is apposed precisely onto the levator surface. At first, the needle passes superiorly to inferiorly (i.e., backhanded) through the inferior skin edge of the incision (Fig. 59.7). A second bite is then taken medially to laterally through raising a fraction of the levator surface tissue (approximately 1 mm) on the level of the superior limit of the tarsus (Figs. 59.8, 59.9). When a single knot is made, the patient is asked to open the eyes to ensure adequate eversion of the eyelashes. The angle of the eyelashes should be oriented slightly over 90° to the upper-eyelid skin surface when gazing. If this criterion is met, then one of the suture tails is pulled outward far enough to allow for a rollover of the incised skin edge, much like that of a cuff on a shirt sleeve or pant leg (Fig. 59.10). The folded skin is then tied down to the levator surface with three square knots. The long suture tails are trimmed down to the knot, and the knot is then buried inside the rolled skin edge. At this time, this fixation suture acts as the initial point of retraction, and the retracted skin margin of the lower incision shows a flying gullwing-shaped outline. And then another reversed gullwing-shaped fold appears in both directions on the levator surface (Fig. 59.11). These two gullwing-shaped folds make a figure-of-eight outline, and this serves as the landmark for placing the rest of the fixation sutures. After placing the first fixation suture on one side, attention is paid to the contralateral side, and the same technique for skin-to levator aponeurosis fixation is conducted. Both lid creases are then inspected for symmetry. After the first fixation suture has been placed on each side, the remaining six skin-to-levator aponeurosis fixation sutures with 7-0 nylon are placed over each eyelid for a total of 14 independent sutures in an alternating tandem fashion to ensure maximum symmetry. In the end, three interrupted skin closure sutures are placed over each lid using the same 7-0 nylon suture, and these sutures are removed on the third postoperative day.

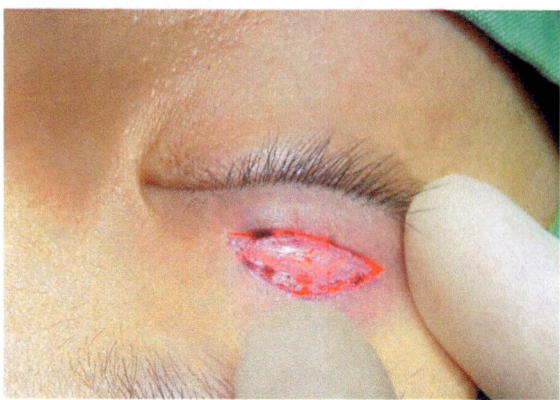

Fig. 59.3 As the eyelid skin and muscle are incised, the orbital septum is exposed

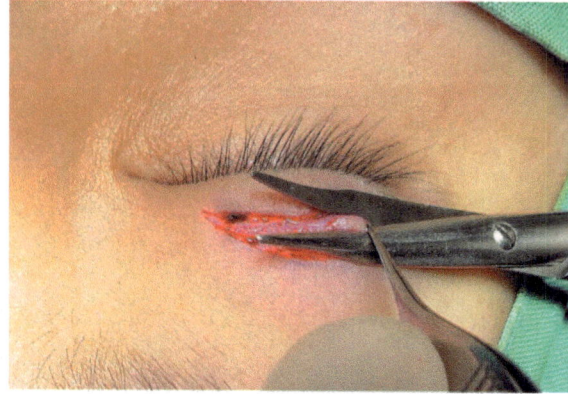

Fig. 59.4 The utmost lateral aspect of the orbital septum is picked up with fine-toothed forceps, and a small orbital-septal fenestration is created with fine tenotomy scissors

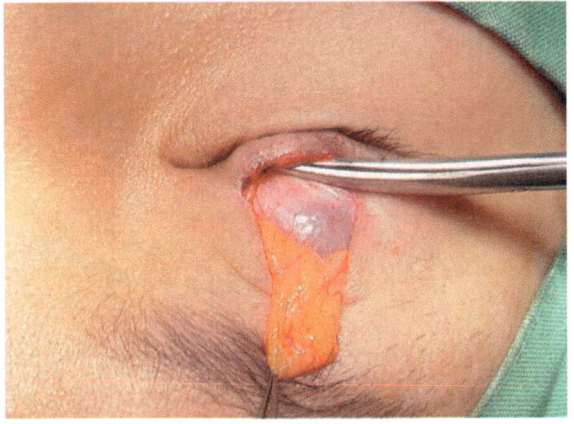

Fig. 59.5 The orbital septum is safely transected laterally to medially along the entire incision length to expose the levator aponeurosis. And the glistening silky white levator surface and the orbital fat are then exposed

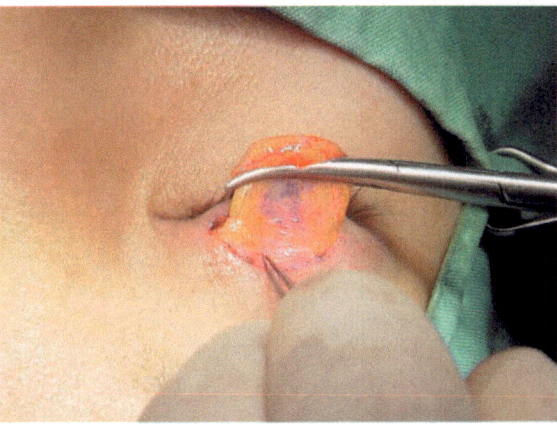

Fig. 59.6 The amount of fat to be excised is estimated about 10 mm above its exposed base. The clamped fat is removed and cauterized

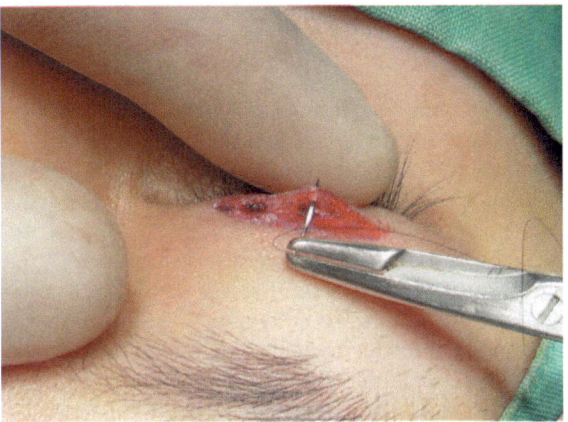

Fig. 59.7 A single 7-0 nylon suture is passed through the middle of the incision to capture the full thickness of the skin. In addition, the suture must also capture 0.5 mm of the epidermal outer surface by supporting the wound edge with the non-dominant index finger as well

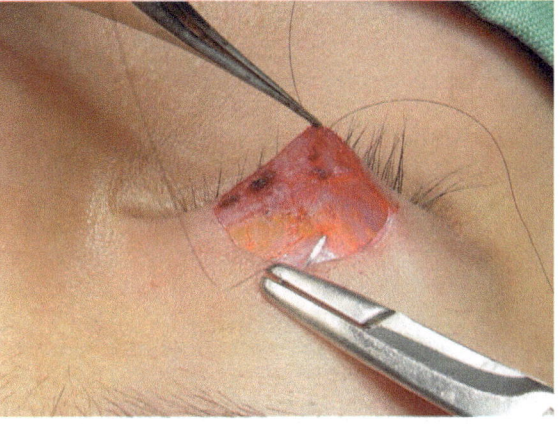

Fig. 59.8 The second bite is taken medially to laterally through raising a fraction of the levator surface tissue (approximately 1 mm) on the level of the superior limit of the tarsus. The author's most important philosophy of the skin-to-levator aponeurosis fixation concerns the raising of a small bite of the epidermis: the levator surface must be apposed by the cornified epidermal surface 0.5 mm from the incised inferior skin edge so that the epidermal cornified cells act as a foreign body on the levator tissue to ensure thinner but more secure adhesion

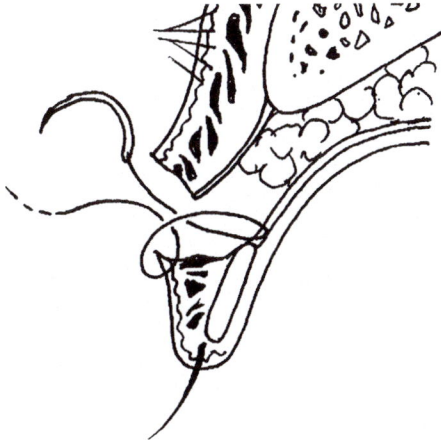

Fig. 59.9 A sagittal section of the upper eyelid showing the skin-to-levator aponeurosis fixation suture

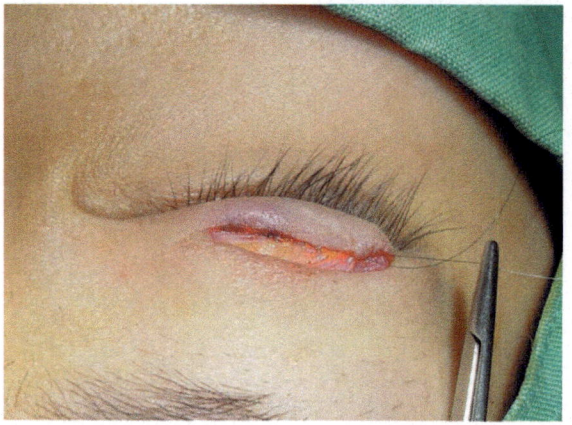

Fig. 59.10 One of the suture tails is pulled laterally far enough to allow for a rollover of the incised skin edge much like that of a cuff on a shirt sleeve or pant leg. This epidermal rolling over will help to appose the epidermal dead cells exactly to the live levator surface

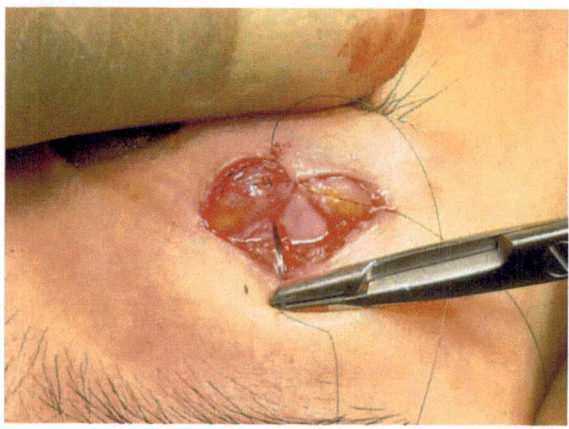

Fig. 59.11 A properly placed first levator–skin fixation suture will be followed by a figure-of-eight crease, configured with the lower incision line and the retracted levator aponeurosis, that will serve as the landmark for placing the rest of the fixation sutures

59.3
Waikiki Full-Incision Technique for the Aged Patient

The pretarsal skin is pulled up cephalically with the non-dominant finger to the point of slight eyelash eversion, and a dot is marked at a height of 7–8 mm superior to the ciliary margin at the level of the pupil. The inferior incision line is drawn on the pretarsal skin along the natural fine crease (where the dot is included) starting from the point 5 mm lateral to the level of the medial canthal angle and proceeding laterally to the level of lateral orbital rim. A curved wire is used to find the natural curve of the inferior incision line. A dot and line are marked on the contralateral crease in the same fashion. The palpebral redundant skin is pinched with forceps superior to the line and the patient is instructed to open and close the eyes to determine the maximal amount of skin that can be excised. And the superior incision line is drawn as done in conventional full-incision blepharoplasty.

A solution of 2% lidocaine with 1:100,000 epinephrine is used for anesthesia. About 1.0 ml of anesthetic with a 30-gauge insulin needle per side is infiltrated. At least 10 min is needed to pass to achieve maximal hemostasis and anesthesia.

An incision is made on both sides with a CO_2 laser. The power setting is same as for the partial-incision technique. Hemostasis is also achieved by defocusing the laser beam, but needle-point Bovie electrocautery can be used in the event of active bleeding.

Skin and underlying subcutaneous tissues are excised as marked, and a strip of orbicularis oculi muscle is excised above the level of the tarsal plate, exposing the orbital septum. The orbital septum is then incised along the full length of the incision from end to end until the underlying orbital fat is exposed. The underlying levator aponeurosis is then exposed.

Bilateral orbital fat pads are excised as done in the partial-incision technique. If any prolapsed medial fat is noted, then it should be removed. A 2–3-mm strip of pretarsal orbicularis oculi muscle and/or pretarsal adipose tissue, adjacent to the inferior incision line, is excised depending on the bulkiness of the pretarsal skin and muscle.

The skin-to-levator aponeurosis fixation is done as in the partial-incision technique.

Continuous running closure sutures are placed over each lid using the same 7-0 nylon suture, and these sutures are removed on the third to fifth postoperative days (Figs. 59.12, 59.13).

59.4
Discussion

The author's partial-incision technique (so-called limited-incision method, small-incision method or partial-incision method) offers an ideal balance between the full-incision and the suture methods. The limited incision that spans only about one third of the total eyelid length offers a rapid and reliable method for double-eyelid creation and limits postoperative edema and risk of scarring [1]. The partial-incision technique is suitable for younger Asian individuals who are in their teenage years and 20s. It is an effective procedure in properly se-

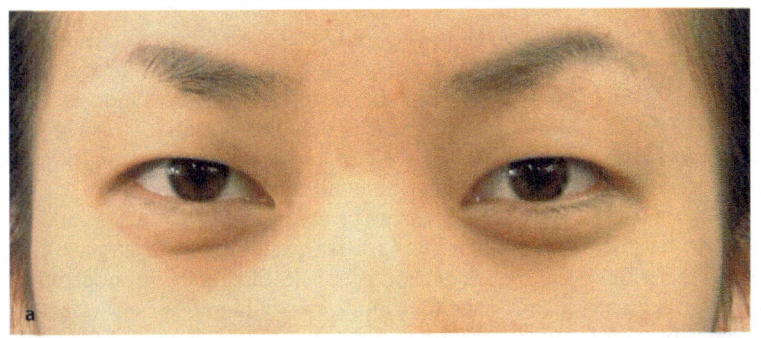

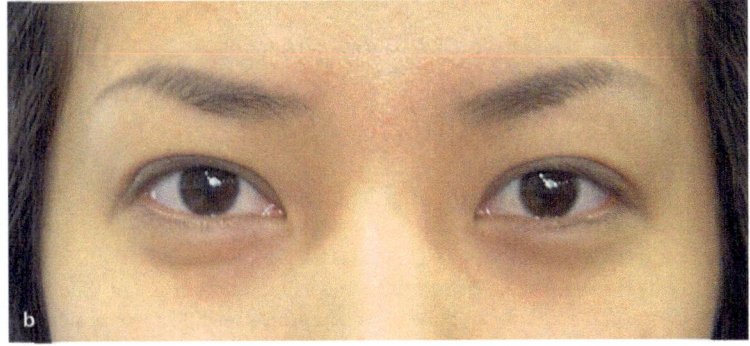

Fig. 59.12 a Preoperative view of a 22-year-old female patient with minimal upper-lid fat and a relatively wide palpebral fissure. **b** Postoperative view 2 months after double-eyelid creation using a partial-incision method. The crease height is relatively fixed in size

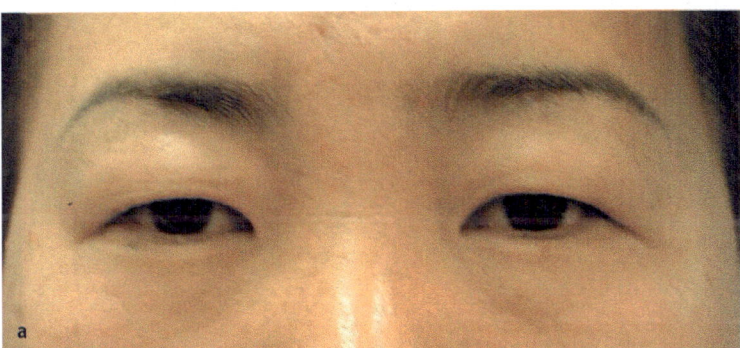

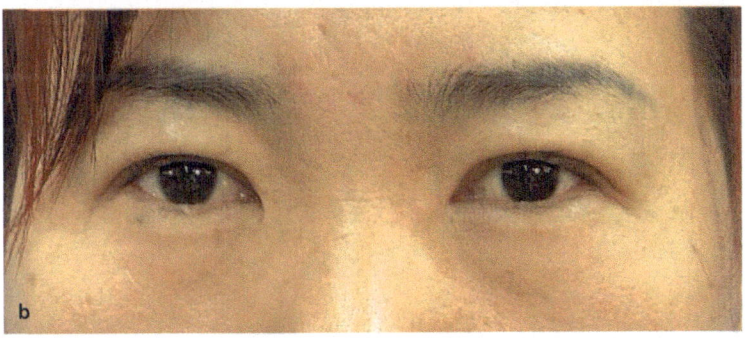

Fig. 59.13 a Preoperative view of a 42-year-old female patient with remarkable upper-lid fat and palpebral skin redundancy. **b** Postoperative view 3 months after double-eyelid creation using a full-incision method. The crease height is relatively fixed in size

lected patients with relatively thin palpebral skin. If the patient shows excessive orbital fat and/or skin redundancy, then a full-incision method may be warranted.

The concept of the skin-to-levator aponeurosis fixation is very important to understand Asian blepharoplasty in the creation of a double eyelid. The author's partial-incision technique for the creation of double eyelids follows Sayoc's hypothesis [2] that levator aponeurosis fibers inserting into eyelid skin play a major role the in creation of the double eyelid [3], and the author's principle involves the direct apposing of the skin to the levator aponeurosis without any interfering tissues between them by fixation of the skin and the levator aponeurosis by placing the inferior epidermal edge precisely onto the levator surface. Cells of the epidermal stratum corneum are dead cells and act as a foreign body when positioned in contact with living tissue. If the cornified epidermal dead cells could provoke a stable adhesion and fixation between skin and the levator aponeurosis, surgeons could do the skin-to-levator aponeurosis fixation by capturing the epidermal skin edge including cornified dead cells instead of capturing the dermomuscularis tissue and, finally, expect to reduce the width of adhesion and ensure a more natural look of the crease line than through a full-incision method. When placing the skin-to-levator aponeurosis fixation suture, the needle should capture not only the dermosubcutis but also the adjacent epidermis 0.5–1.0 mm from the incised skin edge to appose the cornified cells of the stratum corneum precisely onto the levator surface. This stimulates a foreign-body reaction to allow the formation of a stable adhesion. The author has applied this principle, the so-called Waikiki technique, to obtain secure adhesion of the lid crease for the creation of double eyelids either by partial-incision or full-incision blepharoplasty.

The author's underlying principle for skin-to levator aponeurosis fixation and adhesion can also be applied to full-length incisional methods. After the redundant skin of the upper eyelid has been removed adequately, the surgical process is the same as in the partial-incision technique. The skin-to-levator aponeurosis fixation sutures are placed only in the middle third of the fully incised line. Skin closure is then made on the full-length incision with continuous suture.

The CO_2 laser can be used to make an incision and to achieve hemostasis when performing the surgery. The CO_2 laser contributes to minimizing the intraoperative hemorrhage (becoming nearly bloodless) and shortening the total operation time.

References

1. McCurdy JA Jr, Lam SM. Cosmetic surgery of the Asian face (2nd edition). New York: Thieme 2005
2. Sayoc BT. Absence of superior palpebral fold in slit eyes; an anatomic and physiologic explanation. Am J Ophthalmol 1956;42(2):298–300
3. Cheng J, Xu FZ. Anatomic microstructure of the upper eyelid in the Oriental double eyelid. Plast Reconstr Surg 2001;107(7):1665–1668
4. Baker SS, Muenzler WS, Small RG, Leonard JE. Carbon dioxide laser blepharoplasty. Ophthalmology 1984;91(3): 238–244

CHAPTER 60

Blepharoplasty Techniques in Asians

60

Dae-Hwan Park, Young Kyoon Kim

60.1
Introduction

There are definite differences between the upper-eyelid anatomy of the Asian and of the Caucasian (Table 60.1).

The double-eyelid operation is classified into:
1. Non-incision method
   (a) Non-buried-suture method
   (b) Buried-suture method
2. Partial-incision method
   (a) Non-buried-suture method (fixation to tarsus or levator aponeurosis)
   (b) Buried-suture method (fixation to tarsus or levator aponeurosis)
3. Incision method

60.2
Non-Incision Method

The non-incision method cannot be used in patients with too much fat because the fat cannot be removed. The procedure has a short recovery time and minimal complications.

In the non-buried-suture technique, there is fixation of the skin at the level of the tarsus (Fig. 60.1). The eyelid crease depends on the position (height) of the deep portion of the suture (Fig. 60.2). The suture can be partially exposed at the side of the conjunctiva or the

suture can be within the palpebral tissue. Figure 60.3 shows the results of the operation.

Several buried-suture methods are available: Maruo's technique (Figs. 60.4, 60.5), Harada and Kawamoto's method (Fig. 60.6), Umezawa's method (Fig. 60.7), Muto's technique (Figs. 60.8, 60.9), Boo-Chai's method (Figs. 60.10, 60.11). Multiple buried sutures can be placed (Fig. 60.12).

60.3
Partial-Incision Method

The partial-incision method can have fat removed with a minimal incision. There is a short recovery time and minimal complications.

The partial-incision method can be classified as
1. Single partial incision: about 5–15-mm incision at the midline
2. Multiple partial incisions: about 2-mm incision at multiple points

The partial-incision technique with multiple incisions requires small incisions at the upper eyelid and exposure of the orbital septum, dissecting the orbital septum, incising the septum and exposing the orbital fat. The fat is removed carefully and the lateral bulging is then decreased (Fig. 60.13).

Double eyelids are made with full thickness tarsus–dermis buried sutures (Figs. 60.14, 60.15).

Table 60.1 Difference between upper-eyelid anatomy of Asians and Caucasians

Anatomic feature	Caucasian eyelid	Asian eyelid
Preseptal fat pad location	Preseptal	Preseptal and pretarsal
Septum–levator fusion point	Above tarsus	As low as the pretarsal plane
Tarsal height	9–10.5 mm	6.5–8.0 mm
Medial lid crease origin	Medial eyelid	Medial canthus
Presence of crease	100%	50%

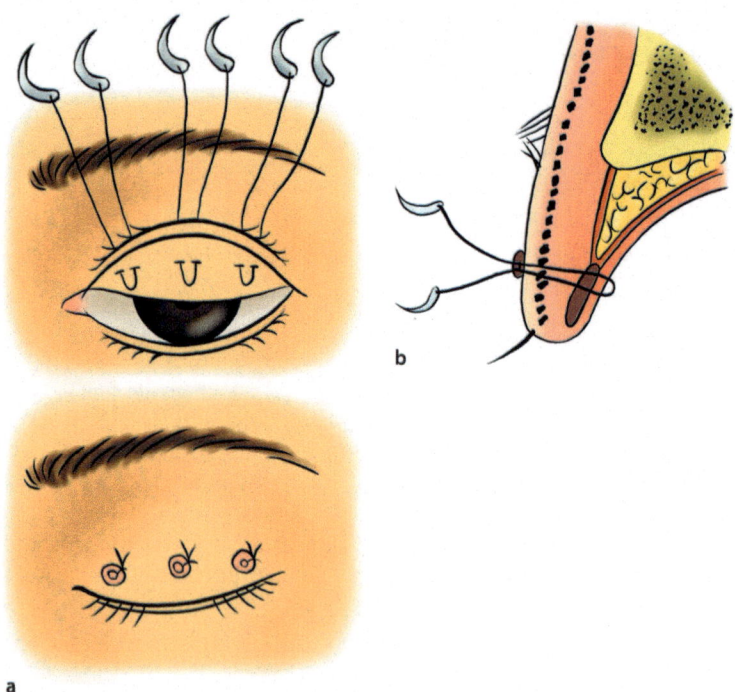

Fig. 60.1 a Fixation at tarsus level. **b** Position of suture

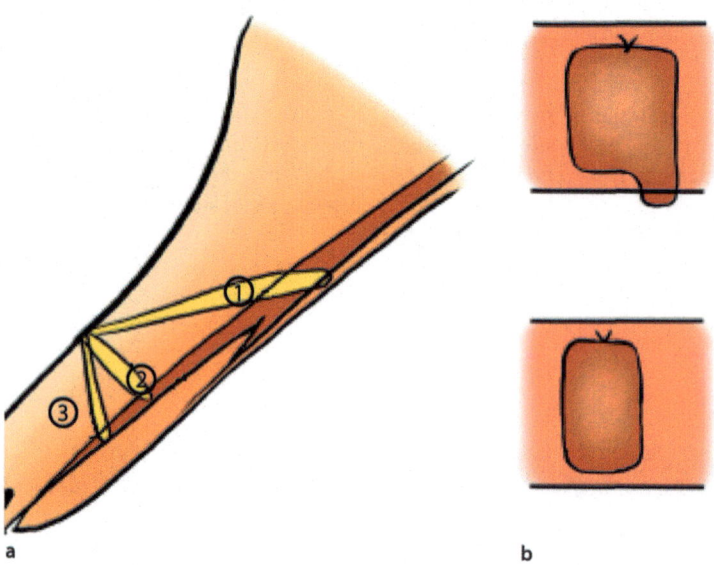

Fig. 60.2 a Eyelid crease level depends on the position of the buried sutures. *1* Suture at the levator aponeurosis to form a higher fold. *2* Suture at the same position of the tarsal plate. *3* Suture at the lower tarsal plate to form a lower fold. **b** Shape of buried suture. *a* Exposing part of the suture at the side of the conjunctiva. *b* Buried suture within palpebral tissue

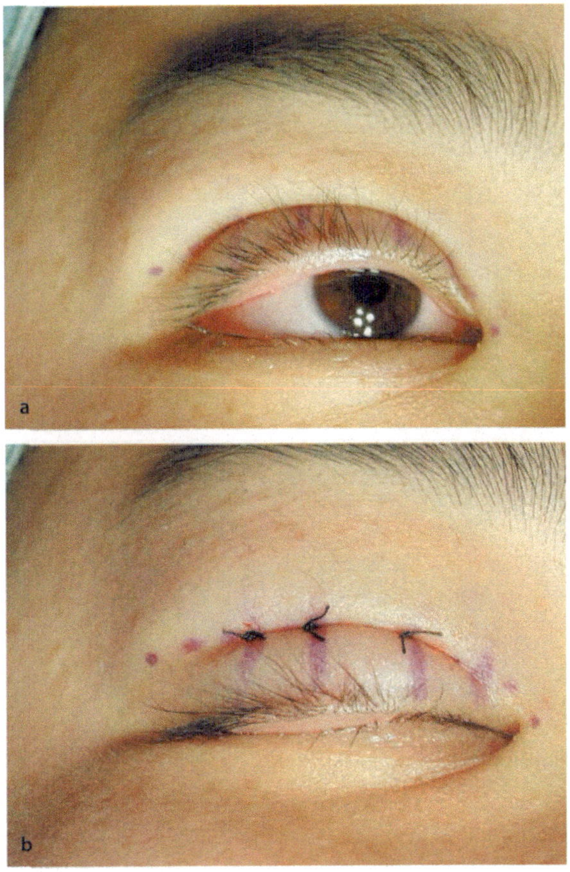

Fig. 60.3 Double-eyelid operation by the non-incision and non-buried-suture method. **a** Preoperatively. **b** Postoperatively

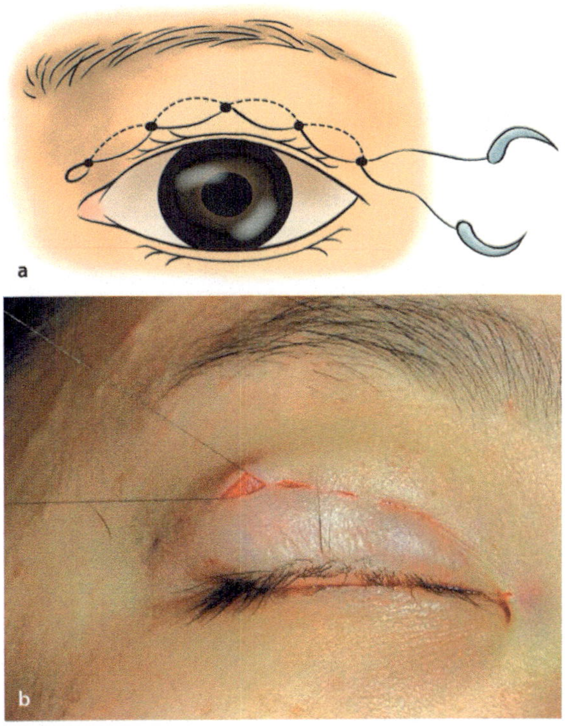

Fig. 60.4 Maruo's buried-suture method. **a** The *solid line* is the tarsal plate and the *dotted line* is the ligature of 5.0 or 6.0 catgut, silk, or nylon. **b** Final closure

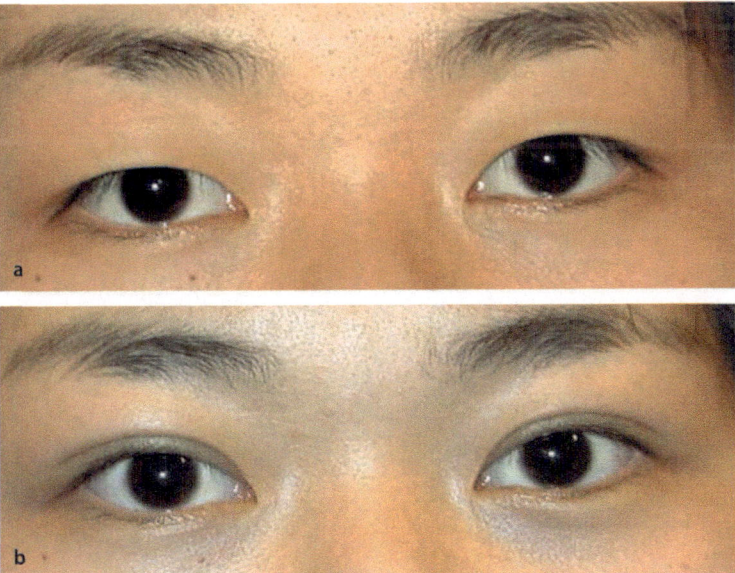

Fig. 60.5 Maruo's technique. **a** Preoperatively. **b** Postoperatively

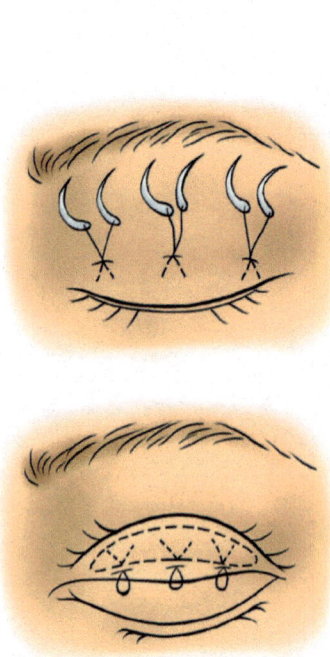

Fig 60.6 Harada and Kawamoto's method

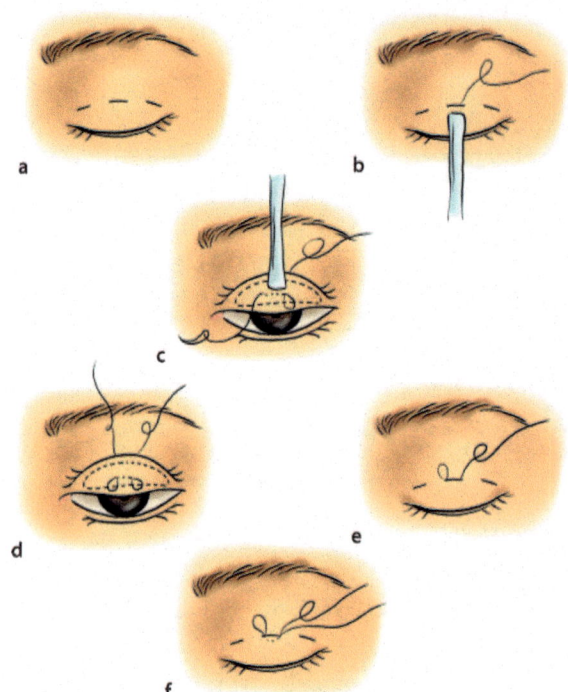

Fig. 60.7 Umezawa's method

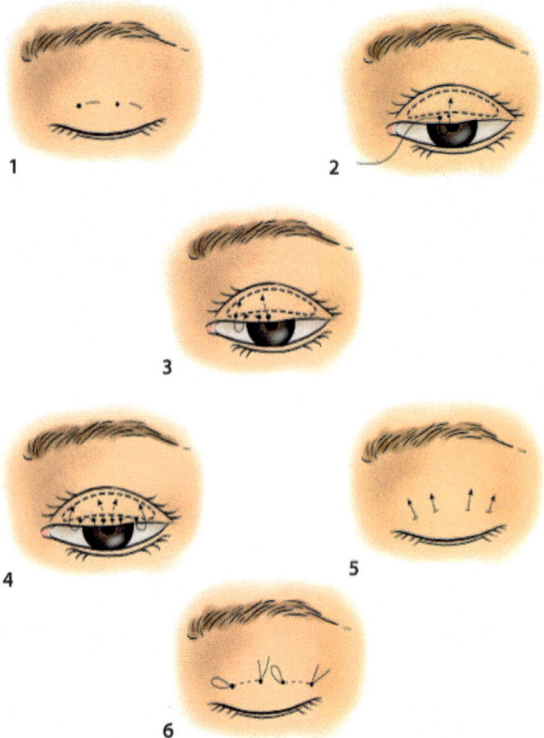

Fig. 60.8 Muto's technique

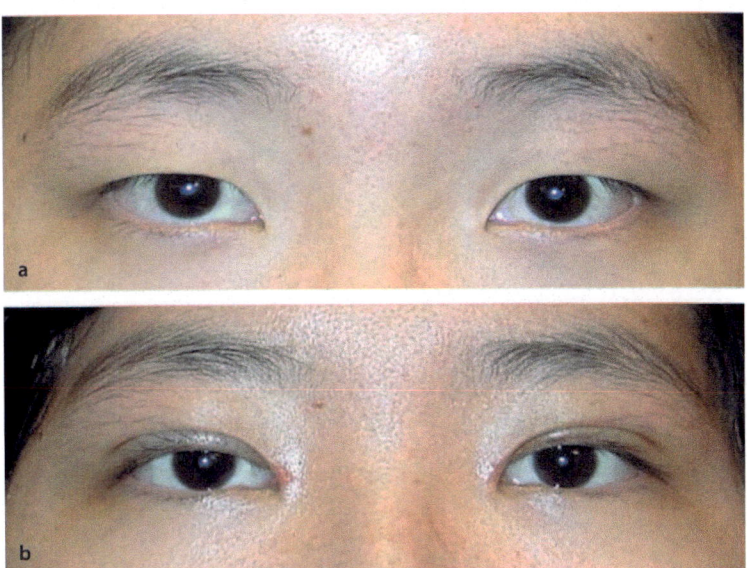

Fig. 60.9 Muto's method. **a** Preoperatively. **b** Postoperatively

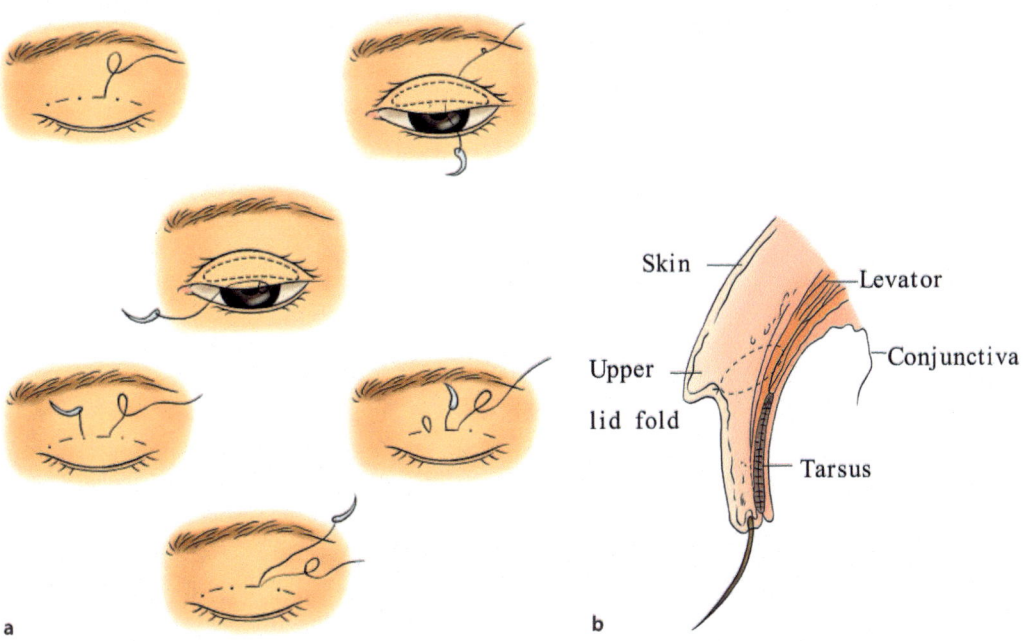

Fig. 60.10 Boo-Chai's method. **a** On the side of conjunctiva, pass through the upper end of tarsal plate. **b** *Dotted line* is buried position of buried suture.

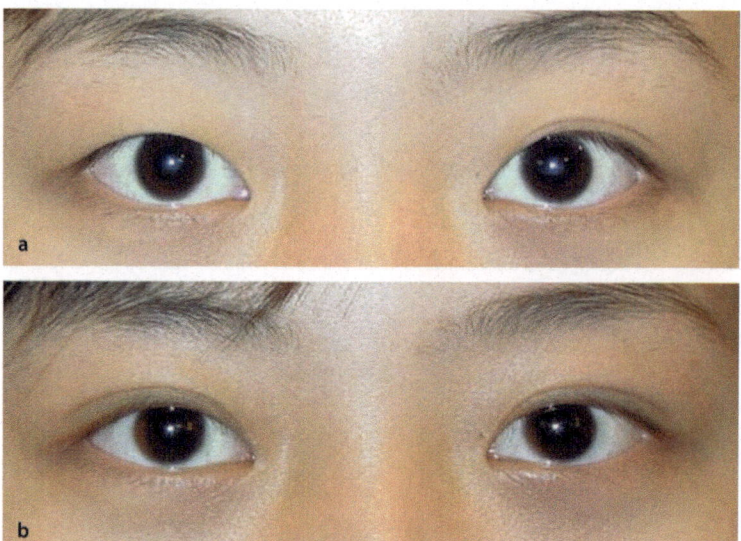

Fig. 60.11 Boo-Chai's method. **a** Preoperatively. **b** Postoperatively

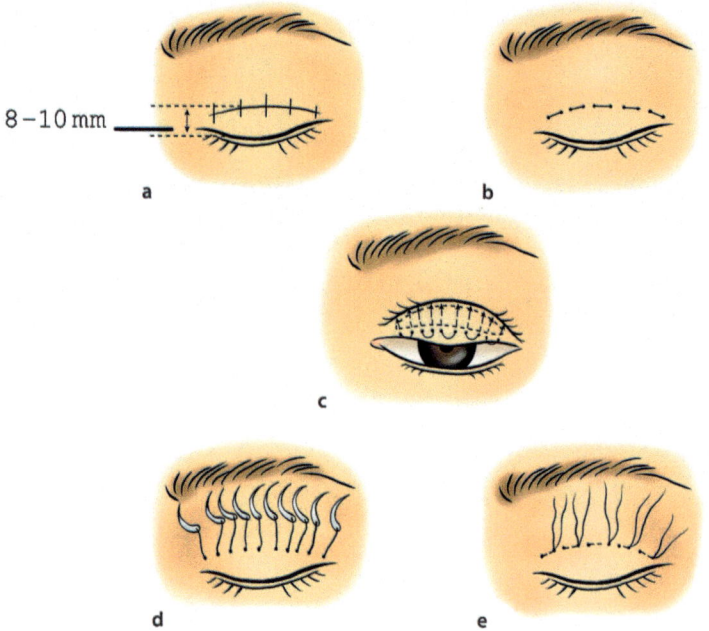

Fig. 60.12 Buried-suture method using more buried sutures. **a** Mark and sign of double eyelid. **b** Distance of thread in and out: 3, 3, 4, 2, and 3 mm. **c** A 6-0 nylon suture passing through just above the level of the tarsal plate on the side of the conjunctiva but put under the conjunctiva, non-exposed thread. **d** Pull-out on the surface of marked skin. **e** Sutures tied

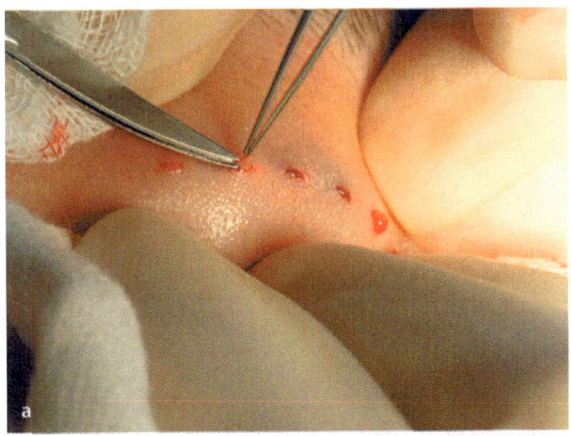

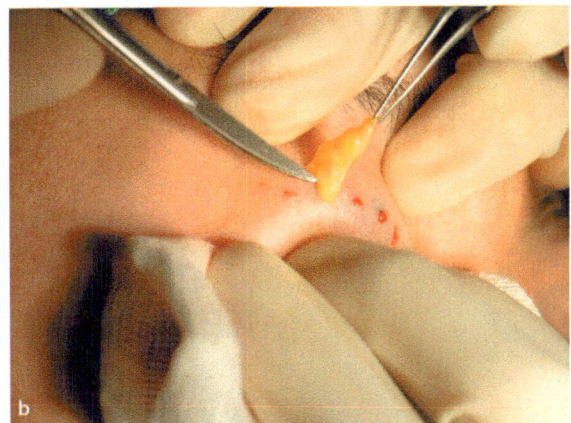

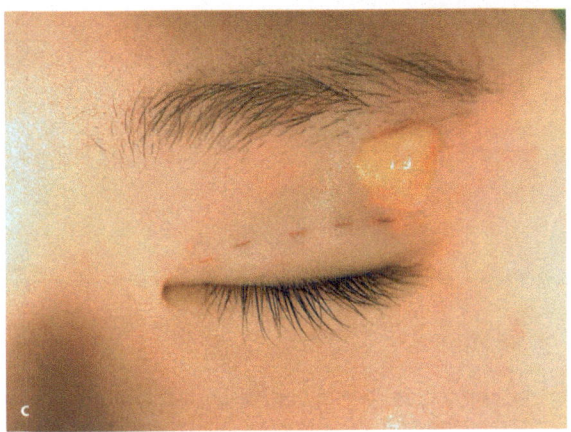

Fig. 60.13 Fat removal. **a** Small incisions at the upper eyelid and exposure of the orbital septum. **b** After the septum has been dissected through small partial-incision sites, the septum is incised and the orbital fat is exposed externally. **c** The fat is removed carefully and lateral bulging is then decreased

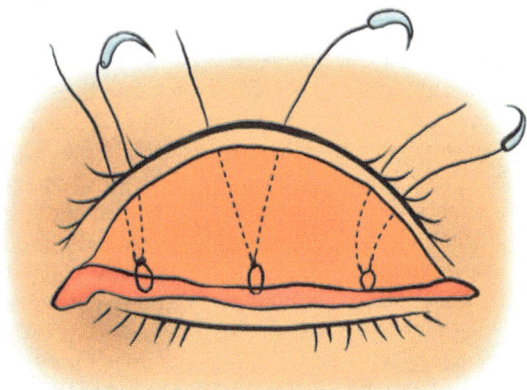

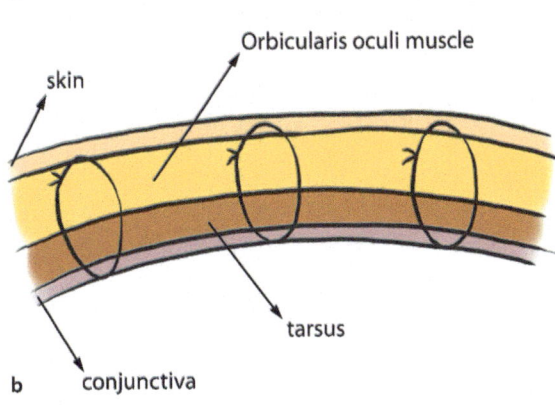

Fig. 60.14 a Double eyelids are made with full thickness tarsus–dermis buried sutures. **b** Transverse section of full-thickness tarsus–dermis buried suture on the upper eyelid

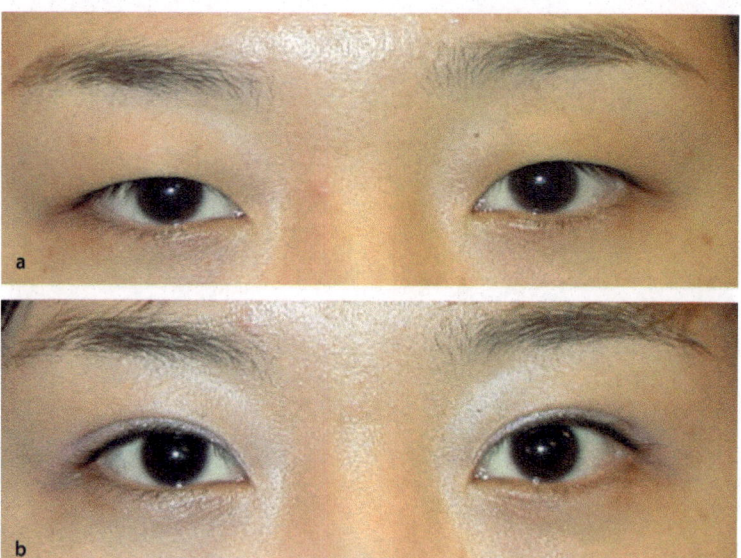

Fig. 60.15 Double eyelids. **a** Preoperatively. **b** Postoperatively

60.4
Incision Method

The incision method can be performed in patients with too much fat since the fat can be removed. There is a longer recovery time but minimal complications.

Indications for the incision method include:

1. Dermatochalasia alone
2. Dermatochalasia with fatty prolapse
3. Dermatochalasia with ptosis
4. Asymmetric eyelids
5. For making prominent double eyelids
6. In the case of scar in upper eyelids
7. Reoperation cases (in complication cases of the non-incision method)

The incision methods are classified as "buried or non-buried" suture and "fixation level" (Figs. 60.16, 60.17). Park's technique involves buried sutures at three to five points and fixation to the superior tarsal plate and aponeurosis (Fig. 60.18). The results are excellent (Figs. 60.19–60.21).

60.5
Complications

In the immediate postoperative period, the complications that may be encountered include corneal exposure or dryness, chemosis, hemorrhage and hematoma with ecchymosis and anterior hematoma or posterior hematoma and retrobular hemorrhage, cellulitis and abscess (Fig. 60.22), inadvertent globe penetration, or eyelid slough. In the intermediate postoperative period, the complications may include orbicularis abnormality with hypertrophy or adhesions, lacrimal system dysfunction, dry eye, medial canthal deformity, diplopia and extraocular muscle movement disorder, and exposure keratinopathy from incomplete eyelid closure. In the late postoperative period, the possible complications include ptosis, ectropion, sunken eyelid resulting from aggressive fat resection, asymmetries (Fig. 60.23), inclusion cyst or suture tunnels, lagophthalmos, hypertrophic scarring, disappearance of double eyelid or shallowness (Fig. 60.24), and high fold and low fold.

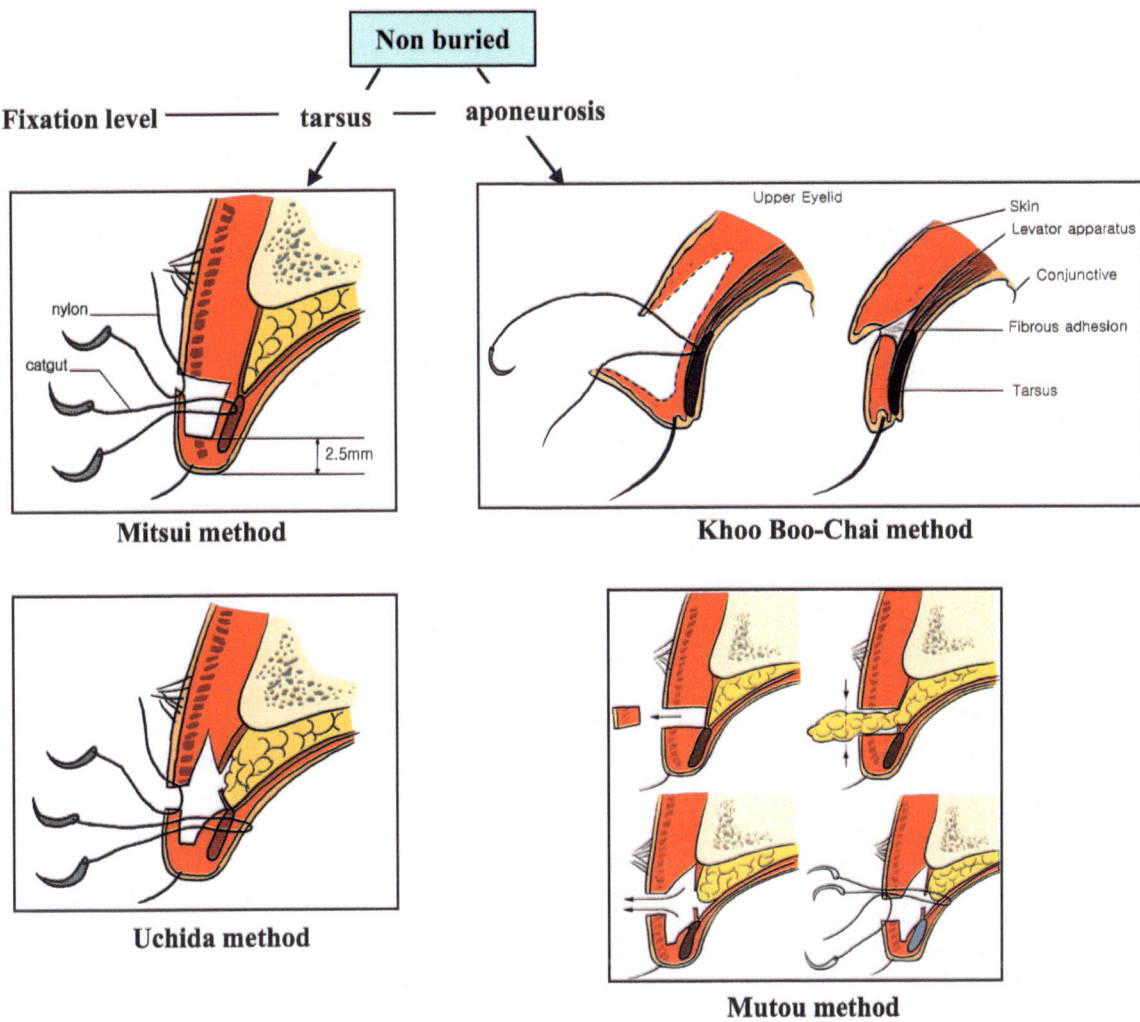

Fig. 60.16 Non-buried method

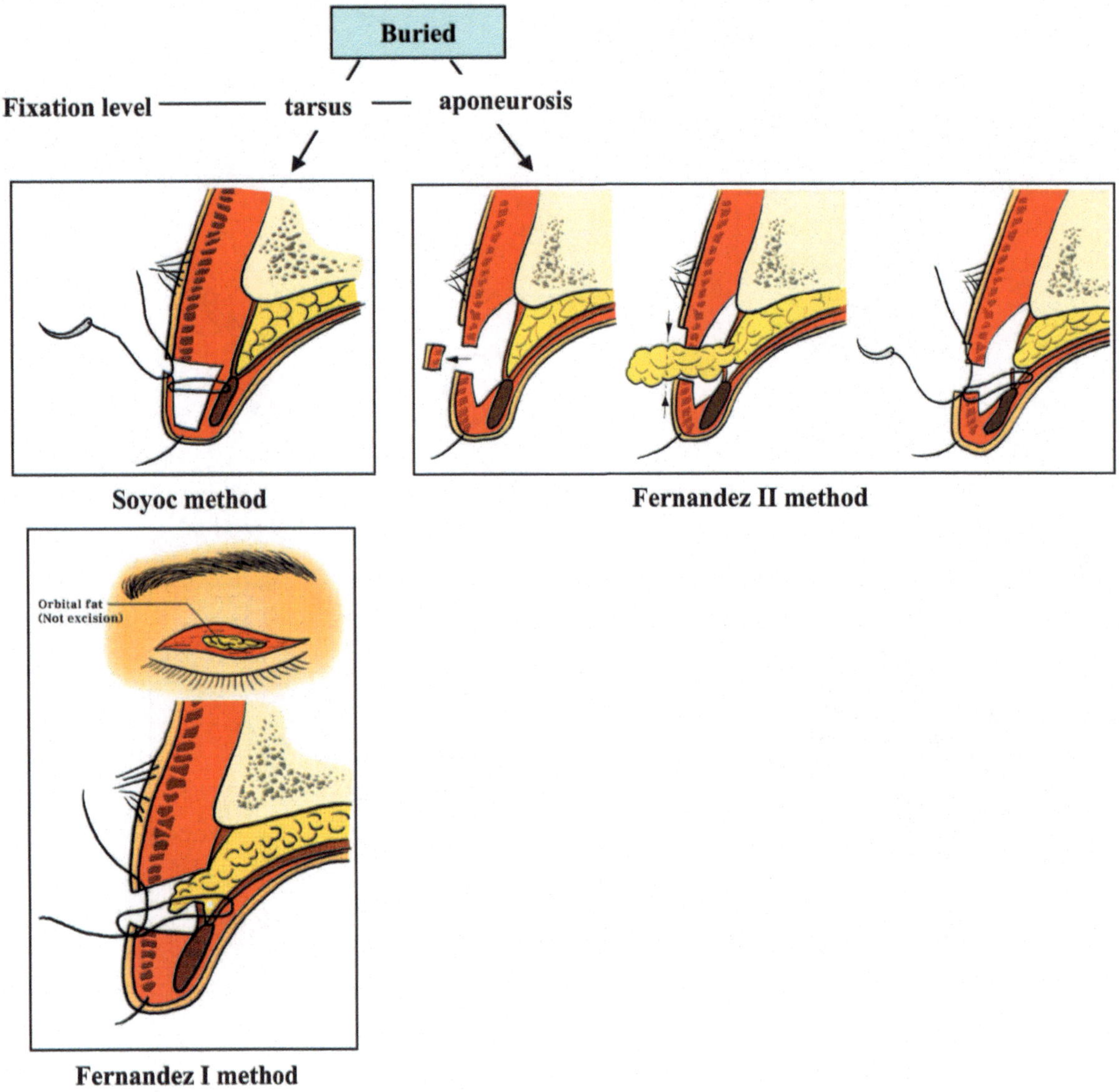

Buried

Fixation level ——— tarsus ——— aponeurosis

Soyoc method

Fernandez II method

Orbital fat
(Not excision)

Fernandez I method

Fig. 60.17 Buried method

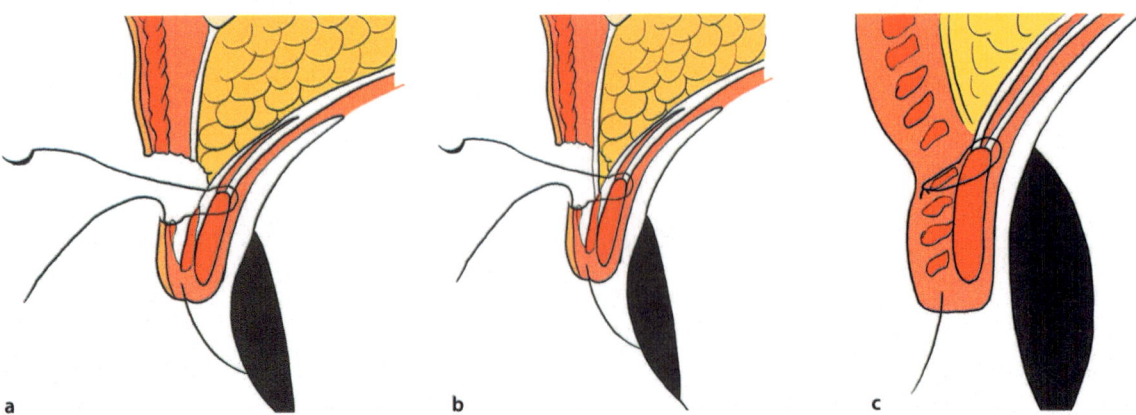

Fig. 60.18 a Septum opened. **b** Sometimes the septum does not open. **c** Completed suturing. **d,e** *see next page*

a   b   c

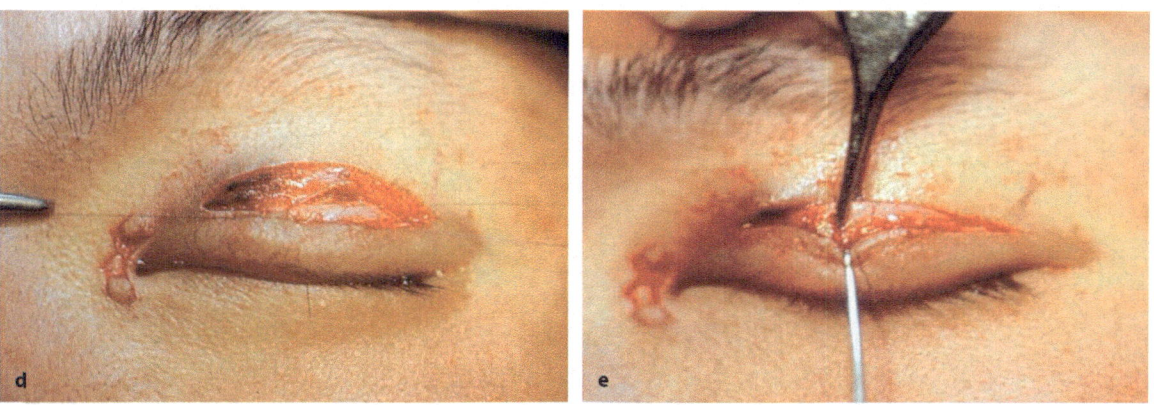

Fig. 60.18 *(Continued)* **d,e** Non-absorbable suture at three to five points

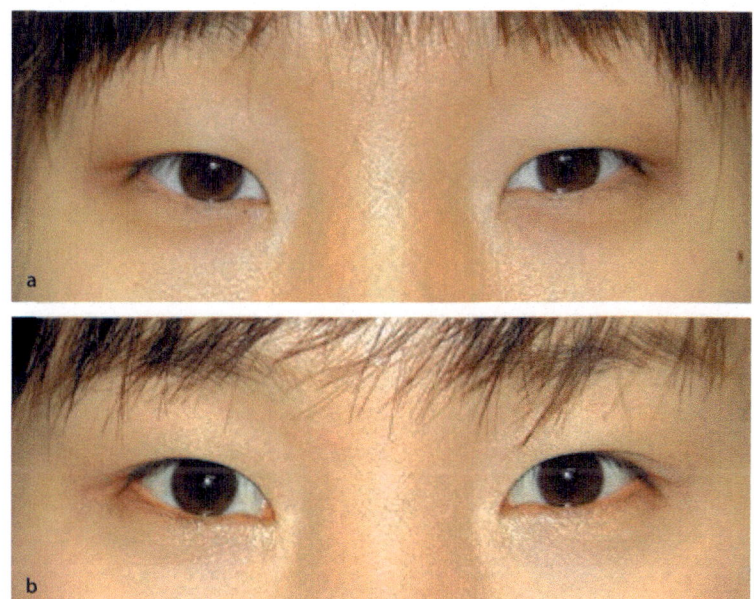

Fig. 60.19 Incision method. **a** Preoperatively. **b** Postoperatively

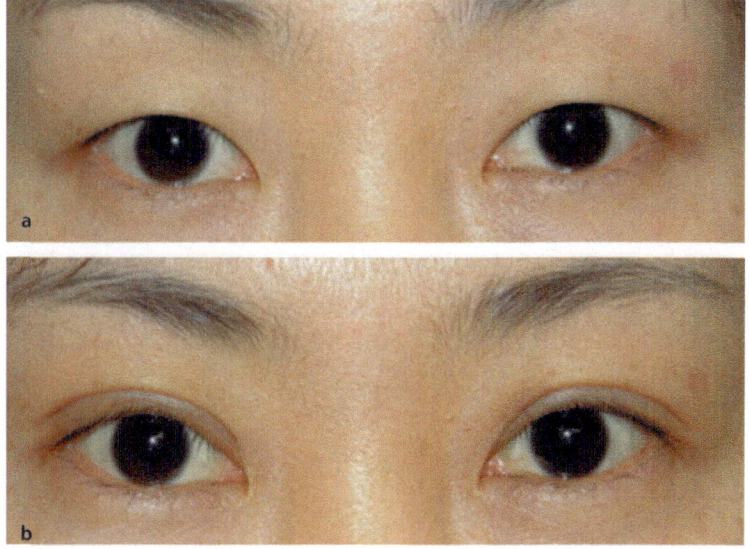

Fig. 60.20 Incision method. **a** Preoperatively. **b** Postoperatively

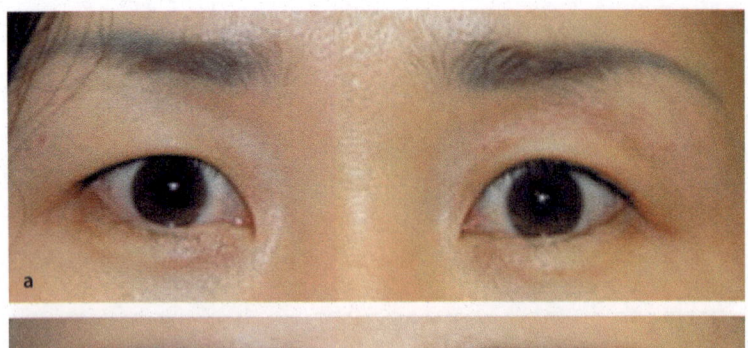

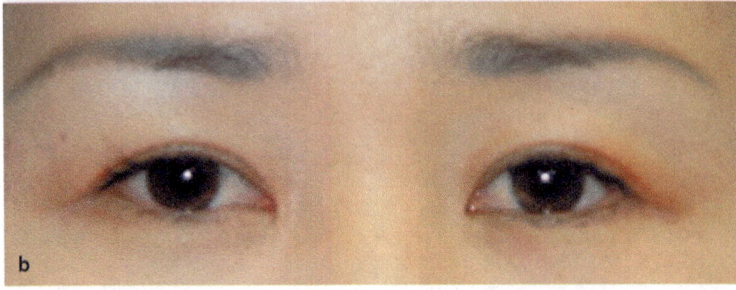

Fig. 60.21 Incision method. **a** Preoperatively. **b** Postoperatively

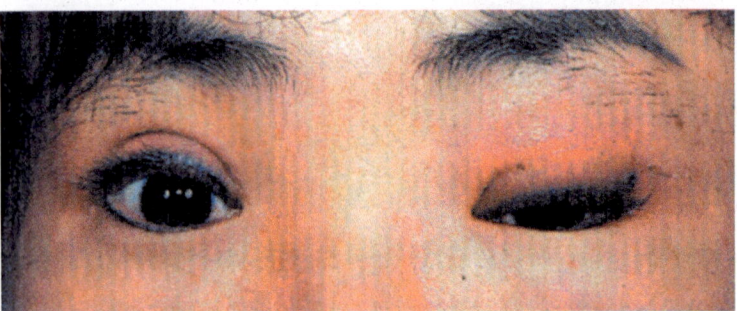

Fig. 60.22 Abscess

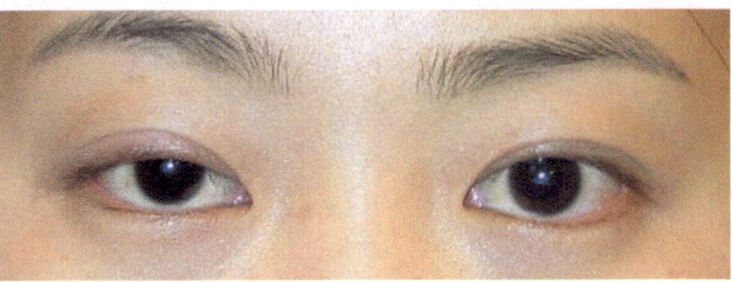

Fig. 60.23 Asymmetry

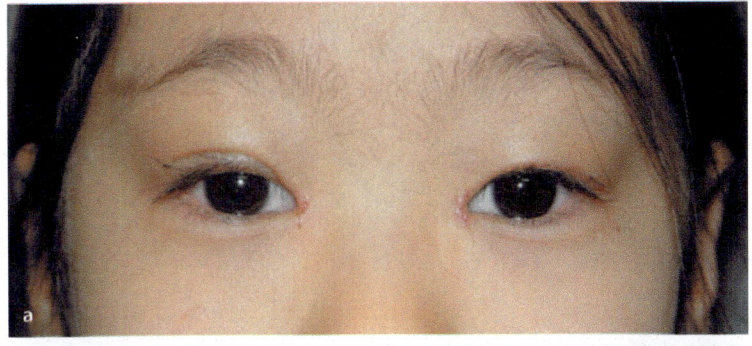

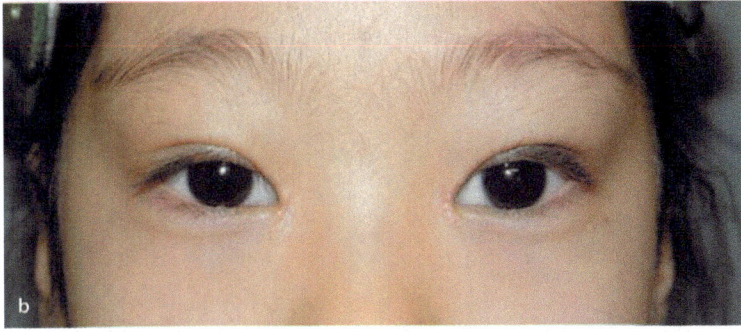

Fig. 60.24 a Disappearance of the fold line on the left side. **b** After revision

60.6
Postoperative Regimen

Ice-pack compresses are used for 1–2 days and bed rest is for 24 h. No reading, viewing of television, computer use, or computer-gaming is allowed. Wound and facial hygiene, dressing, and application of antibiotic ointment for 7 days are undertaken. Hot spas or swimming, strenuous activities, or workout for at least 1 week should be avoided as should aspirin or anything containing ibuprofen. Steroids are not routinely prescribed.

CHAPTER 61

Transconjunctival Approach to Lower-Lid Blepharoplasty

Guy G. Massry

61.1
Introduction

Transconjunctival refers to a surgical approach to handling lower-eyelid fat. There are a variety of adjunctive techniques (canthoplasty, skin pinch, muscle strap) which may be included in surgery which warrant cutaneous incisions and muscle manipulation.

Subperiosteal fat repositioning [1–3] is the author's preferred method of cosmetic lower-lid rejuvenation as the incidence of lower-lid hollowness (skeletonized look) is reduced [1]. With aging there is a change in the lower-lid–cheek continuum. Lower-lid fat becomes more prominent and the cheek descends [4]. This combination of changes leads to a groove overlying the inferior orbital rim which is referred to as the tear trough. This technique uses native fat to fill in the tear trough (nasojugal fold).

61.2
Surgical Technique

In cases of fat repositioning, the tear trough is demarcated preoperatively. In addition, the amount of nasal and central fat to be repositioned is assessed. The lateral fat is rarely repositioned as the amount of fat present is generally not adequate to fill the lateral orbital rim depression.

As opposed to patient discomfort with upper-lid blepharoplasty, potential patient discomfort is much more prevalent with lower-lid surgery. This is especially true if fat is repositioned during surgery. Lower-lid blepharoplasty, without intravenous sedation, when fat is cauterized or excised only, is performed in patients who have the disposition to tolerate the procedure. The success of a cosmetic practice is primarily dependent on customer service and patient satisfaction. The assurance of patient comfort during surgery is paramount to maintaining patient happiness.

For procedures performed under injections of local anesthesia only, patients are pretreated with 5–10 mg of Valium per os depending on the patient's history of sedative use, patient weight, and patient anxiety. A drop of tetracaine is then instilled into the lower cul-de-sacs of each eye. A small piece of cotton torn off the tip of a cotton-tipped applicator is soaked with the same tetracaine drops and this tetracaine pledget is placed into the lower cul-de-sacs and the patient closes the eyes. This is called a "tetracaine bath." After 5 min the tetracaine pledgets are removed. This technique has allowed injection of local anesthetic in the majority of patients without discomfort. In patients receiving intravenous sedation the tetracaine is not necessary since sedation and anxiolytics negate the need for significant preinjection conjunctival anesthesia.

Two to 3 ml of 1% Xylocaine with 1:100,000 epinephrine is injected transconjunctivally after distracting the lower lid inferiorly with the index finger while simultaneously compressing (balloting) the globe through the upper eyelid. This maneuver pushes the inferior cul-de-sac forward while also making it more prominent, increasing the surface area of injectable conjunctiva. After injection, the lower lid becomes more prominent and the skin blanches within a few minutes. The balloting maneuver is repeated and the conjunctiva and lower-lid retractors are incised 5 mm below the tarsus from the puncta nasally to the most temporal portion of the lower lid. It is important to incise tissue 5 mm below the tarsus as this level is inferior to the tarsus enough to access the fat pads without violating the septum. Incisions that are too low should be avoided as this may lead to persistent chemosis postoperatively. The depth of the incision (its end point) is when fat is exposed.

The conjunctiva is engaged with retractors and with a 4-0 silk suture and the suture is secured under tension to the head drape with a hemostat. This accomplishes a number of things. First, the cornea is protected by the conjunctiva and retractors and, second, the lower-lid tissues are placed on stretch, which improves exposure. Finally, with the lower lid pulled down with a Desmarres retractor, the small surgical space is enlarged significantly. A cotton-tipped applicator is used to bluntly dissect inferiorly to the orbital rim. This allows the fat pads and inferior oblique muscle to be delineated. The tip of the nasal fat pad is grasped and decapitated. The fat pad then bulges forward with its borders becoming apparent.

The same is done for the middle fat pad. The fat pads are bluntly dissected from the inferior oblique muscle to ensure that it will be undisturbed when manipulating the fat pads. The temporal fat pad is then exposed with the same technique. Lockwood's ligament separates the middle from the temporal fat pad. Every attempt is made to preserve this ligament (typically dense in persons under 50, and more attenuated thereafter) as it is a support structure for the globe. When fat is only to be excised, all three pads are reduced at this point. The fat is cut flush with the orbital rim without pushing on the eye. If more fat is excised there is a strong tendency toward postoperative hollowness.

In cases of repositioning fat, the nasal and central fat pads are bluntly dissected from the inferior oblique muscle. All connective tissue attachments are severed. The fat pads are held with toothed forceps at their tips and one fat pad is pulled while allowing the other to recess, and then the process is reversed (Fig. 61.1). This demonstrates that the fat pads can move freely beneath and around the inferior oblique muscle. This is called the "shoeshine sign," because it mimics the inverse of shining a shoe. The ends of each fat pedicle are grasped and the pedicle is splayed open to identify the width of the area. This can be filled in with fat (Fig. 61.2). The transconjunctival surface of the lower lid and all tissue over the orbital inferiorly are retracted exposing the periosteum at the arcus marginalis (Fig. 61.3). A cotton-tipped applicator is used to brush the suborbicularis fat inferiorly further exposing suborbital rim periosteum. The periosteum is incised with the cutting mode of an electrocautery unit from just temporal to where the tear trough begins to the most nasal aspect of the orbital rim. A Freer elevator is used to elevate the periosteum from

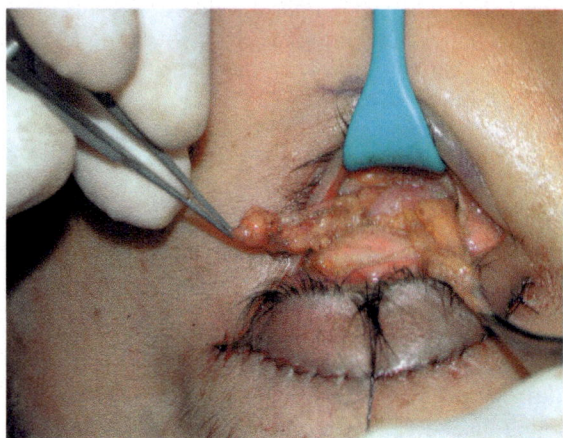

Fig. 61.1 One fat pad is retracted while allowing the other to recess, and then the process is reversed. This demonstrates that the fat pads can move freely beneath and around the inferior oblique muscle

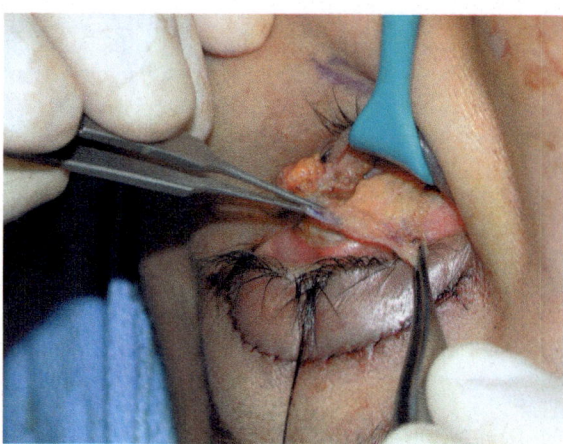

Fig. 61.2 The end of each fat pedicle is grasped and the pedicle is splayed open to identify the width of the area that can be filled with fat

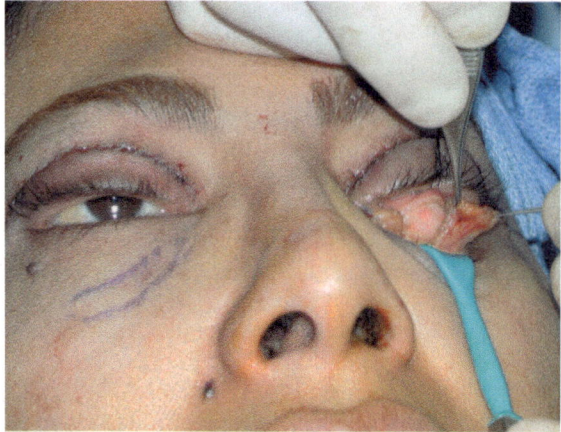

Fig. 61.3 The transconjunctival surface of the lower lid and all the tissue over the orbital inferiorly are retracted exposing the periosteum at the arcus marginalis

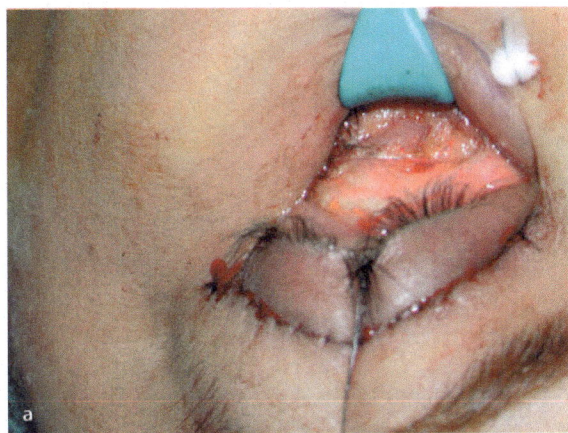
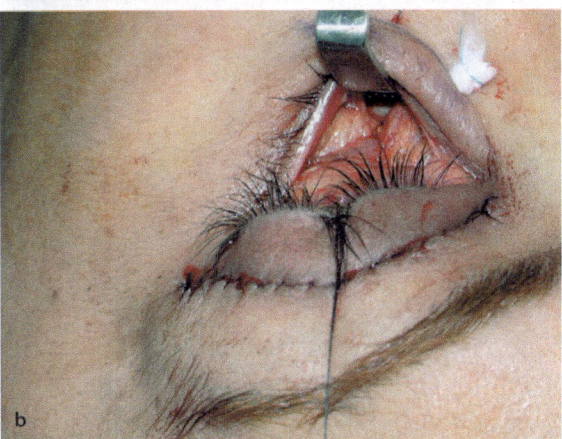

Fig. 61.4 a The suture is tied over a cotton bolster, allowing repositioning and fixation of the fat pedicle over the tear trough. **b** This step is repeated for the central fat pedicle

the face of the maxilla for approximately 15 mm. Dissection is carried around the infraorbital neurovascular bundle. It is not uncommon to experience significant bleeding during this part of surgery. For this reason, the subperiosteal pockets are packed with cotton pledgets soaked in 1:10,000 epinephrine.

The other eye is now approached and the pledgets are allowed to take effect. Surgery on the first eye is completed only after the point of pledgeting the opposite eye. The pledgets are removed and typically there is a dry pocket. A 4-0 Prolene suture on an FS-2 needle is inserted through the skin into the nasal pocket, fed through the fat pedicle and then the suture is brought through the pocket and out of the skin. The suture is tied over a cotton bolster (Fig. 61.4), thus repositioning and fixating the fat pedicle over the tear trough. This step is repeated for the central fat pedicle. Forced ductions are performed to ensure free movement and the wound is allowed to heal by secondary intent.

61.3
Postoperative Care

Patients are instructed to apply ice compresses every hour (for 10 min) while awake for the first 48 h after surgery. It is suggested to sleep as upright as possible for the first week after surgery. I typically recommend two or three pillows. A topical antibiotic steroid drop is applied three times a day for 1 week. In fat repositioning cases an oral steroid preparation (Medrol dose pack) is prescribed and the Prolene sutures and cotton bolsters are removed 4–5 days after surgery.

61.4
Complications

Surgical complications for fat excision versus repositioning are similar. They typically include excessive bruising and swelling, chemosis, and subconjunctival hemorrhage. An overcorrection or an undercorrection of fat reduction can occur. This can lead to persistent fat prominence or hollowness. This is less common with fat repositioning cases. When fat is repositioned, complications unique to this procedure can occur. These include diplopia (beyond the immediate postoperative period), fat granulomas, prolonged edema and chemosis, and tear-trough irregularities. Diplopia is typically transient and related to edema or inferior oblique trauma. This is usually treated with higher-dose oral steroids which are tapered over a 10-day period. This generally allows all cases to resolve over this time period. Fat granulomas are rare, less than 5% of cases, and are treated with intralesional injections of low-dose and concentration steroids (0.1 ml of 5 mg/ml Kenalog). The granulomas usually resolve with one or two injections given 2–3 weeks apart. A granuloma has been encountered that needed surgical excision. Prolonged edema and chemosis is treated with higher-dose steroids.

61.5
Discussion

For the past 5 years the author has rarely excised fat from lower lids (in less than 5% of cases). This is a highly reproducible and reliable surgery with high patient satisfaction (Figs. 61.5, 61.6). The following are the essential points to keep in mind when considering this surgery:
1. There is a high learning curve to the surgery.
2. Watching a number of procedures before attempting the technique is important.
3. The surgical space is small so experience with standard transconjunctival surgery is helpful.
4. There is a risk of diplopia, so be careful dissecting around the inferior oblique muscle.

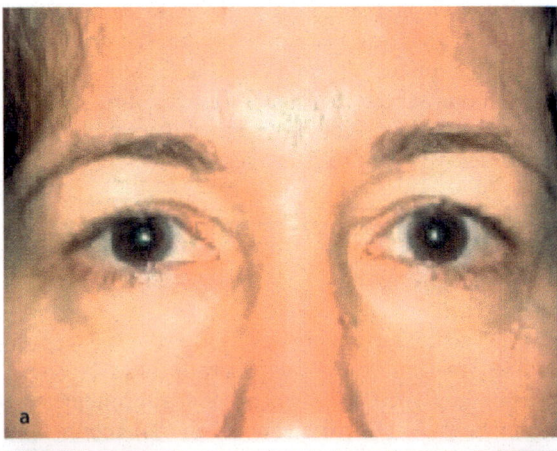

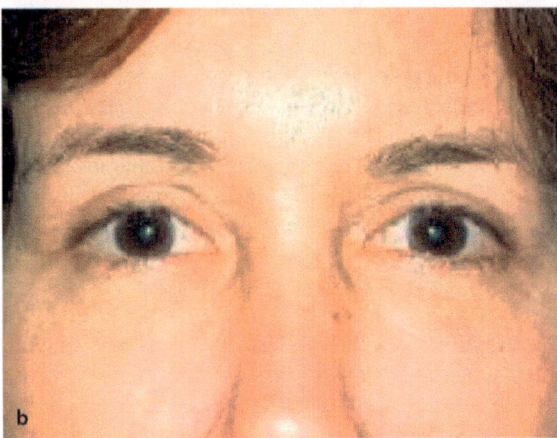

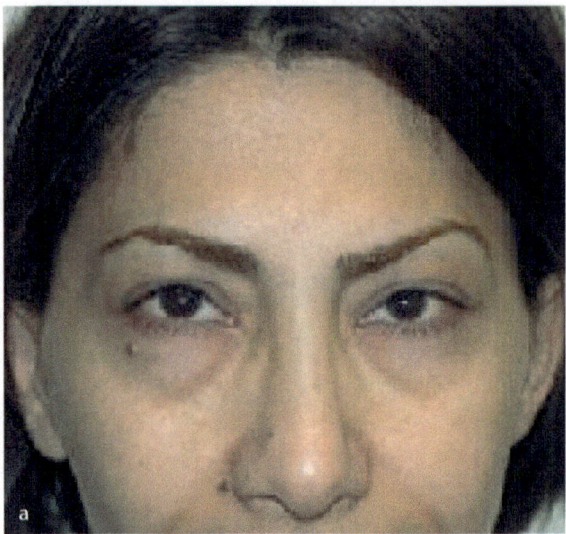

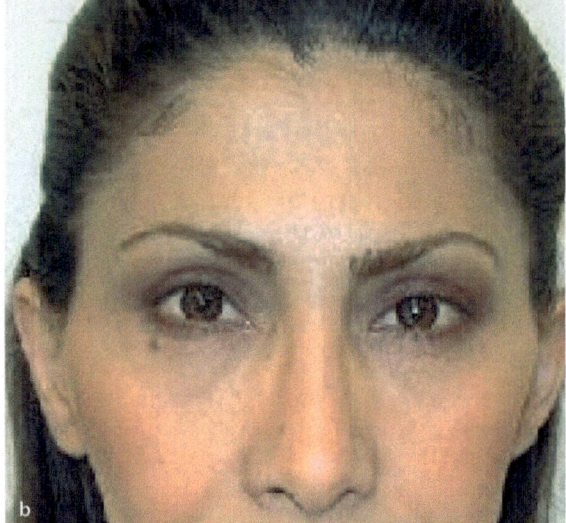

Fig. 61.5 a Preoperatively. **b** Six months after the lower lid fat repositioning procedure. Note reduction of lower lid fat herniation and effacement of the tear trough

Fig. 61.6 a Preoperatively. **b** One year postoperatively following lower lid fat repositioning

References

1. Nassif PS. Lower blepharoplasty: transconjunctival blepharoplasty. Facial Plast Surg Clin North Am 2005:13(4):553–559

2. Hamra ST. Arcus marginalis release and orbital fat repositioning in midface rejuvenation. Plastic Reconstr Surg 1995;92(6):354–362

3. Hamra ST. The role of orbital fat preservation in facial aesthetic surgery. A new concept. Clin Plast Surg 1996;23(1):17–28

4. Edelstein C, Goldberg RA, Shorr N, Balch KC. Transconjunctival approach to the arcus marginalis release. In: Unfavorable Results of Eyelid and Lachrymal Surgery. Mauriello JA (Ed.), Boston, Butterworth Heinemann 2000:20–25

CHAPTER 62

A Clinical Guide to Estimate the Skin Resection in Upper Blepharoplasties

62

Pierre F. Fournier

62.1
Introduction

The author initially obtained the information on this subject from Paule Regnault in Montreal, Canada.

During an upper cosmetic blepharoplasty, the estimation of the skin resection is usually done using the "pinch technique" [1]. It is satisfactory in many cases but quite often skin excess remains in the immediate follow-up and the patients are not fully satisfied and request an "additional touch-up." Many prudent aesthetic surgeons prefer to remove "less" than to remove "too much" and doing a touch-up is better than having a patient unable to close his/her eyelids.

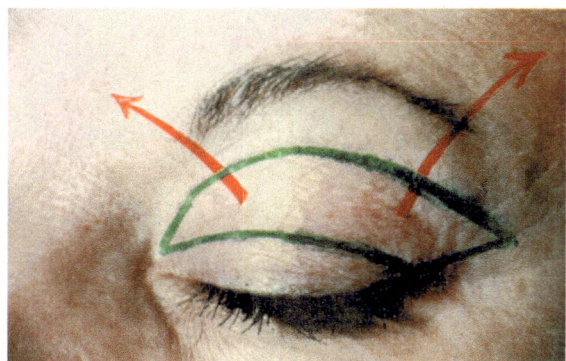

Fig. 62.1 Markings for skin excision of the eyelid

62.2
Appearance of the Skin

It is evident that the skin excess of the upper lid has a special appearance and by "sight" it is easy to estimate the amount of skin to remove to obtain a good result (Fig. 62.1) [2, 3]. The skin excess most often has a special color and a special texture. The color is brown or brownish, is more or less evident in different patients, and is less invisible when the skin is clear. This pigmentation does not exist in some patients.

To demonstrate this pigmented skin, it is necessary to stretch the skin of the upper eyelid between two fingers and then three zones of different color between the line of the eyelashes and the eyebrow can be seen. The lower one, as an arch extending from the eyelashes until the upper limit of the upper tarsal plate, is clear; the upper one, below the eyebrows, is also clear; and another one, between the other two, is pigmented, corresponding to the skin excess.

It is rare that the pigmentation is not evident. The texture of this skin is very special in all individuals, even in children. It has a granular appearance, made of many small bumps evenly disseminated, like grains of sand. Such a granular appearance is not always apparent. It is easy to evidence it by light friction of the skin with gauze. Such small bumps look like very small cysts and their presence is constant and faithfully reveals the amount of skin to be removed. Such an appearance does

not exist laterally but is only on the eyelid. It is a guide when doing the lateral skin resection. This microcystic skin is more pigmented than neighboring skin. This is paradoxical as it is not exposed to the surrounding light. It is believed that this pigmentation is provoked by the friction of the skin on itself as is seen in other places on the body: axillae, submammary sulcus, and inner thighs. The microbumps seem to be sweat or sebaceous glands that are always in great number when there is friction on the skin making the rubbing of the skin on itself easier. Histological findings have confirmed this explanation.

Women have three zones that are very visible. Men have only two, the lower one is clear and the upper one is pigmented. The pigmentation does not exist when reaching the eyebrows. The upper third zone is created artificially by women who depilate.

62.3
Discussion

This guide is only one more element of security during the estimation of the amount of skin to be resected. The punch technique can check that this guide is excellent. Excess removal as well as insufficient removal are avoided. The skin with the best pigmentation for transfer, if there is excess removal, is scrotal skin.

Another advantage is that the scar is in a good position, right in the depth of the suprapalpebral sulcus and not higher or lower, visible on leaving a strip of pigmented skin above or below it, even if the right amount of skin has been resected. It is surprising that such a "trick" is not better known and is not mentioned in books on aesthetic surgery.

References

1. Spira M.: Dark pigmented line in blepharoplasty. In: Regnault P., Daniel R.K. (Eds.), Aesthetic Surgery: Principles and Techniques, Boston, Little Brown, 1984:329
2. Fournier F.P., Otteni F.: Blépharoplasties esthétiques et voie transconjonctivale. In: Faivre J. Zenatti C. (Eds.), Chirurgie Esthétique 1980, Direction Scientifique, Paris, Maloine 1980:237
3. Fournier F.P.: Un guide clinique pour évaluer la peau en excès dans les blépharoplasties cosmétiques supérieures. In: Faivre J., Zenatti C. (Eds.), Chirurgie Esthétique 1980, Direction Scientifique, Paris, Maloine 1980:197

CHAPTER 63

A Frequent Complication of Aesthetic Blepharoplasty: the Surgical Round Eye

63

Pierre F. Fournier

63.1
Introduction

The Caucasian eye may have two different palpebral openings. Most often, it is almond-shaped. The transversal axis measured from the inner to the outer canthus is about 30 mm long and the most important height is from 12 to 15 mm. In another case, the height of the palpebral opening may be more important than in the previous case in relation to the transversal axis, giving the so-called aspect of "the round eye."

In an almond-shaped eye, around the iris, no sclera is visible, while in the round eye, the sclera is more or less important (scleral show). The round eye, which is a normal eye, is considered less beautiful than the almond-shaped eye and for ages makeup has been used to make it look like an almond-shaped eye.

It is evident that if a patient wanting to have a blepharoplasty has a round eye preoperatively, he/she will have a round eye postoperatively. The complication that we are describing is the change of shape that may happen after a blepharoplasty with a patient having an almond-shaped eye before the operation and having a round eye after the operation (Fig. 63.1). This aspect may be described using the words "fish eye", "cow eye", etc. Obviously, the patient suffers aesthetic damage which is evident. Sometimes, he/she may be satisfied with the result, claiming that he/she had again his/her child eyes, as in children the round eye is normal.

The aesthetic complication seems to be ignored in books on aesthetic surgery and in many books a round eye is described as an excellent result by renowned aesthetic surgeons. This shape of the postoperative round eye generally does not appear immediately after the operation. It happens during the following months. It is not associated with an ectropion, or is associated very exceptionally.

63.2
What Are the Causes of this Postoperative Round Eye?

Two opposing forces are responsible: an upper one and a lower one, the most important:
1. Too much skin or too many skin muscles have been resected on the lower lid.
2. Contraction of the scars (upper and lower).

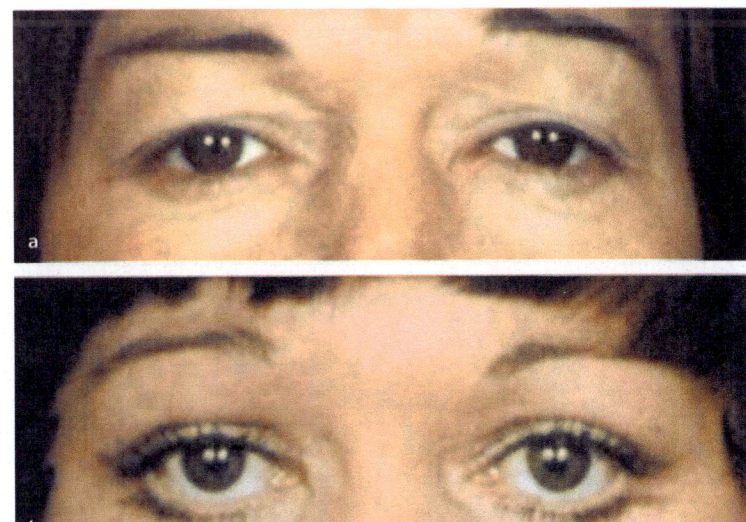

Fig. 63.1 a Patient preoperatively. **b** Round eye postoperatively

3. The weight of the cheeks in the standing position in the immediate postoperative period in some patients who needed, at the same time that they needed blepharoplasty, a cervicofacial lift. This weight has the consequence of giving an inappropriate apposition of the skin on the orbicularis oculi muscle.

4. The operative trauma on the orbicularis oculi muscle.

5. The trauma of the small nerves of the facial branches supplying the orbicularis oculi muscle. This may happen when the surgeon removes the fat excess through only one incision, from one canthus to the other. It seems better to remove the fat excess through three small openings above each fatty hernia, dissociating the orbicularis oculi muscle fibers with fine forceps or using the skin muscle flap incision. The trauma of the small nerves and of the orbicularis oculi muscle will be much less important.

6. Too much important fatty resection of the three hernias.

7. Hypotonia of the orbicularis oculi muscle in mature patients. This hypotonia is easily demonstrated by this test: when the lower lid is depressed inferiorly with the index finger, with the patient in the upright position, the palpebral borders remains distant from the eyeball and cannot go back to touch it if the patient does not blink.

8. Using sunglasses postoperatively for a long time may give hypotonia of the orbicularis oculi muscle as the normal contractions of the eyelids are diminished because the normal light reflex is affected (12 normal contractions per minute).

9. The most important cause seems to be the fact that the skin of the lower lid, which is the thinnest of the body, behaves a skin graft and contracts like a skin graft. This contraction happening slowly postoperatively explains why the round eye is seen in the late follow-up. The skin flap technique should decrease the frequency of this complication, but round eyes are also part of this technique.

10. Techniques connecting upper and lower palpebral incisions may increase the frequency of this complication from the circular scar contraction which may be seen and which is well known after colostomies or transpositions of the navel. This complication is generally forever.

Sometimes a postoperative round eye may be transitory and we have seen several cases with patients continuously using sunglasses, either by habit or postoperatively to camouflage this round eye that they dislike, and if this aspect does not increase, it at least remains unchanged. We are sure that sunglasses should be avoided as soon as ecchymosis and swelling have disappeared. Sunglasses used for a long time may result in weakness of the orbicularis oculi muscle as the number of contractions is decreased, strongly affecting the normal light reflex. There are some cases of round eye disappearing after a few weeks, after the patient stopped using sunglasses. Cases of unilateral permanent round eye have been seen. If in the follow-up a round eye is starting, energetic and repeated contractions of the orbicularis oculi muscle for a long time may avoid or attenuate this complication. The patient places the tips of his/her two index fingers one on each external angle of the palpebral aperture and gently stretches this area. Still stretching, the patient contracts the eyelids energetically 20 or 30 times. This maneuver is repeated three times per day, for several weeks. This maneuver is advised routinely by the author. The patients have to start 1 month after the operation when the healing is satisfactory. Postoperatively, the patient should uses glasses for his/her eyesight and should place the glasses on the bridge of the nose close to middle of the dorsum and not on the root of the nose. When a patient needs a blepharoplasty and has a round eye preoperatively, he/she should be informed about this aesthetic anomaly if he/she is not aware of it and preoperative photographs are indispensable as in any other case of aesthetic surgery. The skin resection should be minimal in such a case or should not performed at all in the lower eyelid. The transconjunctival approach gives satisfactory results and a round eye is never seen as a complication.

63.3
Conclusions

Shifting from an almond-shaped eye to a round eye after a cosmetic blepharoplasty is aesthetic damage and quite often the patient is unhappy with this result. This complication may be less common if the skin muscle flap is used. The nonuse of sunglasses is a must postoperatively except during the first week or 10 days. Contractions of the eyelids starting after 1 month are recommended for 2 months after any case of cosmetic blepharoplasty.

Suggested Reading

1. Fournier P.F. Complications of blepharoplasties, Second International Symposium on Plastic and Reconstructive Surgery of the Head and Neck, Chicago, 8–13 June 1975

2. Fournier P.F. Complicaciones de las blefaroplastias, Tercer Congreso Argentino de Cirugia Esthetica, 12–14 November 1975

3. Fournier P.F. Una complicacion precuente de la blefaroplastia estetica: el ojo redondo. Cirug Estét1979;4(1):6

4. Fournier P.F. Une complication fréquente de la blépharoplastie esthétique : l'œil rond. In: Faivre J., Zenatti C. (Eds.) Chirurgie Esthétique 1980, Direction Scientifique, Paris, Maloine 1980:255

CHAPTER 64

Complications of Blepharoplasty

64

Melvin A. Shiffman, Young-Kyoon Kim

64.1
Introduction

Blepharoplasty surgery is not without risks. The surgeon should be aware of the possible complications and understand how to prevent, diagnosis in a timely fashion, and treat these problems.

64.2
Complications

64.2.1
Asymmetry

Asymmetry is the result of unequal removal of skin in the upper eyelid, unrecognized unilateral brow ptosis, or failure to form symmetric lid creases. Surgical touchup may be required to remove more skin from one side or eyebrow elevation from the low side. The lower skin crease may need to be elevated to the level of the opposite side as long as it is not above 10 mm from the lid margin.

64.2.2
Bleeding

Causes of bleeding include:
1. Surgical technique
2. Aspirin or non-steroidal anti-inflammatory drugs
3. Hypertension
4. Anticoagulation drugs (coumadin)
5. Blood dyscrasia
6. History of easy bruising

64.2.3
Chemosis

Chemosis is excessive edema of the conjunctiva (Figs. 64.1, 64.2). This may occur from physical (conjuctival incision, irritation from swabs or gauze pads) or chemical trauma (antibacterial agents used to sterilize the skin). This will usually subside without treatment in a few days.

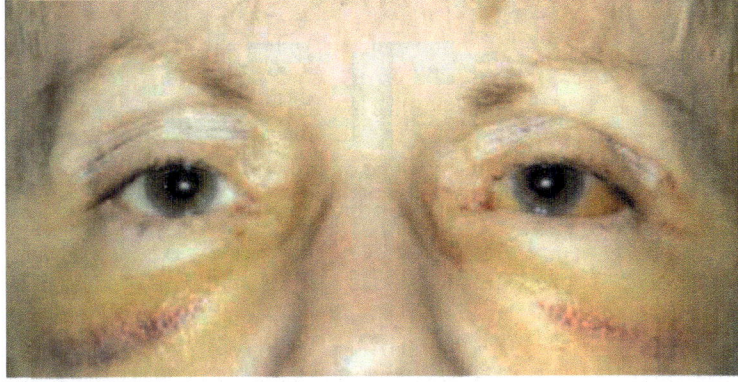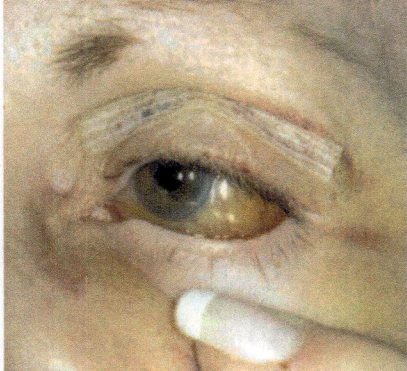

Fig. 64.1 Two days after subconjunctival lower blepharoplasty with chemosis of the left eye

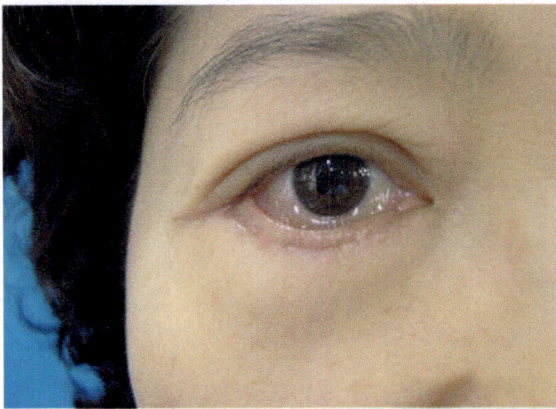
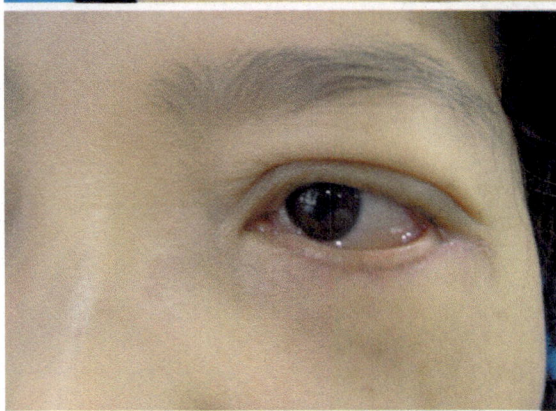

Fig. 64.2 Bilateral chemosis following bilateral lower blepharoplasty

64.2.4
Dehiscence

The skin of either eyelid may disrupt if sutures are removed too soon and skin tape is not applied. These wounds will usually heal secondarily with very little scarring.

64.2.5
Dellen

Dellen consists of saucer-shaped excavations of the periphery of the cornea usually due to insufficiency of the limbic circulation. This problem may appear after excessive chemosis, lid retraction, or from chemical burns (skin antiseptic getting into eyes). Treatment consists of artificial tears and ointments. Patching the eye closed may be helpful but the regrowth of epithelium must be carefully and frequently observed to make sure regrowth has not stopped. The use of topical steroids is controversial but they should not be used for more than 7 days.

64.2.6
Diplopia

Temporary diplopia can occur from local anesthetic diffusion involving the extraocular muscles. This resolves without treatment usually within a few hours.

Persistent diplopia may be due to injury of the inferior oblique, superior oblique, or inferior rectus muscle during fat removal [1]. It is possible for contracture to occur from edema and hemorrhage into the muscle sheath [2]. There is increased risk of injury in secondary blepharoplasties.

Avoidance of diplopia requires careful hemostasis, avoiding injury to the muscles during fat resection, and avoiding traction on the fat pad prior to resection.

64.2.7
Dry Eye Syndrome

Preoperative screening that includes Schirmer testing may forewarn about the possibility of postoperative problems. A preoperative history of laser-assisted in situ keratomileusis (LASIK) surgery should be a warning that dry eye may already be present.

Blepharoplasty may widen the palpebral fissure causing dry eye in patients with unrecognized preoperative borderline tear production. Most dry eye syndromes following blepharoplasty are temporary and need artificial tears applied on a regular basis (hourly to every 4 h) for relief of discomfort.

Lid lag and ectropion after blepharoplasty may result in dry eye as well as other problems.

64.2.8
Ectropion

The most common causes of ectropion are excessive skin excision, closure under tension, or failure to recognize preoperative horizontal laxity (Fig. 64.3). Other causes of ectropion include scarring of the skin to the orbital rim or underlying musculature, orbicularis paresis, or inflammation in the fat pockets. Flat malar eminences may predispose to ectropion because of inadequate support to the lower lid.

Mild ectropion within the first week postoperatively can be relieved by removal of the suture and teasing open the wound. The wound will heal secondarily and the scar, after contracture and softening, will heal almost as thin as the usual incision. Scarring needs exploration of the scar and detachment from the orbital rim and underlying muscle. Missed horizontal laxity requires resection of the excess lid usually with lateral canthopexy.

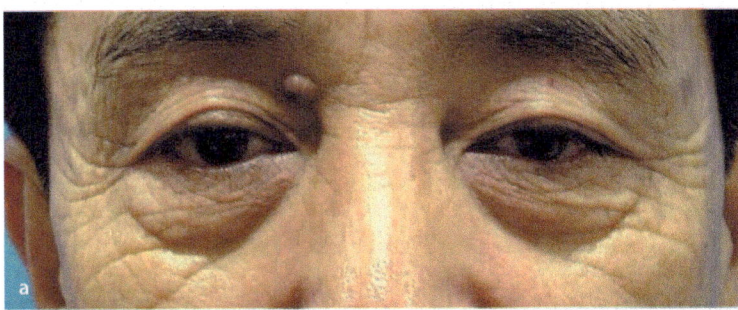
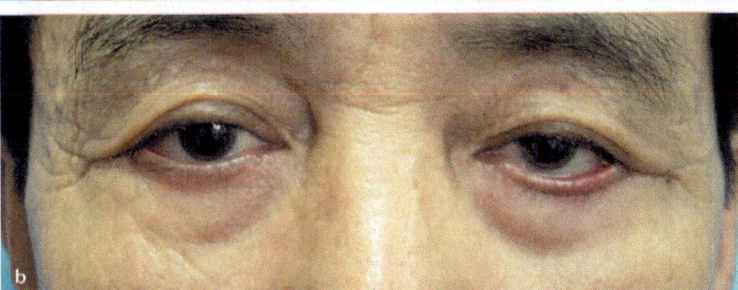

Fig. 64.3 **a** Preoperatively. **b** Four weeks postoperatively with ectropion of the left eye

Round eye deformity is essentially a variation of ectropion and is treated in the same manner.

64.2.9
Excessive Fat Pad Removal

Excessive fat resection in the upper eyelid results in a deep sulcus, while in the lower eyelid it results in a cosmetically poor shallow appearance. Surgical repair has been suggested with overlapping small flaps of orbicularis muscle [3] or buried dermal grafts [4] that tend to lose 25% of their bulk over time. Treatment is best with autologous fat transfer using very small amounts with very fine needles (1.0–1.5-mm diameter) and repeating if necessary.

64.2.10
Inclusion Cyst

Inclusion cysts may occur from invagination of the skin when suturing. This usually requires a very small excision of the cyst in the scar.

64.2.11
Infection

Infection is rare. Inflammation may be treated with topical steroids and any infection should be treated with appropriate antibiotic ointment.

64.2.12
Keratitis

Punctate epithelial keratopathy can occur with corneal exposure from lagophthalmus or from chemical exposure such as with skin antiseptics. Artificial tears or ophthalmic ointments will help. Patching of the eye may be necessary, especially if keratitis is painful.

64.2.13
Lagophthalmos

Mild lagophthalmos immediately after surgery is usually from edema and local anesthetic. This will resolve without treatment, except for lubrication of the eye. Excessive skin excision of the upper and/or lower eyelid can result in lid lag or from incorporation of the orbital septum in the lid closure. Surgical repair may be required if there is excessive skin resection or incorporation of the orbital septum.

64.2.14
Pain

Corneal ulcerations from chemical exposure or from accidental rubbing of the cornea with a gauze pad or swab can be quite painful. They are best treated with patching until the pain subsides. Ophthalmic ointment is also soothing.

64.2.15
Pigmentation

Hemosiderin deposits from bruising will usually resolve over several months but may last for 1 year. Pigmentation of the lower eyelids may be present before surgery and should be recorded in the medical record with photographs. After blepharoplasty, this pigmentation may be more prominent and annoying to the patient.

64.2.16
Ptosis

Ptosis can be present prior to blepharoplasty and this should be recorded in the medical record especially with photographs. Some patients may not have recognized the problem until it is pointed out by the physician.

Temporary ptosis may result from lid edema and may last a few days. Stretching secondary to edema and hematoma can damage the levator aponeurosis or injury can occur to the levator during skin muscle resection where the fibers of the levator merge with the tarsal plate, septum, and orbicularis muscle [5].

64.2.17
Residual Fat Pad

In the lower eyelid the lateral fat pocket may be missed as well as the medial pocket of both upper and lower lids. The lid incision may have to be reopened and more complete resection performed.

64.2.18
Scar

Prominent scarring is unusual especially if the scar falls into a natural skin crease. A slightly thickened scar can be treated with injection of small amounts of steroid. If the scar is unsightly, surgical revision may be necessary.

64.2.19
Sinus Tract

If sutures are left in too long after blepharoplasty, they may cause ingrowth of epithelium into the suture tract and result in a sinus tract. This may need excision.

64.2.20
Suture Exposure

If permanent sutures are used in the subcuticular area for closure, the suture may erode through and become visible. This is best treated by removal of the suture.

64.2.21
Swelling

Persistent swelling may last a few weeks. Early use of ice packs will reduce the amount of swelling significantly.

64.2.22
Visual Loss

Forty case of blindness have been reported in 98,514 surgeries (0.04%) [6]. Most frequently reported is blindness from retrobulbar hemorrhage from inadequately cauterized orbital fat or from rebound vasodilatation from uncauterized blood vessels after the vasoconstrictive effect of the epinephrine wears off. The hemorrhage increases intraorbital pressure that may cause central retinal artery occlusion or ischemia of the optic nerve [7, 8].

Careful examination of the tissues for any small oozing prior to wound closure will help prevent the problem. Having the patient use ice packs on the eyes and avoiding strenuous activities for a few days after surgery are helpful in prevention. Emergency relief of the retrobulbar pressure is mandatory by immediate exploration of the wound, control of bleeders, and removal of clots.

References

1. Harley, R.D., Nelson, L.B., Flanagan, J.C., Calhoun, J.H.: Ocular motility disturbances following cosmetic blepharoplasty. Arch Ophthalmol 1986;104(4):542–5446
2. Hayworth, R.S., Lisman, R.D., Muchnick, R.S., Smith, B.: Diplopia following blepharoplasty. Ann Ophthalmol 1984;16(5):448–451
3. Tenzel, R.R.: Surgical treatment of complications of cosmetic blepharoplasty. Clin Plast Surg 1978(5):517–523
4. Wojno, T., Tenzel, R.R.: Dermis grafts in socket reconstruction. Ophthal Plast Reconstr Surg 1986(2):7–14
5. Baylis, H.I., Sutcliffe, T., Fett, D.R.: Levator injury during blepharoplasty. Arch Ophthalmol 1984;102(4):570–571
6. DeMere, M., Wood, T., Austin, W.: Eye complications with blepharoplasty or other eyelid surgery. Plast Reconstr Surg 1974;53(6):634–637
7. Moser, M.H., DiPirro, E., McCoy, F.J.: Sudden blindness following blepharoplasty. Report of seven cases. Plast Reconstr Surg 1973;51(4):364–370
8. Putterman, A.M.: Temporary blindness after cosmetic blepharoplasty. Am J Ophthalmol 1975;80(6):1081–1083

Chapter 65

Surgery for Prominent Ears

65

Curtis Perry

65.1
Introduction

Ear prominence is the most common congenital deformity. Correcting the prominent ear is usually a very gratifying procedure for both the patient and the surgeon (Fig. 65.1). The goal of otoplasty therefore is to reposition the ear so that the ear occupies a closer angle to the skull while maintaining a natural appearance. A natural appearance is one with smooth curves without sharp angles, step-offs or irregularities, with a sufficiently deep postauricular sulcus.

65.2
Anatomy

Close inspection of the ear reveals a rather complex structure (Fig. 65.2). There is no aesthetic ideal or, for that matter, a standard for what constitutes a normal ear. It is also instructive for the surgeon to continually observe the diversity of appearance in individuals who are considered "normal," i.e., individuals who have no concern about the appearance of their ears.

The two structures that contribute principally to prominence are the antihelix and the concha. Some degree of insufficient folding of the antihelix is almost always seen. Folding of the antihelix may be entirely absent. The concha may be excessively deep or set at an excessively open angle to the mastoid, or both. In addition to the prominence of the cartilaginous structures, the lobule may also protrude.

65.3
Consultation

Otoplasty is performed in teenagers and adults, and is commonly performed in children. Traditionally, age 5 or 6 when the child is about to first start school has been advocated as the preferred time. Age 8, when the ear has reached nearly full growth but is still very flexible, has also been advocated [1]. However, children are starting day care and preschool at much earlier ages. This fact combined with increased awareness and expectations of parents means that much younger children are presenting for evaluation. A review of patients having had the surgery under of the age of 4 concluded the procedure

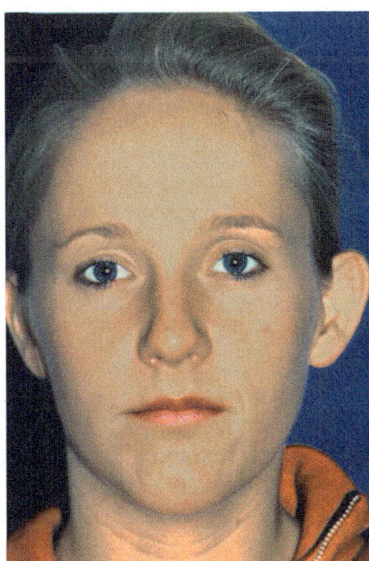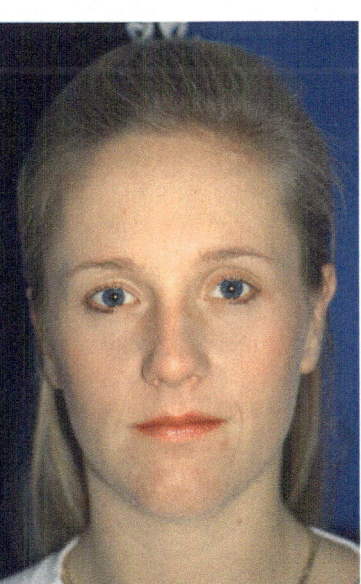

Fig. 65.1 Twenty-two year-old patient. *Left*: Preoperatively. *Right*: Twenty-one days after surgery

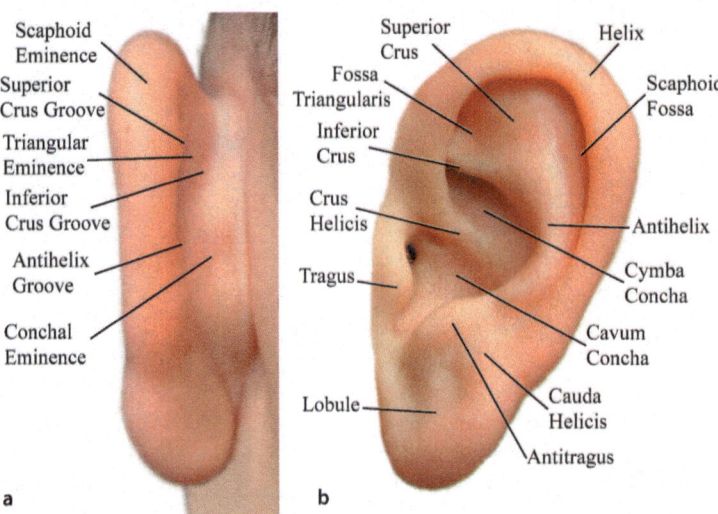

Scaphoid Eminence
Superior Crus Groove
Triangular Eminence
Inferior Crus Groove
Antihelix Groove
Conchal Eminence

Superior Crus
Fossa Triangularis
Inferior Crus
Crus Helicis
Tragus
Lobule

Helix
Scaphoid Fossa
Antihelix
Cymba Concha
Cavum Concha
Cauda Helicis
Antitragus

a   b

Fig. 65.2 Surface anatomy of the external ear. **a** Features of the lateral (anterior) surface. **b** Features of the medial (posterior) surface

could safely be performed in that age group [2]. Follow-up in this study was up to 7.5 years. However, Furnas [3] reported that performing the procedure in children as young as 1 year old often resulted in the need for revision surgery years later. It would seem prudent for the surgeon to advise those considering the procedure under the age of 6 that they may have an increased probability of revision surgery once full growth has been attained.

The consultation is the same as for any other patient seeking cosmetic surgery in that it begins with a detailed medical history followed by a careful interview of the patient. If children are old enough they should be able to express an understanding that the process will entail a surgery, a recovery with some discomfort, and the goal that the ears will be less prominent. As with any cosmetic procedure, parents and adult patients should have realistic expectations concerning the procedure, recovery, and goals.

The next step is a careful evaluation of the patient. The age of the patient will suggest the strength and rigidity of the cartilage; however, age is not absolute. The thickness and resilience of the cartilage can differ substantially between individuals of the same age. There may even be significant variation between sides in the same individual; therefore, palpation to test exactly how the cartilage of each ear "gives" when folded is critical to planning the surgery. While the cartilage is being tested, a careful assessment as to the cause of the prominence is made. The two structures that contribute to prominence are the antihelix and the concha. Some degree of insufficient folding of the antihelix is almost always seen. The concha may be excessively deep or set at an excessively open angle to the mastoid, or both. The degree of prominence of the lobule is also noted.

Discussion of the goals and nature of the surgery with the patient is then done. A prospective patient needs to be educated that there is no normal standard for ears and that a wide range of appearances of ears is acceptable. Asymmetry in patients presenting for prominent ears is common. Often the request is to make the more prominent ear the same as the other. As when the patient is informed about surgery on any paired body part, it is carefully explained to the patient that while the goal is to improve symmetry, perfect symmetry is never possible. In otoplasty surgery it is useful to think of symmetry as having two meanings. One is the degree of offset or prominence the ear has relative to a specific part of the head when compared with the other side. The other is the appearance of the ear when viewed from the side due to its structures such as the helix and antihelix. Patients are typically concerned with the first of these types of symmetry in the preoperative consultations. They may not consider or they may take for granted the second type of symmetry and scrutinize the structure of each ear for symmetry only after the surgery. It is important to discuss both "types" of symmetry preoperatively with the patient. This is especially important if the ears are profoundly asymmetrical with one ear having rudimentary or complete lack of helical and/or antihelical folding. These individuals should be instructed that there will be differences in the side appearance postoperatively (Fig. 65.3). In terms of the degree of symmetry for prominence from the head, it is explained that "normal" individuals often vary by two 2–3 mm and that while the goal is to have good symmetry at the conclusion of the procedure, final variation within this range should be acceptable.

As with any cosmetic procedure, patients seeking otoplasty are often very concerned about the appearance of any scars secondary to the procedure. Procedures that "hide" the incision on the posterior side have an advantage at least from most patients' perspective.

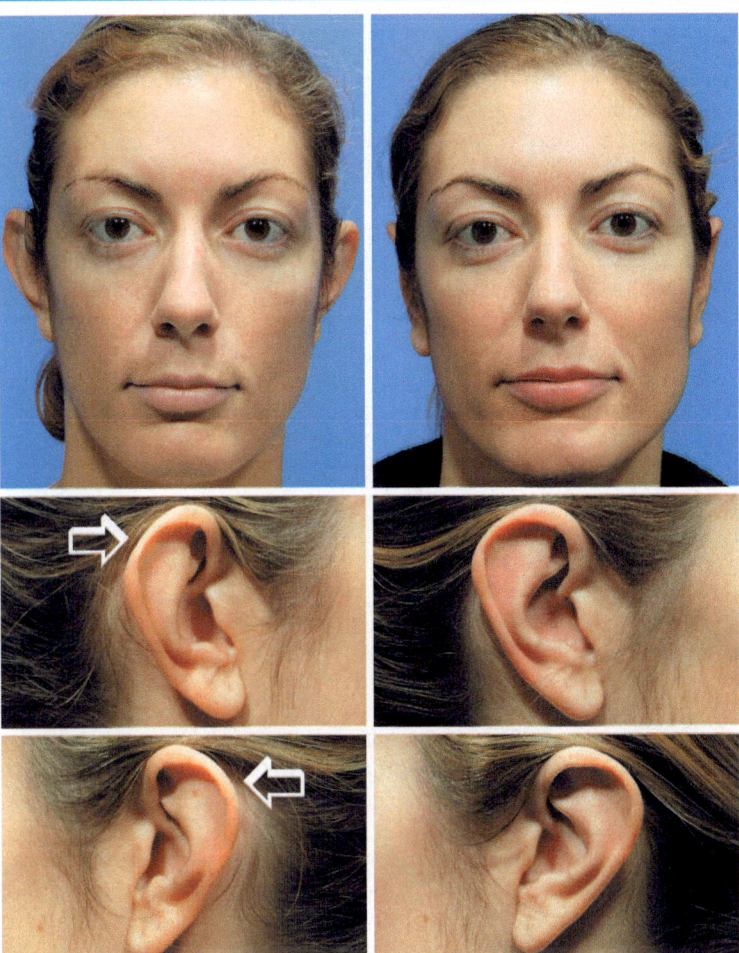

Fig. 65.3 In addition to ear prominence, the helix of the right ear is less developed than that of the left. Minor asymmetries such as this may not be noticed by the patient until the patient scrutinizes the postoperative results. The surgeon should discuss such findings as part of the preoperative consultation

65.4 Anesthesia

Otoplasty may be performed using general anesthesia or any degree of sedation. Many patients do well with no sedation. When minimal or no sedation is planned, the patient is fully informed as to what to expect for the upcoming procedure. It is explained that the local infiltration will sting or burn for approximately 1 min on each side while the infiltration is performed around the ear, after which there will be no further discomfort whatsoever. When this has been carefully explained, many patients, except for the youngest children, will agree and cooperate fully even though they are alert throughout the procedure.

65.5 Surgical Techniques

A multitude of procedures have been published since Ely [4] first described excision of cartilage and skin for the correction of prominent ears in 1881. Surgical techniques can be divided into two basic strategies: incision techniques that rely on incision and sometimes excision of cartilage to allow for repositioning and reducing of the ear structure, and bending techniques in which no incision is made and the cartilage is curved to create the desired positioning. Bending of the cartilage is accomplished by scoring and/or pulling the cartilage into position using sutures. This dichotomy is somewhat oversimplified because many techniques that emphasize incisions may bend cartilage at a specific location, and bending techniques that are based on anterior scoring may use cartilage incisions for access.

The most basic incision/excision technique is incision along the rim of the concha (Fig. 65.4). Once this incision has been made, a fusiform-shaped portion of conchal cartilage may also be excised to reduce the projection of the concha. Since there is now no resistance from the cartilage, medialization of the ear is then accomplished by excising redundant skin at the posterior incision and simply closing the skin. This incision can be combined with relaxing incisions in the fossa triangularis, scaphoid fossa, and at the apex of the antihelical fold (Fig. 65.5). These incisions can also be used in conjunction with abrasion to weaken the posterior antihelical fold. Sutures through the cartilage are then used to control the bend of the antihelical fold [5].

The advantage of incision techniques is that the anatomical changes produced are very precise and the recurrence rate is extremely low. The disadvantage is the surgeon must be very exact with the incision as there will be few or no options for revision. Another disadvantage is that unnatural sharp, crenellated edges, ridges, and step-offs may be created which will lead to an operated-on appearance. Many variations of incision procedures have been proposed to reduce these problems yet maintain the advantage of removing all resistance to repositioning that the complete incision of cartilage affords. One example consists of excising a fusiform skin island on the posterior surface conforming to the desired position on the antihelical fold (Fig. 65.6). An incision through the cartilage is made along the planned summit of the antihelix. Each edge of the incision then has a very fine bevel incised into it to cause it to curl. The two curled edges are then overlapped, creating a curved antihelical fold [6].

The principal bending technique was described fully by Mustarde [7] in 1963. Placement of the new antihelical fold is determined. Next, multiple mattress sutures are placed to fold the cartilage (Fig. 65.7). There are several key points to this procedure. The first is that the mattress sutures should pass through the entire thickness of the cartilage and the anterior perichondrium. The mattress sutures should be placed 7–8 mm from either side of the summit line of the antihelical fold. The skin incision is to be made in the posterior sulcus so that it is as far away from the mattress sutures as possible and never overlying the mattress sutures. Only 3-0 white silk on a reverse cutting needle should be used as the mattress suture. This material allows for a very small knot with ends cut on the knot. Mustarde [8, 9]. Stated that in 30 years of performing this procedure and applying these principles he never had a problem with suture fistula.

Bending techniques may also employ weakening of the cartilage by scoring, rasping, or abrading its surface without completely incising through the cartilage. Gibson and Davis [10] demonstrated that, owing to its cytoarchitecture, cartilage possesses natural internal springs. Scoring one side of cartilage cuts the contracting springs on that side, allowing the internal springs of the other side to contract. This principle has been applied to scoring the anterior surface antihelix. It has been proposed that anterior scoring alone may be sufficient to create the desired bending on the antihelix [11, 12]. Mustarde sutures may also be used [13]. A disadvantage of anterior scoring is that to gain access either an anterior skin incision or a through-cartilage incision from a posterior skin incision must be used. The anterior skin incision has the obvious concern of being placed on the more visible side of the ear. A through-cartilage incision creates the same potential for problems as any of the previously described incision procedures. Further, treating the anterior surface of cartilage has the potential for creating irregularities on the visible side of the cartilage.

Weakening the posterior side of the antihelix may be criticized as being nonphysiologic owing to the discoveries of Gibson and Davis [10]. However, ear cartilage is much more fibrous and pliable than nasal cartilage. The combination of weakening of the cartilage by rasping or abrading, using Mustarde mattress sutures, and the fibrous fixation secondary to healing more than overcomes the forces demonstrated by Gibson and Davis.

Bending techniques alone are not sufficient when the concha is a major contributor to ear prominence. When this occurs some form of concha "setback" must be employed. The easiest method is to simply remove soft tissue immediately deep and slightly posterior to the concha. This creates a deeper cup for the concha to rest in, thereby reducing its projection. Care must be taken that the concha does not slide forward and constrict the external meatus. Mattress sutures passing from the concha to the mastoid periosteum are commonly used to maximize compression of the concha to the mastoid and prevent slippage forward [14]. If even more setback is needed, shaving excision of the cartilage from the posterior conchal surface is then performed. The scalpel is oriented parallel to the tangent of the concha and a thin shaving of cartilage is removed. After each pass the degree of setback is reassessed by positioning the concha within its mastoid "cup." Multiple prominent areas may be excised in this fashion. Even full-thickness excision of cartilage can be achieved without any evidence of step-off owing to the fact that the orientation of the blade ensures that the entire edge of the excision is beveled. Excision continues until the desired degree of setback is obtained. With this technique, very extreme degrees of conchal projection can be corrected without any evidence of surgery (R. Webster 1986, personal communication).

Bending techniques are more popular and typically produce more gradual curves, creating a more natural appearance. An important advantage of Mustarde sutures is that, if the appearance is not as anticipated after their placement, the sutures can easily be removed and new sutures placed in different positions as required. The principal disadvantage of bending procedures is a higher recurrence rate because the cartilage retains part or all of its resilience [15]. Typically there is dependence on suture fixation for results. With some degree of tension on the sutures, suture extrusion and suture granuloma are cited as problems. It is important to remember that overly aggressive weakening of the cartilage can produce a tight fold that creates the same unnatural appearance as is the concern with cartilage incision procedures.

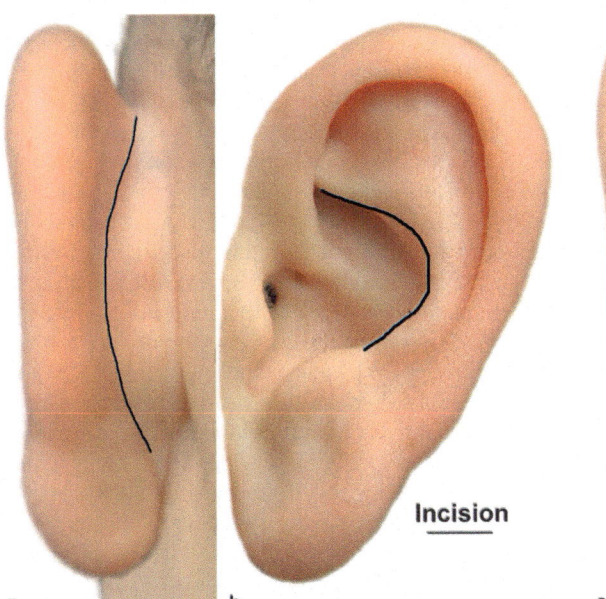

Fig. 65.4 Incision with possible excision of conchal cartilage. **a** Skin incision. A fusiform skin island can be created instead of the simple incision and/or skin can be excised prior to closure as needed. **b** Cartilage treatment. Incision along the conchal rim; excision of the concha can also be performed to decrease projection of the concha

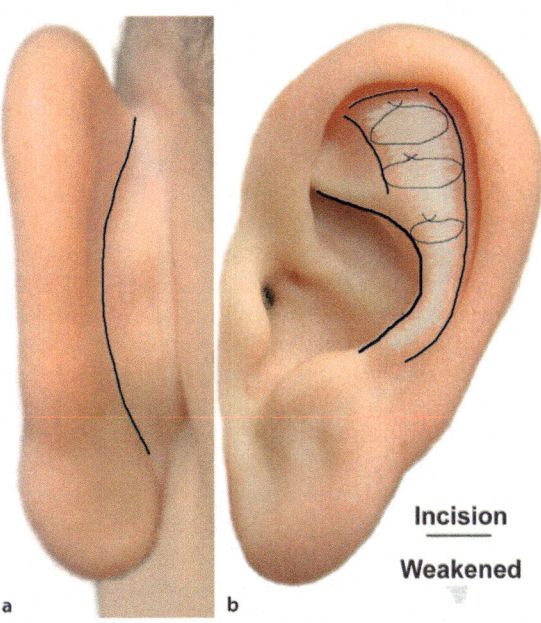

Fig. 65.5 Converse incision procedure. **a** Skin incision. A fusiform skin island can be created instead of the simple incision and/or skin can be excised prior to closure as needed. **b** Cartilage treatment. Multiple incisions with posterior weakening of cartilage along the antihelix. Posterior suturing is performed for stabilization of the antihelix

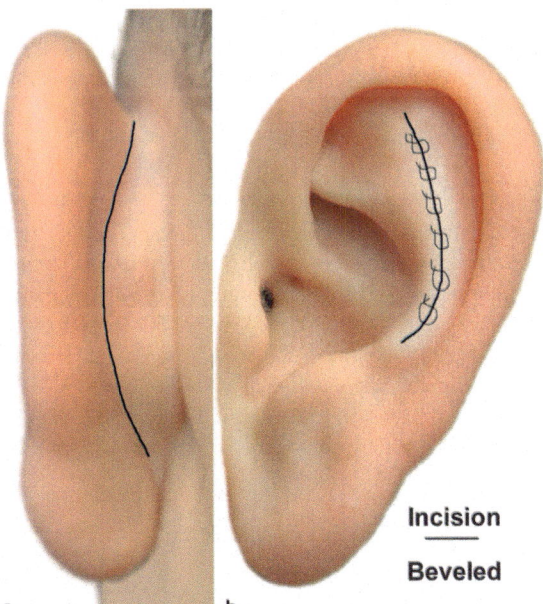

Fig. 65.6 Cartilage incision with beveled edges. **a** Skin incision. A fusiform skin island can be created instead of the simple incision and/or skin can be excised as needed prior to closure. **b** Cartilage treatment. Incision along the summit of the antihelix; each side of the incision is then beveled to create a curl. Curled edges are then overlapped and sutured

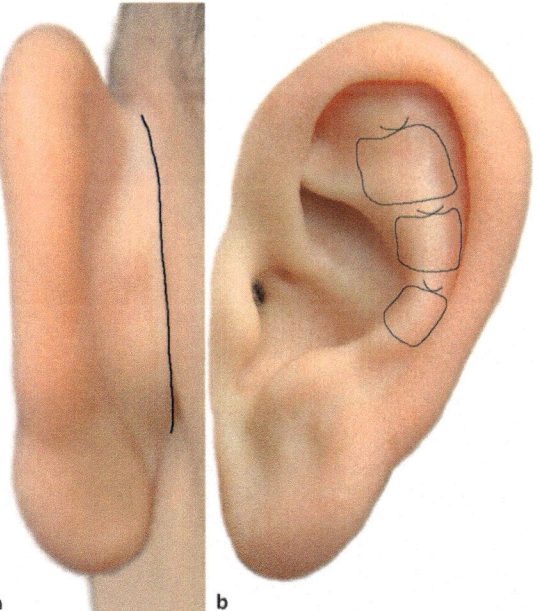

Fig. 65.7 Mustarde technique. **a** Skin incision is placed at the sulcus to avoid the incision overlapping mattress sutures. A fusiform skin island can be created instead of the simple incision and/or skin can be excised prior to closure as needed. **b** Cartilage treatment. Mattress sutures spanning 7–8 mm from either side of the summit of the antihelix

65.6
Author's Technique

The patient is sterilely prepared and draped to include both ears. Each ear is then infiltrated circumferentially with 4–5 ml of 1% lidocaine with epinephrine buffered with bicarbonate. After sufficient time to maximize vasoconstriction, the initial incision is made in the posterior sulcus (Fig. 65.8). If concha setback is planned, an initial conservative skin excision is included. The incision is usually a fusiform shape unless it was determined preoperatively that the projection of the lobule needs to be reduced as well. In that case the inferior end of the fusiform incision will end with a triangle at the superior lobule oriented at right angles to the axis of the main excision. Undermining then proceeds laterally, exposing the antihelix. If concha setback is planned, undermining is also performed medial to the incision to elevate the concha. Hemostasis is achieved with bipolar cautery to minimize inflammation of the cartilage.

Attention is then turned to shaping the antihelical fold. Most adults will require some weakening of this cartilage to create a new fold. Gentle rasping or abrading is all that is required. Upon inspecting the lateral surface, the surgeon determines the location of the and marks this by placing two or three 25-gauge needles at the midpoint of the fold. The ear is then positioned and three to five Mustarde mattress sutures are placed along the course of the fold, then tightened to create the desired degree of folding.

Usually some degree of concha setback is also performed. Even if an acceptable degree of projection from the head can be achieved solely by folding the antihelix, the author feels that particularly in adults with stiffer cartilage a more natural look will be achieved by being a little less aggressive in folding the antihelix and combining this with some degree of concha setback (Fig. 65.9). Sufficient setback can usually be accomplished by removing any soft tissue from the mastoid that is immediately deep and also slightly posterior to the initial position of the concha. This allows the concha to be positioned not only medially but also slightly posteriorly to prevent narrowing of the meatus. Usually two or three sutures are used to maintain position. If further setback is needed, planing excision of the posterior prominences of the concha is then performed.

If needed, further skin is removed; however, care is taken to avoid tension on the closure. The procedure is performed on the other side with careful comparison, including measuring the distance from the head at two or three locations to obtain symmetry. Closure is performed using a running 5-0 nylon suture.

The decrease in prominence is overcorrected by 2–3 mm. The patient has been fully informed preoperatively of this slight overcorrection. It has been explained that the cartilage has memory and even though it is weakened at the time of surgery and supported in the new positioning with sutures, there will be a tendency for the cartilage to return to its preoperative position. Interestingly, most patients are so concerned with reducing the prominence they are immediately accepting of the overcorrection.

Soft gauze is then conformed to the external ear and a standard compression wrap is then applied. This initial bandage is typically left in place for 72 h. Once it has been removed, the patient is instructed to wear a nightly wrap over the ears for 3–4 weeks. The external sutures are removed at 1 week.

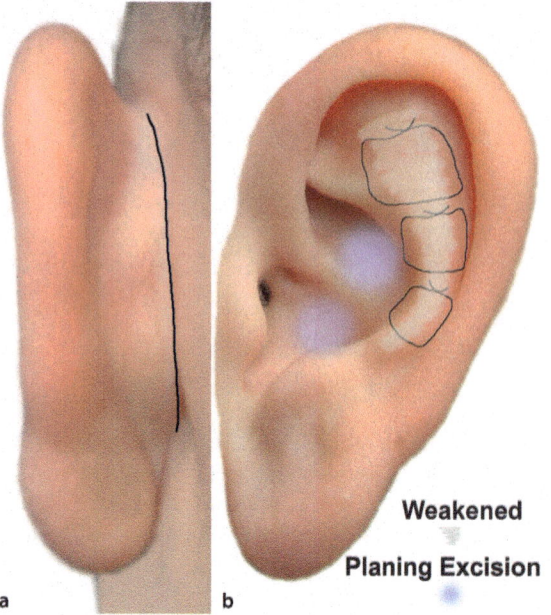

Weakened

Planing Excision

a   b

Fig. 65.8 Author's technique. **a** Skin incision placed at the sulcus to avoid the incision overlapping mattress sutures. A fusiform skin island can be created instead of the simple incision and/or skin can be excised prior to closure as needed. **b** Cartilage treatment. Weakening of the posterior surface of cartilage as needed by abrading or rasping. Mattress sutures spanning 7–8 mm from either side of the summit of the antihelix. Planing (shave) excision of the prominence(s) of the posterior concha is performed as needed

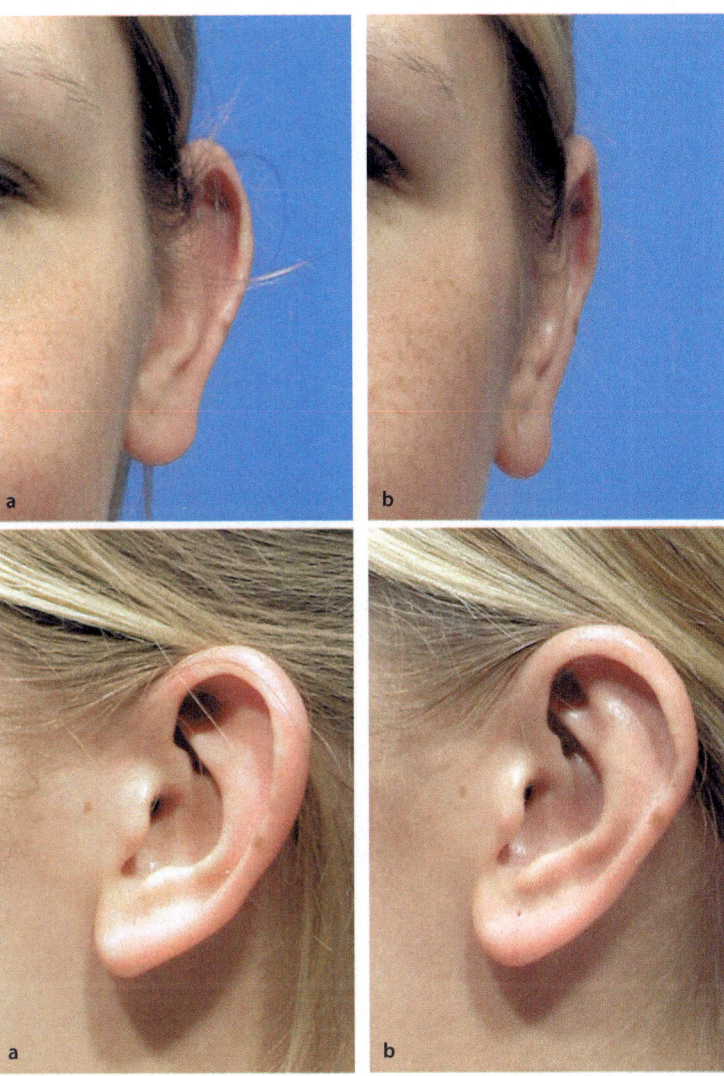

Fig. 65.9 **a** Preoperatively. **b** Three months after surgery combining folding of the antihelical fold with moderate concha setback created good positioning with pleasing natural contours in this 25-year-old patient

65.7
Summary

Otoplasty is a procedure with a high degree of satisfaction for both patient and surgeon. As with any cosmetic procedure, realistic patient expectations and careful preoperative planning are the foundation for good results. Surgical techniques should not only reposition the auricle but also strive for the most natural appearance possible.

References

1. Emery BE: Otoplasty. Facial Plast Surg Clin 2001; 9(1):147–157
2. Gosain AK, Kumar A, Huang G: Prominent ears in children younger than four years of age: what is the appropriate timing for otoplasty? Plast Reconstr Surg. 2004;114(5):1042–1067
3. Furnas DW: Otoplasty for prominent ears. Clin Plast Surg 2002(2):29;273–288
4. Ely ET: An operation for prominence of the auricles. Arch Otol 1881;10:975.
5. LaTrenta GS: Otoplasty. In Aesthetic Plastic Surgery. Rees TD, LaTrenta GS (Eds), Philadelphia, Saunders 1994:891–924
6. Nachlas NE, Duncan D, Trail M: Otoplasty. Arch Otol 1970;91(1):44–49
7. Mustarde JC: The correction of prominent ears using simple mattress sutures. Br J Plast Surg 1963;16:170–178
8. Bull TR, Mustarde JC: Mustarde technique and otoplasty. Facial Plast Surg 1985;2(2):101–107
9. Mustarde JC: Commentary. Facial Plast Surg 1985;2 (2):108

10. Gibson T, Davis WB: The distortion of autogenous cartilage grafts: its cause and prevention. Br J Plast Surg 1958;10:257–274

11. Stenstroem SJ: A "natural" technique for correction of congenitally prominent ears. Plast Reconstr Surg 1963;32:508–518

12. Dicio D, Castagnetti F, Baldassarre S: Otoplasty: anterior abrasion of ear cartilage with dermabrader. Aesthet Plast Surg 2003;27(6):466–471

13. Nolst Trenite GJ: A modified anterior scoring technique. Facial Plast Surg 1994;10(3):255–266

14. Furnas DW: Otoplasty for prominent ears. Clin Plast Surg 2002;29(2):273–288, viii

CHAPTER 66

Nasal Tip Rotation

Phillip R. Langsdon

66

66.1
Introduction

The nasal tip is a three-dimensional structure. Projection, width, and angle of rotation impact appearance. This cartilaginous component of the nose is composed of the lower lateral cartilage and is influenced by the more cephalic components, such as the upper lateral cartilage and bony vault. Internally, the septum supports the overlying structures. Cartilage strength and skin thickness play a large role in the shape of the tip.

66.2
Technique

Tip position is usually determined by analyzing the nasolabial angle; the angle formed by the nasal columella and the lip—95–105° in women and 90–95° in men usually provides a pleasing tip angle. There are several procedures that can be used to affect tip rotation. The technique selected, however, depends on the diagnosis. Every patient is different and there is no single technique that will tackle all of the anatomical obstacles. Of course there are realistic limits to what can be accomplished and proper patient selection is important in terms of both anatomic considerations as well as psychological considerations.

Exposure to the nasal tip can be undertaken with either an internal or an external (open) approach. For the internal approach, I use an "intercartilaginous incision" (between the upper and the lower lateral cartilage) that connects to a "transfixion incision." There is also a "marginal incision" that follows the caudal margin of the lower lateral cartilage and extends over onto the columella, just on the anterior margin of the medial crus and continues about half the length of the columella. Scissors are then used to free up the lower lateral cartilage and it is "delivered" so that the bipedicled flap of cartilage and lining mucosa can be examined, and then treated.

The author uses the external (open) approach with most revision cases as well as the very twisted or asymmetric nasal tip. With this technique, an inverted "V" "transcolumellar" incision is made and this

is connected to a "marginal incision" (as previously described). The nasal skin is then dissected free with scissors until the tip complex is exposed.

The author tends to conserve as much cartilage as possible and minimize cartilaginous incisions as much as possible. We will begin with the most conservative approaches and progress to the most complex.

66.2.1
Complete Strip

With this technique the integrity of the lower lateral cartilage is preserved throughout the length of the cartilage; from the medial crus to the most lateral portion of the lateral crus (Fig. 66.1). Only a cephalic trim is used to reduce the bulk of the cartilage. Today, I tend to remove less cartilage than I did 20 years ago and I leave at the least a minimum of 7 mm in width of the lateral crus. This technique can reduce tip volume or bulbosity and allow for some rotation.

66.2.2
Alteration of the Medial Crus or the Lateral Crus

When the medial crus or the lateral crus of the lower lateral cartilages is too long for the nose, it impacts tip position. If the lateral crus is too long, the nose may appear ptotic. If severe tension is present, no amount of cephalic trim will allow rotation. Reduction of the most lateral component of the lateral crus will reduce the downward forces and allow the tip to rotate superiorly.

A problem that can occur by reducing the lateral portion of the lateral tip is a collapse of the lateral alar wall into the nose. Techniques that reduce the lateral crus to allow rotation of the tip have been used for decades. The "rim strip" is an effective procedure; however, it can result in alar collapse and airway compromise in some patients. As a result, procedures designed to effectively reduce the lateral crus by excising a segment of the crus midway between the dome and the lateral extent and then reconstruction of the crus by suturing the divided edges back together have also been utilized. However, this technique also has the potential to result in alar col-

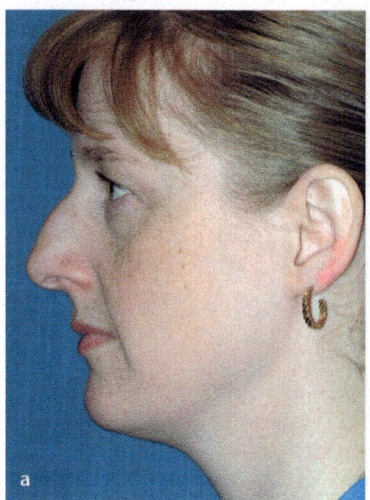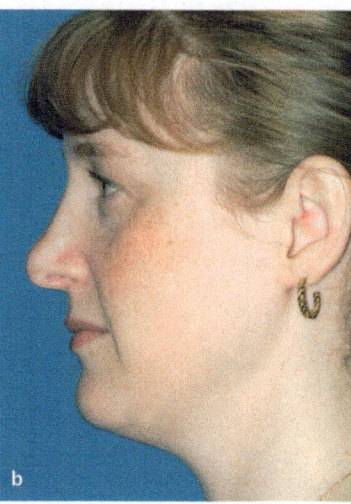

Fig. 66.1 a Preoperatively. **b** Postoperatively following complete strip and removal of excess septal cartilage and nasal spine

lapse and airway compromise because it may create a weak point at the division site.

Another way to reduce the length of the lateral crus is with a technique developed by the author over 18 years ago.

The "lateral crural slide" is performed by dissecting a pocket lateral to the most lateral portion of the lateral crus. This creates room for the lateral crus to slide laterally and superiorly, therefore reducing the downward force from the lower lateral cartilage. If more rotation is required, the mucosa can be dissected free from the internal surface of the most lateral portion of the crus. This technique allows rotation without the collapse that can result from procedures that remove or divide cartilage.

The length of the medial crus can impact rotation as well. If it is too long or strong it can prevent derotation. Segmental resection with repair can allow for a shortening of the medial crus and the effect of rotation in some cases. On the other hand, a strong medial crus aids rotation. Added length of the medial crus can create the effect of superior rotation of the tip. This can be accomplished with a structural cartilage graft added between the feet of the medial crura.

66.2.3
Dome Division Techniques

Another approach to rotation of the tip is to divide the domes. It the lengths of the medial and lateral crural components are not an issue, then the creation of a pivot point may allow movement of the tip. The lower lateral cartilage is a continuous structure from the feet of the medial crus to the most lateral extent of the lateral crus.

If the lateral crus is preventing a superior rotation, its opposition to rotation can be removed by dividing the lower lateral cartilage at the dome. The medial crus then becomes free to rotate superiorly. The lateral crus in the area of the dome can be shortened to accommodate the new tip position if necessary. I routinely secure the divided dome with 5-0 Vicryl suture. Although Vicryl is absorbed over time, it allows fibrosis to occur, securing the cartilage indefinitely.

On occasion the tip may appear ptotic because of a relatively short medial crus, rather than a long lateral crus. In this instance, dome division, lateral to the dome creates the opportunity to "borrow" some of the lateral crus (just lateral to the preoperative dome). The "borrowed" cartilage (which is still continuous with the dome and medial crus) can be rotated anteriorly and secured to the corresponding "borrowed" lateral crus from the opposite lower lateral cartilage. A firm septal cartilaginous graft can be placed between the medial crural and "borrowed" components to add strength. This technique adds length to the medial crus, while at the same time freeing the medial crural components for free superior rotation of the tip.

66.2.4
Tip Grafting

Adding cartilage to the altered or unaltered lower cartilaginous components can create the illusion of superior tip rotation and/or projection. A shield type cartilage graft can be fashioned from septal or ear cartilage. This is then sutured to the medial crus and dome. This effectively adds to the structural components of the lower cartilage support system.

66.3
Impact of Cephalic Components

No matter what technique is selected to rotate the tip, consideration must be given to the cephalic components. If the upper lateral cartilages are long, and prevent the intended upward rotation of the selected tip technique, then they might need to be shortened. The caudal septum may also prevent upward rotation and should be addressed in selected situations. Removal of excess membranous portion of the septum (that portion which does not contain cartilage, between the end of the cartilaginous septum and the medial crural cartilage) may add superior support to rotated tip components.

66.4
Impact of Caudal Components

The ligaments between the cartilage domes of the tip cartilage and the ligaments of the "feet" or most proximal portion of the medial crus provide tip support. Weakening of these components might derotate the tip or allow some settling of a tip that is too projected. Excess nasal spine may overproject the medial crural component of the nose and may give the appearance of a short upper lip. Removal or reduction may allow some settling of the medial crural component of the tip, and it may lengthen the upper lip.

66.5
Conclusions

Several methods are used to handle the task of nasal tip rotation. There are challenges as well. Every patient is anatomically different. The cartilage, skin, and the surrounding components of the nose and maxilla must all be analyzed before selecting the technique deemed most likely to accomplish the task at hand. Rhinoplasty requires significant expertise and can challenge even the most experienced surgeon.

CHAPTER 67

Section of the Depressor Septi Nasi Muscle to Lift the Nasal Tip

67

Pierre F. Fournier

67.1 Introduction

Most of the muscles of the nose are elevators with only one antagonist, the depressor septi nasi muscle. In aging over time the tip of the nose droops. In other individuals, the nasolabial angle is much less that the 110° that is accepted as a nice angle. Sectioning the depressor septi nasi muscles will slightly lift the nose in most individuals (Fig. 67.1). After sectioning, the levators will increase their pull and will improve the nasolabial angle by a few degrees [1–4].

An anatomic study of the depressor septi nasi muscles shows three variations of the depressor septi nasi [4]. Type I depressor septi nasi muscles are visible and identifiable and can be traced to full interdigitation from their origin at the medial crural plate. Type II muscles are visible and identifiable but demonstrate little or no interdigitation with the orbicularis. Type III includes cases in which no, or only a rudimentary, depressor septi nasi muscle is visible.

67.2 Physiology

During smiling or when talking the tip of the nose goes downward.

67.3 Anatomy

The depressor septi nasi is a small muscle that is an expansion of the orbicularis oris. There is one head of the muscle on each side of the midline. This muscle is not shown in all anatomy books.

Transection of the depressor will stabilize the tip of the nose in rhinoplasty and will improve the "parrot beak" deformity.

67.4 Technique

67.4.1 Anesthesia

Infiltration with a few milliliters of local anesthetic consisting of 1% Xylocaine with 1:200,000 epinephrine is enough.

67.4.2 Muscle Sectioning

The goal is to section the two heads through one incision made on one side of the columella nostril angle (Fig. 67.2). The incision is made 0.5 mm inside the medial

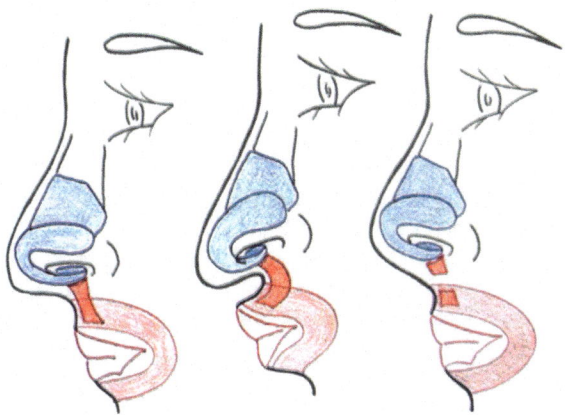

Fig. 67.1 Anatomy of the depressor septi nasi muscle

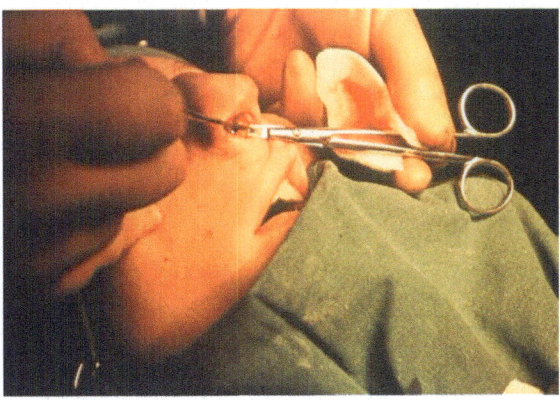

Fig. 67.2 Sectioning of the muscle following exposure

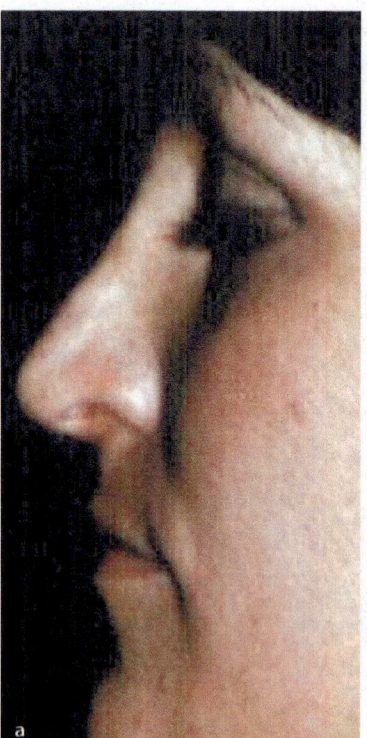
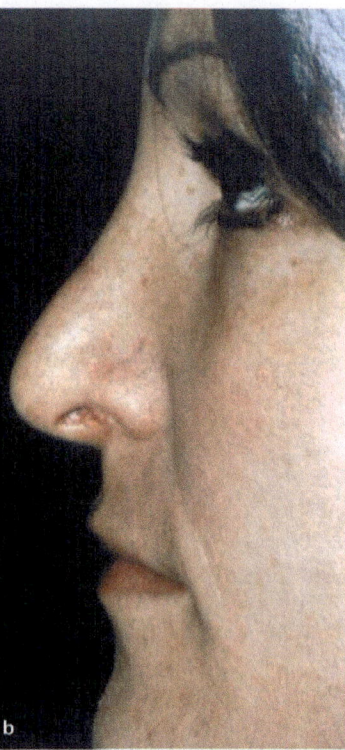

Fig. 67.3 a Preoperative patient with a low nasal tip. **b** Postoperatively after sectioning of the depressor septi nasi muscle

angle of the nostril close to the columella. Small curved scissors are used for dissection under the skin. The tip is pushed to reach the opposite side of the nostril and the dissection is completed with a half turn of the scissors and drawing back to the incision. This exposes the two portions of the depressor muscle. The muscle may be small or large and should be transected completely with a scalpel. Hemostasis is achieved and then the would closed with one suture.

67.5
Complications

There is the possiblity of infection or bleeding, but these complications have not been seen by the author. Reattachment of the muscles can be prevented by suturing the ends of the cut muscle together [5, 6].

67.6
Conclusions

Transection of the complete depressor septi nasi muscle is a simple method for raising the hanging nasal tip resulting from aging or for a "parrot beak" deformity (Fig.

67.3). The procedure may be used alone or with other cosmetic operations of the nose or face.

References

1. Fred, G.B.: Role od depressor septi nasi muscle in rhinoplasty. AMA Arch Otolaryngol 1955;62(1):37–41
2. Furukawa, M.A.: Management of musculus depressor septi nasi in rhinoplasty. Transaction of the Fourth International Congress of Plastic Reconstructive Surgery, Rome, October 1967
3. Mahe, E., Camblin, J.: Musculus depressor septi nasi. Study of its action and the role played in its resection during the post-operative course of cosmetic rhinoplasties. Ann Chir Plast 1974;19(3):257–264
4. Rohrich, R.J., Huynh, B., Muzaffar, A. R., Adams, W.P. Jr., Robinson, J.B.: Importance of the depressor septi nasi muscle in rhinoplasty: anatomic and clinical application. Plast Reconstr Surg 2000;105(1):376–383
5. Mahe, E., Camblin, J.: Le muscle depresseur de la pointe. Ann Chir Plast 1974;19:257
6. Mahe, E, Camblin, J.: A resection du muscle depresseur de la pointe dans les rhinoplasties esthetique. Ann Otolaryngol Chir Cervicofac 1975;92:381

CHAPTER 68

Complications of Rhinoplasty

68

Melvin A. Shiffman

68.1
Introduction

As with any cosmetic procedure, rhinoplasty is associated with a number of risks and complications.

68.2
Complications

68.2.1
Anosmia

Altered sense of smell is rare since the olfactory area is located high in the nasal cavity. Temporary anosmia may last 6–18 months [1, 2].

68.2.2
Asymmetry

Asymmetry is a common problem arising from rhinoplasty and is usually from irregularities or excessive removal of the alar cartilages (Fig. 68.1). Irregularities of the cartilage may need to be secondarily trimmed.

68.2.3
Boxed Tip

The boxed tip may require resection of the alar dome. Resection must be accurate and conservative if the skin is thin.

68.2.4
Callus Formation

A bony callus can form at the site of hump resection (Fig. 68.2). This may be prevented by thorough removal of bone dust, periosteal tags, or blood clots. Treatment requires rasping of the irregularities or repeat osteotomy [3].

68.2.5
Drooping Tip

The drooping tip is usually the result of inadequate trimming of the upper lateral and alar cartilages or their not being sutured in a proper relationship to the shortened caudal margin of the septum. Droop may occur if exces-

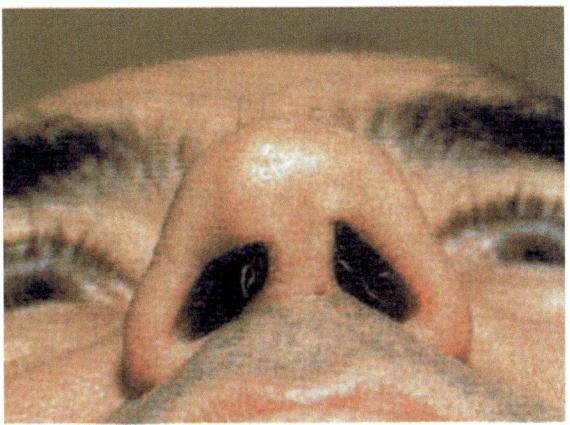

Fig. 68.1 Asymmetry

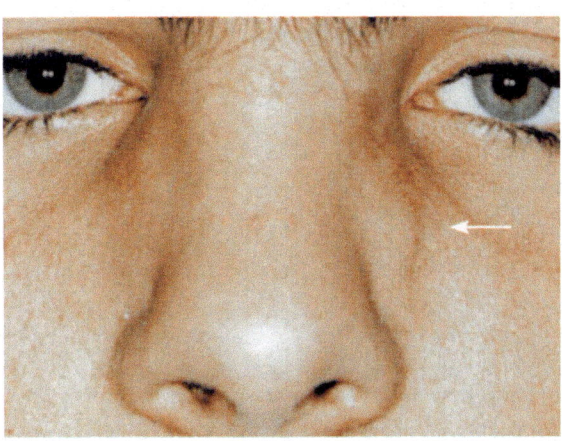

Fig. 68.2 Callus formation

sive hump is removed or if the nose has been shortened without tilting the tip upward. Loss of skin contractility in older patients may contribute to the drooped tip.

Correction may require shortening of the upper lateral cartilages or approximating them to the alar cartilages. The medial crura may have to be fixed to the caudal septal cartilage.

68.2.6
Hanging Columella

Convexity or roundness of the caudal margin of the medial crura of the alar cartilages may appear after rhinoplasty. This can be corrected by marginal incisions in the columella and trimming of the rounded cartilages and, at times, the lining [3].

68.2.7
Hemorrhage

Hemorrhage or epistaxis is the most common complication of rhinoplasty. Bleeding usually occurs within the first 48 h following surgery [4] but can occur at 10–14 days after surgery when the eschar along the incision lines separates.

Causes of bleeding include:
1. Surgical technique
2. Aspirin or non-steroidal anti-inflammatory drugs
3. Hypertension
4. Anticoagulation drugs (coumadin)
5. Blood dyscrasia
6. History of easy bruising

A hematoma may result that can cause distortion of the nasal tip or displace the alar cartilages. Prompt treatment is essential for septal hematoma that can lead to nasal obstruction or septal perforation.

When there is vigorous bleeding, the nasal pack should be removed and the clots suctioned out. Any bleeders should be identified and compressed with epinephrine-soaked cotton pads. The nose can then be repacked.

68.2.8
Infection

Infection is rare and prophylactic antibiotics are not usually necessary. If infection occurs there should be prompt treatment with antibiotics and warm compresses.

Veins from the nose, emissary veins, go directly into the sagittal sinus; therefore, infections should be treated in a timely fashion. If persistent headache occurs after an infection of the nose, sagittal sinus thrombosis should be considered.

68.2.9
Lacrimal Apparatus Injury

Lateral osteotomy may injure the lacrimal sac [5]. Although it is usually temporary, there may be permanent damage (very rare).

68.2.10
Nasal Obstruction

Most patients experience temporary partial nasal obstruction following rhinoplasty from edema and crusting. Patients with allergic disorders or vasomotor rhinitis may have symptoms of nasal obstruction postoperatively from vasomotor rhinitis [6]. This can be treated with intranasal intramuscular injection of corticosteroids [7].

68.2.11
Retraction of the Columella

Excessive removal of the inferior or caudal margin of the septum or excessive removal of the membranous septum or the medial crura can result in retraction of the columella. Correction for a minor deformity includes a septal cartilage implant if sufficient lateral crus or alar cartilage is present or other lengthening procedures [8, 9].

68.2.12
Saddle Deformity

Saddle deformity is usually the result of overresection of cartilages (Fig. 68.3). Correction requires cartilage grafts.

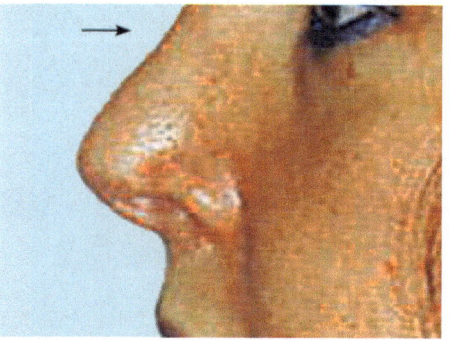

Fig. 68.3 Overresection resulting in a saddle nose

68.2.13
Septal Perforation

Sepal perforation is mainly caused by excessive mucous resection and unrecognized septal hematoma. Antibiotics for early treatment of nasal infection will reduce the incidence of septal perforation. Local or buccal mucosa flaps may be necessary if the patient is symptomatic.

References

1. Champion, R.: Anosmia associated with corrective rhinoplasty. Br J Plast Surg 1966;19(2):182–185
2. Goldwyn, R.M., Shore, S.: The effects of submucous resection and rhinoplasty on the sense of smell. Plast Reconstr Surg 1968;41(5):427–432
3. Rees, T.D., Baker, D.C.: Complications of aesthetic facial surgery. In Complications of Head and Neck Surgery, Conley, J.J. (ed), Philadelphia, Saunders 1979:401–447
4. Rees, T.D., Wood-Smith, D.: Cosmetic Facial Surgery. Philadelphia, Saunders 1973
5. Flowers, R.S., Anderson, R.: Injury to the lacrimal apparatus during rhinoplasty. Plast Reconstr Surg 1968;42(6):577–581
6. Beekhuis, G.J.: Nasal obstruction after rhinoplasty: etiology and techniques for correction. Laryngoscope 1976;86(4):540–548
7. Baker, D.C., Strauss, R.B.: The physiologic treatment of nasal obstruction. Clin Plast Surg 1977;4(1):121–130
8. Millard, D.R.: Columella lengthening by a forked flap. Plast Reconstr Surg 1958;22(5):454–457
9. Marcks, T.M., Trevaskis, A.E., Payne, M.J.: Elongation of columella by flap transfer and Z-plasty. Plast Reconstr Surg 1957;22(5):454–473

CHAPTER 69

Partial Removal of the Buccal Fat

69

Pierre F. Fournier

69.1
Introduction

The oval shape of the face may be lost on its lower portion, on both sides of the face in young, mature, or old people. This aesthetic defect is named "jowls." Jowls may be of different kinds:

1. They may be due to a pure buccal fat ptosis without subcutaneous fat accumulation and this is treated by buccal fat extraction only.
2. Buccal fat ptosis may be associated with a localized fatty subcutaneous accumulation and buccal fat extraction has to be associated with liposuction of this fatty accumulation also responsible for these jowls.
3. Another kind of jowls may be due only to a localized subcutaneous accumulation of fat and this aesthetic anomaly is treated by localized liposuction.
4. Finally jowls may be due to a simple localized or generalized skin excess on the lower face without localized subcutaneous fat accumulation or buccal fat ptosis (pseudojowls or false jowls).

The treatment will be a cervicofacial lift, APTOS threads, or a curl lift. No removal of buccal fat may result in residual jowls (Fig. 69.1). An accurate diagnosis of the aesthetic anomaly is important.

migrate downwards and be responsible for "real jowls" associated or not with a localized fat accumulation (Fig. 69.3).

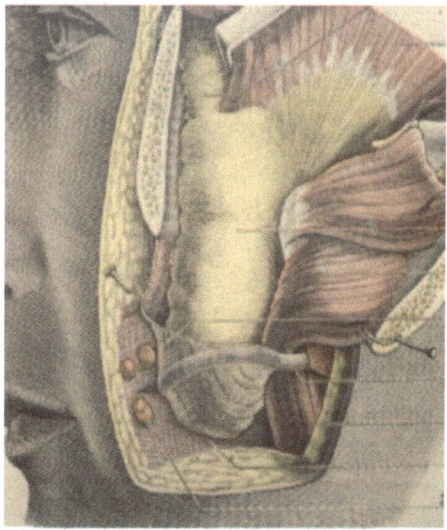

Fig. 69.2 The lower part of the buccal fat is at the level of the labial commissure

69.2
Anatomy

The buccal fat is in the buccal space between two muscles: the masseter and the buccinator (Fig. 69.2). It may

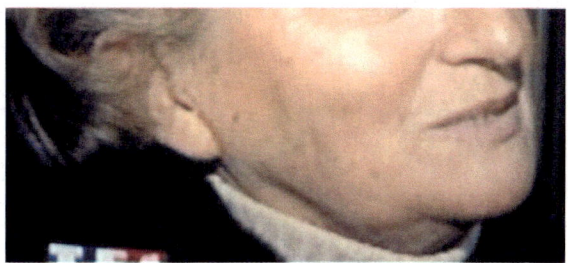

Fig. 69.1 Results of facelift without removal of buccal fat. The jowls are still there

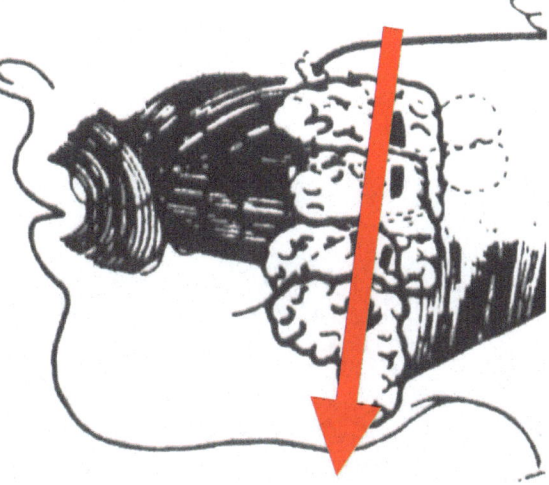

Fig. 69.3 Ptosis of the buccal fat

This buccal fat is surrounded by a fibrous tissue capsule. Removing this buccal fat during facelifting or through a small incision near of the ear is difficult and may be hazardous, while through the mouth it is an easy and not a hazardous operation.

69.3
Technique

The buccal fat extraction may be performed during a cervicofacial lifting or as an isolated procedure.

There are six steps:

1. Marking
2. Anesthesia
3. Incision
4. Grasping of the buccal fat
5. Extraction
6. Suture

The area to be injected on the lower cheek is marked (Fig. 69.4). The local anesthesia consisting of 1% lido-caine with 1:200,000 epinephrine is injected—8–10 ml is enough for one side. The gingivobuccal sulcus around the sixth upper tooth and the lower part of the cheek is infiltrated.

A 1-cm incision is made in the gingivobuccal sulcus at the level of the sixth upper tooth (we count six teeth from the midline). The capsule is broken with the tip of artery forceps or with the tip of the plastic tube containing a needle. The assistant has to retract the commissures of the mouth and push gently externally on the cheek to lift the buccal fat.

The tip of the plastic tube of the cap of a needle is sectioned and the end which is cut is mounted on a 10-ml syringe (Fig. 69.5). This plastic tube is pushed in the incision vertically and the surgeon pulls on the plunger of the syringe. The plastic tube is removed slowly and is filled with fat. The surgeon now has to grasp with Adson forceps the emerging buccal fat when it is visible through the incision (Fig. 69.6). The extraction is carried out with precautions using two Adson forceps. Teasing gently the buccal fat is necessary. Artery forceps clamp the lower part of the visible buccal fat and sectioning is performed

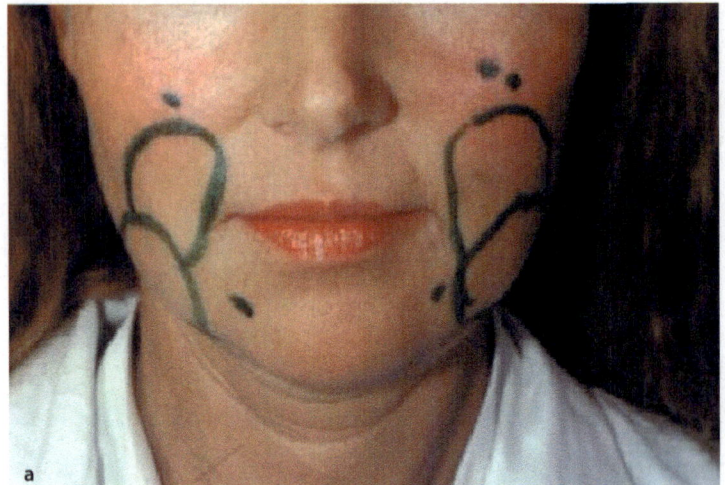
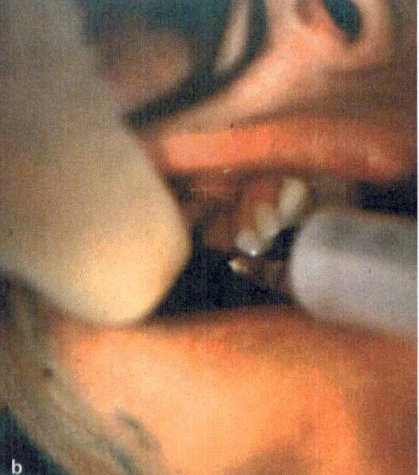

Fig. 69.4 Areas marked for anesthesia. **a** External. **b** Internal

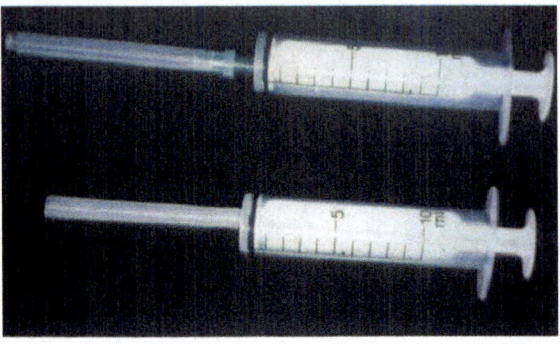

Fig. 69.5 The upper syringe has an uncut plastic tube and is used for perforation of the capsule. The lower syringe has the tip of the plastic tube cut for the first step of the extraction: the grasping of the buccal fat

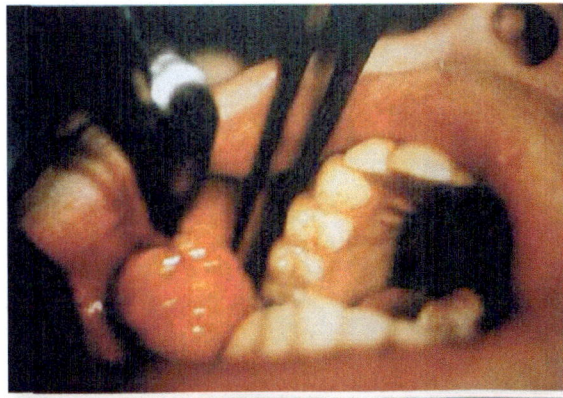

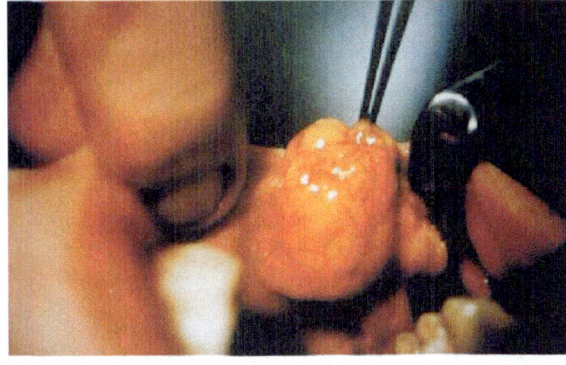

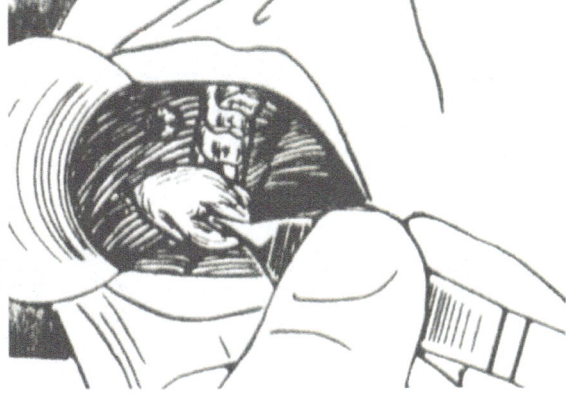

Fig. 69.6 Extraction with Adson forceps

along the artery forceps using small curved scissors. The buccal fat is withdrawn completely. The artery forceps are removed after 1 min and packing is placed between the check and the upper teeth, for 10 minutes.

The same operation is performed on the other side, immediately. The incision may be left open or sutured with a resorbable suture if desired. Packing is applied for 10 min (Fig. 69.7). A moderate-pressure dressing is applied around the head. After 10 min, the two packings are removed as well as the dressing around the head.

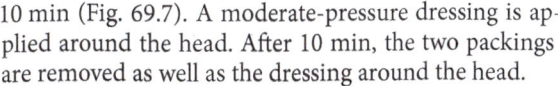

69.4
Postoperatively

Antibiotics are given routinely for 5 days as well as anti-inflammatory tablets.

This operation may also be performed before or after a cervicofacial lifting, but usually after. To grasp the buccal fat, it is also possible to use a small cannula connected to a suction pump, instead of using the syringe technique.

69.5
Complications

Bleeding is easily controlled by pressure. We have seen one mild case of infection treated by antibiotics.

It may be sometimes difficult to grasp the buccal fat if the assistant is not pressing gently on the cheek. Repositioning of this buccal fat has been done by some authors with APTOS threads or through a curl lift.

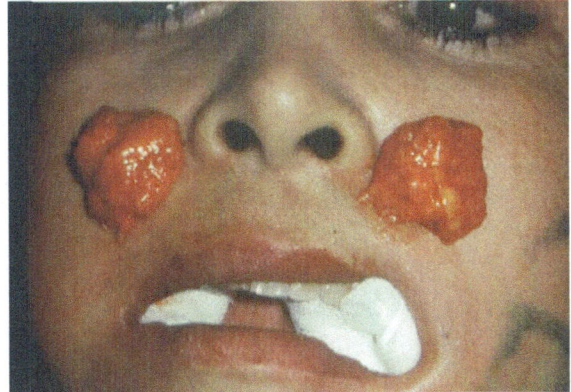

Fig. 69.7 Packing for 10 min

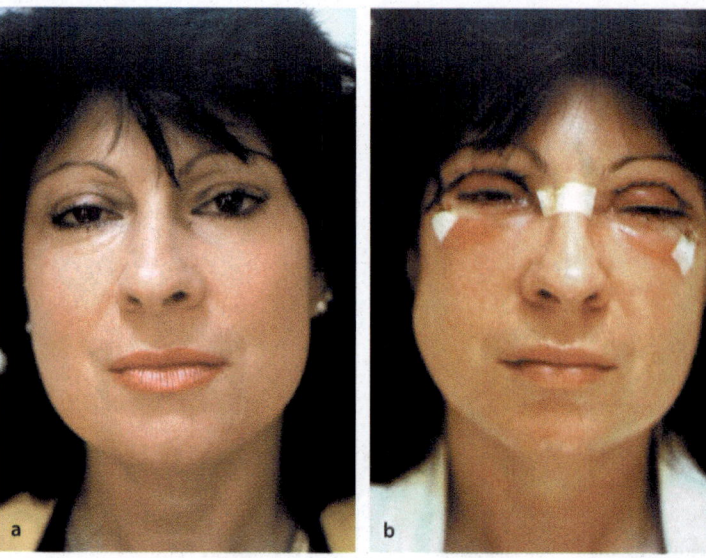

Fig. 69.8 **a** Before. **b** After removal of buccal fat

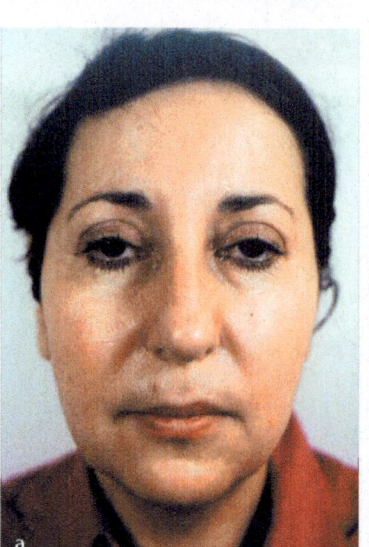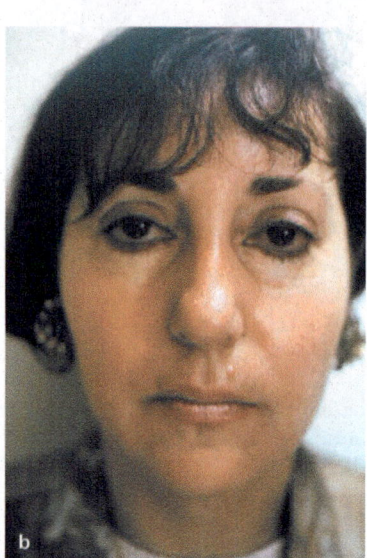

Fig. 69.9 **a** Before. **b** After removal of buccal fat

69.6
Conclusions

The results are excellent with the simple removal of buccal fat (Figs. 69.8, 69.9) [1, 2]. Quite often an unaccounted moderate weight loss may be seen after this operation.

References

1. Newman J., Nguyen A., Anderson R.: Liposuction of the buccal fat pad. Am J Cosmet Surg 1986;3(1):43–52
2. Newman J., Levin J.: "Jowling": introduction of a new surgical treatment for the jowl. In Liposculpture: The Syringe Technique. Fournier, P.F. (Ed.), Paris, Arnette Blackwell 1991:205–211

CHAPTER 70

Anatomy and Surgical Approaches to the Midface Lift

70

Omer Refik Ozerdem, Patricio Andrades, Luis O. Vasconez, Jorge de la Torre

70.1
Surgical Anatomy

Knowledge of the anatomic layers of the face, their contents, and their relationship with each other is of paramount importance to perform effective midface lifting and to minimize the complications. According to Stuzin et. al. [1] the facial soft tissue is composed of skin, subcutaneous fat, the superficial musculoaponeurotic system (SMAS), mimetic muscle, deep facial fascia (parotid masseteric fascia), and the plane containing the facial nerve, the parotid duct, and the buccal fat pad.

Mitz and Peyronie [2] defined "the superficial muscular (since they sometimes detected muscular fibers within the fibrous layer in histological sections) and aponeurotic system (SMAS)" in their cadaver studies. They detailed the relationship of this structure with the adjacent structures. They found that the SMAS is the interposition layer between the subcutaneous fat layers. The superficial fat layer is composed of small fat lobules divided by the small fibrous septa that attach the SMAS to the dermis. The deeper fat layer lies between the facial muscles and is not divided by such fibrous septa. The SMAS continues with the frontalis muscle superiorly and the platysma muscle inferiorly. It is adherent to the deeper parotid fascia in the pretragal area, and becomes a separate layer 1–2 cm anteriorly. The superficial parotid gland and the parotid fascia protect the motor branches of the facial nerve, thus these branches are deeper to the SMAS. However, sensory branches originate from the anterior cervical plexus located superficial to the SMAS in the parotid area. The main vessels that are located deeper to the SMAS send perforators to the subdermal vascular network through the SMAS as consistent with the findings of Whetzel and Mathes [3]. Superiorly the SMAS crosses the zygomatic arch superficially. The temporal motor branch is deeper and the sensory branches are superficial to it. Inferiorly, at the nasolabial level the SMAS is very thin, and it is separated from the dermis by a large amount of fat [2].

The SMAS layer overlying the parotid is thicker than that of the masseter and the buccal fat pad, and contains fibers of the lip elevators at the malar region [1, 2]. Mitz and Peyronie [2] stated that the SMAS is stretched superiorly by the frontal, superficial temporal, and orbicularis oculi muscles, and inferiorly by the platysma. They pointed out that each facial expression is the reflection of the multiple mimic muscles that was transmitted to the skin by the SMAS via vertical fibrous septa. Ozerdem et al. [4] stated the differences between the flat muscles of the face and the skeletal muscles as the origin and insertion on the skin and soft tissues, the absence of the enveloping fascia, and the ability of contraction of the portions that give rise to a multitude of facial expressions. Most of the mimic muscles (platysma, orbicularis oculi, zygomaticus major and minor, risorius) lie superficial to the facial nerve, receiving their innervation from their deep surfaces [1]. The buccinator, the levator anguli oris, and the mentalis muscle lie deeper, posterior to the plane of the facial nerve branches, receiving their innervation from their superficial surface [1]. The superficial fascia invests the superficial mimic muscles. As Stuzin et al. [1] described: "By investing, we mean that the superficial fascia not only is identified along the superficial surface of these muscles, but also lines their deep surfaces." Certain deeper mimic muscles do not have fascial investiture [1].

The deep temporal fascia (fascia proprium), which is the extension of the pericranium, is divided into superficial (the innominate fascia) and deep layers above the zygomatic arch [5]. Between and deeper to these layers are the temporal fat pads [6–8]. The innominate fascia blends with the zygomatic arch periosteum, whereas the deep layer extends as the parotid masseteric fascia below the arch [5]. The deep temporal fat pad continues beneath the zygomatic arch and blends with the buccal fat pad [7, 8]. The extension of the galea aponeurotica and the superficial temporal fascia below the zygomatic arch is the superficial fascia of the face and the neck [1, 2, 7]. The deep facial fascia overlies the different structures and is named with respect to these structures [1]. It is referred to as the parotid capsule or the investing parotid fascia at the parotid area and masseteric fascia anteriorly where it overlies the masseter muscle [1, 9]. Anterior to the masseter, it overlies the buccal space [8].

Stuzin et al. [1] pointed out the significant variation of anatomic descriptions of facial fascial anatomy such as those of Jost and Levet [10] and Yousif et al. [11, 12] Jost and Levet [10] opposed the findings of the Mitz and Peyronie [2] on the basis of their cadaveric human as well as lower mammal dissections and histological examinations, and previous embryological data. They rejected the concept of the SMAS and accepted the superficial fascia as a histologic structure rather than an anatomic one. As a result they indicated the parotid fascia as the only solid layer between the skin and the parotid. They advocated that not the superficial fascia (SMAS) but the parotid fascia includes the muscle fibers and is the continuation of the platysma muscle. They called the parotid fascia the primitive platysma, mentioning the fibrotic regression of the platysma from lower mammals to humans. The superficial fascia and a layer of fat tissue overlie the parotid fascia, and the deep fascia actually underlies the parotid. They thought that the masseteric fascia that lies between the parotid fascia and the masseter muscle is the continuation of the deep fascia anterior to the parotid, and Stensen's duct is located between the deep fascia and the parotid fascia [10].

In contrast to Mitz and Peyronie [2], and Yousif et al. [11, 12] advocated that the superficial fascia and the SMAS are distinct layers, with the former overlying the latter. However, they supported Mitz and Peyronie's SMAS concept and that the SMAS blends with the platysma. They named the superficial fascia the "fascial-fatty layer" that crosses the nasolabial fold and the zygomatic arch. This layer thickens in the cheek region as a tissue composed of fat and fibrous septa forming a honeycomb pattern of dermal insertions that they called the cheek mass (malar fat pad). They advocated that the temporoparietal fascia blends with the deep fascia above the zygomatic arch, and the SMAS blends with the deep subcutaneous tissue superior to the parotid, the fascia-fatty layer becoming the only layer between the skin and the zygomatic arch periosteum. In the parotid region, they observed the SMAS is in close relation to the parotid and they suggested that the thin layer that lies between them is the parotid fascia. Inferiorly the SMAS crosses the nasolabial fold and blends with the superficial orbicularis oris, and superiorly it blends with the superficial fibers of the preorbital orbicularis oculi muscle, which is overlaid by the fascial-fatty layer [11, 12].

Furnas [13] defined four retaining ligaments of the cheek that support the skin in normal anatomic position: two travel between the bone and the dermis (the zygomatic and mandibular ligaments) and the others travel between the SMAS and the dermis (the platysma auricular ligament and the anterior platysma cutaneous ligaments). These are important for being anatomic landmarks and the osteocutaneous types are important for having a tethering effect that must be interrupted to obtain an effective face lifting. The zygomatic ligament (McGregor's patch) localizes at or near the anterior border of the zygomatic arch, 4.5 cm in front of the tragus. It travels from the zygomatic bone to the dermis with an accompanying artery and a sensory nerve. One of the zygomatic motor branches lies deep and inferior to

this ligament. Furnas advocated this ligament should be divided to manage the severe cheek skin laxity. McGregor stated that beyond this patch is the loose fat that includes branches of the facial nerve and the parotid duct, which could be injured during dissection (as cited by Furnas). The mandibular ligament is located at the anterior third of the mandibular body traveling between the bone and the dermis with an accompanying artery and a sensory nerve. This ligament prevents sagging so that behind it is the anterior margin of the jowls. Furnas stated that division of this ligament provides more effective management of the submental area and access to this area without the need of a submental incision. The platysma auricular ligament localizes on the inferior auricular region, over the parotid with the accompanying great auricular nerve branches. It serves as a surgical guide to the posterosuperior border of the platysma, avoiding facial motor branches. The anterior platysma cutaneous ligaments travel between the anterior platysma and the middle and anterior cheek skin. Furnas warned that these ligaments may cause anatomic disorientation that may lead to perforation of the skin during dissection. He advised sectioning of these ligaments to avoid dimpling.

Stuzin et al. [1] stated two types of relationship between the superficial and deep facial fascia layers. First is the areolar plane between the SMAS and the parotid masseteric fascia within the midface that offers easier dissection. A similar relationship exists between the deep and the superficial temporal fascia superiorly, and between the platysma and the strap muscles inferiorly. Second are the dense attachments between these layers that are seen along the zygomatic arch, overlying the parotid gland and along the anterior border of the masseter (the masseteric cutaneous ligaments). They classified the retaining ligaments as the osteocutaneous ligaments that travel between the bone and the dermis, and the supporting ligaments that represent the condensation of the deep and the superficial layers fixing them to the deeper layers such as the parotid and the masseter. The mandibular and zygomatic ligaments belong to the first group, and the parotid cutaneous and the masseteric cutaneous ligaments to the latter. Observing that the ligaments that were called platysma cutaneous ligaments by Furnas previously originate along the anterior border of the masseter, Stuzin et al. proposed the term "the masseteric cutaneous ligament." They stated that this ligamentous system supports the soft tissue of the medial cheek superiorly over the mandibular body. Yousif and Mendelson [12] later observed such dense ligamentous attachments at the level of the infraorbital ridge, superior to the orbital ligament.

Just below the zygoma, deeper to the deep facial fascia, is the buccal pocket, which includes the buccal branches of the facial nerve, buccal fat pad (Bichat's fat), the parotid duct, and the attendant buccal blood vessels [1, 2, 9, 14]. The motor branches of the facial nerve penetrate the parotid masseteric fascia to innervate the mimic muscles [1]. The mandibular branch lies deeper in the mandibular area, offering a safe dissection plane deeper to the SMAS and the platysma [2]. The frontal motor branches leave the parotid gland just caudal to the zygomatic arch and cross this arch within the temporoparietal fascia, the same plane as with the superficial temporal artery, and then enter the frontalis muscle at the level of the superior orbital rim [1, 7]. They are located halfway between the line that connects the lateral canthus to the helical rim of the ear [14]. The locations of the facial nerve branches are taken into consideration during face lifting dissection. Mitz and Peyronie [2], taking the thin space beneath the SMAS into consideration, recommended subcutaneous dissection at the zygomatic arch level [2]. Stuzin et al. [1] recommended a dissection plane superficial to the deep temporalis fascia, and then deeper to its deep layer 2 cm above the zygomatic arch to avoid the frontal branch. Hamra [15] advised dissection superficial to the parotid masseteric fascia and the elevators of the lip to avoid the motor branches (note that these muscles receive their motor branches from underneath, as stated above) while describing his deep plane rhytidectomy.

Whetzel and Mathes [3] performed a study on cadavers to obtain more information about the arterial anatomy of the face. According to their findings there are 11 anatomically distinct territories on the head that receive a primary vascular supply from these arteries: the transverse facial, submental, zygomaticoorbital, anterior auricular, posterior auricular, occipital, supratrochlear, frontal branch and parietal branch of the superficial temporal, superior labial, and inferior labial arteries. There are three distinct arterial vascularizations of the head: (1) the facial and infraorbital arteries supply the anterior face via multiple, small-caliber musculocutaneous perforators; (2) the transverse facial, submental, and zygomaticoorbital arteries supply the lateral face via sparse, isolated, and large-caliber fasciocutaneous perforators with constant sites of locations; and (3) the occipital, superficial temporal, and posterior auricular arteries supply the scalp via dense, small-caliber fasciocutaneous perforators. Lateral to the nasolabial region is the transition zone of the anterior and lateral vascular regions. The facial artery courses deep to or through the mimic muscles and gives off numerous musculocutaneous perforators to the dermis. The fascial cutaneous perforator of the lateral facial artery passes from the masseteric fascia to the dermis of the lateral face through the SMAS. The authors commented on the basis of their studies that lateral dissection in face lifting operation makes the flap supplied by the anteriorly localized musculocutaneous perforators, and that sub-SMAS dissection would not enhance the vascularity, but would enhance preservation of the specific arterial perforators on the lateral face that would not limit the mobility of the flap [3].

The midface includes various fat layers which have surgical significance: the intraorbital fat, the suborbicularis oculi fat (SOOF), the malar fat pad, and Bichat's fat (buccal fat pad). These are excised, plicated, repositioned, or suspended in various techniques and with respect to the needs of patients in midfacial rejuvenation. The intraorbital fat is located behind the orbital septum and causes lower-eyelid bags with the sagging septum [16, 17]. De Cordier et al. [18] defined the malar fat pad as a triangular subcutaneous tissue, whose base sits on the nasolabial fold and whose apex reaches to the malar eminence. Aiache and Ramirez [19] used the term SOOF to define the malar bags or the malar fat pads. The SOOF is located below the lateral half of the infraorbital rim, behind the orbicularis oculi muscle, and superficial to the periosteum [19]. Furnas [17] preferred using the term "the malar mound" rather than "malar bags" or "malar pads" and defined it as the skin-fat bulging and projection at the malar eminence. He described its borders as two folds superiorly and inferiorly that become more prominent in older patients as a result of lax skin, as well as the medial angle formed by converging of these folds. The higher fold is the orbit–cheek fold, which is the combination of the nasojugal fold medially and the malar fold laterally [17, 20]. Furnas [17] observed that a line of fusion of the superficial and deep facial fascias that attaches to the orbital rim forms this fold. The lower fold is the midcheek fold that extends upward and obliquely from the zygomatic ligament level to the medial canthus [17]. The peripheral fibers of the orbicularis oculi are present at the base of the malar mound [17]. Here the muscle is located between the subcutaneous cheek fat and the SOOF, which are connected to each other through the fenestrations between the muscle fibers. The subcutaneous fat and the SOOF blend inferiorly when the muscle traverses only the cephalad portion of the malar mound [17].

Stuzin et al. [8] gave detailed information about the buccal fat pad and cheek contouring with intraoral partial excision of this structure. The buccal fat pad consists of a body and extensions named buccal, deep temporal, superficial temporal, and pterygoid. The facial vessels, the parotid gland, and the anterior border of the masseter, and the mandibular retromolar region make the borders of this structure. The corpus that lies along the posterior maxilla and the upper fibers of the buccinator muscle, and the buccal extension that locates between the parotid duct and the buccinator muscle make the contour of the cheek. The body extends to the pterygomaxillary fissure, where it is in close relationship with the maxillary artery and the maxillary division of the trigeminal nerve. The deep temporal extension travels underneath the zygomatic arch overlying the temporalis muscle as stated above. It also extends posterior to the lateral orbital wall and along the greater wing of the sphenoid bone. The superficial temporal fat pad, which is located between the layers of the deep temporal fascia, is actually anatomically distinct from the buccal fat pad. The pterygoid extension is in close relationship with the pterygoid muscles, inner mandibular ramus, mandibular neurovascular bundle, and the lingual nerve [19].

70.2
Changes in the Aging Face

The anatomic changes in the aging face should be understood profoundly to manage them effectively [21]. Flat muscle activation on the face causes wrinkling of the overlying skin. In young individuals, who have elastic skin, this wrinkling is temporary, whereas in older individuals, who have lost the elasticity of the skin, the wrinkles (or the folds) become permanent [4]. Other factors that contribute to the development of the wrinkles are solar damage, dry weather, progressive loss of some facial fat, and degeneration of the connective tissue [21].

Yousif [21] found that midfacial soft tissue descends inferiorly, laterally, and anteriorly. He pointed out that since the most anterior part of the malar fat is the most distant part of the face away from the constant skeleton, it descends the greatest distance. The other reason is that in contrast to the other parts of the face that are supported by the activity of the mimic muscles, the cheek area is supported by the retaining ligaments that attenuate with time, as stated already. Stuzin et al. [1] also stated that the aging face develops as a result of attenuated facial retaining ligaments and dermal elastosis. Attenuation of the malar ligaments results in malar descent, causing the nasolabial fold to become more accentuated [1]. Attenuation of the masseteric cutaneous ligament leads to descent of the medial cheek, causing the jowls [1]. They advocated that management of the aging face should be directed to these changes.

Hamra [22] described three main ptotic deep anatomic elements that are seen in addition to the skin changes with aging. First are the jowls or the broken mandibular line that develops with ptosis of the platysma muscle. Second is the enhanced distance between the ciliary margin and the malar crescent, which he defined as the inferior border of the orbicularis oculi muscle. The malar crescent descends as a result of attenuated orbicularis oculi muscle. And third are the deepened nasolabial fold and the depressed cheek that develop as a result of ptosis of the cheek fat. He addressed all these three changes in his method "the composite rhytidectomy." Yousif [21] stated that the nasolabial fold does not change nor deepen, and it is the descending of the cheek that makes the difference between the nasolabial fold of youth and age.

There are important changes on the lower lid and the infraorbital area. Goldberg et al. [23] found that there are various causes responsible for the eyelid bags. The most common factors are orbital fat prolapse, lower-lid elasticity, and tear-trough deformity. They stated that these factors become more prominent with age. Aiache and Ramirez [19] stated the causes of the malar bags as the inferior palpebral edema, subcutaneous fat excess, skin relaxation, and the herniation of the SOOF at the malar level. Furnas [16, 17] defined the festoons as the overlapping folds of the orbicularis oculi muscle that are suspended from canthus to canthus as a result of attenuation of the muscle and laxity of the attachments between the muscle and the deep fascia with aging. They contributed to the baggy eyelids. Furnas [16, 17] classified the festoons with respect to their locations and contents. They may appear on the upper or lower lid. The lower-lid festoons are classified as pretarsal, preseptal, orbital, and malar. They may contain only muscle (pure skin–muscle festoons) or muscle with fat tissue that originated from the bulging preaponeurotic orbital fat or the SOOF. In some cases a cutaneous dewlap develops as a result of attenuation of the muscle–skin connection. The folds make the borders of the malar mound become more prominent as a result of lax skin with aging as mentioned above [17].

The changes around the perioral area include elongation of the upper lip resulting in loss of symmetry and convexity, thinning of vermilion with loss of shape, commissural drooping and sad pleats, and formation of radial lines from the vermilion extending onto the upper and lower lips. The changes on the nose include involution of the sebaceous glands and thinning of the skin and drooping of the tip. These changes should be addressed by means of adjuvant procedures to improve the overall result [24].

70.3
Midface Lifting Methods

We (unpublished data) reviewed the evolution of the cervicofacial lifting operations chronologically and used a classification in a technical aspect. We respect this classification, dividing the technical descriptions into the following sections: skin excisions without undermining, minilifts, and classic subcutaneous lifting; the sub-SMAS plane face lifting; the subperiosteal face lifting; the management of the nasolabial fold and the suspension methods, and the periorbital rejuvenation.

70.3.1
Skin Excision without Undermining, Minilifts, and Classic Subcutaneous Face Lifting

Early attempts at face-lifting procedures consisted of skin excision and primary repair without skin undermining (Fig. 70.1) [25–34]. These have been called minilifting procedures. Holländer, Lexer, and Joseph stated in the 1920s and 1930s that they performed their

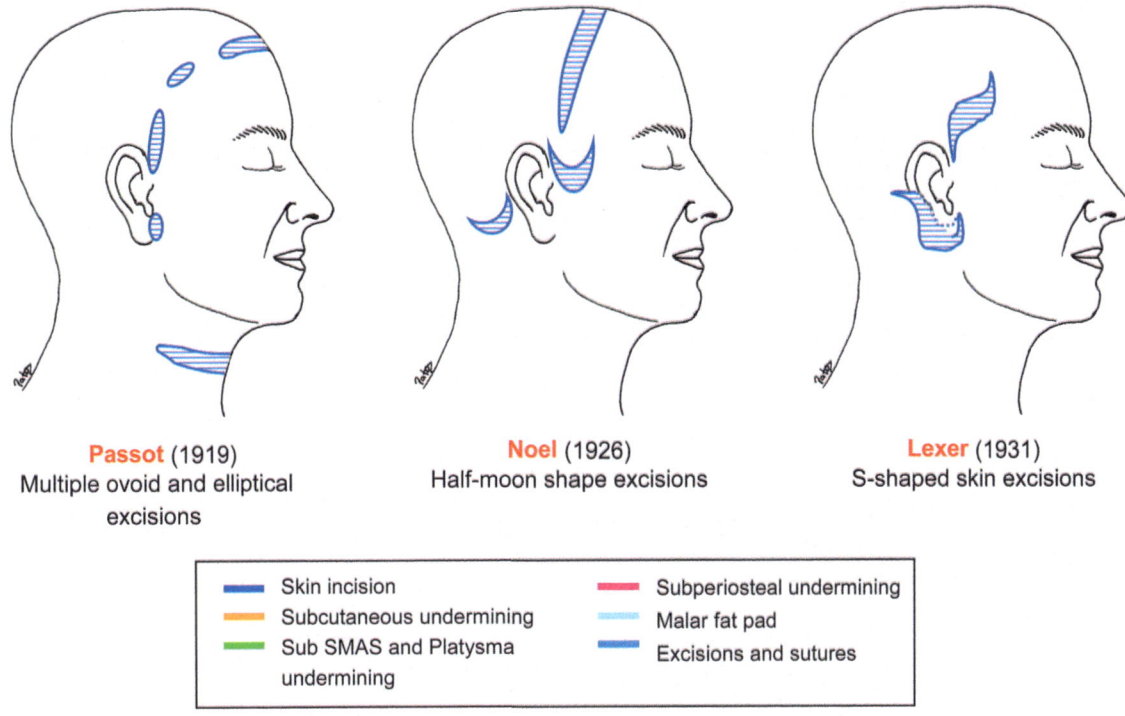

Passot (1919)
Multiple ovoid and elliptical excisions

Noel (1926)
Half-moon shape excisions

Lexer (1931)
S-shaped skin excisions

▬ Skin incision	▬ Subperiosteal undermining
▬ Subcutaneous undermining	▬ Malar fat pad
▬ Sub SMAS and Platysma undermining	▬ Excisions and sutures

Fig. 70.1 Skin excision only without undermining

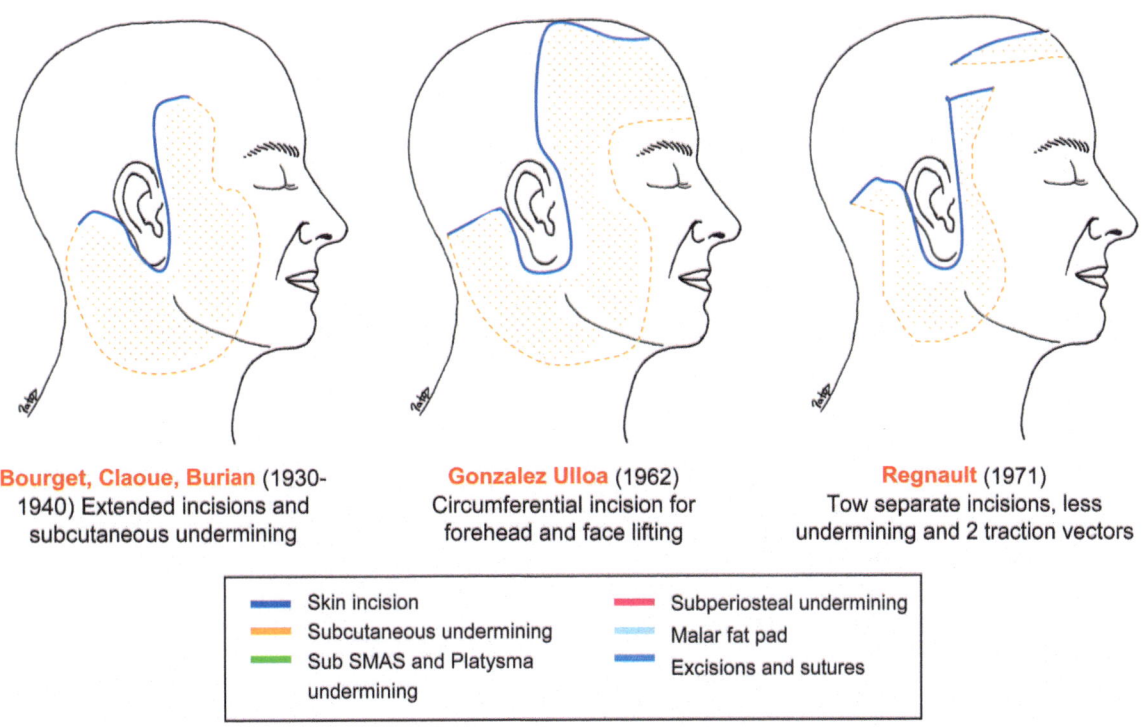

Bourget, Claoue, Burian (1930-1940) Extended incisions and subcutaneous undermining

Gonzalez Ulloa (1962)
Circumferential incision for forehead and face lifting

Regnault (1971)
Tow separate incisions, less undermining and 2 traction vectors

▬ Skin incision	▬ Subperiosteal undermining
▬ Subcutaneous undermining	▬ Malar fat pad
▬ Sub SMAS and Platysma undermining	▬ Excisions and sutures

Fig. 70.2 Classic methods: extended incisions plus skin undermining

first operations at the beginning of the twentieth century. However, Miller and Kolle were the first to have their methods published, in 1906 and 1911, respectively. Passot, Bettman, Bourget, and Noël were the other pioneers of midface lifting in the first half of the twentieth century. They carried out different shapes of excisions (ellipsoid, S-shape, ovoid, crescent, etc.) and concealed them at the frontal hairline, inside the temporal hair, and behind and in front of the ear. Holländer used a longer incision that included the preauricular, infralobular, and lateral neck skin areas to obtain more effective results. Passot limited his incisions to the sideburns for men and to the long hair fall in the women. Bettman was probably the first to employ an incision similar to the one that is used today. His incision started from the temporal area and included the preauricular, infralobular, and postlobular areas. Bourget concealed the preauricular incision on the tragus. His incision continued around the earlobe in a V-fashion, ascended on the retroauricular furrow, then angled onto the mastoid, and finally extended through the hairline.

In the 1920s and 1930s, some surgeons extended their incisions and began to perform subcutaneous undermining to obtain long-lasting results leading to the classic subcutaneous face-lifting period (Fig. 70.2) [26, 30, 31, 33]. Bames, Stein, Joseph, and Bourget were some of the pioneers in this period. Bames performed limited subcutaneous dissection in the 1920s, whereas Claoue and Burian used extended undermining. Bourget extended the dissection as near as possible to the nasolabial fold and the neck.

Gonzales-Ulloa [35] performed dissection at the frontal, midfacial, and cervical areas after a long incision that started behind the frontal hairline and extended to the temporal area, preauricular furrow, retroauricular sulcus (that united with the temporal incision completing a circle around the pinna), and the occipital scalp. After wide dissection he pulled out the tissues in different vectors with respect to the effects of the gravitational force on each region, and then excised the excess tissue.

70.3.2
Sub-SMAS-Plane Face Lifting

Classic subcutaneous face lifting was the main method until the 1970s. One of the disadvantages of the minilifts and the subcutaneous face-lifting methods is that they address only the skin laxity, neglecting the ptosis of the deeper layers [22]. The subcutaneous face lifting does not offer an effective improvement, and carries high risk of tight or drawn-out appearance because of lateral traction [18]. Skoog's [36] introduction of his method "two layer shift" in his book in 1974 heralded a new period (Fig. 70.3). He briefly carried out limited subcutaneous dissection after temporal and preauricular incisions and then entered deeper to the superficial fascia of the face at the level of the anterior border of the masseter and continued his dissection through the nasolabial fold. After postauricular incision he carried out subcutaneous incision to the sternocleidomastoid and submandibular level (avoiding the facial nerve), after which he entered the subplatysmal level. He applied traction to the subcutaneous facial fascia and to the platysma in a posterior and superior direction and fixed these tissues to the masseteric and mastoid fascias, respectively. By doing this, he tried to correct the jowls and the nasolabial fold, provide fullness for the cheeks, and advance the skin and subcutaneous tissue further without tension. He stated the advantages of his operation as more even distribution of the tissues when compared with previously performed plication of the deeper tissues, and less hematoma and scarring but more permanent results when compared with subcutaneous face lifting.

Mitz and Peyronie [2] originated the term SMAS with their anatomic studies in 1976 as mentioned already. They pointed out that fibrous connections between the SMAS and the dermis are divided during subcutaneous face-lifting procedure that could be avoided with sub-SMAS dissection. They stated effective lifting of the skin and the anterior muscles, and even stretching of the oral commissures with dissection, traction, and posterior fixation of the SMAS.

Skoog's method in addition to the anatomic studies of Mitz and Peyronie led Owsley [37] to employ sub-SMAS–platysma dissection (Fig. 70.3). He elevated the SMAS from the zygomatic arch down to the neck at the subplatysmal level, avoiding the marginal mandibular nerve at the mandibular level. The SMAS was then fixed to the pretragal area.

Lemmon and Hamra [38] modified Skoog's technique by adding cervical subcutaneous dissection, submental lipectomy, and submandibular lipectomy in selected cases.

Additionally, they did not extend the dissection to the level of nasolabial fold because it did not produce further improvement.

Hamra [15, 22, 39–42] later modified this sub-SMAS face-lifting method with more effective methods and developed the triplane dissection, the deep-plane dissection, and the composite rhytidectomy methods (Fig. 70.3). He limited sub-SMAS dissection below the malar eminence, and performed subcutaneous dissection in a great part of the midface and the neck to obtain longer-lasting results and to avoid the operated-on appearance of the neck often seen after subplatysmal dissection (the triplane dissection). In order to improve the nasolabial fold, for which he stated that Skoog's method was not very effective, he developed the deep-plane dissection. He created a musculocutaneous flap after limited skin dissection and sub-SMAS dissection at the level of malar eminence, the jawline and beyond the nasolabial fold, and suspended the flap to the superficial temporal fascia. He later added suborbicularis oculi dissection via subciliary incision to suspend it in a medial and superior direction and named this technique "the composite rhytidectomy." As a result he was able to manage the jowls, nasolabial fold, and the malar crescent. He also added repositioning of the inferior-lid fat pad and canthopexy operations, when needed.

Hamra [43], commenting on the findings of Whetzel and Mathes [3] regarding the arterial anatomy of the face stated that a bipedicle flap based on the platysma and the orbicularis oculi muscles is elevated in composite rhytidectomy, ensuring a richer blood supply than seen with the subcutaneous lifting methods through the perforators to the skin by preserving the attachments of the platysma muscle and the facial artery. This vascular advantage enabled the surgeon to apply more tension on the flap that could not be done in the subcutaneous lifting methods.

Connell and Semlacher [44] introduced Connell's method of "contemporary deep-layer facial rejuvenation" in 1997 after using it on more than 1,500 patients with satisfactory results. He limited the subcutaneous dissection to preserve the anterior SMAS and dermis connection lateral to the nasolabial fold to obtain the desired effect on the nasolabial fold, upper lip, and corner of the mouth with later traction of the SMAS. He created a SMAS flap with a horizontal incision at the level of (or just above or beyond it) the zygomatic arch that extended from the malar eminence to the pretragal area, and a vertical incision that extended from the posterior end of the horizontal incision to the level of the anterior sternocleidomastoid muscle. He then pulled the flap superiorly and posteriorly around the malar pivot point and fixed it. He further divided a horizontal segment from the superior part of the SMAS flap and suspended it to the lateral temporal and periorbital tissues when more improvement was needed for the midface; or he divided a vertical segment from the posterior part of the flap and suspended it to the mastoid fascia when more improvement was needed on the neck.

Stuzin et al. [1, 45, 46] performed extended SMAS dissection far enough to release the parotid gland and the zygomatic and superior masseteric ligaments and to elevate and suspend the malar fat pad especially in patients with prominent nasolabial folds (Fig. 70.3). Stuzin carried out more limited skin dissection to preserve the attachments between the skin and the SMAS that would allow the surgeon to reelevate the facial skin through SMAS rotation. He named his method "the extended SMAS dissection technique." He stressed the importance of leaving a thick enough layer on the SMAS to obtain an adequately strong tissue for suspension, to give more fullness to the malar area. In case of a thin SMAS, he rolled the excess tissue onto itself to provide a thickened layer for fixation as suggested by Lambros. He later began to put a Vicryl mesh graft inside the

roll to obtain extra strength. He pointed out that aging changes occur in the face in different vectors and added that the extended SMAS dissection technique enables one to lift these tissues separately in different directions. The main advantages of this were suspension of the skin a bit more lateral than the SMAS so as not to cause misdirected facial rhytids and to allow the surgeon to redrape the individual layers with respect to the specific needs of the patient, since every patient ages differently in terms of both the degree of skin aging and the direction of the facial fat descent. He stated that the disadvantage of subcutaneous face lifting is that it results in an unnatural, tight, mask appearance and it distorted temporal hairlines after overrotation of the skin flap, and that it is not an anatomic approach to correct descended facial fat by traction of the skin flap.

In the extended SMAS dissection technique the skin incision starts at the temporal hair and continues on to the preauricular and postauricular areas [45]. The subcutaneous flap is elevated to the level of the malar area, followed by SMAS dissection. Below the zygomatic arch is the horizontal limb of the SMAS incision that extends to the lateral canthus from the zygomatic body; beyond the level of the lateral canthus the incision is angled inferiorly toward the alar base in order to prepare the malar fat flap. The vertical limb is performed preauricularly and extended inferiorly below the mandible. Sub-SMAS dissection remains superficial to the orbicularis oculi, zygomaticus minor and major, and the elevators of the upper lip since these muscles are innervated from below. The underlying tissues, the parotid and the deep facial fascia, protect the motor branches of the facial nerve. Dissection is carried on until all the retaining ligaments, which restrict the transfer of the desired pulling force, have been divided. Then the SMAS is pulled in a perpendicular direction of the nasolabial fold and fixed to the zygomatic buttress. The superiorly suspended SMAS corrects the jowls; additionally the preauricular SMAS is transposed posterior to the ear to improve the submental and submandibular regions.

Although he stated that there was little morbidity with his method, Stuzin pointed out the transition of the cheek and malar SMAS as the most difficult portion of the dissection because the fascia is too thin at this location and the atypically superficial course of the zygomatic motor branches in some patients (approximately 5%) makes these structures susceptible to injury during the dissection.

Jost and Levet [10] criticized the dissection below the superficial fascia (sub-SMAS), because it provides a thin fatty flap. Alternatively, they advocated dissection below the parotid fascia (primitive platysma) to obtain a stronger, thicker flap with protection of the facial motor branches. Their recommendations were based on their cadaver and histology studies.

Baker [48] also criticized extensive SMAS dissection plication methods; the first method in terms of pos-

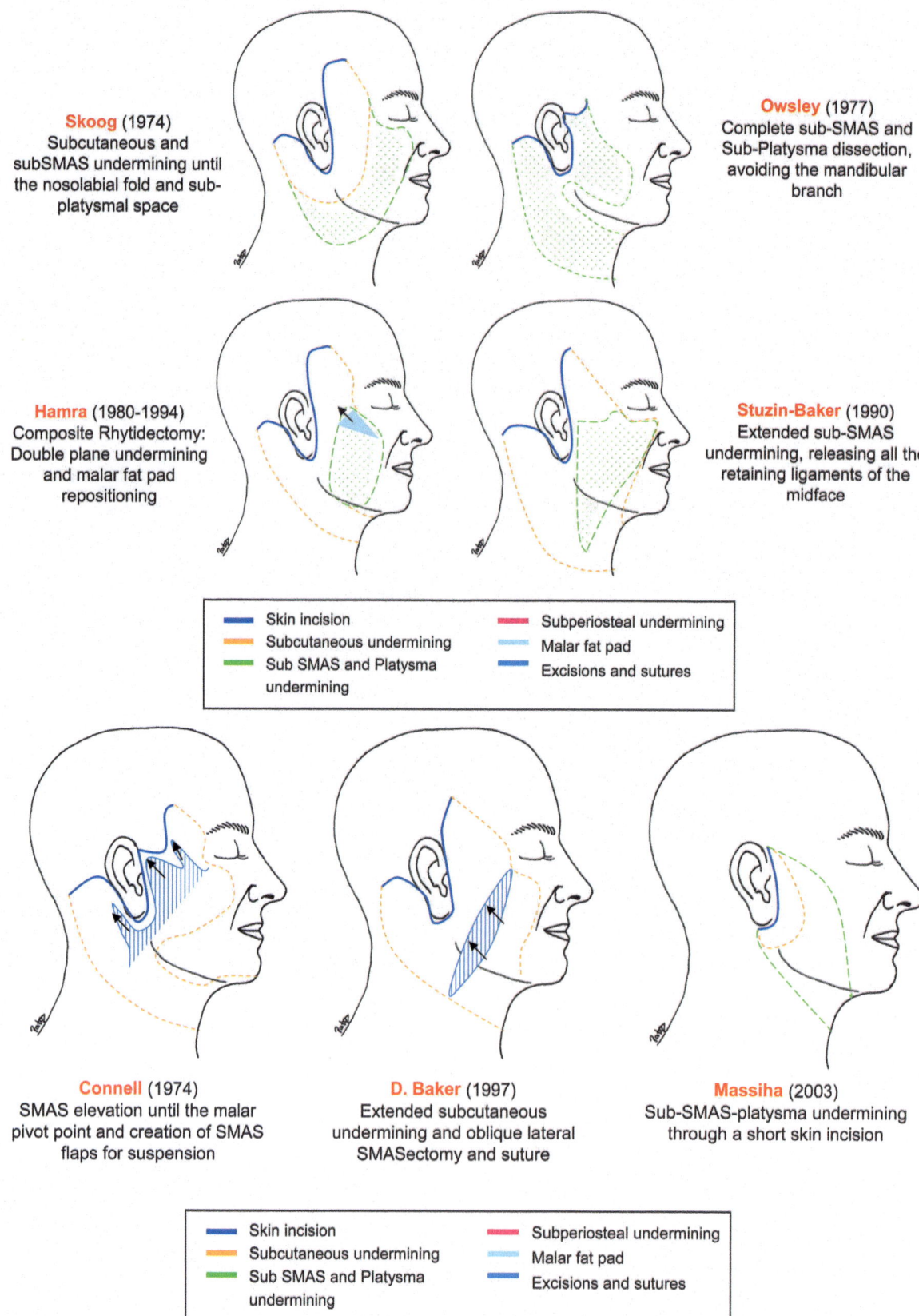

Skoog (1974)
Subcutaneous and subSMAS undermining until the nosolabial fold and sub-platysmal space

Owsley (1977)
Complete sub-SMAS and Sub-Platysma dissection, avoiding the mandibular branch

Hamra (1980-1994)
Composite Rhytidectomy: Double plane undermining and malar fat pad repositioning

Stuzin-Baker (1990)
Extended sub-SMAS undermining, releasing all the retaining ligaments of the midface

▬ Skin incision	▬ Subperiosteal undermining
▬ Subcutaneous undermining	▬ Malar fat pad
▬ Sub SMAS and Platysma undermining	▬ Excisions and sutures

Connell (1974)
SMAS elevation until the malar pivot point and creation of SMAS flaps for suspension

D. Baker (1997)
Extended subcutaneous undermining and oblique lateral SMASectomy and suture

Massiha (2003)
Sub-SMAS-platysma undermining through a short skin incision

▬ Skin incision	▬ Subperiosteal undermining
▬ Subcutaneous undermining	▬ Malar fat pad
▬ Sub SMAS and Platysma undermining	▬ Excisions and sutures

Fig. 70.3 The subcutaneous musculoaponeurotic system (SMAS) era

sible injury to the facial nerve branches and thinning out of the SMAS anteriorly that makes it fragile and a poor substrate for holding the tension, and the second method in terms of application of tension on the more stable posterior part of the fascia. He proposed excising a portion of the SMAS on the lateral aspect of the parotid to avoid the motor branches and then advancement and fixation of the more mobile anterior SMAS to the more stable posterior part without undermining. He introduced his method as "the lateral SMASectomy."

"The short scar face lift and extended SMAS dissection technique" that was described by Massiha [49] relies on a short skin incision with limited subcutaneous dissection to avoid dog-ears to be removed and to protect the dermal–SMAS connections, and on the extensive sub-SMAS and platysma dissection for correction of the aging deformities. The skin incision was started at the sideburn and extended more or less with respect to the needs of the patient to the postlobule area.

70.3.3
Subperiosteal Face Lifting, Mask Lift

The subperiosteal face-lifting period started at the end of the 1970s and in the 1980s, pioneered by Tessier [50], Hinderer et al. [51], Psillakis et al. [52], and Ortiz-Monasterio et al. [54] and contributed to the craniofacial methods (Fig. 70.4). Tessier [50] and Psillakis et al. [52] first dissected the frontal, periorbital, and zygomatic areas subperiosteally after coronal incision. Psillakis et al. [52] extended the subperiosteal dissection to the midface. Studying cadavers, they proposed the term "the anterior face SMAS fixation" referring to fixation of the SMAS and the muscles to the underlying bone. They advocated release of this fixation for effective lifting. After coronal incision, they performed subgaleal dissection through the supraorbital area, from which they carried on with subperiosteal dissection. They extended the subperiosteal dissection to the infraorital foramen, the medial third of the zygomatic arches, and the level of the nasolabial fold, and then fixed the dissected tissues to the deep temporal fascia. Ortiz-Monasterio et al. [53, 54] solved the problem of the horizontal or anti-Mongoloid eye slant problem with repositioning of the lateral canthus.

Some authors used lower-lid incisions to reach the midface subperiosteally [55–58]. Hester et al. [56, 57] in their centrofacial approach method created a subperiosteal cheek flap that included the SMAS, the SOOF, the malar fat pad, and the orbicularis oculi via a subciliary approach and after the subperiosteal dissection. They pulled this flap vertically and fixed it to the deep temporal fascia. Gunter and Hackney [58] in contrast excised the periosteum at the borders of the dissection, creating a composite flap, and fixed it to the lateral orbital rim in order to avoid canthopexy or canthoplasty operations.

Hobar and Flood [59] used temporal and intraoral incisions to elevate the midfacial tissues subperiosteally. They suspended the SOOF and fixed it to the deep temporal fascia. By doing this, they avoided lower-lid incisions, and consequently the accompanying potential lower-lid problems.

Ramirez et al. [60] described their open method, "the extended subperiosteal face lift," in 1991. They stressed the high probability of facial branch injury with Tessier's and Psillakis' the subperiosteal face-lifting methods of Tessier and Psillakis et al. They criticized the method of Psillakis et al. for limited dissection on the zygomatic arch that resulted in limited lifting and for using the periorbital fibrofatty tissues that would risk the zygomatic branches of the facial nerve.

After coronal or modified hairline incision, Hobar and Flood [60] dissected subperiosteally in the frontal area. In the temporal region, they dissected superficial to the deep temporal fascia. They first entered into the fat pad between the layers of the temporalis fascia proprium, and then behind the deep layer of this fascia above the zygomatic arch. Arriving at the arch with further dissection, they again incised the fascia proprium and the periosteum of the arch. With addition of the intraoral incision, they dissected a wide area of the midface, including a part of the masseter fascia. Then they advanced the coronal flap, lifting the midfacial structures, and anchored the temporalis muscle fascia on the flap to the temporal fascia behind the fascial incision (rather than suspending the periorbital soft tissue). They also added limited subcutaneous dissection on the parotid area and the neck, when needed. They compared the complications that they observed in their cases with Tessier's ($n = 15$), Psillakis et al.'s ($n = 45$), and their own ($n = 28$) methods. They observed total nerve injury rates of 20, 11, and 0% with these methods, respectively.

Ortiz-Monasterio [61], discussing the presentation of Ramirez et al. concerning their extended subperiosteal face lift method, recommended this procedure for younger patients who have sagging around the orbitozygomatic area. He advocated the necessity of the addition of the preauricular and neck incisions for older patients.

Heinrichs and Kaidi [62] criticized the dissection of Ramirez et al. [60] on the temporal region for being too bloody and for possible temporal fat atrophy. After temporal scalp incision they completed subtemporoparietal fascia dissection to the level of the V1 vein level above the zygomatic arch, after which they exposed the posterior arch through a back-cut in the SMAS and subcutaneous tissue immediately anterior to the tragus. Further subperiosteal dissection of the arch provided connection to the midfacial subperiosteal dissection that was previously carried out via an intraoral or subciliary incision. The second difference in their method was that they created a temporal SMAS–galea flap at the

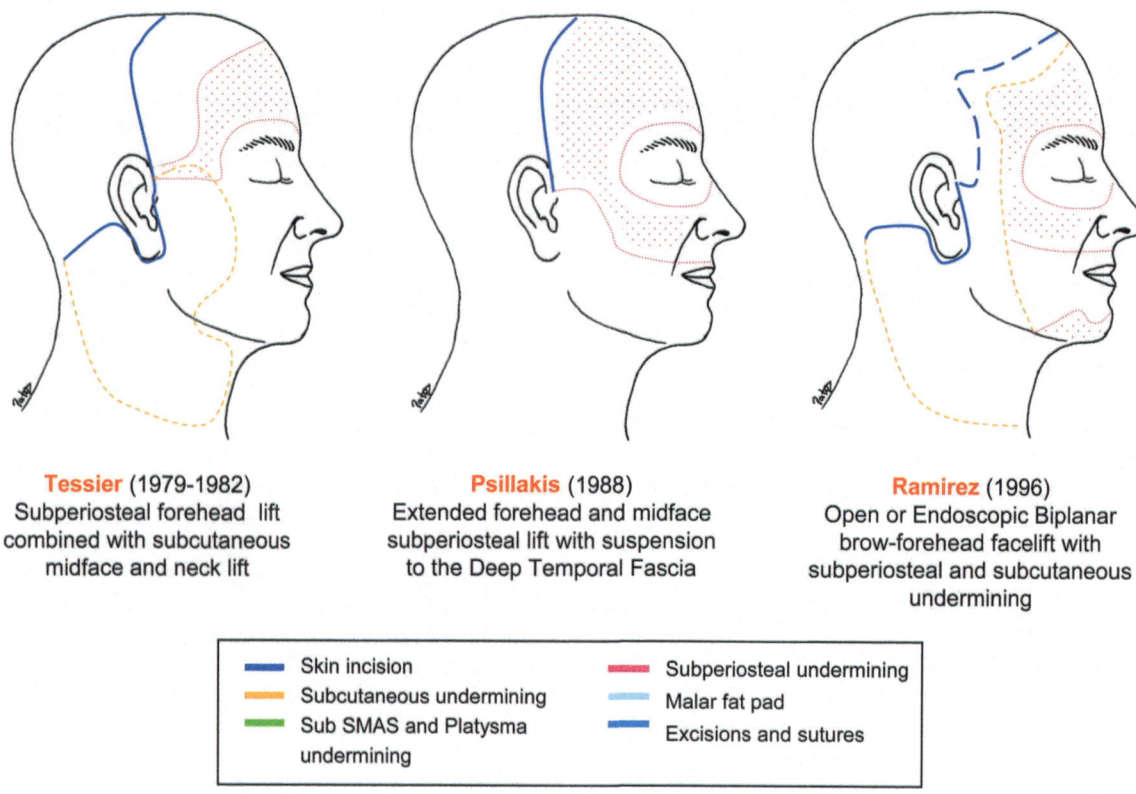

Tessier (1979-1982)
Subperiosteal forehead lift
combined with subcutaneous
midface and neck lift

Psillakis (1988)
Extended forehead and midface
subperiosteal lift with suspension
to the Deep Temporal Fascia

Ramirez (1996)
Open or Endoscopic Biplanar
brow-forehead facelift with
subperiosteal and subcutaneous
undermining

▬ Skin incision	▬ Subperiosteal undermining
▬ Subcutaneous undermining	▬ Malar fat pad
▬ Sub SMAS and Platysma undermining	▬ Excisions and sutures

Fig. 70.4 The subperiosteal facelift

temporal incision. Then they suspended and fixed the SOOF and the SMAS–galea flap to the deep temporal fascia. They stated that they observed 1% (n = 2) transient frontal branch injury and 0.5% (n = 1) infraorbital nerve paresthesia out of their 200 cases. Other complications included hematoma (1%), asymmetrical smile (1.5%), and facial tics (1%).

70.3.4
Management of the Nasolabial Fold and the Suspension Methods

Various methods have been proposed, including excision of the prominent fat, curettage of the nasolabial fat, and augmentation with dermal grafts [63]. Some authors performed suspension and fixation of the malar fat pad to improve the nasolabial fat [64–76]. Owsley [64] extended his sub-SMAS dissection underneath the malar fat pad to the level of the nasolabial fold. He then suspended and fixed this structure to the fascia over the malar eminence. Robbins et al. [65] used subcutaneous dissection through the line drawn from the lateral canthus to 1–2 cm lateral to the corner of the mouth to expose the malar fat pad and suspended this structure laterally. Collawn et al [66] and de la Torre et al. [67] combined these two methods to eliminate their disad-

vantages (lateral traction of both the skin and the fat pad in the method of Robbins et al. [65] and vertical suspension of the fat pad in spite of lateral traction of the skin in the method of Owsley [64]), exposing the malar fat pad through a subcutaneous dissection and lifting the skin and the malar fat vertically (Fig. 70.5).

Byrd and Andochick [68], in their "the deep temporal lift" method, performed a subgaleal approach to the forehead, a subfascial approach to the temporal region, a subperiosteal approach to the zygomatic arch, and a suborbicularis approach to the orbital rim. Then they suspended the midfacial periosteum and the superficial temporal fascia to the deep temporal fascia.

Finger [69], in contrast to the previous methods that enter the subperiosteal plane through the intraoral or temporal incisions, used the transmalar approach and presented his method as "transmalar subperiosteal midface lift with minimal skin and SMAS dissection." After the subcutaneous dissection, he entered the subperiosteal plane at the level of the zygoma just cephalad to the origins of the zygomaticus muscles by using a periosteal elevator. After subperiosteal undermining of the midface lateral to the infraorbital rim, he suspended and fixed the periosteum to the deep temporal fascia.

Sasaki and Cohen [70] used their specially designed percutaneous suspension sutures and fixed the malar fat to the deep temporal fascia. Sulamanidze et al. [71, 72] used a subcutaneous thread system for the same purpose. The authors, aiming at obtaining a long-lasting improvement, have begun to dissect deeper to the superficial temporal fascia and the malar fat pad via a short temporal incision and to fix the malar fat pad to the deep temporal fascia by using the threads.

Noone [73] combined the SMAS plication, modified lateral SMASectomy, and suspension of the malar fat methods. After subcutaneous dissection he suspended the malar fat pad to the deep temporal fascia by using a thin suture-passing instrument that penetrates the SMAS in a safe space (anterior third of the zygomatic arch) to avoid subcutaneous suspension suture.

Saylan [74, 75] suspended the platysma and the SMAS to the zygomatic arch periosteum with purse-string-type sutures after an S-shaped short scar and limited subcutaneous dissection. Tonnard et al. [76] later modified his method and introduced it as the minimal access cranial suspension—MACS lift. They performed skin incision between the caudal edge of the earlobe and the sideburn followed by limited subcutaneous dissection in the simple MACS technique. They also suspended the platysma and the SMAS, but in contrast to Saylan they did so to the deep temporal fascia. In the extended MACS technique, they continued the subcutaneous dissection over the malar fat pad, and then suspended this tissue with a third suspension suture (Fig. 70.5).

70.3.5
Endoscopic Face Lifting

Endoscopic surgery became available in plastic surgery later than other specialties owing to anatomic limitations Vasconez et al. [77] presented their experiences with endoscopic surgery in 1995. Isse [80–82] also presented his methods in 1990s.

Ramirez [83] classified the subperiosteal face-lifting methods into three types: open, endoscopic, and biplanar. He selected the method with respect to the needs of his patients. He performed open or endoscopic methods or their combination, and also added adjuvant techniques to treat fine wrinkles and solar damage [84–86]. He corrected the central oval face endoscopically and added laser skin therapy for patients in their 30s and 40s who did not need skin excision (the subperiosteal minimally invasive laser endoscopic technique–SMILE) [84–86]. For older patients who need improvement of the peripheral face as well as the central part, he added periauricular and cervical undermining to the procedure, followed by excision of the excess skin (biplanar endoscopic assisted mask face lift—BEAM) [86]. To manage severely damaged skin, he combined the BEAM procedure with laser treatment (biplanar endoscopic and laser assisted with immediate resurfacing—BELAIR) [86].

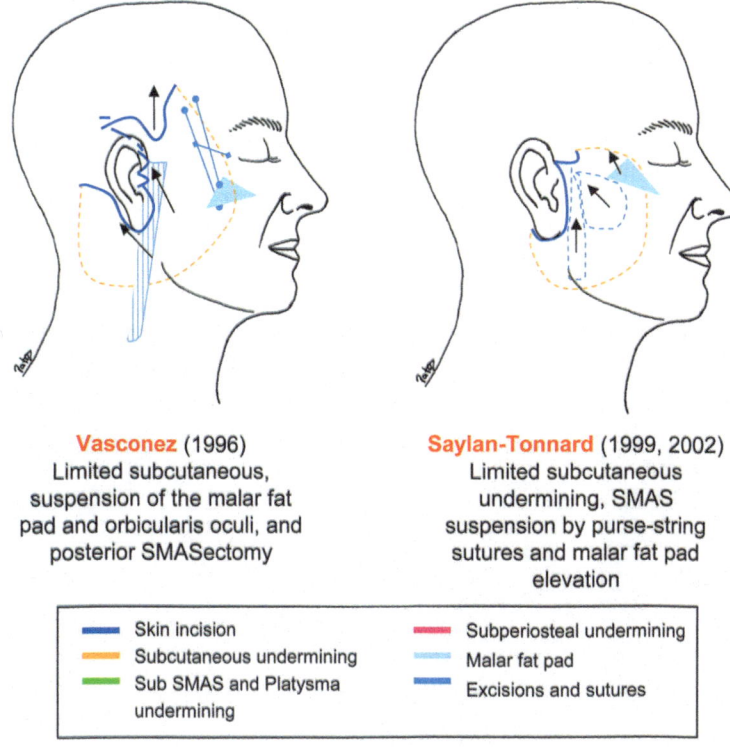

Vasconez (1996)
Limited subcutaneous, suspension of the malar fat pad and orbicularis oculi, and posterior SMASectomy

Saylan-Tonnard (1999, 2002)
Limited subcutaneous undermining, SMAS suspension by purse-string sutures and malar fat pad elevation

— Skin incision	— Subperiosteal undermining
— Subcutaneous undermining	— Malar fat pad
— Sub SMAS and Platysma undermining	— Excisions and sutures

Fig. 70.5 Suspension techniques

Ramirez [87] described his endoscopic method in detail (Fig. 70.6). After temporal slit incision, dissection is performed under endoscopic control. The temporoparietal fascia is undermined to a level 2–3 mm above the zygomatic arch, where dissection continues under the intermediate temporal fascia and the periosteum. Two thirds of, or occasionally all, the zygomatic arch is undermined subperiosteally entering the midface. After an inverted-V-shaped upper buccal sulcus incision, the maxilla and malar bones are exposed with subperiosteal dissection. Further dissection to undermine the lateral zygoma and the masseter fascia is carried out with the aid of the endocope. Dissection is carried on toward the inferior and lateral orbital rims, preserving the zygomaticofacial nerve. The intraorbital fat is fixated or repositioned when needed (i.e., severe tear-trough deformity) after the arcus marginalis has been released and the orbital septum has been transected through the intraoral incision. The excess intraorbital fat can also be excised transconjunctivally. Then the SOOF and the cheek fat are grasped with sutures that are passed through the temporal region. Bichat's fat pad is exposed through the superomedial wall of the buccal space with further dissection intraorally. It is released from the fascial layer of the wall of the buccal space to avoid the traction of the neurovascular structures. It is also grasped with a suture that is passed through the temporal region. All the sutures that are used to grasp the SOOF, cheek fat, and Bichat's fat as well as the superficial temporal fascia are suspended and sutured to the deep temporal fascia. He repaired the intraoral incision in a V–Y fashion for tensionless closure.

Ramirez [87] stated that his endoscopic method decreases the probability of nerve injury significantly when compared with the open techniques and that he had not observed lower-eyelid problem in his cases. Another advantage is that since the superficial tissues are not manipulated, it is possible to employ adjuvant techniques such as lipoinjection.

70.4
Periorbital Rejuvenation

Furnas [16, 17] recommended excision or plication of the orbicularis oculi followed by fixation to the lateral orbital periosteum to treat the festoons. He later gave up the plication method and proposed "the split level flap method." After subciliary incision, he developed a musculocutaneous flap medially and a cutaneous flap laterally. These planes intersected each other centrally, where they were divided by the orbicularis oculi muscle. He excised the excess skin and muscle laterally and fixed the tissues to the periosteum. He trimmed the fat off the skin flap to manage the malar mounds.

The orbicularis oculi muscle has been manipulated to improve the periorbital area. Skoog [36] in his two-layer shift method split, splayed out, and sutured the lateral portion of the muscle. Aston [88] also elevated the muscle, pulled it posterosuperiorly, and then fixed it to the superficial temporal fascia. Connell and Marten [89] reached the muscle after subcutaneous dissection and then transected the inferolateral part of the muscle before its suspension superoposteriorly. McCord et al. [90] considering that the sagging cheek fat is connected to the orbicularis oculi muscle with the SMAS elevated the midface by draping the muscle upward and fixed it to the lateral orbital perosteum or the deep temporal fascia.

70.5
The Authors' Preferred Method (Vasconez)

General anesthesia is preferred. After infiltration of local anesthetic, the incision starts 1–2 cm above the eyebrows and a few millimeters behind the temporal hairline, beveling anteriorly for subsequent hair growth (Fig. 70.6). It follows the contour of the sideburn and is then directed anteriorly toward the preauricular area, making an an-

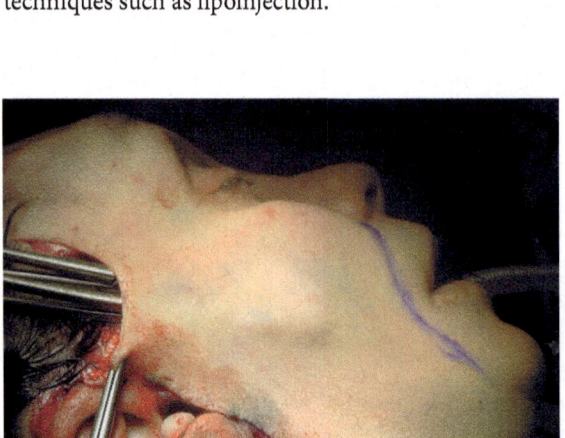
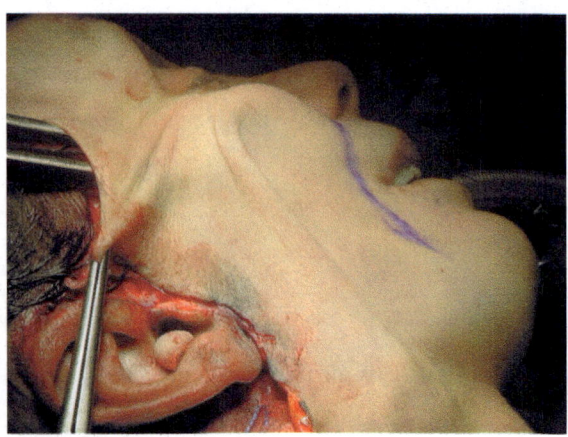

Fig. 70.6 Incision and endoscopic dissection

gle above the ear as a transverse wedge excision. This excision and subsequent repair with the sutures elevate the ear, which has descended with aging. A preauricular incision is made in a fashion of three crescents; each reflects the contour of the helix, tragus, and the lobule. Then the incision turns around the lobule, and extends upward on the concha just adjacent to the postauricular sulcus. At the level of the tragus, the incision is directed to the occipital scalp. The incisions can be tailored to the specific needs of the patients. For example, it is not necessary to extend the incision on the postauricular sulcus, if cervicoplasty is not part of the procedure.

Subcutaneous dissection is the next step. A thin skin flap that contains only a small amount of subcutaneous fat is undermined, keeping the dissection plane superficial to the malar fat pad and the orbicularis oculi muscle. This undermining is extended to the line that is drawn vertically downward starting at the lateral eyebrow and the lateral canthus. As a result, the attachments of the malar fat pad with the overlying skin between the aforementioned line and the nasolabial fold and with the underlying SMAS are preserved, which is important for elevation of the corner of the mouth with subsequent malar fat traction. The inferior extent of the dissection is tailored with respect to the needs of the patient. Should cervicoplasty be added to the procedure, the dissection extends below the mandible.

After subcutaneous dissection, the malar fat pad is grasped beyond the zygoma and traction is applied vertically, elevating the corner of the mouth, improving the nasolabial fold and the jowls. Figure 70.6 shows the intraoperative pictures demonstrating the difference for the midface: before and after the malar fat traction. The malar fat pad is fixed to the superficial temporal fascia with 3-0 Monocryl sutures at the level of the hairline incision to avoid the frontal motor branch. The honeycomb fibrous network content of the malar fat pad [11, 12] makes this fixation stable enough. The lateral preseptal orbicularis oculi muscle is also grasped and traction is applied superolaterally. It is also fixed to the superficial temporal fascia.

SMASectomy is usually added to the procedure, especially when improvement of the neck and the jawline is desired. Excision starts at the arch level and extends

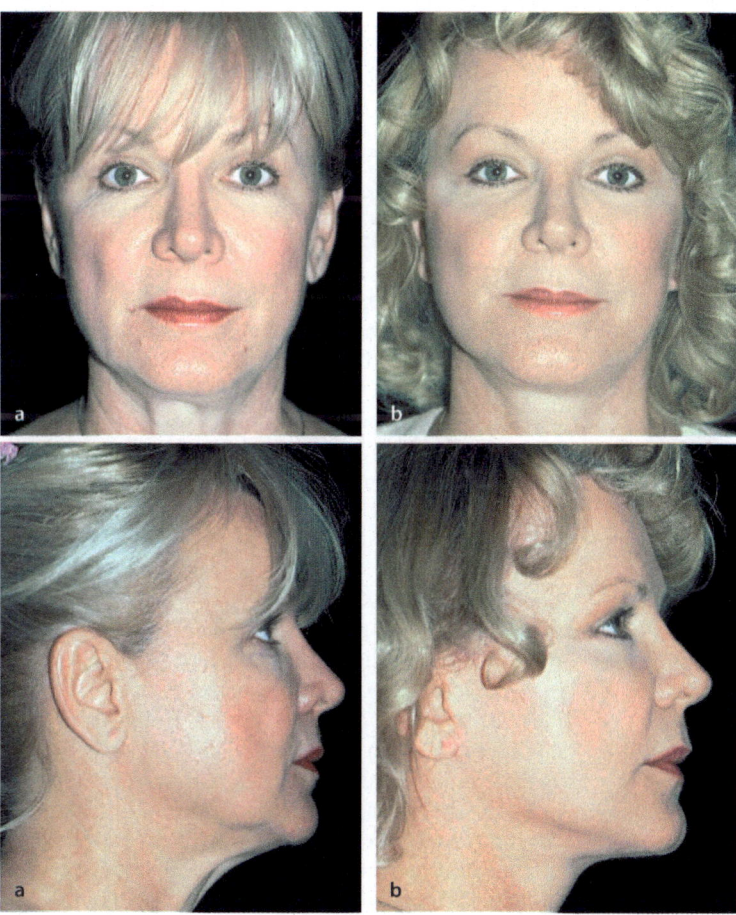

Fig. 70.7 a Preoperatively. **b** Postoperatively

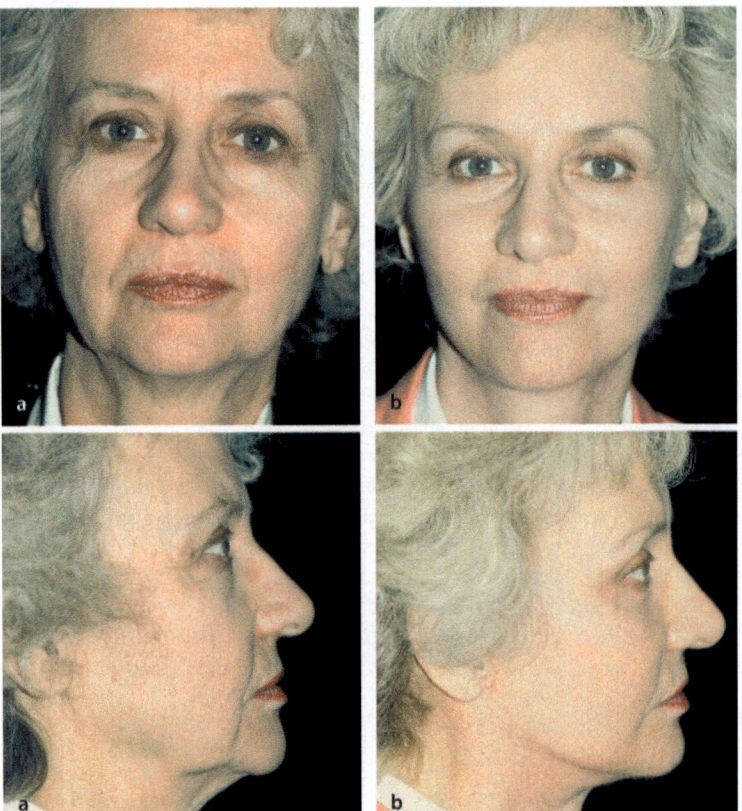

Fig. 70.8 **a** Preoperatively. **b** Postoperatively

inferoposteriorly toward the neck. A meticulous dissection is important to avoid injury of the external jugular vein. The SMAS is then pulled superoposteriorly and fixed with 3-0 Monocryl sutures. The suture below the ear is placed posteriorly to avoid the postauricular nerve.

Vertical traction is applied on the skin flap at the end of the procedure. The excess skin is excised very carefully to avoid tight closure. Because of malar fat suspension the skin can be draped and tailored without tension.

Figures 70.7 and 70.8 show preoperative and postoperative patients who underwent cervicofacial lifting and blepharoplasty operations.

De Cordier et al. [18] reviewed 472 cases with midface lifting and malar fat elevation between the years 1994 and 2000 at the University of Alabama at Birmingham. Concomitant procedures in descending order were SMAS excision and tightening (93%, $n = 437$), submental lipectomy and platysma plication (87%, $n = 410$), forehead lift (72%, $n = 339$), lower blepharoplasty (51%, $n = 243$), upper blepharoplasty (45%, $n = 214$), and limited SMAS excision and plication (4%, $n = 19$).

They classified the undesirable outcomes as malpositioned malar fat pads (3%, $n = 14$), skin dimpling (2.8%, $n = 13$), persistent marionette lines (2.1%, $n = 10$), asymmetric nasolabial folds (1.9%, $n = 9$), and persistent jowl lines (0.6%, $n = 3$).

The most common postoperative complication was scar hypertrophy (postauricular 10.2%, $n = 48$, and preauricular 5.1%, $n = 24$). Other complications in descending order were hematoma (7%, $n = 33$), facial telangiectasias (3.6%, $n = 17$), stitch abscess (3.2%, $n = 15$), neck hyperpigmentation (2.8%, $n = 13$), skin necrosis (postauricular 1.7%, $n = 8$, and preauricular 1.1%, $n = 5$), preauricular dysesthesia (0.6%, $n = 3$), temporal alopecia (0.6%, $n = 3$), and pixie ear (0.2%, $n = 1$). Of these complications in only one case was the hematoma significant enough to warrant drainage in the operating room. Skin necrosis was insignificant in all cases that healed secondarily. They observed temporary facial nerve weakness in 16 cases (3.4%), frontal and mandibular branches in seven cases (1.5%) for each, and zygomatic branch and buccal branches in one case (0.2%) for each. There was no ectropion problem in cases with concomitant lower blepharoplasty. They commented that performing the conservative blepharoplasty prior to the midface lifting and frost sutures avoids this complication.

References

1. Stuzin JM, Baker TJ, Gordon HL. The relationship of the superficial and deep facial fascias: relevance to rhytidectomy and aging. Plast Reconstr Surg 1992;89(3):441–449

2. Mitz V, Peyronie M. The superficial musculo-aponeurotic system (SMAS) in the parotid and cheek area. Plast Reconstr Surg 1976;58(1):80–88

3. Whetzel TP, Mathes SJ. Arterial anatomy of the face: an analysis of vascular territories and perforating cutaneous vessels. Plast Reconstr Surg 1992;89(4):591–603

4. Ozerdem OR, Vasconez LO, de la Torre J. Upper face-lifting. Facial Plast Surg Clin North Am 2006;14(3):159–165

5. Heinrichs HL, Kaidi A. Subperiosteal face lift: a 200-case, 4-year review. Plast Reconstr Surg 1998;102(3):843–855.

6. Ramirez OM, Robertson KM. Update in endoscopic rejuvenation. Facial Plast Surg Clin North Am 2002;10(1):37–51

7. Stuzin JM, Wagstrom L, Kawamato H, Wolfe SA. Anatomy of the frontal branch of the facial nerve: the significance of the temporal fat pad. Plast Reconstr Surg 1989;83(2):265–271

8. Stuzin JM, Wagstrom L, Kawamoto HK, Baker TJ, Wolfe SA. The anatomy and clinical applications of the buccal fat pad. Plast Reconstr Surg 1990;85(1):29–37

9. Ruess W, Owsley JQ. The anatomy of the skin and fascial layers of the face in aesthetic surgery. Clin Plast Surg 1987;14(4):677–682

10. Jost G, Levet Y. Parotid fascia and face lifting: a critical evaluation of the SMAS concept. Plast Reconstr Surg 1984;74(1):42–51

11. Yousif NJ, Gosain A, Matloub HS, Sanger, JR, Madiedo, G, Larson DL. The nasolabial fold: an anatomic and histologic reappraisal. Plast Reconstr Surg 1994;93(1):60–69

12. Yousif NJ, Mendelson BC. Anatomy of the midface. Clin Plast Surg 1995;22(2):227–240

13. Furnas DW. The retaining ligaments of the cheek. Plast Reconstr Surg 1989;83(1):11–16

14. Peterson RA, Johnston DL. Facile identification of the facial nerve branches. Clin Plast Surg 1987;14(4):785–788

15. Hamra ST. The deep-plane rhytidectomy. Plast Reconstr Surg 1990;86(1):53–61

16. Furnas DW. Festoons of orbicularis muscle as a cause of baggy eyelids. Plast Reconstr Surg 1978;61(4):540–546

17. Furnas DW. Festoons, mounds, and bags of the eyelids and cheek. Clin Plast Surg 1993;20(2):367–385

18. De Cordier BC, de la Torre JI, Al-Hakeem MS, Rosenberg, LZ, Costa-Ferreira, A, Gardner, PM, Fix, RJ, Vasconez, LO. Rejuvenation of the midface by elevating the malar fat pad: review of technique, cases, and complications. Plast Reconstr Surg 2002;110(6):1526–1536

19. Aiache A, Ramirez OM. The suborbicularis oculi fat pads: an anatomic and clinical study. Plast Reconstr Surg 1995;95(1):37–42

20. Jelks GW, Jelks EB. The influence of orbital and eyelid anatomy on the palpebral aperture. Clin Plast Surg 1991;18(1):183–195

21. Yousif NJ. Changes of the midface with age. Clin Plast Surg 1995;22(2):213–226

22. Hamra ST. Composite rhytidectomy. Plast Reconstr Surg 1992;90(1):1–13

23. Goldberg RA, McCann JD, Fiaschetti D, Ben Simon GJ. What causes eyelid bags? Analysis of 114 consecutive patients. Plast Reconstr Surg 2005;115(5):1395–1402

24. Gamboa-Bobadilla M, Ozerdem OR, Vasconez LO. Adjunctive surgical procedures to improve the facelift results. In: Reoperative Aesthetic & Reconstructive Plastic Surgery, Grotting JC (Ed.), Quality Medical Publishing, St. Louis, Missouri 2006:347–376

25. Rees TD, Aston SJ. Blepharoplasty and facialplasty. In: McCarthy JG (Ed.), Plastic Surgery, Philadelphia, Saunders 1990:2320–2415

26. Rees TD. Blepharoplasty. In: Rees TD (Ed.), Aesthetic Plastic Surgery, Philadelphia, Saunders 1980:459–582

27. Rogers BO. A brief history of cosmetic surgery. Surg Clin North Am 1971;51(2):265–288

28. Rogers BO. A chronologic history of cosmetic surgery. Bull N Y Acad Med 1971;47(3):265–302

29. Mulliken JB. Biographical sketch of Charles Conrad Miller, "featural surgeon". Plast Reconstr Surg 1977;59(2):175–184

30. Gonzales-Ulloa M. The history of rhytidectomy. Aesthet Plast Surg 1980;4:1–45

31. Paul MD. The evolution of the brow lift in aesthetic plastic surgery. Plast Reconstr Surg 2001;108(5):1409–1424

32. May H. Erich Lexer, a biographical sketch. Plast Reconstr Surg 1962;29:141–152

33. Rogers BO. The development of aesthetic plastic surgery: a history. Aesthet Plast Surg 1976;1:3–24

34. Regnault P, Stephenson KL. Dr. Suzanne Noël. First woman to do aesthetic surgery. Plast Reconstr Surg 1971;48(2):133–138

35. Gonzales-Ulloa M. Facial wrinkles. Integral elimination. Plast Reconstr Surg 1962;29:658–673

36. Skoog T. Plastic Surgery—New Methods and Refinements. Philadelphia, Saunders 1974

37. Owsley JQ. Platysma-fascial rhytidectomy: a preliminary report. Plast Reconstr Surg 1977;60(6):843–850

38. Lemmon ML, Hamra ST. Skoog rhytidectomy: a five-year experience with 577 patients. Plast Reconstr Surg. 1980;65(3):283–297

39. Hamra ST. The tri-plane face lift dissection. Ann Plast Surg 1984;12(3):268–274

40. Hamra ST. Repositioning the orbicularis oculi muscle in the composite rhytidectomy. Plast Reconstr Surg 1992;90(1):14–22

41. Hamra ST. Composite rhytidectomy. Finesse and refinements in technique. Clin Plast Surg 1997;24(2):337–346

42. Hamra ST. Arcus marginalis release and orbital fat preservation in midface rejuvenation. Plast Reconstr Surg 1995;96(2):354–362

43. Hamra ST. Discussion. For "Arterial anatomy of the face: an analysis of vascular territories and perforating cutaneous vessels" by Whetzel TP, Mathes SJ. Plast

Reconstr Surg 1992;89(4):591-603. Plast Reconstr Surg 1992;89(4):604–605

44. Connell BF, Semlacher R. Contemporary deep layer facial rejuvenation. Plast Reconstr Surg 1997;100(6):1513–1523

45. Stuzin JM, Baker TJ, Gordon HL, Baker TM. Extended SMAS dissection as an approach to midface rejuvenation. Clin Plast Surg 1995;22(2):295–311

46. Stuzin JM, Baker TJ, Baker TM. Refinements in face lifting: enhanced facial contour using vicryl mesh incorporated into SMAS fixation. Plast Reconstr Surg. 2000;105(1):290–301

47. Baker D. Rhytidectomy with lateral SMASectomy. Facial Plast Surg 2000;16(3):209–213

48. Baker D. Lateral SMASectomy. Plast Reconstr Surg. 1997;100(2):509–513

49. Massiha H. Short-scar face lift with extended SMAS platysma dissection and lifting and limited skin undermining. Plast Reconstr Surg 2003;112(2):663–669

50. Tessier P. Subperiosteal face-lift. Ann Chir Plast Esthet 1989;34(3):193–197

51. Hinderer UT, Urriolagoitia F, Vildosola R. The blepharo-periorbitoplasty: Anatomical basis. Ann Plast Surg 1987;18(5):437–453

52. Psillakis JM, Rumley TO, Camargos A. Subperiosteal approach as an improved concept for correction of the aging face. Plast Reconstr Surg 1988;82(3):383–394

53. Ortiz-Monasterio, F. Aesthetic surgery of the facial skeleton: The forehead. Clin Plast Surg 1991;18(1):19–27

54. Ortiz Monasterio, F, Barrera G, Olmedo A. The coronal incision in rhytidectomy—the brow lift. Clin Plast Surg 1978;5(1):167–179

55. Paul MD, Calvert JW, Evans GR. The evolution of the midface lift in aesthetic plastic surgery. Plast Reconstr Surg 2006;117(6):1809–1827

56. Hester TR, Codner MA, McCord CD. The "centrofacial" approach for correction of facial aging using the transblepharoplasty subperiosteal cheek lift. Aesthet Surg J 1996;16:51–58

57. Hester TR, Codner MA, McCord C, Nahai F, Gianopoulos A. Evolution of technique of the direct transblepharoplasty approach for the correction of lower lid and midfacial aging: maximizing results and minimizing complications in a 5-year experience. Plast Reconstr Surg 2000;105(1):393–406

58. Gunter JP, Hackney FL. A simplified transblepharoplasty subperiosteal cheek lift. Plast Reconstr Surg 1999;103(7):2029–2035

59. Hobar PC, Flood J. Subperiosteal rejuvenation of the midface and periorbital area: a simplified approach. Plast Reconstr Surg 1999;104(3):842–851

60. Ramirez OM, Maillard GF, Musolas A. The extended subperiosteal facelift: a definitive soft-tissue remodeling for facial rejuvenation. Plast Reconstr Surg 1991;88(2):227–236

61. Ortiz-Monasterio F. Discussion: The extended subperiosteal facelift: A definitive soft-tissue remodeling for facial rejuvenation. By Ramirez OM, Maillard GF, Musolas A. Plast Reconstr Surg 1991;88(2):227–236. Plast Reconstr Surg 1991;88(2):237–238

62. Heinrichs HL, Kaidi AA. Subperiosteal face lift: a 200-case, 4-year review. Plast Reconstr Surg 1998;102(3):843–855

63. Larson DL. An historical glimpse of the evolution of rhytidectomy. Clin Plast Surg 1995;22(2):207–212

64. Owsley JQ. Lifting the malar fat pad for correction of prominent nasolabial folds. Plast Reconstr Surg 1993;91(3):463–474

65. Robbins LB, Brothers DB, Marshall DM. Anterior SMAS plication for the treatment of prominent nasomandibular folds and restoration of normal cheek contour. Plast Reconstr Surg 1995;96(6):1279–1287

66. Collawn SS, Vasconez LO, Gamboa M et al. Subcutaneous approach for elevation of the malar fat pad through a pre-hairline incision. Plast Reconstr Surg 1996;97(4):836–841

67. de la Torre JI, Rosenberg LZ, De Cordier BC, Gardner PM, Fix RJ, Vasconez LO. Clinical analysis of malar fat pad re-elevation. Ann Plast Surg 2003;50(3):244–248

68. Byrd HS, Andochick SE. The deep temporal lift: a multiplanar, lateral brow, temporal, and upper face lift. Plast Reconstr Surg 1996;97(5):928–937

69. Finger ER. A 5-year study of the transmalar subperiosteal midface lift with minimal skin and superficial musculoaponeurotic system dissection: a durable, natural-appearing lift with less surgery and recovery time. Plast Reconstr Surg 2001;107(5):1273–1283

70. Sasaki GH, Cohen AT. Meloplication of the malar fat pads by percutaneous cable-suture technique for midface rejuvenation: outcome study (392 cases, 6 years' experience). Plast Reconstr Surg 2002;110(2):635–654

71. Sulamanidze MA, Fournier PF, Paikidze TK, Saulamanidze,GM. Removal of facial soft tissue ptosis with special threads. Dermatol Surg 2002;28(5):367–371

72. Sulamanidze MA, Paikidze TK, Sulemanidze GM. Facial lifting with "APTOS" threads: featherlift. Otolaryngol Clin North Am 2005;38(5):1109–1117

73. Noone RB. Suture suspension malarplasty with SMAS plication and modified SMASectomy: a simplified approach to midface lifting. Plast Reconstr Surg 2006;117(3):792–803

74. Saylan Z. The S-lift: Less is more. Aesthet Surg J 1999;19:406

75. Saylan Z. Purse string-formed plication of the SMAS with fixation to the zygomatic bone. Plast Reconstr Surg 2002;110(2):667–671

76. Tonnard P, Verpaele A, Monstrey S, Van Landuyt K, Blondeel P, Hamdi M, Matton G. Minimal access cranial suspension lift: A modified S-lift. Plast Reconstr Surg 2002;109(6):2074–2086

77. Vasconez LO, Core GB, Oslin B. Endoscopy in plastic surgery. An overview. Clin Plast Surg 1995;22(4):585–589

78. Howard PS, Gardner PM, Vasconez LO, Core GB. Complications in endoscopic plastic surgery. Clin Plast Surg 1995;22(4):791–796

79. Core GB, Vasconez LO, Graham HD 3rd. Endoscopic browlift. Clin Plast Surg 1995;22(4):619–631

80. Isse NG. Endoscopic facial rejuvenation: endoforehead, the functional lift. Case reports. Aesthet Plast Surg 1994;18:21–29

81. Isse NG. Endoscopic forehead lift. Evolution and update. Clin Plast Surg 1995;22(4):661–673

82. Isse NG. Endoscopic facial rejuvenation. Clin Plast Surg 1997;24(2):213–231

83. Ramirez OM. Classification of facial rejuvenation techniques based on the subperiosteal approach and ancillary procedures. Plast Reconstr Surg 1996;97(1):45–55

84. Ramirez OM. Endoscopic subperiosteal browlift and facelift. Plast Surg Clin 1995;22(2):639–660

85. Ramirez OM. High-tech facelift. Aesthet Plast Surg 1998;22(5):318–328

86. Ramirez OM, Pozner JN. Subperiosteal minimally invasive laser endoscopic rhytidectomy: the SMILE facelift. Aesthet Plast Surg 1996;20(6):463–470

87. Ramirez OM. Three-dimensional endoscopic midface enhancement: a personal quest for the ideal cheek rejuvenation. Plast Reconstr Surg 2002;109(1):329–340

88. Aston JA. Orbicularis oculi muscle flaps: a technique to reduce crow's feet and lateral canthal skin folds. Plast Reconstr Surg 1980;65(2):206–216

89. Connell BF, Marten TJ. Surgical correction of the Crow's deformity. Clin Plast Surg 1993;20(2):295–302

90. McCord C, Codner, MA, Hester TR. Redraping the inferior orbicularis arc. Plast Reconstr Surg 1998;102(7):2471–2479

CHAPTER 71

Section of the Frenulum of the Upper Lip

71

Pierre F. Fournier

71.1
Introduction

The white portion of the upper lip may have a short distance between the Cupid bow and the opening of nostrils. The upper teeth are seen very little during a smile or at rest. A moderate but notable very noticeable elongation may be obtained by a section of the frenulum (Fig. 71.1) of the upper lip on all its length.

71.2
Technique

Local anaesthesia (1% lidocaine with 1:200,000 epinephrine) is used by injection under the frenulum. The frenulum is sectioned on all its length with a no. 11 blade. Following hemostasis the lip is left nonsutured.

71.3
Complications

During the healing period there may be slight discomfort.

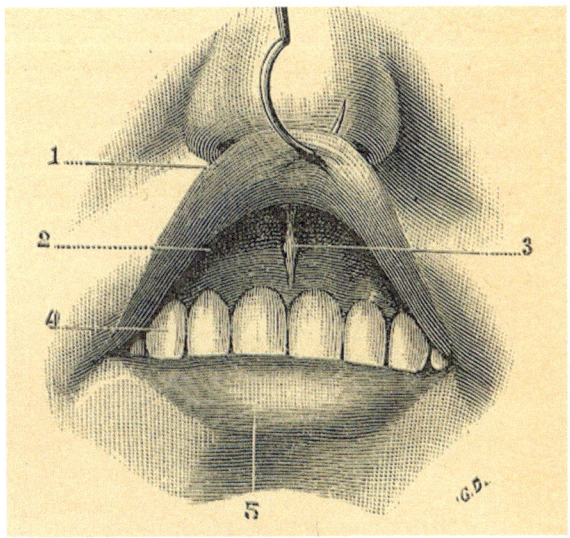

Fig. 70.1 Frenulum (3)

71.4
Results

The healing occurs after 2 weeks and there is always a visible improvement of the surface of this upper white lip as well of its height, during the smile with more teeth surface visible (Fig. 71.2).

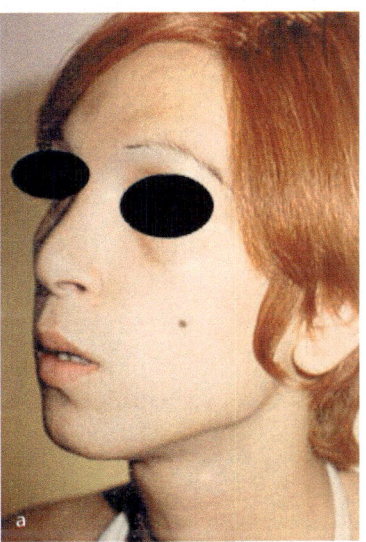

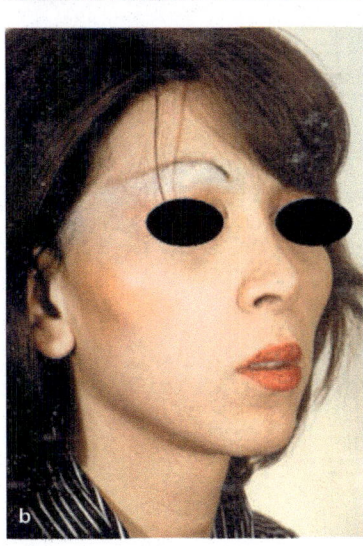

Fig. 70.2 a Preoperatively. **b** Postoperative sectioning of the frenulum

71.5
Conclusion

A Z-plasty of the frenulum allows elongation of the upper lip [1].

Reference

1. de Souza Pinto, E.B.: Importance of the depressor septi nasi muscle in rhinoplasty: Anatomic study and clinical application. Plast Reconstr Surg 2000;105(1):385–388

CHAPTER 72

Surgical Treatment of the Senile Upper Lip 72

Jorge Orlando Guerrissi

72.1
Introduction

The tissue alterations that appear as a consequence of the aging face affect not only the lids, cheek, and the forehead but also the upper lip [1, 2]. The lengthening and the shape deformities of the upper lip are not only the most important senile alterations but are also the most evident aesthetic senile changes [3].

It is necessary to analyze the youthful lip to understand the changes that occur in the aged lip. In the juvenile lip, the vermilion border forms a soft "M" whose two peaks correspond to philtral ridges. The concavity of the youthful lip turns into convexity and elongation in the old one. Also, there is a central full mass, the midline tubercle. The height of the upper lip at its midline is about 7–8 mm, the two peaks increasing to between 9 and 10 mm.

The vermilion border follows an S-shaped curve or an almost straight line toward the corner of the mouth [3] . The following alterations may appear in the upper lip in the process of aging (Fig. 72.1):

1. Vertical wrinkles
2. Reduction in height of the vermilion border with lengthening of the skin area of the lip
3. Disappearance of Cupid's bow
4. The remaining vermilion border losing not only height but also youth and grace

Relaxation of the soft facial tissue such as the skin, muscle and subcutaneous tissue, aponeurosis and the atrophy of the maxilla are the causes of the aesthetic deformities in the senile upper lip. These alterations in the height and volume of the upper lip are usually the consequence of aging, but they may appear in youth as a consequence of hereditary factors.

With aging, the pouting and seductive lips of youth are converted to thin lips and much bulk disappears. A special senile change is the mimetic wrinkles, which are due to contraction of the superficial fibers of the orbicularis oris muscle [4].

This chapter describes the surgical technique for correcting the lengthening and the thickening of the vermilion, reshaping the border and Cupid's bow, and eliminating the wrinkles in the upper lip.

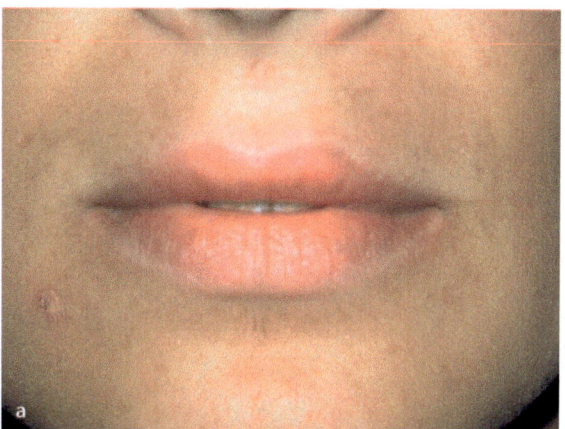
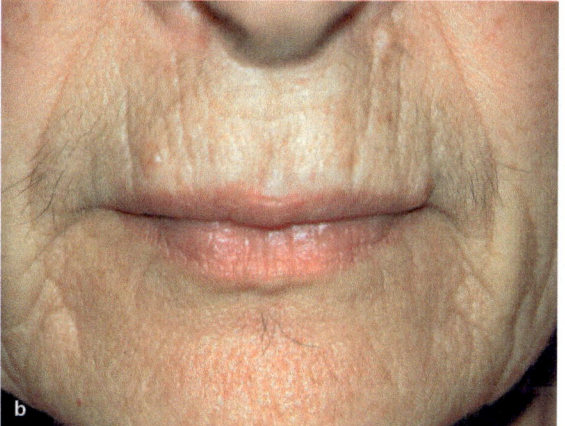

Fig. 72.1 **a** Proportions and size of the juvenile lip. **b** Changes in the senile lip: elongation of the skin area, decrease in the height of the vermilion and vertical wrinkles

72.2
Materials and Methods

From 1998 to 2002, 56 women, ranging in age from 40 to 73 years, were treated at the Service of Plastic Surgery of Argerich Hospital, Buenos Aires, Argentina, for aesthetic senile changes on the upper lip. The most important senile deformities were the decrease of the height of the vermilion and Cupid's bow alteration in 25 patients (44.6%), fine vertical wrinkles in ten patients

(17.8%), loss of lip volume in ten patients (17.8%) and a combination of deformities in 11 patients (19.8%).

Treatment of these aesthetic lip changes was basically performed by means of different techniques:

1. Lip contouring and Cupid's bow reconstruction.
2. Dermabrasion.
3. Lip augmentation with fat injection, dermal-fat graft, Gore-Tex and AlloDerm implants.

In 11 patients who presented both loss of height of the vermilion and Cupid's bow and vertical wrinkles, the surgical technique also permitted the elimination of vertical wrinkles of the upper lip.

72.3
Surgical Technique

The surgical technique has three fundamental steps: (1) preoperative planning, (2) surgical technique and (3) postoperative control.

72.3.1
Preoperative Planning

In the preoperative planning, it is important to identify the cardinal points of the upper lip. The existing and the new vermilion border must be marked (Fig. 72.2). The new peaks should be placed a few millimeters above the existing ones. Usually, the new peaks are placed 2–4 mm higher than the original ones. An additional 1 mm is added for overcorrection, since the new vermilion border will always droop downward by about 1–1.5 mm in 6 months' time [5]. The lateral limits of the incision need to extend beyond the commissure.

72.3.2
Perioperative Treatment

Either local or general anesthesia may be used. In either case it is necessary to infiltrate the operating field with 2% lidocaine with epinephrine because this produces not only local anesthesia but also constriction of the minor arterial vessels.

A strip of the skin on the vermilion border is deepithelialized (Fig. 72.3). The remaining dermal flap will then be buried in the pocket, with this procedure being performed by undermining the skin of the upper lip (Fig. 72.4). The flap is fixed to the orbicularis oris muscle by means of fine resorbable sutures (Fig. 72.5).

The dermal flap has the following advantages:

1. Inclusion under the skin–vermilion union produces a more bulbous and youthful appearance of the lip.
2. The flap could act like a "barrier" interposing between the skin and the orbicularis oris muscle, avoiding skin wrinkles when muscle contraction is produced.
3. It permits firm fixation of the new vermilion.

As the fresh vermilion edge is advanced up into its new position, the central point of the lip tilts forward [5–7]. The incision is closed by means of interrupted 5-0 or 6-0 silk or nylon sutures and they are removed after 7 days (Fig. 72.6).

72.3.3
Postoperative Control

The postoperative period permits a strict evaluation not only of the changes achieved but also of scar evolution. Lipstick is used in the immediate postoperative period because makeup enhances the beauty of the new lip.

This technique was utilized in 36 patients but the follow-up was in 26 patients (90%) and ranged from 1 to 5 years. All 26 patients were evaluated objectively for

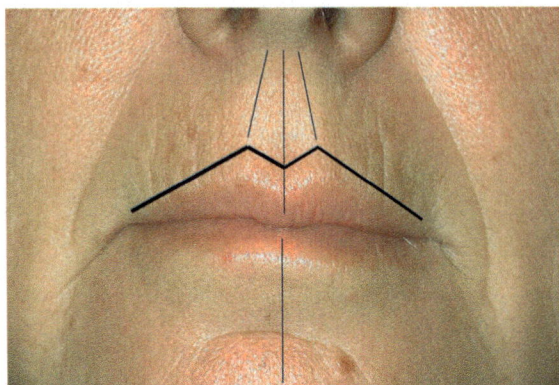

Fig. 72.2 The exact drawing of the new vermilion border is the principal preoperative step

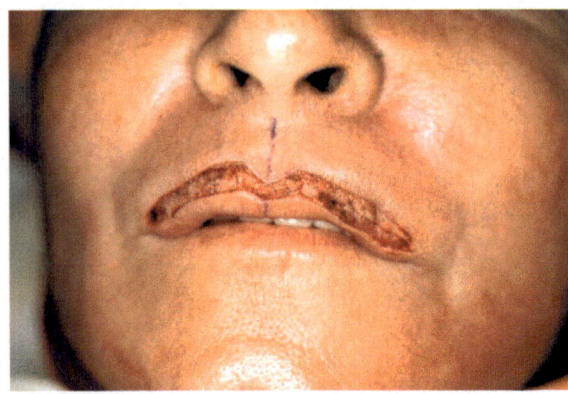

Fig. 72.3 A strip of the skin on the vermilion border is deepithelialized

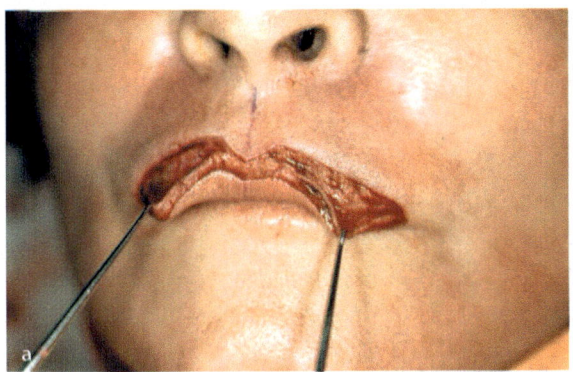

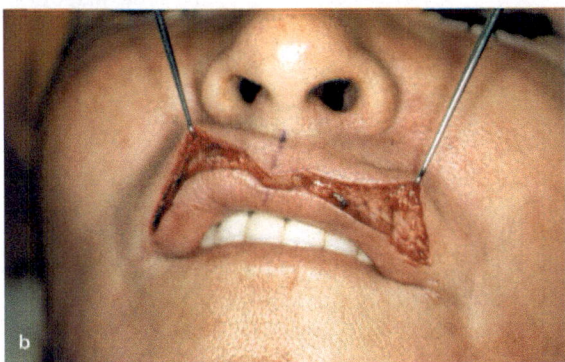

Fig. 72.4 a The dermal flap of the resected skin on the vermilion border is raised. **b** It will be buried in the undermined area of the skin of the upper lip

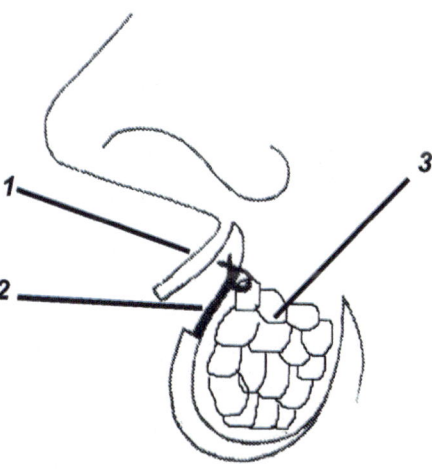

Fig. 72.5 The pocket performed under skin of the lip (*1*) is fixed the dermal flap (*2*), which is fixed to the orbicularis oris muscle (*3*)

symmetry of the vermilion border, thickening of the lip, attractive curved Cupid's bow and quality of mouth and lip movements, and subjectively as to their own opinion (Figs. 72.7, 72.8).

Inflammatory milia and cicatricial bridge were the most common postoperative complications; six patients

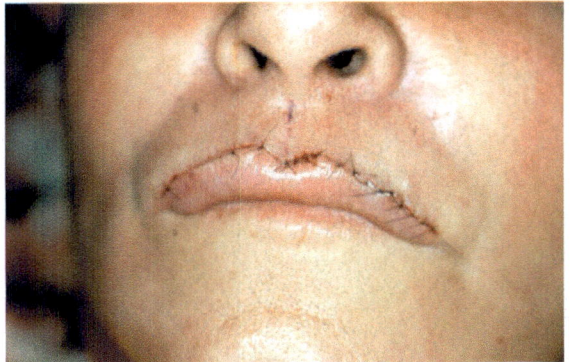

Fig. 72.6 A 6-0 silk suture is used to close the incision

(10.7%) presented a cicatricial bridge with light skin retraction at the vermilion border and lip movement difficulties. Both complications were temporary and self-resolving and resolved in 2–3 months after surgery.

The results were satisfactory to the author and all patients.

72.4 Dermabrasion

No chemical peeling was performed in the perioral area. Dermabrasion was more predictable in the author's experience. Dermabrasion was performed with sandpaper used manually with different grain sizes. The hand of the surgeon permitted recognition of the depth of the surgical maneuvers and level of the abrasion.

This technique was applied to 26 patients. In ten patients (17.8%) only dermabrasion was used and in 16 patients (82.2%) the surgical technique of lip and Cupid's bow reconstruction was utilized.

Hypopigmentation of the skin was the complication most frequently observed but 6–9 weeks after surgery the preoperative color of the skin returned.

72.5 Augmentation of the Upper Lip

In the treatment of senile upper lip one of the most important goals is to restore the bulk of the upper lip and to enhance the protrusion. Different augmentation techniques can be used [8]:
1. Surgical rearrangement of tissue
2. Fat injection
3. Dermal fat graft, AlloDerm and Gore-Tex

Ten patients (17.8%) were treated with the technique based on the use of a dermal flap buried in the undermined skin of the upper lip and the results were aesthetically satisfactory.

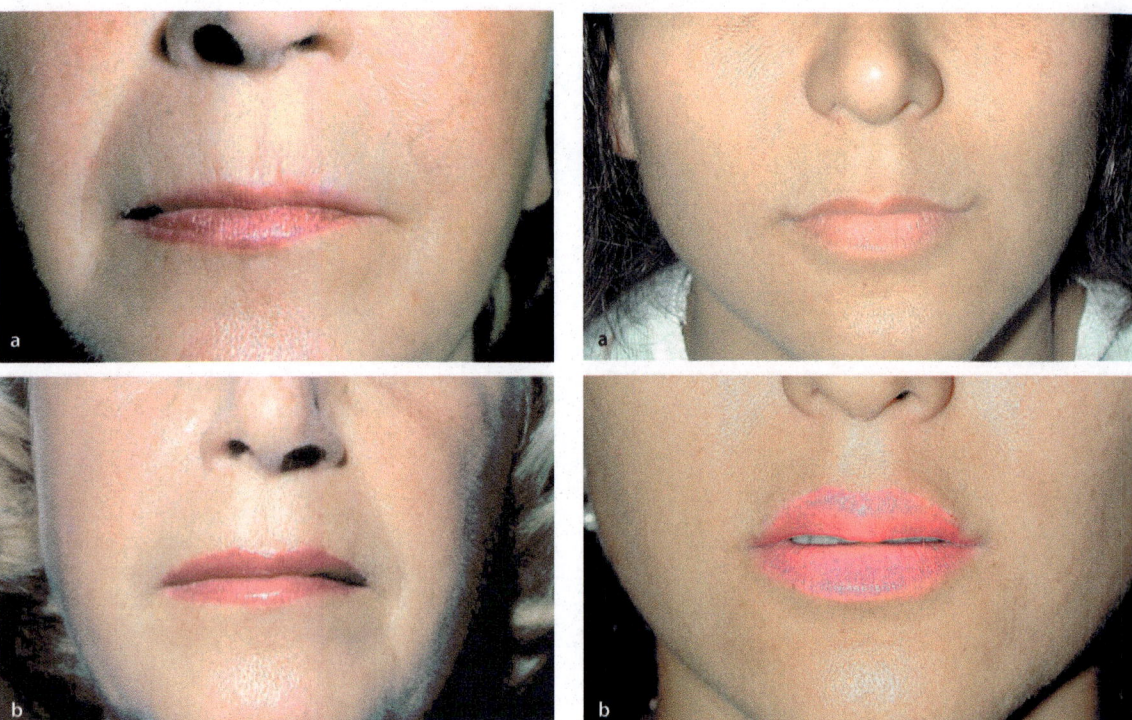

Fig. 72.7 **a** Preoperative senile changes in the upper lip. **b** Four-year postoperative view

Fig. 72.8 **a** Preoperatively showing lip changes. **b** Eight months postoperatively

The material used for lip augmentation was fat aspirated from abdomen or thigh areas; this filler material was only used in four cases and after surgical treatment in two cases.

When the simultaneous lip augmentation technique was used, the materials were placed under both the vermilion border and the dermal flap.

Patient satisfaction was higher when the injection of filler was made after reshaping the vermilion. This gave a more youthful and appealing appearance by defining the red bow.

72.6
Discussion

Diverse surgical techniques have been described for the correction of aesthetic deformities of the upper lip produced not only by aging but also by sequelae of congenital malformations, trauma or tumor resection. The inner flaps, usually the V–Y advancement flaps, or Z-plasty are the most common [9].

In 1932, Gillies and Kilner [6] described an operation for the correction of secondary deformities in unilateral harelip with the following steps: (1) scar resection and (2) new Cupid's bow. Meyer and Rheims [7] performed correction of the aged upper lip by means of

skin resection by undermining of the skin and mucosa and placing a fascial graft under the advanced mucosal membrane. Di Giuseppe [10], in 1988, enhanced the projection of the upper lip by inserting a strip of dermis and fat through the intramuscular plane.

Delerm and Elbaz [11] and Farmand and Seiler [12] proposed different endobuccal approaches for modification of both the upper lip and the floor of the nasal fossa.

The surgical technique described in 1993 by Guerrissi and Sanchez Izquierdo [13] allows correction of the senile changes that occur in the upper lip. It has minimal morbidity and few complications, and most of these are temporary and self-resolved. In our series, only six patients (10.7%) had complications. The scar is hidden in the natural new vermilion border and can be covered easily with the use of lipstick. Most patients accept a youthful lip with a thin scar that may be camouflaged by makeup. The procedure must have a planned and exact surgical technique. To prevent an asymmetrical incision and other complications; the operation must be performed patiently. The surgical procedure can not only correct alterations of the vermilion border but can also eliminate 2–4 mm of the lower portion of the vertical wrinkles near the vermilion border.

One of the more evident stigmata of the senile lip is the increase in the skin area and the consequent lip elongation. These problems can be corrected with the skin resection.

The distance between the nose and vermilion border is shortened. The postoperative use of lipstick is important, because the correctly delineated vermilion border contributes to better results.

Resurfacing techniques improved only the wrinkling, which is part of the lip's aging process. When deep dermabrasion permitted the elimination of 100% of the wrinkling, it was accompanied by the possibility of hypopigmentation and scarring. The area to be dermabraded usually includes from the base of the nose to the skin of the chin, and laterally beyond each nasolabial fold; some patients require only treatment of the upper lip. The deeper dermabrasion should be performed by dermabrading as deeply as necessary to eliminate wrinkles; care should be taken to stretch the skin. Once the redness has disappeared, the results have been pleasing both to the patients and to the surgeon.

Hypopigmentation was evident in four cases as consequence of deep dermabrasion. One of them remained without change 12 months after surgery. No other complications were observed [6].

Lip augmentation was performed using the above-described surgical technique by means of a dermal flap buried in the undermined skin of the upper lip. The results were aesthetically satisfactory in the ten cases treated with this technique In six patients (60%) the lip augmentation was performed only by means of the surgical technique described and in four others (40%) this was combined with fat injection.

Lipofilling was only performed beneath the vermilion border, enhancing the protrusion and bulk. Fat is an ideal filler material, though it does not maintain its original volume and eventually becomes absorbed (between 40 and 60% in our hands) in 2–6 months. To counteract the absorption of the fat, it is necessary to overcorrect the patient's lip, though the patient must be forewarned that more than one injection of fat may be necessary in a different surgical procedure.

Most of the aging changes can be corrected by means of the surgical technique described by the author [13]. In the author's initial series of 19 patients operated upon from 1993 through 1998, a slight lack of vermilion border height and decreasing of the thickness of the lip was observed in 26% of patients after 4 years. Continuous senile changes and gravitational effects are the logical causes. Homologous and heterologous materials used at the same time as surgical treatment have been useful for correcting these problems [14].

In our experience there was more patient satisfaction when lip augmentation was performed after surgical reshaping of the vermilion. This gave a more youthful and appealing look by defining a red bow.

72.7
Conclusions

Senile changes in the upper lip produce not only alterations in the length and shape of the vermilion border but also elongation of the skin area, vertical wrinkles and loss of volume of the lip. Treatment of these aesthetic lips changes is basically performed by means of the author's surgical technique [13]. Other techniques must be used combining dermabrasion and lip augmentation by use of homologous and heterologous materials.

The surgical techniques must be exact and performed patiently. The complications are usually temporary and not serious. The results are satisfactory for patients and surgeons.

References

1. Gonzalez UM: The aging upper lip. In Transaction of the Sixth International Congress of Plastic and Reconstructive Surgery, Marchac D, Hueston T (Eds). Paris, Masson 1975:443–446

2. Converse JM: Aesthetic surgery for the aging face.. In Reconstructive Plastic Surgery, Converse JM (Ed), 2nd Ed. Philadelphia, Saunders 1977:1868–1929

3. Fanous N. Correction of thin lips. "Lip lift." Plast Reconstr Surg 1984;74(1):33–41

4. Lipham WJ: Anatomía pertinente de la musculatura facial. In Aplicaciones Clínicas y Cosméticas de la Toxina Botulínica, Lipham WJ (Ed). Caracas, Amolca 2004:12–19

5. Millard DR Jr: Philtrum contouring and cupid's bow reconstruction. In Cleft Craft: The Evolution of Its Surgery: Bilateral and Rare Deformities, Millard DR Jr (Ed). Boston, Little, Brown. 1957:439–451

6. Gillies H, Kilner TP: Hare-lip: Operation for the correction of secondary deformities. Lancet 1932;2:1369

7. Meyer R, Rheims DM: Chirurgie esthetique peribuccale Ann Chir Plast Esthet 1989;34(4):328–333

8. Austin HW, Weston GW: Rejuvenation of the aging mouth. Clin Plast Surg 1992;19(2):511–524

9. Pitanguy I: Ancillary procedures in face lifting. Clin Plast Surg 1978;5(1):51–69

10. Di Giuseppe A: Innesti dermoadiposi per la correzione di difetti di proiezione del labbro superiore. Rev Ital Cir Plast 1988;20:377

11. Delerm A, Elbaz JS. Cheiloplastie des levres minces: Proposition d'une technique. Ann Chir Plast Esthet 1975;20(2):243–249

12. Farmand M, Seiler HF: Korrertur des schmalen lippenrots: Lippenroteversion versus Gillies operation. Fortschr Kiefer Ges 1989;34:114–117

13. Guerrissi JO, Sanchez Izquierdo L: An approach to the senile upper lip. Plast Reconstr Surg 1993;92(6):1187–1191

14. Guerrissi JO: Surgical treatment of the senile upper lip. Long-term follow-up. Plast Reconstr Surg 2000;106(4):938–940

Chapter 73

Correction of the Gummy Smile

Pierre F. Fournier

73.1
Introduction

Normally, in the function of the smile, the lips are retracted and elevated to expose a portion of the upper incisor teeth. In some cases, the lip retraction is too extreme and it exposes all of the incisors plus a large portion of gum above. This produces the so-called horse smile or gummy smile (Fig. 73.1), the correction of which was described by Rubinstein and Kostianovsky [1]. The operation is a relatively simple one that can be performed on an outpatient basis or in a well-equipped office. The results obtained are good.

73.2
Surgical Technique

73.2.1
Marking

The lips are retracted and the mucous membrane is dried thoroughly. A marking pencil is used to draw a line across the gum approximately 3–4 mm above the upper anterior teeth, from the medial bicuspid on one side to the same position on the opposite side. A second line is then drawn along the mucous membrane inside the lip—exactly where it would touch the line on the gum. Finally, the two lines are connected at each end in the design of an elliptical incision (Fig. 73.2).

73.2.2
Anesthesia

Local anaesthesia is produced by injecting 1% lidocaine (with epinephrine) along the gingival-labial sulcus and into the gum over the upper anterior teeth.

73.2.3
Technique

The upper lip is retracted with two traction sutures (Fig. 73.3). A no.15 blade is used to excise an elliptical (or hexagonal-shaped) piece of tissue, going through

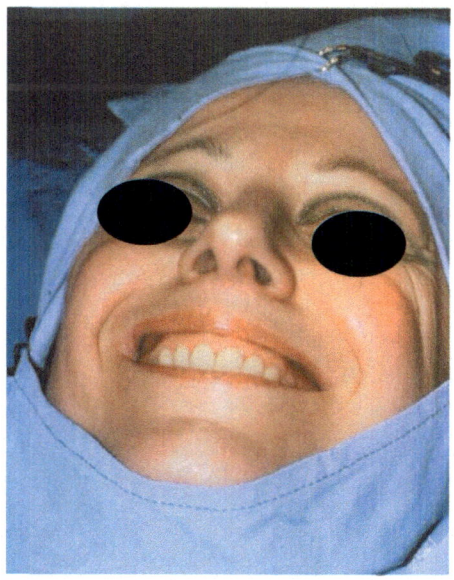

Fig. 73.1 The gummy smile

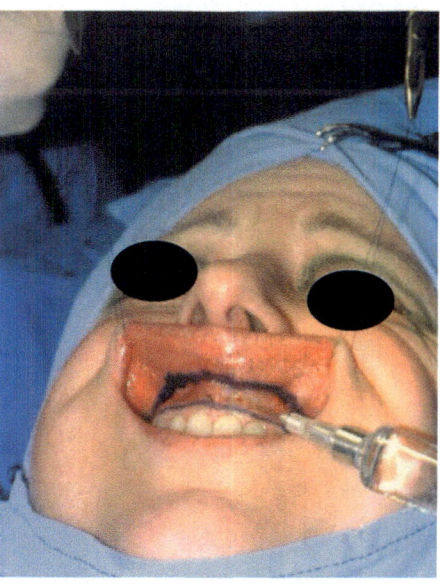

Fig. 73.2 Line marked and anesthesia injected

the mucoperiosteum on the gum side and through the full thickness of the labial mucosa. Undermining the labial mucosa as deep as 1 cm is necessary on all the incision lines (Fig. 73.4). Bleeding is controlled by electrocoagulation. Then a suture is placed in the midline of the gum edge, between the two upper central incisors and through the middle of the incision margin on the labial mucosa and they are approximated. The remaining portions of the mucosa and gum are approximated by progressively bisecting the intervals with 4/0 non-absorbable sutures (Fig. 73.5). A pressure dressing is applied for 1 h.

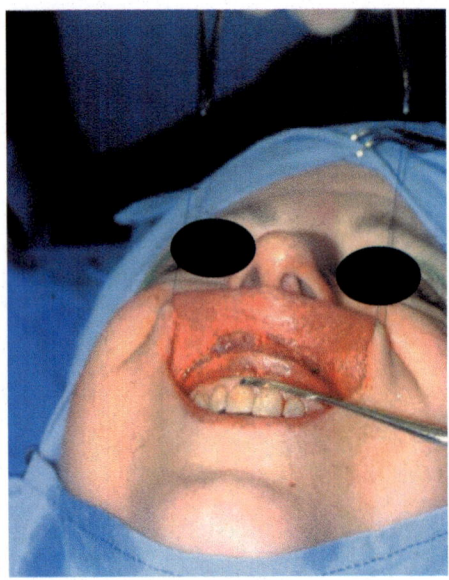

Fig. 73.3 The upper lip is retracted with two traction sutures

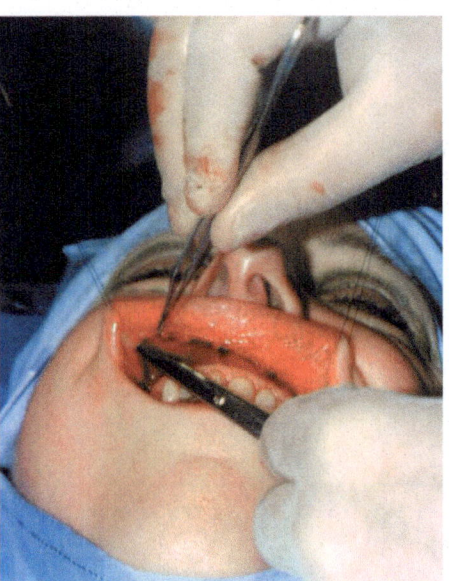

Fig. 73.4 Undermining of the labial mucosa as deep as 1 cm is necessary on all the incision lines

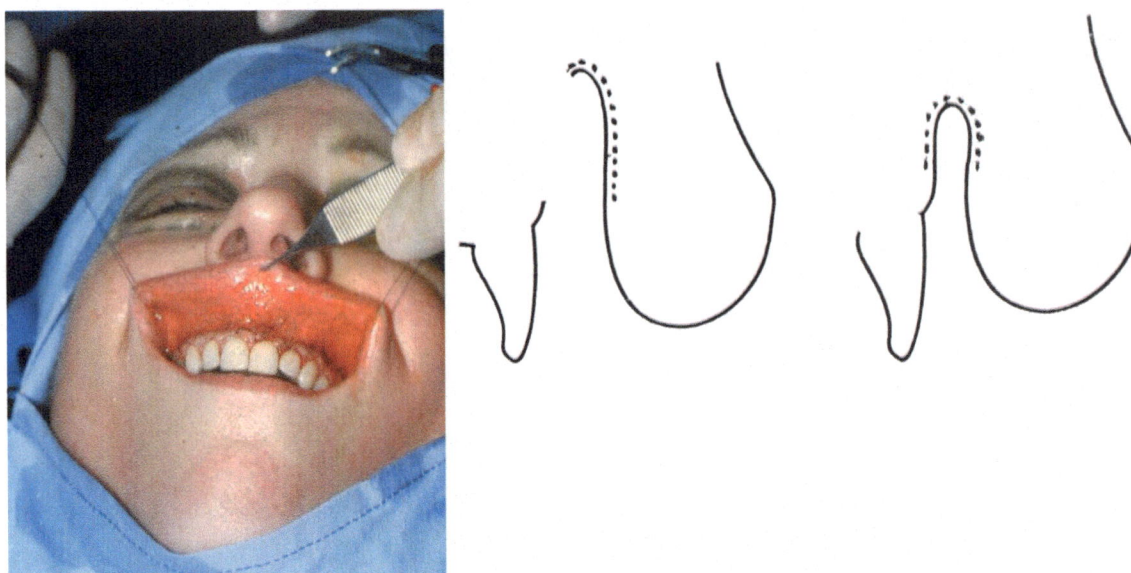

Fig. 73.5 The mucosa and gum are approximated by progressively bisecting the intervals with 4/0 non-absorbable sutures

73.2.4
Postoperatively

Antibiotics are given. The patient is kept on a liquid diet for 1 day and is allowed to resume normal habits. The sutures are removed about the sixth day. Usually, there is a minimal amount of postoperative swelling, provided adequate hemostasis was achieved.

73.3
Results

The results are immediate (Figs. 73.6, 73.7). The height of the incision on the gum above the teeth will determine the amount of correction obtained. If a great deal of correction is needed, the incision should be low on the gum.

73.4
Complications

Recurrence may be seen in some cases as well as incomplete correction; but no abnormal appearance of the upper lip when smiling has been seen. We have not seen cases of infection or abnormal bleeding.

73.5
Comment

If there is gross overbite or overgrowth of the upper jaw, bone surgery may be required. This operation is for moderate "gummy smile."

Others techniques have been described [2–4]:

1. Section of the levator muscles through the mouth.

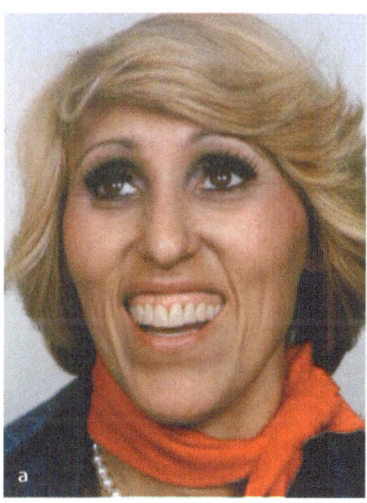
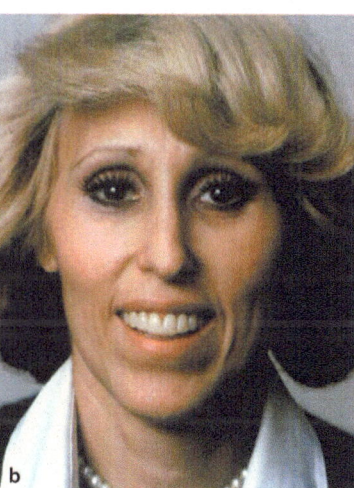

Fig. 73.6 a Before. **b** Following excision

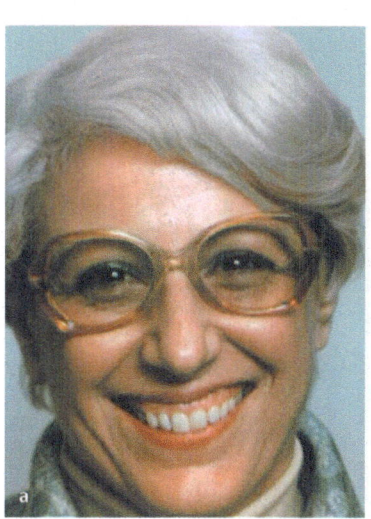
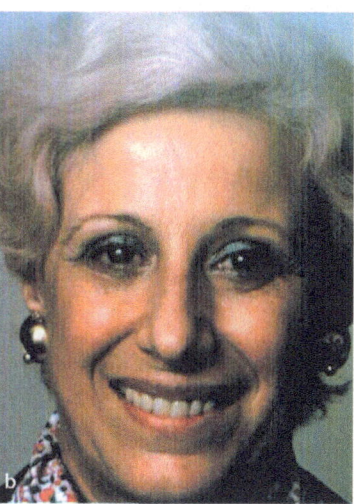

Fig. 73.7 a Before. **b** Following excision

2. Section of the levator muscles through an incision in the alar sulcus.
3. Botulinum toxin injection is used widely. The results last a few months.

73.6
Conclusion

A simple operation on the upper gums is possible to correct a moderate "gummy smile."

References

1. Rubinstein, A., Kostianovsky, A.: Cosmetic surgery for the malformation of the laugh: original technique. Prensa Méd Argent 1973;60:952
2. Litton, C., Fournier, P.: Simple Surgical Correction of the "Gummy smile." Presented at the Annual Meeting Society for Aesthetic Plastic Surgery, San Francisco, 10 May 1978
3. Miskinyar, S.A.: A new method for correcting a gummy smile. Plast Reconstr Surg 1983;72:397
4. Dong, M.D.: Dong's hyperplastic gingival removing operation. Presentation at Congress Aesthetic Surgery, Korea 2004

CHAPTER 74

Surgical Correction of the Aging Lip

74

Pierre F. Fournier

74.1
Introduction

The aging lip may have lines, wrinkles, and pigmentations and often the distance between the base of the columella and the Cupid's bow is increased owing to laxity of the skin or loss of volume. The Cupid's bow then appears flat.

The purpose of the surgical procedure is to shorten the distance between the base of the columella and the Cupid's bow, to restore the normal surface of the upper lip, and to restore the normal curve of the Cupid's bow. The procedure is also helpful in individuals with a "hidden smile" where the upper teeth do not show when smiling.

74.2
Technique

The skin is first marked longitudinally and in an undulating fashion from the lateral edge of the base of the nose to the other (Fig. 74.1). The skin is excised (Fig. 74.2) and hemostasis secured. Slight undermining of the lower lip is performed. The skin is carefully approximated with a running suture or with subdermal sutures (Fig. 74.3).

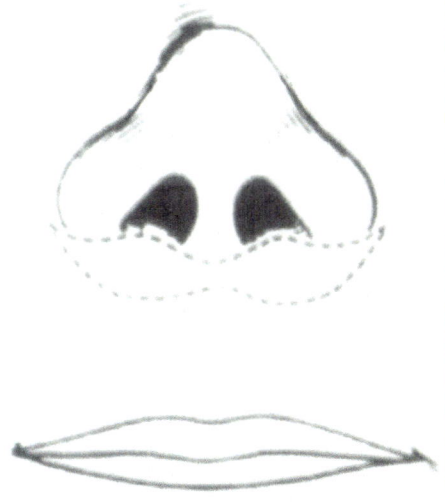

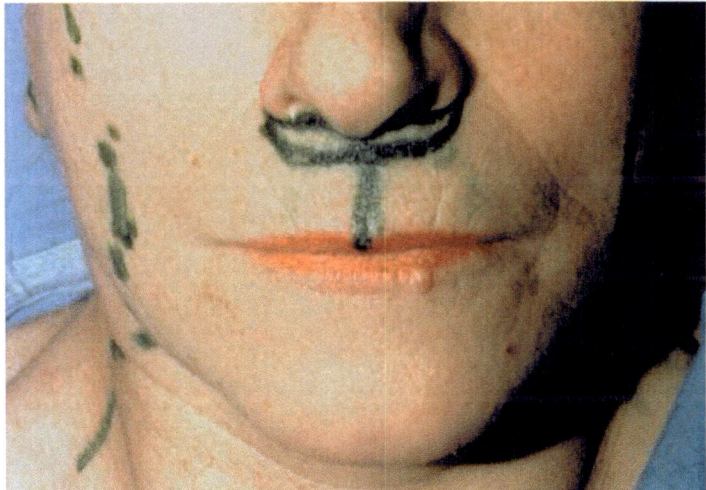

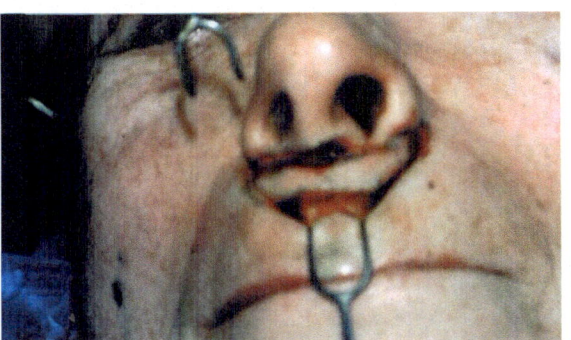

Fig. 74.1 Marking for skin excision

Fig. 74.2 Excision of skin

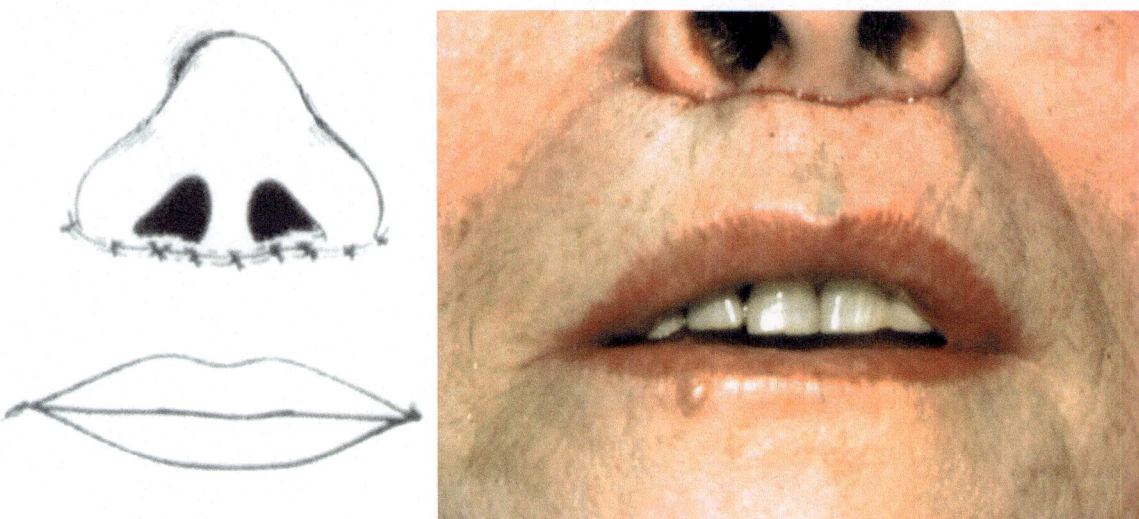

Fig. 74.3 Final suture closure

74.3
Complications

The theoretical complications are scarring, bleeding, asymmetry, and infection.

74.4
Conclusions

Simple skin excision in the upper lip at the inferior border of the nose can shorten the distance between the base of the columella and the Cupid's bow, restore the normal surface of the upper lip, and restore the normal curve of the Cupid's bow. The procedure is also helpful in individuals with a "hidden smile" where the upper teeth do not show when smiling.

Chapter 75

Three-Dimensional Sculpting of the Human Face Using Anatomic Contour Design Alloplastic Facial Implants

75

Edward O. Terino

75.1
Introduction

Within the last three decades, as the demand for aesthetic facial surgery has increased, surgeons have been challenged to discover effective methods that are safe, ethical, and scientifically sound. This experimentation is yielding new knowledge and vastly improved techniques. The author has used the techniques to augment alloplastically the malar midface and premandible regions over the past 15 years.

By altering the facial skeleton, the surgeon can create profound aesthetic changes. The emotional and psychological impact on the patient is powerful and complex. Before undertaking such surgery, it is essential that the surgeon understand the basic aesthetic principles of facial form and skeletal balance. They must be the cornerstone in any preoperative planning. Once the surgeon understands these principles, the technical implementation should be uncomplicated.

When you look at a person is your attention generally focused on his or her lips, eyes, eyebrows, and hair? Yet these are merely the adornment for the basic facial framework. What really determines the extent of a person's attractiveness is the skeletal mass of the face, the configuration of its bones, and the unique volumetric contours they create. The skin and subcutaneous tissues are the "canvas of the face." When distributed over the facial framework in a smooth manner, they present a youthful appearance. As years go by, this canvas becomes coarse and wrinkled, and loosening occurs. The face then takes on an image of age. In youth, the lips are considered beautiful when they are well defined, full, and sensuous, with' a prominent "Cupid's bow." The eyes are considered attractive when there is a medial to lateral tilt of the palpebral fissures, producing a "doe-eyed" or "almond-shaped" configuration. Eyebrows also become an accented feature when they are well demarcated and arch slightly at the junction of the lateral two thirds and one third. The facial pattern formed by these features is enveloped within the skin and is framed by a background of hair, which contributes abundant, multi-varied nuances of color and texture.

75.2
Effect of Altering the Facial Skeleton

When the surgeon alters the bony architecture of the face, he or she can create a new and dramatic visage. Although persons are clearly identifiable by the individuality displayed by their adorning features, i.e., lips, eyes, nose, and eyebrows, these take on a new and different aspect with a change in the bony architecture. Balance in bone structure is what gives the form of the face its maximum attractiveness called beauty.

75.3
Interrelationships of the Facial Promontories

Three major promontories determine a person's facial contours. In order of importance, they are the nose, the two malar zygomatic eminences, and the chin–jawline (Fig. 75.1). The supraorbital ridges, which constitute a fourth promontory, are of less significance. By altering the interrelationships of the three prominences, the surgeon can create or restore facial harmony, balance, and beauty.

Diminution or enhancement of any one of the three promontories directly and inversely affects the aesthetic importance of the others. As nasal significance is reduced, the malar projection and mandible assume a more important role. By accenting the malar cheekbone complex, the surgeon diminishes the significance of the nose and chin. By enhancing both the mandibular and the malar areas, the surgeon will effectively reduce the relative magnitude of the nose (Fig. 75.2). The architectural laws of nature dictate that the strength and volume characteristics of each promontory affect their relative balance with each other. Simultaneous changes in more than one of these anatomic elements have even greater significance than when one alone is altered.

Facial aesthetics, then, is basically the art and science of achieving a balance in all three elements of facial skeletal anatomy. The surgeon can accomplish this balance by using alloplastic implants; altering their size, shape, and design, and controlling their position. Recent advances in these parameters now make it possible for the surgeon to make subtle or dramatic changes in the facial promontories with ease and predictability (Fig. 75.3). Although the supraorbital ridges, the fourth promontory, are of minor significance, some individuals may require reduction or augmentation in this region as well.

Over the past decades, aesthetic facial surgery has evolved for the aging patient as well. Surgical procedures have gone from simple skin-tightening techniques to removal or addition of subcutaneous fat, and more recently to lifting or plication of the submuscular aponeurotic system as well as suspension techniques of the upper face and midface.

The restructuring of all these layers still has many limitations. There are patients with round, full, fleshy facial contours and an abundance of subcutaneous fat that rarely appear beautiful by contemporary standards. And there are lean-faced individuals with a tendency

to a long facial contour who have inadequate skeletal promontories in the malar or mandibular regions or both, and who also possess midfacial, submalar deficiency volume and imbalance. Both extremes of these facial types, as well as innumerable patients who have varying combinations, can be significantly improved by rearranging the balance of their skeletal promontories with alloplastic onlay techniques.

Contour surgery of the facial skeleton is further complemented by associated techniques of lateral canthal sling, revision rhinoplasty, and lip augmentation (Fig. 75.4). It is time, however, that aesthetic surgery places more emphasis on alteration of skeletal structure as the basic foundation for these traditional and anatomically incorrect two-dimensional operations.

Onlay alloplastic implantations of the facial skeleton are used not only for aesthetic purposes, but also for reconstruction of accident injuries and postsurgical deformities from tumor ablation.

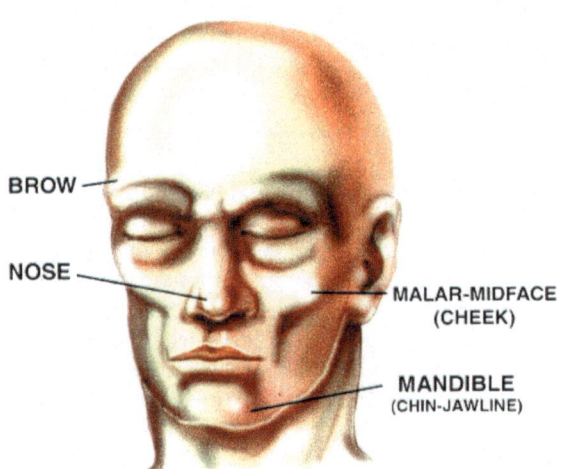

Fig. 75.1 Facial architecture illustrating major promontories of mass and volume: the nose, malar-midface, and mandible jawline

BROW

NOSE

MALAR-MIDFACE
(CHEEK)

MANDIBLE
(CHIN-JAWLINE)

FACIAL ARCHITECTURE

• THE MAJOR PROMONTORIES
OF MASS AND VOLUME

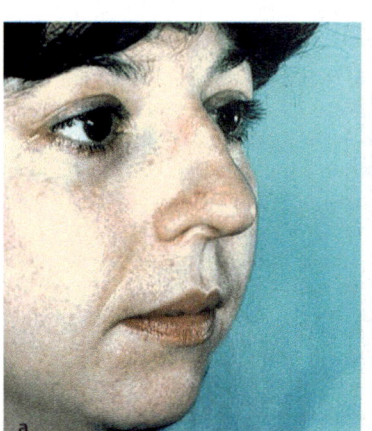
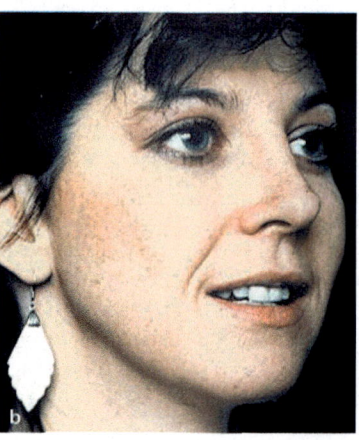

Fig. 75.2 a Preoperatively. **b** Dramatic improvement in facial balance and aesthetic appearance from reshaping the nose and its volume as well as enhancing the volume of the lower-third chin–jawline aesthetic segment. Platysma plication and sculpting as well as submental fat removal were also performed

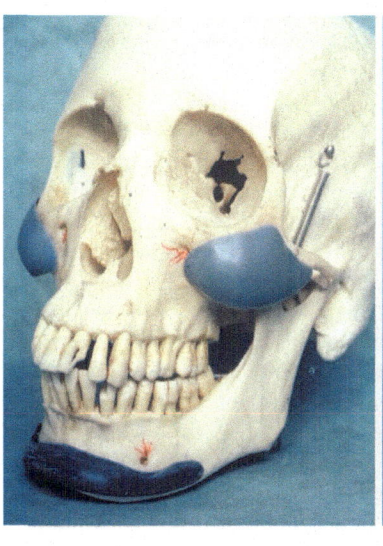
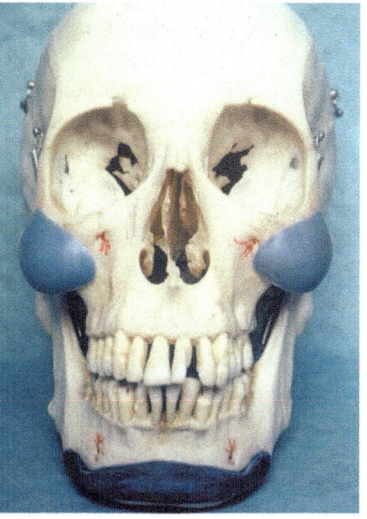
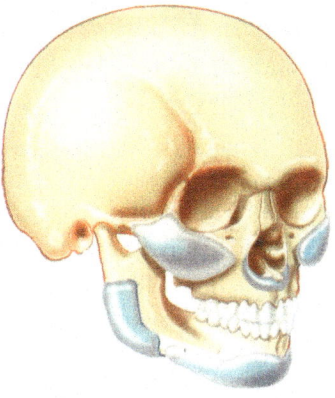

ANATOMIC STYLE IMPLANTS ARE COMMERCIALLY AVAILABLE FOR MID-FACE PREMANDIBLE AND PREMAXILLARY MODIFICATIONS

Fig. 75.3 Anatomic-style implants designed in the 1980s by the author to imitate natural bony and soft-tissue contours in malar-midface and premandible regions

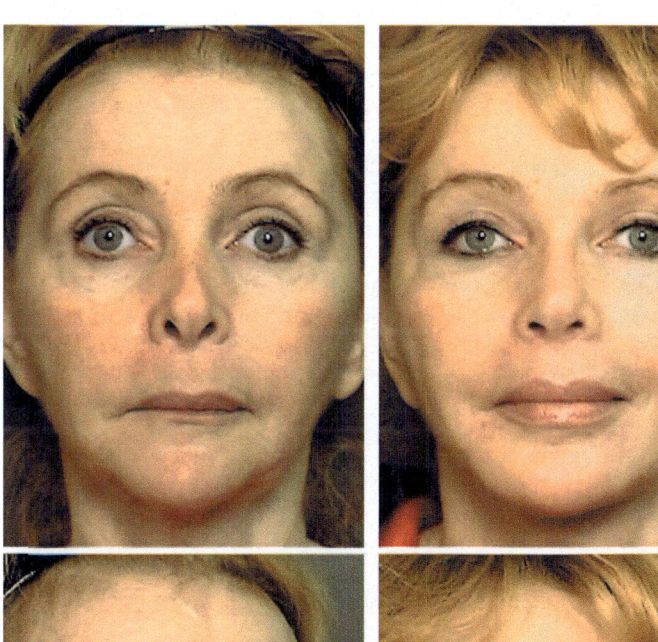
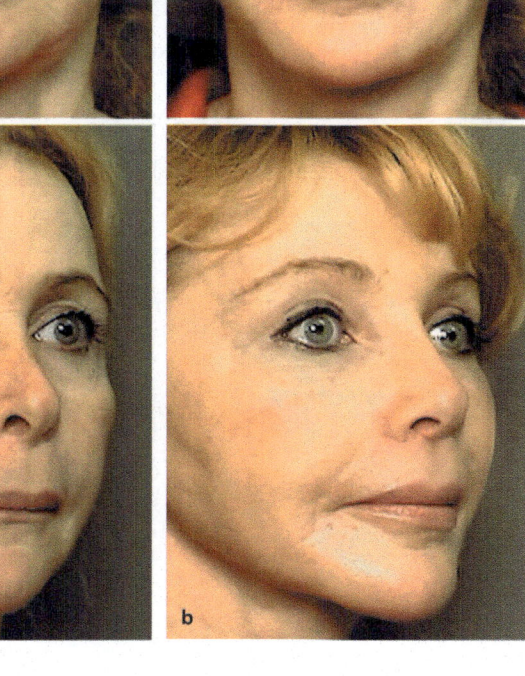

Fig. 75.4 **a** Preoperative 58-year-old female patient. **b** Postoperative upper midface suspension ("SOMME" lift), malar augmentation of zone 1 and SM5 with medium 3-mm malar shells, palpebral shape contouring with a lateral canthal sling, revision rhinoplasty, Alloderm lip augmentation, and chin augmentation with Terino Extended Anatomical chin implant, size large

75.4
Zonal Anatomy of the Malar and Premandible Regions

That part of the facial skeleton which, when appropriately augmented, produces an aesthetic change in the contour of the cheek and midface is called the "malar space." To determine the most aesthetic augmentation to select for that space, it is useful to perceive the malar region as five distinct anatomic zones (Fig. 75.5).

Zone 1, the largest area, includes the major portion of the malar bone and the first third of the zygomatic arch. Augmentation of this entire zone produces the greatest volumetric filling of the cheek and also maximizes the projection of the maxillary eminence.

Zone 2, the second most important site, overlies the middle third of the zygomatic arch. Enhancement of this zone along with zone 1 increases the accentuation of the cheekbone laterally, giving a broader dimension to the upper third of the face, thereby creating a high, arched appearance. This change of contour is particularly useful for individuals with a narrow upper face or a long-face syndrome (Fig. 75.6). When, however, zones 1 and 2 are augmented in excess, an abnormal and unattractive protuberance may result.

Zone 3 is the paranasal area, which lies medial to the infraorbital foramen and nerve. A line drawn vertically down from the infraorbital foramen marks the medial extent of the usual dissection for malar augmentation. This line also represents the lateral border of zone 3. When paranasal augmentation occurs, zone 3 creates a medial fullness of the face, often in the upper nasolabial area, which can be unattractive or can produce a "chipmunk-cheek" effect. The skin and subcutaneous tissues are thin in that region; consequently, any implant placed there must be perfectly sculptured and tapered. Augmentation of zone 3 is indicated for certain reconstructive purposes, following trauma or other heredity deficiencies. Zone 3 along with the entire lower orbital rim and suborbital region constitute an important area to augment with an implant to alter the unattractive hollowness of aging or a recessive inferior orbital rim deficiency (Fig. 75.7).

Zone 4 overlies the posterior third of the zygomatic arch. Augmentation in this area is never needed. It would produce an unnatural appearance. Moreover, dissection here may be dangerous, because the tissues overlying the bone are quite adherent, making it very possible to injure the zygomaticotemporal or orbicularis oculi branches of the facial nerve, and even the capsule of the temporomandibular joint. Symptoms and deformities have been observed that resulted from operations in this area.

Zone 5, the submalar zone or "submalar triangle," is bounded posteriorly by the masseter muscle tendinous origins and anteriorly by the canine fossa region of the maxilla. The superior boundary of zone 5 is the inferior bony margin of the malar eminence, which constitutes the first two thirds of the zygomatic arch. The medial extent of the submalar space ends at the lateral border of the nasolabial mound and sulcus. Its anterior limit is bounded by the inferomedial portion of the roof of the entire malar space. It contains the overlying facial musculature, fat, skin, and subcutaneous tissues of the midface region. The inferior border is the selected lower limit of the natural dissection plane that separates the masseter from the overlying facial musculature. To create midface fullness, aug-

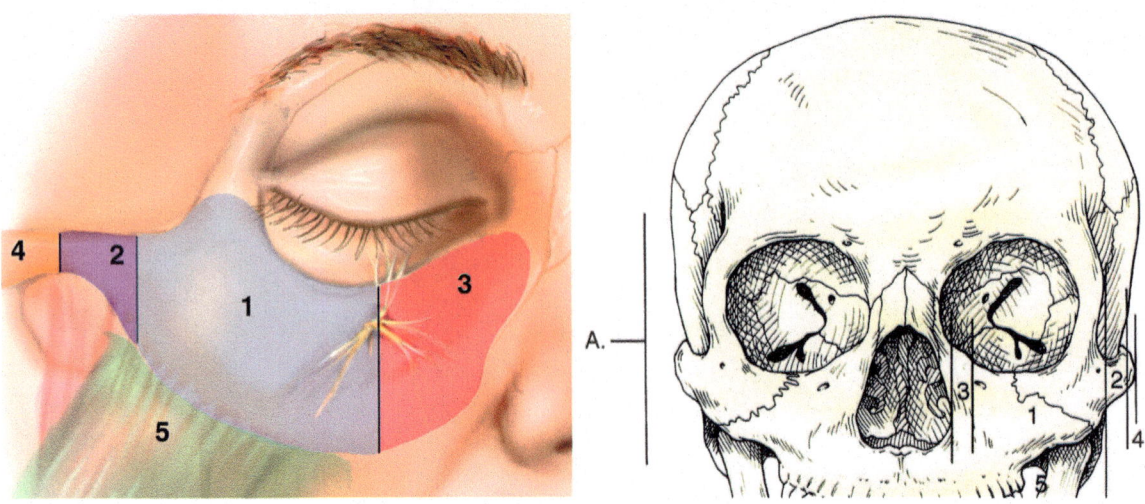

Fig. 75.5 Anatomic facial contour zones of the midface

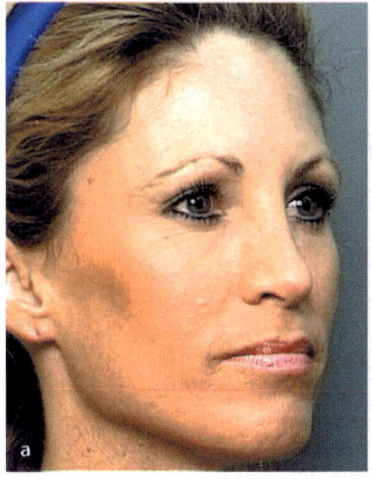
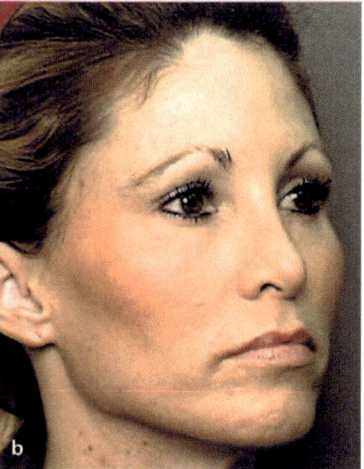

Fig. 75.6 a Preoperative patient with "long face syndrome." **b** Postoperative improvement by volume augmentation of malar zones 1 and 2, expanding upper midface diameter as well as an anatomic chin implant augmentation, which also helps to shorten the appearance of the face and chin

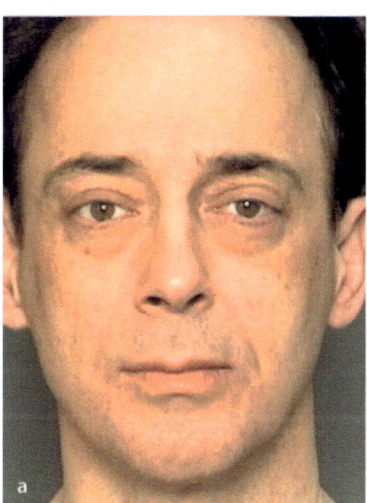
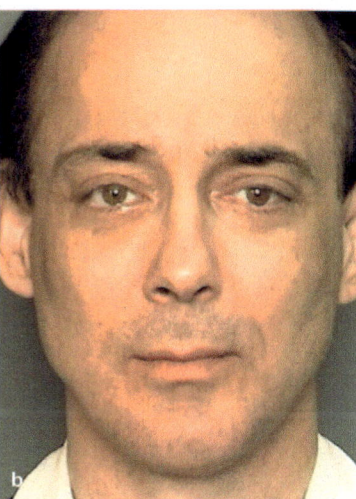

Fig. 75.7 a Preoperatively. **b** Ten months postoperatively following suborbital malar tear-trough augmentation for severe "negative vector" orbit. The patient also had a chin implant and angle of mandible augmentation

mentation within the sulcus that this lower-limit dissection creates is required.

Natural aging, as well as inherited tendencies, causes soft-tissue deficiency to develop in the inframalar midface region. This is accentuated by the superior overhanging prominence of the solid maxillary malar eminence, as well as by the medial and downward sagging of the nasolabial mound. The result is a midface sulcus, or depression, that overlies this submalar zone. In many individuals, midface atrophy creates a tired, drawn, and haggard appearance as early as the third and fourth decade of life. Augmentation within the submalar zone, beneath the soft-tissue sulcus, can bring back a fuller, rounder, and more youthful contour.

A solid implant in the submalar zone recreates the patient's maxillary architecture by effectively adding to the vertical length of the malar bone down from the lateral canthal region into the midcheek. The all-encompassing "malar shell" implant, which the author of this chapter developed over the past 25 years, goes beyond the submalar concept by augmenting both the entire malar bone and the submalar region into a completely united full, round cheek.

By understanding the five zones of the facial anatomy and their interrelationships, the surgeon can vary cheek shapes to accommodate individual patients. Success is determined by appropriate choice of size and shape of the implant and knowledge of which zone or zones to augment.

75.5
Zonal Anatomy of the Premandibular Space

Techniques for chin augmentation have been amplified by extending the shape and size of the traditional, centrally placed implant to provide more lateral and posterior alteration of the chin contour. Oval chin implants have traditionally been placed between the mental foramina (Fig. 75.8). Implants placed only into this central segment often produce an abnormal and unattractive, round, central protuberance. Moreover, displacement of the origins of the mentalis muscle by traditional chin implant surgery may permit a downward dislocation of the overlying soft-tissue mound and musculature, thereby creating a "witch's chin" or "drooping chin" deformity. This is particularly accentuated in a patient who possesses an inherited

round, globular, and protuberant central soft-tissue chin mound. It becomes even more undesirable aesthetically if, in the process of aging, he or she develops an adjacent lateral soft-tissue sulcus between the central chin mound and the sagging, more lateral jowl elements. This sulcus is known as the "marionette groove" or the "anterior mandibular sulcus."

To achieve greater success in chin augmentation, "premandible space" may be perceived. The premandible space is that anatomic region of the lower face which, when variously augmented, creates significant changes in the shape and volume of the lower third of the face and jawline. This region can be configured into four functional anatomic zones (Fig. 75.9).

Extending the premandible space laterally into the middle half of the horizontal ramus, and the region of the oblique line, enables the surgeon to define a midlat-

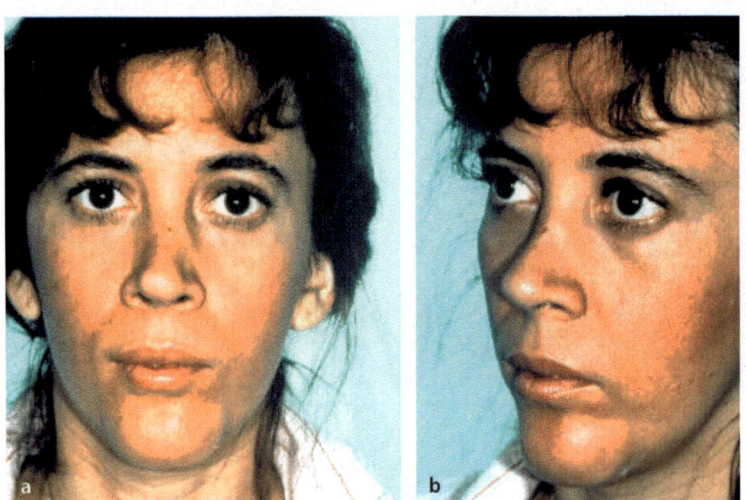

Fig. 75.8 a Preoperative patient with traditional chin implants that have been placed centrally between the mental foramina. This often produces an unattractive central abnormal, rounded protuberance. **b** Postoperatively

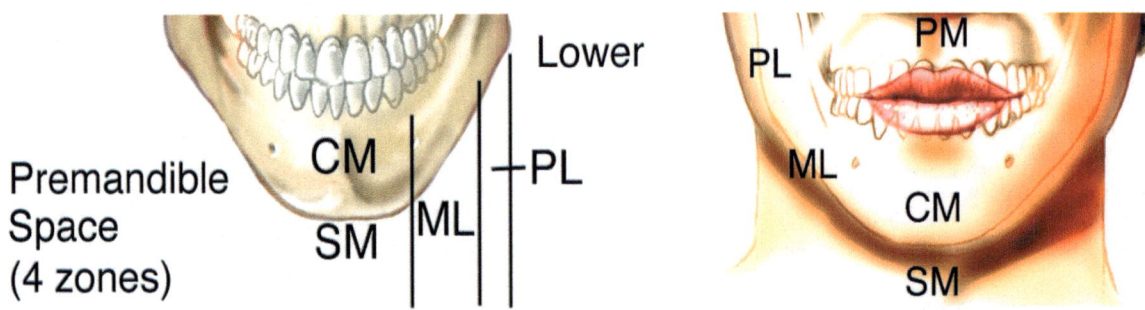

Fig. 75.9 There are four anatomic zones within the premandible space that can be augmented to correct specific regional contours for the lower aesthetic mandibular facial segment

eral zone of the mandible. Augmentation of this zone, in addition to the central mentum, creates a chin–jawline contour that is anatomically natural (Fig. 75.10). This embodies the principle of the "extended anatomic contour" implants designed by the author. Augmentation within the midlateral zone, and even further into the more posterior part of the mandible, creates broadening and definition of the mid and posterior aspects of the jawline (Fig. 75.11).

The posterolateral segment of the premandibular space overlies the posterior half of the horizontal ramus, extending back from the oblique line and including the angle of the mandible and its ascending ramus. Augmentation of this zone creates a broadening of the face and a more sculptured definition of the posterior jawline.

The fourth and final premandibular zone resides beneath the inferior border of the mandible and is called the submandibular zone. Traditional chin implants have lacked the ability to extend deficient mandibles in a vertical direction. The newer implants, however, have been designed to wrap around the bony margin of the mandible and to increase the vertical height of the face from the lower lip to the inferior chinline, thereby augmenting the submandibular zone (Fig. 75.12).

By augmentation of both the lateral portion of this zone and the midlateral zone, it is possible to improve or correct the anterior mandibular sulcus, otherwise known as the marionette groove (Fig. 75.13) or prejowl sulcus. This is the region of the mental nerve where the anterior mandibular ligament restricts the down and forward descent of the lower-cheek issues during the aging process.

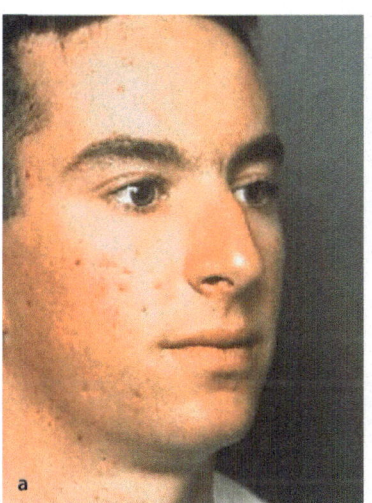
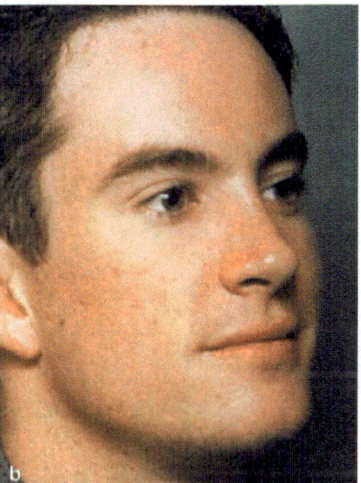

Fig. 75.10 a Preoperative 24-year-old male patient. **b** Postoperatively with a more aesthetic attractive facial balance from rhinoplasty and chin and angle of jaw augmentation

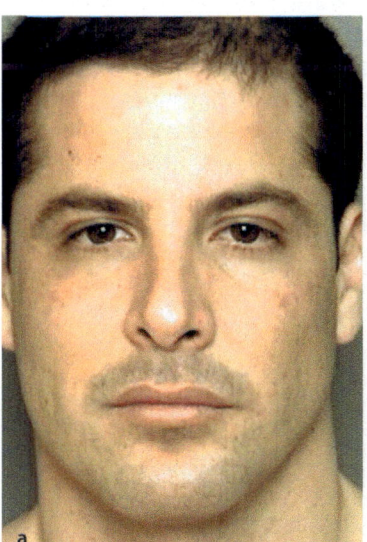
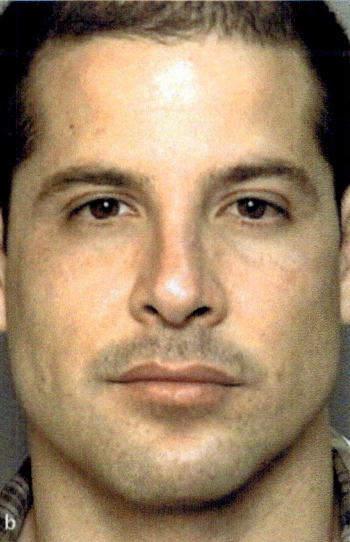

Fig. 75.11 Jawline enhancement is frequently requested by men. **a** Preoperatively. **b** Six months postoperatively after placement of an angle of jaw implant

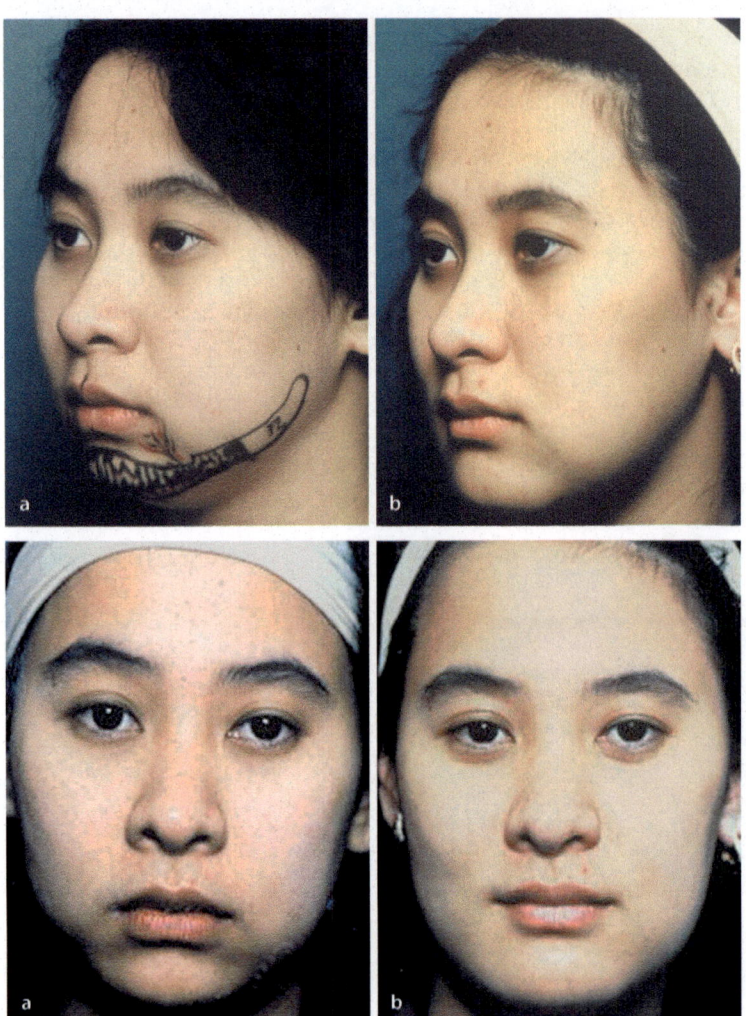

Fig. 75.12 a Preoperative patient with severe lower facial aesthetic segment deficiency. **b** Two years postoperatively after submandibular augmentation with a vertical extension implant

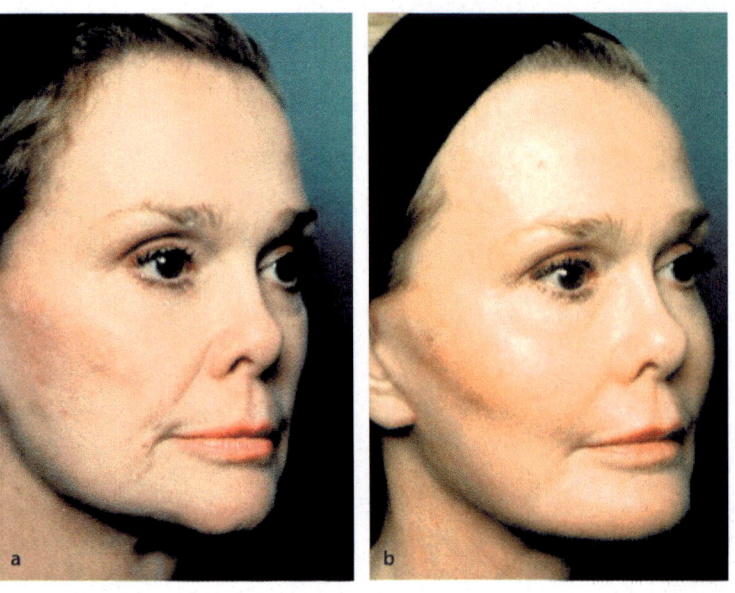

Fig. 75.13 a Preoperative patient with "witch's chin" deformity. **b** One year postoperatively following a rhytidectomy, malar-submalar volume augmentation, and prejowl augmentation using a vertical extension implant to correct the aging, tired appearance of her face

75.6
Qualities of Ideal Facial Implants

The shape of implants is the critical factor in imitating facial anatomy. When appropriate implants have been selected, the potential for mobility and malposition is almost negligible. Ideal implants should be easily implantable, nonpalpable, readily exchangeable, malleable, conformable, acceptable to the body, resistant to infection, and modifiable by the surgeon (Table 75.1).

When placed directly on bone, smooth silicone implants become rapidly fixed and securely surrounded by fibrosis and capsule formation. They can be removed readily and exchanged when necessary or desirable. On the other hand, porous implants that permit ingrowth (such as Medpore and Porex), fenestrated implants, and implants with Dacron backing have a consistent, predictable, and significant incidence of infection. They are also significantly more difficult to exchange or modify.

Silastic implants can survive the onset of inflammation and gross purulence, whereas infected porous implants must always be removed. If inflammation, cellulitis, or abscess should occur, such reaction can be corrected promptly and adequately with antibiotics and perhaps even drainage techniques. However, surgeons should not complacently expect this cure in all cases. Indeed, some disastrous consequences have been reported from facial implant infections. Nevertheless, the fact that silicone facial implants provide a margin of safety from tissue contamination does offer the surgeon a very significant advantage.

Technical limitations in the use of facial implants still prevail, because differential augmentation and alteration of the facial skeleton are still in an early phase of development. Consequently, in choosing the correct size, shape, and placement of implants, the surgeon must rely solely on his or her own judgment and artistic perspective. In the near future, computerized technology may be able to design and manufacture implants and customize them to the needs of individual patients. Currently, physician and patient dissatisfaction with results constitutes the major problem associated with facial implant augmentation.

The success of recent anatomic facial implants is also, in large part, due to their conformability to the facial skeleton. Implants are being produced whose posterior aspect is accurately molded to the shape and form of the human skull, both in the malar and in the premandible regions. The expansion of implant size and shape to volumetrically fit the dimensions of the face effectively minimizes movability and malposition.

To be inserted through small apertures in the soft-tissue envelope of the face, facial implants must have malleability and compressibility. With the current use of larger implants, these two qualities have become even more important. Often implants of 10–20 cm² need to be placed onto the malar bone or the mandible of the

Table 75.1 Comparison of ideal qualities of the most commonly used facial implant materials

Ideal qualities	Silastic	Proplast	Other
Exchangeable	+ - - -	+	-
Conformable	+ + - +	+ +	+ +
Modifiable	+ + +	+ + + +	-
Host acceptable	+ + + +	+ +	+ +
Nonpalpable	+ + +	+	+
Insertable	+ + + +	+ + +	+ +

facial skeleton. Silicone rubber implants, fabricated into a suitable medium-grade consistency, make it possible to perform this procedure with ease.

Finally, the ready modifiability of silicone implants works in the surgeon's favor when a formidable barrier is encountered during the operation. Instead of enforcing a traumatic dissection upon an area of anatomy where nerve damage is imminent, the surgeon can easily diminish the implants or alter their configuration with a scalpel without affecting the resulting contour.

75.7
Preoperative Planning

Preoperative planning for all plastic and reconstructive surgery is the determining factor for achieving successful results. For aesthetic surgery, such planning must include accurate and definitive communication with the patient, whose perceptions and expectations the surgeon must understand completely.

For traditional surgery on aging patients, communication about their needs and wishes is relatively simple: They wish to have their youthful contours and facial features restored as completely as possible. With the passing years, individuals accommodate to the slow, gradual changes that take place in the soft-tissue contours of their faces. The limited technical results of routine two-dimensional tightening techniques from traditional facial aesthetic surgery are therefore acceptable to them, because they do produce some significant visible albeit limited postoperative improvements.

Current three-dimensional techniques for altering facial contours and facial promontories go beyond routine surgery in that they can radically change a patient's inherited anatomic configuration. Following facial implant surgery, patients experience much improved visual and perceptual images of themselves and permanently for the rest of their lives.

Although aesthetic surgery has an assortment of tools, such as cephalometrics, the "zero meridian" concept, CEMAX, magnetic resonance imaging, and computer-imaging techniques, precise implementation of facial form remains difficult, at best. Before the surgeon attempts an alloplastic facial contour alteration, it is imperative that he or she knows exactly what facial image the patient desires. Frequently, patients like strong, bold, well-defined features and classic contours. The author requests his patients to modify photographs of themselves and bring them in, or to provide, from fashion magazines or other sources, examples of facial contours that they admire, namely, faces that they feel look similar to their own but are more attractive in the pertinent skeletal areas. Contrary to standard residency teaching, this procedure clarifies this author's understanding of his patient's expectations by giving him an invaluable visual image to discuss.

Most patients have very precise visual images of the facial contours they wish to emulate. When they do not, it is easy to discover that their expectations cannot be met. Surgeons should not undertake what they are not sure they can accomplish.

This author finds computer imaging technology to be indispensable in determining what precise change a patient is looking for.

During patient consultations, it is important to focus on specific details of zonal anatomy, because the surgeon must decide which anatomic zones to augment. He or she must determine whether enhancement should occur mostly in malar zones 1 or 2, or whether it is submalar zone roundness and fullness that the patient is seeking. Similarly, he or she must distinguish between the contour produced by enhancing the posterolateral aspect of the jawline and those achieved by augmenting the anterior, midlateral, central, and even the vertical dimensions of the mandible.

Multiple consultations with the patient are important. On the morning of surgery, time spent in marking, measuring, and discussing details with the patient is invaluable. Finally, by drawing the configurations of the pertinent regional and zonal designs on the patient's face, the surgeon is provided with guidelines for accurately performing the intraoperative surgical dissection.

75.8
Suggestions for Operative Technique

With regard to operative technique, this author offers the following suggestions:

1. Stay on bone. Placement of implants on bone or not creates a firm and secure attachment to the skeleton. Capsule contracture has not been seen with anatomic implants. Perhaps this is because of their solid consistency, or the inability of the capsule to exert constricting forces when the implant is directly on bone. This accords with the observations on breast augmentation, namely, that total submuscular placement of breast prostheses has an exceptionally low rate of capsule contracture, presumably because they are placed directly on the skeletal plane of the rib cage.

2. Be gentle in elevating the soft tissues from the malar and premandible regions. When there is adequate infiltration of local anesthetic agents, the tissue planes separate easily and without forceful trauma. Two areas that present the most difficulty and also the greatest danger for nerve damage are (a) just beneath and around the mental foramen during surgery for premandible augmentation and (b) above and below the middle third of the bony zygomatic arch. Avoid excessive trauma. Excessive trauma can produce mental nerve symptoms, transient or prolonged, but rarely permanent. Paresis or paralysis of the zygomaticus, the orbicularis oculi, and even the frontalis muscle can occur. Such damage is usually temporary, but in rare cases it can be permanent.

3. Expand the dissection space adequately in either the malar or the premandible regions to accommodate the chosen prostheses comfortably. Elevation of the soft tissues into areas adjacent to bone should be done with a blunt-edged elevator and, again, as gently as possible. Anatomically contoured implants of adequate size and shape present very few problems in malposition or mobility because they fill the space comfortably and hold their position by virtue of their contoured posterior surface and their fixation to bone.

4. Minimize bleeding by using both local and general anesthesia. A "dry operative field" is essential for accurate visualization, precise dissection, and proper placement, the three critical factors in avoiding potential problems with hematoma, seroma, infection, inaccurate placement, and nerve damage. Maintenance of the systolic blood pressure between 90 and 110 provides optimal hemostasis in combination with infiltration of a dilute 0.2% lidocaine solution containing 1:800,000 epinephrine. Clonidine, 0.2 mg by mouth, is also given immediately preoperatively to stabilize the hemodynamics of the patient's blood pressure and pulse (Table 75.2).

Table 75.2 Ideal anesthesia for alloplastic facial contouring

General anesthesia	Local anesthesia
Maintain systolic blood pressure at 90–110	0.2% lidocaine solution
0.2 mg Clonidine prior to surgery	1:800,000 epinephrine
	Generous tissue infiltration into malar and or premandible space (20–30 ml each)

75.9 Technical Details

Once the basic principles of dissection have been understood, the remaining technical aspects of facial implantation in the malar, midface, and premandible region are straightforward.

As with augmentation mammoplasty, the anatomic space required for the implant remains the same, regardless of which incisional approach and entrance wound is used (Fig. 75.14). The maneuvers to achieve accurate implant placement and positioning vary very little for the different approaches. The most important decision, of course, should be made prior to the operation, namely, the choice of implant size and shape.

The various routes for entering the malar space, including the submalar region, are as follows: (1) intraoral, (2) lower blepharoplasty (subcilial), (3) rhytidectomv, (4) zygomaticotemporal, and (5) transcoronal and (6) transconjunctival.

The intraoral route has been the traditional and most frequent approach to maxillary malar and midface augmentation. This author uses an L-shaped incision with 1-cm limbs, made through the mucosa and in a vertically oblique direction. It is located over the anterior buttress of the maxilla, just above the canine tooth and approximately 2.5 cm medial to the orifice of Stensen's duct (Fig. 75.15).

A subperiosteal, spatula-shaped elevator with a 1-cm-wide blade is thrust directly under the orbicularis oris

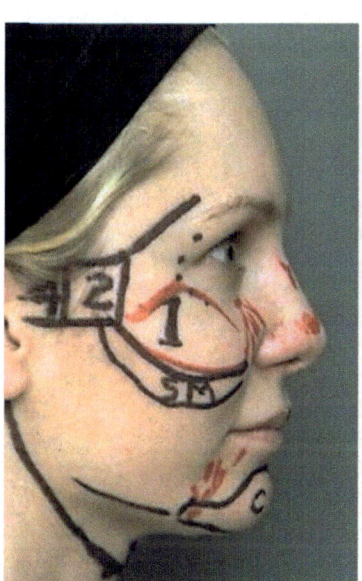
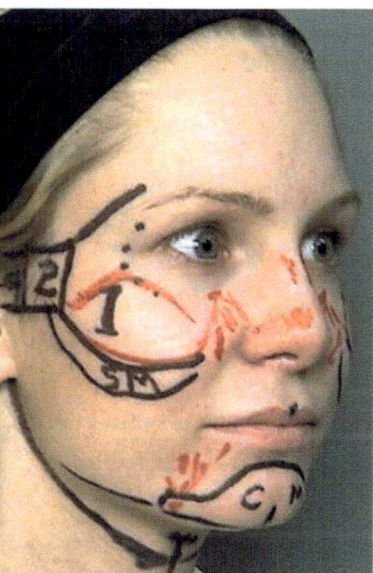

Fig. 75.14 Preoperative markings are made on all patients' faces the morning of surgery to outline their zonal anatomy and bone structure

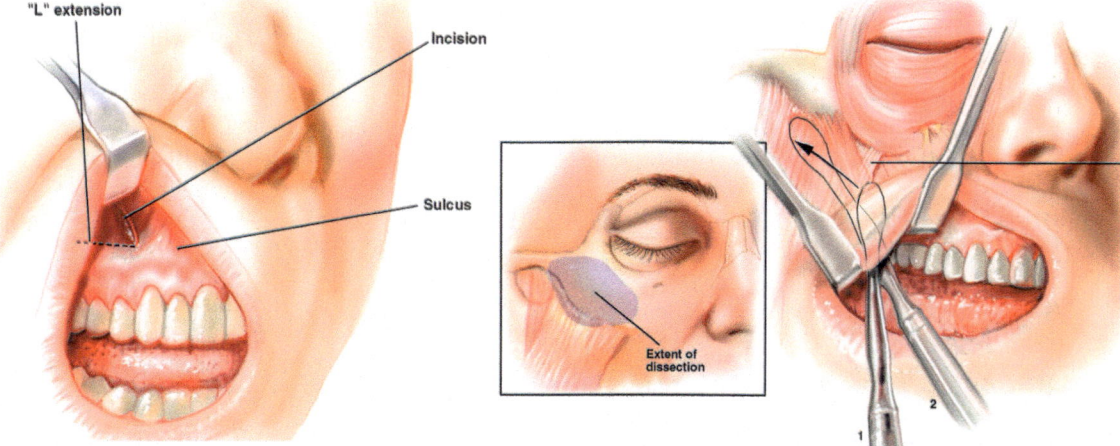

Fig. 75.15 An intraoral approach for placement of a malar implant can be used to dissect the proper space and identify and visualize the internal anatomy for proper placement

muscle onto bone in a vertical orientation at the inferior base of the maxillary buttress, in the apex of the gingival-buccal sulcus. The overlying soft tissues are swept obliquely upward over the maxillary eminence by maintaining the elevator directly on bone. The elevator should always remain on the bony margin along the inferior border of the malar eminence and zygomatic arch. Manual palpation of the previously marked zonal design of the malar space anatomy on the skin is performed, while the underlying elevator mobilizes the tissues directly from the bone (Fig. 75.16).

This maneuver includes palpating the orbital rim and the upper and lower borders of the zygoma as the elevator dissects the subperiosteal space within these areas. A lighted fiberoptic Aufricht retractor confirms the anatomic dissection.

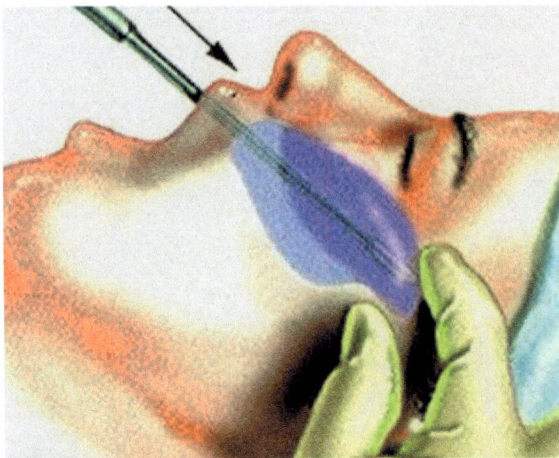

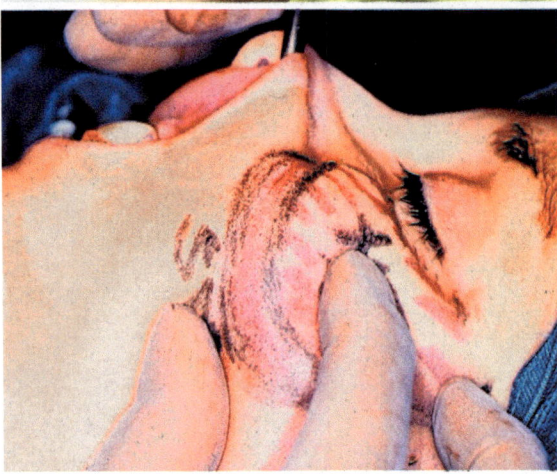

Fig. 75.16 Malar shell augmentation by the intraoral route showing elevation of the soft tissues over the malar region by staying on the bone with an elevator and controlling the space between the index finger and thumb

Once bony margins have been reached, further space expansion is performed only by means of a rounded, blunter spatula elevator. No dissection should occur into the soft tissues with a penetrating and forceful motion. No dissection should occur directly into the area of the infraorbital nerve. When desired, the periosteum may be mobilized, both lateral and inferior to the infraorbital foramen, with a careful scraping motion until the nerve and foramen are visualized. This is indicated for suborbital tear-trough implant.

Frequent irrigation is performed with antibiotic solution (50,000 U/l bacitracin or 1 g/l Ancef in normal saline).

Once the space has been mobilized, the chosen implant is introduced with a long, curved, serrated clamp placed transversely across the upper end of the implant and inserted into the posterior zygomatic tunnel while two 10-in. needles swedged on a 2-0 Prolene suture (Ethibond) are placed from inside to outside the temporal region and tied over a large tonsil sponge. Should buckling of the implant occur, correct positioning can be ensured by using Russian forceps, in combination with a spatula periosteal elevator, passed both anterior and posterior to the implant. Fiberoptic Aufricht retractors are used to illuminate the interior of the space, reveal the internal anatomy, and confirm the correct position of the implant.

In the submalar zone, the soft tissues are swept off the shiny, white, glistening, fibrous tendon of the masseter muscle in an inferior and outward direction. This opens up the submalar space for approximately 1–2 cm, depending on the desired choice of cheek shape and the corresponding implant necessary to achieve it (Fig. 75.17). When augmented by a total malar shell implant, the submalar or inframalar region exhibits a lower, rounder facial contour. This occurs by volumetric filling of the midface in the submalar triangle.

When adequate anesthesia techniques are used, the intraoral approach permits excellent visualization of the skeletal anatomy and musculature. This exposure facilitates accurate implant placement into zones 1, 2, and 5 (submandibular zone). It permits the surgeon to place a spatula elevator above and below the implant to make certain that its edges are not buckled or that the zygomatic extension of the implant is not curled. It is not necessary to visualize the infraorbital nerve, but it is easy to do so when indicated, or when an implant is used for the suborbital region.

Complications from the intraoral approach include dysesthesias from damage to the infraorbital nerve or motor dysfunction of the orbicularis oris musculature. Nerve symptoms may be attributed to transection of small branches in the lip during the incision, direct damage to the major nerve bundle during dissection, or pressure impingement on the nerve from the implant. These complications, however, are rare and almost non-

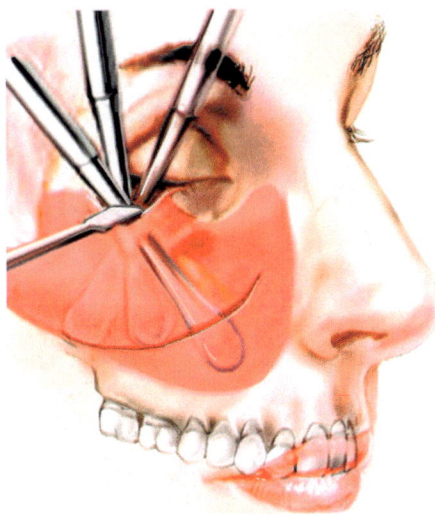

Fig. 75.17 Vertical subperiosteal midface suspension. The surgical dissection involves degloving not only the maxilla but down over the masseter muscle to the buccal fat pad and the gingival-buccal sulcus. Implants are easily positioned to improve deficiencies in zones 1, 2, 3 and SM5

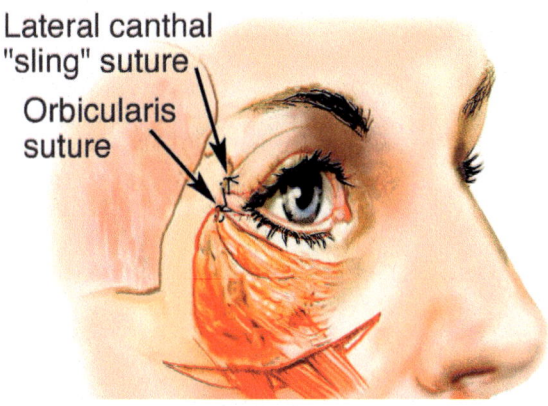

Fig. 75.18 The lateral canthopexy sling technique with a second suture securing the orbicularis oculi muscle to the lateral orbital periosteum

existent when the previously stated guidelines to dissection are applied.

Closure of the oblique intraoral incision is secure because the muscle pillars of the zygomaticus, which overlie the maxillary buttress, can be firmly reapproximated with sutures to provide a sturdy two-layer closure. Traditional transverse incisions through these muscles produce traumatic transection, resulting in transient and perhaps even permanent damage to muscle function. This can inhibit normal lip elevation.

75.10
Subcilliary Blepharoplasty Approach

In the subcilial blepharoplasty approach, an incision is made 3 mm below the lashline, and limited in its lateral extension to avoid scars in the lateral canthal region. This approach may be used either in conjunction with routine blepharoplasty or as an independent route of entry for a malar implant. When used for implant placement alone, the incision is limited to a length of 10–15 mm. It is designed only in the middle to lateral third of the lower eyelid, in the subcilliary region. There is no contamination by intraoral organisms with this incision. Moreover, the dissection inferiorly develops no floor weakness. Instead, it provides a sturdy shelf upon which the implant rests.

During the dissection, the infraorbital nerve is also intentionally avoided. An incision is made in the peri-

osteum 3–4 mm anterior to the orbital rim along its lateral aspect, to obviate potential adhesions that may result in ectropion and lower-lid contracture. A skin flap should never be used, because it always shrinks and predisposes to eyelid retraction and ectropion. By utilizing a skin–muscle flap approach, however, there should be no trauma to the orbicularis oculi muscle.

Excessive muscle damage, with bleeding into lid tissues, stimulates fibrosis and contracture within the middle lamella of the lower eyelid, producing ectropion. Standard lateral canthopexy techniques are used to minimize this possibility (Fig. 75.18). Resection of skin and muscle flap should be conservative, i.e., minimal to no excision, because of additional traction exerted on the lower eyelid from the volume expansion caused by the implant under the malar tissues.

The greatest advantage of the subcilial blepharoplasty approach is the opportunity for correct positioning. The surgeon is able to directly observe the relationship of the implant to the inferior orbital rim. The greatest disadvantage of this approach is the potential for creating morbid distortions of the eyelid anatomy, as described previously.

75.11
The Rhytidectomy Approach

Zone 1 of the malar region is a safe zone for penetration through the superficial musculoaponeurotic system

(SMAS) into the malar space. There are no significant branches of the facial nerve in that region. Once the rhytidectomy flap has been elevated over zones 1 and 2, the roof of the malar space can be directly penetrated through the SMAS with a small, sharp elevator onto the malar bone. This may be done either medial or lateral to the zygomaticus origins. The seventh nerve branches leading to the frontalis muscle run more proximal over the middle third of the zygomatic arch, and the motor nerve to the orbicularis oculi is more superior. By creating a transverse aperture that parallels facial nerve fibers, there is minimal risk of impairing the motor function. Once the bone level has been reached, a standard subperiosteal dissection and expansion of the malar space are accomplished as described previously (Fig. 75.19). It is important to remember that dissection backward along the zygomatic arch is necessary to position a malar shell implant comfortably and correctly without a buckling of the lateral tail.

Rhytidectomy insertion offers two advantages: (1) a sterile and readily accessible entry wound and (2) a reasonable opportunity for accurate placement with direct observation and palpation (Fig. 75.20).

The author has not used this approach frequently. Nevertheless, because it provides great accuracy in placement and minimal occurrence of asymmetries, it should be seriously evaluated by all surgeons who undertake malarplasty.

75.12
Basic Principles for Augmentation

The basic principles for augmenting the maxillary-midface (malar) and premandible spaces are the same. When applied properly to either region, successful augmentation with few serious or permanent complications should result.

Implants that fill the upper and lateral malar zygomatic areas of zones 1 and 2 create a sharp, high, and angular appearance. Implants that augment the lower aspect of these zones down into submalar zone 5 create a lower, full, round cheek form. Implants that can produce either type of facial contour are now available in varying sizes and shapes.

To augment only the submalar zone, one isolated

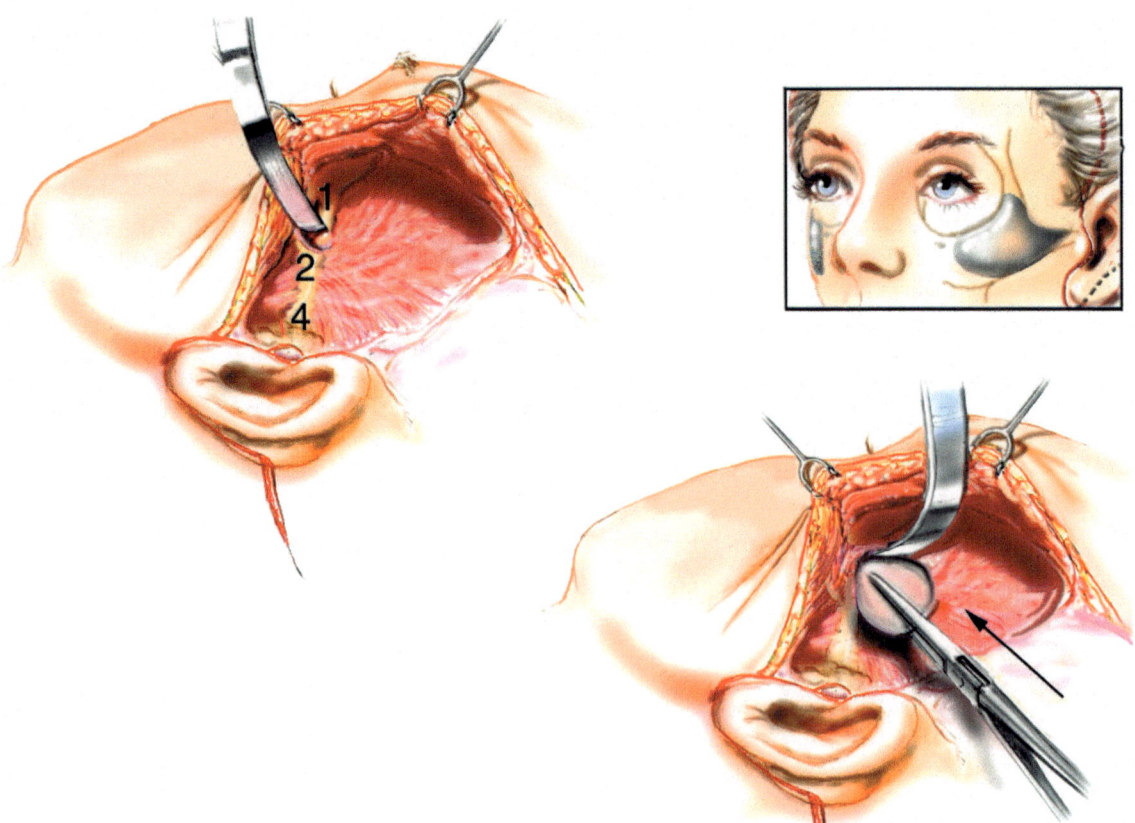

Fig. 75.19 A rhytidectomy insertion of a malar implant is performed by penetrating the soft tissues at the lateral margin of zone 2 over the malar–zygomatic junction. The dissection is routinely performed on the subperiosteal plane. No facial nerve branches are endangered

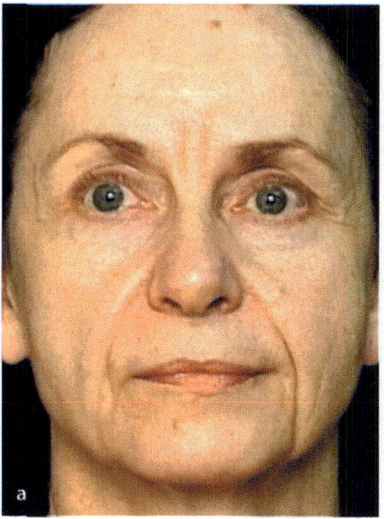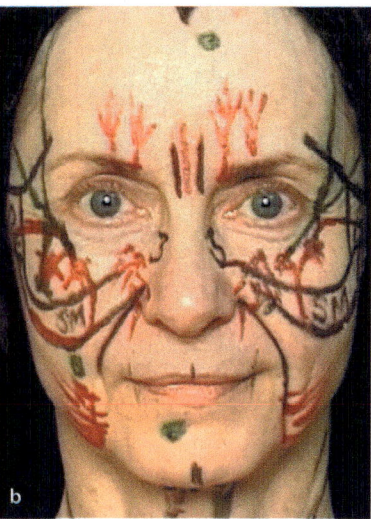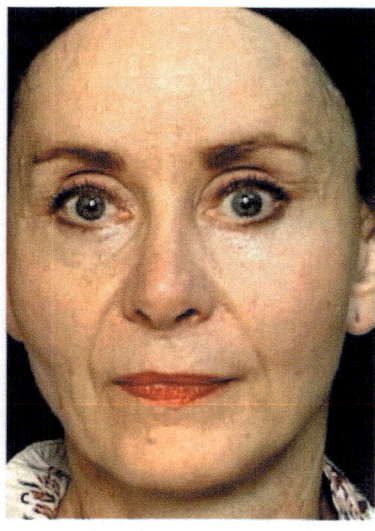

Fig. 75.20 a Preoperative 62-year-old female patient. **b** Postoperative facial contouring consisting of upper midfacial suspension, lateral brow and temple contouring, palpebral eye shaping, malar augmentation, rhinoplasty, and rhytidectomy of the lower face and neck

alloplastic implant is needed. Routinely, this implant is placed through an intraoral approach, and with full visualization of the masseteric tendinous floor upon which it must lie. A submalar implant is basically an anatomic extension of the patient's malar zygomatic bone. Depending upon the thickness that has been chosen (up to 6 mm), this implant adds volume to canine fossa, as well as along the medial and inferior aspect of the patient's virgin bony malar zygomatic eminence. It specifically increases midfacial malar cheek contour medially and inferiorly, provided that the patient already has adequate upper malar zygomatic volume in zones 1 and 2. The anatomic "submalar triangle" (submandibular zone 5) can be variably filled by altering the thickness of the implant.

75.13
Techniques to Ensure Accuracy of Placement

The basic shape of anatomically contoured malar and premandible implants has been designed to fit the facial skeleton. By virtue of their size and the configuration of their posterior surface, these implants have limited capacity for rotational malposition. Accuracy of position is more important in the malar region than in the premandible region. The soft tissues of the central mentum and midlateral zones are usually thick enough to obscure a mild malposition or rotational deformity. In the midlateral zone, where the subcutaneous tissues overlie the mandible, just anterior to the thick volume of the masseter muscle, the posterior tail of the implant

may be significantly prominent, either visually or by palpation. This can be troublesome to the patient, even though a slightly abnormal position may be nearly imperceptible. For these reasons the author's Silastic implants are manufactured with thinly tapered margins that are nearly nonpalpable.

Malposition of an implant is not difficult to correct, but it requires a redissection of the standard premandible space so that the implant can be manually replaced in correct position. Although it is possible to use suture fixation of the implant either percutaneously or intraorally, this author has not found these methods necessary. Fenestration of the implants either peripherally or centrally, as well as texturing of them, may minimize rotational displacement. This problem may be due to dissection of an asymmetric space, along with abnormal placement at the very outset.

Accurate placement of malar implants can be ensured by visually relating the external position of the implant to the internal anatomy. As mentioned previously, the intraoral approach, using fiberoptic instrumentation and adequate anesthesia techniques, facilitates such visualization. The surgeon can create further security by suturing the malar or submalar implant anteriorly to the fibers of the masseter tendon. If placed posterolaterally, the implant can be secured by traction sutures through the implant tail. This can be accomplished by means of 2-0 Surgibond arthroscopy sutures armed on 10-in. needles, which are used to penetrate transcutaneously and posteriorly from within the malar space to behind the temporal hairline (Fig. 75.21). The sutures are tied over a

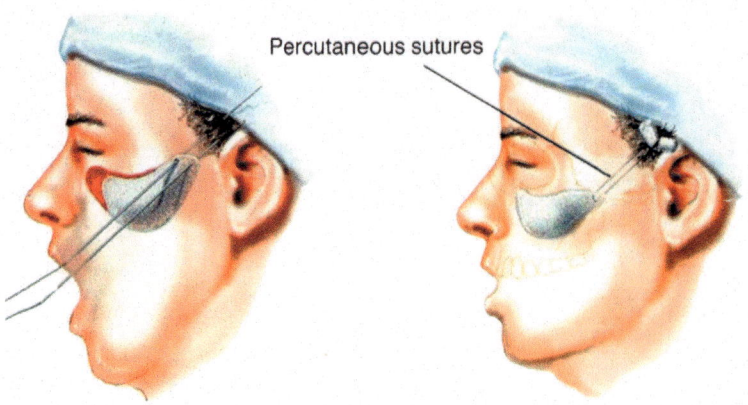

Percutaneous sutures

Fig. 75.21 The long-needle percutaneous fixation technique for malar implants

tonsil sponge for 2 or 3 days. Although not absolutely necessary, this technique appears to provide a small percentage of extra precision necessary to "guarantee" symmetric positioning.

The subcilial blepharoplasty approach, as has already been mentioned, also offers the surgeon an opportunity to visually supervise placement and confirm the accuracy of positioning.

75.14
Premandible Augmentation

Extending a centrally placed implant into the midlateral and posterolateral zones requires only a dissection along the inferior mandibular border into the "safe zone" posterior to the mental nerve. There is a significant constriction and adherence of the tissues to the bone surrounding the mental foramen called the mandibular ligament. Once these have been released, dissection of the tissues from the posterolateral zone occurs easily.

Although operations to augment the central mandible for aesthetic purposes have existed for 60 years, and plastic surgeons have well understood the advantages of improved nasomentum profile relationships, it is only within the last 30 years that methods have been developed for augmenting the premandible by extending central chin implants over a larger surface area as well as their being designed anatomically. These techniques also make it possible to alter the shape and size of the midlateral and posterior aspects of the mandible, and even to lengthen the submandibular segment vertically.

Access to the premandible space can be achieved by either the standard intraoral route or the submental route. This author uses the submental approach exclusively for operations that require additional surgery in the submental and submandibular region, such as liposculpturing and platysmal contouring (Fig. 75.22).

In both approaches, the incisions are transverse and 2 cm long. The intraoral transverse incision is through mucosa only. The mentalis muscles are then divided vertically through their midline raphe to avoid transaction of the muscle bellies and total detachment from

their bony origins (Fig. 75.23). This aperture provides direct access downward onto the bony plane and eliminates the muscle weakening that occurs with customary transaction methods. Incisions that transact muscle fibers not only lead to inadequate closure but also may create weakness and laxity of the mentalis muscle, thereby contributing to a potential for chin ptosis. Ptosis of the mentalis musculature and soft-tissue mound of the central mentum is described in the literature as one of the controversial aspects of alloplastic implants. Indeed, the possibility for deformities, such as central drooping and "witch's chin," does exist. They can be prevented, however, by using the previously described vertical entrance wound and securely approximating the mentalis muscle pillars during closure. The mentalis muscle can easily stretch to accommodate the introduction easily of large, extended anatomic implants.

By adhering to the principle of subperiosteal elevation on bone, the muscle attachments are elevated from their origins along the inferior margin of the mandible. This area does not endanger the mental nerve. The mandibular branch of facial nerve VII does, however, cross just anterior to the midportion of the mandible in the midlateral zone. Consequently, it is important not to traumatize the tissues that overlie and constitute the roof of the premandible space in that region. The mental nerve and foramen can vary in number and location. Reported anatomic variations consist of multiple foramina existing between 1.5 and 4.5 cm from the midline in a certain percentage of individuals. The bony configuration of the foramen, however, directs the mental nerve in a superior path upward into the lower lip. Dissections that remain inferior to the foramen and along the lower border of the mandible avoid significant danger of nerve damage.

In one operation, the author inadvertently placed a premandible implant superior to the mental nerves bilaterally. The immediate result was compression symptoms in the form of anesthesia of the lower lip. Unfortunately, other facial procedures performed at the same time (rhytidectomy and blepharoplasty) obscured the diagnosis until the swelling had diminished. The implant was repositioned beneath the nerves on the ninth postoperative day. Replacement of an implant or repositioning can easily be done within the first 10–14 days. By applying the basic principles of wound healing taught during residency, the surgeon is able to re-enter the premandible or malar space to replace or reposition implants prior to the rapid increase in wound tensile strength, which occurs from 14 to 21 days after the operation. Dysesthesias and paresthesias in small or sometimes larger areas of distribution of the mental nerve are not common following alloplastic chin and premandible augmentation. The symptoms are usually temporary and subside within 4–6 weeks.

Clinically, there appears to be a definite correlation between the occurrence of nerve symptoms and the degree of difficulty that the surgeon experiences in placing the implant. There is no correlation, however, with the size and shape of the implant. Extended alloplastic anatomic-contoured implants contain specific notches designed to avoid pressure around the mental foramen. They provide for normal variations in the location of

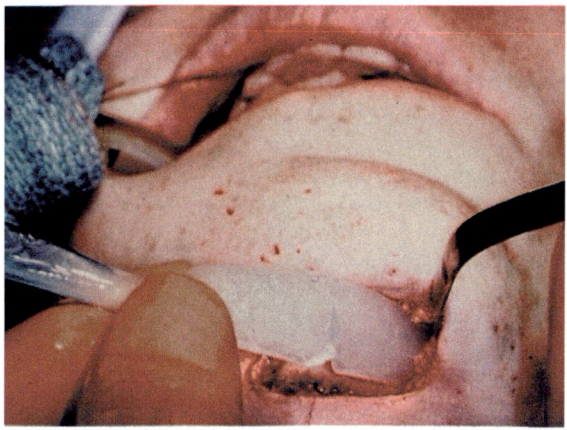
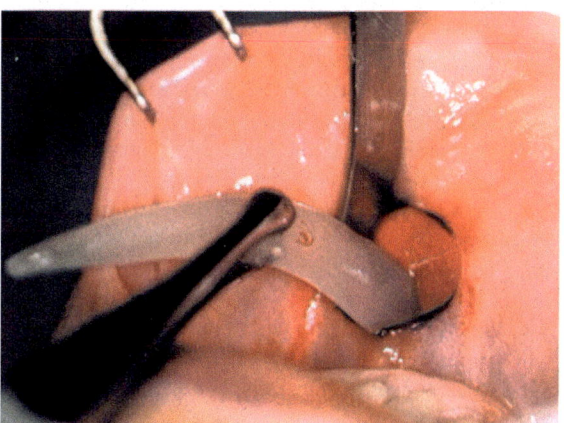

Fig. 75.22 Chin implants can be placed by either the submental or the intraoral route

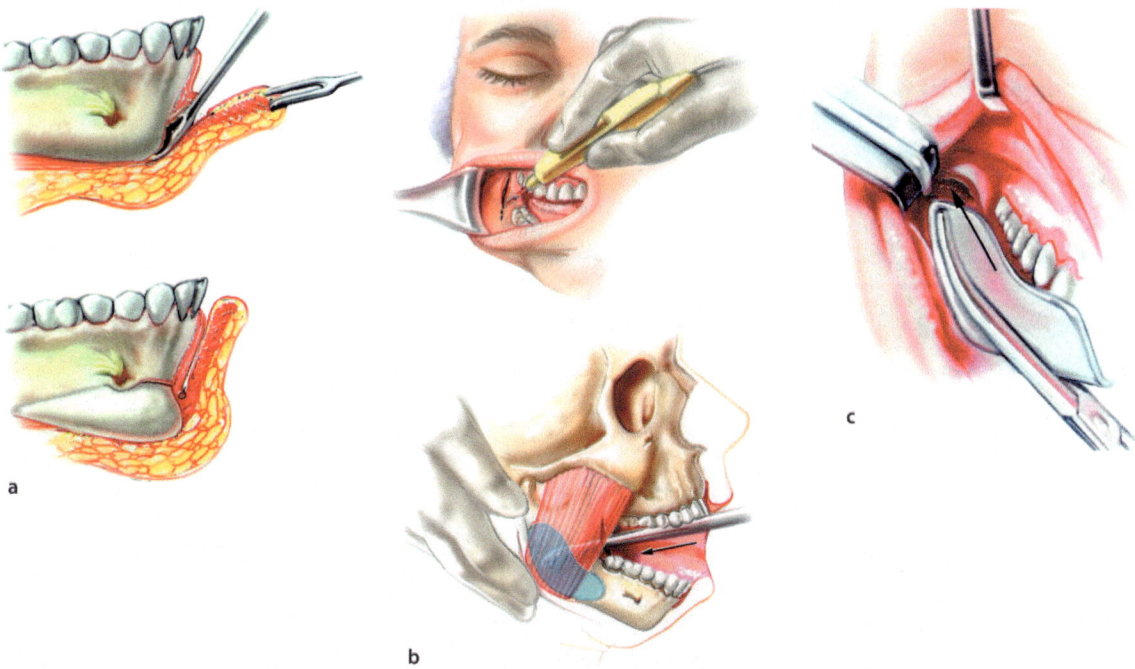

Fig. 75.23 a Intraoral placement of anatomic chin implant subperiosteally and by dissecting vertically between the two heads of the mentalis muscle. **b** A 3-cm intraoral incision is made just posterior to the molar teeth. A subperiosteal space is created, inserting the masseter from the inferior posterior border, and angle of the mandible, as well as on its anterior surface extending up the ascending ramus. **c** Mandibular angle implant insertion using a curved clamp and placing it in an upward and posterior position over the mandibular angle and ascending ramus

the mental foramen, which is 8–10 mm up from the lower mandibular margin.

Additional incisions may be made posterior to the mental nerve to accurately place lateral mandibular bars and implants that extend into the midlateral and posterolateral zones. A 3-cm horizontal mucosal incision made in front of the first molar, followed by direct penetration through the muscle onto the mandibular bone, allows access to, and easy dissection of, the premandible space beneath. This aperture assists accurate placement of the mandibular angle implant and also facilitates positioning the posterior extensions of other implants to augment simultaneously the central mentum and the midlateral zones anteriorly.

The integrity of the mental nerve and easy positioning of the implant beneath it can be ensured through fiberoptic techniques. A narrow, malleable ribbon retractor is utilized to distract the soft tissues for the placement of premandible implants into their tunnels. To position a long, extended premandible implant, a tunnel or space must be created that is longer posteriorly than the length of the implant. The implant can then be inserted from the central incision far into one side and then be folded upon itself to be introduced into the opposite mandibular tunnel. Careful palpation, lateral positioning, and observing the central marking of the implant directly over the central mental protuberance are keys to accurate placement.

Posterolateral implants are placed through either a midlateral incision or a posterolateral incision. The posterolateral incision is transverse and is located approximately 1.5–2 cm anterior and adjacent to the angle of the mandible. Appropriate space for placement is created by making a direct dissection onto bone and subperiosteally beneath the masseter muscle (Fig. 75.23).

A curved elevator is used to dissect around onto the internal and posterior aspects of the ascending ramus in the angle region. In this way, implants designed to fit securely around the angle of the mandible can be accurately positioned. As with all facial implant incisions, a two-layer closure of muscle and mucosa is optimal.

75.15
Choosing Premandible Implants

Implants can be designed to augment every zone of the premandible space. There is very little indication for a central mentum implant. Central implants except for large customized "square front" implants almost always creates a central mound deformity with an adjacent "anterior mandibular sulcus" and potential "witch's chin" or "drooping" appearance (Fig. 75.24). Anterior widening and broadness are achieved when the implant is extended into the midlateral zone. Volumetric expansion of the midlateral and posterolateral zones creates widening of the lower-third facial contour in those premandible zones. The angle of the jaw can be markedly accentuated with a posterior mandibular implant. Heretofore, osteotomies have been used to lengthen the vertical dimensions of the lower facial segment from the nasal spine to the mentum. Now implants have been designed that wrap around the inferior margin of the mandible in the central mentum and midlateral zones to augment and enhance the vertical dimension of the face by 3–5 mm (Fig. 75.24). These implants can produce profound improvement. They also help to correct the anterior mandibular sulcus or "marionette groove" of the aging face.

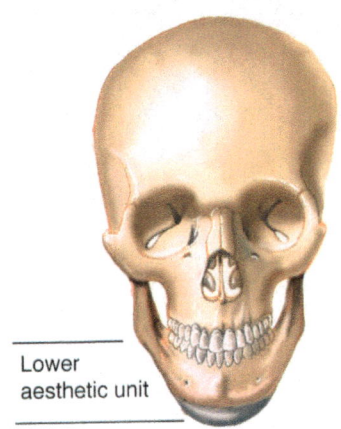

Lower
aesthetic unit

**Submandibular Implant Lengthens Face
in the Vertical Dimension**

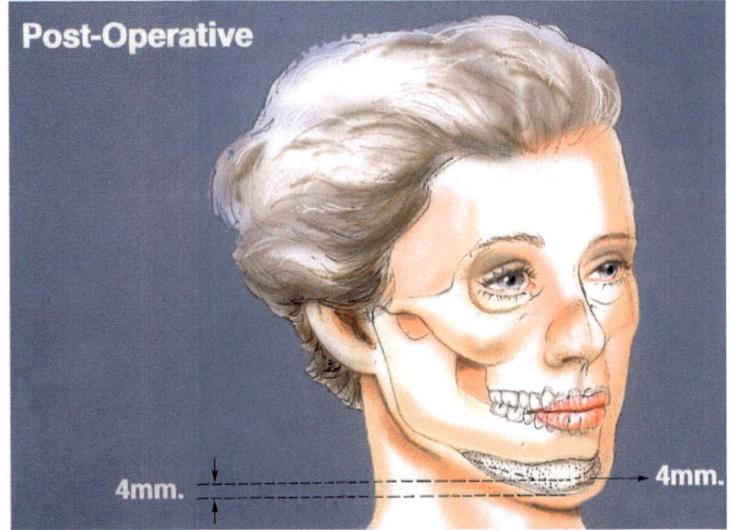

Fig. 75.24 Position of a vertical extension submandibular implant and its dimensions, which produce augmentation of 4 mm of anterior and downward projection

75.16
Conclusions

Infinite variations in facial contour can now be achieved with alloplastic facial implants. By utilizing basic techniques and concepts of zonal anatomy, we can augment the facial skeleton with a minimum of complications. Paramount in determining facial cotour and in minimizing the patient's dissatisfaction is the choice of the size and shape of the implant.

Implants are available or can be customized by the surgeon to create a variety of contours and to fulfill almost any need CEMAX and magnetic resonance imaging computer technology are leading to the manufacture of customized implants with which the surgeon can optimally improve each patient's aesthetic or reconstructive facial balance.

Historically, skin elevation and tightening provided the only remedies for the aging face. In the 1970s and 1980s, the evolution of aesthetic facial surgery created techniques for fat sculpturing and liposuction. SMAS techniques developed by Skoog and improved by others like Peterson, Connell, and Guerrerosantos provided significant advances in rhytidectomy. Midface suspension procedures as promoted by Ramirez, Hester, and others added another attempt at aesthetic alterations with improved contours.

Skeletal augmentation, however, now represents the final chapter for improvement of facial contours. By modifying the skeletal framework, it is possible to alter inherited facial images, as well as to correct the deterioration, sagging, and diminution of facial tissue mass that comes with age. Progress in implant development is continuing. Implants are being designed for the temporal region; the supraorbital, lateral orbital, and frontal ridges; the medial infraorbital groove; and the nasojugal sulcus.

There is now virtually no aspect of the facial skeleton that cannot be augmented satisfactorily. It can truthfully be said that alloplastic implants are the "open sesame" of aesthetic surgery—the door by which almost magical facial changes can be made, depending upon the imagination and skill of the surgeon.

Suggested Reading

1. Gonzales-Ulloa M: Building out of the malar prominences an addition to rhytidectomy. Plast Reconstr Surg 1974;53(3):293–296
2. Gonzalez-Ulloa M: Planning for the integral correction of the human profile. J Int Coll Surg 1961;36:364–373
3. Guerrero-Santos J: The role of the platysma muscle in rhytidoplasty. Clin Plast Surg 1978;5(1):29–49
4. Hinderer U: Malar implants for improvement of the facial appearance. Plast Reconstr Surg 1975;56(2):157–165
5. Millard RD: Chin implants. Plast Reconstr Surg 1953;13:70
6. Pitanguy I: Augmentation mentoplasty. Plast Reconstr Surg 1968;42(5):460–464
7. Ramirez OM: The subperiosteal rhytidectomy: The third generation face lift. Ann Plast Surg 1992;28(3):218–232
8. Safian J: Progress in nasal and chin augmentation. Plast Reconstr Surg 1966;37(5):446–452
9. Terino EO: Complications of chin & malar augmentation. In Peck G (ed): Complications and Problems in Aesthetic Plastic Surgery. New York, Gower Medical 1991:62–63
10. Terino EO: Malar, mandible and chin augmentation by alloplastic techniques. In: Ousterhout D (ed): Aesthetic Contouring of the Cranial Facial Skeleton. Boston, Little, Brown 1991:109–115
11. Terino EO: Alloplastic facial contouring: Surgery of the fourth plane. Aesthet Plast Surg 1992;16(3):195–212
12. Terino EO: Unique mandibular implants including lateral and posterior angle implants. Facial Plast Surg Clin N Am 1994;2(3):311–328
13. Tessier P: The definitive plastic surgical treatment of the severe facial deformities of craniofacial dysostosis. Crouzon's and Apert's Diseases. Plast Reconstr Surg 1971;48(5):419–442

CHAPTER 76

Chin Augmentation

Harry Mittelman, David S. Chrzanowski, Jared Spencer

76.1
Introduction

Chin augmentation with alloplastic implants has been established for over 40 years. The popularity of this procedure has grown owing to a better understanding of the anatomy and aging process of the mandible and an increase in diversity of alloplastic implants which have been more artistically designed for fit, form, and function.

Facial beauty and balance is due in part to a balanced proportion of the chin with the remainder of the face and a straight, youthful, full jawline as the central mentum transitions into the midlateral mandible. The beauty of a strong jawline has been depicted by some of the great artists of the past. In both men and women, a strong jawline gives the illusion of power, strength, confidence, aesthetic balance, and beauty. A weak, receding chin conveys an illusion of negative attributes, such as weak character, combined with a lack of proper facial proportions, resulting in a lack of optimal beauty.

Although chin implantation may seem to be a minor procedure, it is vital for facial beauty and balance. The number of choices for mandibular augmentation may quickly overwhelm a surgeon, since the quality of the surgical result is due in part to selection of the proper implant. However, when one understands the genetic differences in mandibles and particularly the aging process of the mandible, that selection process can be more straightforward. It is possible to fulfill 98% of the needs of the facial plastic surgeon using a small number of alloplastic extended mandibular implants. No aesthetic surgical procedure in the surgeons' armamentarium yields as much benefit for as little time and effort as augmentation of the mandible with the properly chosen alloplastic implant.

76.2
Anatomy

The basic anatomy of the mandible is familiar to the facial aesthetic surgeon, but some points are worth emphasizing. The mental foramen transmits a portion of the third division of the trigeminal nerve, which supplies sensation to the lower lip and chin. The neurovascular bundle, which is surrounded by a tough sheath, exits the mental foramen, and travels in a superior direction.

The location of the mental foramina was described in an anatomic study, showing 50% of humans with their mental foramen below their second mandibular premolar, 25% between their first and second premolar, and 25% posterior to their second premolar [1]. In the typical young adult mandible, the mental foramen is located approximately halfway between the alveolar ridge and the inferior border of the mandible, and approximately 25 mm lateral to the midline, with a range of 20–30 mm [2]. In children, the mental foramen lies closer to the inferior border of the mandible, and slightly more anterior. During the aging process, atrophy of the alveolar ridge causes the foramen to lie in a relatively more superior position, since the distance to the inferior border of the mandible is fairly constant. Even in the aging mandible, there is generally a distance of more than 8 mm between the mental foramen and the inferior border of the mandible at the site of the muscular attachments.

The position of the mental foramina in the aging mandible is important for the facial aesthetic surgeon to understand. This anatomy clearly dictates that the surgeon must dissect carefully when creating a pocket for the implant that is below the mental foramen yet immediately above the muscular attachments at the inferior border of the mandible. Generally, one has approximately 10 mm of space in this area. Properly designed implants should have a vertical height of 6–8 mm when placed into this area.

Because of the superior direction the neurovascular bundle takes when leaving the mental foramen, an elevator used in this space may touch the sheath, and may stretch it to some degree; however, it would be difficult to transect this structure. Although the surgeon has a greater safety factor because of this anatomy, one must still use caution when elevating this lateral pocket for placement of the implant.

Teeth occlusion is another factor to consider in evaluation of the chin. Angle described classes of occlusion of the mandible. In Angle class I occlusion, the mesobuccal cusp of the maxillary first molar abuts the buccal groove of the mandibular first molar. Class II occlusion occurs when the maxilla is relatively more anterior and the mandible is relatively more posterior. Class III occlusion occurs when the maxilla is relatively more posterior and the mandible is relatively more anterior [3]. Chin augmentation with alloplastic implants does not affect mandibular occlusion, but this is an important assessment in determining the proper treatment for mandibular augmentation. Occlusive problems may be better addressed by orthognathic surgery.

76.3
Preoperative Assessment

76.3.1
Patient Evaluation

The basics tenets of facial proportions have been summarized by Powell and Humphreys [4], and include frontal and lateral examination of the face. On frontal view, anatomical landmarks determine the lower third of the face, which extends from the subnasale, the junction of the columella and the lip aesthetic units, to the menton, the most inferior portion of the chin. The lower third of the face can be further subdivided into the upper portion from subnasale to stomion superiorus, the wet–dry border of the upper lip, and the lower portion from stomion inferiorus, the wet–dry portion of the lower lip, to the menton. The ideal proportion exists when the upper portion of the lower third of the face is half the vertical height of the lower portion. With aging, there is loss of the vertical height of the mandible, and therefore a loss of ideal proportion. In addition, the soft tissues overlying the mandible often display some laxity as well as atrophy. This results in creation of a prejowl sulcus.

On lateral view, the pogonion is the most anterior projection of the chin. The ideal location of the pogo-nion is noted when a vertical line is dropped perpendicular to the Frankfort plane from the vermilion of the lower lip [5]. If a patient has Angle class I occlusion, and the pogonion is posterior to this line, the patient has a hypoplastic mentum. While a man's ideal pogonion position is at this vertical line, a woman's ideal position may lay 1–2 mm posterior to this line.

A hypoplastic mentum may be the result of microgenia, which is a small chin that results from underdevelopment of the mandibular symphysis, or from micrognathia, which is a result of hypoplasia of various parts of the jaw. Mandibular augmentation is usually performed for microgenia or mild cases of micrognathia. It is critical to evaluate the patient's mandibular occlusion, with alloplastic augmentation considered in those individuals with normal or near-normal occlusion.

Although congenital factors contribute to development of a hypoplastic mentum, the development of a prejowl sulcus is primarily due to the aging process. Loss of elasticity, and therefore aging, is most notable in the skin and soft tissues of the eyelids, cheeks, and submentum. However, a subtle change also occurs in the area immediately anterior to the jowl, which can have an important effect on facial appearance. A combination of progressive atrophy of the soft tissue and gradual resorption of bone of the inferior edge of the mandible in the area immediately anterior to the jowls [6] causes the development of a groove between the chin and the remainder of the body of the mandible. This is known as the prejowl sulcus (Fig. 76.1) [7]. With time, the prejowl sulcus can become part of the commissure–mandibular groove, or "marionette line", drawing further attention to this area of facial aging.

Chin augmentation is not always a standalone procedure. Mandibular implants are often placed in conjunction with rhinoplasty or rhytidectomy procedures. Therefore, when a patient seeks consultation for improvement in their nasal contour or their submental

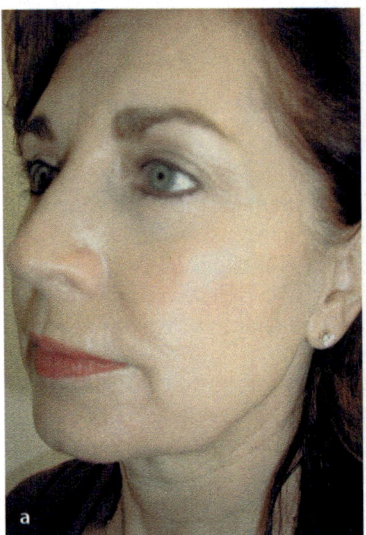 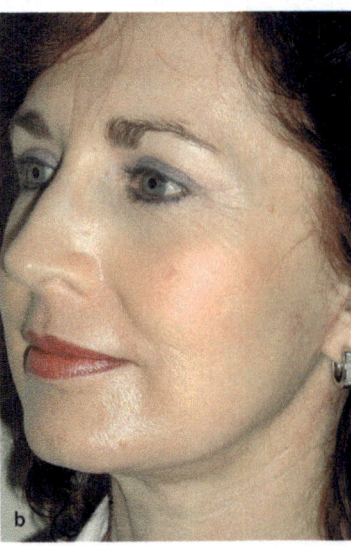

Fig. 76.1 a Preoperative patient with a prejowl sulcus secondary to aging. **b** Postoperative view of same patient following placement of a Mittelman prejowl implant with face–neck lift

area, the astute facial aesthetic surgeon must also consider the importance of projection of the chin or irregularity of the jawline in the prejowl sulcus.

Preoperative photography with a minimum of frontal, lateral, and oblique views is important for photodocumentation and is useful for preoperative planning for implant sizing. Care must be taken to position the patient in the Frankfort plane for all photography. Computer imaging may be especially useful in discussing chin augmentation with the patient with a hypoplastic mentum, especially with the patient who did not seek improvement in this area at the initial consultation. It is also of fundamental importance to assess the patient for preoperative symmetry. Sometimes asymmetry of the jawline may be emphasized after placement of a mandibular implant.

76.3.2
Implant Selection

Both the implant composition and its shape are important factors for proper selection of an implant to meet the needs of the patient. The ideal material for mandibular implantation should have the right consistency, flexibility, and firmness for ease of implantation [8]. In addition it should be non-reactive, resistant to infection, and stable after placement. However, if needed it should be readily removable. The ideal implant should also be easily manufactured and reproducible so that limited resizing needs to be done by the surgeon at the time of the operation. The only alloplastic material that meets almost all of these criteria is a solid, but flexible silicone elastic polymer (Silastic).

Silastic is made of a polymer that can be varied in its number of chains to alter its consistency in order to provide the optimal material in terms of softness and flexibility. The body accepts the material, forming a fibrous capsule that surrounds it, without distorting the implant. Fenestrated Silastic implants may be further stabilized by tissue ingrowth. Silastic may be commercially manufactured to particular sizes and shapes with the aid of computer-aided design technology. These preformed implants may be easily customized by the surgeon in the operating room if indicated by trimming the edges with conventional instruments.
Expanded poly(tetrafluoroethylene) (Gore-Tex, Gore, Flagstaff, AZ, USA) is another material available for mandibular augmentation. The senior author feels that there is limited ingrowth with Gore-Tex implants, which can make their removal, when necessary, slightly more difficult than removal of Silastic implants; however, these implants are still felt to be an acceptable choice by the senior author. Another available material for chin augmentation is polyethylene, or Medpore (Gore). This material is rigid and very difficult to shape. Its rigidity necessitates splitting the implant in half and reapproximating the edges in order to place the implant through

an incision of acceptable size. Medpore permits fibrous ingrowth and is difficult to remove. For these reasons, in the opinion of the senior author, it is not an acceptable choice for chin augmentation.

Selection of one of the many commercially available Silastic mandibular implants can be confusing. The first decision must be the use of an extended mandibular implant rather than a central chin implant. Central chin augmentation results in an unnatural, non-anatomic, pointed chin and undefined jawline. The implants frequently change position and become asymmetrical. Properly designed extended mandibular implants have tapered ends, which provide a smooth transition from the central mentum to the lateral mandible with preservation of the natural jawline.

The three best-researched and most commonly used implants are the extended anatomical mandibular implant (four sizes), the Flowers chin implants (standard, vertical, anterior tilt, and posterior tilt), and the Mittelman prejowl–chin implants (four sizes). All three of these implants provide a slightly different configuration and philosophy, but all give excellent results. The extended anatomical mandibular implant gives uniform augmentation of the prejowl area with varying degrees of central chin augmentation. The Flowers mandibular implants provide a variation in the tilt of the implant at the central mentum with a tapered extension along the mandible beneath the mental foramen.

The Mittelman prejowl–chin implant provides four variations in the size of central mentum augmentation with a comparable four variations in thickness in its lateral extensions, which provide increasing augmentation to the prejowl area. In addition, the Mittelman prejowl implant (without chin/mentum augmentation) is designed with a very thin strip of Silastic in the central third over the mentum, with its thickness situated over the prejowl sulcus. Therefore, it provides four increasing amounts of augmentation to the prejowl area with no augmentation to the central mentum. This implant is an important adjunct for the facelift patient who has adequate chin projection but who has a prominent prejowl sulcus. In another modification of the extended anatomical chin implant by Terino [9], a more squared anterior projection has been designed that is particularly helpful in achieving a more prominent anterior projection, especially suitable for some male patients.

Silastic implants can be of varying firmness or durometer. Softer implants are more flexible and can be placed more easily in smaller incisions. They are also more conforming to the underlying mandible and cause less bony resorption. The senior author prefers Silastic implants with a medium durometer for mandibular augmentation. Fenestrations, which can aid fixation of the implant with the overlying tissue, are included in some extended mandibular implants and all Mittelman prejowl–chin implants and Mittelman prejowl implants.

Table 76.1 Treatment options for mandibular augmentation

Approach	Advantages	Disadvantages
Submental incision	Same submental incision used for submentoplasty/face–neck lift procedure	External scar
	More precise implant positioning	May deepen submental crease when incision not designed properly
	Lower risk of implant migration	
Intraoral incision	Well-camouflaged scar	Less precise implant positioning
		Higher risk of implant migration

76.4 Surgical Technique

76.4.1 Approach

Chin implants may be placed via an intraoral incision or through a submental approach. The intraoral approach avoids an external scar, but implant placement is less precise, with a greater chance of implant malpositioning (Table 76.1). The senior author feels that the submental incision is well hidden, and that the benefits of precise placement afforded by the submental approach will outweigh the well-camouflaged scar.

76.4.2 Initial Dissection

The author's setup for this operation includes a double-hook skin retractor, a scalpel, cautery, an 8-mm ribbon retractor, a 6- and an 8-mm periosteal elevator, two straight clamps, and a gentamicin saline solution (40 mg gentamicin in 100 ml normal saline) to bathe the implant and instruments prior to allograft placement. The submental incision is generally placed immediately anterior to the submental crease, since placement of the incision inside the crease may result in a more depressed scar (Fig. 76.2).

After the submental incision, sharp dissection is carried deep through the soft tissue, muscle, and periosteum just superior to the inferior border of the mandible. Care is taken to ensure the scalpel blade is perpendicular to the tissues and not beveled, which would lead to placement of a periosteal incision too high or too low on the mandible. The length of the skin–soft tissue–muscle–periosteum incision is about 3–4 cm. The periosteum is dissected free for several millimeters inferiorly and approximately 2 cm superiorly to expose the central mentum (Fig. 76.3). Next, dissection continues laterally in the subperiosteal plane between the muscular attachments at the inferior border of the mandible and the mental nerve superiorly (Fig. 76.4). With the right hand holding the dissector, the left "smart" hand

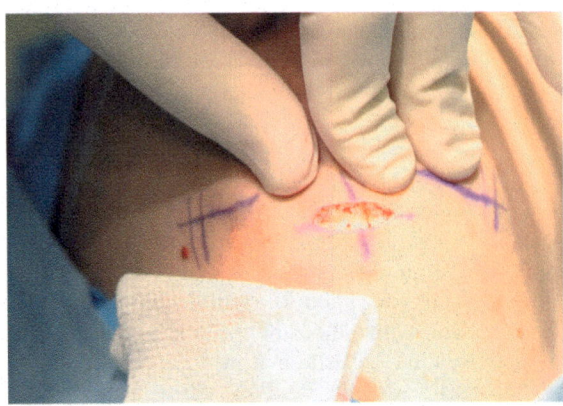

Fig. 76.2 Incision just anterior to the submental crease to prevent depression of scar

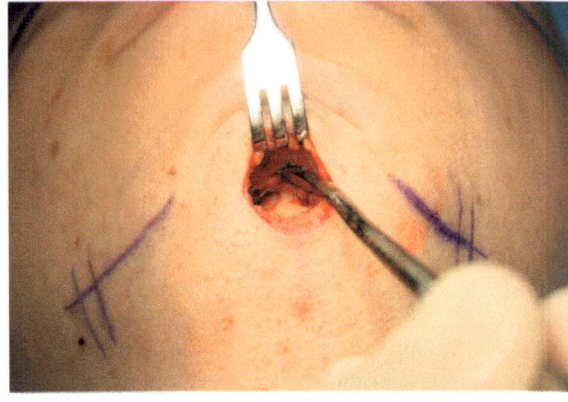

Fig. 76.3 Creation of a central subperiosteal pocket

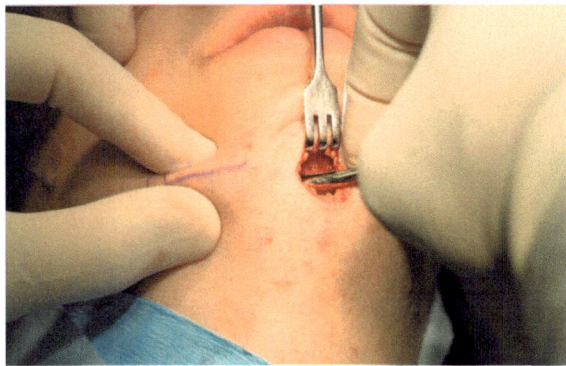

Fig. 76.4 The pocket is extended laterally 6–7 cm from the midline along the inferior border of the mandible. Care is taken to not disrupt the mental nerve superior to the pocket

76.4.3
Implant Preparation and Placement

After the lateral pockets have been developed, the implant is removed from the gentamicin solution and placed in the subperiosteal pocket. All instruments used, including the gloved fingers of the surgeons hands, are dipped in the antibiotic solution to further prevent infection. After the right half of the implant has been placed in the pocket, the left half of the implant is guided with clamps and retractors into the left pocket, by folding the implant acutely on itself (Fig. 76.5). After placement, the implant is checked for smoothness against the mandible, and for absence of lateral fullness that may signal folding or "curling" of its edges on implantation.

In cases when a large or extralarge implant is used, it is not uncommon for the implant to be cut in the center to allow independent placement of each half of the implant (Fig. 76.6). The implant is then sutured at the midline following placement of the two halves. Some authors advocate leaving a central portion of intact periosteum on the mandible, in order to decrease mandibular resorption in this area by the implant (Fig. 76.7). However, the senior author generally undermines the periosteum. Resorption does occur but does not appear to be clinically significant.

protects the nerve of the mental foramen and helps the surgeon guide the instrument externally along the inferior border of the mandible. This helps to prevent excursions above the intended dissection pocket. Lateral dissection should extend approximately 6–7 cm from the midline. Technique CDs can be obtained from implant manufacturers without cost and are most helpful to the surgeon.

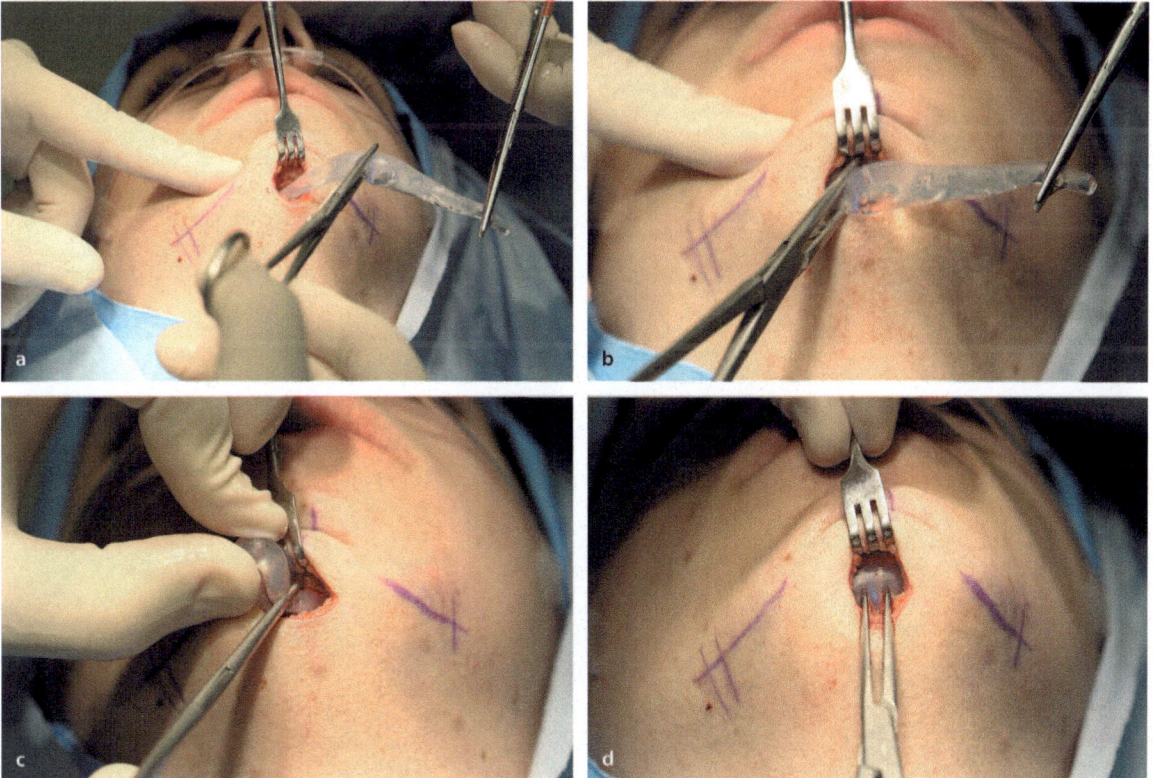

Fig. 76.5 **a** Two straight clamps are used to guide the implant into the right lateral pocket first. **b** The assistant holds the left half to help prevent contact and potential contamination with the skin. **c** The implant is folded on itself and placed into the left pocket. **d** Midline placement is confirmed with the implant's vertical blue line

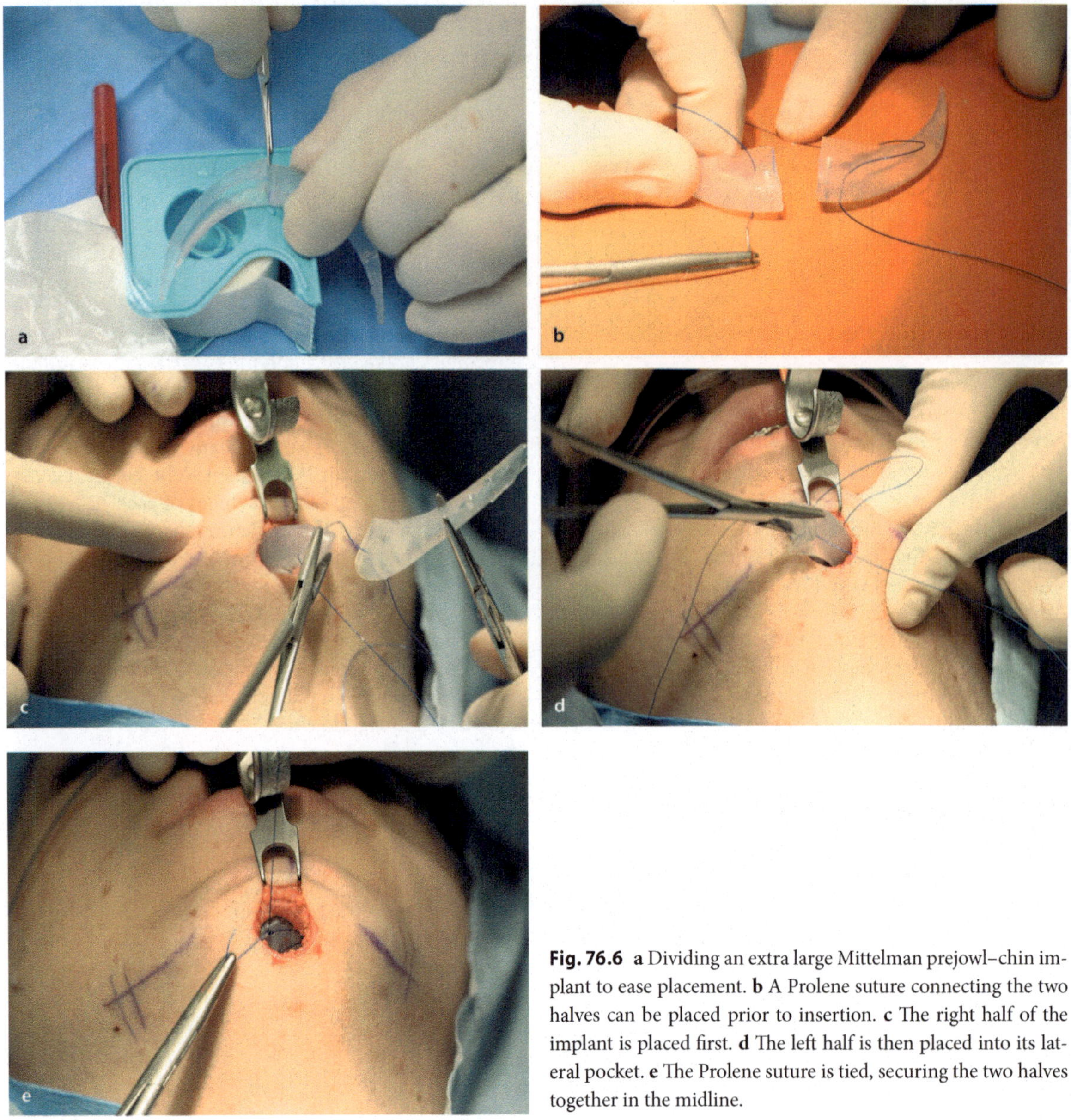

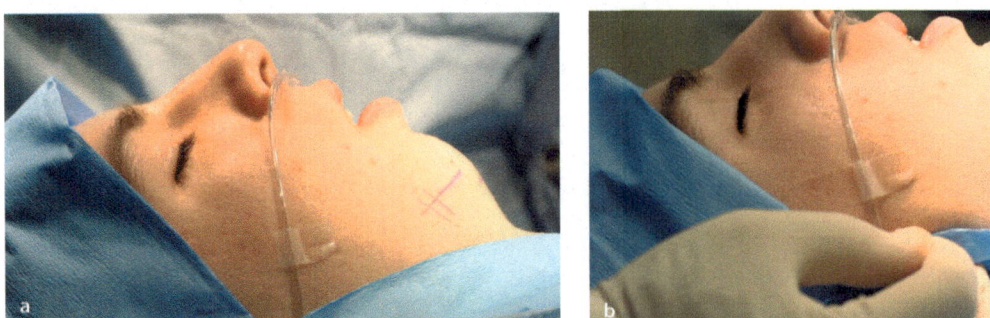

Fig. 76.6 **a** Dividing an extra large Mittelman prejowl–chin implant to ease placement. **b** A Prolene suture connecting the two halves can be placed prior to insertion. **c** The right half of the implant is placed first. **d** The left half is then placed into its lateral pocket. **e** The Prolene suture is tied, securing the two halves together in the midline.

Fig. 76.7 **a** A 16 year-old male patient with hypoplastic mentum just prior to mandibular augmentation. **b** The same patient after placement of an extralarge Mittelman prejowl–chin implant

If difficulty is encountered during insertion of the implant after a pocket was created, the surgeon must identify where the obstruction lies. This may be due to failure of extending the dissection laterally enough. More commonly, the obstruction is found immediately lateral to the central dissection zone, since the implant is still prominent in its vertical height in that location as it tapers from the center to the lateral extensions. This is the location of the anterior mandibular ligament, which is more resistant to elevation in some patients.

76.4.4
Implant Stabilization and Incision Closure

The Mittelman implants have multiple fenestrations present that allow tissue ingrowth to further stabilize the implant. The implant is also marked with a blue line in the center, assisting the surgeon in symmetrical placement of the implant. Prolene sutures can be used to secure all implants to the periosteum. The overlying muscle and soft tissue are closed over the implant. A meticulous closure of the skin follows, using vertical mattress sutures. A sterile dressing is then placed over the incision.

76.5
Postoperative Care

Patients receiving alloplastic implants are always placed on preoperative and postoperative antibiotics. Cephalexin, 500 mg per os, is given the morning of surgery and continued for 5 days postoperatively, in those who are not allergic to the medication. A dressing is used when chin augmentation is performed concurrently with rhytidectomy, and it is removed 24 h after surgery. Patients who have chin augmentation without facelift surgery generally do not need a compressive dressing. Sutures in the submentum are removed between 4 and 7 days postoperatively, and the incision is taped with sterile strips for about 1 week following removal of sutures.

76.6
Complications

Fortunately, the number of complications from placement of alloplastic mandibular implants is small and most commonly temporary. When complications occur, they are usually easily treatable. In the case of improper implant selection or patient preference, the implant may be exchanged for a different size or removed in a relatively simple procedure.

It is estimated from the literature that 4–5% of procedures may result in infection. However, the incidence of infection is lowered dramatically in the author's hands by the use of sterile technique and the incorporation of intraoperative gentamicin solution to bathe all instruments, the alloplastic implant, and the surgically created subperiosteal pockets prior to implantation. It is also important to place the patient on prophylactic antibiotics before and after the procedure. When infection does occur, it usually entails removing the implant, waiting for proper healing, and consideration of replacement of the implant at a later time.

Hematoma is a very uncommon complication of this procedure. Migration or extrusion of extended mandibular implants has not been reported. Also, neither skin necrosis from the external approach nor allergy to the silastic component of the implants has been reported.

Sensory alterations are more common and the most important negative sequela of this procedure, and 20–30% of patients may expect some hypesthesia of the mental nerve distribution on one or both sides [2]. This hypesthesia is almost always temporary, and must be discussed with the patient preoperatively. A period of observation for many weeks is indicated before taking any action if the implant was placed properly. Often a "tingle" or "pins-and-needles" sensation will herald the return of sensation to the numb area. Occasionally, a longer-lasting hypesthesia may be the result of improper dissection of the lateral pocket and placement of the implant superior to the mental nerve foramen. In that case, removal of the implant with or without replacement must take place.

Very infrequently, the smile may be temporarily altered as a result of muscular or nerve surgical trauma. Furthermore, a very small percentage of patients may exhibit temporary speech impediments postoperatively, usually lisping, secondary to the effects of swelling or injury to the depressor muscles of the lip. A combination of hypesthesia of the lip and injury to the mentalis or depressor muscles of the lip may cause temporary drooling and slurring of speech. Motor nerve injury to the marginal mandibular branch of the facial nerve is extremely rare and has almost always been temporary [2].

Bony resorption deep to the implant has been reported since the 1960s, but without significant clinical effects [10]. The softer Silastic implants tend to resorb less bone than the harder ones. Larger implants may cause greater absorption than smaller ones owing to the greater degree of pressure between the implant and bony cortex from the tighter fit.

Resorption tends to occur in the first 12 months and is self-limiting if the implant is properly positioned. It is possible that a small amount of resorption actually stabilizes the implant further over the following years. The soft-tissue profile of the chin tends to remain stable despite this process. No pain or dental erosion has been reported as a result. If the implant is removed, the area of bony resorption may regenerate to some degree.

Visual or palpable projections along the lateralmost portion of the extended mandibular implants may occur owing to capsular formation around the implant, or possibly as a result of infolding of the edge of the implant. This is especially true of the extremely thin, pliable edges of the extended anatomical chin implants. Frequently, gentle massaging over these areas will resolve the problem. Rarely, the implant needs to be removed and the pocket expanded and the implant repositioned. A pocket that was initially too small for correct placement of the extended mandibular implant will cause the feathered edges of the implant to fold on themselves. This problem is usually noted within the first few weeks following the procedure.

Asymmetry may occur owing to improper identification of the patient's preoperative mandibular asymmetry or owing to improper placement of the implant. The surgeon must be aware of any preoperative asymmetry and discuss this with the patient before the procedure. If asymmetry is due to improper placement, the lateral pocket can be dissected and the implant repositioned in the proper position.

76.7
Future Considerations

Mandibular contouring with alloplastic implants is a valuable tool, which allows the facial aesthetic surgeon to improve balance and restore youth to the patient's jawline. Although Gore-Tex and Silastic are proven, reliable materials for use in mandibular allograft surgery, new materials are continually being developed in order to find a more ideal facial aesthetic implant.

References

1. Hollinshead WH. Anatomy for Surgeons: The Head and Neck. Philadelphia, Harper & Row, 1982
2. Mittelman H, Newmann J. Aesthetic Mandibular Implants. Facial Plastic and Reconstructive Surgery. Papel, I. (Ed.), New York, Thieme 2002
3. Angle EH. Some studies in occlusion. Angle Orthod. 1968;38(1):79–81
4. Powell N, Humphreys B. Proportions of the Aesthetic Face. New York, Thieme-Stratton 1984
5. Gonzalez-Ulloa M. A quantum method for the appreciation of the morphology of the face. Plast Reconstr Surg. 1964;34:241–246
6. Anderson JE. Grant's Atlas of Anatomy. Baltimore, Williams & Wilkins 1983
7. Mittelman H. The anatomy of the aging mandible and its importance to facelift surgery. Papel, I. (Ed.), Facial Plastic and Reconstructive Surgery, 2nd edition, New York, Thieme 2002
8. Binder W, Kamer F, Parkes M. Mentoplast—a clinical analysis of alloplastic implants. Laryngoscope. 1981;91(3):381–391
9. Terino EO. Alloplastic facial contouring by zonal principles of skeletal anatomy. Clin Plast Surg. 1992;19(2):487–510
10. Lilla JA, LM, Jobe RP. The long term effects of hard alloplastic implants when put on bone. Plast Recon Surg. 1976;58(1);14–18

CHAPTER 77

Genioplasties for Facial Rejuvenation

Charles D. Hasse

77.1
Introduction

For the most part, the preceding chapters have focused on a spectrum of soft-tissue procedures that can have a profound effect on altering facial form and ultimately improving aesthetics. The vast number of procedures which have been presented make it clear that today's cosmetic surgeon has an extensive armamentarium of techniques available to achieve facial rejuvenation. While patients seeking advice about facial cosmetic surgery often focus on structures such as the nose, the eyes, and the laxity of their skin, the facial cosmetic surgeon's assessment frequently identifies the lower third of the face as an area that can be surgically modified to improve overall facial appearance and harmony.

Like many aesthetic parameters of the face, the concept of the "ideal" chin form has changed with time. The characteristics that are considered aesthetically pleasing vary according to culture, ethnic type, and even historical period. Through art and sculpture, one can visualize the historical patterns regarding chin projection and prominence, vertical proportions, and degree of facial convexity or concavity.

Traditionally, Western society attributes certain personality traits to an individual's facial features [1]. A person with a weak or deficient chin may subconsciously be expected to have a timid, non-athletic, non-aggressive, or non-decisive personality. A weak or retruded chin frequently becomes associated with femininity. An individual with a strong or prognathic chin may be expected to be bold, athletic, aggressive, and decisive. A strong or prominent chin thus becomes associated with masculinity.

Changing fashion, as well as personal preferences of the patient and surgeon alike, play an important role in treatment planning. The surgical techniques for manipulating the chin region have also changed dramatically. Historically, the first sliding osteotomy for correction of a chin deficiency was described in 1942 by Hofer [2], who performed the procedure through an extraoral approach. Today, several surgical options exist for the treatment of chin deformities. Alloplastic chin implants (mentoplasty) and the sliding genioplasty represent the

two currently accepted methods of chin augmentation. Among cosmetic surgeons there is often a debate as to whether alloplastic augmentation or osseous genioplasty is a superior choice for treatment [3]. Obviously, it is important for the surgeon to critically look at the advantages and disadvantages of each approach in the context of the patient's particular needs. Then, the procedure should be chosen which the individual surgeon considers to be the best method in his/her hands for achieving the desired cosmetic result. Regardless of the approach, the symmetry of a patient's face can be significantly improved through osseous movement or augmentation of the mentum. And with this change, facial rejuvenation becomes a reality, and a positive experience for enhancing the well-being of our patients.

77.2
Technique

Excellence in facial rejuvenation techniques requires both a good aesthetic sense and proper surgical technique and preparation. These are skills which can readily be mastered by any well-trained facial cosmetic surgeon. Many facial cosmetic surgeons avoid the genioplasty procedure because it is considered to be technically more difficult, requires longer operating time, or is considered to be potentially more problematic than the augmentation mentoplasty. We refute this mentality emphatically. Any surgeon who is versed in using osseous microsaws should be able to readily achieve the desired cosmetic changes for their patients with little difficulty. The operating time should be a non-issue since it rarely exceeds 60 min. Finally, in our experience, the list of complications, both immediate and long-term, is considerably more extensive when the augmentation mentoplasty is compared with the genioplasty.

Epker and Wolford [4] advocate that in treatment planning for a genioplasty, frontal as well as profile soft-tissue and skeletal morphology must be considered in order to assess the overall objectives to be achieved by the procedure. In simplicity, the surgeon's preoperative assessment must determine what alterations in the transverse, anteroposterior, and vertical dimensions

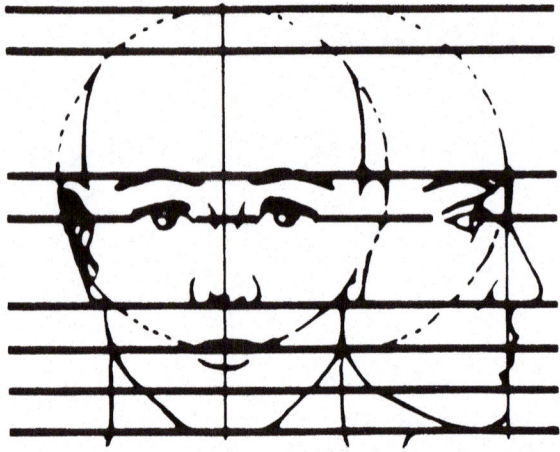

Fig. 77.1 Hasse facial profile analysis
1. The face can be proportionalized into thirds.
2. The lower facial height can be proportionalized into thirds.
3. The face can be proportionalized into halves.
4. A circle drawn from the top of the skull to the lip line, should demarcate the width of the face.

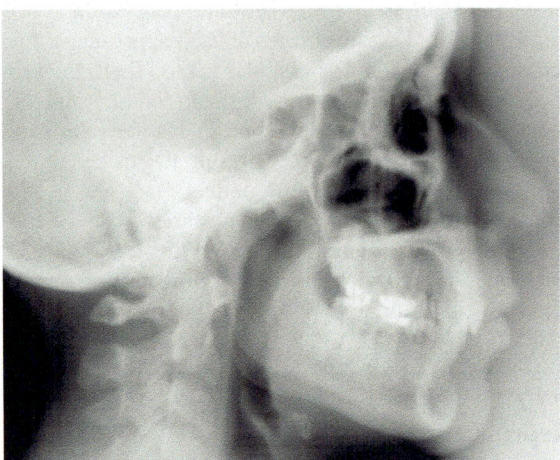

Fig. 77.2 Preoperative lateral cephalometric study with mandible in protrusion during preoperative assessment to estimate the amount of forward bony projection required for optimal aesthetics

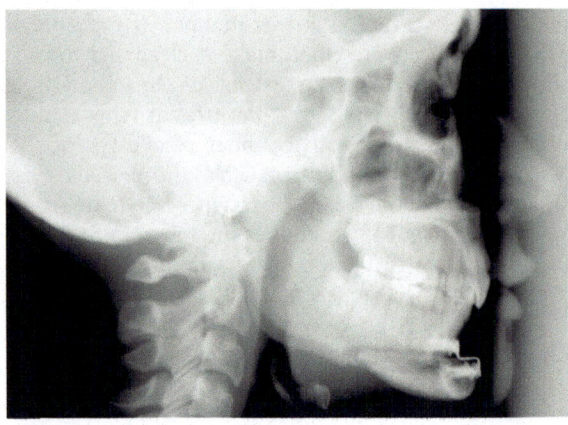

Fig. 77.3 Postoperative lateral cephalometric study. Note lip competency, mentolabial fold, and neck line

are desired and then design an appropriate procedure to achieve these objectives. The use of photographs and quantitative measuring of various facial landmarks can help the surgeon better understand soft-tissue considerations [5]. These, in turn, can be applied to any number of facial profile analysis standards. In 1982, the author introduced the Hasse facial profile analysis [6] (Fig. 77.1), which was an amalgamation of the profileplasty lines of Gonzales-Ulloa [7], combined with our own observations of key proportions of facial symmetry. Regardless of which facial analysis the surgeon favors, the important concept not to be minimized is that in assessing the facial form, the surgeon must have a standard to compare it against.

The use of radiographs is also essential to the necessary assessment for analyzing what can best be accomplishing to achieve optimal facial esthetics (Fig. 77.2). Lateral and anterioposterior cephalometric studies and a panographic X-ray will provide the surgeon with sufficient information to effectively treatment-plan a facial rejuvenation accomplished through osseous surgery (Figs. 77.2, 77.3).

77.3
Standard Genioplasty

Genioplasties can be used to augment, reduce, lengthen, or straighten the external chin [8]. Regardless of the type of genioplasty, the basic surgical approach remains the same. The incision we favor is made in the lower lip with a diathermy knife approximately 15–20 mm from the depth of the vestibule when the lip is extended. Care must be taken to not carry the incision too deep toward the cutaneous surface. The incision is taken down into the orbicularis oris muscle and then directed tangentially toward the bone so that some muscle as well as mucosa remains in the flap adjacent and attached to the dental alveolus. This will allow for a two-layer soft-tissue closure and ensure good superior support to the lip and prevent wound breakdown.

Once the incision has been carried to the bone, the symphysis is degloved by subperiosteal dissection. It is prudent for the surgeon to identify the position of the mental nerves from the preoperative panographic radiograph since their location can be quite variable. The mental nerves are exposed by dissecting posteriorly along the inferior border of the mandible and elevating the mucoperiosteum. Frequently, the subperiosteal dissection can be extended above the neurovascular bundle to gain better exposure, but this is not always necessary. The periosteum around the bundle is then excised for relaxation to minimize retraction tension.

The digastric muscles are cut with the diathermy knife to reduce the muscle tension they otherwise would exert on the osteotomized bone. The geniohyoid muscles remain attached and provide the principal blood supply to the osteotomized segment.

The horizontal osteotomy should be planned out with a few points in mind. Specifically, the surgeon must be cognizant of where the apices of the anterior teeth, particularly the cuspid teeth, lie. It is recommended to leave 4–6 mm of clearance below the cuspids to ensure that the vitality to the anterior teeth is maintained and to allow sufficient room for placement of a fixation plate in the superior segment. Similarly, the position of the mental nerves should be identified and it is advisable to leave about 3 mm of clearance below the foramina to prevent postoperative neurosensory alteration.

The horizontal osteotomy is made with a reciprocating saw blade and is completed through both the labial and lingual cortices. The cut must be made cleanly but judiciously through the lingual cortex. The surgeon

should stop repeatedly and feel his/her way through the bone with the saw blade to ensure that a complete cut is obtained. An incomplete cut can result in a pathological fracture particularly in the area just posterior to the mental foramina. Conversely, too aggressive an approach can result in a significant muscle bleed from the geniohyoids. Following completion of the cut bilaterally, the pedicled inferior segment is mobilized. Any irregularities in the bone cut can be modified by using a reciprocating bone file or a rotary football burr. This will allow good bone-to-bone contact to maximize stability and healing.

The author favors using a six-holed titanium plate with a step (Walter Lorenz, Jacksonville, FL, USA) to stabilize the inferior segment (Fig. 77.4). The plate is secured using screws typically of 7–13 mm in length. The screw length is determined by the anteroposterior dimension of the chin. It is important to have the screw engage the lingual cortex for stability but not extend beyond into the muscle. Generally, the anteroposterior dimension of the symphysis is about 8–15 mm, so advancements of this magnitude can be readily accomplished. The Lorenz plates are marked on the face of the plate with the desired amount of forward movement. Some surgeons have reported good results using resorbable plates but we have not used this method nor seen the need for this approach. Regardless of the method of stability, the presurgical workup determining the desired (predicted) amount of advancement is the key to accomplishing a predictable and aesthetic cosmetic result (Fig. 77.5).

The incision is closed in two or three layers with resorbable sutures. It is recommended to place the first suture of each layer first at the midline to properly align the soft tissues and prevent uneven closure. The deep sutures are placed so as to maximally elevate the lip. Reposition (reattach) the mentalis with interrupted 3-0 Vicryl sutures buried deep. Continue to the mucosal layer with a continuous running or locking stitch. The face and muscles should be supported with an elastoplast dressing. We use 1-in. strips positioned just below

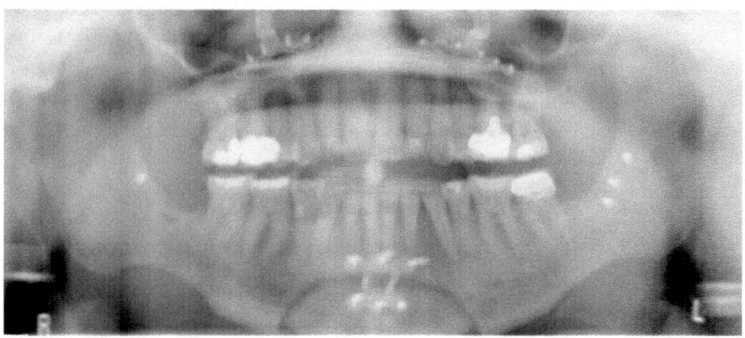

Fig. 77.4 Six-holed titanium plate (Walter Lorenz, Jacksonville, FL, USA)

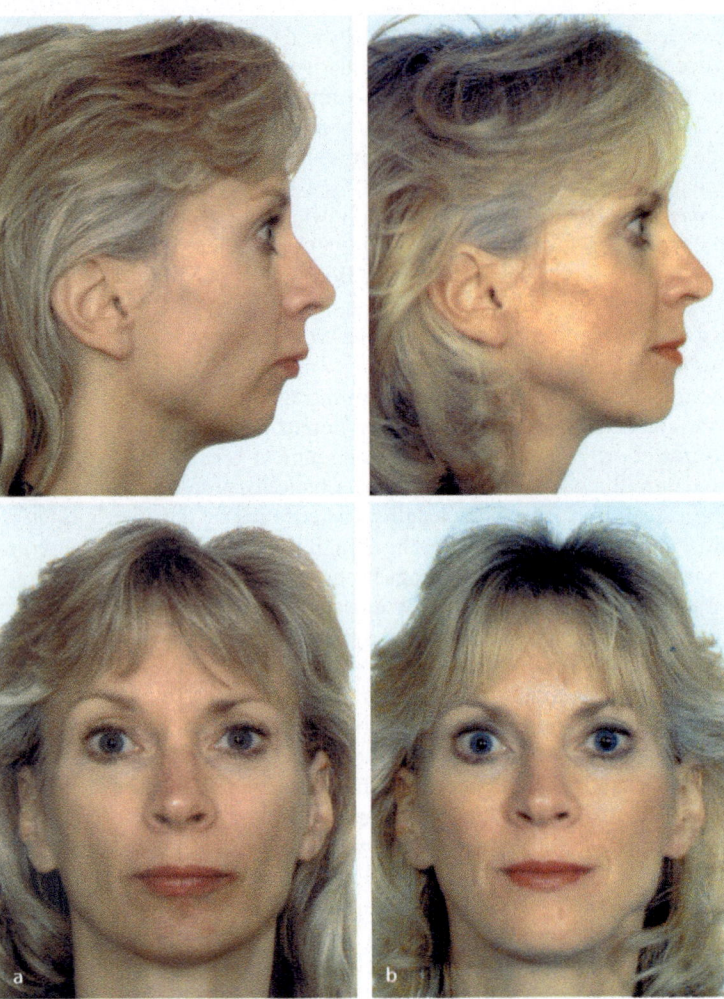

Fig. 77.5 Standard genioplasty. **a** Preoperatively. **b** Postoperatively

the cutaneous border of the lower lip to support the mentalis and associated lip musculature to maintain proper lip form. Additionally, this will minimize the potential for swelling and hematoma formation. Next, a strip of 2-in. elastoplast is placed in a U configuration to support the submental area. Some surgeons favor additional support using a Jobst facioplasty stocking with fluffs. A hot-ice bag is placed inside the Jobst stocking with running continuous laminar water flow set at 40°F for the first hours. This approach will greatly reduce swelling and promote quick clot formation.

77.4
Reduction Genioplasty

In situations where the surgeon has determined that the lower facial height is greater than the mid and upper facial heights or that the anterior projection of the chin is due to macrogenia, then a reduction genioplasty is

the procedure of choice. A reduction genioplasty can effectively decrease the size of the chin vertically, anteroposteriorly, or in both directions as determined by the surgeon's aesthetic sense and facial profile analysis (Fig. 77.6).

The basic technique employed for the standard genioplasty is used with a few modifications. The initial soft-tissue incision is the same except that the anteroinferior aspects of the symphysis is not degloved. Nevertheless, an adequate amount of anterior and inferior periosteum must be reflected in order to allow for sufficient room to make the bony cuts and to provide room for the fixation plate. It is necessary to reflect the periosteum directly below the mental foramen off the inferior border to facilitate completion of the ostectomy through the inferior border.

The midline should be scribed with an oscillating saw blade or a fine-fissured bur as a reference to maintain symmetry. It is further recommended to place vertical reference lines just lateral to and below the cuspid api-

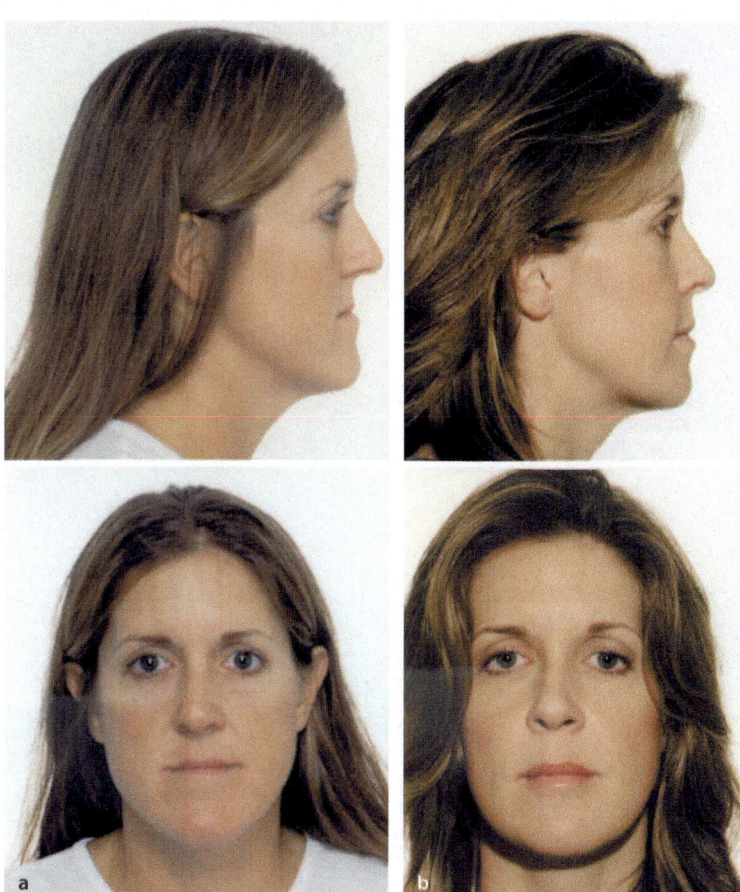

Fig. 77.6 Reduction genioplasty. **a** Preoperatively. **b** Postoperatively

ces to facilitate accurate repositioning of the mobilized inferior segment. With use of Epker bone calipers, the predetermined amount of vertical bone to be removed is outlined and scored prior to cutting. It is recommended to perform the ostectomy as high as possible while maintaining the necessary 4–6 mm of clearance below the root apices of the anterior teeth. With use of a reciprocating saw, the two horizontal osteotomy cuts are made, with the lower cut being completed first. The superior osteotomy is then performed and the bony wedge removed. The attached musculature (geniohyoid and/or genioglossus muscles) should be detached from the wedge using the diathermy knife. The inferior portion of the symphysis with its attached soft tissues is mobilized inferiorly and with good visualization the superior and inferior lingual cortical margins are checked for bony interferences. These are readily removed with a reciprocating bone file or rotary football bur.

The surgeon lines up the midline and lateral reference points prior to fixation. The author advocates using two four-holed titanium plates or two L-shaped plates (Walter Lorenz, Jacksonville, FL, USA) to secure the segment. Titanium plates with a step can be used if the surgeon desires to both reduce the vertical chin dimension but increase the anterior projection. The surgical site is irrigated copiously, the soft tissues are closed in layers as previously described, and the supportive chin dressings are applied. Van Sickels et al. [9] report that with this basic technique a predictable 80–100% soft tissue to osseous change can be obtained, depending on the degree of change in the anteroposterior and vertical directions. Our experience in using this approach in over 200 cases is in agreement with their findings with an average soft tissue to bony change of 86%. Such predictability allows the surgeon to present an accurate and realistic final picture when treatment-planning our patients. Finally, contingent upon the size of the wedge removed and the laxity of the patient's skin, a concomitant submental liposuction procedure or chin tuck may be advisable to complete the facial rejuvenation.

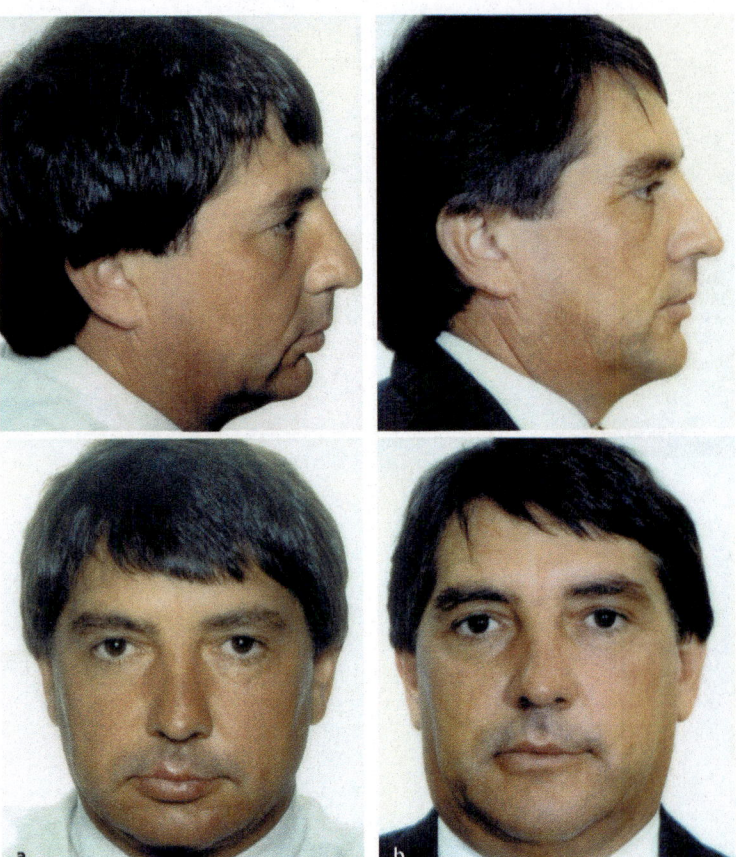

Fig. 77.7 Lengthening genioplasty. **a** Preoperatively. **b** Postoperatively

77.5
Lengthening Genioplasty

The lengthening genioplasty is indicated in clinical situations in which the primary facial deformity is a decreased anterior mandibular vertical dimension. Microgenia is exactly the opposite condition of macrogenia, with the anatomical deformity resulting in a short vertical lower third of the face. This "short face syndrome" can readily be corrected through the use of the standard genioplasty technique modified to accommodate osseous augmentation to increase the lower facial height as determined by facial profile analysis (Fig. 77.7).

After routine exposure of the symphysis through a full-thickness mucoperiosteal incision in the mandibular anterior vestibule and lip, the proposed osteotomy is delineated, midline and lateral reference lines are scored in the bone, and the cut is then completed with a reciprocating saw. In performing the osteotomy, the surgeon should attempt to carry it as far posteriorly as possible. The type of fixation plates that the surgeon selects is contingent upon what is the goal of the procedure. If it is desirous to lengthen the chin in a vertical dimension only, then a plating system without an anterior step is selected. If, however, the surgeon desires to increase the lower facial height vertically and increase the anterior projection of the chin, then a titanium plate with a predetermined step should be selected.

Cortical block grafts are wedged in-between the mobilized inferior segment and the body of the anterior mandible before fixation. Prior to the turn of the century, bone was readily harvested either from the anterior iliac crest or from the tibia to accomplish this purpose. In recent times, processed bone products have been made available to accomplish the lengthening without subjecting the patient to the harvesting procedure, which could have morbidity as well as be both painful and time-consuming.

For lengthening procedures in which the desired vertical increase is 6 mm or less, the author recommends maintaining bony contact in the posterior piece while angulating the anterior piece downward to the desired additional vertical length. The chin is stabilized with a

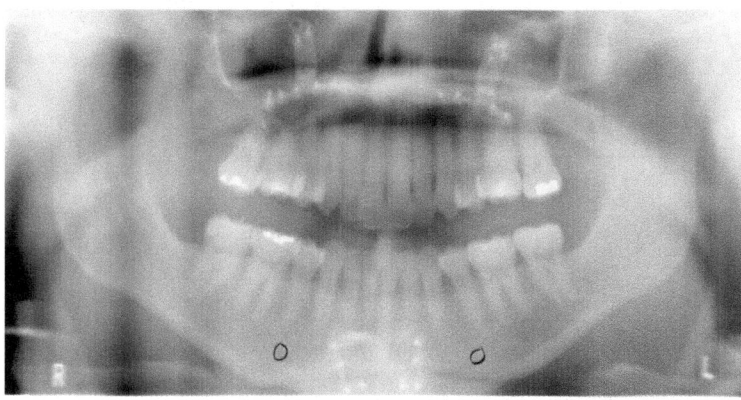

Fig. 77.8 Postoperative panographic radiograph showing lengthening genioplasty stabilized by two L-shaped Lorenz fixation plates

six-hole Lorenz plate (Walter Lorenz, Jacksonville, FL, USA) (Fig. 77.8). The bony gap that is created by tipping the bone downward is then filled in with bone matrix product OrthoBlast II (Isotis Orthobiologics US, Irvine, CA, USA) to allow for rapid healing, stability, contour, and eventual bone ingrowth. OrthoBlast II contains demineralized bone matrix and cancellous bone in a putty or paste medium which provides an osteoconductive scaffold for bone deposition and remodeling.

For vertical lengthening procedures in which the increase is greater than 6 mm, the surgeon should use cortical block grafts of some type for stability. The grafts are wedged between the superior and inferior (mobilized) segments prior to plating the anterior portion of the segments. Instead of harvested corticocancellous bone grafts the surgeon can use banked autogenous bone or a bone matrix product such as Grafton DBM Flex grafts (Osteotech, Eatontown, NJ, USA). The use of OrthoBlast II is recommended to promote osteoinductive and conductive activity, bone fill, contour, and stability.

Upon completion of the lengthening procedure, the wound is closed in layers as previously described with a supportive chin dressing applied, a hot-ice bag, and a Jobst facioplasty stocking. Depending upon the amount of lengthening achieved, it may be difficult to reattach the mentalis muscle over the lengthened chin as desired. Close reapproximation of the muscle is sufficient. Similarly, the soft-tissue mucosa may require a releasing incision to ensure good, tension-free primary closure.

77.6
Straightening Genioplasty

Straightening genioplasty is indicated in any facial rejuvenation case in which there is an asymmetry in the lower facial height which is of a cosmetic nature only

and not a functional problem. Functional problems are best solved by conventional orthognathic surgery techniques and usually result in surgery of the mandibular ramus or body of the mandible.

The predictability of a satisfying cosmetic result is best achieved through careful planning. An anterioposterior cephalometric facial film is essential. Through the use of a profile analysis, the surgeon can determine whether the asymmetry can best be resolved by sliding the chin laterally, or adding bone (modified lengthening technique) to one side or subtracting bone (modified reduction technique) from one side to best achieve facial proportion. Regardless of the surgical approach, Epker and Wolford [4] stress the importance of maintaining the optimum possible amount of soft tissues attached to the inferior segment. This is because cases with pronounced asymmetry have inherent asymmetry of both the bony and the soft-tissue components. If the soft tissues are totally reflected from the inferior border, they will not rotate equally to the osseous change and a soft tissue to bone change will not be achieved, resulting in less than optimal aesthetics.

The principles of the surgical technique are essentially identical as previously described for standard, lengthening, and reduction genioplasties. It is imperative that the surgeon identify where the bony discrepancy lies from his/her preoperative facial profile analysis. In simplicity, the surgeon is performing a lateral sliding genioplasty, a reduction genioplasty, or a lengthening genioplasty on either the right or the left side of the osteotomized menton. The incision is the same, with care taken not to deglove the mandibular symphysis. A horizontal osteotomy is performed after scoring the midline and lateral reference lines. The midpoint of the chin should be aligned with a vertical reference line dropped from subnasale, through the philtrum of the lip and the dental midline provided that these reference points are anatomically centered.

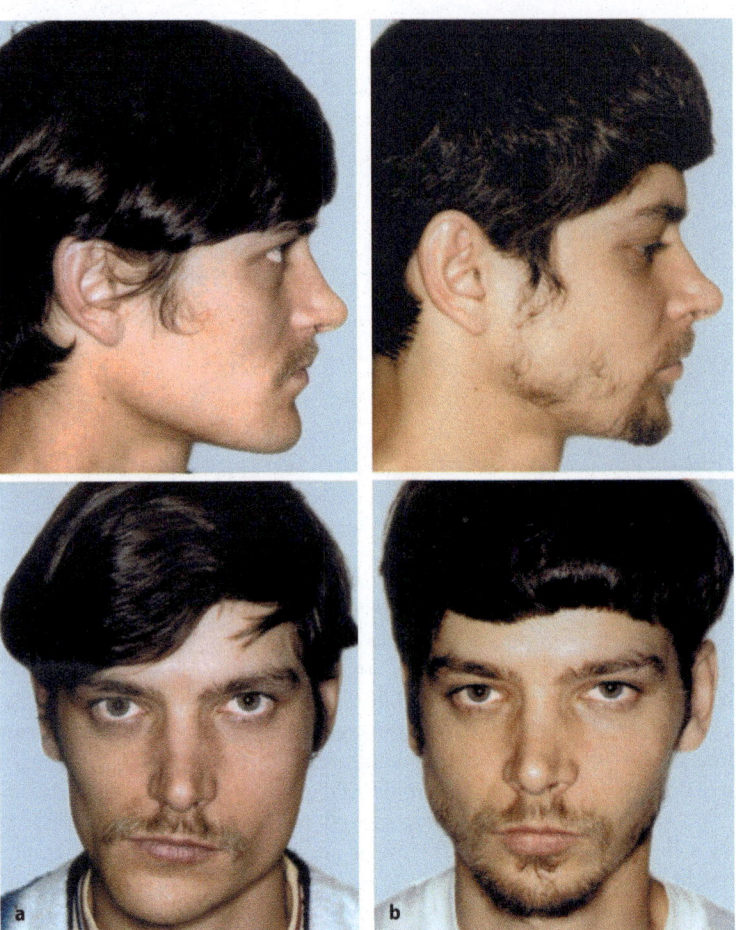

Fig. 77.9 Straightening genioplasty.
a Preoperatively. **b** Postoperatively

The surgeon either adds bone for balance or removes bone through a second osteotomy to create harmony. In some instances a sliding genioplasty is performed with lateral rotation to the midline. In this instance it may be necessary to use a rotary football bur or a reciprocating bone file to trim any excess at the lateral extent. The segment is repositioned and stabilized as previously described. A layered closure is made and supportive chin dressing applied (Fig. 77.9).

77.7
Complications

Neurosensory disturbance of the mental nerve has been reported as the most common complication associated with genioplasty surgery; however, it is generally thought to be transient provided that no major branches of the mental nerve are transected. Karas et al. [10] reported that immediately following surgery 20% of lower lip and 40% of chin sites showed alteration following genioplasty. However, all lip and chin sites were reported to return to preoperative values within 6 months as quantified by static light touch, moving-touch discrimination, and two-point discrimination evaluation. Because of its location, the mental nerve is vulnerable to damage when a genioplasty procedure is done.

Possible causes for neurologic complications include:
- Inadequate exposure secondary to poorly designed or executed soft-tissue dissections.
- Inadequate protection of the mental nerve during the osteotomy cut.
- Excessive retraction or compression around or on the mental nerve.
- Injury to the nerve during the osteotomy at the point where it dips below the foramen.

Other complications reported but rarely encountered are infection, malpositioning of the segment, nonunion or fibrous union of the segments, relapse, and complications with use of the hardware (plate extrusion, fixation screw breakage).

77.8
Discussion

The sliding genioplasty is a time-honored technique that can modify facial form and obtain a proportionality more far reaching result than many of the soft-tissue procedures currently in use for facial rejuvenation. It is more versatile than the mentoplasty, that is, augmentation via alloplastic implant, since mentoplasty procedures are limited to enhancing anterior projection of the chin only. Alloplastic chin implants lack the versatility necessary to achieve three-dimensional positional changes so critical to overall facial proportionality and optimal facial rejuvenation.

In addition, a significant advantage of the genioplasty versus mentoplasty is the preservation of the natural contour of the chin. Furthermore, the disadvantages associated with mentoplasty to augment the contour-deficient profile are numerous [11]:

- Bone erosion beneath the implant
- Mobility of the implant
- Infection
- Unpredictable soft-tissue changes
- Improperly sized implants
- Malpositioning
- Extrusion
- Capsular contracture
- Encapsulation of implant
- Facial scarring
- Neurosensory deficits
- Chin ptosis
- Lower-lip retraction

In spite of these disadvantages, the main advantage to the mentoplasty is that it can readily be performed under local anesthesia. A further advantage to the mentoplasty when performed through a submental facial incision is that it allows for adjunctive procedures such as submental liposuction and effacement of platysmal banding to be performed through it.

However, concomitant genioplasty and submental lipectomy can effectively be accomplished together. The genioplasty is performed as described in our standard fashion. Then, the submental lipectomy is done extraorally through a short transverse skin incision in the submental area. While this approach requires two surgical sites, each site is self-contained and the chance for infection is negligible provided that the surgeon is diligent.

Finally, the genioplasty should be considered as a wonderful adjunct to other cosmetic facial surgery. Chang et al. [12] estimates that correction of poor projection of the chin is desirable in approximately 20% of patients undergoing rhinoplasty and in about 25% of patients having a rhytidectomy. The surgical goals for any given procedure are to create an aesthetically pleasing facial contour. Thus, it is the surgeon's responsibility to educate the patient regarding any deficiency that may exist, and to show how with surgery an overall balanced cosmetic result may be achieved.

77.9
Conclusions

Strauss and Abubaker [13] reported that when comparing augmentation mentoplasty versus genioplasty technique, the genioplasty technique had a slightly better patient satisfaction rating, better soft-tissue predictability, and fewer detrimental postoperative complications. This has been our experience also. While complication rate for either procedure should remain low provided that the surgeon adheres to good surgical technique, the inherent advantages of the genioplasty as a more versatile procedure that can be used to correct any type of chin deformity make it the procedure of choice in most instances of facial rejuvenation. We limit the use of augmentation mentoplasty solely to instances where three-dimensional positional changes of the chin are not essential for overall facial proportionality. In all other clinical situations, the genioplasty remains the procedure of choice to achieve optimal facial aesthetics.

References

1. Bell WH, Gallagher DM: The versatility of genioplasty using a broad pedicle. J Oral Maxillofac Surg 1983;41(2):763–769
2. Hofer O: Operation der pronathie und mikogenia. Dtsch Zahn Mund Kieferheikd 1942;27:81
3. Guyuron B, Raszewski RL: A critical comparison of osteoplastic and alloplastic augmentation genioplasty. Aesthet Plast Surg 1990;14(3):199–206
4. Epker BN, Wolford LM: Dentofacial Deformities: Surgical-Orthodontic Correction . St. Louis, Mosby 1980
5. Schendel SA: Genioplasty: A physiological approach. Ann Plast Surg 1985;14(6):506–514
6. Hasse CD, Morgan DH: Orthognathic Surgery in Diseases of the Temporomandibular Apparatus: A Multidisciplinary Approach. St. Louis, Mosby 1982
7. Gonzalez-Ulloa M, Stevens E: Role of chin correction in profileplasty. Plast Reconstr Surg 1968;41(5):477–486
8. Hinds EC, Kent JN: Genioplasty: The versatility of horizontal osteotomy. J Oral Surg 1969;27(9):690–700
9. Van Sickels JE, Smith CV, Tiner BD, Jones DL: Hard and soft tissue predictability with advancement genioplasties. Oral Surg Oral Med Oral Pathol 1994;77(3):218–221
10. Karas ND, Boyd SB, Sinn DP: Recovery of neurosensory function following orthognathic surgery. J Oral Maxillofac Surg 1990;48(2):124–134

11. Guyuron B: Genioplasty. Boston, Lippincott, Williams & Wilkins 1993

12. Chang EW, Lam SM, Karen, M, Donlevy JL: Sliding genioplasty for correction of chin abnormalities. Arch Facial Plast Surg 2001;3(1):8–15

13. Strauss RA, Abubaker AO: Genioplasty: A case for advancement osteotomy. J Oral Maxillofac Surg 2000;58(7):783–787

CHAPTER 78

Aesthetic Surgery of the Aging Neck: Options and Techniques

Bhupendra C.K. Patel

78.1
Introduction

"I have baggy eyelids," and "I don't like my neck" are, arguably, the commonest complaints one hears from patients seeking facial aesthetic improvements. The latter complaint may be presented as "I am beginning to look like my mother," "I have a fat neck," "I have loose skin in my neck," "I hate my jowls" and other such specific or nonspecific complaints. When pressed to identify the exact changes needing improvement, patients may point to the obtuse cervicomental angle, loose skin, neckbands, presence of jowls and submental fat.

To rejuvenate the aging neck, it is important for the surgeon to have an understanding of normal neck anatomy in youth, the chronological changes that occur in most patients, the anatomy of the aged neck and variations as they apply to gender and race [1, 2].

78.2
Anatomy of the Neck

The ideal youthful profile shows various distinct features (Fig. 78.1). The distinct cervicomental angle is between 105 and 120° (Fig. 78.2). The cervicomental angle is created by a breakpoint between the vertical portion of the neck and the transverse submandibular plane. The junction of the vertical and horizontal portion of the cervicomental angle is at the anterior surface of the hyoid, which is normally at or above the plane of the jaw; therefore, a low hyoid or a recessed mandible may affect the position of the cervicomental angle. The horizontal portion of the neck (transverse submandibular plane) is composed of the mandibular border, subplatysmal fat, digastric muscles, platysma, fat and skin. The digastric muscles, supplied by the mylohyoid branch of the inferior alveolar nerve, are attached superiorly to the medial surface of the parasymphyseal portion of the mandible bilaterally. The muscles course inferolaterally to attach to the lesser cornu of the hyoid bone by way of an aponeurosis. The muscle elevates during deglutination (Fig. 78.3).

On anterior view, the mandible should demarcate the face from the neck as a distinct inferior border, casting a shadow that hides the submandibular glands. This prominent jawline is often described as a "manly jaw" or a "strong jaw". The chin should be prominent, both anteroposteriorly in width and height ("strong chin"). The mandibular angle should be visible; there should be no skin laxity or jowling along the mandibular border.

There is a transition zone between the relatively fixed perioral area and the mobile neck and cheek skin. This transition in the neck is seen at the submental fold, which is barely visible in youth. In adults, with age, it often extends onto the cheeks. There are retaining cutaneous ligaments that originate from the anterior mandibular border, interdigitate among the muscle fibers of platysma and insert onto the skin. The labiomandibular groove forms in front of these ligaments.

The youthful neck has a subcutaneous layer of fat and a subplatysmal layer of fat, but these do not cause any prominence. The layer of subcutaneous fat is just sufficient to hide the underlying cartilaginous structures, although the youthful neck shows the thyroid notch as a gentle indentation, a subthyroid depression and a visible thyroid cartilage. The anterior border of the sternocleidomastoid muscle should be visible extending inferiorly, creating a small depression in the suprasternal notch.

The skin should show no horizontal rhytids or solar elastosis, and no vertical platysmal bands.

An understanding of the anatomy of the superficial musculoaponeurotic system (SMAS) is important when considering rejuvenation of the face or neck [3]. The SMAS is a fibromuscular layer that encompasses and distributes force among the facial mimetic muscles. Superiorly, the SMAS is continuous with the galea and incorporates the superficial temporal fascia (Fig. 78.4). In the parotid region, the SMAS is located superficial to and is distinct from the parotid fascia and peripherally, the branches of the facial nerve exit deep to the SMAS. The SMAS envelops the facial muscles anteriorly and has attachment to muscles in the perioral, nasolabial and periorbital areas. Inferiorly, the SMAS is continuous with the platysma muscle.

The platysma (Greek for "plate") is the vestigial remnant of the panniculous carnosus of animals. It is a quadrangular sheet of muscle, which originates on the fascia of the pectoralis major muscle and ascends to three main points of insertion. The most anterior fibers decussate in the midline to a variable extent and for variable levels below the chin and insert into the mentum. The central fibers insert into the body of the mandible and the more posterior fibers turn anteriorly and blend closely with the fibers of the risorius muscle, the depressor anguli oris and mentalis muscles (Fig. 78.5).

Aging tends to splay the fibers laterally, diminishing the effects of this muscle on the midline and increasing the cervicomental angle. Immediately overlying the platysma is the subcutaneous fat and skin. The cervical branch of the facial nerve innervates the platysma: the main lower branch exits the parotid and enters the deep surface of the platysma. The upper twigs of the cervical branch and the lower twigs of the marginal branch intermingle before the marginal mandibular branch of the facial nerve passes on to supply the depressor anguli oris and risorius. This nerve is at or just inferior to the portion of the mandible traversed by the facial artery (Fig. 78.7).

Platysmal bands seen in the necks of patients represent the medial edge of the platysma or lateral pleats caused by laxity of the platysma muscle and its investing fascia. Asking the patient to tense the platysma muscle will identify the bands as pleats or a true medial edge of the muscle. It was thought these bands simply represented loose platysma; however, the fact that the bands respond well to botulinum toxin injections indicates that these are tonic bands with the contracting folds bowstringing across the concave neck. Many procedures have been described for the management of these bands: lateral advancement of the SMAS, direct excision, anterior plication, platysmal notching, creation of muscle flaps and Z-plasty of the muscle.

Owsley [4] noted that some of his patients that only had lateral incisions and a SMAS–platysma tightening procedure developed recurrence of neckbands. In these patients, he subsequently notched the muscle at the site of the cervicomandibular groove. If only a lateral approach is used to tighten the platysma, subsequent tissue relaxation may result in recurrent bands. The best option is to suture the platysma at the midline and release, if necessary, at the level of the cricoid.

Vistnes and Souther [5] derived several basic anatomic principles based upon anatomic considerations of the platysma:

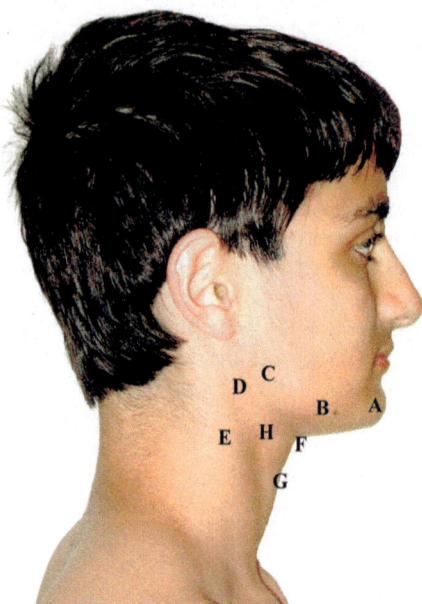

Fig. 78.1 Defining features of a youthful neck: *A* pronounced chin level or just anterior to the line drawn from the lower lip in men and just behind in women; *B* well-defined mandibular border with a submandibular shadow; *C* well-defined mandibular angle; *D* a distinct depression between the anterior border of the sternocleidomastoid muscle and the mandible; *E* a distinct sternocleidomastoid muscle; *F* a distinct cervicomental angle; *G* prominence of the thyroid cartilage. The skin is smooth with an absence of platysmal bands

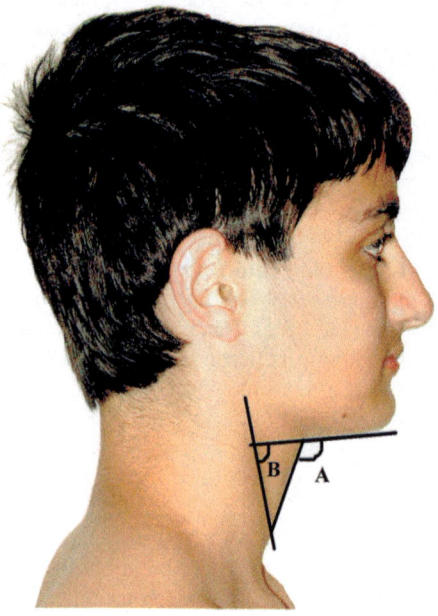

Fig. 78.2 The two angles useful in assessing a neck: *A* the cervicomental angle which should be between 105 and 120°; *B* the sternocleidomastoid-mandibular angles should be less than 90°

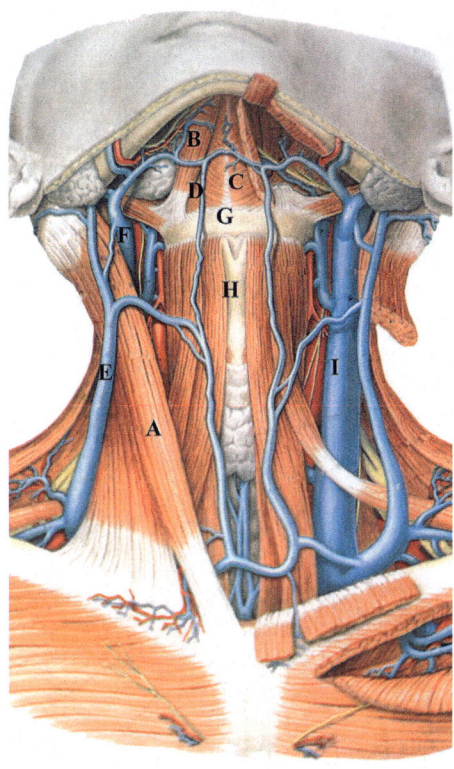

Fig. 78.3 Anatomy of the neck deep to the platysma: *A* sternocleidomastoid muscle; *B* digastric muscle; *C* mylohyoid muscle; *D* anterior jugular vein (runs just under and lateral to the medial edge of the platysma); *E* external jugular vein; *F* internal jugular vein; *G* hyoid; *H* thyroid cartilage; *I* internal jugular vein

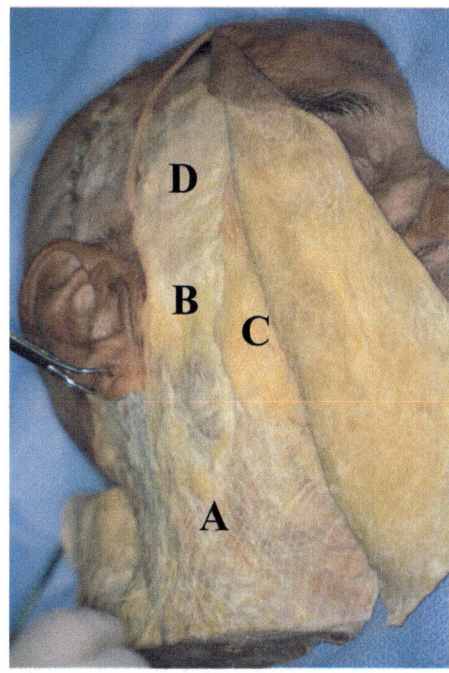

Fig. 78.4 The superficial musculoaponeurotic system (SMAS) and its relations: *A* platysma; *B* the SMAS; *C* malar fat pad; *D* superficial temporal fascia. Skin and subcutaneous fat have been elevated

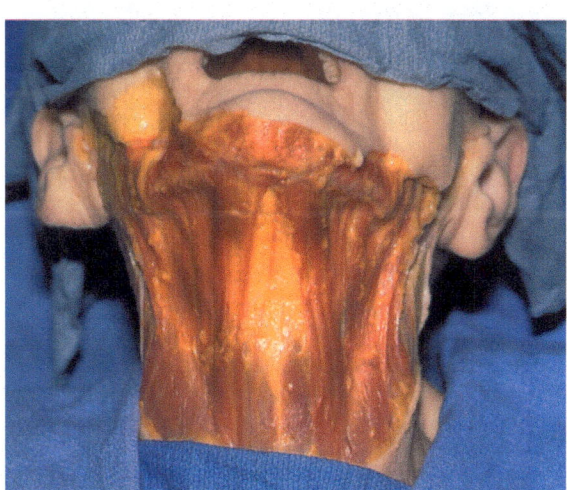

Fig. 78.5 The platysma. Note that only the very superior portion of the platysma decussates in this elderly patient. This decussation is variable. The platysma continues over the edge of the mandible to interdigitate with the risorius muscle, the depressor anguli oris and mentalis muscles. Note the separation of the medial fibers exposing the subplatysmal fat in front of the thyroid cartilage. Excessive sculpting of this neck fat will result in a skeletonized neck

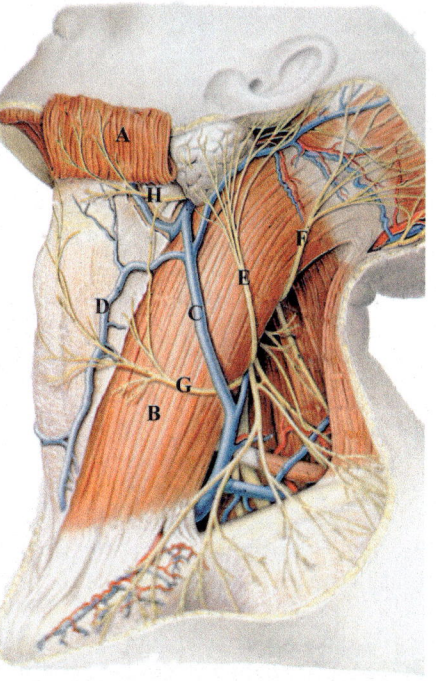

Fig. 78.6 Lateral anatomy of the neck deep to the platysma: *A* platysma; *B* sternocleidomastoid muscle; *C* external jugular vein; *D* anterior jugular vein; *E* greater auricular nerve; *F* lesser occipital nerve; *G* transverse cervical nerve; *H* cervical branch of the facial nerve

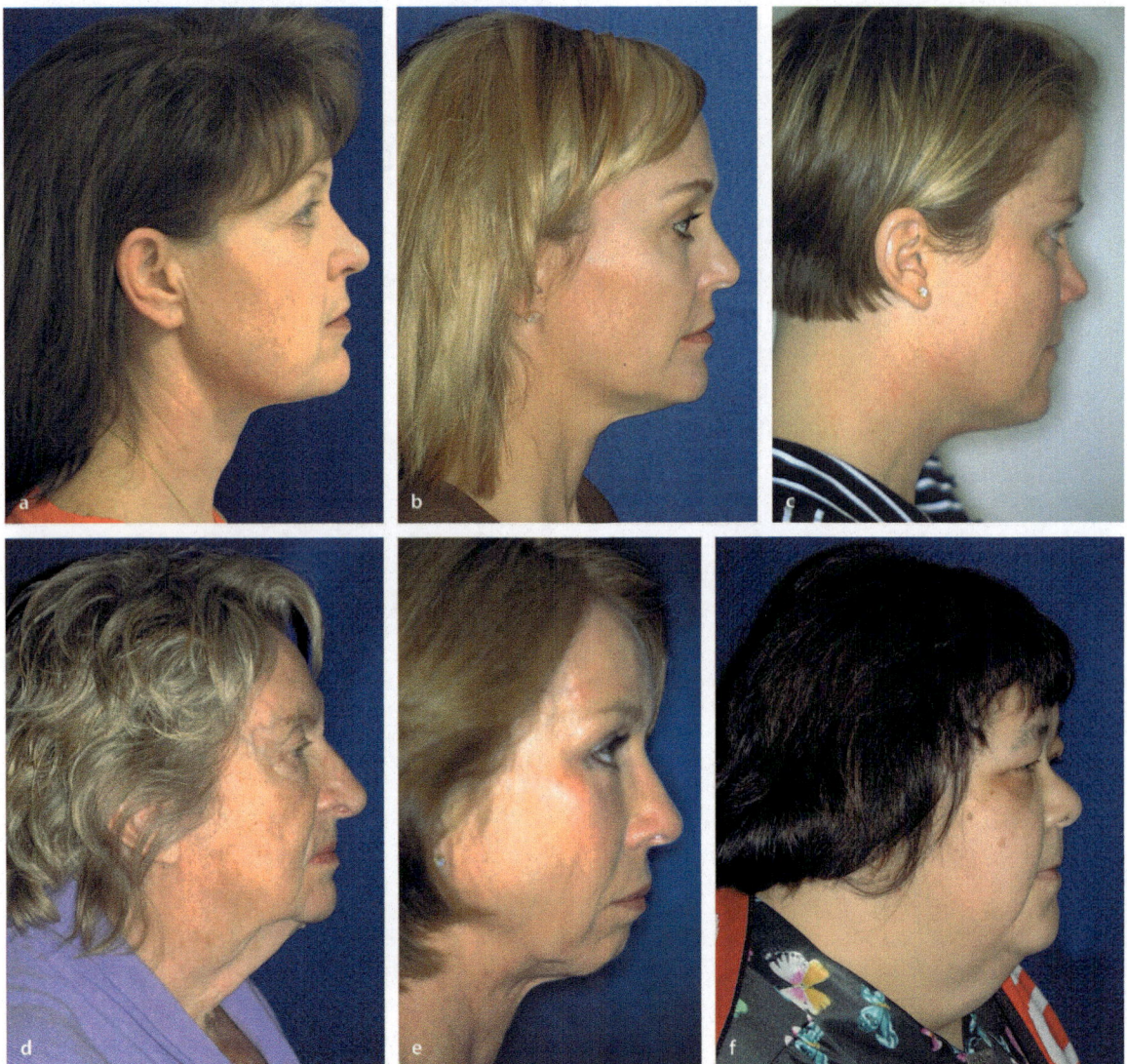

Fig. 78.7 Dedo classification of the neck. **a** Class I: well-defined mental angle with little submental fat, good skin and platysma tone. **b** Class II: early laxity of cervical skin without significant submental fat or loss of platysma tone. **c** Class III: subcutaneous layer of fat. **d** Class IV: platysmal abnormality is the predominant change but there may also be preplatysmal and subplatysmal fat. **e** Class V: retrognathia. **f** Class VI: abnormally low hyoid. This type of patient has a "short neck" although excess fat may disguise a normally placed hyoid

1. The platysma is intimately attached to the skin by fibrous septa, which must be completely separated to mobilize the skin independently of the platysma muscle. Because of this relationship, redundancy of the skin usually implies redundancy of the platysma muscle.

2. If changing the direction of its fibers tightens the platysma, the change in vector forces may affect other muscles. For example, if the platysma is pulled posteriorly, the anterior fibers will be distracted so they do not firmly decussate. The anterior fibers inserting on the mandible will not be affected but the fibers inserting on the risorius can result in an abnormal smile.

3. If the anterior fibers do not decussate, prominent vertical bands in the anterior neck may form. The submandibular fat pad and submandibular glands will not be well supported and may become ptotic, blunting the contour between the neck and face. Treatment requires approximation of the medial borders of the platysma.

4. Transection of the cervical branch of the facial nerve may have a detrimental effect on some people with a "full denture" smile if the platysma acts as a significant depressor of the lower lip.

78.3
Classification of the Aging Neck

Surgical correction of the aging neck requires precise diagnosis of the pathologic anatomy causing the cosmetic deformity. Factors such as age, skin quality, fat deposition, muscle anatomy and skeletal support all influence the surgical plan. In 1980, Dedo [6] proposed a classification system of the neck based on anatomic layers (Fig. 78.7):

- Class I. A well-defined mental angle, little submental fat, good skin and platysma tone.
- Class II. Laxity of the cervical skin without significant submental fat or loss of platysma tone. The skin must be redraped so wide undermining is required but a submental incision is usually not needed. A standard rhytidectomy with plication of the SMAS–platysma complex is usually all that is required.
- Class III. A layer of subcutaneous fat, which is either genetic or acquired. Liposuction is usually required to improve the cervical contour.
- Class IV. Patients have varying degrees of platysma abnormality, which must be diagnosed by voluntary facial grimacing. This is usually evident as anterior cervical cording, but it may be difficult to assess the platysma owing to fat accumulation. These patients require some form of surgical manipulation of the platysma.
- Class V. Patients have retrognathia: they require mentoplasty or advancement genioplasty.
- Class VI. Patients have an abnormally low hyoid position. Patients with abnormally low hyoids (normal is at C4) need to be counseled preoperatively because there are currently no effective procedures to elevate the hyoid and their surgical results will likely be less than optimal.

Although this classification is useful, many patients will have more than one class of deformity. We generally document each specific anatomical change in the neck and note its contribution to neck abnormalities. Ellenbogen and Karlin [7] in 1980 and Giampapa et al. [8, 9] have superbly illustrated this approach.

78.4
Aims of Neck Rejuvenation

The essential aims of neck rejuvenation are:

- To create a sharper cervicomental angle (of 105–120) with a visible subhyoid depression (creates the appearance of a long, thin neck).
- To improve platysmal bands.
- To create a visible thyroid cartilage bulge (excessive visibility in a woman can create a masculine neck).
- To enhance the definition and perceived length of the mandibular border.
- To enhance the definition and sharpness of the mandibular angle.
- To enhance the anterior sternocleidomastoid muscle border.
- To enhance the prominence, height and width of the chin.
- To improve labiomandibular folds.
- To improve jowls.

78.5
Examination of the Neck

The patient is examined in a well-lit area and the following anatomic points are evaluated:

1. Cervicomental angle depth (includes assessment of submental fat and bands).
2. Skin. Examine the skin for a preoperative crepe-paper appearance: this is the best predictor of failure of suction-assisted lipectomy without a face lift.
3. Creases. Note any deep permanent, horizontal and oblique creases: even with an efficient cervicofacial rhytidectomy, these bands will be impossible to eradicate. Superficial laser treatment may be needed following surgery for these.
4. Tone and elasticity. Perform the snap-back test of the neck skin by pulling the skin down caudally to assess tone and elasticity: in the presence of poor tone and elasticity, it should be pointed out to the patient that even with a cervicofacial rhytidectomy, some degree of laxity will return following surgery.
5. Skin changes. Perform the pinch test for laxity to assess postoperative "cervical ectropion": if present, it may be a contraindication to minimally invasive neck rejuvenation techniques. Skin changes are not caused just by laxity but may be affected by hormonal changes, dehydration, damage by UV-A and UV-B radiation and other factors that cannot entirely be helped by tightening the skin.
6. Subcutaneous midline cervical fat. Perform the sausage test: longitudinal midline fullness with palpation or squeezing of the cervical midline is the best indication for proceeding with lipectomy.
7. Fat and muscle. Palpate subcutaneous fullness in the neck with tensing of the platysma muscle to distinguish between fat and thick muscle. Subplatysmal fat is filled with connective tissue and, unlike softer preplatysmal fat, is very fibrous. Observe the quantity and location of subcutaneous fat Perform the pinch test for subcutaneous thickness of more than 1.5 cm.
8. SMAS. The lower face is pulled upward to see if there is any improvement in the lax tissues of the neck. If so, a cervicofacial rhytidectomy may be necessary. Ptosis of the upper third of the neck may be an indication of laxity of the SMAS. Examine the patient with the movement of the head up and down and side-to-side.

9. Platysma. The neck is examined for cervical fullness without bands, visible bands without animation or active platysmal bands that are active with animation.
10. Hyoid–thyroid complex location (Fig. 78.8). If this complex is low, an optimal result may not be obtained [10].
11. Mandible. The border definition and the mandibular angle definition are noted. The mental prominence is examined. A line is drawn down from the lower lip. In women, the mentum should be on or slightly behind this line. For men, the mentum should be on or anterior to this line. No neck evaluation is complete without evaluation of the chin.
12. Jowls. The labiomandibular groove and fold prominence (jowling) should be examined.
13. Neck width. The neck width should be examined and compared with the width of the neck on photographs of the patient from younger days. Increase in neck width is associated with muscle laxity, collapse of the cervical spine and an increase in subcutaneous and submental fat deposits.
14. Submandibular gland. Examine for submandibular gland fullness.
15. Asymmetries. Carefully note asymmetries in the chart. Photographs of the face and neck are taken: anteroposterior, oblique and lateral views. Any asymmetries or local deformities are photographed.

78.6
Preoperative Discussion

The patient's own photographs and their present appearance are compared and the changes are explained.

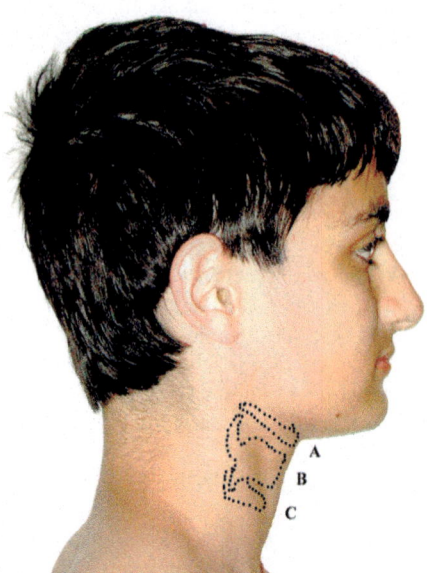

Fig. 78.8 *A* Hyoid bone, *B* thyroid cartilage, *C* cricoid cartilage

Examples of other patients with similar changes are shown with preoperative and postoperative appearances. It is stressed that these are simply examples and not a palette from which to choose a particular result. On the basis of the assessment, patients are shown the alternative techniques available and the best technique suitable for them. The best surgical option may not be the best one for the patient because of personal choices (does not want a face lift, cost) or medical conditions.

78.7
Neck Rejuvenation Techniques

Conventional SMAS techniques have been considered the gold standard in cervicofacial rhytidectomy [11]. Particular issues, however, are not completely corrected by SMAS plication, imbrication or excision techniques. The two areas in question are the drooping midface and the obtuse cervicomental angle.

Using almost any technique, it is not uncommon to see progressive tightening of the skin in the submandibular region over a 6–12-month period in patients with significant preoperative cervical skin laxity. The final result may not be achieved for 1 year.

Although the literature describes many variations, three main approaches are used for minimally invasive neck rejuvenation:
1. Cervical supraplatysmal liposuction.
2. Wide supraplatysmal undermining, direct excision of subplatysmal fat, approximation of platysmal edges, with or without lateral support.
3. Supraplatysmal suspension sutures from mastoid to mastoid.

78.7.1
Cervical Supraplatysmal Liposuction

78.7.1.1
Aims of Liposuction

The surgical goal is a balanced youthful facial profile.

78.7.1.2
The Ideal Candidate for Closed Liposuction

Traditionally, it has been stated that neck liposuction should be reserved for younger patients who possess good skin tone to allow skin contraction and adherence [12]. While this remains essentially true, patients may not be candidates for a face lift because of medical conditions. Some patients may refuse a face lift because of recovery time or cost or the refusal may reflect regional variations on views of face lifts. We have found that in many patients who would not strictly fall into the liposuction group, the use of liposuction, with or without other ancillary techniques, may give very gratifying results [13–15].

78.7.1.3
Examination

The neck should be palpated with the platysma alternately tensed and relaxed. This will give a good idea of the distribution of the fat in the subcutaneous and subplatysmal spaces. To identify patients who would respond well to liposuction, Illouz has suggested that the distance between the ear lobe and the chin tip is measured. If the skin distension is less than 15% of its length, liposuction is indicated. More than 20% distension requires a face lift. However, this does not take into account the fact that the skin of the neck will recontour itself over the newly formed cervicomental area. Although a fatty neck appears to have too much skin, when the cervicomental angle is augmented and a concavity is created, more skin is required to fill this deeper angle.

78.7.1.4
Technique

Preoperative marking is performed with the patient in the sitting position. A topographic map is drawn using the pinch test. The markings should take into account asymmetry of fat distribution, which is common. Submaxillary gland fullness is noted. The mandibular border and the anterior palpated border of the sternocleidomastoid muscles are marked.

Entry Sites for Liposuction

Traditionally, liposuction has been performed via a central incision in the middle of the submental groove. Incisions behind the lobules were added, "when needed". We find the use of two entry points at either end of the submental groove, approximately 1 cm from the midline, to be more useful when suctioning the jowls and along the mandibular border. This avoids injury to the marginal mandibular branch of the facial nerve. A subcutaneous liposuction of the jowl can be safely performed through one of these submental incisions. The rest of the neck can also be efficiently suctioned through these two incisions. We also, routinely use the incisions behind the lobules. We undermine below the retroauricular incisions in front of the sternocleidomastoid muscle to avoid entry of the cannula below the platysma muscle.

The entry sites are injected with 1% lidocaine and 1:200,000 epinephrine. We use a pair of curved Steven's scissors to create the correct plane between the subdermal fat and the deeper region where liposuction should be performed. A liposuction tumescence mixture is injected via the four entry points into the space created with scissors, using the infusion cannula and a 60-ml syringe. The infusion cannula allows creation of the plane within which liposuction will be performed. Prior to the use of tumescence, it had been noted that pretunneling (blunt dissection without the use of suction) was often helpful in releasing dermal attachments of the platysma muscle. We find the use of the infusion cannula with creation of spaces between the dermal attachments to be just as useful. Injection of the fluid in this manner and subsequent liposuction results in a cheeselike cavity with platysmal-dermal attachments intact. Secondary contracture results in better definition of the neck, avoiding a wrinkled appearance of the skin.

A 2.4-mm liposuction cannula is inserted through the incisions while performing the pinch test to find an appropriate depth for liposuction. Passages of the cannula are made in the center of the topographic bull's eye. Fewer passages of the cannula are performed at the edges of the bull's eye, producing feathering along the edges. This allows aspiration of the neck, the jowl and the mandibular border without having to go deep (Fig. 78.9). Closed liposuction should not be used for manipulation of subplatysmal fat.

End Point

There is no true end point to the liposuction that can be measured. The aim should be to stop once an adequate

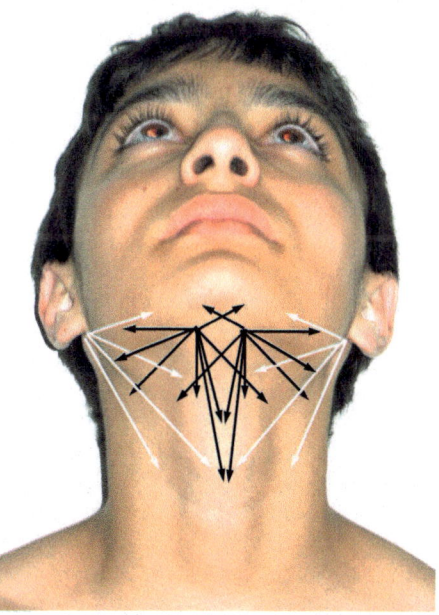

Fig. 78.9 Placement of the incisions for liposuction. Using two incisions at either end of the submental groove allows efficient liposuction with the passage of the cannula crossing those made through the other sites. These points of entry also allow safe liposuction of the jowls

reduction in the thickness in the fat has been achieved. At the end of the liposuction, the neck generally looks the same as it did before the liposuction fluid was injected. The palm of the hand is used on the neck and the jawline as one performs suction to allow assessment of the position of the cannula as well as to assess the degree of fat removal. Running the cannula over the skin confirms the presence of a smooth contour. In the cervical region, a pinch-and-roll test result of less than 1 cm over the entire region that has been treated is usually found at completion.

We prefer the hand aspiration technique as it gives more accurate control over the liposuction. It is important to use a small cannula and not to use liposuction close to the dermis.

Faces become square as they age, with the jowl fat making the lower corners of the square. Treatment of the jowl fat makes the face oval again. The jowl fat seems to spill over the edge of the mandible. It is uncertain if the jowl is formed by cheek fat that has fallen because of relaxation of the masseteric-cutaneous ligaments and that has been arrested by the perioral cutaneous ligament system. If that is the case, moving the SMAS up and pulling the skin superolaterally will improve the jowl, as has been found in the commonest form of cervicofacial rhytidectomy that involves SMAS manipulation. However, when elevation with the SMAS alone is relied upon, it has been noted that the jowl returns postoperatively. Therefore, we elevate the jowl, when necessary, and then diminish its volume with suction.

Some of the jowl fat is probably an absolute excess of localized facial fat, the "love handles" of the face; these need direct sculpting. Virtually all patients who need neck contouring, with or without face lift, need to have jowl contouring as well. Contouring only the neck makes the jowl fat look more obvious. Excessive liposuction should be avoided in the jowl. In the jowl, tunneling without applying suction will contribute to an improvement in the jowl contour. If the neck liposuction and jowl liposuction are being performed together with midface lifting, the liposuction is completed first to allow appropriate cephalic movement of the jowl and mandibular skin as the midface is lifted.

The plastic surgery dictum "not what you take, but what you leave" is particularly relevant when dealing with neck liposculpture. What the surgeon leaves, in an open or closed procedure, is considerably more than what at last remains. Millard suggested that at least 5 mm of subcutaneous fat should be left in the neck (giving a thickness of 1 cm on the pinch test). The contoured neck should be left undercorrected at the conclusion of the procedure. After liposuction, there is invariably a discontinuous degree of undermining of the subcutaneous tissues. The liposuction process creates tunnels, which "heal" with colonization by fibroblasts and myofibroblasts. Following closed liposuction, swelling in the retained fat will persist for a number of weeks. The very

act of instrumentation sets into motion a cascade of events—scarring, fat necrosis, liquefaction, absorption and lipocide. Secondary contraction results with contraction of the subcutaneous tissues. The overlying skin, which is elastic, responds by retraction. It has been estimated that skin retraction of approximately one tenth of its length can be expected. A skin flap that is elevated but not sutured undergoes a retraction of between one tenth and one seventh [15].

Another reason to leave a healthy layer of subcutaneous fat behind is the fact that, invariably, platysmal bands will worsen over time. The dictum "think about your patient at 1 month, 1 year, 10 years and 30 years" applies to neck liposuction. The patient is likely to seek further treatment when the platysmal bands become apparent. A lack of fat would make it difficult to manipulate the platysma effectively.

The mandibular border may be enhanced by performing suction-assisted lipectomy above and below the mandibular border, leaving a strip of subcutaneous fat along the bony border. Some surgeons augment the mandibular border with fillers such as Radiesse. Alloplastic implants may be considered to augment relatively hypoplastic mandibles.

Dressing

Foam and a chinstrap are used to provide compression while keeping the skin smooth by providing upward traction. If edema results in skin that is not stretched, persistent unsightly irregularities may result. The patient is encouraged to sleep with the head up and with the neck in extension to prevent formation of a neck crease. A chinstrap is worn for 24 h and then every night for 2 weeks. Firm areas are hand-massaged with a circular motion using vitamin E cream for 5–10 min each day. External ultrasound massage may also be performed.

78.7.1.5
Limitations of Liposuction

In patients older than 65 years, liposuction alone is unlikely to give satisfactory results, as most of these patients will have platysmal bands and substantial skin laxity. In patients with more than just preplatysmal fat, even with the best technique, recreation of a visible subhyoid depression and a visible thyroid cartilage bulge may be difficult using liposuction alone. Liposuction is most successful in improving the submandibular border and a more visible anterior sternocleidomastoid muscle border.

Male patients exhibit fewer irregularities than women because of their thicker skin. Conversely, they demonstrate a comparably less acute cervicomental angle and less defined jawline.

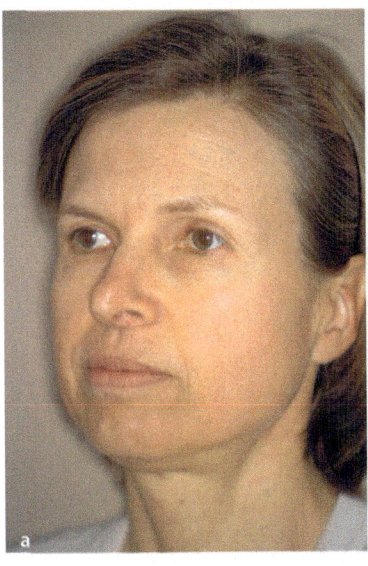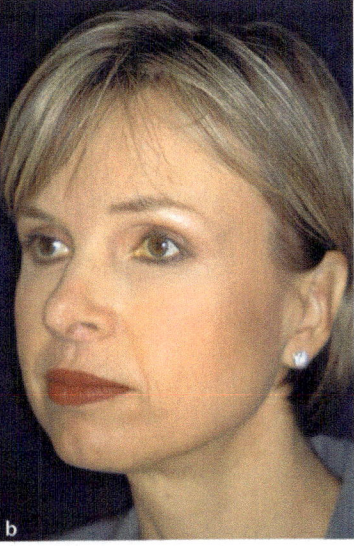

Fig. 78.10 **a** Female patient in her mid-40s presented with submental fat, no platysmal folds, some fullness over the submandibular gland and a slightly weak mandibular border. She has a good thyroid prominence and a well-defined sternocleidomastoid muscle. **b** Four years after an endoscopic brow lift, upper and lower blepharoplasty, endoscopic cheek lifts and neck liposuction and direct excision of submental fat via a submental incision. The mandibular border definition has improved, as has the cervicomental angle. The fullness over the submandibular gland was actually fat and not the gland

Although closed liposuction is used in most patients, some patients will have an isolated collection of submental fat, which may be resected directly via a submental incision (Fig. 78.10).

78.7.1.6
Contraindications for Suction-Assisted Lipectomy

Contraindications are:

1. Cepe-paper appearance of the skin.
2. Marked laxity of the skin. However, this is a relative contraindication. We have found, as have others [16], that many patients will be delighted with an improvement in the jawline, even if the excess skin remains (Fig. 78.11). Some patients, once informed that the cervicomental angle cannot be recreated with liposuction alone when they have excess skin laxity, will be delighted to just see an improvement in the convexity of the neck skin caused by fat.
3. Marked oblique angle between chin and neck with minimal subcutaneous fullness.
4. Older patient desiring maximal improvement.
5. Multiple deep horizontal and oblique neck creases.
6. Severe jowling.
7. Patients older than 65 years (relative contraindication).

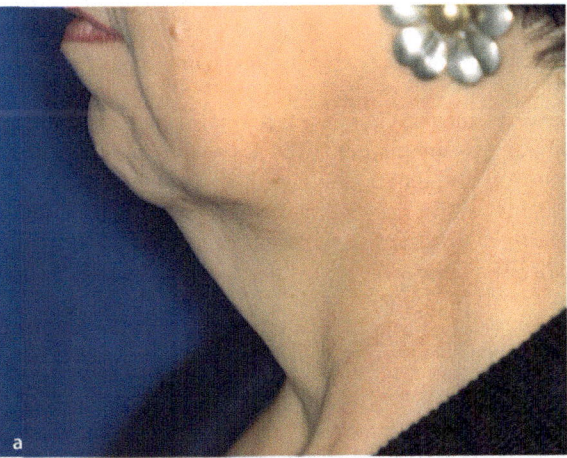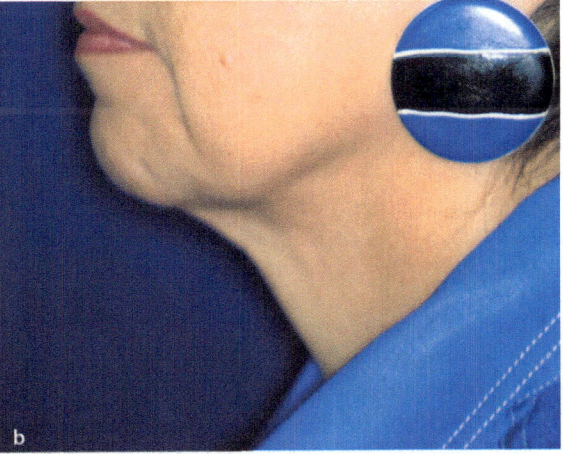

Fig. 78.11 **a** This female patient, in her late 50s, has jowls, platysmal folds, marked cervical skin laxity and poor cervical skin tone. There is complete loss of her mandibular border and angle and she has a moderately weak mentum. The best procedure for such a patient would be a cervicofacial rhytidectomy with skin, platysma and SMAS manipulation. However she chose to undergo just liposuction and insertion of a suspension suture. **b** One year after surgery. Even though there is the expected loose skin and underlying revealed platysmal bands, the recontouring of the skin is quite acceptable. She now has a better mandibular border and a concavity between the mandible and the anterior border of the sternocleidomastoid muscle

78.7.1.7
Complications of Liposuction

Pittman and Teimourian [17] found that the highest incidence of undesired sequelae of liposuction occurred in the neck (30%).

Dillerud [18] found that male patients registered 5 times more (15%) dissatisfaction than female patients (2.8%) who underwent suction lipectomy (this included all areas of the body, not just the neck). Careful preoperative patient selection and avoidance of overresection are vital. Also, as the neck may take several months to achieve its final result, preoperative explanations become vital. Patients may complain of insufficient fat removal when the surgeon feels the removal is adequate. We stress that an undercorrected neck is a desirable result as an overcorrected neck would be difficult to correct. It is not uncommon for minor touchups to be performed on patients. We generally wait at least 6 months before performing such touchups as tissue change may take 6 months or longer.

With the use of tumescent fluid, use of blunt cannulas, attention to the depth of liposuction and use of postoperative compression dressings, hematomas and seromas are uncommon after neck liposuction. A drain may be inserted at the end of the procedure if there is significant collection of fluid, especially if a sharp dissection of the neck has been necessary. Hematoma and seroma formation may lead to irregularities and hyperpigmentation.

Platysmal bands may be exposed after liposuction. In some patients, occult platysmal bands are exposed once the liposuction has been completed. These may need plication and lateral elevation.

Overly aggressive central liposuction may create skin adhesions to the underlying muscle. Similar irregularities may occur in the jowl, necessitating microlipoinfiltration to correct the deformities. Waviness and asymmetry are other contour complications. Contour irregularities are very difficult to correct. Excessive fat removal from the cervical area can create a "cobra" deformity.

The submandibular gland may become obvious after liposuction in the presence of previous ptosis. Although repositioning of ptotic submandibular glands has been described, we prefer not to perform this surgery. We generally aim to leave enough of a fat layer over the gland so as to not make the glands obvious. The presence of prominent submandibular glands is pointed out to the patient prior to surgery.

Most patients will notice a decrease in sensation in the treated areas. Most of the sensation returns within 3 months; however, some sensory change may persist for as long as 1 year.

78.7.1.8
Advantages and Disadvantages of Cervical Liposuction

Advantages are:
1. Less risk for patients with medical problems.
2. Less risk of skin slough among smokers.
3. Less invasive.
4. Less costly.
5. Less scarring.
6. Less pain.
7. Shorter recovery.
8. Less dissection.
9. Less risk of nerve injury.
10. Less risk of hematoma.
11. Only option for some patients: shorter procedure and less anesthesia.

Disadvantages are:
1. Not applicable for older patients with severe cervical and platysmal laxity.
2. Unsightly skin irregularities may result.
3. Secondary platysmaplasty and skin lift may be required.
4. Lipectomy may expose platysmal bands.
5. Inferior results.

78.7.2
Platysmaplasty

Manipulation of the platysma has been called many names: corset platysmaplasty, muscle slings, SMAS–platysma slings, etc. [19–24]. The principle of a platysmaplasty is to recreate the tight horizontal neck contour and the deep cervicomental angle of youth by approximating the splayed central platysmal edges, and, in some patients, elevating and tightening the SMAS–platysma complex laterally and superiorly. Therefore, platysmaplasty is often combined with a cervicofacial rhytidectomy. When done as an isolated neck procedure, platysmaplasty may be done with or without liposuction of the neck. We almost always perform at least a conservative liposuction. Also, in most of our patients, we often use the suspension suture in combination with the platysmaplasty.

78.7.2.1
Indications

Platysmaplasty is best used when patients have marked platysmal bands or when there is a substantial amount of preplatysmal and subplatysmal fat together with platysmal laxity. Some patients will need skin resection, either with a cervicofacial rhytidectomy if there is significant lower facial and SMAS laxity or direct retroauricular skin excision (Fig. 78.12).

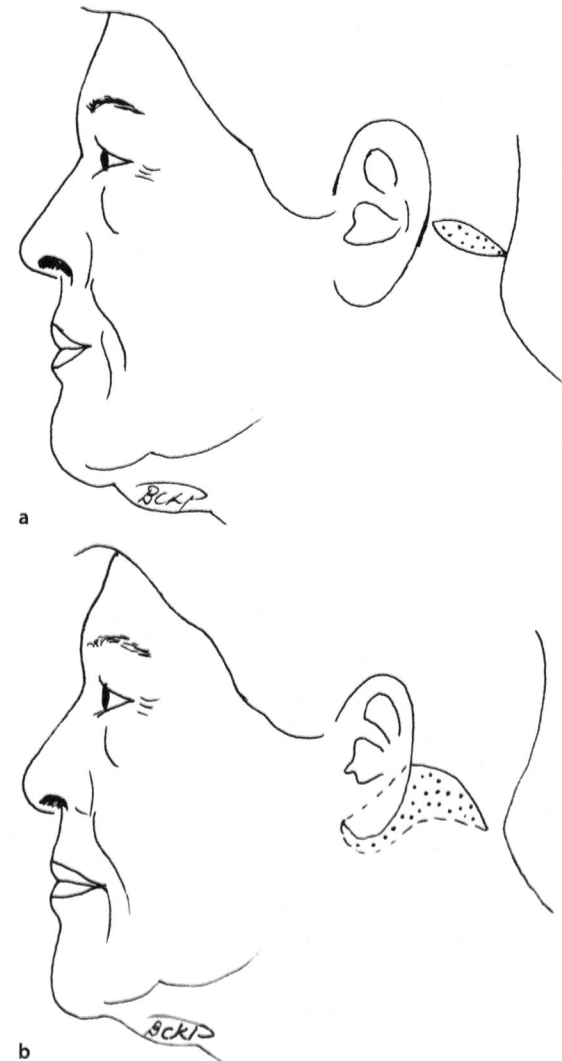

Fig. 78.12 a Preoperatively with excess cervical skin. **b** Following skin resection by using one of these two incisions. We prefer the incision illustrated in **b** as it allows better rearrangement of the excess skin and allows better control of dog-ears. The incision may be carried further forward into the preauricular area if significant jowl skin needs to be addressed

78.7.2.2
Technique

A submental mark, 3–3.5 cm long, is made just behind the natural submental crease with the patient sitting up. Local anesthesia is injected and the incision made. The skin and fat anteriorly are retracted with a 1-cm double-hook while lifting the inferior submental skin and fat with a long retractor. A surgical fiberoptic headlight and long, insulated coagulation forceps are used.

A postauricular incision is made in the form of an ellipse to take up redundant skin. This ellipse can be enlarged as necessary. The skin is dissected off the platysma and off the anterior border of the sternocleidomastoid muscle. We use a combination of suctioning and long dissecting scissors. The skin and fat are raised as a composite, ensuring that excessive fat is not removed from the skin flap. Through the submental incision, the central portion of the neck skin flap is undermined almost down to the suprasternal notch in the midline and connected with the lateral undermined area on each side.

The subplatysmal space between the digastrics is shaped like a box. It is bounded laterally by the digastrics, superiorly by the mylohyoid and inferiorly by the platysma. Lateral to the digastrics, one finds fat for a small distance, until the submaxillary glands are encountered. Suturing of the digastric muscles together has been suggested to enhance the angle and help create a more concave or flat submental triangle. We have found that sutures will rarely hold when applied to the digastric muscles.

The central, usually nondecussating platysma muscle edges are cleared of fat all the way down the front of the neck. The submental area between the digastric muscles is examined. In the presence of excess fat, a judicious resection of fat between the digastric muscles is performed. The anterior jugular vein runs vertically in the fat just under the medial platysmal edge on each side. Subplatysmal fat is very vascular and somewhat fibrous. The edges of the medial platysma can be retracted using long right-angled hemostats. Some surgeons recommend removing subplatysmal fat in the submental and perihyoid area and also further caudally from over the thyroid cartilage. The advantage of judiciously removing such subplatysmal fat is that a well-defined hyoid angle can be obtained even in patients thought to have a low hyoid. However, the risk is that the neck will look too skeletonized if excess fat is removed.

The author does not take fat more superiorly than the most inferior point of the digastric muscles. The space between the digastric muscles is leveled but not hollowed. Excessive removal of fat from the submental space will make the platysma stick to the digastrics and the mylohyoid, if it has been exposed. This may occur many months after surgery. One can differentiate an exposed digastric muscle from a recurrent platysmal band by position (the digastric muscle will end just lateral and superior to the thyroid cartilage) and the fact that a platysmal band will animate with grimacing whereas a digastric muscle will not.

The medial platysmal edges should meet without tension. If not, the medial borders are freed from the tethering fascia under the muscle. Some patients will have widely separated muscle edges or the platysma may be stiff and inelastic. Broad undermining of the muscle inferiorly and cutting the fibrous filaments on the undersurface are necessary to release the muscle and allow the two platysma halves to stretch and slide together easily. Unless the two sides can be brought together with minimal tension, there is a good chance that sutures will pull out, resulting in recurrence of the muscle bands and a midline interplatysmal depression.

A 4-0 Vicryl suture on a taper needle takes a bite of platysma just outside each opposing muscle edge and the suture is securely tied with an inverted knot. A continuous suture is then run downward, taking small bites along or just lateral to each medial platysmal edge. The suture is applied as far down the neck as possible and certainly below the thyroid cartilage (Fig. 78.13). If there is skin puckering, the adhesions between the platysma and skin need to be released. A second row of sutures is then inserted by taking bites of platysma outside the first seam, producing a smoother and tighter second seam. After the first row of sutures has been placed, there may be a bowstring look to the platysma: this usually disappears with the second row of sutures and the platysma sinks into the hyoid concavity. If there is redundancy of the platysma on either side of the midline just behind the jaw, buried 4-0 Vicryl sutures are used in an oblique line to imbricate the excess muscle inward.

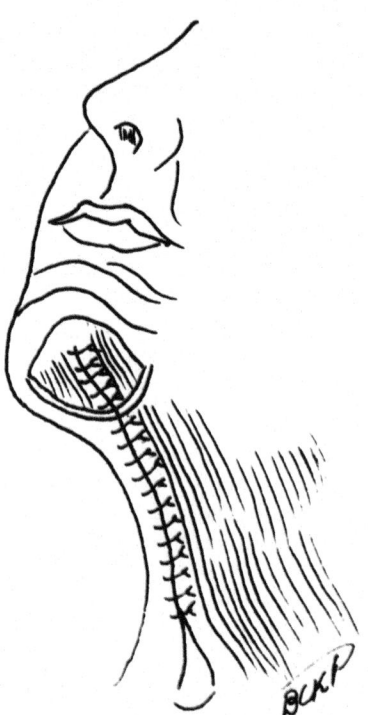

Fig. 78.13 Central platysmal plication. Interrupted or continuous sutures may be used

In a secondary neck lift when a previous face lift has been performed, the medial platysmal bands may not approximate even with extensive undermining. In such patients, anteriorly based platysmal flaps are created by performing horizontal releasing incisions low down the platysma. This will allow the medial edges of the platysma to be rotated and approximated.

In patients with a marked turkey goblet neck, extensive undermining of the skin, removal of preplatysmal and subplatysmal fat and a corset platysmaplasty will allow the excess skin to recontour itself in the newly created cervicomental angle. A small amount of skin may be excised in the postauricular area in the form of an ellipse.

78.7.2.3
Variations of the Corset Platysmaplasty

While some surgeons perform the corset platysmaplasty aggressively in the midline with several layers of sutures [22] others believe that only a lateral pull on the platysma and SMAS is necessary to recreate the neck anatomy [11]. We have tried both techniques and found that most of our patients will need a combination of liposuction, a central corset platysmaplasty, insertion of a suspension suture and some retroauricular skin excision. When a patient needs SMAS–platysma manipulation because of lower facial and jowl laxity, we will still perform a central platysmal plication, with or without use of a suspension suture. It is rare for us to perform just a central corset platysmaplasty.

78.7.2.4
Complications

Excessive tightening may pull down the platysma at the mandibular margin lowering the jowl further. In such cases, direct liposuction of the fat within the jowl and repositioning of the skin with an appropriate facial procedure should be performed. Also, a subcutaneous dissection all the way up to and just above the mandibular border should decrease the chance of such a lowering of the jowls.

The sutures may be palpable in the midline if excessive fat is removed from the preplatysmal plane.

A deep hollow between the digastric muscles may appear months later if excess subplatysmal fat is removed.

The forward rotation of the platysma may bring the submandibular glands forward, making them more prominent compared with the preoperative status. In such cases, imbrication of the platysma over the glands described above may help to make them less prominent.

Using just anterior platysmal sutures without lateral support will cause a recurrence of bands, often lateral to the suture line centrally.

78.7.3
The Suspension-Suture Technique

The principle of this technique is to recreate the cervicomental angle and display the mandibular border by invaginating neck tissues from the midline to the mastoid. Although Giampapa refined and popularized the suspension-suture technique in the 1990s [25], others had used it in one form or another over the preceding three decades [26–29].

78.7.3.1
Indications

This technique works best for patients with a poorly defined cervicomental angle. The skin is of moderate thickness, there is no evidence of significant midfacial descent and no significant jowl formation. The suspension-suture technique is most useful when combined with a central platysmaplasty: the suspension suture defines the mandibular border, while the platysmaplasty corrects the cervical bands. When combined with judicious skin excision, the results can be very gratifying. Giampapa has shown impressive long-term results with this technique [8, 9, 30]. Liposuction is also often used in combination with the suspension-suture technique.

This technique will not work well in patients with very thin or sun-damaged skin as the loss of elasticity limits the skin's ability to conform to the new cervicomental angle.

78.7.3.2
Technique

The patient is marked in the sitting position. Markings on the neck include the sternocleidomastoid muscles, external jugular veins, platysmal bands, jowls, mastoid tip and mandibular border. The sites of the submental and postauricular incisions are marked, as is the site of the new cervicomental angle and the intended submandibular path of the suspension suture.

After general anesthesia or monitored sedation anesthesia has been induced, 1% lidocaine with 1:200,000 epinephrine is injected in the submental and postauricular regions. When general anesthesia is used, the endotracheal tube is not draped to facilitate movement during surgery.

The submental incision is made just posterior to the first submental crease. The lateral margins of the incision are directed posteriorly, away from the mandibular border to minimize visibility of the scar. The incision length varies depending on the particular situation, but can be as long as 4 cm. Closure with buried 5-0 Vicryl subcuticular sutures will not leave any suture marks. Tumescent liposuction fluid is injected in the submental area and the jowls.

A liposuction cannula is used for preplatysmal liposuction, undermining the skin flap to the level of the thyroid notch inferiorly and as far as the external jugular vein laterally. In some cases, preplatysmal fat is excised under direct vision using face-lift scissors. Specific attention needs to be paid to the fat pocket lying medial to the platysmal edges, overlying the anterior bellies of the digastric muscles. This fat is removed judiciously. It usually contains several small vessels, which bleed vigorously; bipolar cautery needs to be used. The medial edges of the platysma are sutured using 3-0 or 4-0 Mersilene, Ethibond or Vicryl sutures. Occasionally, we divide the platysma transversely for 1–2 cm at the predetermined level of the cervicomental angle if necessary. Suturing the midline platysma narrows the width of the neck.

A 2-0 Gore-Tex or Mersilene suture is next placed across the platysma muscle at the previously approximated edges. The two sutures cross each other (Fig. 78.14). The interlocking suture allows for a superior and internal vector that elevates the platysma muscle into its new position, usually immediately above the hyoid. The needles are removed from the suture ends and the sutures are brought out through the submental incision.

The author uses two variations of the suspension suture. The first is used to obtain support of the submandibular glands. The suture is passed through the platysma over the submandibular gland (Fig. 78.15). Giampapa has suggested another modification of the suspension suture to create a loop immediately before placement of the suture through the mastoid fascia (Fig. 78.16). A small bite of the sternocleidomastoid muscle is taken immediately below the angle of the mandible and a second bite is taken, creating a loop with the suture. The other suture is passed through the loop, allowing a more defined angle to be formed.

A small ellipse of skin is excised posterior to the postauricular crease in the mastoid region to access the mastoid periosteum. This ellipse of skin may be larger in patients with significant laxity or prominent jowling. In some patients, we bring this ellipse just anterior to the lobule, allowing tightening of the neck without creation of dog-ears. A preplatysmal liposuction is performed from these incisions to join the submental incision. Care is taken to avoid tunneling in a subplatysmal plane, which could potentially cause marginal mandibular nerve injury or injury to the facial vessels. The sutures are passed from the submental to the retroauricular incisions using the liposuction cannula. A free needle is used to secure the suture to the mastoid periosteum. Care is taken not to allow the suture to ride forward and over the mandibular angle, as this will give the neck an unnatural creased appearance at the angle of the mandible. If the suture is too low, a hanging submental pouch will result. The suture is tied on the left with the patient's face turned toward the right (Fig. 78.17). The procedure is repeated in a similar fashion on the contralateral side. Adjustment of the tension

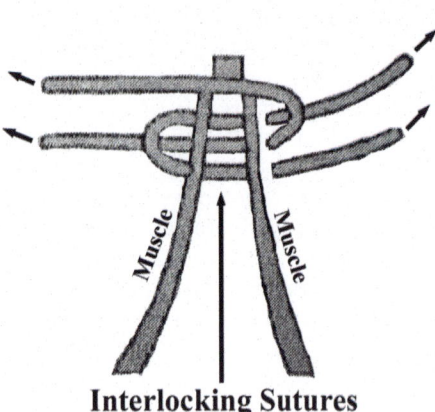

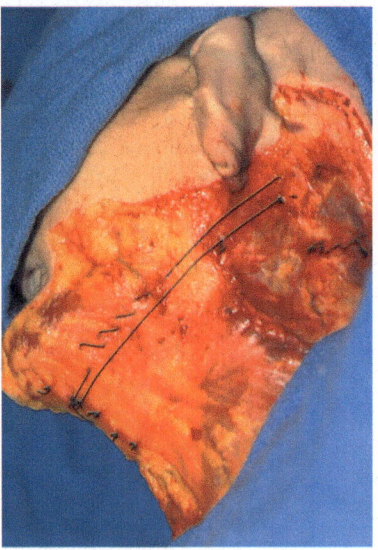

Fig. 78.14 Interlocking sutures placed after the platysma has been sutured in the midline

Fig. 78.15 Cadaver showing technique of suspension-suture placement. The anterior platysmal borders have been approximated and the interlocking sutures placed leading up to each mastoid. In the presence of a pronounced submandibular gland, we pick the platysma over the gland as shown

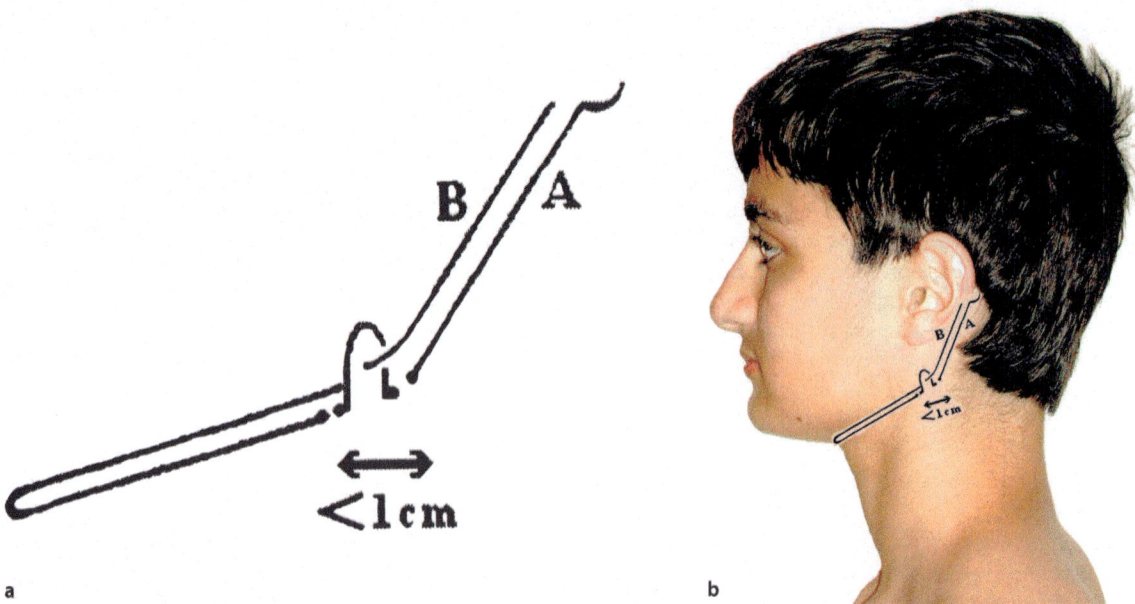

a

b

Fig. 78.16 a The Giampapa modification where a loop 1 cm wide placed over the sternocleidomastoid allows better definition of the mandibular border. **b** Placement of the suture. Placing this suture requires a larger retroauricular incision

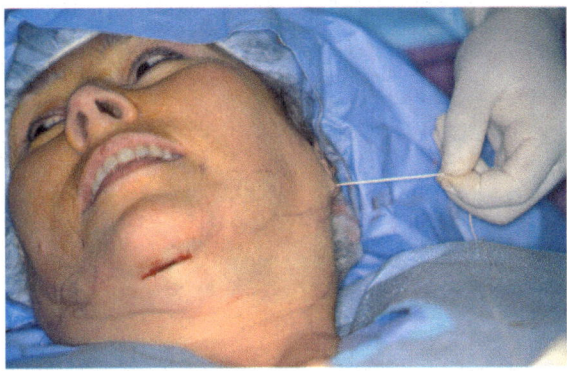

Fig. 78.17 The suture is tied over the mastoid fascia with the patient looking in the opposite direction. When performed under sedation, the patient may sit up to assess the effect of the suture

on this suture allows for adjustment of the angle depth from mild to moderate. Individual anatomy will dictate how much improvement may be achieved. Defatting of the supraplatysmal and subplatysmal fat may also enhance this angle or help it remain soft. The wounds are irrigated with bacitracin solution. The deep portion of the posterior incision is closed in two layers with 4-0 polyglactin sutures to ensure that the Mersilene knot does not spit. The skin is closed with 6-0 Nylon sutures. The chin is augmented to increase the depth of the cervicomental angle when a weak mentum is present.

A small amount of skin may excised from the posterior edge of the submental incision. A 7-mm round drain is placed when bleeding is a concern; the skin margins are approximated with buried interrupted 5-0 Vicryl sutures and a running subcuticular 4-0 polypropylene suture is used for dermal closure. The wound is supported with a strip of Reston foam (3M, Maplewood, MN, USA) held in place with a Kling roll (Johnson and Johnson, Arlington, TX, USA) and a Velcro chinstrap. Patients are instructed to wear the compression dressing as much as possible for the first 4–5 days and then wear the chinstrap at night for an additional 7–10 days.

78.7.3.3
Mental Prominence

A naturally prominent chin projection contributes to the overall length and beauty of an aesthetically balanced neck. Chin augmentation or sliding genioplasties yield good results and may help prevent skin from becoming redundant in the submental area. Other options include fat and long-term fillers. Most patients undergoing the suspension-suture technique will need such adjuvant procedures.

78.7.3.4
Complications

Too much tightening or overtightening of the suture may result in the "overcorrected neck". If the sutures are overtightened, the patient may complain of pain. Malposition of the sutures will result in unnatural creases. Uneven tightening may lead to asymmetry. Granuloma at the suture insertion over the mastoid fascia with exposure of the suture may occur.

78.7.3.5
Advantages

Advantages are:
1. Less invasive than a full cervicofacial rhytidectomy.
2. Limited incisions and undermining.
3. Preauricular area is spared of surgical manipulation.
4. Avoids posterior movement of the hair-bearing areas.

78.8
Midface Lift Combined with Neck Procedures

When performing an extended endoscopic midface lift, the direction of the lift superiorly and superolaterally can help improve the jawline and the jowl (Fig. 78.18).

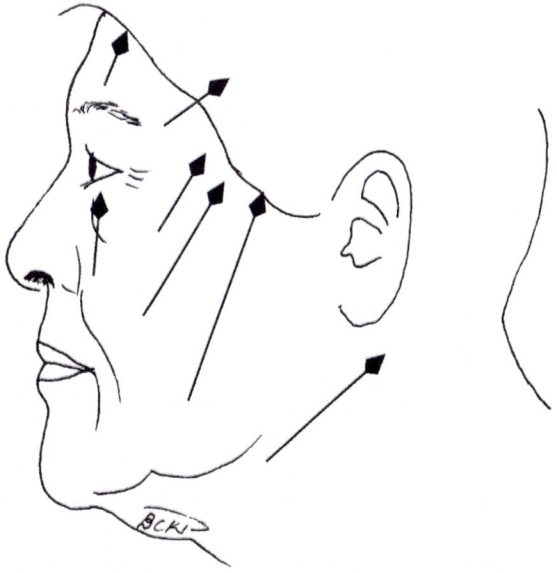

Fig. 78.18 An extended endoscopic midface lift with appropriately applied vectors as shown will help improve some lower facial laxity, including the jowls. When combined with liposuction of the neck and suspension suture application, the results can be very reasonable

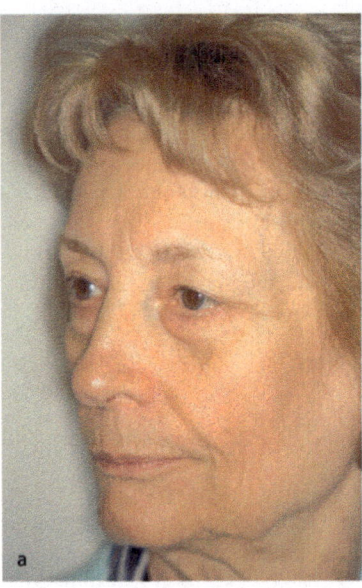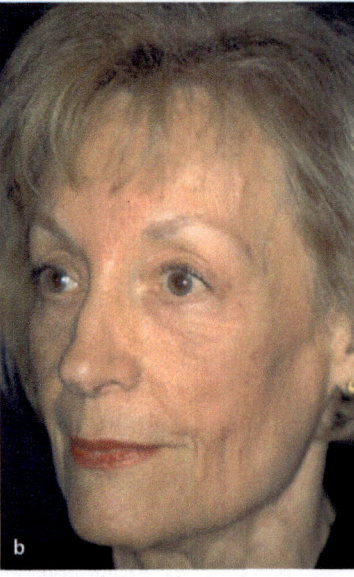

Fig. 78.19 a Female patient, in her early 60s, presented with jowls, poor mandibular definition and neck platysmal bands. She did not want any treatment to the neck. **b** Five months after endoscopic brow lift, upper and lower blepharoplasty, and extended endoscopic cheek lift. Other than isolated jowl liposuction and the supero-temporal component to the midface lift, no neck procedure was performed. Note the moderate improvement in the jowls. The platysmal bands are still present as no treatment was directed toward these

When an endoscopic midface lift is combined with neck liposuction with or without suspension sutures, a very reasonable improvement in the jawline can be achieved. (Fig. 78.19). In these cases, the neck procedures and liposuction are completed first.

78.9
Management of the Labiomandibular Groove and Fold (Jowl)

The labiomandibular groove and fold are difficult to improve when a cervicofacial rhytidectomy is not performed. In addition to placement of the neck suspension suture, the jowl area is suctioned from the submental incision and from the postauricular incision. This results in skin contracture in a superolateral direction, especially when combined with a superotemporally directed endoscopic cheek lift. When the suspension suture is used with liposuction and with lateral skin excision, there will be some flattening of the labiomandibular fold which can be further helped with fat grafting in the groove. It has been suggested that the depressor labii muscle may be released via a small intraoral incision and subperiosteal dissection to alleviate the downward-turned corners of the mouth and prominent mandibular folds but we have not utilized this. In addition to the neck suspension sutures, superotemporal lifting with barbed sutures may help with residual jowls but the longevity of this approach remains to be determined.

Even though an impressive degree of skin redraping will occur after liposuction and neck suspension suture insertion (Fig. 78.20), these techniques are not a substitute for appropriate skin resection. In the presence of pronounced jowling, the suture-suspension platys-

maplasty should be combined with a formal rhytidectomy for optimal improvement and for achievement of a more balanced overall face and neck area.

78.10
Direct Excision of Excess Skin

When addressing loose skin in the neck, the principles of redraping, redistributing and resecting apply. In some male patients with thick, sebaceous, inelastic skin with platysmal bands, direct resection of the lax skin and plication of the platysmal bands may be performed to lengthen the vertical length and shorten the horizontal length. Care must be taken not to resect too much skin as the jowl skin can otherwise be pulled downward. Closure should be meticulous to prevent prominent scars (Fig. 78.21).

78.11
Other Minimally Invasive Techniques

The skin of the neck and chest damaged by aging and sun exposeurewill have a combination of horizontal creases, poikiloderma of Civatte, keratoses and changes in texture. None of the surgical procedures discussed will effectively address these changes. Poikiloderma of Civatte will respond to intense pulsed light (wavelength from 515 to 1200 nm) or flashlamp-pumped pulsed dye laser treatments (585 and 595 nm). The carbon dioxide laser does not give acceptable results when used on the neck with a significant risk of scarring. Various radiofrequency devices are becoming available which heat the deeper layers of the skin. This technology continues to evolve as the results are not entirely predictable and

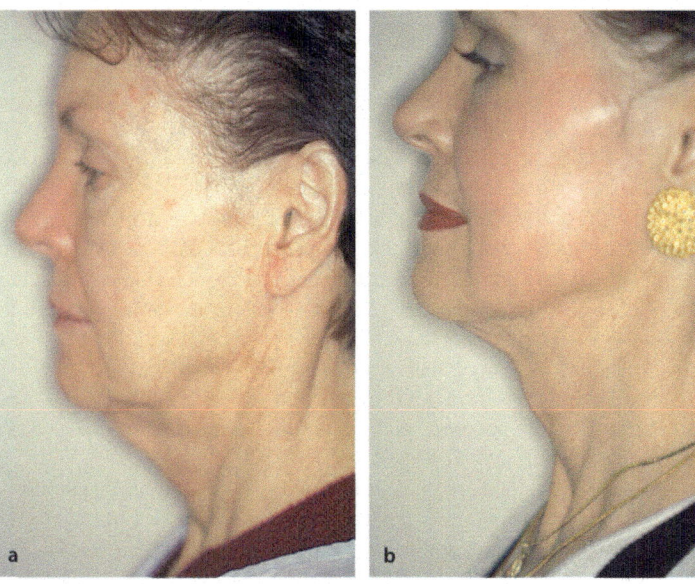

Fig. 78.20 **a** Female patient, in her mid-60s, with lower facial and cervical skin laxity, jowls, loss of definition of the mandible and platysmal bands. An ideal candidate for a cervicofacial rhytidectomy. **b** One year after an extended endoscopic midface lift, platysmal plication centrally and insertion of a suspension cervical suture. Note that there are still platysmal bands although there is an improvement in the jowls, the mandibular definition and the definition between the sternocleidomastoid and the mandible. The cervicomental angle is improved but not ideal. In such patients, there is no substitute for appropriate skin excision (which was not performed in this patient)

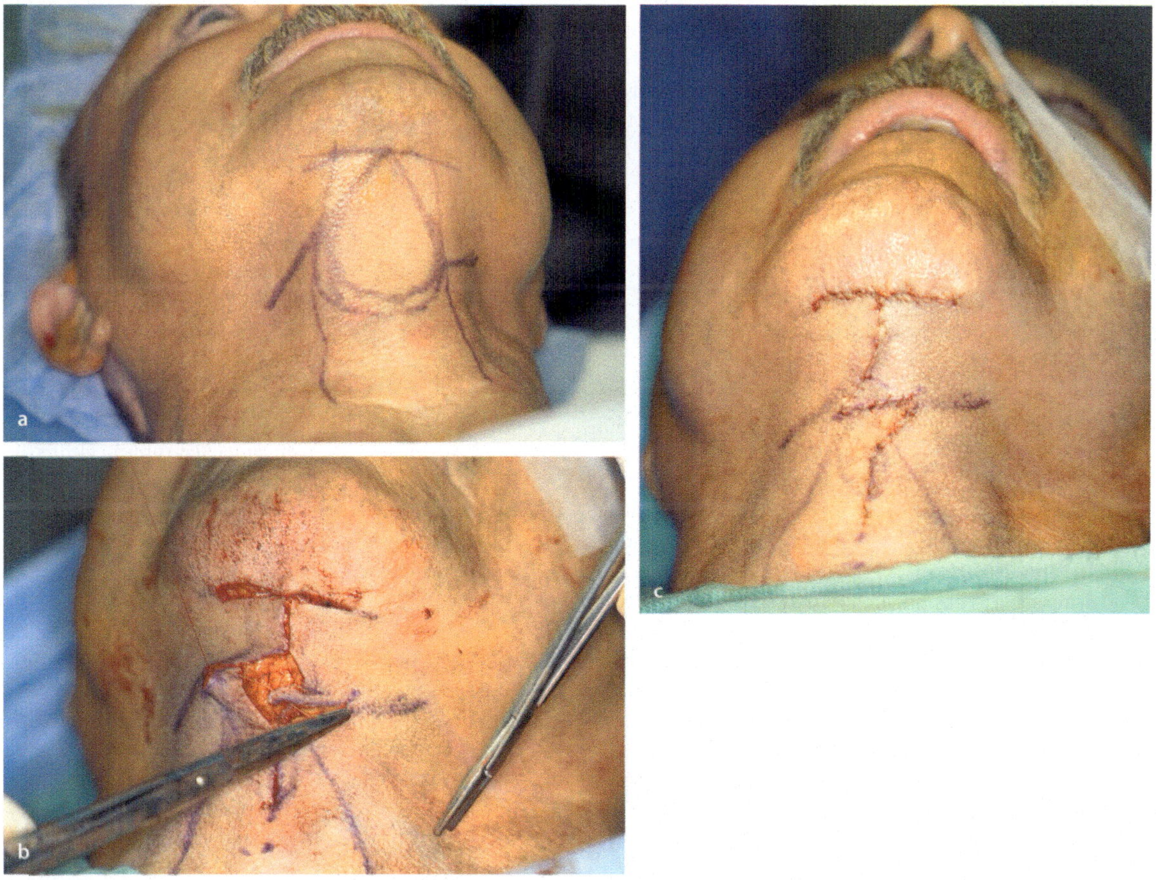

Fig. 78.21 In some men with thick sebaceous lax skin when a cervicofacial rhytidectomy is not acceptable to the patient, direct excision may be used. **a** The markings include the submental crease, platysmal bands and an oval resection of skin as shown. A Z-plasty is marked so as to increase the vertical length and shorten the horizontal length of the neck skin. **b** After the central oval has been excised and the platysmal bands have been sutured (with liposuction as indicated), the flaps are transposed. **c** Meticulous closure

the duration of any improvement is unknown. Some of the newer nonablative lasers show promise but the results need to be reviewed over an extended period of time before widespread applicability can be recommended.

Effective management of the aging neck depends upon a careful review of the changes in each of the anatomical parts and application of the most appropriate procedures.

Acknowledgement

Supported in part by a grant from Research to Prevent Blindness, New York, to the Department of Ophthalmology, University of Utah.

References

1. Dedo D. The aging neck. In Bailey B (ed): Head & Neck Surgery-Otolaryngology, ed. 2. Philadelphia, Lippincott-Raven 1998:2717–2732

2. Watson D. Submentoplasty. Facial Plast Surg Clin North Am 2005;13(3):459–467

3. Ghassemi A, Prescher A, Riediger D, Axer H. Anatomy of the SMAS revisited. Aesthet Plast Surg 2003;27:258–64

4. Owsley JQ. Face lifting: problems, solutions, and an outcome study. Plast Reconstr Surg 2000;105(1):302–313

5. Vistnes LM, Souther SG. The platysma muscle. Anatomic considerations for aesthetic surgery of the anterior neck. Clin Plast Surg 1983;10(3):441–448

6. Dedo D. A preoperative classification of the neck for cervicofacial rhytidectomy. Laryngoscope 1980;90(11 Pt 1):1894–1896

7. Ellenbogen R, Karlin JV. Visual criteria for success in restoring the youthful neck. Plast Reconstr Surg 1980;66(6):826–838

8. Giampapa V, Bitzos I, Ramirez O, Granick M. Suture suspension platysmaplasty for neck rejuvenation revisited: technical fine points for improving outcomes. Aesthet Plast Surg 2005;29(5):341–350

9. Giampapa V, Bitzos I, Ramirez O, Granick M. Long-term results of suture suspension platysmaplasty for neck rejuvenation: a 13-year follow-up evaluation. Aesthet Plast Surg 2005;29(5):332–340

10. Guyuron B. Problem neck, hyoid bone, and submental myotomy. Plast Reconstr Surg 1992;90(5):830–837

11. Owsley JQ. Face lift. Plast Reconstr Surg 1997;100(2):514–519

12. Singer R. Improvement of the "young" fatty neck. Plast Reconstr Surg 1984;73(4):582–589

13. Hetter GP. Improved results with closed facial suction. Clin Plast Surg. 1989;16(2):319–332

14. Lambros V. Fat contouring in the face and neck. Clin Plast Surg 1992;19(2):401–414

15. Illouz Y, Flageul G. Isolated cervicofacial liposuction in facial rejuvenation. Perspect Plast Surg 1996;10:95–106

16. Gryskiewicz J.M. Submental suction-assisted lipectomy without platysmaplasty: pushing the (skin) envelope to avoid a face lift for unsuitable candidates. Plast Reconstr Surg 2003;112(5):1393–1405

17. Pitman GH, Teimourian B. Suction lipectomy: complications and results by survey. Plast Reconstr Surg 1985;76(1):65–72

18. Dillerud E. Suction lipoplasty: a report on complications, undesired results, and patient satisfaction based on 3511 procedures. Plast Reconstr Surg 1991;88(2):239–246

19. Connell BF. Contouring the neck in rhytidectomy by lipectomy and a muscle sling. Plast Reconstr Surg 1978;61(3):376–383

20. Connell BF, Gaan A. Surgical correction of aesthetic contour problems in the neck. Clin Plast Surg 1983;10(3):491–505

21. Caplin DA, Prendville S. Modifications in rejuvenation of the aging neck. Facial Plast Surg Clin North Am 2002;10(1):77–86

22. Feldman JJ. Corset platysmaplasty. Clin Plast Surg 1992;19(2):369–382

23. McKinney P. The management of platysma bands. Plast Reconstr Surg 1996;98(6):999–1006

24. McKinney P. Management of platysma bands. Plast Reconstr Surg 2002;110(3):982–984

25. Giampapa VC, DiBernardo BE. Neck recontouring with suture suspension and liposuction: an alternative for the early rhytidectomy candidate. Aesthet Plast Surg 1995;19(3):217–223

26. Guerrerosantos J. Neck lift: simplified surgical technique, refinements, and clinical classification. Clin Plast Surg 1983;10(3):379–404

27. Guerrero-Santos J, Espaillat L, Morales F. Muscular lift in cervical rhytidoplasty. Plast Reconstr Surg 1974;54(2):127–130

28. Guerrerosantos J. Surgical correction of the fatty fallen neck. Ann Plast Surg 1979;2(5):389–396

29. Webster RC, Smith RC, Smith KF. Face lift, part 5:suspending sutures for platysma cording. Head Neck Surg 1984;6(4):870–879

30. Giampapa VC. Suture suspension technique offers predictable, long-lasting neck rejuvenation. Aesthet Surg J 2000;20:253–255

CHAPTER 79

Algorithm for Neck Rejuvenation

George Bitar, Vincent Giampapa

79.1
Introduction

"I want to look better, but I don't want a full facelift". That is a statement a plastic surgeon hears frequently from a patient. What can a plastic surgeon offer a patient who wants a significant facial rejuvenation but does not want a full facelift? In a world where there is a new technique being advertised everyday on TV, or in high-end magazines, about looking younger with minimal downtime, it is more important than ever to get educated as plastic surgeons and to educate the public on what to realistically expect. No one procedure is perfect for every patient. The neck and the jaw line show the early signs of facial aging, so achieving a youthful neck line is a very critical step in facial rejuvenation.

Many techniques have been described to perform neck lifts as an isolated procedure or in conjunction with a rhytidectomy [1–5]. In 1973 Guerrero-Santos et al. [2] described the muscular lift. Feldman [3, 4] described the corset platysmaplasty in 1989. In 1990 Giampapa developed the concept of the suture-suspension neck lift. He started performing the suture-suspension neck lift in open facelift patients. It later evolved into a closed neck lift approach. In the following years, the suture-suspension neck-lift technique underwent many technical changes and improvements. Conrad et al. [5] described the Gore-Tex suspension cervical fascial rhytidectomy. In 1995 an article by Giampapa and Di Bernardo [6] was published on neck recontouring with a new technique involving the use of platysmal resection and the use of two interlocking permanent sutures through a subcutaneous tunnel immediately below the submandibular border running from the midline to the mastoid bony fascia, creating an artificial ligament, which may be responsible for the positive long-term effects of this procedure. This is combined with liposuction of the neck to achieve the desired result. The postoperative course included dressings for 7 days.

The addition of the fibrin sealant to suture-suspension neck lifts, in 2001, by Giampapa and Bitar [7] proved to be a very valuable improvement in decreasing the rates of hematomas, seromas, ecchymosis, edema, and postoperative discomfort. Recently, articles on the technical points in refinement of the neck lift technique by Giampapa et al. [8], as well as a 13-year follow-up study on suture-suspension neck lifts by Giampapa et al. [9], have served as a continued effort to improve on this versatile technique.

79.2
Technique

79.2.1
Classification of Neck Types

It is important to evaluate the individual anatomy of each patient's neck and select the treatment accordingly. The following neck classifications include most neck types and are a valuable tool in order to address the key anatomical points and the treatment approach:

1. Class I deformity (Fig. 79.1)
   (a) No midface laxity
   (b) Mild platysmal laxity
   (c) Mild submental fat

These patients are the best candidates for the suture-suspension platysmaplasty technique and demonstrate excellent early, as well as long-term, results. Some people with a class I neck elect to have liposuction only. The advantage of liposuction only may be reduction of cost, quicker recovery, less invasive surgery, and fewer incisions. The disadvantage is the lack of a dramatic improvement secondary to the suture-suspension platysmaplasty and skin excision that is performed in a neck lift, but not in a liposuction of the neck solely.

2. Class II deformity (Fig. 79.2)
   (a) Mild midface laxity/mild jowling
   (b) Moderate subplatysmal fat

The treatment of a class II neck is suture-suspension platysmaplasty with plication of the platysma muscle and submental and/or subplatysmal fat removal with moderate liposuction, as well as appropriate postauricular skin excision. These patients exhibit excellent early and long-term results and respond well with excellent skin contraction and improvement in neck contour.

3. Class III deformity (Fig. 79.3)
   (a) Moderate midface laxity and prominent jowling

(b) Moderate platysmal laxity
(c) Moderate submental fat

The treatment is suture-suspension technique with resection of a portion of the anterior medial bands of the platysma muscle with vigorous suction of the submental and/or subplatysmal fat, and removal with direct excision of the subplatysmal fat. Postauricular skin resection is more extensive in a class III neck. These patients exhibit a good result and respond well with good skin contraction to the anterior cervical and lateral neck. Correction of jowling is usually not complete with this technique alone, and other ancillary techniques may need to be employed.

4. Class IV deformity (Fig. 79.4)
   (a) Midface laxity and prominent jowling with extensive labial mandibular deformities
   (b) Moderate to severe platysmal laxity

(c) Severe submental fat and subcutaneous laxity in the lower portion of the neck

The treatment is a rhytidectomy with complete undermining of the cervical mental area along with anterior midface skin. Although suture suspension can be utilized for the platysmaplasty portion of the rhytidectomy, a more extensive procedure needs to be undertaken for the best results.

Occasionally, a patient who has a class IV neck cannot have a full facelift for medical reasons, financial reasons, or other personal reasons. In this situation, the patient needs to be told explicitly that a neck lift will not yield results similar to those of a facelift. Also, adding ancillary procedures to the midface such as fat grafting or implants may improve the result and need to be discussed with the patient to the extent of the surgeon's expertise.

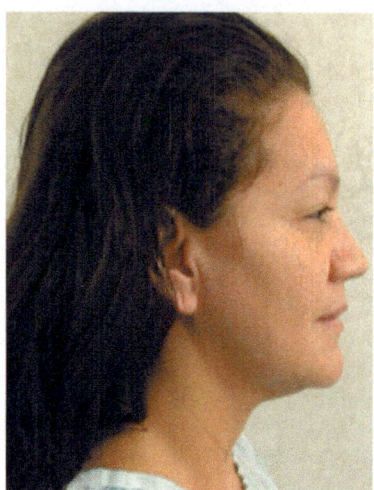

Fig. 79.1 Class I deformity

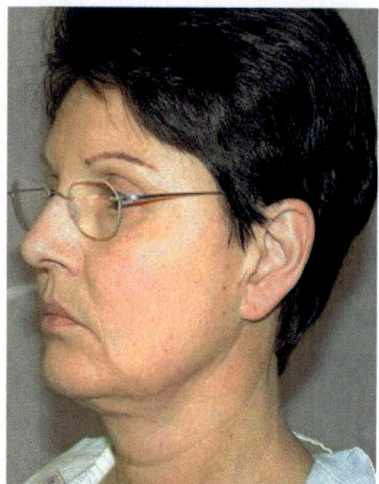

Fig. 79.2 Class II deformity

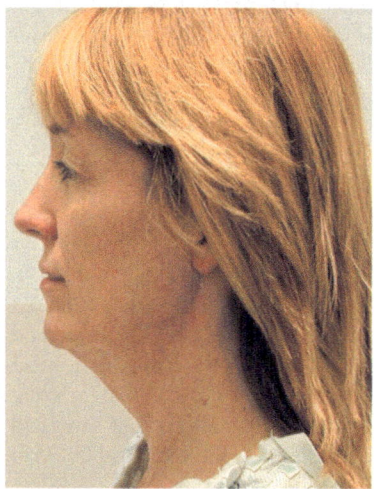

Fig. 79.3 Class III deformity

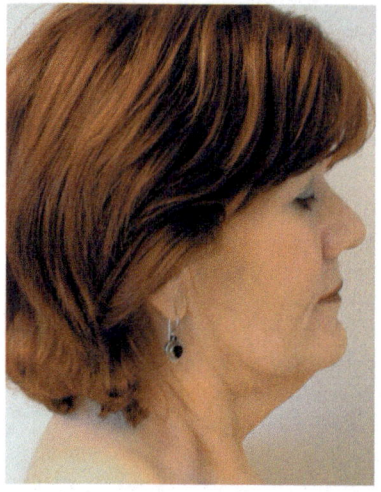

Fig. 79.4 Class IV deformity

79.2.2
The Six Basic Points of the Neck Evaluation

Ellenbogen and Karlin [10] originally discussed the five youthful neck criteria:
1. Acute cervicomental angle (between 105 and 120°)
2. Distinct inferior mandible border
3. Subhyoid depression
4. A visible thyroid cartilage
5. A visible anterior sternocleidomastoid border

The suture-suspension platysmaplasty technique addresses the first three criteria. In men, a visible thyroid cartilage contour gives a desirable masculine look, but in a woman, a surgeon has to be careful not to lose the feminine appearance of the neck. Furthermore, a visible anterior border of the sternocleidomastoid border can be achieved with the right suctioning technique.

A specific numerical protocol was designed in order to identify all of the important points of the neck anatomy that undergo the most modification with aging. Additionally, these are the points on which the surgical techniques focus, as described below, and that are utilized presently when evaluating a prospective patient for neck rejuvenation. Those points are:
1. Cervicomental angle depth
2. Mandibular border definition
3. Mandibular angle definition
4. Labiomandibular fold prominence (jowling)
5. Mental prominence
6. Neck width

79.2.3
The Suture-Suspension Platysmaplasty Technique

79.2.3.1
Preoperative Assessment

It is essential to explain to the patient what a neck lift can accomplish [11], and what it cannot accomplish. Limitations, risks, benefits, and what to expect in the postoperative course are discussed at length. Usually a patient comes because they want an improvement in their neck but do not want a full facelift. The main indication for a suture-suspension neck lift is a poorly defined cervicomental angle and mandibular border, which is common with the aging process. This loss of definition is due to the aging process and the loss of key hormones that occur with the aging process, which causes loss of skin tone, loss of muscle tone, and reduced muscle fiber density. A poor definition of the submandibular border is evident from a side view, when looking at a face and seeing the cheek blending into the side of the neck. In short, contour loss is a stigma of an aging face. In order to properly evaluate a patient for a neck lift procedure, it is important to evaluate the

midface, jaw line, and neck. Next a suitable operative plan is formulated.

Midface Evaluation

Evaluating the midface is very important for a potential neck lift patient. Minimal laxity to midface structures is important in achieving a good neck lift. At the initial consultation, it should be made clear to the patient that a neck lift is not the procedure of choice to improve the jowls or the nasolabial folds. We usually pinch the patients' jowls to remind them, physically, that this area will not be improved with a neck lift. This point cannot be overemphasized because patients may feel that they will get all the benefits of a facelift with a neck lift, but with "less surgery". That is not true, especially if the patient has significant jowling. A neck lift is meant to make a new cervicomental angle and new definition, but is it not a substitute for a facelift, especially when addressing the jowls in a person with significant midface laxity. There is the occasional patient who comes back after surgery and says, "My neck looks great, but what about this" (pointing to the jowls), and we, as surgeons, remind them of discussing that specific point preoperatively. They acknowledge that fact when they remember the preoperative pinch to that area!

Jaw Line Evaluation

One of the goals of a neck lift is to recreate the mandibular contour by repositioning the platysma and tucking it underneath the border of the mandible. With a wider and more prominent jaw, we obtain better results. One of the initial questions in a consultation is, "Does the patient have a nice, full, wide jaw, or is it narrow?" If the patient has a narrow jaw, the results are not going to be as dramatic as in an individual with a wide jaw. Patients of Romanian or Slavic descent who have wide jaws do very well with a neck lift. Northern Europeans with narrow faces or Latin Americans with smaller facial features may not have as good a result. Of course these are generalities and exceptions are found.

Neck Evaluation

In order to evaluate the neck with the patient in an interactive manner, we suggest taking a long Q-Tip, or something long and thin, and pressing against the neck line to show how deep the cervicomental angle is, i.e., the distance between the anteriormost tip of the mentum and the thyroid cartilage. This maneuver done in front of the mirror will show the patient the amount of realistic improvement expected from a neck lift. In people with a narrow neck, even the best neck lift may not yield a dramatic improvement if the patient's expectations are unrealistic. In evaluating the neck, attention needs to be given to the amount of fat, its distribution in the neck, platysmal laxity, and skin laxity [12]. Categorizing the neck as in classes I–IV will aid in determining what procedure is offered to the patient.

Neck Lift or Facelift?

There are, of course, patients for whom a neck lift is not appropriate, and a full facelift is the procedure of choice. The appropriate way to handle these patients is to be firm about the fact that they will need a full facelift if they would like reasonable improvement. If there are other matters which prompt them to have a neck lift instead, such as health issues, financial considerations, or other reasons, then they need to know that their results with a neck lift will be suboptimal.

An important question a patient may ask is, "If I do my neck now, can I do my upper face later?" The patient should be given the option to have the neck lift done now and the face later, when the neck does not need to be redone. Performing a facelift as the initial procedure is another option. We, as surgeons, can give our patients what they want in stages, keeping the incisions acceptable, by doing a neck lift first, and a midface lift later. We believe that patients like to have options given to them. Cosmetic surgery patients on the whole are smart, educated people, and should have the appropriate information to decide on what surgery suits them, not the surgeon.

Suture-Suspension Platysmaplasty Indications

The procedure described here may be an additional procedure in the plastic surgeon's armamentarium for treating the aging neck. An appropriate candidate for this procedure should meet some of the following criteria (Fig. 79.5):
1. Poorly defined cervical mental angle.
2. Poorly defined submandibular border.

3. Absence of laxity in the midface structures (since no tightening of the underlying superficial musculoaponeurotic system fibers and facial muscles in the midface is accomplished through this procedure).
4. Mild to moderate amount of jowling and neck fat (those with large amounts of neck and jowl fat will find some soft-tissue irregularities if this procedure is used alone in lieu of a facelift).
5. Unwillingness or inability to undergo a full facelift.

Patients who previously would have been considered "early rhytidectomy candidates", i.e., with a class I or a class II neck, seem to the ideal candidates. Men have found this technique to be an excellent option to avoid preauricular incisions with the multiple problems associated with the beard and hair-baring areas, which are repositioned posteriorly onto the tragus when the standard facelift incision is used. Furthermore, the platysmaplasty portion of this procedure can be performed during primary and secondary rhytidectomies for treating fatty necks and acute cervicomental angles which have been difficult to correct with previous surgical procedures.

Advantages of the Suture-Suspension Technique for Neck Contouring

1. Excellent option for male patients who want a nicely contoured neck and jaw without a facelift.
2. Quick recovery of 5–10 days compared with a facelift.
3. Little chance of nerve damage or soft-tissue loss, since the neck does not have the abundance of motor nerves that the face has, and the skin undermining is less than in a facelift.
4. No preauricular or hair-baring area incisions are involved.
5. Can be used during both primary and secondary rhytidectomy for the difficult neck in the obtuse cervicomental angle patients.
6. Good option for treating the prolapsed submandibular gland deformity.

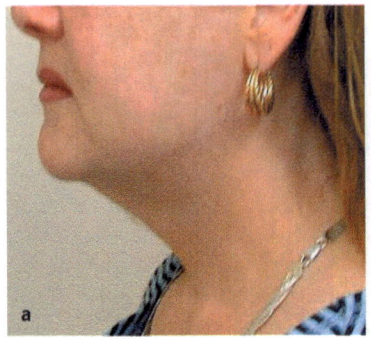 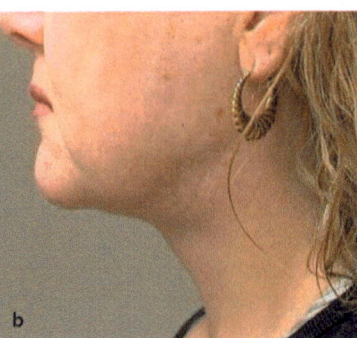

Fig. 79.5 Suture suspension indication. **a** Before. **b** After

79.2.3.2
Surgical Technique

Patients should get medical and psychiatric clearance when appropriate before proceeding to surgery. It is a good idea to give prospective patients references of people who have had the surgery and consented to be used as references, so the prospective patient may contact them by phone and ask them questions. After the patient is ready for surgery, the immediate preoperative preparation commences. Optimizing a patient for surgery is done differently by different surgeons. Some useful steps have been to place patients on vitamin K and Arnica for 5 days preoperatively, requesting that the patients stop taking aspirin and aspirin products for 10 days, and that they abstain from smoking for 2 weeks preoperatively and 2 weeks postoperatively.

Surgical Marking

The patient is marked in the holding area in the supine position (Fig. 79.6). First, a midline line is drawn. Next, the mandible contour is marked and a line parallel and 1.5 cm inferior to the mandible border is also marked to create the subcutaneous tunnel. The submental curvilinear incision and the inferior border of the dissection are then marked. The inferior border depends on the individual's neck laxity. Finally, the postauricular ellipse of skin to be incised is marked. The extent of that ellipse, similar to the lower border of dissection, depends on the skin laxity in the lateral neck.

Surgical Prep

The patient is initially given prophylactic antibiotics, deep venous thrombosis prophylaxis, and is intubated with either general anesthesia or intravenous sedation given as a surgeon's choice. The table is turned 180°, and the arms of the patient are tucked to the side. The submandibular area, postauricular area, and lower neck are infiltrated in a fashion similar to a rhytidectomy with about 75–150 ml on each side with tumescent solution for a total of 150–300 ml (500 ml of saline, 50 ml of 1% plain lidocaine, and 1 ampule of 1:10,000 epinephrine). The patient is then prepped in the usual sterile fashion and draped with a head and a full body drape while the tumescent fluid is allowed to take effect. Men may need to be injected with more tumescent solution than women because of the increase in blood supply to the neck hair follicles and thicker muscles.

Suction-Assisted Lipectomy

After the tumescent solution has taken effect, the neck is liposuctioned initially with 2–3-mm spatulated cannulas and finally with a 4-mm liposuction spatulated cannula. The area of the submandibular tunnel is suctioned along its dermal surface with the 4-mm cannula facing the dermis. This maneuver helps encourage skin contraction in this area. Specific areas such as the anterior border of the sternocleidomastoid, the jowls, and the angle of the mandible are liposuctioned in the appropriate patient. The inferior border of the liposuction

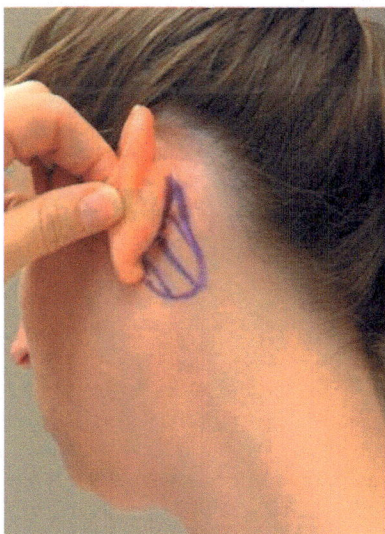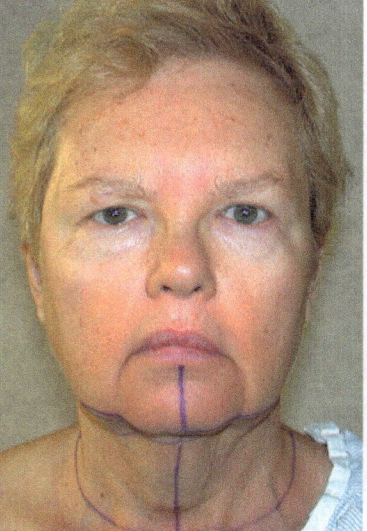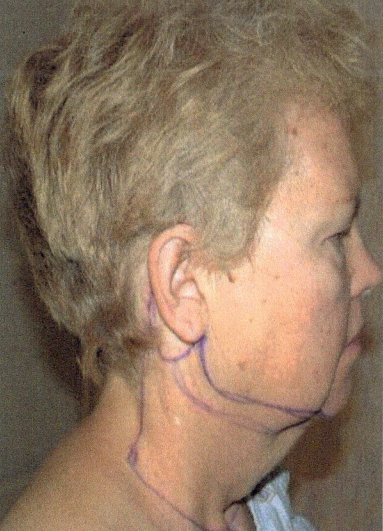

Fig. 79.6 Surgical marking

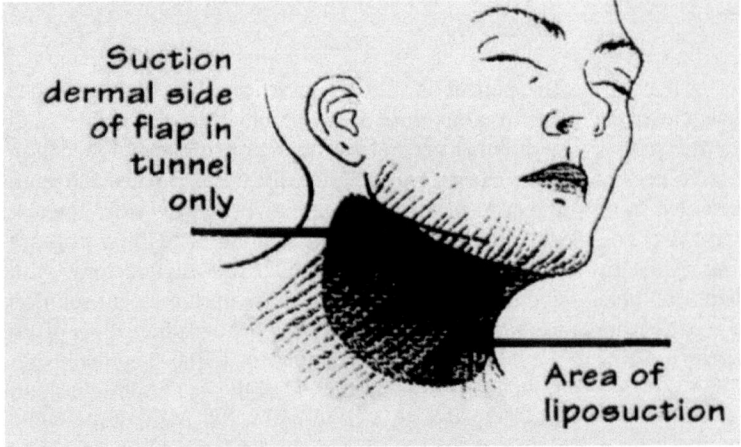

Fig. 79.7 At times, the whole extent of the neck needs to be suctioned if there is a significant fatty layer (i.e., in class III or class IV neck deformities)

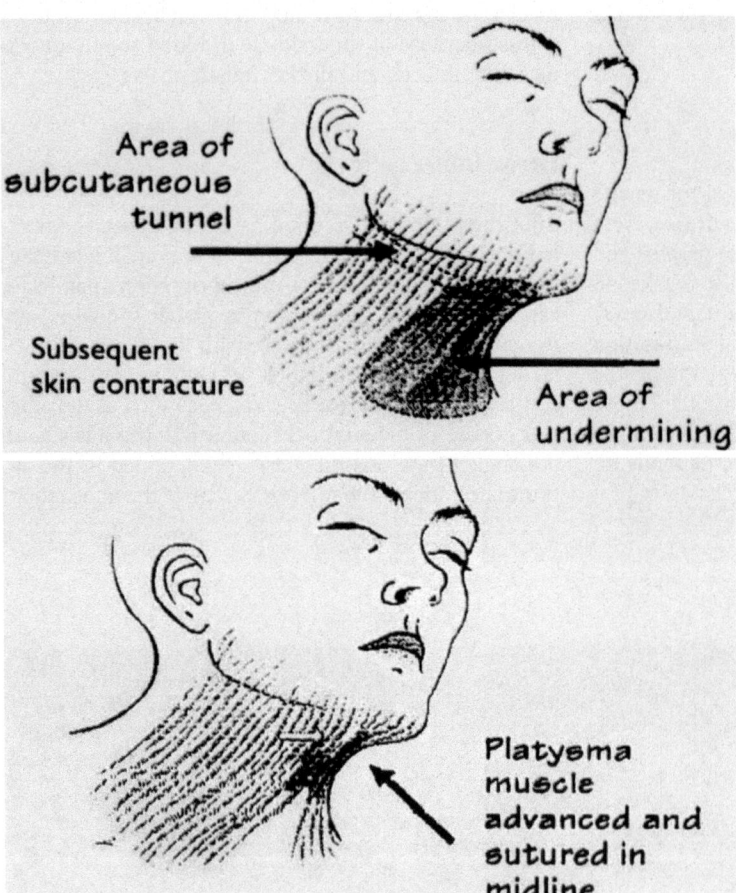

Fig. 79.8 Management of the platysma muscle

area depends on the amount of fat in the lower aspect of the neck. At times, the whole extent of the neck needs to be suctioned if there is a significant fatty layer (i.e., in class III or class IV neck deformities) (Fig. 79.7).

Management of the Platysma Muscle

A midline curvilinear submental incision is made in the horizontal crease, and the skin immediately overlying the platysma muscles is elevated with facelift scissors (Fig. 79.8). A curvilinear incision seems to heal better than a straight incision after scar contraction. Excess subplatysmal fatty tissue is excised under direct visualization with a lighted retractor. The platysmal border in the midline is sometimes resected, if there is significant laxity, in a triangular fashion, and the platysmal borders are cauterized. Prominent platysmal bands are transected for approximately 2–3 cm on each side of the platysmal border or are imbricated at the midline with

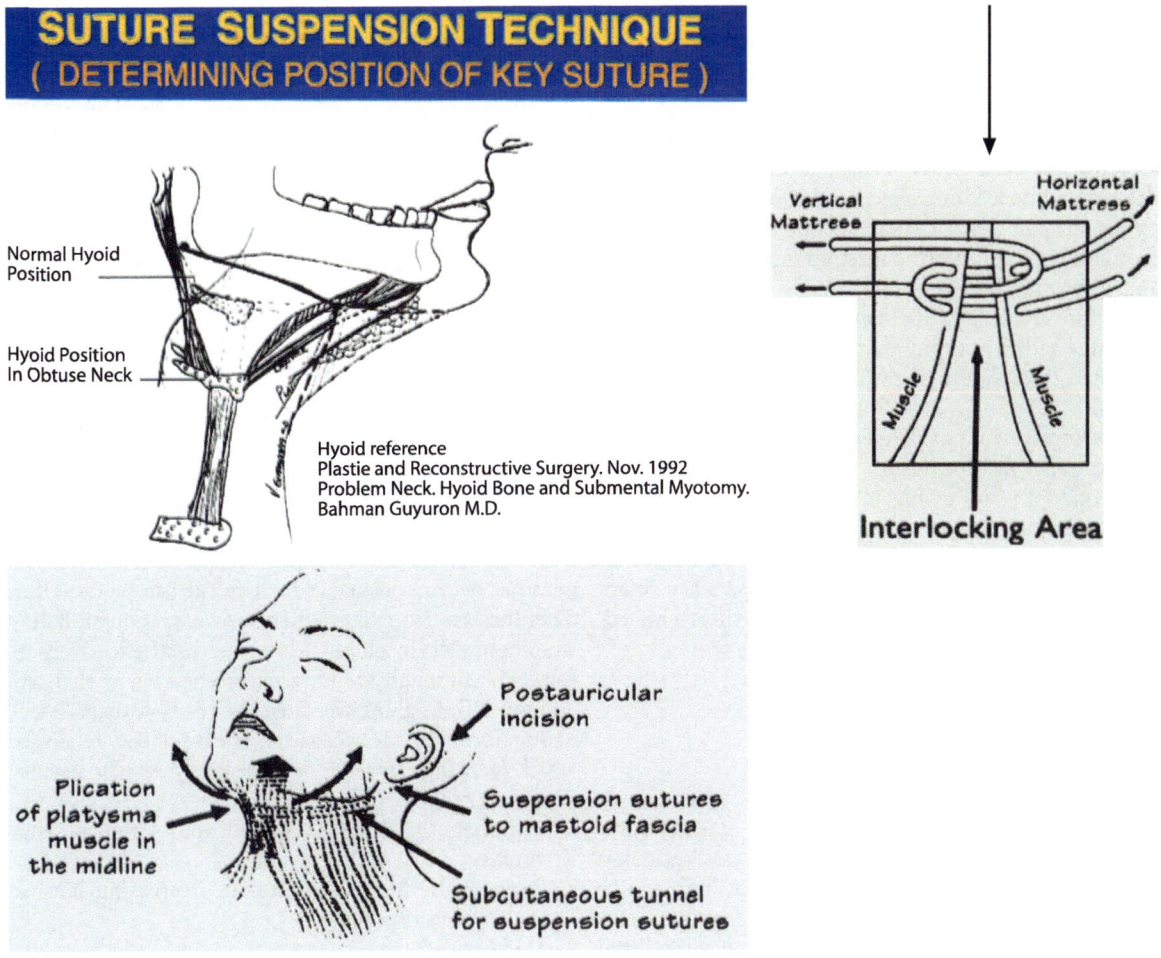

SUTURE SUSPENSION TECHNIQUE
(DETERMINING POSITION OF KEY SUTURE)

Normal Hyoid
Position

Hyoid Position
In Obtuse Neck

Hyoid reference
Plastie and Reconstructive Surgery. Nov. 1992
Problem Neck. Hyoid Bone and Submental Myotomy.
Bahman Guyuron M.D.

Vertical
Mattress

Horizontal
Mattress

Muscle   Muscle

Interlocking Area

Postauricular
incision

Plication
of platysma
muscle in
the midline

Suspension sutures
to mastoid fascia

Subcutaneous tunnel
for suspension sutures

Fig. 79.9 Suture-suspension technique

buried 4-0 Prolene sutures. This technique reapproximates and shortens the width of the platysma muscle, thus decreasing the width of the neck.

The Interlocking Suture Placement

At the depth desired to create the new cervicomental angle, usually the hyoid bone, a 3-0 Prolene suture (and an 0 Prolene suture in men) is placed in a horizontal mattress fashion from right to left, including both borders of the platysma muscle. Another similar suture is placed from left to right in a vertical mattress style interlocking with the first suture. The ends of both sutures are taken out through the submental incision and the sutures are clamped separately with a Webster needle holder to avoid weakening the suture (Fig. 79.9).

The postauricular skin on each side is identified and an ellipse of skin is excised. This maneuver eliminates the redundant skin from the neck in an easily hidden incision and allows better access to the underlying mastoid fascia. The skin between the mastoid area and the submental area is then undermined to connect to the previously made tunnel. A long curved hemostat is placed at the postauricular sulcus and exits through the tunnel at the submental incision. The left suture is grasped by the instrument and taken through the submandibular tunnel. Then, the suture is sutured deep into the mastoid fascia while the patient's face is turned towards the opposite side and maximally extended. The suture is then tied just enough so that the platysma muscle is tucked up underneath the border of the mandible. Similarly, the vertical mattress suture is tied to the right mastoid. The suspension sutures result in a superior and internal vector force that creates the new cervicomental angle and defines the submandibular border. The inherent properties of soft-tissue contraction allow the overlying skin to adapt to the new muscle positions.

The Submandibular Angle Loop Suture

An important technical fine point that evolved over the last 13 years is the submandibular angle loop suture [8]. This involves securing the non-absorbable interlocking suture under the area of the angle of the mandible at the anterior sternocleidomastoid border, before suturing it on the mastoid fascia. After the loop has been created, the suture is secured at the mastoid process periosteum, and it is critical to keep the tension of the interlocking suture moderate. The suture should be placed on each side of the mastoid fascia while the patient's face is turned towards the opposite side and maximally extended.

The angle loop suture creates a more natural and anatomically pleasing result. Additionally, it creates a "hinge mechanism", owing to its geometry, which decreases the suture tension, especially when the patient turns the neck sideways. This eliminates the chance of "overcorrection", and the feeling of tightness that a small percentage of patients experienced before this technical modification was introduced.

Skin Excision

Usually, only small amount of skin needs to be excised in the form of an elliptical skin strip that extends from the ear lobule area to the midlevel of the postauricular sulcus. It is important to understand that although a fatty neck appears to have too much skin that this is, in essence, an illusion. In reality, a full neck has too little skin rather than too much, owing to the fact that when the cervicomental angle is augmented, and a concavity is subsequently created, more skin is required to fill this

deeper angle (Fig. 79.10). Patients with very redundant skin need more excised but with care to avoid skin tension and a subsequent "pixie ear" deformity.

After the interlocking sutures have been placed and before closing the incisions, the fibrin sealant is sprayed under the skin flaps. Next, the postauricular incisions are closed. The submental incision is then closed. Paper tape is used to dress the neck followed by either foam or ABD dressings. Usually, dressings are placed over the skin, along with a Velcro overhead strap for support.

Tissue Fibrin Sealant

To improve the recovery phase of the suture-suspension technique, a fibrin tissue sealant (Fig. 79.11), which may be applied in the subcutaneous tunnel, is used, in lieu of surgical drains [7]. In 2001, the Tisseel Vapor Heated (VH) fibrin sealant, a sealant prepared from human plasma, became available for clinical use in the USA. Bioadhesives from the patients' own cryoprecipitate—autologous fibrin glues—have been used effectively in surgery. Although we have experience using such autologous fibrin glues, we chose the ready-to-use Tisseel tissue fibrin sealant because of its ease of use, relatively quick learning curve, and consistently reliable results. The goals of the sealant are to:

- Eliminate the dead space and avoid seromas/hematomas
- Support the healing process by decreasing tension on the incision sites
- Decrease edema
- Promote hemostasis
- Eliminate postoperative wrinkling or rippling of the skin

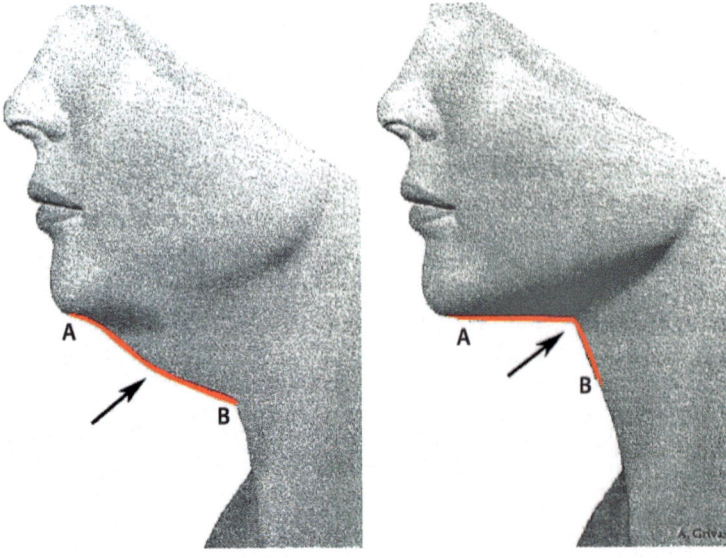

Fig. 79.10 In reality, a full neck has too little skin rather than too much, owing to the fact that when the cervicomental angle is augmented, and a concavity is subsequently created, more skin is required to fill this deeper angle

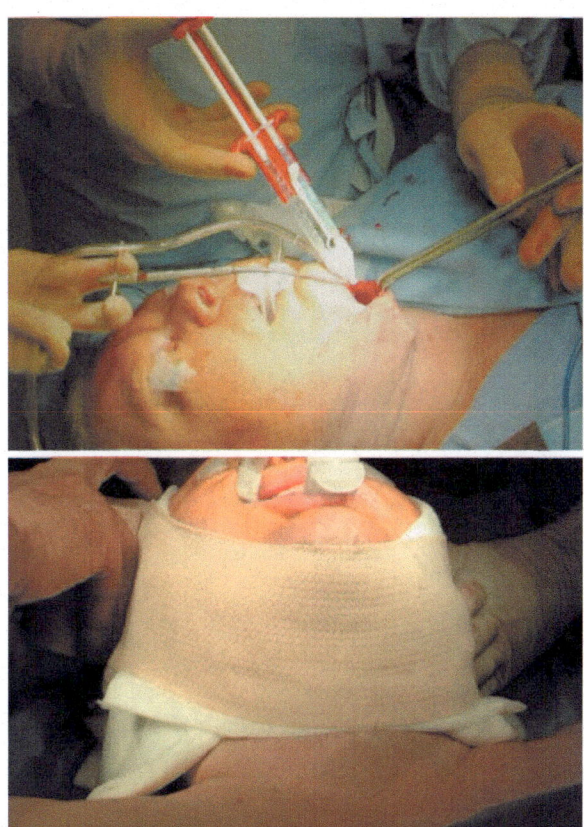

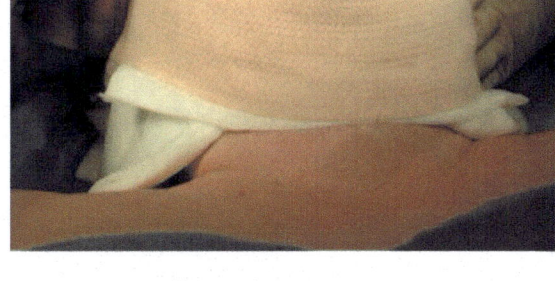

Fig. 79.11 Tissue fibrin sealant

Application of the Fibrin Sealant

After excellent hemostasis has been achieved, the fibrin sealant is applied. On the side table, the fibrin sealant is prepared simultaneously, or reconstituted, in two separate syringes. One syringe contains the sealer protein concentrate dried powder mixed with the fibrinolysis inhibitor solution, to make the Tisseel solution. The other syringe holds the human thrombin, which is freeze-dried and mixed with the calcium chloride solution, to form the thrombin solution. Once the reconstitution has taken place, the Tisseel fibrin sealant must be used within 4 h.

The two syringes are mounted on a Duploject applicator. The fibrin sealant is then sprayed, simultaneously, into the pockets, in thin layers, for 60 s, the time required for the liquid sealant to activate. Gentle manual pressure is applied over the neck skin, with the surgeon's fingers spread evenly over the whole neck, to prevent pooling of the fibrin sealant to any given area. Such pooling may result in overlying skin necrosis, hematomas, seromas, or skin wrinkling, caused by interruption of the vascular supply to the overlying dermis. Pressure is applied for 3 min, the time required for the fibrin sealant to solidify. Past potential complications

of rippling or fluid collections are avoided because the skin flaps adhere immediately to the underlying tissues. The incisions are then closed, and dressings are applied.

79.2.3.3
Postoperative Care

Postoperative care is minimal. Patients are kept on oral pain medications for 3–5 days and antibiotics for 1 week. They are instructed to keep their head elevated while sleeping. The dressings and the paper tape are removed after 48 h. Male patients are advised not to shave for 7–10 days after the operation, to avoid trauma to the neck flaps. Patients are instructed to resume activities of daily living in 2–3 days and strenuous activity, including exercise, in 3–4 weeks.

79.3
Selective Neck Enhancement/Addressing the Six Basic Points

After the basic procedure has been described, it is important to explore each anatomical aspect of the neck,

The Six Key Points to Consider in Evaluation of The Neck.

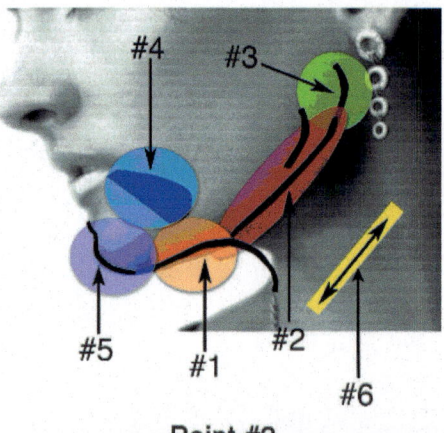

Point #1

Depth of Cervical Mental Angle

Deficiency Corrected by:
1. Adjusting Tension of interlocking suspention sutures
2. Defatting Supra and Subplatysmal Space
3. Suturing Digastric muscles together
4. Transecting Platysmal Borders

Point #2

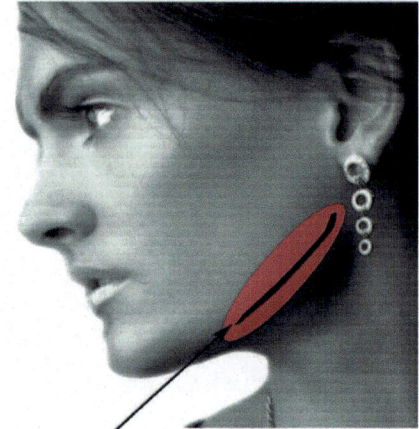

Mandibular Border Definition

Deficiency Corrected by:
1. SAL above and below border of Mandibular (leave strip SubQ. fat along bony border)
2. Fat Grafting to Mandibular border.
3. Long term fillers Radiance™.

Point #3

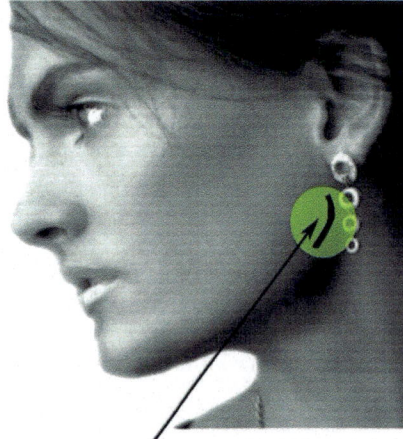

Madibular Angle Definition

Deficiency Corrected by:
1. Loop Suture elevation of SMAS
2. Fat grafting into Masseter
3. Long term fillers Radiance™ etc .
4. Alloplastic augmentation (mandibular angle implant)

Point #4

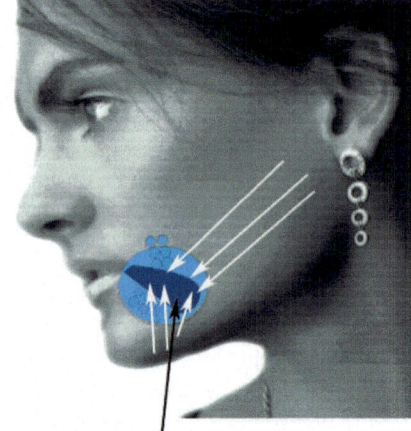

Labial Mandibular Fold Prominence

Deformity Corrected by:
1. SAL from Submental and Post aurocular approaches.
2. Camoflage fat grafting.
3. Depressor Labii muscle release.
4. Contour threads ("featherlift" sutures)

Fig. 79.12 Six key points to consider in evaluation of the neck

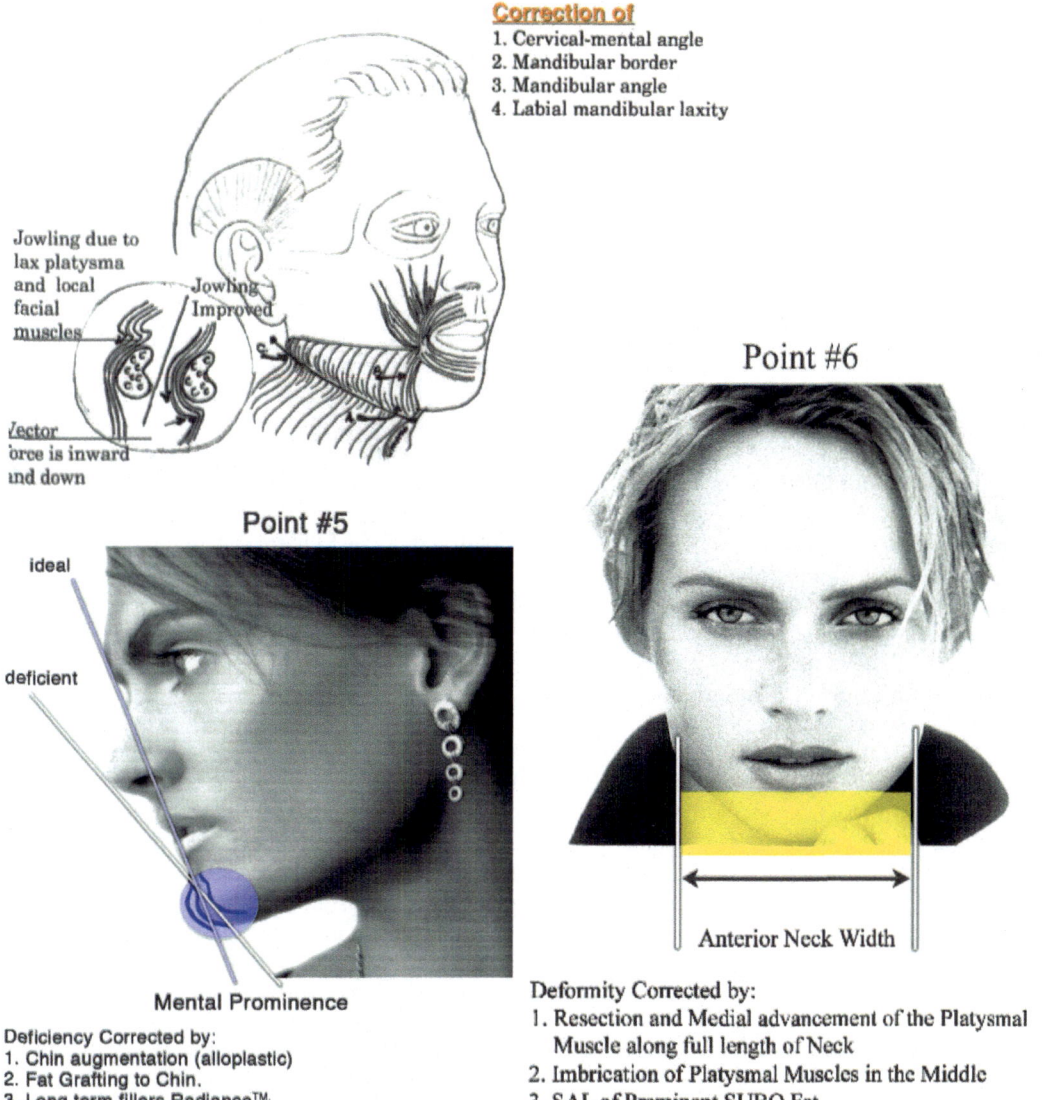

Correction of
1. Cervical-mental angle
2. Mandibular border
3. Mandibular angle
4. Labial mandibular laxity

Jowling due to lax platysma and local facial muscles

Jowling Improved

Vector force is inward and down

Point #5

Point #6

ideal

deficient

Mental Prominence

Anterior Neck Width

Deficiency Corrected by:
1. Chin augmentation (alloplastic)
2. Fat Grafting to Chin.
3. Long term fillers Radiance™

Deformity Corrected by:
1. Resection and Medial advancement of the Platysmal Muscle along full length of Neck
2. Imbrication of Platysmal Muscles in the Middle
3. SAL of Preminent SUBQ Fat

Fig. 79.12 *(Continued)* Six key points to consider in evaluation of the neck

and address it individually, to get the overall perception of a youthful and aesthetically pleasing neck [8]. The observation of the aging neck shows evidence of many factors contributing to its loss of shape and contour. These anatomical changes have been described over the years and include loss of tone of the dermal elastic fibers with sagging of the skin, ptosis of the soft tissues of the neck and chin, banding of the platysma muscles at the anterior neck, elimination of the anterior sternocleidomastoid border, increased fat deposition, bone resorption, submandibular gland protrusion, and others. Additionally, during the aging process the cervical spine collapses.

This, in essence, not only shortens the height of the neck, but is subsequently responsible for creating an increased width in the anterior dimension of the neck.

The key anatomical points utilized clinically when evaluating and surgically treating the aging neck are the following (Fig. 79.12):
1. Cervicomental angle depth
2. Mandibular border definition
3. Mandibular angle definition
4. Labiomandibular fold prominence (jowling)
5. Mental prominence
6. Neck width

79.4
Results and Complications

79.4.1
Results

Neck-lift patients have ranged in age from the early 30s to the late 70s, both male and female. Some patients had simultaneous procedures, such as chin augmentation, fat grafting, or blepharoplasties, along with the suture-suspension technique and fibrin sealant. The "recovery time", that is the time necessary to return to activities of daily living and be cosmetically inconspicuous at work and at home, has been reduced to just a few days. The full recovery time is similar to that of the neck recontouring alone without the Tisseel fibrin sealant. It requires 6 months to allow for soft-tissue contraction to reach its optimal state and for the fine edema resolution to be complete. Before fibrin sealant was used, hematoma/seroma rates, in our experience, were 2–3% in neck lifts performed on the male population and about 1% in neck lifts performed on the female population. Since the fibrin sealant has been used, the rate of hematoma/seroma formation has markedly diminished.

Furthermore, because the bleeding postoperatively is minimized by the sealant, the ecchymosis that our patients have had has been significantly less than in patients on whom the sealant was not used. Other minor and moderate complications experienced infrequently are addressed in the following section. No mortalities or long-term serious complications have been recorded in our patient population.

79.4.2
Avoidance of Complications and Pitfalls

79.4.2.1
Discussing Potential Complications

Honesty is the best policy. It is very important to go over, in detail, the risks of a neck lift and comparing them with those of a facelift. We discuss, with our patients, the risks of hematoma, seroma, skin necrosis, unsightly scars, nerve damage, discomfort from the tightness initially, asymmetry, unsatisfactory results, and the potential for revisional surgery. To get the patients involved in their care makes them active participants who can identify a complication and alert the surgeon in a timely fashion to treat it. Furthermore, it is more effective to explain to patients why smoking can increase the rate of complications, rather that telling them to quit smoking before the surgery. Postoperatively, smokers may develop postauricular skin ischemia, or necrosis, where the skin is under the most tension, so avoidance of surgery until the patient is smoke-free for at least 2 weeks may help in decreasing the rate of complications.

79.4.2.2
Planning the Surgery

A neck lift can be a fairly straightforward procedure with a low rate of complications, but attention to detail is critical. The first step is to draw the markings correctly. The larger the surface area dissected, the more edema, ecchymosis, and chance for a fluid collection, postoperatively.

79.4.2.3
Skin Management

The amount of postauricular skin to be excised is very important. If too much skin is excised, it is difficult to be able to close the incisions without placing the neck under significant tension. If not enough is excised, the neck laxity will not be fully corrected. It is best to err on the side of excising less skin initially and, at the time of closure, resecting more skin, if necessary.

79.4.2.4
Fat Management

If a neck has paucity of fat, liposuction can do more harm than good. It is unnecessary to liposuction or undermine the anterior base of the neck if it is not lax, or if it has a normal amount of adipose tissue. This can create an irregular appearance of the skin and a skeletonized neck look that is unattractive. Equally important is to not suction the lateral base of the neck. Usually it is unnecessary, and may increase risk of hematoma in an area where the adipose layer is thin and the skin adheres to the underlying sternocleidomastoid muscle. A 3 or a 4-mm spatulated cannula can give good results in terms of ease of liposuction and contour regularity. In order to improve the mandibular border, and decrease the jowling, it is important to liposuction both above and below the mandibular border, leaving a strip of subcutaneous fat along the bony mandibular border for highlighting the border itself. This maneuver will accentuate the angle and create an aesthetically pleasing strong jaw line, that is especially desirable in men. We have not had any clinically significant injuries to the marginal mandibular nerve with this technique. It is critical to not overresect the preplatysmal fat at the midline because that can lead to a hollow appearance of the mid anterior neck contour, and is difficult to correct.

79.4.2.5
Platysma Management

It is important to suture the platysmal midline edges with buried permanent sutures, such as 4.0 Prolene. If absorbable sutures are used, when the sutures dissolve, the tension can allow the muscles to spread apart. This action results in losing the tightening effect that the midline sutures have created to narrow the neck width. Secondly, when suturing the two medial edges of the platysma, the suture "bites" should not be taken too wide, thus bunching up the platysma at the midline and creating an undesirable ridge, which people will feel afterwards and be dissatisfied. Thirdly, it is important to allow the artificial ligament-like Prolene suspension suture to be tied at a firm, but not too tight, position, to avoid patients complaining of tightness or a choking feeling. Also, the suspension suture needs to be placed within the mastoid fascia, and not too low on the mastoid, to get the optimal neck contour. Lastly, it is important to bury the Prolene suture knots in the postauricular region with overlying absorbable sutures, where the two ends of the suspension suture are tied to the mastoid fascia to form the artificial sling. If the surgeon does not bury the sutures, the knots in the postauricular region create two masses behind the patient's ears that will cause concern, irritation, or erosion through the skin.

79.4.2.6
Fibrin Sealant

After spraying the sealant, gentle manual pressure should be applied evenly with the surgeon's fingers spread over the whole neck for 3 min, to prevent pooling of the fibrin sealant in any given area and possible skin necrosis of the overlying skin. It is not advisable to spray more than the stated amount of 2–3 ml because then it will be more likely to form pools of the sealant as well.

79.4.2.7
Dressing Placement

The dressings should not be too tight, otherwise, there could be ensuing necrosis of the submental region where the skin has been undermined. One should be able to place two fingers comfortably between the dressings and the skin at the conclusion of the procedure.

79.4.3
Complications

79.4.3.1
Wound Dehiscence

Minor complications, such as a small wound dehiscence, have been treated conservatively with dressing changes and topical antibiotic ointment, with satisfactory resolution.

79.4.3.2
Managing Hematomas/Seromas

Since Tisseel sealant was introduced, the rate of hematoma has been less than 1%. In the case of an immediate postoperative hematoma, drainage is the treatment. If a hematoma forms later, then surgical judgment needs to be exercised. The patient can be taken back to the operating room for drainage, aspirated in the office, or observed, depending on the size of the hematoma and the symptoms. Seromas are usually aspirated in the office.

79.4.3.3
Prolonged "Tightness in the Neck"

It is normal for people to comment about neck tightness, initially, owing to the platysma plication and the suspension suture. If the tightness feeling persists and is excessive, then this is easily alleviated by a small postauricular incision, with the patient under local anesthesia, identification of the suspension suture, cutting one end, and removing the other end. This will alleviate the tightness, but it will also result in a slight decrease in the definition along the cervicomental angle and mandibular borders.

79.4.3.4
Prolonged Skin Contractures

This is most likely to happen to the postauricular scar because the superior skin edge of the incision is longer than the inferior skin edge, as a result of the elliptical skin excision. This can result in "bunched-up skin", initially. If the scar is to be kept postauricular, and not get extended preauricular, one of the hallmarks of the suture-suspension platysmaplasty technique, then this early result is avoidable by not being overly zealous when excising the postauricular skin. If the scar is hypertrophic, then Kenalog injections can be used as well as scar massage. Time will also soften the scars.

79.4.3.5
Asymmetry of the Mouth

This could be due to marginal mandibular nerve neuropraxia, edema, or tension on the platysma muscle, creating a temporary depression at the corners of the mouth for patients who have a platysma–depressor labii connection in their muscular anatomy (less than 1% of all patients). This usually resolves in 2–3 months postoperatively.

79.5
Discussion

After understanding the fundamentals of a suture-suspension platysmaplasty, it is important to address specific situations in which this technique may be used. The basic principals of handling the following types of neck-lift operations will be discussed:

1. Secondary neck lift
2. Rhytidectomy with suture-suspension platysmaplasty
3. Male neck lifts
4. Neck lifts after massive weight loss

Furthermore, in order for a neck lift operation to be yield optimal results, a few ancillary techniques will enhance the neck lift results:

1. Fat grafting
2. Submandibular gland management
3. Chin augmentation

79.5.1
Applications of the Suture-Suspension Neck-Lift Techniques in Different Circumstances

79.5.1.1
Secondary Neck Lift

A patient who had suboptimal results from a prior neck lift may be a good candidate for a secondary neck lift. The aging process and gravity may be other reasons for dissatisfaction. Patients who had undergone a facelift in the preceding years may present to the surgeon's office with photographs of a satisfactory result shortly after the procedure, but are no longer happy. They may also be candidates for a secondary neck lift. A secondary neck lift can be performed to improve the result of a primary neck lift or a facelift. The ideal candidate for a secondary neck lift, after a facelift, is someone who had aesthetically pleasing midface and jowl areas but is dissatisfied with the resultant neck contour.

Common conditions leading to a secondary neck lift are:

1. Excess or ptotic neck skin.
2. Ptotic platysma muscle at the midline (with or without muscle placation).
3. Excess adipose tissue (either because no liposuction was initially performed or because the patient gained weight).

Counseling the Patient

In the preoperative consultation with the patient, it is essential to determine the patient's expectations and reasons for dissatisfaction with the initial operation. It is important to stress that a neck lift is not a facelift; it has limitations when it comes to midface and jowl rejuvenation. Those limitations that made a patient unsatisfied from a primary neck lift may not be addressed with a secondary neck lift and may require a facelift.

Technical Considerations

A secondary neck lift is more challenging in some ways. The anatomy may be more difficult to discern, owing to the previous operation. The skin is more difficult to dissect, owing to lack of adipose tissue, which may make inadvertent "button-holing" of the skin more likely.

In the time period between the initial neck rejuvenation procedure and the secondary neck lift, anatomical differences may have occurred such as increase in adipose content, which would be treated with liposuction or direct excision. If the submandibular glands have prolapsed, or if they had never been addressed in the first procedure, then performing a submandibular gland suspension is recommended. Most commonly, there is excess skin, which should be excised.

In a suture-suspension platysmaplasty, the durability of results depends on the suture, i.e. "artificial ligament", extending between the mastoid fascia of both sides. This suture is permanent and does not change position or migrate over time. Significant improvement may be accomplished in a secondary neck lift by performing a suture-suspension procedure, if one was not performed initially.

Revision of Suture-Suspension Neck Lifts

If a patient who underwent a suture-suspension neck lift is bothered by remaining excess skin, the problem may either be that the initial excision was not aggressive enough, or that laxity of the skin created excess skin with time. In this patient, the initial neck-lift incisions are utilized. Liposuction is performed, if necessary. The skin is elevated and the appropriate amount of skin is excised. If the area undermined is substantial, fibrin sealant may be used. The suspension suture should be intact and does not need to revised.

In a few cases, the subplatysmal fat was overly excised and the patients ended with a concavity in the submental region. In order to correct this deformity, the platysma may need to be retightened at the midline using a non-absorbable suture with buried knots to avoid their palpation or visualization.

79.5.1.2
Rhytidectomy and Suture Suspension of the Neck

The suture-suspension platysmaplasty has proven to be a very important "tool" in neck management when performing a rhytidectomy. This fact is due to the versatility of this technique and the ease of adjustment to different neck types. We have frequently combined the suture-suspension platysmaplasty with both primary and secondary rhytidectomies. The evaluation and decision to perform a suture-suspension platysmaplasty along with a rhytidectomy should be individualized to each patient.

Incision

When combining a rhytidectomy and a suture-suspension platysmaplasty, the posterior neck incision is made and continued around the ear lobes inferiorly, progressing superiorly along the pretragal area, and ending at the superioanterior aspect of the ear or extending higher into the temple, if a temporal lift is to be performed. If the neck laxity is mild to moderate, it is unnecessary to extend the posterior incision into the hairline.

Dissection

There are numerous rhytidectomy techniques, the discussion of which is outside the scope of this chapter. The authors' preference is to perform limited skin undermining and plication of the superficial musculoaponeurotic system as needed.

Platysmal Plication

It is easier to perform a platysmal plication with the elevation of the skin that offers more visibility in a rhytidectomy as opposed to the limited elevation in a neck lift. The management of the neck in a rhytidectomy is comparable to its management in a suture-suspension platysmaplasty, as previously discussed.

Fibrin Sealant

Fibrin sealant can be used in a full rhytidectomy as apposed to drains. It is sprayed under the neck flaps first, until it gels, and is then sprayed in the facial region (under the skin flaps of the cheeks down to the jowls). This two-step approach affords the surgeon control of the areas sprayed and allows the fibrin sealant to gel in a systematic approach.

79.5.1.3
The Male Neck Lift

The suture-suspension technique is an excellent rejuvenation tool for male patients that frequently present to the plastic surgeon's office and report, "I don't want a facelift, I only want this to be gone…" and they hold the submental/neck area with their hand. Men find this

technique especially appealing because the incisions are hidden behind the ears. The stigma of having had a "facelift" does not exist with this technique. Several technical points distinguish a neck lift performed on a man (Fig. 79.13) from that performed on a woman [13]:

- The neck area has a richer blood supply in men than in women because of the blood flow to the hair follicles; therefore, excellent hemostasis should be obtained before closure to avoid a higher risk of hematoma formation.
- Interlocking sutures need to be 0 Prolene sutures, owing to the anatomical nature and the weight of the neck structures in men.
- Attention to the amount of skin excised and the vector of pull for the bilateral neck flaps is important so the hairline, in its new location, will not look artificial.
- Men must be counseled not to shave their necks for a couple of weeks after surgery to avoid injury to the neck flaps with decreased sensation, postoperatively.
- Men must also be counseled to rest after surgery to avoid early complications such as hematoma, especially those with underlying hypertension. Men tend to become more impatient after surgery than women, and are more likely to return to high-energy activities prematurely.

79.5.1.4
Neck Lift After Massive Weight Loss

Obesity as a Health Risk

Obesity is a chronic disease in which there is excess of body adiposity leading to severe secondary health problems. The three components of obesity are genetic, lifestyle, and the aging process. As more societies become affluent with consumption of high caloric food on the rise, and exercise in decline, there is an epidemic of obesity around the world, in certain societies, in adults. A more alarming trend is that recently, in the USA, adolescent and childhood obesity is on the rise as well. Consequently, bariatric surgery has become commonplace, and plastic surgery after massive weight loss is also on a steep rise. A neck-lift procedure is usually part of an overall body-contouring plan for massive weight loss patients [14].

Plastic Surgery After Massive Weight Loss

Surgery following massive weight loss as a result of bariatric surgery is a unique field within plastic surgery, in certain ways. It has aspects of both reconstructive and aesthetic surgery. These patients have some unique characteristics:

1. They all have a history of clinically severe obesity.
2. They have undergone bariatric surgery, typically within the previous 1–4 years.

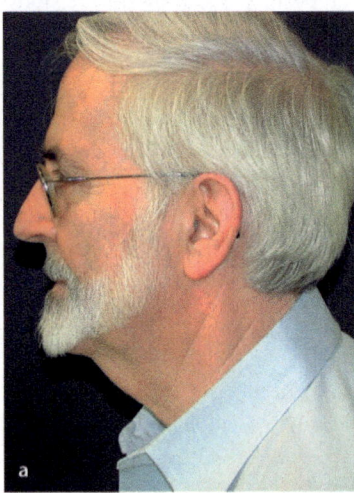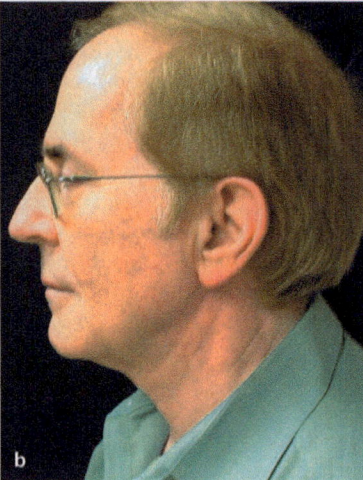

Fig. 79.13 Male neck lift. **a** Before. **b** After

3. They are strongly determined to get rid of their loose skin.
4. The vast majority are women.

For some patients, the decision to undergo bariatric surgery is part of a "new me" plan. They have bariatric surgery, lose weight, want to improve their eating habits and exercise patterns, and lead a healthier lifestyle. Plastic surgery can be at the center of this transformation and can play a very positive role, if utilized appropriately. Changes occur in the process of weight loss with respect to family dynamics, romantic relationships, social interactions, work habits, self-esteem, and other issues unique to each individual patient. The more a plastic surgeon is tuned in to these changes, the better we are able to serve these patients.

Increased Risk in Massive Weight Loss Patients

Neck lifts performed in massive weight loss patients are an essential part of treating the excess skin resulting from the rapid massive weight loss. In order to operate on a patient who has had bariatric surgery, we need to have thorough knowledge of the patient's medical history, and the options to offer him/her. After a patient undergoes a gastric bypass operation with ensuing massive weight loss, medical changes, including the elimination of certain diseases, occur. The physical changes that occur are essentially trading a large body for excess skin, and some other medical conditions that can arise such as:
1. Anemia
2. Poor nutrition (low albumin)

3. Significant skin laxity
4. Decrease in blood supply to tissues
5. Attenuation of the fascia

These risk factors create an increased risk of complications, such as hematomas, skin necrosis, as well as poor skin contraction after a body-contouring operation. The new goals that need to be set for this patient include proper dieting, exercise, and a healthier lifestyle. A neck lift may be part of an overall body-contouring plan for these patients. Deciding when to do the neck lift should be part of the medical consultation.

Considerations in Neck Lifts in Massive Weight Loss Patients

Timing of Surgery

In addition to a routine consultation with a full history and physical examination, massive weight loss patients have certain issues that need to be addressed. The weight loss plateaus at different times after bariatric surgery, generally between 1 and 2 years, so cosmetic surgery, ideally, should not be performed before 18 months, since the patient can regain the weight.

Neck Lift Versus Facelift

The amount of skin and fat that is to be excised needs to be addressed with the patient carefully. These patients have a significant amount of excess skin and fat in the neck region. Even with an aggressive neck lift there still may be laxity of skin 6–12 months later that may lead to unhappiness and the patient seeking a secondary procedure. The patient needs to be reminded that a neck lift will address the laxity of skin and will improve it but it will not yield a perfect result, because of the significant amount of excess skin. These patients should be offered a rhytidectomy, as an alternative, and one should only resort to performing a neck lift if the patient refuses to have a full facelift. The patient needs to be made aware that there is the possibility of additional surgery 6–12 months later, to remove excess skin, if the patient requires "the best result possible"; however, the retightening of the platysma is usually unnecessary at that time.

79.5.1.5
Performing a Neck Lift As Part of a Multiple Procedure Plan

When a massive weight loss patient asks for multiple procedures, the plan is very subjective. Typically, procedures that a patient would ask for are a facelift or neck lift, breast lift, reduction or lift with implants, arm lifts, abdominoplasty or lower-body lifts, and thigh lifts. In counseling the patient, a safe treatment plan has to be conceived after a thorough understanding of the patient's goals. One approach is to discuss, with patients, their priorities. Some patients' priorities are for their face to look more youthful and to get rid of the stigma of weight loss by removing the excess neck skin. Other patients would like to get rid of the excess body skin first, and then address the neck at a later time.

Surgeries on different body parts can be performed during the same operation as long as the time under anesthesia is reasonable and the amount of surgery not excessive. For example, a neck lift can be performed with arm lifts or breast lifts with implants and then, at a later date, further operations on other body parts can be performed.

79.5.2
Technical Considerations

If a patient chooses to have a neck lift as opposed to a facelift, then it needs to be in most cases an extended neck lift. The incision should extend anteriorly to the tragus to be able to liposuction the jowls and excise the skin that is superior to the mandibular border, up to the tragus, and therefore improve the jowl status in this patient.

One consideration with people who have had gastric bypass surgery is that they have a small stomach, and are more likely to have nausea and vomiting with anesthesia, and to retch after surgery. That is an important factor to remember, since these patients may be at a higher propensity of immediate postoperative hemato-

mas as well as late hematomas in the 10–14-day postoperative period, when the fibrin sealant has dissolved and the body is laying down its own fibrin.

79.5.3
Revisional Surgery

Before a revisional surgery is contemplated, the patient needs to be advised that skin laxity can be the cause of a disappointment in a secondary neck lift, no matter how tight the skin is sutured. A revisional surgery can be performed through the existing scars. More liposuction may need to be performed. If there is excess skin, then excising it is appropriate. If the muscles are lax or are in bands, then muscle plication should be performed. Fibrin sealant can be placed and the surgery can proceed as previously described with the primary neck lift.

79.5.4
Ancillary Procedures

79.5.4.1
Fat Grafting

The goal in fat grafting is to inject groups of transplanted fat that are small enough so that blood vessels can grow into the fat cells and nourish them. The fat is harvested from the abdomen with a manual syringe, the "mushroom cannula". The fat is aspirated and then centrifuged to separate all the oil and blood products from the fat. The supernatant fluid and oils are then removed at the side table. The test tubes of fat are then refrigerated in the operating room until the fat is to be injected. Next, the fat is transferred into 3-ml syringes with 18-gauge needles. An 18-gauge needle hole is small enough not to need to be sutured, but the needle diameter is large enough that the fat can be injected easily.

79.5.4.2
Nasolabial Folds and Cheek

The fat is injected in the subcutaneous tissue, mostly at the level of the subcutaneous and dermal plexuses, with excellent blood supply. Caution is used not to squeeze or traumatize the fat unnecessarily, to guarantee the highest rate of fat cell survival. For more volume, rather than filling a fold or a wrinkle, the fat can be injected in the deeper muscle layers. The method of injection is as follows. A stab incision is made in the periform aperture. The nasolabial folds are injected inferior to the subcutaneous tissues and then inferior to the mucosa. The cheeks can be injected with the fat to create a more youthful cheek with a visible prominence.

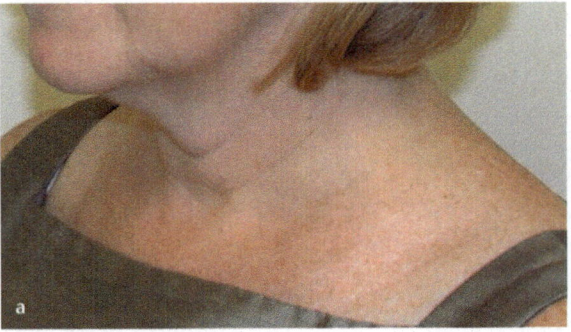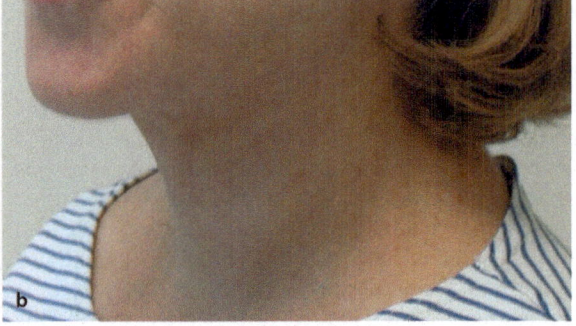

Fig. 79.14 The angle of the mandible can be enhanced by fat grafting. **a** Before. **b** After

79.5.4.3
Mandibular Border and Angle of the Mandible

In order to improve the mandibular border, whether in conjunction with a neck lift operation or as an individual procedure, fat grafting along the border of the mandible gives a noticeable improvement. The angle of the mandible can be enhanced in the same way, especially for narrow mandibles (Fig. 79.14).

79.5.4.4
Labial Mandibular Folds and Lips

A stab at the oral commissure provides access for injecting the upper lips, the lower lips, and the labial mandibular area. To correct the labial mandibular area, when the corners of mouth appear turned down, fat is injected in a crisscross fashion at the corner of the mouth, thus lifting the corners. The lips, and the more inferior aspect of the labial mandibular crease, can then be filled as needed.

79.5.4.5
The Submandibular Glands

Prolapsed or prominent submandibular glands can be a problem and need to be addressed initially with the patient, before the surgery. The patient has to be told that even with a good neck lift technique, if he/she has prolapsed or prominent submandibular glands, the result will not be as good. The submandibular glands need to be pointed out to the patient and a discussion about the attempt to improve the contour should be undertaken preoperatively. To demonstrate the location and size of the submandibular gland, a long Q-Tip is placed at the cervicomental angle and pressed. The patient feels where the submandibular gland is and can see the outline in a mirror. If the submandibular glands are not shown to the patient preoperatively, when the neck laxity may be masking the glands, then the patient may be dissatisfied with a good result because the "bulge" is more evident after the fat has been liposuctioned and the skin and muscles have been tightened.

It is not recommended to resect the submandibular glands, owing to a high complication rate. After the platysmal plication has been performed, the prominent gland prolapses inferiorly. This is called the "hammock effect". If a person sits in a hammock, there is a hanging effect because the weight is great, the hammock is weak, or a combination of both. With the submandibular gland sitting above the platysma, the analogy holds true. When the suspension suture is placed, the muscle is holding up the gland. A 3.0 Prolene suspension suture is sutured to the medial aspect of the platysma fibers, passing inferior to the submandibular gland, and tied to the mastoid fascia through the same tunnel where the suture suspension has been placed. The result is the reinforcement of the weak area and the superior elevation of the submandibular gland.

79.5.4.6
Chin Augmentation

Options for Chin Augmentation

Appropriate chin projection adds tremendously to the overall length and beauty of an aesthetically balanced neck. It also prevents the skin from becoming redundant in the submental area. Cosmetic techniques to augment a deficient or retrusive chin prominence focus primarily around the alloplastic chin implant. The use of sliding geneoplasties, with or without wire fixation, is also an option, but requires significantly more time, effort, and pain with more potential complications. Fat grafting to the chin can moderately enhance the chin prominence as well. Long-term fillers have been utilized with success.

Assessing the Chin Projection

Utilizing a very simple technique, by drawing a vertical line from the glabella down through the upper lip and a second vertical line from the nasal tip to the chin prominence, will help to quickly define whether the chin is normal, hyperplastic, or hypoplastic. A 3–4-mm augmentation is usually recommended. If the implant is 3–4 mm in projection, there is another 2 mm of projection from the soft tissues, which should be enough to balance the chin, except for severe cases of retrusion. That 4–5 mm is enough to take up extra skin and give the female jaw a more aesthetically pleasing profile. With men, it is desirable to have a chin augmentation that surpasses the vertical line beyond the lower lip to give a more masculine look.

Chin Augmentation Technique with K-Wire Fixation

The neck-lift submental incision may be used to insert the chin implant. Cautery and a subperiosteal elevator are used to create the chin implant pocket. The pocket should be wide to decrease the chance of excessive force on the implant, which may lead to capsular formation around the implant and ensuing implant distortion or malpositioning. The implant is then positioned at the edge of the mentum at 45° to give both horizontal and vertical projection. Two 0.035 K-wires are placed through the implant, at about 45° to the implant, which makes them perpendicular to the bone, just into the outer cortex to stabilize the implant. The K-wires are cut off right at the surface of the implant (Fig. 79.15).

Chin Augmentation K-Wire Fixation

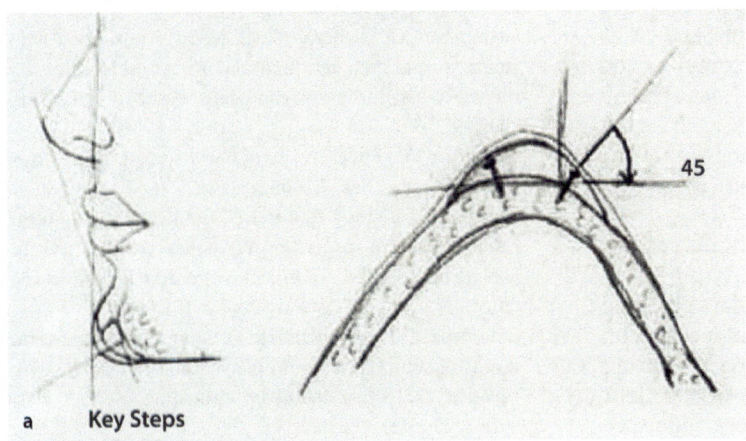

Fig. 79.15 a Chin augmentation with K-wire fixation. **b** Before. **c** After

- Curvilinear submental incision.
- "Extra-wide" subperiosteal pocket (use cautery for dissection).
- K-Wire fixation of implant (adjust appropriate angle of implant) use .035 K-Wires.
- Close pocket in two layers.
- Antibiotic irrigation.

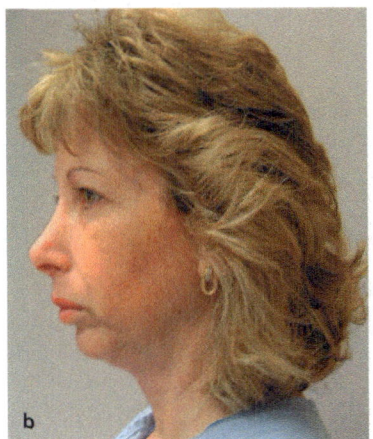

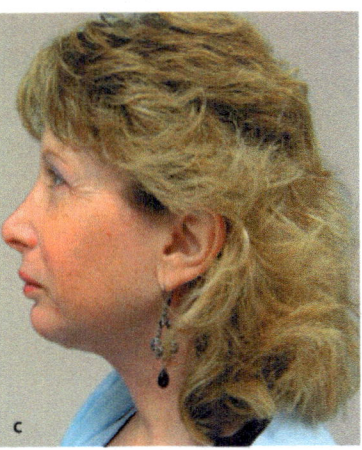

The advantages of this K-wire fixation are several. First, it enables the implant to sit at 45° to the edge of the mentum and give both horizontal and vertical projection with the fixation. Second, it anchors the implant, so it is virtually impossible for the implant to migrate or rotate. Third, it creates two points of interface with the bone, so, theoretically, the whole surface of the implant is not juxtaposed to the bone and can decrease the bony resorption by the implant. We have 5–6 year X-rays on four patients where we do not see any normal bony resorption. The periosteum is then closed by releasing about 5 mm of the muscle, where it joins the mentum. It is then irrigated with a little antibiotic solution before closure. The platysma can be closed over the implant.

79.6
Conclusions and Future Trends

There are many techniques for neck rejuvenation. We have tried to discuss, in detail, one particular technique that we feel is simple, versatile, reproducible, and yields good results. The key to any happy outcome is good communication with the patient and the management of expectations. The technical points that we have discussed serve to guide surgeons performing suture-suspension neck lifts to achieve happiness and consistently good results for their patients.

In our experience with secondary neck lift patients, whether they had a facelift as their primary procedure or a neck lift with suboptimal results, we have observed the patients to be very satisfied after their specific concerns were addressed. This fact underscores the flexibility of the suture-suspension platysmaplasty technique, and its ability to be adjusted to improve a wide spectrum of neck contours, primarily or secondarily.

Someone may choose to have a neck lift and full-face fat grafting as opposed to a facelift for a variety of reasons, including cost, risk, healing time, and ease of postoperative management. It is important for the plastic surgeon who performs neck lifts to be well versed with the ancillary options to provide to a patient.

In recent articles about fine-tuning the suture-suspension techniques to address the six major points as well as the long-term follow-up studies, this neck lift technique has proven to stand the test of time. Future ancillary techniques, such as thread lifts, more permanent fillers, and improved grafted fat survival will undoubtedly enhance the results accomplished with the suture-suspension platysmaplasty.

References

1. Zins JE, Fardo D. The "anterior-only" approach to neck rejuvenation: An alternative to face lift surgery. Plast Reconstr Surg 2005;115(6):1761–1768
2. Guerrero-Santos J, Espaillat L, Morales F.: Muscular lift in a cervical rhytidoplasty. Plast Reconstr Surg 1974;54(2):27–131
3. Feldman J. Corset platysmaplasty. Plast Reconstr Surg 1990;85(3):333–343
4. Feldman JJ. My approach to neck lift. Presented at the Colorado Society of Plastic Surgeons, Denver, April 1995
5. Conrad K, Chapnik JS, Reifen E.: PTFE (Gore-Tex) suspension cervical facial rhytidectomy. Arch Otolaryngol Head Neck Surg 1993;119(6):694–698
6. Giampapa VC, Di Bernardo B. Neck recontouring with suture suspension and liposuction: An alternative for the early rhytidectomy candidate. Aesthet Plast Surg 1995;19(3):217–223
7. Giampapa VC, Bitar GJ. Use of fibrin sealant in neck contouring. Aesthet Surg J 2002;2:5192525
8. Giampapa V, Bitzos I, Ramirez O, Granick M.: Long-term results of suture suspension platysmaplasty for neck rejuvenation revisited: Technical fine points for improving outcomes. Aesthet Plast Surg 2005;29(5):341–350
9. Giampapa V, Bitzos I, Ramirez O, Granick M.: Long-term results of suture suspension platysmaplasty for neck rejuvenation: A 13-year follow-up evaluation. Aesthet Plast Surg 2005;29(5):332–340
10. Ellenbogen R, Karlin V. Visual criteria for success in restoring the youthful neck. Plast Reconstr Surg 1980;66(6):826–837
11. Bitar GJ. Liposuction or lift? An algorithm for neck rejuvenation. Plast Surg Prod 2005;15(9):24–28
12. Bitar GJ, Giampapa VC. The suture suspension neck lift. Plast Surg Prod 2005;15 (10):31–34
13. Bitar GJ. What men want. Plast Surg Prod 2006;16(2) 20–26
14. Bitar GJ, Understanding the characteristics of massive weight loss patients. Plast Surg Prod 2006;16(5):38–44

CHAPTER 80

Cervicoplasty Without Skin Excision

80

Oscar M. Ramírez

80.1
Introduction

Despite the periorbital and nasolabial areas being the structures that are most visible during social engagements and showing the signs of aging at an earlier stage, aging of the neck with or without fat accumulation seems to be the most troublesome to most patients. For this reason, patients request neck rejuvenation as an isolated procedure or as a component of a more comprehensive facial rejuvenation.

The introduction of minimal incision surgery has allowed a younger group of patients to request improvement of their neck contour for rejuvenation or beautification purposes. Liposuction or liposculpting of the neck through puncture wound incisions were probably the first type of minimal incision surgery in the neck. This technique was suitable for young patients with moderate to heavy necks and good skin elasticity. Despite isolated liposuction of the neck becoming commonplace in many practices in the mid to late 1980s and beyond, very few published series on the subject were made during those years.

In 1993, Giampapa at the Annual Meeting of the American Society of Aesthetic Plastic Surgery presented his work on cervicoplasty combining liposuction with the suture-suspension technique. Subsequently, his landmark paper was published in 1995 [1].

During the early years of 1992 and 1993, the author was developing the endoscopic techniques for facial rejuvenation. This took the author to May of 1993, when he performed the first ever reported total facial rejuvenation using endoscopic techniques [2]. Aware of Giampapa's contribution, the author readily introduced the suture-suspension technique of the neck in his endoscopic methods. This procedure was videotaped and presented widely within teaching workshops and national meetings. In 1997, a paper by the author on cervicoplasty without excision was published [3]. This approach has been updated with some variations [4–7].

80.2
Preoperative Evaluation

There are patients in whom these techniques will be long-lasting and durable. In others, this should be considered a mere postponement for the traditional excisional approach. In some, the contour and shape obtained will be comparable to those obtained with excisional techniques. In others, there will be some residual laxity and contour shortcomings. These variable results are dependent on several factors: age, preexisting anatomical and aesthetic configuration, and laxity and quality of the skin. It is important to identify and qualify these factors and to communicate openly to the patient to avoid misunderstandings, frustrations, and unhappiness postoperatively.

There are a few important conditions that are related to the factors affecting the final aesthetic outcome. These are:

1. The younger the patient, the better the contour and skin reaccommodation that can be obtained (age factor).
2. Patients with better skin elasticity independent of age will do better (elasticity factor).
3. Patients with excessive fat accumulation will do better than someone with flaccidity and lack of fat (anatomical factor).
4. Patients with good skeletal support at the gonial angle and chin will have better aesthetic outcome than someone with a poor framework (anatomical/aesthetic factor).
5. Patients with excessive jowls and labiomandibular folds will be better off with an excisional cervicofacial lift unless improvement obtained with the addition of liposuction to these areas would be enough for that particular patient and he/she is willing to accept these residual flaws instead of a lesser surgery with a quicker recovery time (anatomical and psychological factor).

It becomes clear that careful evaluation of the skin elasticity, the absence of or excess fat under the skin or below the muscle layer, the quality of the gonial angle, jawline, and chin projection, and the presence or absence of jowls and/or labial mandibular folds are important steps during the initial consultation. Patients should be made aware of all and each of these components of the facial analysis. The basic surgical strategy, necessary ancillary procedures, and the expected surgical and aesthetic outcome that we predict we will obtain with or without the necessary ancillary procedures should be pointed out to the patient. Careful surgical planning should be made on the basis of this analysis. The surgeon's aesthetic objectives should agree with those of the patient. If the patient's objectives are different or if improvements sought are more on the conservative scale, then the surgical planning should be made accordingly. However, the patient should be made aware of the potential residual flaws if the surgical planning does not match the findings of the anatomical and aesthetic analysis.

Patients in general at the subconscious level wish to have the maximal improvement with minimal surgery. It is up to the surgeon to bring the patient to the conscious reality that this might not be feasible, otherwise the potential for postoperative conflicts and unhappiness might be significantly high. It is also imperative to point out that the potential for complications may increase as the complexity of the surgery increases. The same is true for the time of recovery needed for the patient to return to his/her normal activities.

80.3
Surgical Technique

The cervicoplasty without skin excision has several variants:

1. The Giampapa cervicoplasty with suture suspension. This method is unique not only in how the suture suspension is applied but also in how the neck is contoured. The original technique used a 1-in. submental incision and a 1-in. retroauricular incision on each side. Through these incisions liposuction is done without skin undermining. In the submental area, the borders of the platysma muscles

are identified and an interlocking suture suspension is applied starting from the medial border of each platysma. The two ends of the suture from one side are tunneled to the contralateral mastoid area. These sutures are brought through the incisions in the retroauricular areas. While mild tension is applied to the contralateral suture, the homolateral suture is anchored to the mastoid fascia. Then the contralateral suture is anchored in a similar fashion. Any residual skin excess that results from the pleating effect in the retroauricular area is conservatively excised without extending significantly the length of the original incision (Fig. 80.1 right and Fig. 80.2).

2. The Ramirez cervicoplasty that initially was called the "anterior approach cervicoplasty" differs from the Giampapa technique in several points (Fig. 80.2). The neck is remodeled primarily from the anterior approach. Skin undermining is done in a generous area of the neck, with the limits being the triangle formed by the anterior borders of the sternocleidomastoid muscles. The superficial and deep neck is approached through this submental incision. As described in the original technique, digastric muscle shaving, salivary gland suspension/excision, and subplatysmal fat resection is done through this incision. Two additional incisions are made one behind each ear at the level of the mastoid/occipital scalp hairline. These are made at positions more posterior than the Giampapa incision. These additional incisions are also used for the placement of the anchoring sutures into the upper mastoid fascia in a similar fashion to the Giampapa suture suspension. Most importantly these incisions are used for a wide undermining of the retroauricular skin. This skin undermining is

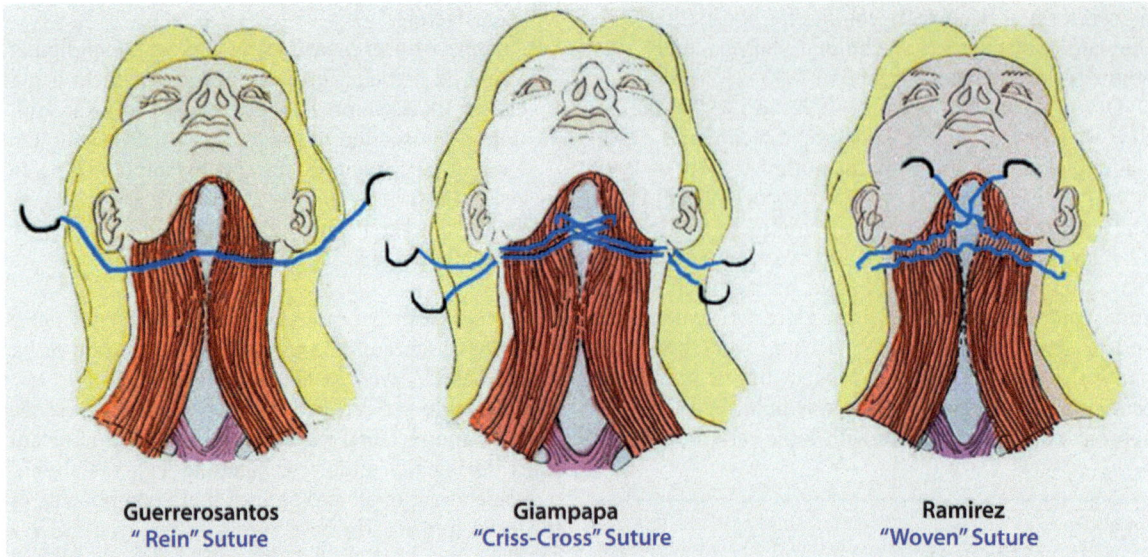

| Guerrerosantos | Giampapa | Ramirez |
| "Rein" Suture | "Criss-Cross" Suture | "Woven" Suture |

Fig. 80.1 Comparative views of the Giampapa and Ramirez suture suspension. Guerrerosantos was the first to use a suture suspension but he did it during open techniques

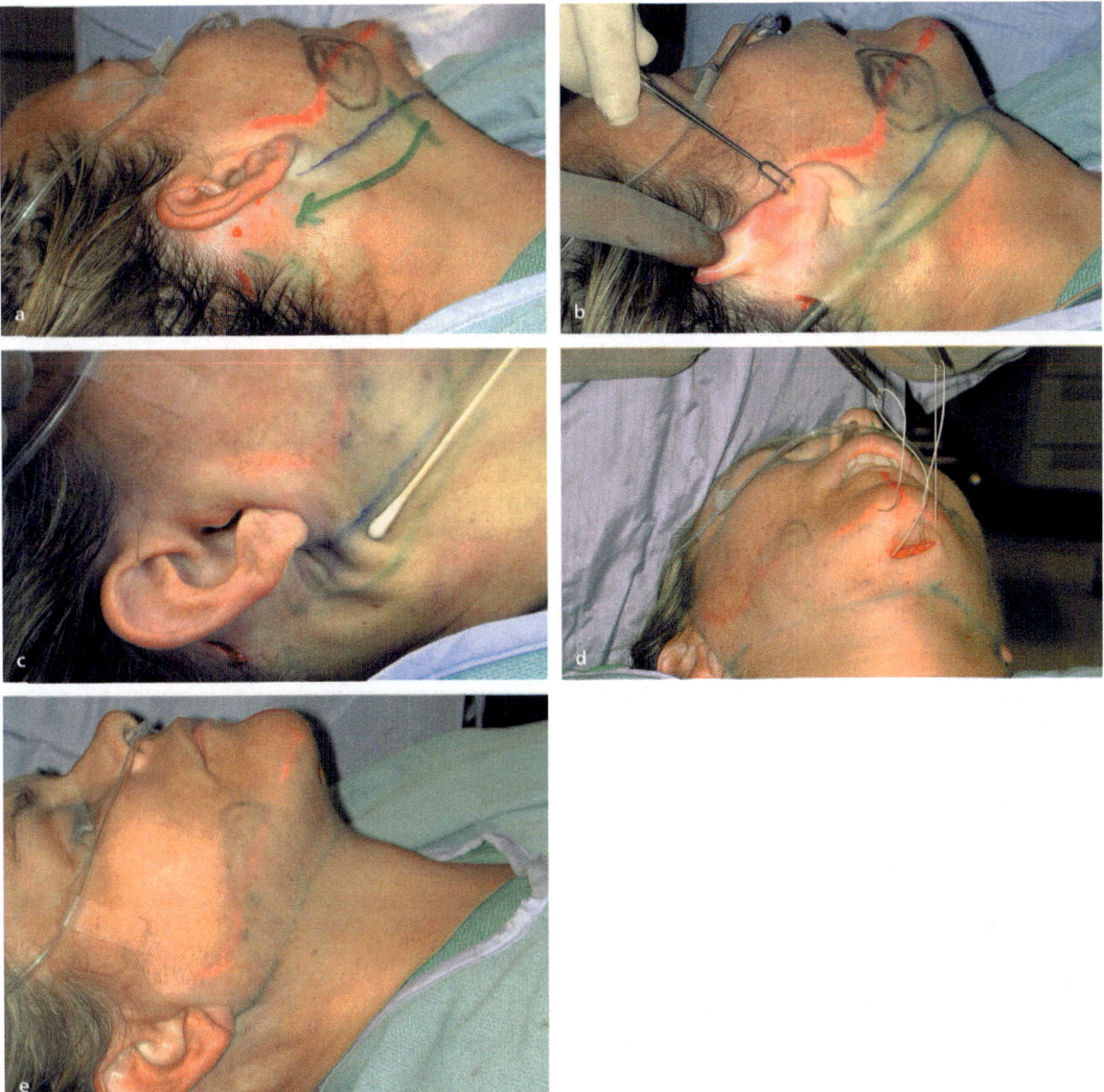

Fig. 80.2 **a** Local anesthetic with epinephrine solution has been injected. Preoperatively, for guiding purposes, several landmarks have been marked: jawline in *red*, jowl in *black*, cervicomental break in *blue*, and the direction of skin redistribution in *green*. **b** Through a 2-cm incision at the occipital hairline a wide subcutaneous dissection with a Ramirez no. 4 elevator is being performed. This will connect with the submental dissection. **c** Observe the skin redistribution toward the retroauricular area. **d** The two ends of the suture suspension (Ramirez variation 2) have been brought through the submental incision after weaving on the platysma and anchoring on the mastoid fascia bilaterally had been done. The knots will be made deep under the medial borders of the platysma. **e** Observe the definition of the cervicomental area, the enhancement of the gonial area, and the correction of the jowl

extended anteriorly and inferiorly over the sterno-cleidomastoid fascia and eventually connected with the area of undermining done via the anterior approach. This way the degree of undermining in the neck is closer in extent to that in the open cervicofacial lift. This continuous undermining will also allow better redistribution of the excessive loose skin of the submental area to the tighter skin in the retroauricular area. The suture suspension is anchored

anteriorly to the borders of the platysma muscle and after the crisscrossing has been done the sutures are weaved into the platysma muscle, effectively pleating and recruiting more muscle to provide support to the salivary gland. The final anchoring can be done on each mastoid area or the suture can be brought back after anchoring into the mastoid area and the knots made in the midline underneath the borders of the platysma to bury the knots as deep as possible.

In terms of support to the salivary gland, I use this for minor degrees of submandibular salivary gland ptosis. Moderate to large degrees of ptosis with salivary gland enlargement might need a deep approach through the submental incision. This would require partial or subtotal salivary gland resection.

In either of the two variations of the cervicoplasty without skin excision, these are the goals to be achieved:
1. Cervical mental angle depth.
2. Definition of the gonial angle.
3. Definition of the mandibular line.
4. Correction of the jowl and labial mandibular fold.
5. Increaseed mental projection.
6. Decreaseed width of the neck.

80.4
Cervicomental Angle Depth

This is created by a combination of liposuction and the application of the interlocking suture suspension. Liposuction or direct lipectomy is done through the incisions previously described. In the Giampapa method this relies mostly on closed liposuction as opposed to the Ramirez method in which there is a minor or larger degrees of undermining that helps to redrape the skin and create the cervicomental angle. Cervical fat can be removed with direct open liposuction using the "vacuum cleaner" technique with the hole of the cannula directed toward the platysma or under direct visualization with long scissors. In the Giampapa method, the multiple discontinuous undermining with the liposuction helps to accommodate the neck skin from a convexity to a concavity. The reaccommodation of the skin in the Ramirez technique is more straightforward. The interlocking suture suspension that is applied uses a 2-0 nylon suture. One side of the platysma at the level of the cricoid is grasped with one suture. The contralateral platysma border is grasped with another 2-0 nylon suture. Both sutures are interlocked in the midline and each double-ended suture is tunneled to the opposite retroauricular area. Here the incision measures between 2.5 and 3 cm. On each side, the suture anchors on the fascia just posterior to the gonial angle and immediately the suture is shifted upward and posteriorly to the hairline incision on the occipital/mastoid area where the sutures are anchored and the knots buried under the mastoid fascia so this will not become palpable. This maneuver defines more the gonial angle and is called the "angle-defining point".

For further definition of the depth of the cervicomental angle, one or more of the components of the deep subplatysmal cervicoplasty are occasionally needed—subplatysmal fat excision, digastric shaving and/or plication, salivary gland partial or subtotal excision—all of this aided by a good corset platysmaplasty.

The mandibular angle can be defined further with the injection of fat into the masseter muscle on its insertion into the gonial angle or via the insertion of a gonial angle implant.

80.5
Mandibular Line Definition

This is also accomplished with the previously described maneuvers. The mandibular line is further defined with liposuction below and above the mandibular line, fat grafting to the deficient areas of the mandibular line, and/or with the insertion of prejowl or extended geniomandibular implants.

80.6
Jowl and Labiomandibular Fold Correction

The jowl and labiomandibular fold are components above the neck but have a significant negative influence on the overall aesthetic appearance of the neck and jawline. Liposuction of these areas with a 2-mm or smaller cannula from the submental incision and through a tiny prelobular puncture wound helps to remodel this area and create a bidirectional tension of skin contraction, tightening the labial mandibular fold and jowl areas. It is important to mention that liposuction should be judicious otherwise rippling and contour irregularities in these areas will develop.

80.7
Mental Protection

A prominent chin helps to create the overall length and beauty of not only the face but also the neck. It also takes up some of the redundant submental skin fullness that frequently is seen following any technique of cervicoplasty, whether this is open or closed. Among the techniques of chin enhancement, fat grafting is probably least effective. Sliding genioplasty and chin implants are effective methods but not all patients are willing to have an osteotomy of the mandible or an alloplastic implant inserted. A simple and effective method is a mentopexy via the same submental incision used for the anterior component of the cervicoplasty or via a separate intraoral incision. A wide subperiosteal dissection of the chin area is done. The chin pad is anchored in an upward position to a bone tunnel made on the symphysis of the chin in the first variant and to the thick soft-tissue cuff left during the intraoral incision. The mentopexy rotates the tissue in the anterosuperior direction. The necessary dissection also releases the origin of the lip depressors and helps to elevate the corner of the mouth. A simple method to diagnose the need for a chin augmentation is the use of Reidel's line with a long-stemmed Q-tip. This line starts in the infralobular portion of the nose, touches the lip, and should touch the pogonium. This is a very visual technique of evaluation and a patient placed in front of a mirror can also see the amount of deficit that is present in his/her case.

80.8
Width of the Neck

The width of the neck is a feature to which very little or no attention has been devoted. There is a marked widening of the neck with aging. This is the result of collapse of the cervical spine, laxity of muscles and ligaments, along with increase of the subcutaneous and fat deposits and redundant skin. The visual effect of a thin neck can be created by plication of the platysma muscle in the midline, by the tension provided by the interlocking suture suspension, and by the redistribution of the skin to the new neck concavity. Although liposuction or direct lipectomy are excellent tools to debulk fat from the neck, a word of caution against overtreating with these modalities is in order because the risk of masculinization of the feminine neck is high. All of these can be done with almost invisible scars (Fig. 80.3).

80.9
Discussion

Comments have been made that the described techniques are too sophisticated and cannot be done by the average surgeon. This is a completely overstated statement. These techniques are based on fundamental anatomic, aesthetic, and surgical principles. There is nothing esoteric about them. The keys to obtain a predictable result are:

1. Patient selection for the specific surgical technique.
2. Maximization of every surgical step to get the best result but avoiding overtreatment.
3. Discussion and clarification of the realistic expectations of the patient.
4. Minimization of complications.

Proper patient evaluation and an adequate surgical recipe for that specific patient's problem are critical. This leads to the issue of consent. The patient should be willing to accept the proposed surgical plan and the potential risks involved as a result of that decision. The common reaction of the patient who is not happy with the surgical results is to claim "she was talked into a surgi-

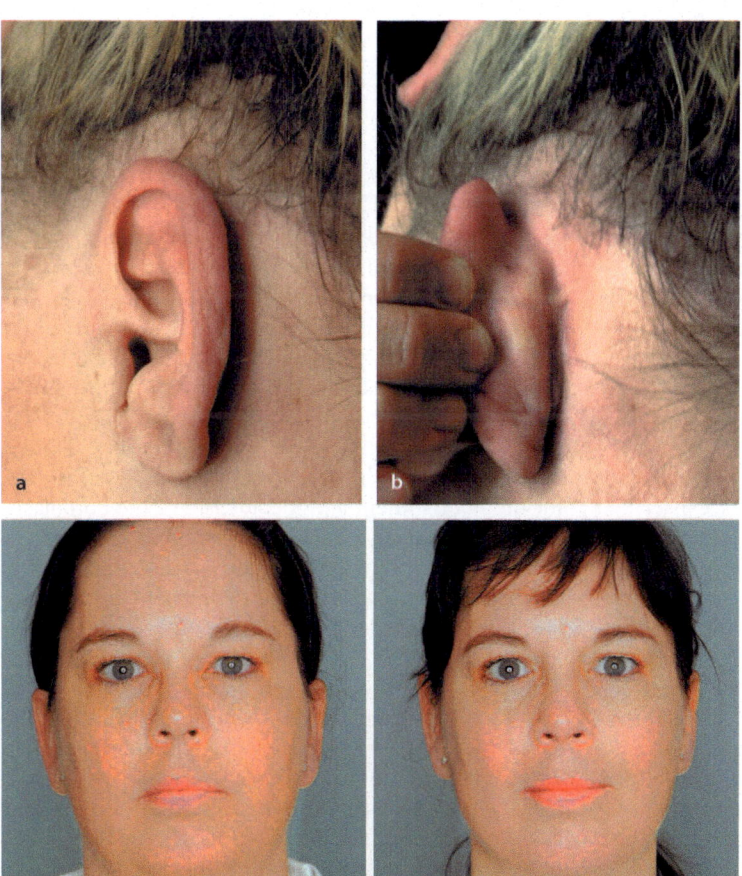

Fig. 80.3 A 40-year-old patient who had only a cervicoplasty without skin excision using the anterior and posterior approach. **a** The incision scar is barely visible even at an early stage (1 month). **b** Even when pulling the ear anteriorly there is no visible scar. **c** *Left*: Preoperatively. *Right*: Postoperatively. Observe the definition of the mandibular line and the apparent and real diminution of the thickness of the neck. *d, e see next page*

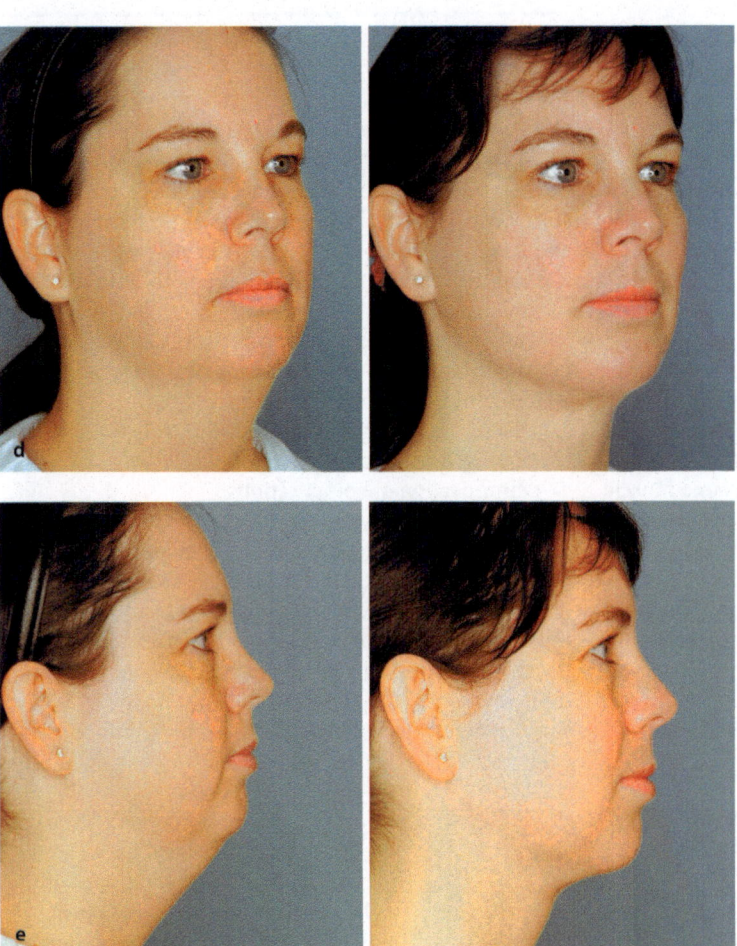

Fig. 80.3 *(Continued)* **d** Observe the outline of the mandibular line and the enhancement of the gonial angle. **e** Observe the depth of the cervicomental angle, the definition of the mandibular line, and the enhancement of the gonial angle

cal procedure that she did not request." At one extreme is the patient who unless he/she is very sophisticated and knowledgeable about the intricacies of the surgical procedures usually has a limited outlook of what a given procedure will achieve. At the other extreme is the surgeon with all of his/her arsenal of procedures trying to do the best for the patient. Many patients think that all "facelifts," in this case "neck lift" procedures, are the same. With the proliferation and advertising of "lunchtime" operations, patients expect that they can return to work in hours or days after surgery. In my view the only "lunchtime" procedures are injection of Botox, temporary fillers, and some non-ablative laser treatments. Anything else is a surgical procedure and will require a lesser or greater degree of recovery time. So the surgical consultation becomes a teaching endeavor and every question that the patient has should be answered to his/her satisfaction. Ultimately, it is the patient, after he/she has been instructed and fully informed, who should make an "informed decision."

There are three types of problems that arise from secondary surgery on patients that have had his/her surgery done somewhere else. The first is contour ir-

regularities secondary to excessive or too superficial liposuction around the neck or jawline. The second is excessive loose skin around the jawline and neck. The third is excessive fullness in the submental and/or the submandibular line. The first problem is due to a surgeon's desire to push the limits of a technique, namely, superficial liposuction. In my experience superficial liposuction should be very limited and should leave enough fat under the subdermal plane. Fat is necessary for the nourishment and metabolism of the fibroblasts of the dermal layer. Skin without the necessary fat tends to look older prematurely, even worse, after surgery, scar tissue may tend to give a cobblestone appearance and different shades of discoloration. Too many surgeons have relied on superficial liposuction for skin contraction but this does not happen predictably and the risk of the complications mentioned is too high. Residual loose skin is most likely due to patient selection. Those patients should have been selected for an excisional type of cervicofacial lift. Excessive fullness in the submental area is usually due to subplatysmal fat accumulation and/or digastric muscle fullness. Submandibular fullness is most likely due to submaxillary salivary gland ptosis and/or hypertrophy. These two last conditions will require a subplatysma deep cervicoplasty to address those problems.

Although most cases will be improved with soft-tissue manipulation alone, many patients will require some sort of skeletal support. The easiest is the use of alloplastic implants. The surgeon should become very proficient with the use of facial implants. Osteotomies on the face are more complicated procedures and should be done by surgeons experienced with these techniques and for more complicated aesthetic problems.

When going from the traditional Giampapa cervicoplasty, to the Ramirez cervicoplasty with his last innovation of complete subcutaneous skin undermining on the neck from the front to the back has added a technological factor that is critical. This is the use of the endoscopic techniques to check for bleeders and to acheive hemostasis with the suction coagulator under endoscopic control. The retroauricular area tends to bleed and in those cases if no endoscope is available the surgeon should be prepared to open a large retroauricular incision and to achieve hemostasis under direct visualization.

80.10
Conclusions

A complete cervicoplasty without skin excision is feasible to perform. In most patients this can be accomplished with excellent aesthetic results and minimal downtime and minimal complications. A systematic and complete aesthetic analysis of the neck and adjacent structures is critical. Patients and surgeons should be aware of the limitations and possibilities of each technique. Thorough familiarity with the anatomy and the intricacies of the surgical techniques is mandatory.

References

1. Giampapa VC, DiBernardo BE. Neck recontouring with suture suspension and liposuction: an alternative for the early rhytidectomy candidate. Aesthet Plast Surg 1995;19(3):217–223
2. Ramirez OM. Endoscopic full face lift. Aesthet Plast Surg 1994;18:363–371
3. Ramirez OM. Cervicoplasty: Non-excisional anterior approach. Plast Reconstr Surg 1997;99:1576–1585
4. Ramirez OM. Cervicoplasty non-excisional anterior approach: Ten year follow-up. Plast Reconstr Surg 2003;111(3):1342–1345
5. Ramirez OM, Robertson KM. Comprehensive approach to rejuvenation of the neck. Facial Plast Surg 2001; 17(2):129–140
6. Giampapa VC, Bitzos I, Ramirez OM, Granick M. Long-term results of the suture suspension platysmaplasty for neck rejuvenation: A 13 year follow-up. Aesthet Plast Surg 2005;29:332–340
7. Giampapa VC, Bitzos I, Ramirez OM, Granick M. Platysmaplasty for neck rejuvenation revisited: Technical fine points to improve outcomes. Aesthet Plast Surg 2005;29:341–350

CHAPTER 81

Cervicoplasty with Hexagonal Excision

Melvin A. Shiffman

81.1
Introduction

The problem of redundant neck skin from aging of the face and neck has been resolved with many different techniques. Full neck lift with or without facelift is the best procedure in some cases. Where there is minor neck skin excess, a modified facelift or S-lift is helpful. Direct excision of skin has been tried with submental incision and a U-shaped or triangular-shaped excision. Platysma tightening either by suturing or with the Giampapa suture [1] may be used in combination with skin excision. A new technique utilizing a "trapdoor" type of hexagonal excision results in a curved scar with less chance of dog-ear than the other forms of excision.

81.2
Surgical Technique

The "trapdoor" form of skin excision consists of a hexagon-shaped area to be removed from the neck, using the pinch technique to determine the extent of resection, starting with an incision in a submental fold. The submental incision (A to F) is extended inferiorly parallel to the mandible for half the distance of the expected excision (A to B and F to E) (Fig. 81.1). The incision is then extended inferiorly at the same angle and distance medially to the base of the "trapdoor" (B to C and E to D). The incision is continued deep into the subcutaneous tissues to the underlying platysma. A pocket is formed at this level inferiorly and laterally approximately 2 cm (Fig. 81.2) or more to allow advancement of the flap for closure. The flap is totally excised (C to D) and the platysma treated by suturing, resection, or incision as usually performed to allow dissipation of platysmal bands and to tighten the neck.

The incision is closed in two layers with 4-0 chromic interrupted sutures in the subcuticular tissues and 5-0 nylon in the skin or as a subcuticular stitch. A is sutured to C and F is sutured to D to form a scar that parallels the mandible at the outer ends. If a dog-ear results, the excess can be excised in an elliptical fashion and since it parallels the mandible, the scar is kept in the neck.

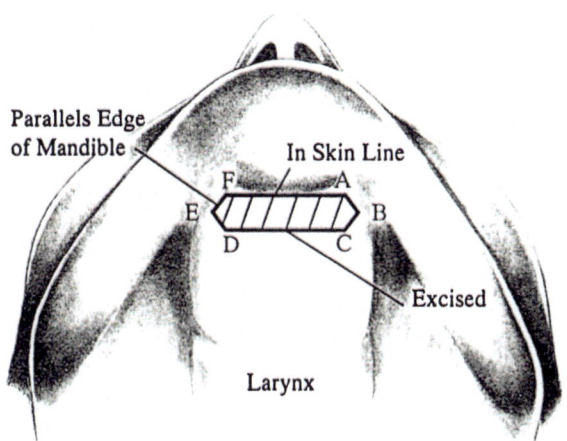

Fig. 81.1 Hexagonal area marked in submental region

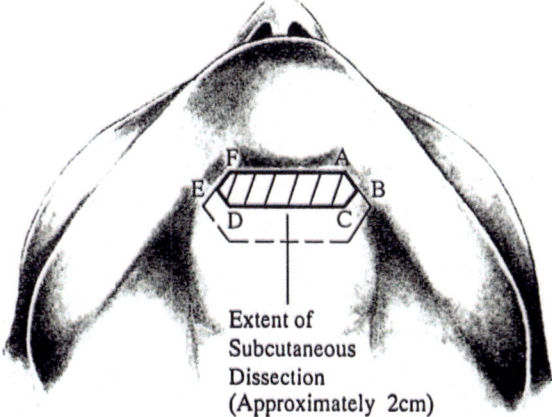

Fig. 81.2 Extent of dissection under the skin flap and above the platysma muscle

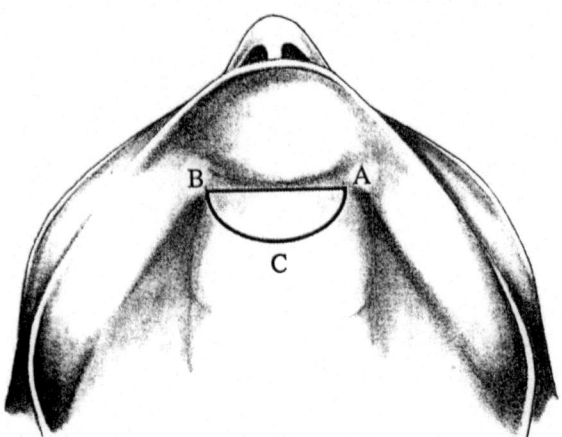

Fig. 81.3 Usual method of resection for loose skin using a U-shaped incision

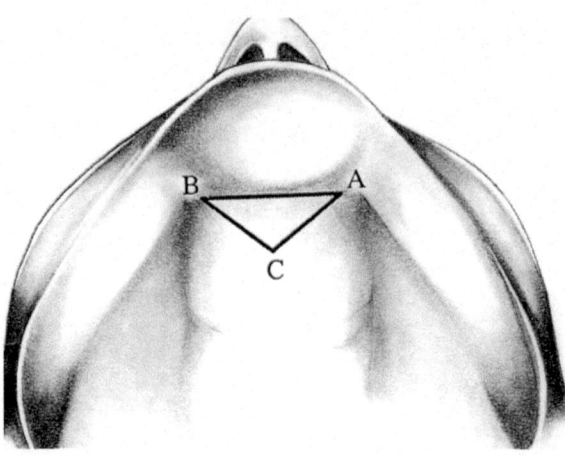

Fig. 81.4 Alternative method of resection for loose skin with a triangular excision. Note that the angles at *A* and *B* are narrower than with the U-shaped excision and will result in less chance for a dog-ear

81.3
Discussion

When skin is excised in the neck in the usual fashion with a U-shaped excision (Fig. 81.3), the ends almost always form dog-ears. Excising the dog-ears with elliptical excisions causes the scar to approach or extend beyond the edge of the mandible, allowing the scar to be visible. With a U excision, the angle is larger than with a triangle excision (Fig. 81.4) and is more likely to cause a dog-ear.

The "trapdoor" excision allows a wide approach to the platysma for tightening of the neck and leaves room for excision of any dog-ear that might occur (Fig. 81.5). The more tissue removed, the more likely there will be a dog-ear.

81.4
Conclusions

The use of a hexagonal submental skin excision allows more skin to be removed in the upper neck than using other techniques. Dog-ears that may result can be treated with elliptical excision with ease since the lateral portions of the incision parallel the mandible.

Reference

1.   Giampapa, V.C., Di Bernardo, B.E.: Neck recontouring with suture suspension and liposuction: an alternative for the early rhytidectomy candidate. Aesthet Plast Surg 1995;19(3):217–223

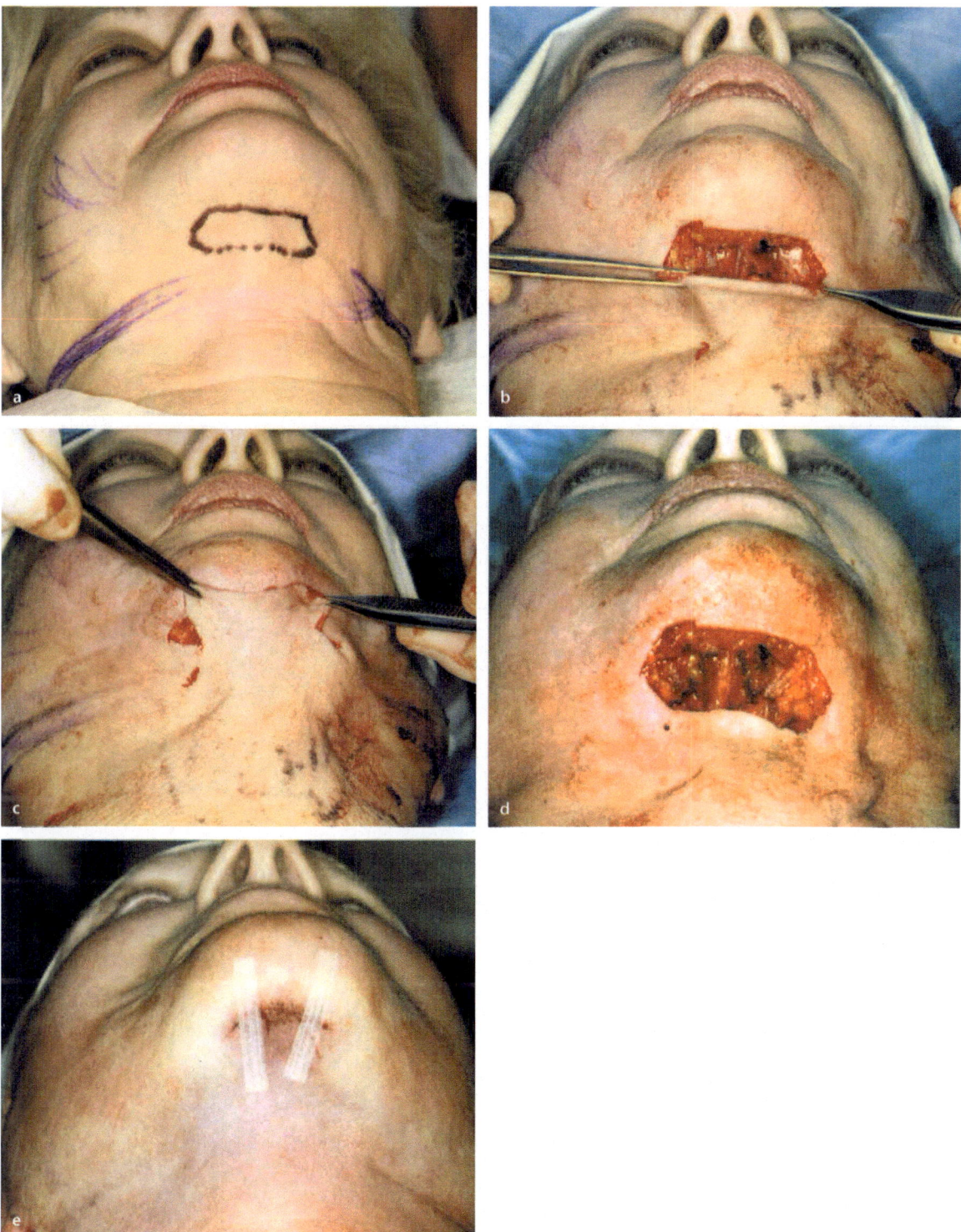

Fig. 81.5 a Preoperative view of excess neck skin with markings for excision and Giampapa stitch. **b** Flap lifted after incision through the marked lines except for the final transverse cut. **c** Flap raised back into the original position. **d** Flap totally excised. **e** Wound suture closed showing the ends of the incision curving parallel with the mandible

CHAPTER 82

Mesh Platsymaplasty

82

Sid J. Mirrafati

82.1
Introduction

There are several techniques and procedures proposed for neck rejuvenation that have less than optimal results for correcting the submental and jowl areas. The problem with the submental area is that the point of the pull is angled and too far away. That is to say behind the ear and the back hairline is distant from the submental area. Therefore, if the surgeon wants to have a natural look to a facelift there will always be some laxity and looseness in the submental area and if the surgeon pulls it too tight to compensate for the distance there will be an unnatural result with a windblown appearance. Patients wish to have a natural appearance.

82.2
Consultation and Patient Selection

During the initial consultation it is important to fully assess the patient for only the mesh platsymaplasty or a neck lift as well as the mesh platsymaplasty. If the patients are good candidates for mesh platsymaplasty alone, the scars will be short, the recovery much faster, and the procedure can be done completely under local anesthesia.

Patients are classified (Table 82.1) to determine which procedure is best suited for the patient:

- Grade IA: There is fullness in the submental area but when pinched between the index finger and the thumb it is 1 cm or less and the area feels firm. This means that there is good adipose tissue under the skin. In this case liposuction alone would be a good treatment option. If the patient would like to be as tight as possible in the neck region, then the mesh platysmaplasty is recommended as well.
- Grade IB: There is up to 1.5 cm looseness in the submental area but there is no firmness, which means there is not much adipose tissue. In these patients liposuction alone would not be a good treatment option. This patient needs mesh platsmaplasty.
- Grade II: When there is up to 3cm of skin with the pinch test, the mesh platysmaplasty is advised.

- Grade III: There is more than 3–4 cm of loose skin in the submental area. These patients will benefit from mesh platsymaplasty and a neck-lift procedure as well. Some patients prefer a suboptimal result with mesh platsymaplasty only to reduce the extended scarring behind the ear and the posterior hairline.
- Grade IV: More than 4 cm of looseness in the submental area as well as looseness below Adam's apple. These patients need mesh platysmaplasty as well as a neck-lift procedure.

Since a foreign substance is to be used, the risks and the complications of mesh placement are discussed with the patient. Patients are told that the mesh is the size of a quarter in the submental area and if they look for it, just like any other implant, they can find it. Most of the time the mesh-platysmaplasty procedure is accompanied by some form of facelift procedure. Although mesh platysmaplasty causes a more defined angle of the jaw it is not a jowl-lift procedure. If a patient has a ptotic or loose jowl, the patient must have some form of facelift. The degree or invasiveness of the facelift depends on the facial muscle ptosis and the expectations of the patient.

Patients should be told that they will feel tightness in their neck for 4–5 weeks postoperatively especially when turning their head.

Table 82.1 Mira classification of neck skin laxity

Grade	Pinch test	Treatment
IA	1.5 cm, firm	Liposuction
IB	1.5 cm, loose	Mesh platysmaplasty
II	1.5–3.0 cm	Mesh platysmaplasty
III	3.0–4.0 cm	Mesh platysmaplasty and possible neck lift
IV	Over 4.0 cm	Mesh platysmaplasty and neck lift

82.3
Surgical Procedure

For the mesh-platysmaplasty procedure alone or combined with a simplified facelift procedure local anesthesia can be used. Preoperative photographs are taken. A good set of preoperative and postoperative photographs can really show patients the changes that they have after the surgery. The preoperative and postoperative photographs should be taken in the same positions with the same lighting. Lateral views should have the patient with the angle of the head to the neck at 90°. Normally when patients have a ptotic submental area or jowl area they try to compensate by stretching out their neck or looking up. This does not show the true hanging or the looseness in the neck area.

The preoperative marking is done with a 1-in. line in the submental crease ending at equal distances from the midline. A line is drawn from the midline to the mastoid area on each side, staying below the angle of the mandible.

The patient is in a supine position and the neck and face areas are prepped and draped in a sterile manner. Because of the use of a foreign object (mesh), special attention should be paid to sterility. Lidocaine (2%) with epinephrine is injected along the markings in the submental area and on each side in the mastoid region. A stab incision is made in the submental crease and behind both ears, and tumescent solution, consisting of 1,000 ml of lactated Ringer's solution with 500 mg of lidocaine and 1/500:000 epinephrine, is injected into the neck and the jowl area.

After proper tumescent injection and waiting for 15–20 min the neck and jowl areas are liposuctioned with a 2-mm Mercedes cannula on a 20-ml syringe that is vented by 5 ml. The neck should not be completely liposuctioned, especially in the submental area, so as to leave enough fat to minimize palpation of the mesh. Care should be taken not to get an indentation in the jowl area during liposuctioning. The liposuction should be done in a crisscross fashion. The surgeon should be wary not to cause pressure injury to the marginal mandibular nerve when liposuctioning the jowl area.

The submental stab incision is extended equally on both sides of the midline (Fig. 82.1). The flap is raised superficial to the platysma (Fig. 82.2), making sure that there is some layer of fat remaining in the subdermal tissues (Fig. 82.3).

Mersiline mesh is cut to shape and size to fit the submental area (Fig. 82.4). It is always safer to cut a smaller piece than a larger one. The purpose of the mesh is to cause scarring and attachment to the skin. The mesh is placed in antibiotic solution (Ancef) and then inserted into the pocket. The surgeon should make sure that the pocket can easily fit the mesh without retraction or folding of the edges (Fig. 82.5).

The Mersiline mesh is sutured to the platysma using 5.0 nylon. The suturing is started at the superior edge on one side and is continued in a running manner to the inferior margin to the superior edge of the opposite side (Fig. 82.6). During the suturing, the surgeon must make sure that there is no retraction of the skin and there is a free space from the edge of the mesh to the pocket.

The head of the patient is turned and a 2.0-cm incision is made behind the ear lobe at the mastoid area. Using Metzenbaum scissors the skin is raised and a pocket is formed on top of the muscle going toward the midline for about 3–4 cm. Through the submental pocket, a 2.0 nylon suture is placed on each side of the mesh, grabbing the mesh and the platysma muscle and making sure it is sutured at the middle of the mesh and below the level of the angle of the mandible. The needle is cut from the suture and with use of a double-ended Keith needle both ends of the suture are passed in the subcutaneous layer to the pocket made over the mastoid bone behind the ear lobe. The surgeon should make sure that the suture is passed below the angle of the mandible and there is no skin retraction along the route of the suture. With use of a free curved needle on one end of the suture, the nylon is sutured to the underlying mastoid periosteum. The surgeon should pull so there is a moderate tension on the suture and there is nice angle created in the jowl area. One should not to pull too much as this might move the mesh off-center. Sometimes some puckering may be present along the mandibular line but this will resolve in time. The same procedure should be repeated on the opposite side. When completed, the mesh is in the center and it is pulling up on the platysma. When everything has healed, the skin will attach to the mesh and will be pulled upward. The surgeon should ensure that there is proper hemostasis and should completely irrigate the pockets with an antibiotic solution. The pocket is then closed in two layers, the subcutaneous and the skin, using the preferred choice of sutures.

A 0.25-in.-thick foam pad is placed extending from one ear to the other and a neck band (ACE wrap) is used to hold the dressing. The neck band should be placed moderately tight but not too tight.

82.4
Postoperative Instructions

82.4.1
Day of Surgery

Patients are advised to start a soft liquid diet such as Jell-O, soup, etc. when they get home and should not eat anything that requires a lot of chewing. About 20 min after eating light food, the patients are advised to start taking pain-relief medication such as Vicodin or Darvocet. Patients may take pain-relief medication every 3–4 h and should not to wait for the pain to become great. This will increase their comfort postopera-

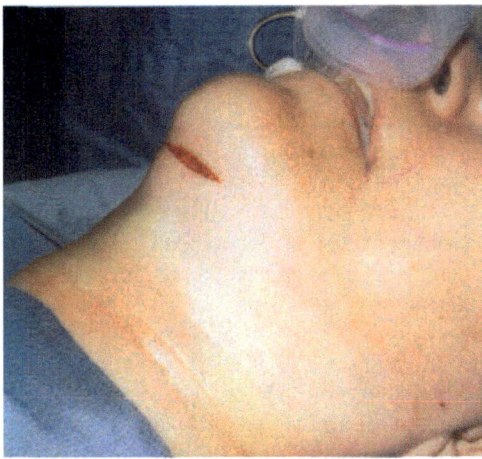

Fig. 82.1 The submental stab incision is extended equally on both sides of the midline

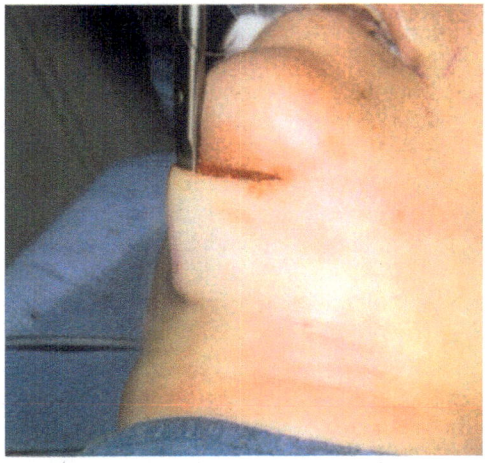

Fig. 82.2 The flap is raised superficial to the platysma

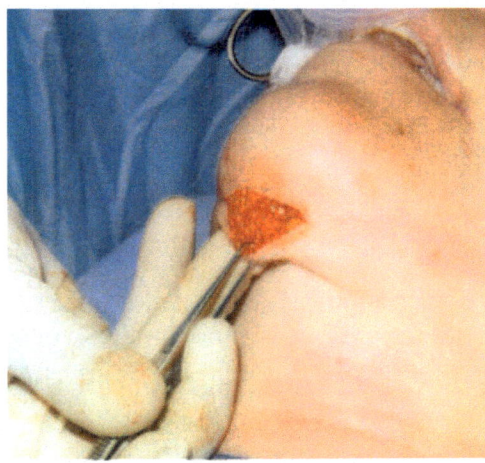

Fig. 82.3 There should be some layer of fat remaining in the subdermal tissues

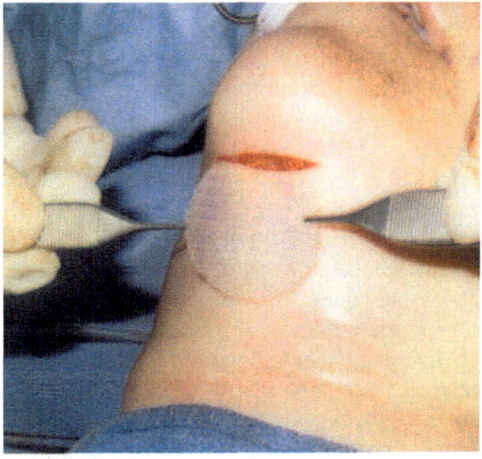

Fig. 82.4 Mersiline mesh is cut to shape and size to fit the submental area

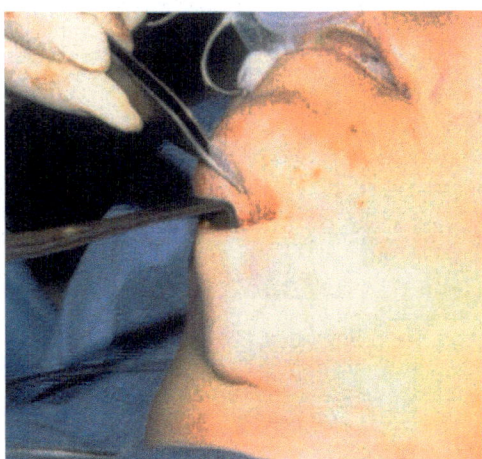

Fig. 82.5 Make sure that the pocket can easily fit the mesh without retraction or folding of the edges

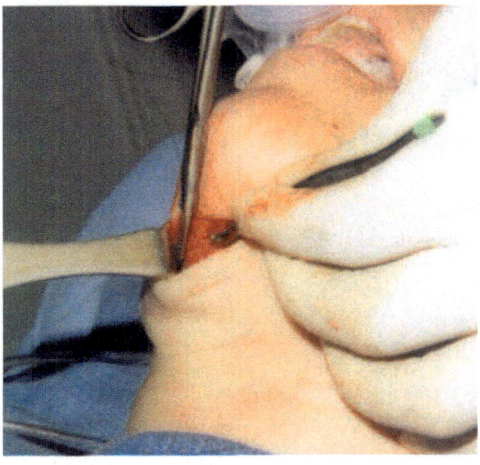

Fig. 82.6 The Mersiline mesh is sutured to the platysma using 5.0 nylon

tively and in turn keep their blood pressure stable and low, which in turn prevents postoperative bleeding and swelling. Patients are advised to continue taking the antibiotic, usually Keflex, and vitamin C, 2,000–3,000 mg/day. Patients are started on a Medrol Dosepack and are given valium (10 mg) to take at night. This will help the patient to sleep better at night and also relaxes the neck muscles from the suspension lift. The head is kept elevated at 33° and a pillow is placed under the knees to take the pressure off the lower back. The patient is not to remove or change the dressings.

82.4.2
Day After Surgery

The patient is seen in the office the day after surgery. The foam and ACE wrap are removed and an adjustable chin binder is applied. This will remain in place for 1–3 days depending on how swollen the area is. The more swelling, the longer the compression should be worn. The binder may be removed to shower and is then put back on. The head is elevated is kept elevated for the next 2 weeks to minimize swelling and bruising.

The incisions under the chin and behind the ears are cleaned twice daily with alcohol and antibiotic ointment applied until the sutures are removed. This will usually be 5 days under the chin and 7–10 days behind the ears.

The patient is to continue prescribed medications and advised not to take aspirin, ibuprofen or vitamin E for a further 2 weeks. Turning the head abruptly, more than 90°, or opening the mouth wide should be avoided for 2 weeks.

Walking is begun the day following surgery but no cardiovascular activities, such as running, are begun for 4–6 weeks. There should be no submersion in water un-til all suture lines have completely healed. This is usually in 4 weeks.

82.5
Complications

In 100 mesh-platysmaplasty procedures there have been three incidents where the submental area became hard with induration scarring. In one case the mesh was larger than the submental area and was extended beyond the mandibular angle. These three patients were treated with injections of Kenalog to the scar tissue followed by ultrasound treatments three times per week for a period of 2–3 weeks. Two of the patients had good results and one patient had the mesh removed as the mesh extended beyond the angle of the mandible. All three of these cases were the first procedures performed and subsequent techniques were modified with smaller sections of surgical mesh.

All patients have been extremely pleased with the final results and are experiencing long-lasting improvement of the neck suspension (Figs. 82.7, 82.8).

There have been no infections or mesh extrusions.

82.6
Discussion

The mesh is sewed to the muscle and because of the characteristic shape and the material of the mesh the tissue on top grows into the mesh and causes scar tissue buildup which will result in a tight adherence. The suspension suture that is passed from either side of the mesh and tied to the mastoid bone causes lifting of the platysma muscle. This in turn causes the lifting of

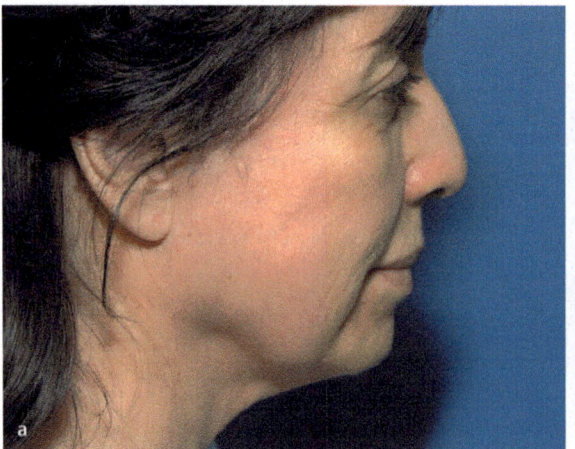 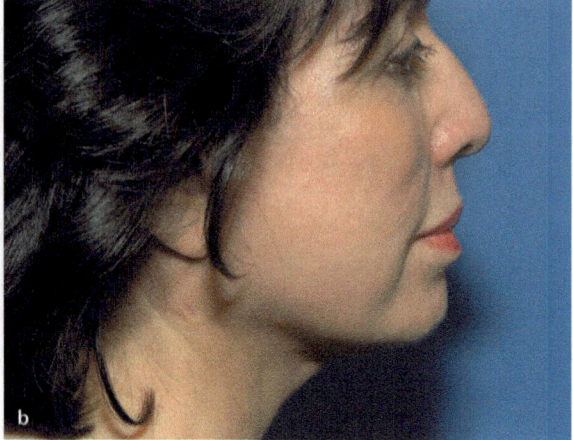

Fig. 82.7 **a** Preoperatively. **b** Postoperatively

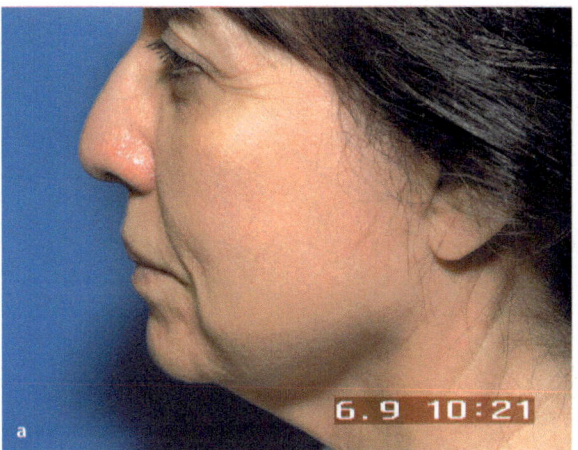 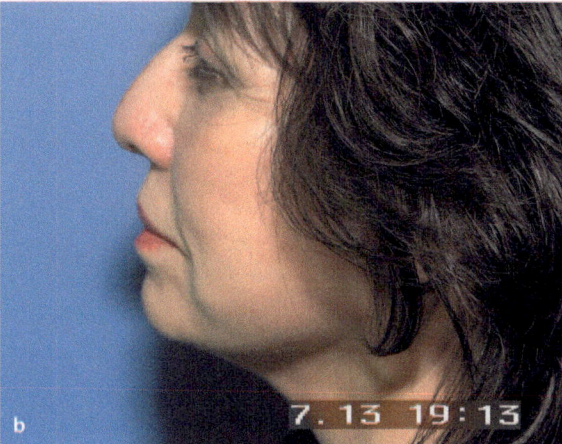

Fig. 82.8 a Preoperatively. **b** Postoperatively

the submental skin because the subdermal tissues will grow into the mesh and adhere to it. This is sort of a clothesline concept, where as the line is pulled tighter the clothes that are hanging on the line are pulled up higher. Doing only mesh platysmaplasty in all patients is not a good idea. Some patients who have much excess skin that is hanging and loose should probably have a neck lift and the mesh platysmaplasty.

82.7 Conclusions

The mesh platysmaplasty has been a very popular procedure with a very high patient satisfaction and patient referrals. The complications have been minimal and simply treated. The technique is fairly safe and can be learned easily. The surgical time is minimal and the procedure can be completely performed under tumescent local anesthesia.

Chapter 83

Adams's Apple Reduction

83

Pierre F. Fournier

83.1
Introduction

Male transsexuals wish to appear as feminine as possible. Many of them request on the face supraorbital ridge reduction (Lintilhac operation), rhinoplasty, and chin reduction and on the neck Adam's apple reduction. It is a simple operation. It was taught to us long ago by Lintilhac, who innovated this technique.

83.2
Technique

Steps in the procedure:
1. Marking
2. Anesthesia
3. Incision
4. Exposure
5. Reduction of the Adam's apple
6. Closure

83.2.1
Marking

A 3-cm horizontal line is marked about 2 cm above the Adam's apple with the patient in the standing position.

83.2.2
Anesthesia

General or local anesthesia with sedation may be used. Local anesthesia is used most of the time with or without sedation. Six to 8 ml of 1% lidocaine and 1:200,000 epinephrine is enough for the skin and strap muscles.

83.2.3
Incision

A no. 11 blade is used to transect the skin and subcutaneous tissues in a skin crease.

83.2.4
Exposure

The strap muscles are incised in the midline and retracted. The retractors are lowered until the Adam's apple is fully visible in the middle of the incision emerging like an iceberg (Fig. 83.1).

83.2.5
Reduction

The Adam's apple has to be stabilized by Adson forceps or with two traction sutures. It is possible to remove the excess of the cartilage in one piece but many surgeons remove the excess volume only by "chips" one by one with a no. 11 or no. 15 blade held horizontally until the excess has been removed giving the desired result (Figs. 83.2, 83.3). Bleeding is controlled by electrocoagulation.

83.2.6
Closure

The strap muscles are sutured with Vicryl® 4/0 and the skin is closed with a subdermal suture (Fig. 83.4). A light dressing is applied for 1 day.

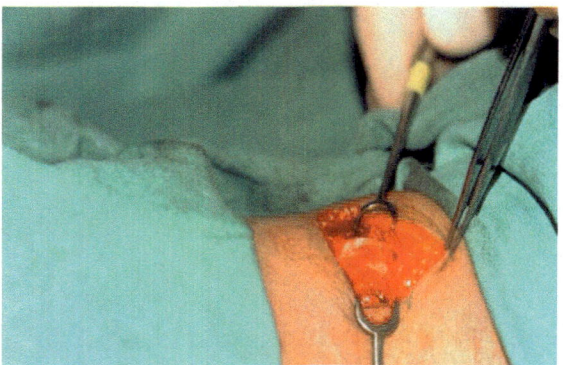

Fig. 83.1 Exposure

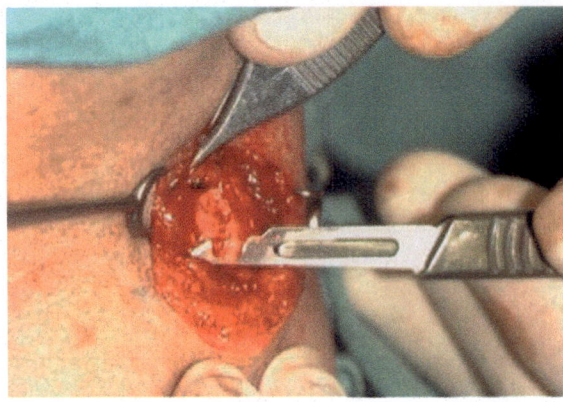

Fig. 83.2 Cartilage resection

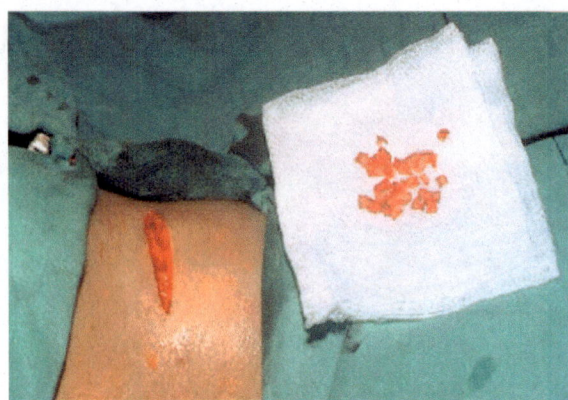

Fig. 83.3 After cartilage resection

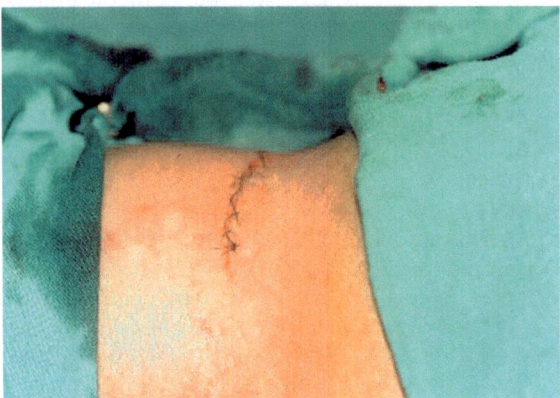

Fig. 83.4 Closure

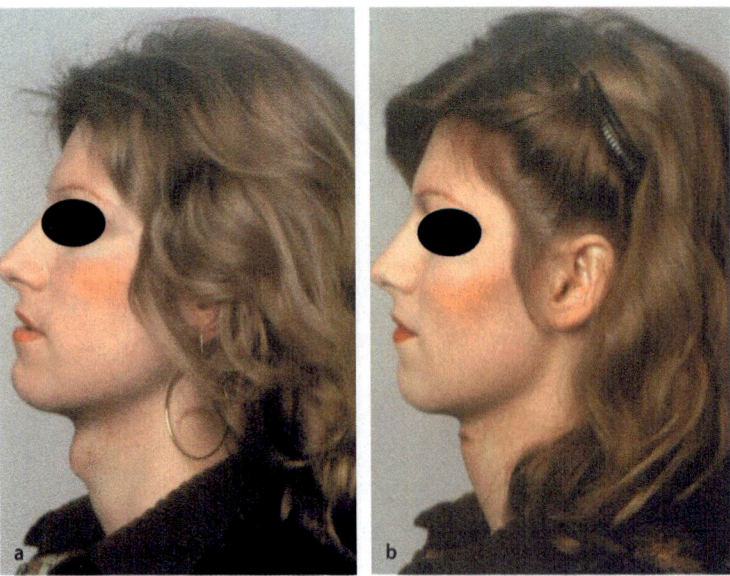

Fig. 83.5 **a** Before. **b** After Adam's apple reduction

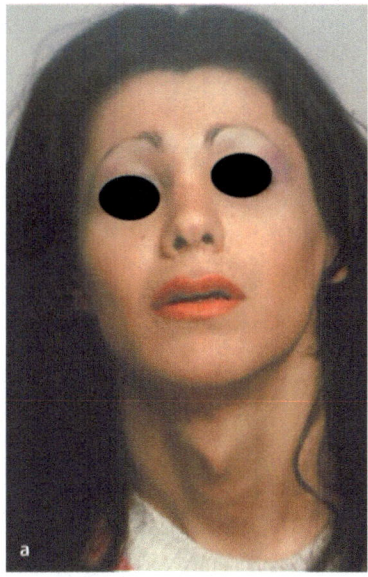 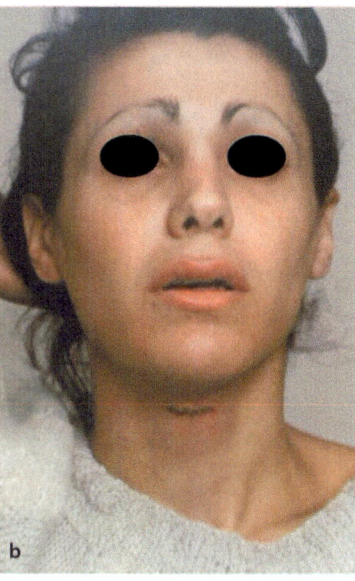

Fig. 83.6 a Before. **b** After Adam's apple reduction

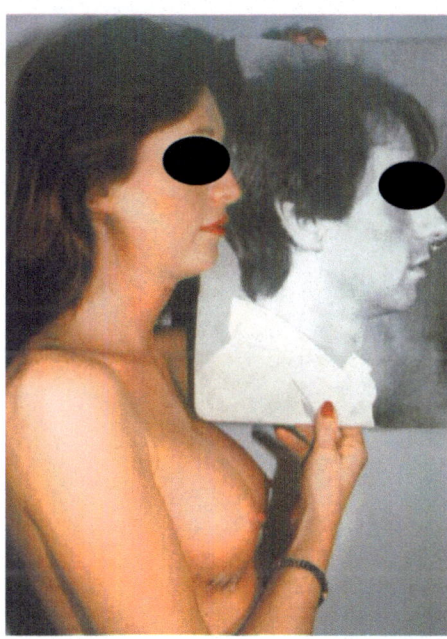

Fig. 83.7 Example of patient who underwent transsexual surgery before surgery and after supraorbital ridge reduction, reduction rhinoplasty, chin reduction, Adam's apple reduction, and breast augmentation

83.3
Postoperative Treatment

Antibiotics are given as well as anti-inflammatories.

83.4
Results

Examples of surgical results are given in Figs. 83.5–83.7.

83.5
Complications

The voice of the patient is not modified. The scar is not visible, being in a high position and of good quality. There have been no cases of infection or of wound disruption.

Part VIII
Medical Legal and Commentary

CHAPTER 84

Medical Legal

Melvin A. Shiffman

84.1
Introduction

The medical legal implications of facial cosmetic procedures are related to:

1. Failure to maintain patient rapport
2. Breach of the standard of care
3. Failure to obtain informed consent
4. Failure to obtain information on significant past medical history
5. Failure to diagnose and/or treat complications in a timely manner
6. Performing procedures not requested

Some of the problems concerning patient rapport can be personality conflicts between physician and patient, unrealistic patient expectations, dysmorphic personality of the patient, and handling the difficult patient.

84.2
Standard of Care

The standard of care is what a reasonably prudent (careful) physician would do under the same or similar circumstances. The court considers expert testimony to establish the standard of care in most instances except if the circumstances are in the purview of a lay person. Also, the court may consider what a responsible minority of physicians would do under the same or similar circumstances. Medical literature may help to establish standard of care.

84.3
Informed Consent

84.3.1
Definition

The patient has the absolute right to receive enough information about his or her diagnosis, proposed treatment, prognosis, and possible risks of proposed therapy and alternatives to enable the patient to make a knowl-

edgeable decision. The patient is the one who makes all the decisions in opposition to the old paternalistic theory that gave the physician complete control over all decisions. A physician would now have to prove that the decision he or she made was because of the patient's inability to make the decision or because there was an extreme emergency.

Other requirements of the "informed consent" doctrine in law require that a complication which was not explained to the patient did in fact occur and that the patient would not have agreed to have the surgery if he or she had been informed of that particular risk or complication.

84.3.2
Legal Definition

In terms of surgical procedures, the patient must have explained to him or her the nature and purpose of any proposed operation or treatment, any viable alternatives, and the material risks and benefits of both. All questions must be answered.

In order for the plaintiff to succeed in a complaint for lack of informed consent, he or she must show:

1. That the risk or complication, which was not explained to him or her, indeed did occur.
2. That if he or she had been informed of that particular risk, he or she would not have consented to the surgical procedure.

There are different means of proof at trial depending upon the jurisdiction (state). The opinion as to what risks are "material" to the patient in order to make his or her decision, under the same or similar circumstances, can be that of:

1. A reasonably prudent physician: This allows a physician to testify as to what is material.
2. A reasonably prudent patient: This allows the jury to decide what a reasonably prudent patient would consider material risks.
3. The plaintiff patient: This places the onus on the plaintiff to decide what would be material risks for him or her.

84.4
Legal Cases

It may help the physician to understand cases in the medical legal context with explanations as to the reason for the court decisions.

The Illinois Appeals Court, in Zalazar vs Vercimak (1994) [1], decided that the subjective (patient) standard is less of an "insurmountable" barrier than the objective standard (reasonably prudent physician or reasonably prudent patient) would be. The court believed that the decision whether to elect cosmetic surgery is personal and third-party testimony as to the decision a reasonably prudent person would make under similar circumstances would be of limited value.

In Parikh vs Cunningham (1986) [2], the plaintiff had signed a release prior to surgery, which authorized the treatment, recited the procedures to be performed, and recited that the risks and consequences had been explained and that no guarantees or assurances had been made as to the results. The court reversed a jury verdict for the defendant physician where the jury instruction stated that a written consent, executed by a person mentally and physically competent to give consent, gave rise to a conclusive presumption of informed consent. The court held that there must be more than just a writing introduced as evidence and that the elements of informed consent must be established.

Comment: The elements of informed consent must include a discussion by the physician or office staff that includes a description of the procedure to be performed, viable alternatives to the procedure, and material risks and benefits of the procedure and the alternatives.

In Largey vs Rothman (1988) [3], the New Jersey Supreme Court adopted the "prudent patient" standard for informed consent. The court held that the disclosure of "material risks" is determined by what a reasonable patient, in what the physician knows or should know to be in the patient's position, would be likely to attach significance to the risk or cluster of risks in deciding whether to forego the proposed therapy or submit to it.

84.4.1
Suggestions for Office

Methods for preventing litigation concerning informed consent are misunderstood by most physicians who are convinced that a patient's signature or initials on a list of risks and complications will forego the problem. You can be assured that every time there is litigation, the patient will testify to the "fact" that the defendant physician did not explain the risks to him or her and that he or she did not read the consent form with all the risks listed despite his or her signature.

The following are recommendations:

1. The physician or office staff should explain all material risks and viable alternatives and their risks and complications and answer all the patient's questions.
2. The medical record should contain the following: "The surgical procedure was explained to the patient and risks and complications were discussed as well as viable alternatives and their risks and complications. All questions were answered."
3. Any witness to the patient's signature or initials concerning information for informed consent should have the following statement above the witness signature: "I requested that the patient read the complete form. I personally observed the patient read the form. The patient stated to me that all the material was read and, after all questions were answered, understood the complete form before signing."
4. Except under special circumstances, the physician should meet with the patient prior to the day of surgery to establish some personal rapport. Sometimes it is not possible to consult with the patient directly before the day of surgery if the patient is from out of town and arrives shortly before the day of surgery. It is usually possible to meet with this type of patient the evening before surgery if the physician is insistent. Remember that it is the physician's ultimate responsibility to establish the relationship and make sure the information necessary for the patient to make a knowledgeable decision has been received and understood. The day of surgery is a relatively poor time to try to explain all that is necessary when the patient is nervous, fearful, and is finding it hard to concentrate on what the physician is trying to explain.

84.4.2
Medications

The patient has the right to know what medications are being given, the purpose of the medication, and the possible risks and complications of the medication. This can usually be done by means of a written explanation describing all the information about the drug or by discussion with the patient by the physician or by other adequately trained health care personnel.

The following are recommendations:

1. The medical record should contain the fact that a discussion about the medication was held or that the patient received written information.
2. Check allergies to drugs.
3. Evaluate need for laboratory studies as per the *Physician's Desk Reference* (PDR).
4. Prescribe for the purposes as set forth in the PDR. If off-label use is decided upon, all the reasons should be set down in the medical record.
5. Prescribe or dispense only in small quantities for the period of time needed.

6. Refills should be recorded in the chart and should be cautiously given especially if it involves a controlled substance. Remember that the physician has the final determination as to how much and how often a medication should be taken. Do not let the patient control the medication prescription. If overuse is detected, then refuse all further refills and record this in the chart or refer to another physician for evaluation specifically for the drug use.

84.4.3
Echavarria vs. Prado: Dade County (FL) Circuit Court, Case No. 01-8503 CA 11.

In *Medical Malpractice Verdicts, Settlements & Experts* 2004;20(4):58–59

The 75-year-old female plaintiff had facelift and revision of upper eyelids. The plaintiff alleged that the right eye did not close, had tears all night, and was swollen in the morning. The defendant claimed that she had senile atrophy of the lacrimal glands that caused "dry eye." This was documented 1 year before the plaintiff's eye surgery. There was a defense verdict.

84.4.4
Mahler vs. Johns Hopkins Hospital: Baltimore City (MD) Circuit Court.

In *Medical Malpractice Verdicts, Settlements & Experts* 2004;20(1):57

The 36-year-old plaintiff had a sliding genioplasty for chin augmentation and malar augmentation in 1993. Corrective surgery of the chin was performed in 1997. The plaintiff alleged that his chin "fell" within 1 h after the 1997 surgery, that there was damage permanent disfigurement of the chin, and that there was permanent nerve damage that caused the lower lip to droop and required the use of a chin support. He also alleged that he was never informed about the potential risks of disfigurement and nerve damage. The defendant claimed that the plaintiff had been informed of the risks and that the plaintiff had unrealistic expectations of what the surgery would accomplish. There was a $550,000 verdict.

84.4.5
Pellot vs. New York City Health and Hospitals Corporation: Kings County (NY) Supreme Court, Index No. 1963/97.

In *Medical Malpractice Verdicts, Settlements & Experts* 2004;20(6):50

The 52-year-old plaintiff had facelift surgery at the defendant hospital. The plaintiff's expert opined that the surgery was improperly performed and that the plaintiff was not properly informed of the risks of "bad visible scarring." The defendant claimed that the plaintiff was properly informed and that the surgery was properly performed. There was a defense verdict.

84.4.6
Hayes vs. Cha: US District Court, District of New Jersey, at Camden.

In *Medical Malpractice Verdicts, Settlements & Experts* 2004;20(5):51–52

The 56-year-old plaintiff underwent facelift surgery in 1995. She developed painful sores on her face that could not be cured with ointments and antibiotics. Six years later she was diagnosed with mycobacterium fortuitum. The plaintiff alleged that unsanitary instruments caused disfiguring infection and that there was failure to keep records on sterilization that was required by state law and professional standards. There was a verdict for $20,000,000.

Comment: The large judgment was the result of a delayed diagnosis of a serious complication as well as failure to keep records required by state law.

84.4.7
Black vs. Staffel: US District Court, Western District of Tennessee, Case No. 01-2841 D BRE.

In *Medical Malpractice Verdicts, Settlements & Experts* 2004;20(9):48

The 57-year-old plaintiff had a Baker–Gordon phenol peel during which the solution spilled onto the Mayo tray. The defendant swabbed the spilled solution onto the plaintiff's face. The plaintiff suffered burns of the neck and face that resulted in permanent cosmetic and nerve damage. The plaintiff alleged that the defendant improperly prepared and applied the solution, failed to make a fresh solution, and that the plaintiff was not an appropriate candidate for the procedure. The plaintiff's expert opined that the phenol and croton oil are highly toxic and not water-soluble, that the solution ingredients must be vigorously agitated into a white milky substance and applied immediately, and that without agitation the mixture will separate into layers in approximately 8 s. The defendant claimed that the plaintiff's injuries were caused by a Neosporin reaction and an unanticipated sensitivity to the chemical peel solution. There was an undisclosed settlement.

Comment: The physician failed to follow simple precautions in the use of a dangerous substance that had spilled. The solution should have been reformulated prior to use.

84.4.8
Dukes vs. Dillinger: Summit County (OH) Common Pleas Court, Case No. 02-03-1682.

In *Medical Malpractice Verdicts, Settlements & Experts* 2004;20(9):48

The 65-year-old plaintiff underwent blepharoplasty performed by the defendant. Following surgery the plaintiff was unable to close her eyelids, leading to damaged and overexposed corneas, with resultant light sensitivity. The plaintiff alleged that the defendant resected too much skin, which resulted in incompetent upper eyelids. The defendant claimed that the result was simply the result of excessive scarring. There was a defense verdict.

84.4.9
Perez vs. Blinski: Dade County (FL) Circuit Court, Case No. 02-7563 CA 15.

In *Medical Malpractice Verdicts, Settlements & Experts* 2004;20(12):39

The 51-year-old plaintiff had a brow lift with a surgical incision in a wrinkle in the plaintiff's forehead, because of profound hair loss. The consent form did not state where the incision would be placed. The plaintiff was displeased with the placement of the scar across his forehead. There was a $65,000 verdict after the defendant admitted liability.

Comment: A forehead incision that might become a visible scar should be carefully explained to the patient and the agreement by the patient for the placement of the incision should have been entered in the medical record in order to protect the physician.

84.4.10
Wolfe vs. Magnat: Kenton County (KY) Circuit Court, Case No. 01-1771.

In *Medical Malpractice Verdicts, Settlements & Experts* 2005;21(4):39

The 47-year-old plaintiff had a trichloracetic acid chemical peel of the face. She sustained swelling and burns that required steroid injections, laser treatments, and a silicone bandage for 6 months. Permanent scarring resulted. The plaintiff alleged negligence of the physician in using an "old" formulation a second time, as another patient suffered burns prior to the plaintiff's treatment, negligence of the pharmacy for changing the mixture and not notifying the physician, and failure of the supplier for failure to provide adequate instructions when switching from weight-to-volume measurement to weight-to-weight measurement, resulting in a 54.3% solution instead of 40%. The verdict was for $500,000, apportioning fault of 40% to the pharmacy, 30% to the physician, and 30% to the supplier.

84.4.11
Moray vs. Watson: Dallas County (TX) District Court, Case No. 02-2243.

In *Medical Malpractice Verdicts, Settlements & Experts* 2005;21(6):38

The plaintiff underwent a facelift with fat transfer to the tear troughs by the defendant. The plaintiff alleged that the troughs were overfilled with fat, resulting in disfigurement, lack of informed consent, misrepresentation of qualifications, and negligence in performing the procedure. There was a verdict for $40,000.

84.4.12
Ocampo vs. Golflies: Cook County (IL) Circuit Court, Case No. 98L-12603.

In *Medical Malpractice Verdicts, Settlements & Experts* 2003;19(2):52

The 35-year-old plaintiff had a silicone implant placed in his nose in 1993 and the implant became dislodged when he was assaulted in 1995. The defendant plastic surgeon removed the silicone implant and replaced it with a Porex implant 1997. The Porex implant was partially removed 10 months later by the defendant after the plaintiff could not become accustomed to the feel of the implant. After this surgery the plaintiff had breathing difficulties due to the lack of support. Another surgeon removed the remainder of the Porex implant and inserted a cartilage graft and his breathing difficulties resolved. The plaintiff alleged that the defendant was negligent in using a synthetic implant for a secondary rhinoplasty, for reoperating in less than 12 months, and for not investigating the plaintiff's problem with alcohol. The defendant claimed that synthetic implants are not the first choice for a secondary rhinoplasty but they were still an option and within the standard of care. The defendant claimed that the plaintiff refused the option of cartilage implant although this was not documented. There was a defense verdict.

84.4.13
Besson vs. Weintraub: New York (NY) Supreme Court, Index No. 120398/00.

In *Medical Malpractice Verdicts, Settlements & Experts* 2003;19(2):52

The 68-year-old plaintiff had facelift, laser resurfacing, and blepharoplasty. After surgery she complained of dry eye and pain and numbness of the neck. The plaintiff alleged that doing the three procedures at once increased the risk of scarring and nerve damage and that she was not informed of these risks. She alleged that the defendant did not take a proper medical history. The defendant claimed that there were no additional risks in performing all three procedures at the same time and the plaintiff failed to disclose that she had a pre-existing dry eye condition. There was a verdict for $1,004,000 that was reduced to $531,116 for 47.1% comparative negligence.

84.4.14
Pienkowski vs. Siemian: Ornage County (FL) Circuit Court, Case No. C1099-7445.

In *Medical Malpractice Verdicts, Settlements & Experts* 2003;19(2):53

The 69-year-old plaintiff had facial chemical peel. Postoperatively she had severe pain and crusts on the face were debrided. She had scarring to her face and ectropion. She discovered also that the defendant performed laser surgery to her eyelids and that she had specifically instructed the defendant not to perform any surgical procedures on her eyes. The plaintiff alleged that aggressive debridement of the eschar caused loss of epithelium and resulted in the scars and ectropion. The defendant claimed that the plaintiff did not adhere to the specific postoperative instructions. There was a $350,000 verdict that was reduced to $175,000 for comparative negligence of the patient of 50%.

Comment: The aggressive removal of eschar (scabs) in a non-infected wound or incision may increase the scarring and delay healing.

84.4.15
Guardado vs. Surgeon: (CA) Superior Court.

In *Medical Malpractice Verdicts, Settlements & Experts* 2003;19(10):55

The 50-year-old plaintiff had blepharoplasty under local anesthesia by the defendant and was sent home later

the same day. She had increased pain and swelling of the left eye and attempted to contact the physician several times. Eventually, the surgeon sent his assistant to the patient's home, where massive swelling of the left eye was noted. The plaintiff was brought to the surgeon's office, at which time the surgeon observed the swelling and began to treat her. The plaintiff's family telephoned "911" and had an ambulance take her to a nearby hospital. She sustained partial blindness of the left eye. The plaintiff alleged negligence in that the defendant did not appreciate the risk of hematoma and did not know how to treat it. The defendant claimed that he met the standard of care and that hematoma was a risk of the procedure. There was a settlement for $300,000.

Comment: Delayed diagnosis and treatment of a complication is a frequent problem in malpractice litigation and is difficult to defend. Complications should be suspected with any complaint and the patient seen if there is any possibility of a serious complication.

84.4.16
Doe vs. Anonymous: Fairfax County (VA) Circuit Court.

In *Medical Malpractice Verdicts, Settlements & Experts* 2003;19(6):52–53

The 20-year-old man had laser hair removal from his back and arms using topical anesthetic cream. When the same topical anesthetic was applied 7 weeks later, the decedent lost consciousness and had decreased respirations. He was in full cardiac arrest by the time the emergency personnel arrived. He could not be resuscitated. The plaintiffs alleged that the defendant failed to recognize the signs of anaphylaxis, failed to treat the anaphylaxis with epinephrine, which would have resulted in a more than 95% chance of successful survival, and that life-saving techniques were not performed in a timely manner. The defendant claimed that the decedent did not suffer anaphylaxis but suffered a sudden cardiovascular collapse from an arrhythmia or other unknown cause and that vomiting prevented the administration of CPR or oxygen and that the decedent's airway was maintained preventing him from aspirating vomitus. There was a $728,000 settlement.

Comment: Every office and physician should be prepared for any acute complication where immediate care is mandatory. The complication should have been diagnosed and treatment started immediately. When cardiac arrest occurred, early intubation was essential to prevent emesis and aspiration.

84.4.17
Samouhi vs. Loria: Nassau County (NY) Supreme Court, Index No. 010315/00.

In *Medical Malpractice Verdicts, Settlements & Experts* 2003;19(5):48

The plaintiff, in his mid-20s, underwent a series of hair transplants by the defendant. Scars occurred with an additional bald spot on the back of the scalp. The plaintiff alleged that the defendant did not allow sufficient time between the graft procedures and the scar revision. There was one incident in which there was only a 3-week interval. The defendant denied any negligence. There was a verdict for $70,000.

Comment: Scars take 6 months to mature and soften. Early repetitive surgery may introduce more scarring and should not be considered in a non-emergency or urgent situation.

84.4.18
McAllister vs. Bundrick: Madison County (AL) Circuit Court, Case No. 00-0636.

In *Medical Malpractice Verdicts, Settlements & Experts* 2003;19(4):45–46

The 61-year-old plaintiff had rhinoplasty and endoscopic brow lift by the defendant. Following the surgery, the plaintiff had symptoms of visual problems and memory loss. Seven months later an MRI scan was performed and revealed a foreign metal object embedded in her skull. At this time the defendant admitted to the plaintiff that a needle had broken off during the rhinoplasty surgery but believed it would cause no problem. The defendant attempted to remove the needle but was unsuccessful. Five days later the needle, having penetrated the brain, was removed by another surgeon. Neurologic symptoms persisted after the surgery. The plaintiff alleged there was negligence in breaking off the needle that was further compounded by the failure to inform the patient, that she should have been referred to a specialist for removal of the object, and that the plaintiff should not have continued with the second surgery (brow lift) but should have referred her to a specialist to remove the needle. The defendant claimed that he did not breach the standard of care and denied that any neurologic injury occurred. There was a verdict for $85,000.

Comment: Breaking of a needle is not in itself a breach of the standard of care. However, failing to inform the patient of the problem (fraudulent concealment) and failure to realize that a sharp object can migrate were breaches of the standard of care.

84.4.19
Gross vs. Barbour: Sarasota County (FL) Circuit, Case No. 2001-CA-012165 NC.

In *Medical Malpractice Verdicts, Settlements & Experts* 2003;19(3):47

The 56-year-old plaintiff had a 10-h surgery consisting of neck lift, mid-facelift, and laser resurfacing. She had persistent swelling, scar formation of the upper and lower eyelids, and was generally unhappy with the results of the surgery. The plaintiff alleged that the defendant was negligent in performing a mid-facelift instead of a conventional facelift and that he had inadequate training and experience. There was a verdict for $2,145,000.

Comment: The performance of a procedure (the mid-facelift) not consented to is a battery and may include punitive damages.

References

1. Zalazar v. Vercimak, 261 Ill.App.3d 250, 199 Ill.Dec. 232, 633 N.E.2d 1223 (Ill.App. 3 Dist. 1993)
2. Parikh v. Cunningham, 493 So. 2d 999 (Fla. 1986)
3. Largey v. Rothman, 540 A. 2d 504 (N.J. 1988)

CHAPTER 85

Editor's Commentary

Melvin A. Shiffman

85.1
Introduction

There are some editorial comments necessary to supplement aspects that may be missing in the text. These are purely this editor's opinions and do not necessarily reflect the opinions of the other editors or the contributors.

85.2
Suture Lifts

1. Barbed suture lifts without tying the sutures to the underlying fascia or galea do not appear to last as long as those suture lifts that are tied to the underlying fascia [1, 2]. Fat will not hold sutures in a stable position. Only 55% of patients are satisfied or highly satisfied [2]. If only one side of the suture is stabilized in the fascia or galea, the portion in the fat will not hold tension for very long (1–2 years). If one considers thread lift as a temporary measure such as botulinum toxin or absorbable injectable fillers, then the patient should be told the average length of time (not the longest possible time) that the improvement will remain.
2. The best situation would be fixation of threads at both ends in stable positions: one end in the fascia and the other end not simply in fat. This will require more research.
3. Non-absorbable sutures used in suture lifts will tend to loosen over time as the material weakens.
4. The barbed threads when inserted through the sharp tip of a needle can develop tears in the thread or reverse direction of the barbs (Fig. 85.1)
5. Absorbable threads have not had a long enough critical evaluation to determine how long the lift lasts, but information from Asia is that they last only 1–2 years. Some of the threads appear rather thick and there are no statistics of the risk of palpable or visible threads in the face. There is no comparison of risks with non-absorbable threads. These threads probably do not maintain the tissues in position with scar once the threads are absorbed.
6. Contour Threads™, at $100 per thread, are too expensive per thread to consider in the long term since they increase costs far beyond the actual value of the threads. That the Food and Drug and Administration (FDA) approves the thread means very little since any thread that is tied is an approved method according to the FDA. The thread barbs are under tension in the subcutaneous tissues that do not appear to hold the position of the skin for more than 1–2 years.
7. There are some threads on the market that have complicated methods for insertion.

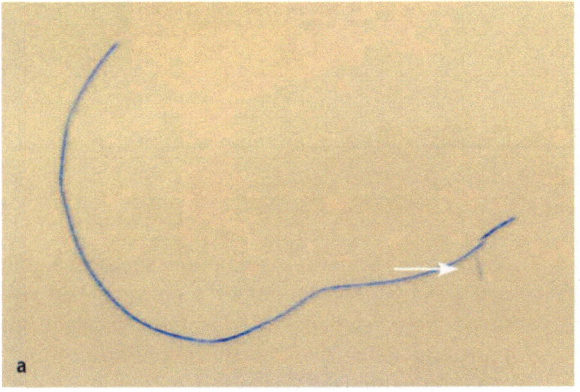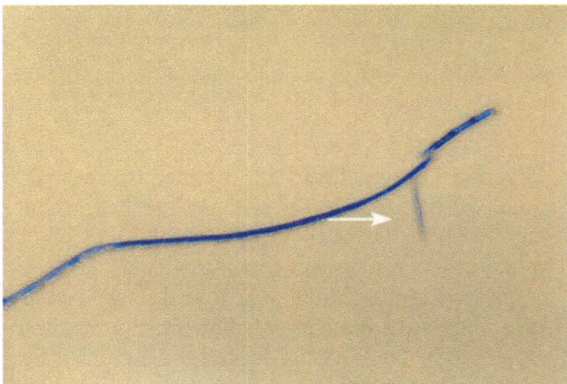

Fig. 85.1 **a** Suture partially cut by needle. *b see next page*

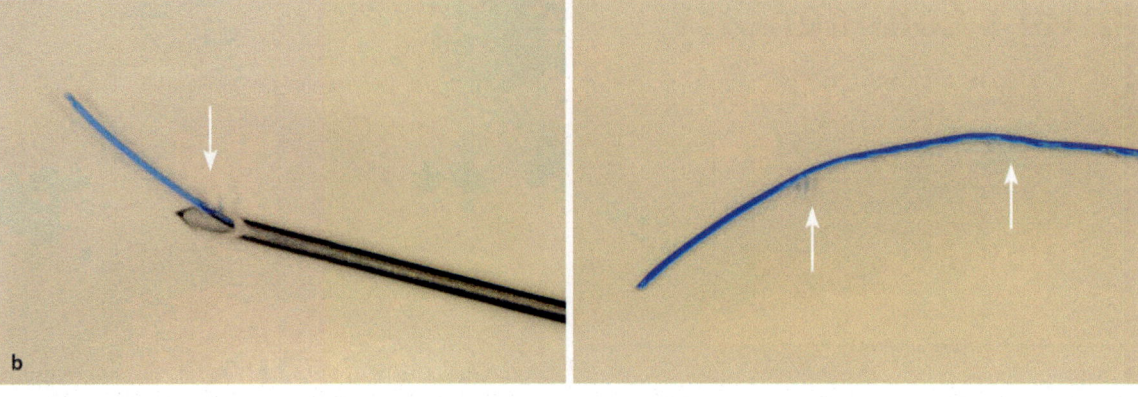

Fig. 85.1 *(Continued)* **b** Barbs reversed in direction by needle

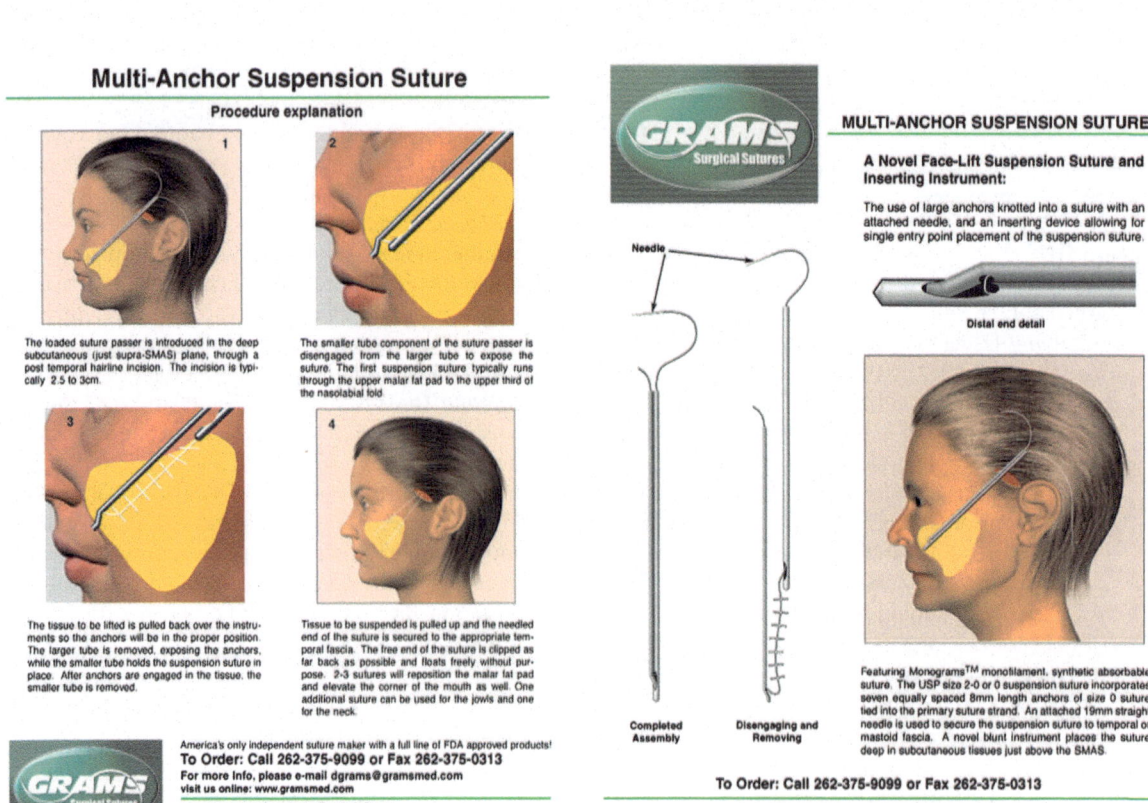

Fig. 85.2 Advertisement of the Multi-Anchor Suspension Suture

8. A recent form of thread lift, invented by Sorin Ermia, combines the thread with an attached needle and inserting device allowing for single entry point placement of the suspension suture (Fig. 85.2).

9. Another recent addition to the threads is the Silhouette Mid-Face Suture, invented by Nicanor Isse and approved by the FDA on 23 October 2006, that uses a cone-shaped piece (resorbable) at various intervals to allow scar to form around the knots and thread (Fig. 85.3).

85.3 Peels

1. Trichloracetic acid (TCA) solution should be prepared weight-to-weight rather than weight-to-volume so the percentages of TCA are consistent (G. Monheit, October 2005, personal communication). Not all companies and pharmacists are aware of this and complications can arise from the difference in the true percentage of TCA.

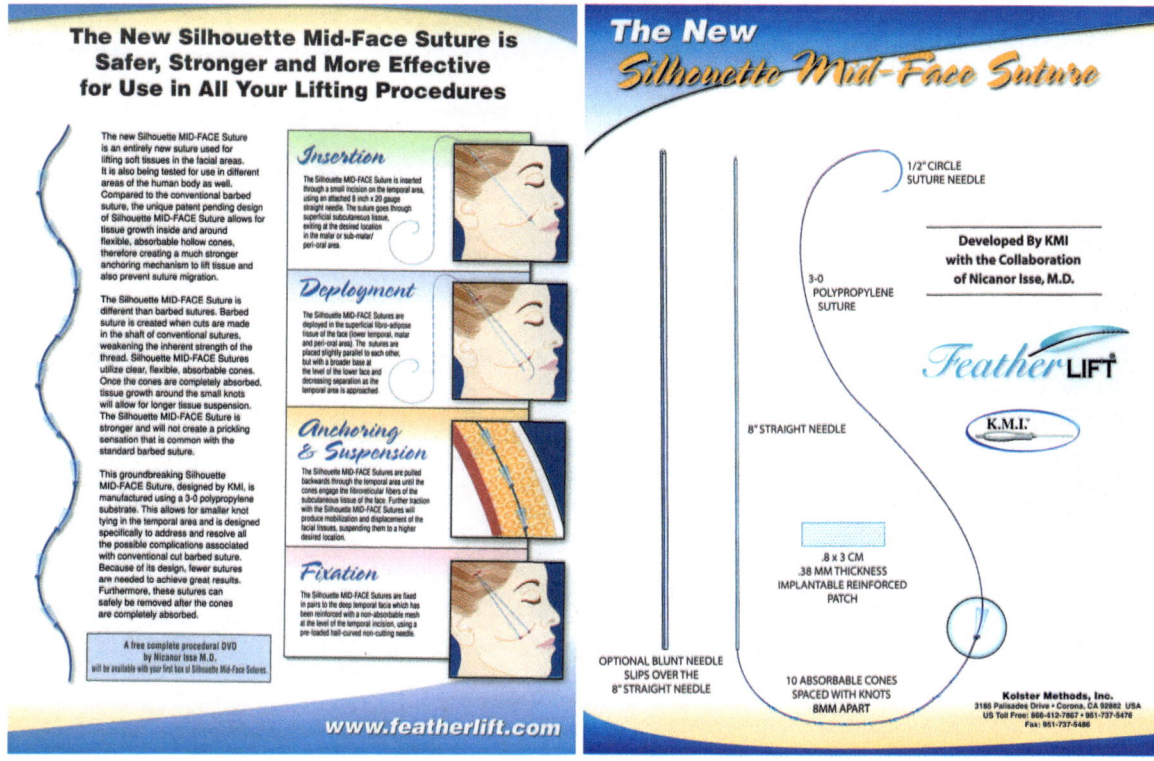

Fig. 85.3 Advertisement for the Silhouette Mid-Face Suture

2. TCA solution maintains potency for 4–5 months after being formulated (G. Monheit, October 2005, personal communication). Placing the solution in a brown bottle and avoiding sunlight prevents discoloration but does not alter the potency.
3. Peels containing phenol should be performed with the patient on continuous electrocardiogram monitoring during application of the solution.

85.4
Facelift

1. Standard facelift principles still apply even with modified facelifts.
2. The pull of the skin should be posterior and superior. The S-lift pulls the platysma superiorly and the parotid fascia into a circle.
3. Absorbable threads in the superficial aponeurotic fascia system will not hold the tissues in position for very long despite any scarring around the suture. The facial skin will revert back to its original position in about 1–2 years.

85.5
General Comments

1. Complication avoidance, timely diagnosis, and treatment are some of the most important aspects of cosmetic surgery.
2. Inform the patient as to the procedure that is advised, any viable alternatives, and the material risks and complications and record in the medical record that the conversation was held on the date that it occurred.
3. Take preoperative and postoperative photographs of all patients undergoing surgery or volume replacement.

References

1. Gagnon, L.: Taking the middle ground: Suture suspension as a facial rejuvenation technique. Cosmet Surg Times Nov/Dec 2005:14
2. Haiavy, J., Leventhal, M.S.: Facial rejuvenation with barbed sutures: A retrospective analysis of technique and results. Am J Cosmet Surg 2005;22(4):239–247

Subject Index